ESSENTIALS of
RUBIN'S PATHOLOGY
FIFTH EDITION

ESSENTIALS of RUBIN'S PATHOLOGY
FIFTH EDITION

EDITORS:

Emanuel Rubin, MD
Gonzalo E. Aponte Distinguished Professor of Pathology
Chairman Emeritus of the Department of Pathology,
Anatomy, and Cell Biology
Jefferson Medical College
Philadelphia, Pennsylvania

Howard M. Reisner, PhD
Professor of Pathology and Laboratory Medicine
Department of Pathology and Laboratory Medicine
The University of North Carolina at Chapel Hill
School of Medicine
Chapel Hill, North Carolina

WITH **44** CONTRIBUTORS
Illustrations by Dimitri Karetnikov, George Barile, and Kathy Jaeger

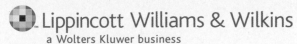
. Lippincott Williams & Wilkins
a Wolters Kluwer business
Philadelphia · Baltimore · New York · London
Buenos Aires · Hong Kong · Sydney · Tokyo

Acquisitions Editor: Betty Sun
Developmental Editor: Kathleen Scogna
Managing Editor: Kelley Squazzo
Copy Editor: Dvora Konstant
Marketing Manager: Emilie Moyer
Associate Production Manager: Kevin P. Johnson
Designer: Risa Clow
Compositor: Maryland Composition, Inc.

Library of Congress Cataloging-in-Publication Data
Essentials of Rubin's pathology / editors, Emanuel Rubin, Howard M. Reisner ; with 44 contributors ; illustrations by Dimitri Karetnikov, George Barile, and Kathy Jaeger. — 5th ed.
    p. ; cm.
  Rev ed. of: Rubin's pathology. 5th ed. c2008.
  Includes bibliographical references and index.
  ISBN-13: 978-0-7817-7324-9
  ISBN-10: 0-7817-7324-5
  1. Pathology. I. Rubin, Emanuel, 1928- II. Reisner, Howard M. III. Rubin's pathology. IV. Title: Rubin's pathology.
  [DNLM: 1. Pathology. QZ 4 E782 2009]
  RB111.E856 2009
  616.07—dc22
                                                                2007036036

ISBN: 978-07817-7324-9

To purchase additional copies of this book, call our customer service department at **(800) 638-3030** or fax orders to **(301) 824-7390**. International customers should call **(301) 714-2324**.

Visit Lippincott Williams & Wilkins on the Internet: http://www.LWW.com. Lippincott Williams & Wilkins customer service representatives are available from 8:30 am to 6:00 pm, EST.

07 08 09 10 11
1 2 3 4 5 6 7 8 9 10

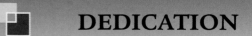

We dedicate this book to our wives and families, whose love and support throughout this endeavor sustained us; to our colleagues, from whom we have learned so much; and to students everywhere, upon whose curiosity and energy the future of medical science depends.

Also to the memories of Fred Zak and Lotte Strauss, who were my first teachers of pathology.
Emanuel Rubin, MD

Cui dono lepidum novum libellum
Arido modo pumice expolitum?
Emily, tibi
Howard M. Reisner, PhD

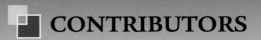

Michael F. Allard, BSc, MD, FRCP(C)
Professor and Cardiovascular Pathologist
Department of Pathology and Laboratory Medicine
University of British Columbia
Senior Scientist
The James Hogg iCAPTURE Centre for Cardiovascular
and Pulmonary Research
St. Paul's Hospital - Providence Health Care
Vancouver, British Columbia, Canada

Mary Beth Beasley, MD
Department of Pathology
Providence Portland Medical Center
Portland, Oregon

Douglas P. Bennett, MD
Clinical Fellow of Infectious Diseases
Department of Medicine
Jefferson Medical College
Philadelphia, Pennsylvania

Marluce Bibbo, MD, ScD
Professor of Pathology
Director of Cytopathology
Department of Pathology, Anatomy, and Cell Biology
Jefferson Medical College
Philadelphia, Pennsylvania

Thomas W. Bouldin, MD
Professor and Vice Chair for Faculty and Trainee
Development
Department of Pathology and Laboratory Medicine
The University of North Carolina at Chapel Hill
School of Medicine
Chapel Hill, North Carolina

Mark Curtis, MD, PhD
Assistant Professor of Pathology, Anatomy, and Cell
Biology
Jefferson Medical College
Philadelphia, Pennsylvania

Ivan Damjanov, MD, PhD
Professor of Pathology
The University of Kansas School of Medicine
Kansas City, Kansas

Giulia De Falco, PhD
Assistant Professor of Human Pathology and Oncology
University of Siena
Siena, Italy

Renee Z. Dintzis, PhD
Associate Professor of Cell Biology
Director of Organ Histology
Johns Hopkins University School of Medicine
Baltimore, Maryland

Hormoz Ehya, MD
Director of Cytopathology of Pathology
Fox Chase Cancer Center
Philadelphia, Pennsylvania

David Elder, MD
Professor of Pathology and Laboratory Medicine
Director of Anatomic Pathology
Hospital of the University of Pennsylvania
Philadelphia, Pennsylvania

Kevin Furlong, DO
Assistant Professor of Clinical Medicine
Division of Endocrinology, Diabetes, and Metabolic
Diseases
Department of Medicine
Jefferson Medical College
Philadelphia, Pennsylvania

Robert M. Genta, MD
Professor of Pathology and Medicine (Gastroenterology)
University of Texas Southwestern Medical Center
Chief, Department of Pathology
Dallas VA Medical Center
Dallas, Texas

Antonio Giordano, MD, PhD
Director
Sbarro Institute for Cancer Research and Molecular
Medicine and Center of Biotechnology
College of Science and Technology
Temple University
Philadelphia, Pennsylvania

Barry Goldstein, MD, PhD
Director, Division of Endocrinology, Diabetes, and
Metabolic Diseases
Department of Medicine
Jefferson Medical College
Philadelphia, Pennsylvania

Avrum I. Gotlieb, MDCM, FRCP(C)
Professor and Chair of Laboratory Medicine and
Pathobiology
University of Toronto
Toronto, Ontario, Canada

Donna E. Hansel, MD, PhD
Associate Staff
Department of Anatomic Pathology
Cleveland Clinic
Cleveland, Ohio

Benjamin Hoch, MD
Assistant Professor of Pathology
Director, Orthopaedic Pathology
Director, ENT Pathology
Mount Sinai School of Medicine
New York, New York

Serge Jabbour, MD, FACP, FACE
Associate Professor
Division of Endocrinology, Diabetes, and Metabolic
Diseases
Department of Medicine
Jefferson Medical College
Philadelphia, Pennsylvania

J. Charles Jennette, MD
Kenneth M. Brinkhous Distinguished Professor and Chair
Department of Pathology and Laboratory Medicine
The University of North Carolina at Chapel Hill
School of Medicine
Chapel Hill, North Carolina

Lawrence C. Kenyon, MD, PhD
Associate Professor of Pathology, Anatomy, and Cell
Biology
Jefferson Medical College
Philadelphia, Pennsylvania

Anthony A. Killeen, MD, PhD
Associate Professor of Clinical Pathology
Department of Laboratory Medicine and Pathology
University of Minnesota
Minneapolis, Minnesota

Robert Kisilevsky, MD, PhD, FRCPC
Professor Emeritus of Pathology and Molecular Medicine
Queen's University
Kingston, Ontario, Canada

Michael J. Klein, MD
Professor of Pathology
Head, Section of Surgical Pathology
University of Alabama School of Medicine
Birmingham, Alabama

Gordon K. Klintworth, MD, PhD
Professor of Pathology and Joseph A.C. Wadsworth
Research
Professor of Ophthalmology
Duke University Medical Center
Durham, North Carolina

Gregory Y. Lauwers, MD
Director, Gastrointestinal Pathology Service
Massachusetts General Hospital
Associate Professor of Pathology
Harvard Medical School
Boston, Massachusetts

Steven McKenzie, MD, PhD
Vice President for Research, Medicine
Thomas Jefferson University
Philadelphia, Pennsylvania

Bruce M. McManus, MD, PhD, FRCPC, FACC, FCAP
Professor of Pathology and Laboratory Medicine
University of British Columbia
Director
The James Hogg iCAPTURE Centre for Cardiovascular
and Pulmonary Research
St. Paul's Hospital-Providence Health Care
Vancouver, British Columbia, Canada

Maria J. Merino-Neumann, MD
Senior Principal Investigator
Laboratory of Pathology
National Cancer Institute
National Institutes of Health
Bethesda, Maryland

Mari Mino-Kenudson, MD
Assistant Professor of Pathology
Harvard Medical School
Assistant in Pathology
Massachusetts General Hospital
Boston, Massachusetts

Frank A. Mitros, MD
Frederic W. Stamler Professor of Anatomical Pathology
Professor of Surgical Pathology
Department of Pathology
University of Iowa College of Medicine
Iowa City, Iowa

Hedwig S. Murphy, MD, PhD
Assistant Professor of Pathology
University of Michigan
Pathologist, Pathology and Laboratory Medicine
Veteran's Affairs Ann Arbor Healthcare System
Ann Arbor, Michigan

George L. Mutter, MD
Associate Professor of Pathology
Harvard Medical School
Department of Pathology
Brigham and Women's Hospital
Boston, Massachusetts

Adeboye O. Osunkoya, MD
Clinical and Research Fellow
Division of Genitourinary Pathology
Department of Pathology
The Johns Hopkins Hospital
Baltimore, Maryland

Roger J. Pomerantz, MD, FACP
President, Tibotec
Senior Vice President, World-Wide Therapeutic
Area Head of Virology
Johnson and Johnson Corporation
Yardley, Pennsylvania

Martha M. Quezado, MD
Chief, Neuropathology Unit
Surgical Pathology Section
Laboratory of Pathology
National Cancer Institute
National Institutes of Health
Bethesda, Maryland

Howard M. Reisner, PhD
Professor of Pathology and Laboratory Medicine
Department of Pathology and Laboratory Medicine
The University of North Carolina at Chapel Hill
School of Medicine
Chapel Hill, North Carolina

Stanley J. Robboy, MD
Professor of Pathology and Obstetrics and Gynecology
Vice Chairman for Diagnostic Services
Duke University Medical Center
Durham, North Carolina

Emanuel Rubin, MD
Gonzalo E. Aponte Distinguished Professor of Pathology
Chairman Emeritus of the Department of Pathology,
Anatomy, and Cell Biology
Jefferson Medical College
Philadelphia, Pennsylvania

Raphael Rubin, MD
Professor of Pathology, Anatomy, and Cell Biology
Jefferson Medical College
Philadelphia, Pennsylvania

Jeffrey E. Saffitz, MD, PhD
Mallinckrodt Professor of Pathology
Harvard Medical School
Chief, Department of Pathology
Beth Israel Deaconess Medical Center
Boston, Massachusetts

Alan L. Schiller, MD
Irene Heinz Given and John LaPorte Given
Professor and Chairman of Pathology
Mount Sinai Medical School
New York, New York

Roland Schwarting, MD
Professor and Chair of Pathology
Cooper University Hospital
Camden, New Jersey

David A. Schwartz, MD, MS (Hyg)
Associate Clinical Professor of Pathology
Vanderbilt University School of Medicine
Nashville, Tennessee

Gregory C. Sephel, PhD
Associate Professor of Pathology
Vanderbilt University Medical Center
Nashville, Tennessee

Craig A. Storm, MD
Assistant Professor of Pathology
Dartmouth-Hitchcock Medical Center
Lebanon, New Hampshire

David S. Strayer, MD, PhD
Professor of Pathology, Anatomy, and Cell Biology
Jefferson Medical College
Philadelphia, Pennsylvania

Ann D. Thor, MD
Professor and Chair of Pathology
University of Colorado Health Sciences Center at
Fitzsimons
Aurora, Colorado

William D. Travis, MD
Attending Thoracic Pathologist
Department of Pathology
Memorial Sloan-Kettering Cancer Center
New York, New York

John Q. Trojanowski, MD, PhD
Professor of Pathology and Laboratory Medicine
University of Pennsylvania School of Medicine
Center for Neurodegenerative Disease Research
Philadelphia, Pennsylvania

Jeffrey S. Warren, MD
Warthin/Weller Endowed Professor and Director
Division of Clinical Pathology
Department of Pathology
University of Michigan Medical School
Ann Arbor, Michigan

Bruce M. Wenig, MD
Professor of Pathology
Albert Einstein College of Medicine
Bronx, New York
Chairman of Pathology and Laboratory Medicine
Beth Israel Medical Center, St. Luke's-Roosevelt Hospital
Center and Long Island College Hospital
New York, New York

Stephen C. Woodward, MD
Professor Emeritus of Pathology
Vanderbilt University Medical Center
Nashville, Tennessee

Robert Yanagawa, PhD
Scholar
Faculty of Medicine
University of Toronto
Toronto, Ontario, Canada

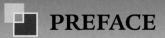
The enthusiastic reception of the prior edition of *Essentials of Rubin's Pathology* motivated us to prepare a new fifth edition. The text is based on the larger fifth edition of *Rubin's Pathology* and provides a summary of contemporary general and systemic pathology. We have omitted most of the discussions of normal anatomy, physiology and histology, as well as the descriptions of less frequently encountered diseases, when such do not teach important fundamental concepts. In addition, the clinical and experimental support for statements in the text have been shortened. Thus, our goal for *Essentials of Rubin's Pathology* is to present the reader with all the key concepts of the evolution and expression of disease and to assign priorities based on the clinical importance and heuristic relevance of the individual disorders. In revising the manuscript we have updated and modified content that is important in achieving our goal.

As in earlier editions, *Essentials of Rubin's Pathology* maintains the tradition of dividing the subject matter into general (Chapters 1–9) and systemic (Chapters 10–30) pathology. The text continues to distinguish between pathogenesis, pathology and clinical features of the various diseases discussed. Throughout the text, key terms and definitions of importance have been highlighted by bullets, italics, bold face and color to add emphasis and aid review. Many of the original drawings and photographs have been revised and new ones have been added.

This edition of *Essentials of Rubin's Pathology* recognizes the expansion of knowledge relevant to pathology into the molecular realm and contains a considerable amount of new material. It should continue to serve the needs of all students of pathology who wish to integrate the concepts of molecular, cellular and tissue based biology with the study of clinical medicine.

Attempting to edit a comprehensive textbook of pathology without missing prior errors, or introducing new ones is like trying to live without sin--worth the effort, but ultimately impossible. The inevitability of human error has not deterred us from the inclusion of new and sometimes still controversial concepts. Some of these will stand the test of time, others will be corrected in the next edition. We stand ready to catch cast stones.

Emanuel Rubin, MD
Howard Reisner, PhD

ACKNOWLEDGMENTS

This fifth edition of *Essentials of Rubin's Pathology* is based on the hard work and insights of all those who made the fifth edition of Rubin's Pathology possible. In addition, the editors would like to to thank the managing and editorial staff at the Lippincott Williams & Wilkins division of Wolters Kluwer Health and in particular Betty Sun, Kelley Squazzo, and Kathleen Scogna for their continuing support. Without their help this volume would not have been possible.

The editors also acknowledge the contributions made by our colleagues who participated in writing previous editions and those who offered suggestions and ideas for the current edition.

Stuart A. Aaronson
Mohammad Alomari
Adam Bagg
Karoly Balogh
Sue Bartow
Hugh Bonner
Patrick J. Buckley
Stephen W. Chensue
Daniel H. Connor
Jeffrey Cossman
John E. Craighead
Mary Cunnane
Joseph C. Fantone

John L. Farber
Gregory N. Fuller
Stanley R. Hamiliton
Terrence J. Harrist
Arthur P. Hays
Robert B. Jennings
Kent J. Johnson
Michael J. Klein
William D. Kocher
Robert J. Kurman
Ernest A. Lack
Antonio Martinez-Hernandez
Wolfgang J. Mergner

Juan Palazzo
Robert O. Peterson
Timothy R. Quinn
Brian Schapiro
Stephen M. Schwartz
Benjamin H. Spargo
Charles Steenbergen, Jr.
Steven L. Teitelbaum
Benjamin F. Trump
Jianzhou Wang
Beverly Y. Wang

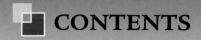

1 Cell Injury

David S. Strayer
Emanuel Rubin

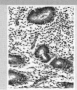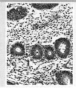

Pathology is the study of structural and functional abnormalities that are expressed as diseases of organs and systems. Classic theories attributed diseases to imbalances or noxious effects of humors on specific organs. In the 19th century, Rudolf Virchow, often referred to as the father of modern pathology, proposed that injury to the smallest living unit of the body, the cell, is the basis of all disease. To this day, clinical and experimental pathology remain rooted in this concept, which is now extended by an increased understanding of the molecular nature of many disease processes.

A living cell must maintain the ability to produce energy, much of which is spent in establishing a barrier between the internal milieu of the cell and a hostile environment. The plasma membrane, associated ion pumps, and receptor molecules serve this purpose.

A cell must also be able to adapt to adverse environmental conditions, such as changes in temperature, solute concentrations, oxygen supply, or the presence of noxious agents, and so on. If an injury exceeds the adaptive capacity of the cell, the cell dies. From this perspective, pathology is the study of cell injury and the expression of a cell's pre-existing capacity to adapt to such injury.

Reactions to Persistent Stress and Cell Injury

Persistent stress often leads to chronic cell injury. Whereas permanent organ injury is associated with the death of individual cells, the cellular response to persistent sublethal injury (whether chemical or physical) reflects adaptation of the cell to a hostile environment. Again, these changes are, for the most part, reversible on discontinuation of the stress. The major adaptive responses are atrophy, hypertrophy, hyperplasia, metaplasia, dysplasia, and intracellular storage of certain endogenous or exogenous materials. In addition, certain forms of neoplasia may follow adaptive responses.

Proteasomes are Key Participants in Cell Homeostasis, Response to Stress, and Adaptation to Altered Extracellular Environment

Cellular homeostasis requires mechanisms that allow the cell to destroy certain proteins selectively. Although there is evidence that more than one such pathway may exist, the best-understood mechanism by which cells target specific proteins for elimination is the ubiquitin (Ub)-proteasomal apparatus.

Proteasomes

The importance of the proteosome is underscored by the fact that it may comprise up to 1% of the total protein of the cell. Proteasomes are evolutionarily highly conserved and are present in all eukaryotic cells. Mutations leading to interference with normal proteasomal function are lethal.

Proteasomes exist in two forms. The 20S proteasomes are important in degradation of oxidized proteins. In 26S proteasomes, ubiquitinated proteins are degraded.

Ub and Ubiquitination

Proteins to be degraded are flagged by attaching small chains of Ub molecules to them, thereby serving to identify proteins to be destroyed.

How Ubiquitination Matters

The importance of ubiquitination and specific protein elimination is fundamental to cellular adaptation to stress and injury. Defective ubiquitination may play a role in several important neurodegenerative diseases. Mutations in parkin, a Ub ligase, and also a related enzyme, are implicated in two hereditary forms of Parkinson disease. Manipulation of ubiquitination may be important in tumor development. Thus, papilloma virus strains that are associated with human cervical cancer (see Chapters 5 and 18) produce increased p53 ubiquitination and accelerate p53 degradation. Impaired ubiquitination may also be involved in some cellular degenerative changes that occur in aging and in some storage diseases.

Atrophy is an Adaptation to Diminished Need or Resources for a Cell's Activities

Clinically, atrophy is often noted as a decrease in size or function of an organ that occurs under pathologic or physiologic circumstances. Therefore, atrophy may result from disuse of skeletal muscle or from loss of trophic signals as part of normal aging. At the level of an individual cell, atrophy may be thought of as an adaptive response, whereby a cell accommodates to changes in its environment while remaining viable. Reduction in an organ's size may reflect reversible cell atrophy or irreversible loss of cells. For example, atrophy of the brain in Alzheimer disease is secondary to extensive cell death; the size of the organ cannot be restored (Fig. 1-1). Atrophy occurs under a variety of conditions:

- **Reduced Functional Demand:** For example, after immobilization of a limb in a cast, muscle cells atrophy, and muscular strength is reduced. When normal activity resumes, the muscle's size and function return.
- **Inadequate Supply of Oxygen:** *Interference with blood supply to tissues is called ischemia.* Although total cessation of oxygen perfusion results in cell death, partial ischemia is often compatible with cell viability. Under such circumstances, cell atrophy is common.

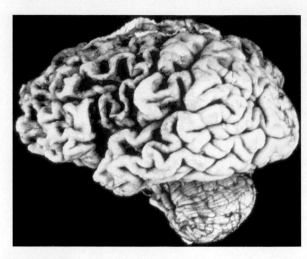

FIGURE 1-1. **Atrophy of the brain.** Marked atrophy of the frontal lobe is noted in this photograph of the brain. The gyri are thinned and the sulci conspicuously widened.

- **Insufficient Nutrients:** Starvation or inadequate nutrition associated with chronic disease leads to cell atrophy, particularly in skeletal muscle.
- **Interruption of Trophic Signals:** The functions of many cells depend on signals transmitted by chemical mediators, of which the endocrine system and neuromuscular transmission are the best examples. Loss of such signals via ablation of an endocrine gland or denervation results in atrophy of the target organ. Atrophy secondary to endocrine insufficiency is not restricted to pathologic conditions. For example, the endometrium atrophies when estrogen levels decrease after menopause (Fig. 1-2).
- **Aging:** The size of all parenchymal organs decreases with age. The size of the brain is invariably decreased, and in the very old, the size of the heart may be so diminished that the term **senile atrophy** has been used.

Hypertrophy is an Increase in Cell Size and Functional Capacity

Hypertrophy is an adaptive change that results in an increase in cellular size to satisfy increased functional demand or trophic signals. In some cases, increased cellular number (hyperplasia, see below) may also result. In organs made of terminally differentiated cells (e.g., heart, skeletal muscle), such adaptive responses are accomplished solely by increased cell size (Fig. 1-3). In other organs (e.g., kidney, thyroid), cell numbers and cell size may both increase. Hypertrophy is associated with an initial increase in the degradation of certain cellular proteins, followed by an increase in the synthesis of proteins needed to meet increased functional demand. Programmed cell death (apoptosis, see below) may be inhibited, thereby resulting in an increase in cell survival.

Hyperplasia is an Increase in the Number of Cells in an Organ or Tissue

Hypertrophy and hyperplasia often occur concurrently. The specific stimuli that induce hyperplasia and the mechanisms by which they act vary greatly from one tissue and cell type to the next. Whatever the stimulus, hyperplasia involves stimulating resting cells (G0) to enter the cell cycle (G1) and then to multiply. This may be a response to an altered endocrine milieu, increased functional demand, or chronic injury. These topics are discussed in Chapters 3 and 5.

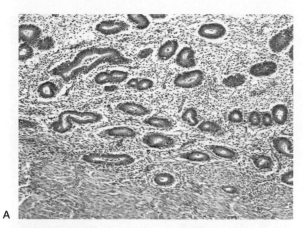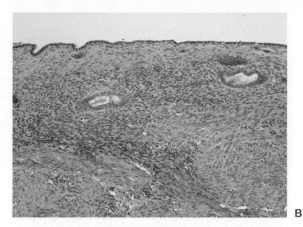

A   B

FIGURE 1-2. **Proliferative endometrium. A.** A section of the uterus from a woman of reproductive age reveals a thick endometrium composed of proliferative glands in an abundant stroma. **B.** The endometrium of a 75-year-old woman (shown at the same magnification) is thin and contains only a few atrophic and cystic glands.

- **Hormonal Stimulation:** Changes in hormone concentrations, whether physiologic or pathologic, can elicit proliferation of responsive cells. The normal increase in estrogens at puberty or early in the menstrual cycle leads to increased numbers of endometrial and uterine stromal cells. Exogenous estrogen administration to postmenopausal women has the same effect. Ectopic hormone production may also result in hyperplasia. Erythropoietin production by renal tumors may lead to hyperplasia of erythrocytes in the bone marrow.
- **Increased Functional Demand:** Hyperplasia, like hypertrophy, may be a response to increased physiologic demand. At high altitudes, low atmospheric oxygen content leads to compensatory hyperplasia of erythrocyte precursors in the bone marrow and increased erythrocytes in the blood (secondary polycythemia). Chronic blood loss, as in excessive menstrual bleeding, also causes hyperplasia of erythrocytic elements.
- **Chronic Injury:** Long-standing inflammation or chronic physical or chemical injury often results in a hyperplastic response. Pressure from ill-fitting shoes causes hyperplasia of the skin of the foot, so-called corns or calluses, which reflects the skin's protective capacity.

Inappropriate hyperplasia can itself be harmful—witness the unpleasant consequences of psoriasis, which is characterized by conspicuous hyperplasia of the skin (Fig. 1-4). Excessive estrogen stimulation, whether from endogenous or exogenous sources, may lead to endometrial hyperplasia.

Metaplasia is Conversion of One Differentiated Cell Type to Another

Metaplasia is usually an adaptive response to chronic persistent injury, in which a tissue assumes the phenotype that provides it with the best protection from the insult. Most commonly, glandular epithelium is replaced by squamous epithelium. Columnar or cuboidal lining cells may be committed to mucus production but may not be adequately resistant to the effects of chronic irritation or a pernicious chemical. For example, prolonged exposure of the bronchial epithelium to tobacco smoke leads to squamous metaplasia. A similar response occurs in the endocervix afflicted by chronic infection (Fig. 1-5).

The process is not restricted to squamous differentiation. When highly acidic gastric contents reflux chronically into the lower esophagus, the squamous epithelium of the esophagus may be replaced by stomach-like glandular mucosa (Barrett epithelium). This can be thought of as an adaptation to protect the esophagus from injury by gastric acid and pepsin, to which the normal gastric mucosa is resistant. Metaplasia may also consist of replacement of one glandular epithelium by another. Metaplasia of transitional epithelium to glandular epithelium occurs when the bladder is chronically inflamed (cystitis glandularis).

Although metaplasia is often adaptive, it is not necessarily innocuous. For example, squamous metaplasia may protect a bronchus from tobacco smoke, but it also impairs mucus production and ciliary clearance. Neoplastic transformation may occur in metaplastic epithelium; cancers of the lung, cervix, stomach, and bladder often arise in such areas. *Metaplasia is usually fully reversible.* If the noxious stimulus is removed (e.g., when one stops smoking), the metaplastic epithelium eventually returns to normal.

Dysplasia is Disordered Growth and Maturation of the Cellular Components of a Tissue

The cells that compose an epithelium normally exhibit uniformity of size, shape, and nuclear structure. Moreover, they are arranged in a regular fashion, as, for example, a squamous epithelium progresses from plump basal cells to flat superficial cells. In dysplasia, this monotonous appearance is disturbed by (1) variation in cell size and shape, (2) nuclear enlargement, irregularity, and hyperchromatism, and (3) disarray in the arrangement of cells within the epithelium (Fig. 1-6). Dysplasia occurs most often in hyper-

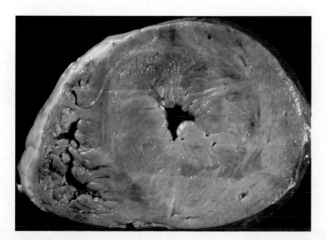

FIGURE 1-3. **Myocardial hypertrophy.** Cross-section of the heart of a patient with long-standing hypertension shows pronounced, concentric left ventricular hypertrophy.

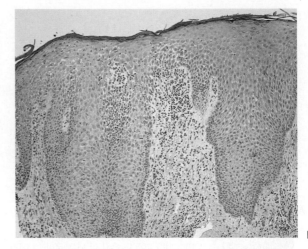

A

B

FIGURE 1-4. **Hyperplasia. A.** Normal epidermis. **B.** Epidermal hyperplasia in psoriasis, shown at the same magnification as in **A.** The epidermis is thickened, owing to an increase in the number of squamous cells.

plastic squamous epithelium, as seen in epidermal actinic keratosis (caused by sunlight) and in areas of squamous metaplasia, such as in the bronchus or the cervix. It is not, however, exclusive to squamous epithelium. Ulcerative colitis, an inflammatory disease of the large intestine, is often complicated by dysplastic changes in the columnar mucosal cells.

Like metaplasia, dysplasia is a response to a persistent injurious influence and will usually regress, for example, on cessation of smoking or the disappearance of human papillomavirus from the cervix. However, it shares many cytologic features with cancer, and the line between the two may be very fine. For example, it may be difficult to distinguish severe dysplasia from early cancer of the cervix. *Dysplasia is preneoplastic, in the sense that it is a necessary stage in the multistep cellular evolution to cancer.* In fact, dysplasia is included in the morphologic classifications of the stages of intraepithelial neoplasia in a variety of organs (e.g., cervix, prostate, bladder). Severe dysplasia is considered an indication for aggressive preventive therapy to cure the underlying cause, eliminate the noxious agent, or surgically remove the offending tissue.

As in the development of cancer (see Chapter 5), dysplasia results from sequential mutations in a proliferating cell population. *Dysplasia is the morphologic expression of the molecular disturbance in growth regulation.* However, unlike cancer cells, dysplastic cells are not entirely autonomous, and with intervention, tissue appearance may still revert to normal.

Mechanisms and Morphology of Cell Injury

All cells have efficient mechanisms to deal with shifts in environmental conditions. Thus, ion channels open or close, harmful chemicals are detoxified, metabolic stores such as fat or glycogen may be mobilized, and catabolic processes may lead to the segregation of internal particulate materials. *It is when environmental changes exceed the cell's capacity to maintain normal homeostasis that cell injury occurs.* If the stress is removed in time or if the cell can withstand the assault, cell injury is reversible, and complete structural and functional integrity is restored. The cell can also be exposed to persistent sublethal stress, as in mechanical irritation of the skin or exposure of the bronchial mucosa to tobacco smoke. In such instances, the cell has time to adapt to reversible injury in a number of ways, each of which has its morphologic counterpart. On the other hand, if the stress is severe, irreversible injury leads to death of the cell. The precise moment at which reversible injury gives way to irreversible injury, the "point of no return," cannot be identified at present.

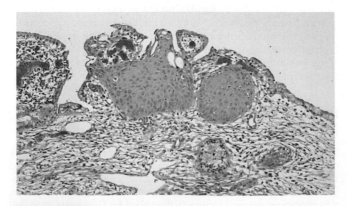

FIGURE 1-5. **Squamous metaplasia.** A section of endocervix shows the normal columnar epithelium at both margins and a focus of squamous metaplasia in the center.

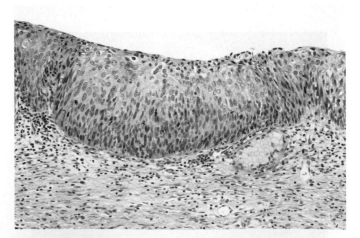

FIGURE 1-6. **Dysplasia.** The dysplastic epithelium of the uterine cervix lacks the normal polarity, and the individual cells show hyperchromatic nuclei, a larger nucleus-to-cytoplasm ratio, and a disorderly arrangement.

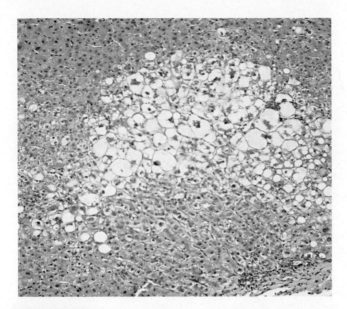

FIGURE 1-7. **Hydropic swelling.** A needle biopsy of the liver of a patient with toxic hepatic injury shows severe hydropic swelling in the centrilobular zone. The affected hepatocytes exhibit central nuclei and cytoplasm distended (ballooned) by excess fluid.

Hydropic Swelling is a Reversible Increase in Cell Volume

Hydropic swelling is characterized by a large, pale cytoplasm and a normally located nucleus (Fig. 1-7). The greater volume reflects an increased water content. Hydropic swelling reflects acute, *reversible* cell injury and may result from such varied causes as chemical and biological toxins, viral or bacterial infections, ischemia, excessive heat or cold, etc.

By electron microscopy, the number of organelles is unchanged, although they appear dispersed in a larger volume. The excess fluid accumulates preferentially in the cisternae of the endoplasmic reticulum, which are conspicuously dilated, presumably because of ionic shifts into this compartment (Fig. 1-8). Hydropic swelling is entirely reversible when the cause is removed.

Hydropic swelling results from impairment of cellular volume regulation, a process that controls ionic concentrations in the cytoplasm. This regulation, particularly for sodium (Na^+), involves three components: (1) the plasma membrane, (2) the plasma membrane Na^+ pump, and (3) the supply of ATP. The plasma membrane imposes a barrier to the flow of Na^+ down a concentration

gradient into the cell and prevents a similar efflux of potassium (K^+) from the cell. The barrier to Na^+ is imperfect, and the relative leakiness to that ion permits its passive entry into the cell. To compensate for this intrusion, the energy-dependent plasma membrane Na^+ pump (Na^+/K^+-ATPase), which is fueled by ATP, extrudes Na^+ from the cell. Injurious agents may interfere with this membrane-regulated process by (1) increasing the permeability of the plasma membrane to Na^+, thereby exceeding the capacity of the pump to extrude Na^+, (2) damaging the pump directly, or (3) interfering with the synthesis of ATP, thereby depriving the pump of its fuel. In any event, the accumulation of Na^+ in the cell leads to an increase in water content to maintain isosmotic conditions; the cell then swells.

Subcellular Changes Occur in Reversibly Injured Cells

- **Endoplasmic Reticulum:** The cisternae of the endoplasmic reticulum are distended by fluid in hydropic swelling. In other forms of acute, reversible cell injury, membrane-bound polysomes may undergo disaggregation and detach from the surface of the rough endoplasmic reticulum.
- **Mitochondria:** In some forms of acute injury, particularly ischemia, mitochondria swell. This enlargement reflects the dissipation of the energy gradient and consequent impairment of mitochondrial volume control. Amorphous densities rich in phospholipid may appear, but these effects are fully reversible on recovery.
- **Plasma Membrane:** Blebs of the cellular plasma membrane—that is, focal extrusions of the cytoplasm—are occasionally noted. These can detach from the membrane into the external environment without the loss of cell viability.
- **Nucleus:** In the nucleus, reversible injury is reflected principally in nucleolar change. The fibrillar and granular components of the nucleolus may segregate. Alternatively, the granular component may be diminished, leaving only a fibrillar core.

These changes in cell organelles (Fig. 1-9) are reflected in functional derangements (e.g., reduced protein synthesis and impaired energy production). *After withdrawal of an acute stress that has led to reversible cell injury, by definition, the cell returns to its normal state.*

Ischemic Cell Injury Usually Results from Obstruction to the Flow of Blood

When tissues are deprived of oxygen, ATP cannot be produced by aerobic metabolism and is instead generated inefficiently by anaerobic metabolism. Ischemia initiates a series of chemical and pH

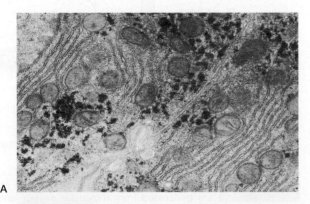

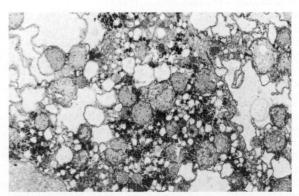

FIGURE 1-8. **Ultrastructure of hydropic swelling of a liver cell. A.** Two apposed normal hepatocytes with tightly organized, parallel arrays of rough endoplasmic reticulum. **B.** Swollen hepatocyte in which the cisternae of the endoplasmic reticulum are dilated by excess fluid.

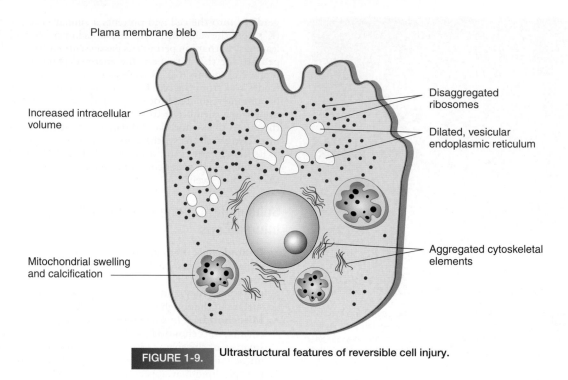

Plama membrane bleb

Increased intracellular volume

Disaggregated ribosomes

Dilated, vesicular endoplasmic reticulum

Aggregated cytoskeletal elements

Mitochondrial swelling and calcification

FIGURE 1-9. Ultrastructural features of reversible cell injury.

imbalances, which are accompanied by enhanced generation of injurious free-radical species. The damage produced by short periods of ischemia tends to be reversible if the circulation is restored. However, cells subjected to long episodes of ischemia become irreversibly injured and die. The mechanisms of cell damage are discussed later.

Oxidative Stress Leads to Cell Injury in Many Organs

For human life, oxygen is both a blessing and a curse. Without it, life is impossible, but oxygen metabolism can produce partially reduced oxygen species that react with virtually any molecule they reach.

Reactive Oxygen Species (ROS)

ROS have been identified as the likely cause of cell injury in many diseases and other damaging events. These include:

- **The inflammatory process** (see Chapter 2)
- **Chemical toxicity**
- **Ionizing radiation** in which injury is the result of the direct formation of hydroxyl ($\cdot$OH) radicals from the radiolysis of water (H_2O)
- **Chemical carcinogenesis**
- **Aging** (see below)

Cells may also be injured when oxygen is present at concentrations greater than normal. The lungs of adults and the eyes of premature newborns were at one time the major targets of such oxygen toxicity (retrolental fibroplasia) until recognized.

Complete reduction of O_2 to H_2O by mitochondrial electron transport involves the transfer of four electrons. There are three partially reduced species that are intermediate between O_2 and H_2O, representing transfers of varying numbers of electrons (Fig. 1-10). They are O_2^-, superoxide (one electron); H_2O_2, hydrogen peroxide (two electrons); and $\cdot$OH, the $\cdot$OH radical (three electrons). For the most part, these ROS are produced principally by

leaks in mitochondrial electron transport, with an additional contribution from the mixed-function oxygenase (P450) system. The major forms of ROS are listed in Table 1-1.

Superoxide

The superoxide anion (O_2^-) is produced principally by leaks in mitochondrial electron transport or as part of the inflammatory response (see Chapter 2). Superoxide and other ROS are the princi-

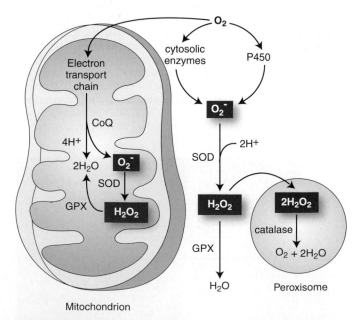

FIGURE 1-10. Mechanisms by which reactive oxygen radicals are generated from molecular oxygen and then detoxified by cellular enzymes. CoQ, coenzyme Q; GPX, glutathione peroxidase; H+, hydrogen ion; H$_2$O, water; H$_2$O$_2$, hydrogen peroxide; O$_2$, oxygen; O$_2^-$ superoxide; SOD, superoxide dismutase.

TABLE 1–1

Reactive Oxygen Species

Molecule	Attributes
Hydrogen peroxide (H_2O_2)	Forms free radicals via Fe^{2+}-catalyzed Fenton reaction
	Diffuses widely within the cell
Superoxide anion (O_2^-)	Generated by leaks in the electron transport chain and some cytosolic reactions
	Produces other ROS
	Does not readily diffuse far from its origin
Hydroxyl radical (•OH)	Generated from H_2O_2 by Fe^{2+}-catalyzed Fenton reaction
	The intracellular radical most responsible for attack on macromolecules
Peroxynitrite (ONOO•)	Formed from the reaction of nitric oxide (NO) with O_2 damages macromolecules
Lipid peroxide radicals (RCOO•)	Organic radicals produced during lipid peroxidation
Hypochlorous acid (HOCl)	Produced by macrophages and neutrophils during respiratory burst that accompanies phagocytosis
	Dissociates to yield hypochlorite radical (OCl^-)

Fe^{2+}, ferrous iron; ROS, reactive oxygen species.

pal effectors of cellular oxidative defenses that destroy pathogens, fragments of necrotic cells, or other phagocytosed material. They may also serve as signaling intermediates that elicit the release of proteolytic and other degradative enzymes (see Chapter 2).

Hydrogen Peroxide

O_2^- anions are catabolized by superoxide dismutase to produce H_2O_2. Hydrogen peroxide is also produced directly by a number of oxidases in cytoplasmic peroxisomes (see Fig. 1-10). By itself, H_2O_2 is not particularly injurious, and it is largely metabolized to H_2O by catalase or glutathione peroxidase in both the cytosol and the mitochondria (see Fig. 1-10). However, when produced in excess, it is converted to highly reactive •OH. In neutrophils, myeloperoxidase transforms H_2O_2 to the potent radical hypochlorite (OCl^-), which is lethal for microorganisms and cells.

Hydroxyl Radical

Hydroxyl radicals (•OH) are formed by (1) the radiolysis of H_2O, (2) the reaction of H_2O_2 with ferrous iron (Fe^{2+}) (Fenton reaction), and (3) the reaction of O_2^- with H_2O_2 (Haber-Weiss reaction). *The •OH radical is the most reactive molecule of ROS, and there are several mechanisms by which it can damage macromolecules.*

- **Lipid Peroxidation:** This process ultimately results in the destruction of the unsaturated fatty acids of phospholipids and a loss of membrane integrity.
- **Protein Interactions:** As a result of oxidative damage caused by •OH, proteins undergo fragmentation, cross-linking, aggregation, and eventually degradation.
- **DNA damage:** DNA is an important target of the •OH. A variety of structural alterations include strand breaks, modified bases, and cross-links between strands. In most cases, the integrity of the genome can be reconstituted by the various DNA

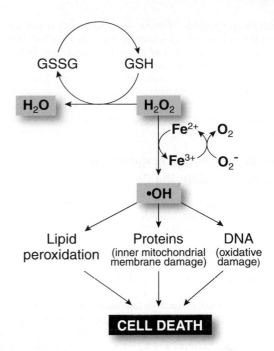

FIGURE 1-11. Mechanisms of cell injury by activated oxygen species. Fe^{2+}, ferrous iron; Fe^{2+}, ferric iron; GSH, glutathione; GSSG, glutathione; H_2O_2, hydrogen peroxide; O_2, oxygen; O_2^-, superoxide anion; •OH, hydroxyl radical.

repair pathways. However, if oxidative damage to DNA is sufficiently extensive, the cell dies.

Figure 1-11 summarizes the mechanisms of cell injury by activated oxygen species.

Cellular Defenses against Oxygen-Free Radicals

Cells manifest potent antioxidant defenses against ROS, including detoxifying enzymes such as superoxide dismutase, catalase and glutathione peroxidase (see above), and exogenous free-radical scavengers such as vitamins C (ascorbate), vitamin E (α-tocopherol), and vitamin A precursors (retinoids)

Ischemia/Reperfusion Injury Reflects Oxidative Stress

Ischemia/reperfusion (I/R) injury is a common clinical problem that arises in occlusive cardiovascular disease, infection, shock, and many other settings. I/R injury reflects the interplay of transient ischemia, consequent tissue damage, and exposure of damaged tissue to the oxygen that arrives when blood flow is re-established (reperfusion). Initially, ischemic cellular damage leads to the generation of free-radical species. Reperfusion then provides abundant molecular O_2 to combine with free radicals to form ROS. The evolution of I/R injury also involves several other factors, including inflammatory mediators (tumor necrosis factor-α [TNF-α], interleukin-1 [IL-1]), platelet-activating factor, nitric oxide synthase (NOS), NO•, intercellular adhesion molecules, and many more.

Reperfusion injury can be put into perspective by emphasizing that there are three different degrees of cell injury, depending on the duration of the ischemia:

- With short periods of ischemia, reperfusion (and, therefore, the resupply of oxygen) completely restores the structural and functional integrity of the cell. Cell injury in this case is completely reversible.

- With longer periods of ischemia, reperfusion is not associated with restoration of cell structure and function but rather with deterioration and death of the cells. In this case, lethal cell injury occurs during the period of reperfusion.
- Lethal cell injury may develop during the period of ischemia itself, in which case reperfusion is not a factor. A longer period of ischemia is needed to produce this third type of cell injury. In this case, cell damage does not depend on the formation of activated oxygen species.

Intracellular Storage Is Retention of Materials Within the Cell

The substances that accumulate may be normal or abnormal, endogenous or exogenous, harmful or innocuous and may act as an indicator of cell injury (Fig 1-12).

- **Degraded phospholipids**, which result from the turnover of endogenous membranes, are stored in lysosomes and may be recycled or remain as insoluble pigments (lipofuscin) (Fig. 1-12D).
- **Substances that cannot be metabolized** accumulate in cells. These include (1) endogenous substrates that are not further processed because a key enzyme is missing (hereditary storage diseases) (see Chapter 6), (2) insoluble endogenous pigments, such as lipofuscin (see above) and melanin (Fig. 1-12 E), (3) aggregates of normal or abnormal proteins, and (4) exogenous particulates (e.g., inhaled silica and carbon or injected tattoo pigments).
- **Overload of normal body constituents**, including iron, copper, and cholesterol, injures a variety of cells.
- **Abnormal proteins** may be toxic when they are retained within a cell. Examples are Lewy bodies in Parkinson disease and mutant α_1-antitrypsin in liver disease (Fig. 1-12 C).

Fat

Abnormal accumulation of fat is most conspicuous in the liver, a subject treated in detail in Chapter 14. When delivery of free fatty acids to the liver is increased, as in diabetes, or when intrahepatic lipid metabolism is disturbed, as in alcoholism, triglycerides accumulate in liver cells. Fatty liver is identified morphologically as lipid globules in the cytoplasm. Other organs, including the heart, kidney, and skeletal muscle, also store fat, as do atherosclerotic plaque macrophage (Fig. 1-12A,B). Fat storage is generally reversible, and there is no evidence that the excess fat by itself interferes with cell function (although such storage may well be associated with disease).

Lipofuscin

Lipofuscin is a mixture of lipids and proteins containing a golden-brown pigment called *ceroid*. Lipofuscin tends to accumulate by accretion of oxidized, cross-linked proteins and is not digestible. It occurs mainly in terminally differentiated cells (neurons and cardiac myocytes) or in cells that cycle infrequently (hepatocytes) (see Fig. 1-12D). It is often more conspicuous in conditions associated with atrophy of an organ.

Melanin

Melanin is an insoluble, brown-black pigment found principally in the epidermal cells of the skin but also in the eye and other organs (see Fig. 1-12E). It is located in intracellular organelles known as *melanosomes* and results from the polymerization of certain oxidation products of tyrosine. The amount of melanin is responsible for the differences in skin color among the various races, as well as the color of the eyes. It serves a protective function, owing to its ability to absorb ultraviolet light. In white persons, exposure to sunlight increases melanin formation (tanning). Melanin is discussed in detail in Chapter 24.

Exogenous Substances

Anthracosis refers to the storage of carbon particles in the lung and regional lymph nodes (Fig. 1-12F). Virtually all urban dwellers inhale particulates of organic carbon generated by the burning of fossil fuels. These particles accumulate in alveolar macrophages and are also transported to hilar and mediastinal lymph nodes, where the indigestible material is stored indefinitely within macrophages. Although the gross appearance of the lungs of persons with anthracosis may be alarming, the condition is innocuous.

Tattoos are the result of the introduction of insoluble metallic and vegetable pigments into the skin, where they are engulfed by dermal macrophages and persist for a lifetime.

Iron and Other Metals

Total body iron may be increased by enhanced intestinal iron absorption, as in some anemias, or by administration of iron-containing erythrocytes in a transfusion. In either case, the excess iron is stored intracellularly as ferritin and hemosiderin (Fig. 1-12G). Increasing the body's total iron content leads to progressive accumulation of hemosiderin (a partially denatured form of ferritin that aggregates easily and is recognized microscopically as yellow-brown granules in the cytoplasm), a condition termed *hemosiderosis*. Intracellular accumulation of iron in hemosiderosis does not usually injure cells. However, if the increase in total body iron is extreme, we speak of **iron overload syndromes** (see Chapter 14), in which iron deposition is so severe that it damages vital organs—particularly the heart, liver, and pancreas. Excessive iron storage in some organs is also associated with an increased risk of cancer. Pulmonary siderosis encountered among certain metal polishers is accompanied by an increased risk of lung cancer. Hereditary hemochromatosis (a genetic abnormality of iron absorption) leads to a higher incidence of liver cancer, as well as cirrhosis and cardiac disease.

Excess accumulation of lead, particularly in children, causes mental retardation and anemia. In Wilson disease, a hereditary disorder of copper metabolism, storage of excess copper in the liver and brain may produce severe chronic disease of those organs.

Calcification is a Normal or Abnormal Process

The deposition of mineral salts of calcium is a normal process in the formation of bone from cartilage. Calcium entry into dead or dying cells occurs, owing to the inability of such cells to maintain a steep calcium gradient. This cellular calcification is not ordinarily visible except as inclusions within mitochondria.

Dystrophic calcification refers to the macroscopic deposition of calcium salts in injured tissues. This type of calcification does not simply reflect an accumulation of calcium derived from the bodies of dead cells. Rather it represents an extracellular deposition of calcium from the circulation or interstitial fluid associated with persistent necrotic tissue. Dystrophic calcification may have no functional consequences, but if it occurs in a crucial location, such as a mitral or aortic valve, it may result in disease.

Metastatic calcification reflects deranged calcium metabolism, in contrast to dystrophic calcification, which has its origin in cell injury. Metastatic calcification is associated with an increased serum calcium concentration (hypercalcemia).

How Exogenous Agents Injure Cells

Ionizing radiation, chemicals, and viral pathogens injure cells by diverse mechanisms, often by direct interactions with and damage to critical cell components. Other agents may require metabolic activation that produces highly reactive free radicals (ROS), or as is the case with ionizing radiation, directly produce reactive •OH radicals. Viruses may subvert intrinsic cell death pathways (apoptotic pathways) to their advantage or provoke immune-mediated injury.

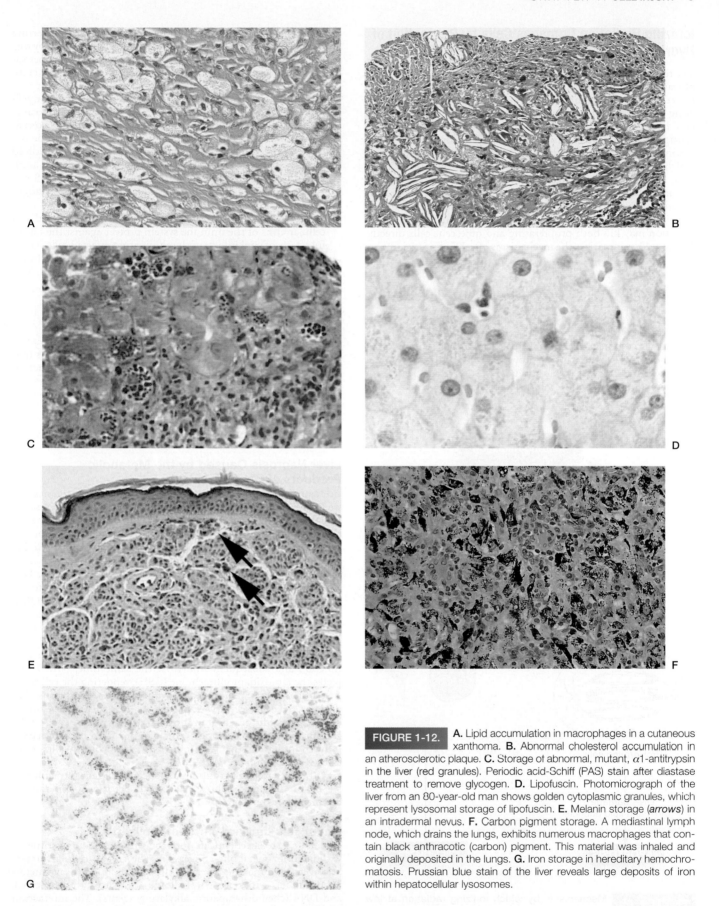

FIGURE 1-12. **A.** Lipid accumulation in macrophages in a cutaneous xanthoma. **B.** Abnormal cholesterol accumulation in an atherosclerotic plaque. **C.** Storage of abnormal, mutant, α1-antitrypsin in the liver (red granules). Periodic acid-Schiff (PAS) stain after diastase treatment to remove glycogen. **D.** Lipofuscin. Photomicrograph of the liver from an 80-year-old man shows golden cytoplasmic granules, which represent lysosomal storage of lipofuscin. **E.** Melanin storage (*arrows*) in an intradermal nevus. **F.** Carbon pigment storage. A mediastinal lymph node, which drains the lungs, exhibits numerous macrophages that contain black anthracotic (carbon) pigment. This material was inhaled and originally deposited in the lungs. **G.** Iron storage in hereditary hemochromatosis. Prussian blue stain of the liver reveals large deposits of iron within hepatocellular lysosomes.

Ionizing Radiation Damages Cells by Production of Hydroxyl Radicals and Direct Mutagenic Effects

The term "*ionizing radiation*" connotes an ability to cause radiolysis of water, thereby directly forming •OH. As noted above, •OH interact with DNA and inhibit DNA replication. For a nonproliferating cell, such as a hepatocyte or a neuron, the inability to divide is of little consequence. For a proliferating cell, however, the prevention of mitosis is a catastrophic loss of function. Once a proliferating cell can no longer divide, it dies by **apoptosis** (see below), which rids the body of those cells that have lost their prime function. Direct mutagenic effects of ionizing radiation on DNA are also important. The cytotoxic effects of ionizing radiation are dose dependent. Whereas exposure to significant amounts of radiation impairs the replicating capacity of cycling cells, massive doses of radiation may kill both proliferating and quiescent cells directly. Figure 1-13 summarizes the mechanisms of cell killing by ionizing radiation.

Viral Cytotoxicity is Direct or Immunologically Mediated

The means by which viruses cause cell injury and death are as diverse as viruses themselves. Unlike bacteria, a virus requires a cellular host to (1) house it; (2) provide enzymes, substrates, and other resources for viral replication; and (3) serve as a source for dissemination when mature virions are ready to be spread to other cells.

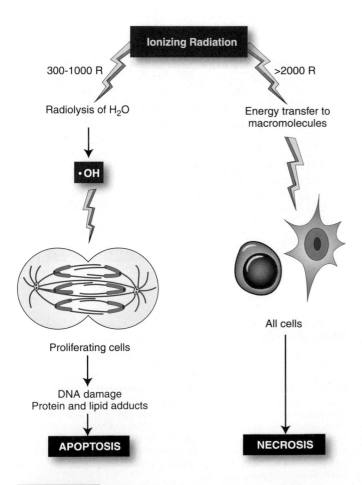

FIGURE 1-13. Mechanisms by which ionizing radiation at low and high doses causes cell death. H_2O, water; •OH, hydroxyl radical; R, rads.

- **Direct Toxicity:** Viruses may injure cells directly by subverting cellular enzymes and depleting the cell's nutrients, thereby disrupting the normal homeostatic mechanisms. The mechanisms underlying virus-induced lysis of cells, however, are complex.
- **Manipulation of Apoptosis (see below):** There are many viral activities that can elicit apoptosis. For example, apoptosis is activated when the cell detects episomal (extrachromosomal) DNA replication. Because viruses must avoid cell death before they have produced infectious progeny, they have evolved mechanisms to counteract this effect by upregulating antiapoptotic proteins and inhibiting proapoptotic ones. Some viruses also encode proteins that induce apoptosis once daughter virions are released.
- **Immunologically mediated cytotoxicity:** Both humoral and cellular arms of the immune system protect against the harmful effects of viral infections by eliminating infected cells. These arms of the immune system eliminate virus-infected cells by inducing apoptosis or by lysing the cell with complement (see Chapter 4).

Chemicals Injure Cells Directly and Indirectly

Innumerable chemicals can damage almost any cell in the body. The science of toxicology attempts to define the mechanisms that determine both target cell specificity and the mechanism of action of such chemicals. Toxic chemicals either (1) are themselves not toxic but are metabolized to yield an ultimate toxin that interacts with the target cell or (2) interact directly with cellular constituents without requiring metabolic activation. Whatever the mechanism, the result is usually necrotic cell death (see below).

Liver Necrosis Caused by the Metabolic Products of Chemicals

Acetaminophen, an important constituent of many analgesics, is a well-studied hepatotoxin, which is metabolized by the mixed-function oxidase system of the endoplasmic reticulum of the hepatocyte and causes liver cell necrosis. The drug is innocuous in recommended doses, but when consumed to excess, it is highly toxic to the liver. Most acetaminophen is enzymatically converted in the liver to nontoxic glucuronide or sulfate metabolites. Less than 5% of acetaminophen is ordinarily metabolized by isoforms of cytochrome P450 to *N*-acetyl-*p*-benzoquinone imine (NAPQI), a highly reactive quinone (Fig. 1-14). However, when large doses of acetaminophen overwhelm the glucuronidation pathway, toxic amounts of NAPQI are formed. The conjugation of NAPQI with sulfhydryl groups on liver proteins causes extensive cellular dysfunction and subsequent injury. At the same time, NAPQI depletes the antioxidant glutathione (GSH), rendering the cell more susceptible to free radical-induced injury. Thus, conditions that deplete GSH, such as starvation, enhance the toxicity of acetaminophen. In addition, acetaminophen toxicity is increased by chronic alcohol consumption, an effect mediated by an ethanol-induced increase in the 3A4 isoform of P450, which results in increased production of NAPQI.

Other hepatotoxic compounds (such as carbon tetrachloride [CCl_4]) produce metabolites that directly peroxidate and damage cell membrane phospholipids.

Chemicals that are Not Metabolized

Directly cytotoxic chemicals interact with cellular constituents without prior metabolic conversion. The critical cellular targets are diverse and include, for example, mitochondria (heavy metals and cyanide), cytoskeleton (phalloidin from toxic mushrooms), and DNA (chemotherapeutic alkylating agents). The interaction of directly cytotoxic chemicals with glutathione (alkylating agents) weakens the cell's antioxidant defenses.

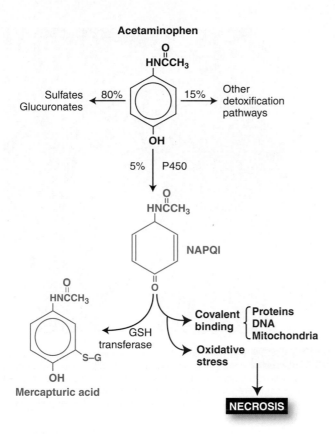

FIGURE 1-14. Chemical reactions involved in acetaminophen hepatotoxicity. GSH, glutathione; NAPQI, *N*-acetyl-*p*-benzoquinone imine.

Abnormal G Protein Activity Leads to Functional Cell Injury

Normal cell function requires the coordination of numerous activating and regulatory signaling cascades. Hereditary or acquired interference with correct signal transduction can result in significant cellular dysfunction, as illustrated by diseases associated with faulty G proteins. Inherited defects in G protein subunits can lead to constitutive activation of the enzyme. In one such hereditary syndrome, endocrine manifestations predominate, including multiple tumors in the pituitary and thyroid glands. Another G protein mutation appears to predominate in many cases of essential hypertension, in which exaggerated activation of G protein signaling results in increased vascular responsiveness to stimuli that cause vasoconstriction. Certain microorganisms (e.g., *Vibrio cholerae* and *Escherichia coli*) produce their effects by elaborating toxins that activate G proteins.

Cell Death

Paradoxically, an organism's survival requires the sacrifice of individual cells. Physiologic cell death is integral to the transformation of embryonic anlagen to fully developed organs. It is also crucial for the regulation of cell numbers in a variety of tissues, including the epidermis, gastrointestinal tract, and hematopoietic system. *Physiological cell death* involves the activation of an internal suicide program, which results in cell killing by a process termed **apoptosis**.

By contrast, *pathologic cell death* is not regulated and is invariably injurious to the organism. It may result from a variety of insults to cellular integrity (e.g., ischemia, burns, and toxins). **Necrosis** occurs when an insult irreversibly interferes with a vital structure or function of an organelle (plasma membrane, mitochondria, etc.) and does not trigger apoptosis. Pathologic cell death, however, can also result from apoptosis, as exemplified by viral infections and ionizing radiation.

Necrosis Results from Exogenous Cell Injury

At the cellular level, necrosis is characterized by cell and organelle swelling, ATP depletion, increased plasma membrane permeability, release of macromolecules, and eventually inflammation. Although the mechanisms responsible for necrosis vary according to the nature of the insult and the organ involved (see above), most instances of necrosis share certain mechanistic similarities.

Whatever the nature of the lethal insult, cell necrosis is heralded by disruption of the permeability barrier function of the plasma membrane. Normally, extracellular concentrations of Na^+ and calcium are orders of magnitude greater than intracellular concentrations. The opposite holds for potassium. The selective ion permeability requires (1) considerable energy, (2) structural integrity of the lipid bilayer, (3) intact ion channel proteins, and (4) normal association of the membrane with cytoskeletal constituents. When one or more of these elements is severely damaged, the resulting disturbance of the internal ionic balance is thought to represent the "point of no return" for the injured cell.

The role of calcium in the pathogenesis of cell death deserves special mention. Ca^{2+} concentration in extracellular fluids is in the millimolar range (10^{-3} M). By contrast, cytosolic Ca^{2+} concentration is 10,000-fold lower, on the order of 10^{-7} M. Many crucial cell functions are exquisitely regulated by minute fluctuations in the cytosolic free calcium concentration. Thus, a massive influx of Ca^{2+} through a damaged plasma membrane ensures the loss of cell viability.

Coagulative Necrosis

Coagulative necrosis refers to light microscopic alterations in a dead or dying cell (Fig. 1-15). The appearance of the necrotic cell has traditionally been termed **coagulative necrosis** because of its similarity to coagulation of proteins that occurs upon heating. However, the usefulness of this historical term today is questionable.

Shortly after a cell's death, its outline is maintained. When stained with the usual combination of hematoxylin and eosin, the cytoplasm of a necrotic cell is more deeply eosinophilic than usual.

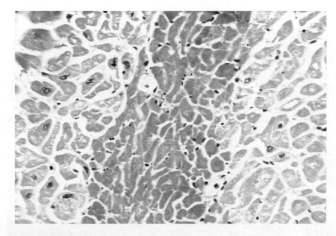

FIGURE 1-15. Coagulative necrosis. Photomicrograph of the heart in a patient with an acute myocardial infarction. In the center, the deeply eosinophilic necrotic cells have lost their nuclei. The necrotic focus is surrounded by paler-staining, viable cardiac myocytes.

In the nucleus, chromatin is initially clumped and then is redistributed along the nuclear membrane. Three morphologic changes follow:

- **Pyknosis:** The nucleus becomes smaller and stains deeply basophilic as chromatin clumping continues.
- **Karyorrhexis:** The pyknotic nucleus breaks up into many smaller fragments scattered about the cytoplasm.
- **Karyolysis:** The pyknotic nucleus may be extruded from the cell or it may manifest progressive loss of chromatin staining.

Early ultrastructural changes in a dying or dead cell reflect an extension of alterations associated with reversible cell injury. In addition to the nuclear changes described above, the dead cell features dilated endoplasmic reticulum, disaggregated ribosomes, swollen and calcified mitochondria, aggregated cytoskeletal elements, and plasma membrane blebs.

After a variable time, depending on the tissue and circumstances, a dead cell is subjected to the lytic activity of intracellular and extracellular enzymes. As a result, the cell disintegrates. This is particularly the case when necrotic cells have elicited an acute inflammatory response (see Chapter 2).

Whereas the morphology of individual cell death tends to be uniform across different cell types, the tissue responses are more variable. This diversity is described by a number of terms that reflect specific histologic patterns that depend upon the organ and the circumstances.

Liquefactive Necrosis

When the rate of dissolution of the necrotic cells is considerably faster than the rate of repair, the resulting morphologic appearance is termed **liquefactive necrosis**. The polymorphonuclear leukocytes of the acute inflammatory reaction contain potent hydrolases capable of digesting dead cells. A sharply localized collection of these acute inflammatory cells, generally in response to bacterial infection, produces rapid cell death and tissue dissolution. The result is often an **abscess** (Fig. 1-16), which is a cavity formed by liquefactive necrosis in a solid tissue. Eventually, an abscess is walled off by a fibrous capsule that contains its contents.

Coagulative necrosis of the brain may occur after cerebral artery occlusion and is followed by rapid dissolution—liquefactive necrosis—of the dead tissue by a mechanism that cannot be attributed to the action of an acute inflammatory response. Liquefactive necrosis of large areas of the central nervous system can lead to an actual cavity or cyst that persists for the rest of the person's life.

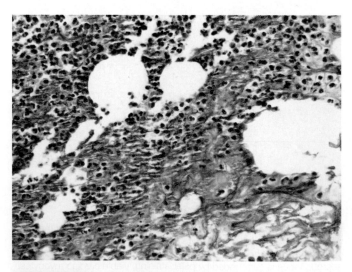

FIGURE 1-16. **Liquefactive necrosis in an abscess of the skin.** The abscess cavity is filled with polymorphonuclear leukocytes.

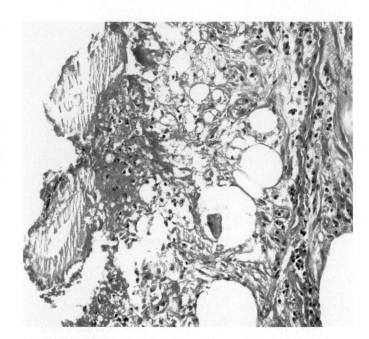

FIGURE 1-17. **Fat necrosis.** A photomicrograph of peripancreatic adipose tissue from a patient with acute pancreatitis shows an island of necrotic adipocytes adjacent to an acutely inflamed area. Fatty acids are precipitated as calcium soaps, which accumulate as amorphous, basophilic deposits at the periphery of the irregular island of necrotic adipocytes.

Fat Necrosis

Fat necrosis specifically affects adipose tissue and most commonly results from pancreatitis or trauma (Fig. 1-17). The unique feature determining this type of necrosis is the presence of triglycerides in adipose tissue. The process begins when digestive enzymes, normally found only in the pancreatic duct and small intestine, are released from injured pancreatic acinar cells and ducts into the extracellular spaces. On extracellular activation, these enzymes digest the pancreas itself as well as surrounding tissues, including adipose cells. Free fatty acids bind calcium and are precipitated as calcium soaps. Grossly, fat necrosis appears as an irregular, chalky white area embedded in otherwise normal adipose tissue. Traumatic fat necrosis is common in the breast, where triglycerides and lipases are released from injured adipocytes as a result of direct cell injury.

Caseous Necrosis

Caseous necrosis is characteristic of tuberculosis. The lesions of tuberculosis are compact aggregates of macrophages and other inflammatory cells termed *granulomas* or *tubercles* (see Chapter 2). In the center of such caseous granulomas, accumulated mononuclear cells that mediate the chronic inflammatory reaction to the offending mycobacteria are killed. The necrotic cells fail to retain their cellular outlines but do not disappear by lysis, as in liquefactive necrosis. Rather, the dead cells persist indefinitely as amorphous, coarsely granular, eosinophilic debris. Grossly, this debris is grayish white, soft, and friable. It resembles clumpy cheese, hence the name **caseous necrosis**. This distinctive type of necrosis is generally attributed to the toxic effects of the mycobacterial cell wall, which contains complex waxes (peptidoglycolipids) that exert potent biological effects.

Necrosis Usually Involves Accumulation of a Number of Intracellular Insults

The processes by which cells undergo death by necrosis vary according to the cause, organ, and cell type. The best-studied and most clinically important example is ischemic necrosis of cardiac myocytes, the leading cause of death in the Western world. The mechanisms underlying the death of cardiac myocytes are in part unique, but the basic processes that are involved are comparable to

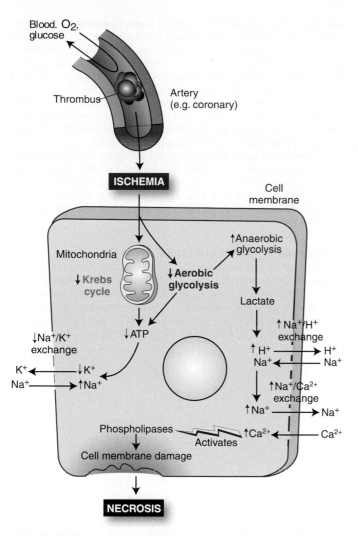

ATP, adenosine triphosphate; Ca^{2+}, calcium ion; H^+, hydrogen ion; K^+, potassium ion; Na^{2+}, sodium ion; O_2, oxygen.

those in other organs. Some of the unfolding events may occur simultaneously; others may be sequential This complex series of events is summarized below (Fig. 1-18).

- **Interruption of blood supply decreases delivery of O_2 and glucose.**
- **Anaerobic glycolysis leads to overproduction of lactate and decreased intracellular pH.**
- **Distortion of the activities of pumps in the plasma membrane as a result of lack of ATP and intracellular acidosis skews the ionic balance of the cell.**
- **Ca^{2+} accumulates in the cell.**
- **Activation of phospholipase A_2 (PLA_2) and proteases by high intracellular Ca^{2+} disrupts the plasma membrane and cytoskeleton, thereby causing cell swelling.**
- **The lack of O_2 impairs mitochondrial electron transport, thereby decreasing ATP synthesis and facilitating production of ROS.**
- **Mitochondrial damage promotes the release of cytochrome c to the cytosol.**
- **The cell dies.**

Ample data from experimental and clinical studies indicate that pharmacologic interference with a number of events involved in the pathogenesis of cell necrosis can preserve cell viability after an ischemic insult. Treatments that increase glucose uptake and redress some of the ionic imbalances may preserve myocyte viability during ischemia.

Apoptosis, or Programmed Cell Death, Refers to a Cellular Suicide Mechanism

Apoptosis is a prearranged pathway of cell death triggered by a variety of specific extracellular and intracellular signals. It is part of the balance between the life and death of cells and determines that a cell dies when it is no longer useful or when it may be harmful to the larger organism. As a self-defense mechanism, cells that are infected with pathogens or in which genomic alterations have occurred are destroyed. In this context, many pathogens have evolved mechanisms to inactivate key components of the apoptotic signaling cascades. Apoptosis detects and destroys cells that harbor dangerous mutations, thereby maintaining genetic consistency and preventing the development of cancer. By contrast, as in the case of infectious agents, successful clones of tumor cells often devise mechanisms to circumvent apoptosis.

The Morphology of Apoptosis

Apoptotic cells are recognized by nuclear fragmentation and pyknosis, generally against a background of viable cells. Importantly, individual cells or small groups of cells undergo apoptosis, whereas necrosis characteristically involves larger geographic areas of cell death. Ultrastructural features of apoptotic cells include (1) nuclear condensation and fragmentation, (2) segregation of cytoplasmic organelles into distinct regions, (3) blebs of the plasma membrane, and (4) membrane-bound cellular fragments, which often lack nuclei (Fig. 1-19).

Cells that have undergone necrotic cell death tend to elicit strong inflammatory responses. Inflammation, however, is not generally seen in the vicinity of apoptotic cells. Mononuclear phagocytes may contain cellular debris from apoptotic cells but recruitment of neutrophils or lymphocytes is uncommon (see Chapter 2). In view of the numerous developmental, physiologic, and protective functions of apoptosis, the lack of inflammation is clearly beneficial to the organism. Apoptosis plays multiple vital roles in normal development and physiology including:

- Pruning of nonpersistent structures (such as interdigital tissue) during development
- Removal of self-reactive clones during the generation of immune diversity
- Removal of mature, senescent, and less functional cells in organs continuously repopulated from stem cells (such as the gastrointestinal mucosa, epidermis, and hematopoietic system)
- Regression of hyperplasia in organs responding to changing trophic signals (such as postmenopausal atrophy of the endometrium)
- Deletion of mutant cells after recognition of irreparable DNA damage, in concert with p53

Apoptosis as a Defense against Dissemination of Infection

When a cell "detects" episomal (extrachromosomal) DNA replication, as in a viral infection, it tends to initiate apoptosis. This effect can be viewed as a means to eliminate infected cells before they

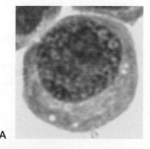
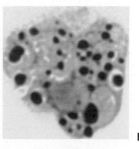

A   B

A viable leukemic cell **(A)** contrasts with an apoptotic cell **(B)** in which the nucleus has undergone condensation and fragmentation.

can spread the virus. Many viruses have evolved protective mechanisms to manipulate cellular apoptosis. Viral gene products that inhibit apoptosis have been identified for many agents, including human immunodeficiency virus, human papillomavirus, adenovirus, and many others. In some cases, these viral proteins bind and inactivate certain cellular proteins (e.g., p53) that are important in signaling apoptosis. In other instances, they may act at various points in the signaling pathways that activate apoptosis.

The Initiation of Apoptosis

Apoptosis is a final effector mechanism that can be initiated by many different stimuli and has signals that are propagated by a number of pathways. Unlike necrosis, apoptosis engages the cell's own signaling cascades. That is, a cell that undergoes apoptosis is an active participant in its own death (suicide). Most intermediate enzymes that transduce proapoptotic signals belong to a family of cysteine proteases called **caspases**.

The best understood initiators of apoptosis at the cell membrane are the binding of TNF-α to its receptor (TNFR) and that of the Fas ligand to its receptor (Fas, or Fas receptor). TNF-α is most often a free cytokine, whereas the Fas ligand is located at the plasma membrane of certain cells, such as cytotoxic effector lymphocytes.

The receptors for TNF-α and the Fas ligand become activated when they bind their ligands. These transmembrane proteins have specific amino acid sequences, termed **death domains**, in their cytoplasmic tails that act as docking sites for death domains of other proteins that participate in the signaling process leading to apoptosis (Fig. 1-20A). After binding to the receptors, the latter proteins activate downstream signaling molecules, especially procaspase-8, which is converted to caspase-8. In turn, caspase-8 initiates an activation cascade of other downstream caspases in the apoptosis pathway. These caspases (3, 6, and 7) activate a number of nuclear enzymes (e.g., polyadenosine diphosphate [ADP]-ribosyl polymerase [PARP]) that mediate the nuclear fragmentation of apoptotic cell death.

Activation of caspase signaling also occurs when killer lymphocytes, mainly cytotoxic T cells, recognize a cell as foreign. These lymphocytes release perforin and granzyme B. Perforin, as its name suggests, punches a hole in the plasma membrane of a target cell, through which granzyme B enters and activates procaspase-8 directly (see Fig. 1-20B).

Apoptosis and Mitochondrial Proteins

The mitochondrial membrane is a key regulator of the balance between cell death and cell survival. Proteins of the Bcl-2 family reside in the mitochondrial inner membrane and are either proapoptotic or anti-apoptotic (prosurvival). The balance between such factors determines the fate of the cell (see Fig. 1-20C). Bcl-2 dimers at the mitochondrial membrane bind the protein Apaf-1. A surfeit of

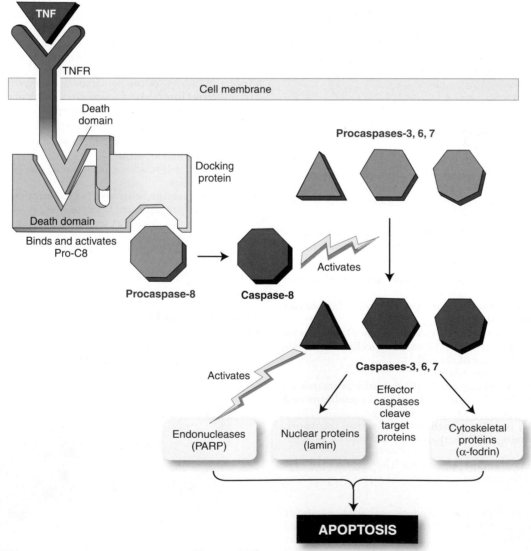

A

FIGURE 1-20. Mechanisms by which apoptosis may be initiated, signaled, and executed. A. Ligand–receptor interactions that lead to caspase activation. TNF, tumor necrosis factor; TNFR, tumor necrosis factor receptor.

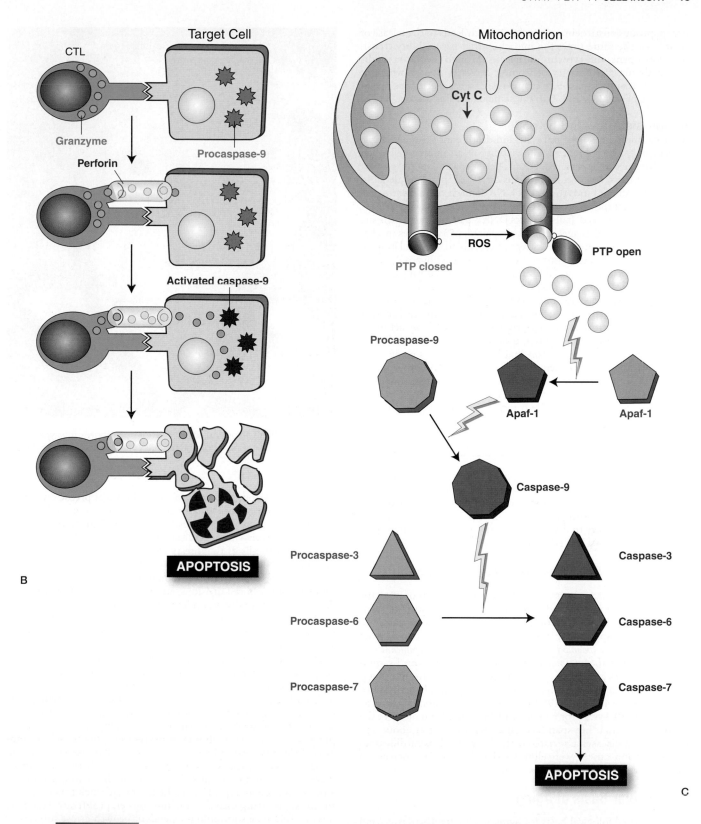

FIGURE 1-20. *Continued.* **B.** Immunologic reactions in which granzyme released by cytotoxic lymphocytes (CTLs) causes apoptosis. **C.** Opening of the mitochondrial permeability transition pore, leading to Apaf-1 activation, thereby triggering the apoptotic cascade. Cyt C, cytochrome C; PTP, permeability transition pore; ROS, reactive oxygen species.

proapoptotic constituents of the Bcl-2 family leads to the release of Apaf-1. At the same time, the mitochondrial permeability transition pore opens, and cytochrome c leaks through the mitochondrial membrane. Cytosolic cytochrome c activates Apaf-1, which in turn converts procaspase-9 to caspase-9. Caspase-9 activates downstream caspases (3, 6, and 7) in the same manner as caspase-8.

Apoptosis Activated by p53

A pivotal molecule in the cell's life-and-death dance is the versatile protein p53, which preserves the viability of an injured cell when DNA damage can be repaired, but propels it toward apoptosis after irreparable harm has occurred (p53 is discussed in greater detail in Chapter 5). After it binds to areas of DNA damage, p53 activates proteins that arrest the cell in stage G1 of the cell cycle, allowing time for DNA repair to proceed. It also directs DNA repair enzymes to the site of injury. If DNA damage cannot be repaired, p53 activates mechanisms that lead to apoptosis. Stress also leads to accumulation of p53. Activation of certain oncogenes, such as *c-myc*, hypoxia, depletion of ribonucleotides, and loss of cell–cell adhesion during oncogenesis all promote p53-dependent apoptotic pathways.

In summary, cells are continually poised between survival and apoptosis: their fate rests on the balance of powerful intracellular and extracellular forces and have signals that constantly act upon and counteract each other. Often, apoptosis functions as a self-protective programmed mechanism that leads to a cell's suicide when its survival may be detrimental to the organism. At other times, apoptosis is a pathologic process that contributes to many disorders, especially degenerative diseases. Thus, pharmacologic manipulation of apoptosis is an active frontier of drug development.

Biological Aging

Aging must be distinguished from mortality on the one hand and from disease on the other. Death is a random event; an aged person who does not succumb to the most common cause of death will die from the second, third, or tenth most common cause. Although the increased vulnerability to disease among the elderly is an interesting problem, disease itself is entirely distinct from aging.

Maximal Life Span Has Remained Unchanged

Millennia ago, the psalmist sang of a natural life span of 70 years, which with vigor may extend to 80. By contrast, it is estimated that the usual age at death of Neolithic humans was 20 to 25 years, and the average life span today in some regions is often barely 10 years more. *Interestingly, the maximum life span attained is not significantly altered by a protected environment.* With improved safety and sanitation, antibiotics and other drugs, and better diagnostic and therapeutic methods, the age-adjusted death rate in the United States has declined by 40% since 1970. In 2004, life expectancy at the time of birth was 80.4 years for females and 75.2 years for males. Yet the maximum human life span has remained constant at about 110 years. Even if diseases associated with old age, such as cardiovascular disease and cancer, were eliminated, only a modest increase in average life expectancy would be seen.

The Cellular Basis of Aging

Although the biological basis for aging is obscure, there is general agreement that its cause lies at the cellular level. Various theories of cellular aging have been proposed, but the evidence adduced for each is at best indirect. Support for the concept of a genetically programmed life span comes from studies of replicating cells in tissue culture. Unlike cancer cells, normal cells in tissue culture have a limited capacity to replicate at about 50 population doublings. If they are exposed to an oncogenic virus or a chemical carcinogen, they may continue to replicate; in a sense, they become immortal. A rough correlation between the number of population doublings in fibroblasts and life span has been reported in several species. Moreover, cells ob-

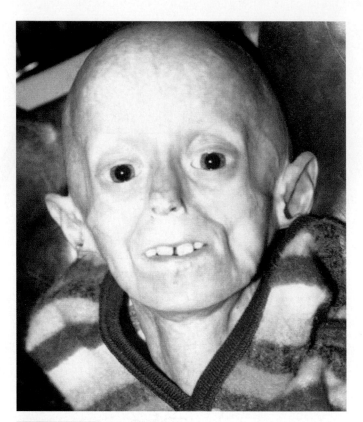

FIGURE 1-21. **Progeria.** A 10-year-old girl shows the typical features of premature aging associated with progeria.

tained from persons afflicted with a syndrome of precocious aging, such as progeria (see below), also display a reduced number of population doublings in vitro. However, there is no demonstrable age-related change in vivo in the replicative capacity of rapidly cycling cells (e.g., epithelial cells of the intestine), leaving one with an apparent paradox. Cellular senescence in vitro is also a dominant genetic trait. Thus, hybrids between normal human cells in vitro, which exhibit a limited number of cell divisions, and immortalized cells with an indefinite capacity to divide, undergo senescence.

An attractive explanation for cell senescence in vitro centers on the genetic elements at the tips of chromosomes, termed **telomeres**. These are series of short repetitive nucleotide sequences (2,000 in human chromosomes). Because DNA polymerase cannot copy the linear chromosomes all the way to the tip, the telomeres tend to shorten with each cell division until a critical diminution in size interferes with replication. Thus, telomere shortening acts as a molecular clock that produces senescence after a defined number of cell divisions in vitro. Most eukaryotic cells have the potential to express a ribonucleoprotein enzyme termed **telomerase**, which can extend chromosome ends. Expression of telomerase can reverse the senescent phenotype in vitro, and can be demonstrated in immortalized cells, but at the cost of producing a tumor-like phenotype. Hence, the telomeric clock functions as a tumor-suppressing mechanism, limiting cell proliferative capacity in vivo. Telomere shortening-dependent growth arrest suppresses tumorigenesis but at the cost of contributing to aging.

Genetic Factors Influence Aging

In humans, the modest correlation in longevity between related persons, the excellent concordance of life span among identical twins, and the presence of heritable disease associated with accelerated aging (progeria) lend credence to the concept that aging is influenced by genetic factors. One of the most striking of such genetic diseases is Hutchinson-Guilford progeria, in which the entire

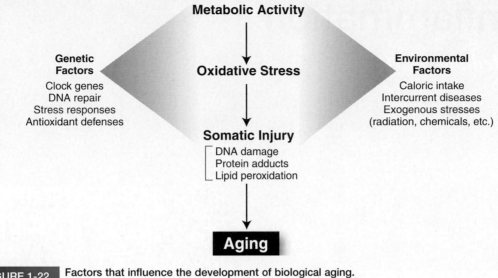

FIGURE 1-22. Factors that influence the development of biological aging.

process of aging, including features such as male-pattern baldness, cataracts, and coronary artery disease, is compressed into a span of less than 10 years (Fig. 1-21). The cause of this form of progeria is a mutation in the LMNA gene; its product is a protein termed lamin A, and the mutant form of this protein is termed progerin. This abnormal protein accumulates in the nucleus from one cell generation to the next, thereby interfering with the structural integrity and organization of the nucleus. A variety of additional mutations of the LMNA gene (termed "laminopathies"), as well as defects of other genes, are associated with the progeric phenotype.

Aging May Reflect Accumulated Somatic Damage

Oxidative stress is an invariable consequence of life in an atmosphere rich in oxygen. An important hypothesis holds that the loss of function that is characteristic of aging is caused by progressive and irreversible accrual of molecular oxidative damage. The rate of generation of ROS correlates with an organism's overall metabolic rate. The theory that aging is related to oxidative stress is based on several observations: (1) larger animals usually live longer than smaller ones; (2) metabolic rate is inversely related to body size (the larger the animal, the lower the metabolic rate); and (3) generation of activated oxygen species correlates inversely with body size. Additional evidence for progressive oxidative damage with aging is the deposition of oxidized aggregated proteins and lipofuscin pigment, principally in postmitotic cells of organs such as the brain, heart, and liver (see above) and the accumulation of hydroxyl radical-mediated damage to mitochondrial DNA. Aerobic respiration in mitochondria is the richest source of ROS in the cell.

Summary Hypothesis of Aging

Current evidence supports the notion that *although aging is under some measure of genetic control, it is unlikely that a predetermined genetic program for aging exists* (Fig. 1-22). It is likely that the combined effects of a number of genes eventually lead to the accumulation of somatic mutations, deficiencies in DNA repair, the accretion of oxidative damage to macromolecules, and a variety of other defects in cell function, all culminating in the progressive failure of homeostatic mechanisms characteristic of aging. As Maimonides said in the 12th century, "The same forces that operate in the birth and temporal existence of man also operate in his destruction and death."

2 Inflammation

Hedwig S. Murphy

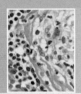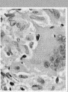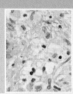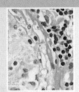

Inflammation is the response to injury of a tissue and its microcirculation *and is characterized by the elaboration of inflammatory mediators as well as the movement of fluid and leukocytes from the blood into extravascular tissues. Inflammation localizes and eliminates microorganisms, damaged cells, and foreign particles, paving the way for a return to normal structure and function.*

The clinical signs of inflammation, recognized in Egyptian medical texts before 1000 BC, were codified as the four cardinal signs of inflammation: ***rubor*** *(redness),* ***calor*** *(heat),* ***tumor*** *(swelling), and* ***dolor*** *(pain) by the Roman encyclopedist Aulus Celsus in the*

second century AD. These features correspond to the inflammatory events of vasodilation, edema, and tissue damage. A fifth sign, ***functio laesa*** *(loss of function), was added in the 19th century by Rudolf Virchow, who recognized inflammation as a response to tissue injury.*

Overview of Inflammation

Inflammation is best viewed as an ongoing process that can be divided into phases.

- **Initiation** results in a stereotypic, immediate response termed **acute inflammation**. The acute response is characterized by the rapid flooding of the injured tissue with fluid, coagulation factors, cytokines, chemokines, platelets and inflammatory cells, and neutrophils in particular (Fig. 2-1).

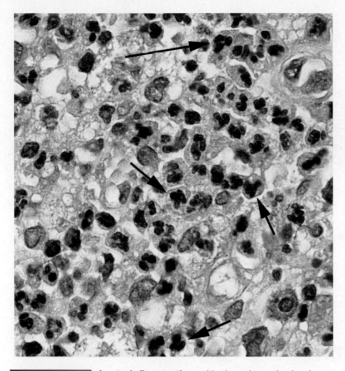

FIGURE 2-1. **Acute inflammation** with densely packed polymorphonuclear neutrophils (PMNs) with multilobed nuclei (*arrows*).

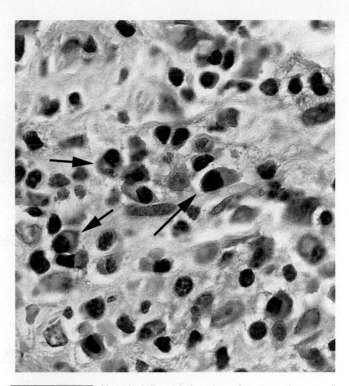

FIGURE 2-2. **Chronic inflammation.** Lymphocytes, plasma cells (*arrows*), and a few macrophages are present.

- **Amplification** depends upon the extent of injury and the activation of mediators such as kinins and complement components. Additional leukocytes and macrophages are recruited to the area.
- **Destruction** of the inciting agent by phagocytosis and enzymatic or nonenzymatic processes reduces or eliminates foreign material or infectious organisms. At the same time, damaged tissue components are also removed, paving the way for repair to begin (see Chapter 3).
- **Termination** of the inflammatory response is mediated by intrinsic anti-inflammatory mechanisms that limit tissue damage and allow for either restoration of tissue, with return to normal physiological function, or repair and the development of a scar in place of normal tissue.

Certain types of injury trigger a sustained inflammatory response associated with the inability to clear injured tissue and foreign agents. Such a persistent response (which often has an immune component) is termed **chronic inflammation**. Chronic inflammatory infiltrates are composed largely of lymphocytes, plasma cells, and macrophages and often have an immune component (Fig. 2-2). Acute and chronic inflammatory infiltrates often coexist.

Acute Inflammation: Vascular Events

Among the earliest responses to tissue injury are alterations in the anatomy and function of the microvasculature, which may promote edema (see Figs. 2-3 and 2-4). These responses include:

1. **Transient vasoconstriction of arterioles** at the site of injury is the earliest vascular response to mild skin injury. This process is mediated by both neurogenic and chemical mediator systems and usually resolves within seconds to minutes.
2. **Vasodilation of precapillary arterioles** then increases blood flow to the tissue, a condition known as **hyperemia**.

Vasodilation is caused by the release of specific mediators and is responsible for redness and warmth at sites of tissue injury.

3. **An increase in endothelial cell barrier permeability** results in edema. Loss of fluid from intravascular compartments as blood passes through capillary venules leads to local stasis and plugging of dilated small vessels with erythrocytes. These changes are reversible following mild injury: within several minutes to hours, the extravascular fluid is cleared through lymphatics.

The vascular response to injury is a dynamic event that involves sequential physiological and pathological changes. **Vasoactive mediators**, originating from both plasma and cellular sources, are generated at sites of tissue injury (see Fig. 2-4). These mediators bind to specific receptors on vascular endothelial and smooth muscle cells, causing vasoconstriction or vasodilation. Proximal to capillaries, vasodilation of arterioles increases blood flow and can exacerbate fluid leakage into the tissue. Distally, vasoconstriction of postcapillary venules increases capillary bed hydrostatic pressure, potentiating edema formation. By contrast, vasodilation of venules decreases capillary hydrostatic pressure and inhibits movement of fluid into extravascular spaces.

After injury, vasoactive mediators bind specific receptors on endothelial cells, causing endothelial cell contraction and gap formation, a reversible process (see Fig. 2-3B). This break in the endothelial barrier leads to extravasation (leakage) of intravascular fluids into the extravascular space. Mild direct injury to the endothelium results in a biphasic response: an early change in permeability occurs within 30 minutes after injury, followed by a second increase in vascular permeability after 3 to 5 hours. When damage is severe, exudation of intravascular fluid into the extravascular compartment increases progressively, peaking 3 to 4 hours after injury.

Severe direct injury to the endothelium, such as is caused by burns or caustic chemicals, may result in irreversible damage. In such cases, the endothelium separates from the basement membrane, resulting in cell blebbing (blisters or bubbles between the

A NORMAL VENULE

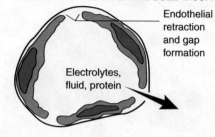

Basement membrane

Endothelial cell

Tight junction

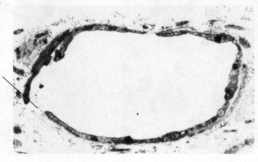

B VASOACTIVE MEDIATOR-INDUCED INJURY

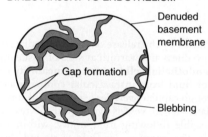

Endothelial retraction and gap formation

Electrolytes, fluid, protein

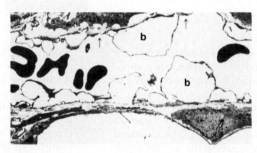

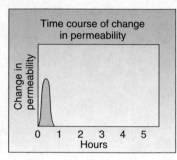

Time course of change in permeability

C DIRECT INJURY TO ENDOTHELIUM

Denuded basement membrane

Gap formation

Blebbing

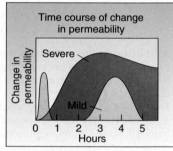

Time course of change in permeability

Severe

Mild

FIGURE 2-3. **Responses of the microvasculature to injury. A.** The wall of the normal venule is sealed by tight junctions between adjacent endothelial cells. **B.** During mild vasoactive mediator-induced injury, the endothelial cells separate and permit the passage of the fluid constituents of the blood. **C.** With severe direct injury, the endothelial cells form blebs (*b*) and separate from the underlying basement membrane. Areas of denuded basement membrane (*arrows*) allow a prolonged escape of fluid elements from the microvasculature.

endothelium and the basement membrane). This leaves areas of basement membrane naked (see Fig. 2-3C), thereby disrupting the barrier between the intravascular and extravascular spaces.

Several definitions are important for understanding the vascular components of inflammation:

- **Edema** is the accumulation of fluid within the extravascular compartment and interstitial tissues.
- A **transudate** is edema fluid with a low protein content (specific gravity <1.015). Transudates tend to occur in noninflammatory conditions, where the endothelial barrier remains intact and prevents the loss of large molecules from the vasculature.
- An **exudate** is edema fluid with a high protein concentration (specific gravity >1.015), which frequently contains inflammatory cells. Exudates are observed early in acute inflammatory reactions and are produced by mild injuries, such as sunburn or traumatic blisters.
- A **fibrinous exudate** contains large amounts of fibrin as a result of activation of the coagulation system. When a fibrinous exudate occurs on a serosal surface, such as the pleura or pericardium, it is referred to as "fibrinous pleuritis" or "fibrinous pericarditis."

- **A purulent exudate or effusion** contains prominent cellular components. It is frequently associated with pathological conditions such as pyogenic bacterial infections, in which the predominant cell type is the polymorphonuclear neutrophil (PMN).

Plasma-Derived Mediators of Inflammation

Numerous chemical mediators are integral to the initiation, amplification, and termination of inflammatory processes (Fig. 2-4). Cell- and plasma-derived mediators work in concert to activate cells by (1) binding specific receptors, (2) recruiting cells to sites of injury, and (3) stimulating the release of additional soluble mediators. These mediators themselves are relatively short-lived, or are inhibited by intrinsic mechanisms, effectively turning off the response and allowing the process to resolve. Cell-derived mediators are considered below.

Plasma contains the elements of three major enzyme cascades, each composed of a series of proteases. Sequential activation of proteases results in release of important chemical mediators.

SOURCE   MEDIATOR

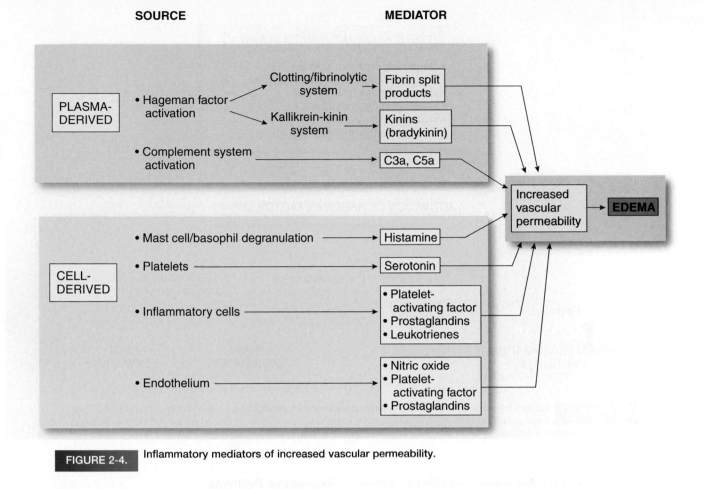

FIGURE 2-4. Inflammatory mediators of increased vascular permeability.

These interrelated systems include (1) **the coagulation cascade and fibrinolytic system**, (2) **kinin generation**, and (3) the **complement system** (Fig. 2-4). The coagulation cascade is discussed in Chapters 10 and 20; the kinin and complement systems are presented here.

Hageman Factor is a Key Source of Vasoactive Mediators

Hageman factor (clotting factor XII) is generated within the plasma and is activated by exposure to negatively charged surfaces such as basement membranes, proteolytic enzymes, bacterial lipopolysaccharides, and foreign materials. This key component triggers activation of additional plasma protease systems that are important in inflammation, including (1) the "intrinsic" coagulation cascade, (2) fibrinolysis with the concomitant elaboration of plasmin and plasmin-derived bioactive peptides, (3) generation of kallikrein and subsequent production of kinins, and (4) activation of the alternate complement pathway (see Fig. 2-5).

Kinins Amplify the Inflammatory Response

Kinins are potent inflammatory agents formed in plasma and tissue by the action of serine protease kallikreins on specific plasma glycoproteins termed **kininogens**. **Bradykinin** and related peptides regulate multiple physiological processes, including blood pressure, contraction and relaxation of smooth muscle, plasma extravasation, cell migration, inflammatory cell activation, and inflammatory-mediated pain responses. Kinins amplify the inflammatory response by stimulating local tissue cells and inflammatory cells to generate additional mediators, including prostanoids, cytokines (especially tumor necrosis factor-α [TNF-

α] and interleukins), and nitric oxide (NO•). Kinins are rapidly degraded to inactive products by kininases and, therefore, have rapid and short-lived functions.

Complement is Activated Through Three Pathways to Form the Membrane Attack Complex (MAC)

The complement system is a group of proteins found in plasma and on cell surfaces, whose primary function is defense against microbes. The physiological activities of the complement system include (1) defense against pyogenic bacterial infection by opsonization, chemotaxis, activation of leukocytes and lysis of bacteria and cells; (2) bridging innate and adaptive immunity for defense against microbial agents by augmenting antibody responses and enhancing immunological memory; and (3) disposal of immune products and products of inflammatory injury by clearance of immune complexes from tissues and removal of apoptotic cells.

The endpoint of complement activation is the formation of the MAC and cell lysis. The cleavage products generated at each step of the way catalyze the next step in the cascade and have additional properties that render them important inflammatory molecules (Fig. 2-6):

• **Anaphylatoxins** (C3a, C4a, C5a): These proinflammatory molecules mediate smooth-muscle contraction and increase vascular permeability.
• **Opsonins** (C3b, iC3b): Bacterial opsonization is the process by which a specific molecule (e.g., IgG or C3b) binds to the surface of the bacterium. The process enhances phagocytosis by enabling receptors on phagocytic cell membranes (e.g., Fc receptor or C3b receptor) to recognize and bind the opsonized bac-

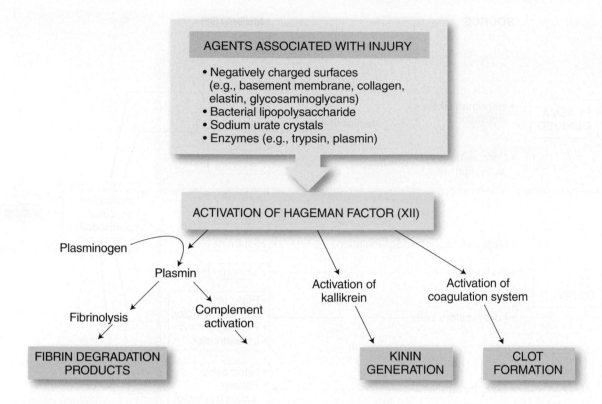

FIGURE 2-5. **Hageman factor activation and inflammatory mediator production.** Hageman factor activation is a key event leading to conversion of plasminogen to plasmin, resulting in generation of fibrin split products and active complement products. Activation of kallikrein produces kinins, and activation of the coagulation system results in clot formation.

terium. Viruses, parasites, and transformed cells also activate complement by similar mechanisms, an effect that leads to their inactivation or death.

- **Proinflammatory molecules** (MAC, C5a): These chemotactic factors also activate leukocytes and tissue cells to generate oxidants and cytokines and induce degranulation of mast cells and basophils.

The complement system is activated by three convergent pathways termed **classical, mannose-binding lectin (MBL)**, and **alternative pathways** (see Fig. 2-6).

The Classical Pathway
Activators of the classical pathway include antigen-antibody (Ag-Ab) complexes, products of bacteria and viruses, proteases, urate crystals, apoptotic cells, and polyanions (polynucleotides). The proteins of this pathway are C1 through C9, the nomenclature following the historical order of discovery. Ag-Ab complexes activate C1, initiating a cascade that leads to formation of the MAC, which proceeds as shown in Figure 2-6.

The Mannose-Binding Pathway
The mannose- or lectin-binding pathway has some components in common with the classical pathway. It is initiated by the binding of microbes bearing terminal mannose groups to **mannose-binding lectin**, a member of the family of calcium-dependent lectins, termed the **collectins**. This multifunctional acute-phase protein has properties similar to those of immunoglobulin M (IgM) antibody (binds to a wide range of oligosaccharide structures), IgG (interacts with phagocytic receptors), and C1q. This last property enables it to interact with either C1r-C1s or with a serine protease called MASP (MBL-associated serine protease) to activate complement (see Fig. 2-6).

Alternative Pathway
The alternative pathway is initiated by derivative products of microorganisms, such as endotoxin (from bacterial cell surfaces), zymosan (yeast cell walls), polysaccharides, viruses, tumor cells, and foreign materials. Proteins of the alternative pathway are called "factors," followed by a letter. Activation of the alternative pathway occurs at the level of C3 activation to produce small amounts of C3b, which become covalently bound to carbohydrates and proteins on microbial cell surfaces (see Fig. 2-6).

The Complement System and Disease
The importance of an intact and appropriately regulated complement system is exemplified in persons who have acquired or congenital deficiencies of specific complement components or regulatory proteins. Such patients have an increased susceptibility to infectious agents, and in some cases, a propensity for autoimmune diseases associated with circulating immune complexes.

Cell-Derived Mediators of Inflammation

Circulating platelets, basophils, PMNs, endothelial cells, monocyte/macrophages, tissue mast cells, and the injured tissue itself are all potential cellular sources of vasoactive mediators. In general, these mediators are (1) derived from metabolism of phospholipids and arachidonic acid (e.g., prostaglandins, thromboxanes, leukotrienes, lipoxins, platelet-activating factor [PAF]), (2) preformed and stored in cytoplasmic granules (e.g., histamine, serotonin, lysosomal hydrolases), or (3) derived from altered production of normal regulators of vascular function (e.g., NO•).

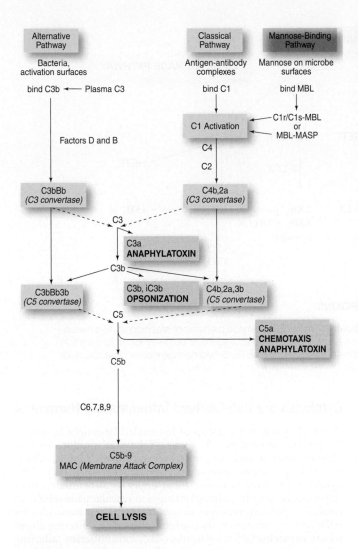

TABLE 2–1	
Biological Activities of Arachidonic Acid Metabolites	
Metabolite	**Biological Activity**
PGE_2, PGD_2	Induce vasodilation, bronchodilation, inhibit inflammatory cell function
PGI_2	Induces vasodilation, bronchodilation, inhibits inflammatory cell function
$PGF_{2\alpha}$	Induces vasodilation, bronchoconstriction
TXA_2	Induces vasoconstriction, bronchoconstriction, enhances inflammatory cell functions (especially platelets)
LTB_4	Chemotactic for phagocytic cells, stimulates phagocytic cell adherence, enhances microvascular permeability
LTC_4, LTD_4, LTE_4	Induce smooth muscle contraction, constrict pulmonary airways, increase microvascular permeability

PG, prostaglandin; TXA_2, thromboxane A_2; LT, leukotriene.

FIGURE 2-6. **Complement activation.** The alternative, classical, and mannose-binding pathways lead to generation of the complement cascade of inflammatory mediators and cell lysis by the membrane attack complex (MAC). MBL, mannose-binding lectin; MBL MASP, MBL-associated serine protease.

Arachidonic Acid and Platelet-Activating Factor are Derived from Membrane Phospholipids

Phospholipids and fatty acid derivatives released from plasma membranes are metabolized into mediators and homeostatic regulators by inflammatory cells and injured tissues. As part of a complex regulatory network, prostanoids, leukotrienes and lipoxin (derivatives of arachidonic acid), both promote and inhibit inflammation (Table 2-1).

Arachidonic Acid

Depending on the specific inflammatory cell and the nature of the stimulus, activated cells generate arachidonic acid by one of two pathways, involving either stimulus-induced activation of phospholipase A_2 (PLA_2) or phospholipase C. Once generated, arachidonic acid is further metabolized through two pathways: (1) **cyclooxygenation**, with subsequent production of prostaglandins and thromboxanes; and (2) **lipoxygenation**, to form leukotrienes and lipoxins (Fig. 2-7).

Corticosteroids are widely used to suppress the tissue destruction associated with many inflammatory diseases. These drugs induce synthesis of an inhibitor of PLA_2 and block release of arachidonic acid in inflammatory cells. Although corticosteroids (e.g., prednisone) are widely used to suppress inflammatory responses, their prolonged administration can have significant harmful effects, including increased risk of infection, damage to connective tissue, and adrenal gland atrophy.

Platelet-Activating Factor (PAF)

Another potent inflammatory mediator derived from membrane phospholipids is PAF, synthesized by virtually all activated inflammatory cells, endothelial cells, and injured tissue cells. PAF is derived from membrane phospholipids by the PLA_2 pathway. During inflammatory and allergic responses, PAF stimulates platelets, neutrophils, monocyte/macrophages, endothelial cells, and vascular smooth muscle cells. PAF induces platelet aggregation and degranulation at sites of tissue injury and enhances the release of serotonin, thereby causing changes in vascular permeability. The molecule is also an extremely potent vasodilator, augmenting permeability of the microvasculature at sites of tissue injury.

Prostanoids, Leukotrienes, and Lipoxins are Biologically Active Metabolites of Arachidonic Acid

Prostanoids

Arachidonic acid is further metabolized by cyclooxygenases 1 and 2 (COX 1, COX-2) to generate prostanoids (see Fig. 2-7). **COX-1** is constitutively expressed by most cells and increases upon cell activation. It is a key enzyme in the synthesis of prostaglandins, which in turn (1) protect the gastrointestinal mucosal lining, (2) regulate water/electrolyte balance, (3) stimulate platelet aggregation to maintain normal hemostasis, and (4) maintain resistance to thrombosis on vascular endothelial cell surfaces. **COX-2** expression is generally low or undetectable but takes over as the major source of prostanoids as inflammation progresses. Both COX isoforms generate prostaglandin H (PGH_2), which is then the substrate for the production of prosta-

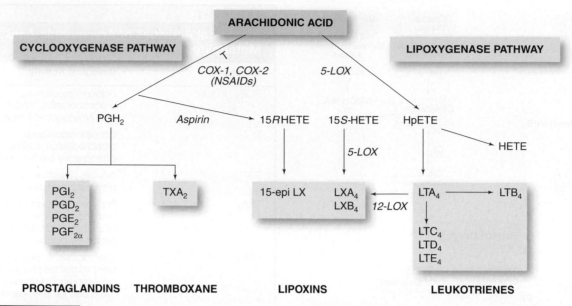

FIGURE 2-7. **Biologically active arachidonic acid metabolites.** The cyclooxygenase pathway of arachidonic acid metabolism generates prostaglandins (PG) and thromboxane (TXA$_2$). The lipoxygenase pathway forms lipoxins (LX) and leukotrienes (LT); COX, cyclooxygenase; HETE, hydroxyeicosatetraenoic acid; HpETE, 5-hydroperoxyeicosatetraenoic acid; NSAIDs, nonsteroidal anti-inflammatory drugs.

cyclins (PGI$_2$), PGD$_2$, PGE$_2$, PGF$_{2\alpha}$, and TXA$_2$ (thromboxane). The profile of prostaglandin production (i.e., the quantity and variety produced during inflammation) depends in part on the cells present and their activation state (see Table 2-1). *Inhibition of COX is one mechanism by which nonsteroidal anti-inflammatory drugs (NSAIDs), including aspirin, indomethacin, and ibuprofen, exert their potent analgesic and anti-inflammatory effects.* NSAIDS block COX-2–induced formation of prostaglandins, thereby mitigating pain and inflammation. However, they also inhibit COX-1 and lead to adverse effects on the stomach and kidneys. This complication led to the development of COX-2–specific inhibitors (see Fig. 2-7).

Leukotrienes

Slow-reacting substance of anaphylaxis has long been recognized as a smooth muscle stimulant and mediator of hypersensitivity reactions. It is, in fact, a mixture of leukotrienes, the second major family of derivatives of arachidonic acid (see Fig. 2-7 and Table 2-1). Leukotriene A$_4$ (LTA$_4$) serves as a precursor to several other leukotrienes. LTB$_4$ is a major product of neutrophils as well as certain macrophage populations and has potent chemotactic activity for neutrophils, monocytes, and macrophages. In other cell types, especially mast cells, basophils and macrophages, LTC$_4$, LTD$_4$, and LTE$_4$ are produced. These three cysteinyl-leukotrienes (1) stimulate smooth-muscle contraction, (2) enhance vascular permeability, and (3) are responsible for the development of many of the clinical symptoms associated with allergic-type reactions, notably asthma. Leukotrienes exert their action through high-affinity specific receptors, which may prove to be important targets of drug therapy.

Lipoxins

Lipoxins, the third class of proinflammatory products of arachidonic acid, are synthesized by platelets and neutrophils within the vascular lumen in a manner dependent on cell–cell interactions (see Fig. 2-7). Neutrophil LTA$_4$ serves as a source for platelet-dependent synthesis of lipoxins. Monocytes, eosinophils, and airway epithelial cells generate 15S-hydroxyeicosatetraenoic acid (15S-HETE), which is taken up by neutrophils and converted to lipoxins.

Cytokines are Cell-Derived Inflammatory Hormones

Cytokines constitute a group of low-molecular-weight hormone-like proteins secreted by cells. Many cytokines are produced at sites of inflammation, including interleukins, growth factors, colony-stimulating factors, interferons, and chemokines (Fig. 2-8). Cytokines produced at sites of tissue injury regulate inflammatory responses, ranging from initial changes in vascular permeability to resolution and restoration of tissue integrity. These molecules are inflammatory hormones that exhibit **autocrine** (affecting themselves), **paracrine** (affecting nearby cells), and **endocrine** (affecting cells in other tissues) functions. *Through production of cytokines, macrophages are pivotal in orchestrating tissue inflammatory responses.* **Lipopolysaccharide** (LPS), a molecule derived from the outer cell membrane of gram-negative bacteria, is one of the most potent activators of macrophages, as well as of endothelial cells and leukocytes (Fig. 2-9). LPS activates cells via specific receptors, either directly or after binding a serum LPS-binding protein (LBP). It is a potent stimulus for the production of TNF-α and interleukins (IL-1, IL-6, IL-8, IL-12, and others). Macrophage-derived cytokines modulate endothelial cell leukocyte adhesion (TNF-α), leukocyte recruitment (IL-8), the acute phase response (IL-6, IL-1), and immune functions (IL-1, IL-6, IL-12).

Interleukins

IL-1 and TNF-α, produced by macrophages, as well as other cells, are central to the development and amplification of inflammatory responses. These cytokines activate endothelial cells to express adhesion molecules and release cytokines, chemokines, and reactive oxygen species (ROS) (see below). TNF-α induces priming and aggregation of neutrophils. IL-1 and TNF-α are also among the mediators of fever, catabolism of muscle, shifts in protein synthesis, and hemodynamic effects associated with inflammatory states (see Fig. 2-9). IFN-γ, another potent stimulus for macrophage activation and cytokine production, is produced by a subset of T lymphocytes as part of the immune response (see Chapter 4).

Chemokine Structure and Function

Chemokines direct cell migration (a process termed **chemotaxis**). The accumulation of inflammatory cells at sites of tissue

Interleukins	Growth Factors	Chemokines	Interferons	Pro-Inflammatory Cytokines
IL-1 IL-6 IL-8 IL-13 IL-10	GM-CSF M-CSF	CC CXC XC CX3C	IFNα IFNβ IFNγ	TNFα
• Inflammatory cell activation	• Macrophage • Bactericidal activity • NK and dendritic cell function	• Leukocyte chemotaxis • Leukocyte activation	• Antiviral • Leukocyte activation	• Fever • Anorexia • Shock • Cytotoxicity • Cytokine induction • Activation of endothelial cells and tissue cells

FIGURE 2-8. **Cytokines important in inflammation.** GM-CSF, granulocyte macrophage-colony stimulating factor; IL, interleukin; NK, natural killer; IFN, interferon; TNF, tumor necrosis factor.

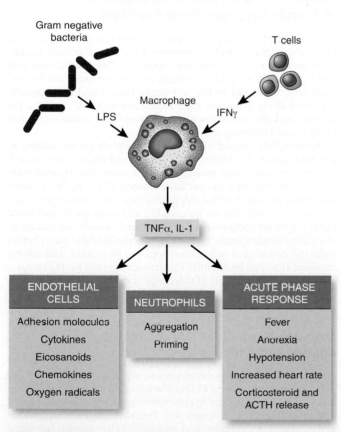

FIGURE 2-9. **Central role of interleukin (IL)-1 and tumor necrosis factor (TNF)-α in inflammation.** Lipopolysaccharide (LPS) and IFN-γ activate macrophages to release inflammatory cytokines, principally IL-1 and TNF-α, responsible for directing local and systemic inflammatory responses. ACTH, adrenocorticotropic hormone.

injury requires their migration from the vascular space into extravascular tissue. Chemokines are a large class of cytokines (over 50 known members) that regulate leukocyte trafficking in inflammation and immunity. For example, chemokines are important chemotactic factors for PMNs in acute inflammation (see later).

Chemokines are small molecules that interact with G-protein coupled receptors on target cells. These secreted proteins are produced by a variety of cell types, either constitutively or after induction, and differ widely in biological action. This diversity is based on specific cell types targeted, specific receptor activation, and differences in intracellular signaling.

Two functional classes of chemokines have been distinguished, namely inflammatory chemokines and homing chemokines. **Inflammatory** chemokines are produced in response to bacterial toxins and inflammatory cytokines (especially IL-1, TNF-α, and IFN-γ) by a variety of tissue cells, as well as leukocytes themselves. **Homing** chemokines are constitutively expressed and upregulated during disease states, they direct trafficking and homing of lymphocytes and dendritic cells to lymphoid tissues during an immune response (see Chapter 4).

Chemokines function as immobilized or soluble molecules that generate a chemotactic gradient by binding to proteoglycans of the extracellular matrix or to cell surfaces. As a result, high concentrations of chemokines persist at sites of tissue injury. Specific receptors on the surface of the migrating leukocytes bind the matrix-bound chemokines and associated adhesion molecules, which tend to move cells along the chemotactic gradient to the site of injury. This process of responding to a matrix-bound chemoattractant is termed **haptotaxis**. As soluble molecules, chemokines control leukocyte motility and localization within extravascular tissues by establishing a chemotactic gradient. The multiplicity and combination of chemokine receptors on cells allows an extensive variety in biological function. Neutrophils, monocytes, eosinophils, and basophils share some receptors but express other receptors exclusively. Thus, specific chemokine combinations can recruit selective cell populations.

Reactive Oxygen Species are Signal-Transducing, Bactericidal, and Cytotoxic Molecules

ROS are chemically reactive molecules derived from molecular oxygen. Normally, they are rapidly inactivated, but when generated inappropriately, they can be cytotoxic (see Chapter 1). ROS create **oxidative stress** by activating signal-transduction pathways and combining with proteins, lipids, and DNA. Leukocyte-derived ROS, released within phagosomes, are bactericidal. ROS important in inflammation include superoxide (O_2^-), nitric oxide (NO•), hydrogen peroxide (H_2O_2), and hydroxyl radical (•OH) (Fig. 2-10) (see below and Chapter 1).

Cells of Inflammation

Leukocytes are the major cellular components of the inflammatory response and include neutrophils, T and B lymphocytes, monocytes, macrophages, eosinophils, mast cells, and basophils. Specific functions are associated with each of these cell types, but such functions overlap and vary as inflammation progresses. In addition, local tissue cells interact with one another and with inflammatory cells, in a continuous response to injury and infection.

Neutrophils are the Major Cellular Participants in Acute Inflammation

The PMN is the major cellular participant in acute inflammation. It has granulated cytoplasm and a nucleus with two to four lobes. PMNs are stored in the bone marrow, circulate in the blood, and rapidly accumulate at sites of injury or infection (Fig. 2-11A). They are activated in response to phagocytic stimuli, cytokines, chemotactic mediators or antigen–antibody complexes, which bind specific receptors on their surface membrane. In tissues, PMNs phagocytose invading microbes and dead tissue (see below). Once they are recruited into tissue, they do not re-enter the circulation.

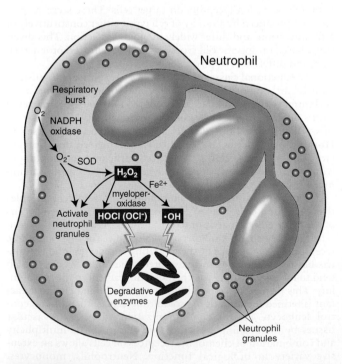

Generation of reactive oxygen species in neutrophils as a result of phagocytosis of bacteria. Fe^{2+}, ferrous iron; H_2O_2, hydrogen peroxide; HOCl, hypochlorous acid; NADPH, nicotinamide adenine dinucleotide phosphate; OCl^-, hypochlorite radical; •OH, hydroxyl radical; SOD, superoxide dismutase.

Endothelial Cells Line Blood Vessels

Endothelial cells comprise a monolayer of cells lining blood vessels and help to separate intra- and extravascular spaces. They produce agents that maintain blood vessel patency and also vasodilators and vasoconstrictors that regulate vascular tone. Injury to a vessel wall interrupts the endothelial barrier and exposes a local procoagulant signal (Fig. 2-11B).

Endothelial cells are gatekeepers in inflammatory cell recruitment: they can promote or inhibit tissue perfusion and the influx of inflammatory cells. Inflammatory agents, such as bradykinin and histamine, endotoxin and cytokines, induce endothelial cells to reveal adhesion molecules that (1) anchor and activate leukocytes, (2) present major histocompatibility complex (MHC) class I and II molecules, and (3) generate cytokines and important vasoactive and inflammatory mediators.

Monocyte/Macrophages are Important in Acute and Chronic Inflammation

Circulating monocytes (Fig. 2-11C) have a single lobed or kidney-shaped nucleus. They are derived from the bone marrow and can exit the circulation to migrate into tissue and become resident macrophages. In response to inflammatory mediators, they accumulate at sites of acute inflammation where they ingest and process microbes. Monocyte/macrophages produce potent vasoactive mediators, including prostaglandins and leukotrienes, PAF, and inflammatory cytokines. These cells are especially important for maintaining chronic inflammation.

Mast Cells and Basophils are Important in Allergic Hypersensitivity Reactions

Mast cell products play an important role in regulating vascular permeability and bronchial smooth muscle tone, especially in allergic hypersensitivity reactions (see Chapter 4). Granulated mast cells and basophils (Fig. 2-11D) contain cell surface receptors for IgE. Mast cells are found in the connective tissues and are especially prevalent along lung and gastrointestinal mucosal surfaces, the dermis, and the microvasculature. Basophils circulate in small numbers and can migrate into tissue.

When IgE-sensitized mast cells or basophils are stimulated by antigens, physical agonists such as cold and trauma, or cationic proteins, inflammatory mediators in the dense cytoplasmic granules are secreted into extracellular tissues. These bodies contain acid mucopolysaccharides (including heparin), serine proteases, chemotactic mediators for neutrophils and eosinophils, and histamine, a primary mediator of early increased vascular permeability. Histamine binds specific H_1 receptors in the vascular wall, thereby inducing endothelial cell contraction, gap formation, and edema, an effect that can be inhibited pharmacologically by H_1-receptor antagonists. Stimulation of mast cells and basophils also leads to the release of products of arachidonic acid metabolism and cytokines, such as TNF-α and IL-4.

Eosinophils are Important in Defense Against Parasites

Eosinophils circulate in the blood and are recruited to tissues in a manner similar to that of PMNs. They are characteristic of IgE-mediated reactions, such as hypersensitivity, allergic, and asthmatic responses (Fig. 2-12A). Eosinophils contain leukotrienes and PAF, as well as acid phosphatase and peroxidase. They express IgA receptors and exhibit large granules that contain eosinophil major basic protein, both of which are involved in defense against parasites.

Platelets Play a Role in Normal Hemostasis

Platelets play a primary role in normal hemostasis and in initiating and regulating clot formation (see Chapter 20). They are

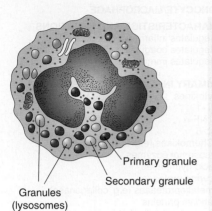
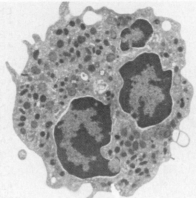

Granules
(lysosomes)

Primary granule

Secondary granule

A

POLYMORPHONUCLEAR LEUKOCYTES

CHARACTERISTICS AND FUNCTIONS
- Central to acute inflammation
- Phagocytosis of microorganisms and tissue debris
- Mediates tissue injury

PRIMARY INFLAMMATORY MEDIATORS
- Reactive oxygen metabolites
- Lysosomal granule contents

Primary granules	**Secondary granules**
Myeloperoxidase	Lysozyme
Lysozyme	Lactoferrin
Defensins	Collagenase
Bactericidal/permeability	Complement activator
increasing protein	Phospholipase A$_2$
Elastase	CD11b/CD18
Cathepsins Protease 3	CD11c/CD18
Glucuronidase	Laminin
Mannosidase	
Phospholipase A2	**Tertiary granules**
	Gelatinase
	Plasminogen activator
	Cathepsins
	Glucuronidase
	Mannosidase

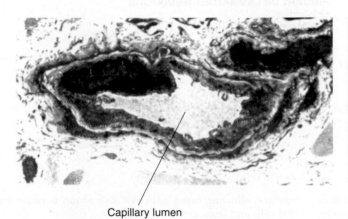

B

Capillary lumen

ENDOTHELIAL CELLS

CHARACTERISTICS AND FUNCTIONS
- Maintains vascular integrity
- Regulates platelet aggregation
- Regulates vascular contraction and relaxation
- Mediates leukocyte recruitment in inflammation

PRIMARY INFLAMMATORY MEDIATORS
- von Willebrand factor
- Nitric oxide
- Endothelins
- Prostanoids

FIGURE 2-11. Cells of inflammation: morphology and function. **A.** Neutrophil. **B.** Endothelial cell

sources of inflammatory mediators, including potent vasoactive substances and growth factors that modulate mesenchymal cell proliferation (Fig. 2-12B). The platelet is small (2 μm in diameter), lacks a nucleus, and contains three distinct kinds of inclusions:

- dense granules, rich in serotonin, histamine, calcium and adenosine diphosphate (ADP)
- α granules, containing fibrinogen, coagulation proteins, platelet-derived growth factor, and other peptides and proteins
- lysosomes, which sequester acid hydrolases

Platelets adhere, aggregate, and degranulate when they contact fibrillar collagen (e.g., after vascular injury that exposes extracellular matrix [ECM] proteins) or thrombin (after activation of the coagulation system).

Leukocyte Recruitment in Acute Inflammation

One of the essential features of acute inflammation is the accumulation of leukocytes, particularly PMNs, in affected tissues. Leukocytes adhere to vascular endothelium, where they become activated. They then flatten and migrate from the vasculature through the endothelial cell layer into surrounding tissue. In the extravascular tissue, PMNs ingest foreign material, microbes, and dead tissue.

Leukocyte Adhesion to Endothelium Results from Interaction of Complementary Adhesion Molecules

Leukocyte recruitment to the postcapillary venules begins with the interaction of leukocytes with endothelial cell selectins, which are redistributed to endothelial cell surfaces during activation. This interaction, called **tethering**, slows leukocytes in the blood flow (Fig. 2-13). Leukocytes then move along the vascular endothelial cell surface with a saltatory movement, termed **rolling**. PMNs become activated by proximity to the endothelium and by inflammatory mediators, and adhere strongly to intercellular adhesion molecules on the endothelium (leukocyte **arrest**). As endothelial cells separate, leukocytes **transmigrate** through the vessel wall and, under the influence of chemotactic factors, they migrate through extravascular tissue to the site of injury.

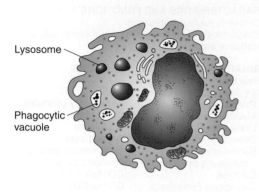

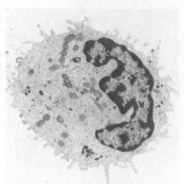

MONOCYTE/MACROPHAGE

CHARACTERISTICS AND FUNCTIONS
• Regulates inflammatory response
• Regulates coagulation/fibrinolytic pathway
• Regulates immune response (see Chapt. 4)

PRIMARY INFLAMMATORY MEDIATORS
• cytokines
  -IL-1
  -TNF-α
  -IL-6
  -Chemokines (e.g. IL-8, MCP-1)
• lysosomal enzymes
  -acid hydrolases
  -serine proteases
  -metalloproteases (e.g. collagenase)
• cationic proteins
• prostaglandins/leukotrienes
• plasminogen activator
• procoagulant activity
• oxygen metabolite formation

Lysosome

Phagocytic
vacuole

C

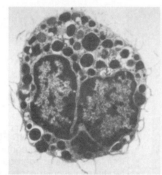

MAST CELL (BASOPHILS)

CHARACTERISTICS AND FUNCTIONS
• Binds IgE molecules
• Contains electron-dense granules

PRIMARY INFLAMMATORY MEDIATORS
• Histamine
• Leukotrienes (LTC, LTD, LTE)
• Platelet activating factor
• Eosinophil chemotactic factors
• Cytokines (e.g., TNF-α IL-4)

D

FIGURE 2-11. *Continued.* **C.** Monocyte/macrophage. **D.** Mast cell. IL, interleukin; MCP-1, monocyte chemoattractant protein-1; TNF-α, tumor necrosis factor-α.

The events involved in leukocyte recruitment are regulated as follows: (1) Inflammatory mediators stimulate resident tissue cells, including vascular endothelial cells; (2) Adhesion molecules are expressed on vascular endothelial cell surfaces and bind to reciprocal molecules on the surfaces of circulating leukocytes; and (3) Chemotactic factors attract leukocytes along a chemical gradient to the site of injury.

Adhesion Molecules

Four molecular families of adhesion molecules are involved in leukocyte recruitment: selectins, addressins, integrins, and members of the immunoglobulin super family.

Selectins

The selectin family (part of the C-type, calcium-dependent lectin group) includes P-selectin, E-selectin, and L-selectin, expressed on the surface of platelets, endothelial cells, and leukocytes, respectively. Selectins share a similar molecular structure, which includes a chain of transmembrane glycoproteins with an extracellular carbohydrate-binding domain specific for sialylated oligosaccharides. The last is the sialyl-Lewis X moiety on addressins, the binding of which allows rapid attachment and rolling of cells.

P-selectin (CD62P, GMP-140, PADGEM) is preformed and stored within Weibel-Palade bodies of endothelial cells and α-granules of platelets. On stimulation with histamine, thrombin, or specific inflammatory cytokines, P-selectin is rapidly transported to the cell surface, where it binds to sialyl-Lewis X on leukocyte surfaces. Preformed P-selectin can be delivered quickly to the cell

surface, allowing rapid adhesive interaction between endothelial cells and leukocytes.

E-selectin (CD62E, ELAM-1) is not normally expressed on endothelial cell surfaces but is induced by inflammatory mediators, such as cytokines or bacterial LPS. E-selectin mediates the adhesion of neutrophils, monocytes, and certain lymphocytes via binding to molecules that contain Lewis X.

L-selectin (CD62L, LAM-1, Leu-8) is expressed on many types of leukocytes. It was originally defined as the "homing receptor" for lymphocytes. It binds lymphocytes to high endothelial venules in lymphoid tissue, thereby regulating their trafficking through this tissue. L-selectin binds glycan-bearing cell adhesion molecule-1 (GlyCAM-1), mucosal addressin cell adhesion molecule-1 (MadCAM-1), and CD34.

Addressins

Vascular addressins are mucin-like glycoproteins, including GlyCAM-1, P-selectin glycoprotein-1 (PSGL-1), E-selectin ligand 1 (ESL-1), and CD34. They possess sialyl-Lewis X, which binds the lectin domain of selectins. Addressins are expressed at leukocyte and endothelial surfaces. They regulate the localization of subpopulations of leukocytes and are involved in lymphocyte activation.

Integrins

Chemokines, lipid mediators, and proinflammatory molecules activate cells to express the integrin family of adhesion molecules (see Chapter 3). Integrins have transmembrane α and β chains arranged as heterodimers. They participate in cell–cell interactions and cell–ECM binding. Very late activation (VLA) molecules include

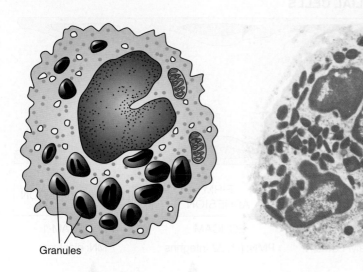

A

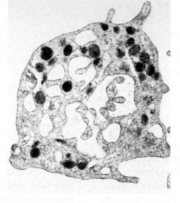

B

EOSINOPHILS
CHARACTERISTICS AND FUNCTIONS
* Associated with:
  - Allergic reactions
  - Parasite-associated inflammatory reactions
  - Chronic inflammation
* Modulate mast cell-mediated reactions

PRIMARY INFLAMMATORY MEDIATORS
* Reactive oxygen metabolites
* Lysosomal granule enzymes
  (primary crystalloid granules)
  - Major basic protein
  - Eosinophil cationic protein
  - Eosinophil peroxidase
  - Acid phosphatase
  - β-glucuronidase
  - Arylsulfatase B
  - Histaminase
* Phospholipase D
* Prostaglandins of E series
* Cytokines

PLATELETS
CHARACTERISTICS AND FUNCTIONS
* Thrombosis; promote clot formation
* Regulates permeability
* Regulate proliferative response of
  mesenchymal cells

PRIMARY INFLAMMATORY MEDIATORS
* Dense granules
  - Serotonin
  - Ca^{2+}
  - ADP
* α-granules
  - Cationic proteins
  - Fibrinogen and coagulation proteins
  - Platelet-derived growth factor (PDGF)
* Lysosomes
  - Acid hydrolases
* Thromboxane A_2

FIGURE 2-12. **More cells of inflammation: morphology and function. A.** Eosinophil. **B.** Platelet. ADP, adenosine diphosphate.

VLA-4 ($\alpha4\beta1$) on leukocytes and lymphocytes that bind VCAM-1 (an immunoglobulin-domain-bearing molecule) on endothelial cells. The $\beta2$ integrins (CD18) form molecules by association with α integrin chains: $\alpha_1\beta_2$ (also called CD11a/CD18 or LFA-1) and $\alpha_m\beta_2$ (also termed CR3, CD11b/CD18 or Mac-1) bind to both ICAM-1 and ICAM-2 (also members of the Ig domain-bearing family, see below). Leukocyte integrins exist in a low-affinity state, but are converted to a high-affinity state when these cells are activated.

Immunoglobulin Superfamily
Adhesion molecules of the immunoglobulin (Ig) superfamily include ICAM-1, ICAM-2, and VCAM-1, all of which interact with integrins on leukocytes to mediate recruitment. They are expressed at the surfaces of cytokine-stimulated endothelial cells and some leukocytes, as well as certain epithelial cells, such as pulmonary alveolar cells.

Recruitment of Leukocytes
Tethering, rolling, and firm adhesion are prerequisites for recruitment of leukocytes from the circulation into tissues. For a rolling cell to adhere, there must first be a selectin-dependent reduction in rolling velocity. The early increase in rolling depends on P-se-

lectin, whereas cytokine-induced E-selectin initiates early adhesion. Integrin family members function cooperatively with selectins to facilitate rolling and subsequent firm adhesion of leukocytes. Leukocyte integrin binding to the Ig superfamily of ligands expressed on vascular endothelium further retards leukocytes, increasing the length of exposure of each leukocyte to endothelium. At the same time, engagement of adhesion molecules activates intracellular signal transduction. As a result, leukocytes and vascular endothelial cells are further activated, with subsequent upregulation of L-selectin and integrin binding. The net result is firm adhesion (see Fig. 2-13).

Chemotactic Molecules Direct Neutrophils to Sites of Injury

Leukocytes must be accurately positioned at sites of inflammatory injury to carry out their biological functions. For specific subsets of leukocytes to arrive in a timely fashion, they must receive specific directions. *Leukocytes are guided through vascular and extravascular spaces by a complex interaction of attractants, repellants, and adhesion molecules.* **Chemotaxis** is the dynamic and energy-dependent process of directed cell migration. Blood leukocytes are recruited by chemoattractants released by endothelial cells. They then migrate from the en-

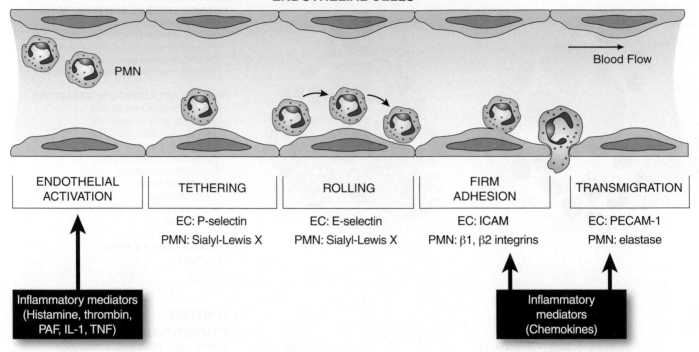

ENDOTHELIAL CELLS

ENDOTHELIAL ACTIVATION	TETHERING	ROLLING	FIRM ADHESION	TRANSMIGRATION
	EC: P-selectin	EC: E-selectin	EC: ICAM	EC: PECAM-1
	PMN: Sialyl-Lewis X	PMN: Sialyl-Lewis X	PMN: β1, β2 integrins	PMN: elastase

Inflammatory mediators (Histamine, thrombin, PAF, IL-1, TNF)

Inflammatory mediators (Chemokines)

FIGURE 2-13. **Neutrophil adhesion and extravasation.** Inflammatory mediators activate endothelial cells to increase expression of adhesion molecules. Sialyl Lewis X on neutrophil PSGL-1 and ESL-1 binds to P- and E-selectins to facilitate tethering and rolling of neutrophils. Increased integrins on activated neutrophils bind to ICAM-1 on endothelial cells to form a firm attachment. Endothelial cell attachments to one another are released, and neutrophils then pass between separated cells to enter the tissue. EC, endothelial cell; ICAM, intercellular adhesion molecule; IL, interleukin; PAF, platelet activating factor; PMN, polymorphonuclear neutrophil; TNF, tumor necrosis factor.

dothelium toward the target tissue, down a gradient of one chemoattractant in response to a second more distal chemoattractant gradient. During migration, the cell extends a pseudopod toward increasing chemokine concentrations. At the leading front of the pseudopod, marked changes in levels of intracellular calcium are associated with the assembly and contraction of cytoskeleton proteins. This process draws the remaining tail of the cell along the chemical gradient. Neutrophils must integrate the various signals to arrive at the appropriate site at the correct time to perform their assigned tasks. The most important chemotactic factors for PMNs are:

- C5a, derived from complement
- Bacterial and mitochondrial products, particularly low-molecular-weight N-formylated peptides (such as N-formyl-methionyl-leucyl-phenylalanine)
- Products of arachidonic acid metabolism, especially LTB$_4$
- Chemokines

Chemotactic factors for other cell types, including lymphocytes, basophils, and eosinophils, are also produced at sites of tissue injury and may be secreted by activated endothelial cells, tissue parenchymal cells, or other inflammatory cells. They include PAF, transforming growth factor-β (TGF-β), neutrophilic cationic proteins, and lymphokines. *The cocktail of chemokines presented within a tissue largely determines the type of leukocyte attracted to the site.* Cells arriving at their destination must then be able to stop in the target tissue. Contact guidance, regulated adhesion, or inhibitory signals may determine the final arrest of specific cells in particular tissue locations.

Leukocytes Traverse the Endothelial Cell Barrier to Gain Access to the Tissue

Leukocytes adherent to the vascular endothelium emigrate by **paracellular diapedesis**, (i.e., passing between adjacent endothelial cells). Responding to chemokine gradients, neutrophils extend

pseudopods and insinuate themselves between the cells and out of the vascular space. Vascular endothelial cells are connected by tight junctions and adherens junctions. CD31 (platelet endothelial cell adhesion molecule) is expressed on endothelial cell surfaces and binds to itself to keep cells together. These junctions separate under the influence of inflammatory mediators, intracellular signals generated by adhesion molecule engagement, and signals from the adherent neutrophils. Neutrophils mobilize elastase to their pseudopod membranes, inducing endothelial cell retraction and separation at the advancing edge of the neutrophil. Neutrophils also induce increases in intracellular calcium in endothelial cells, to which the endothelial cells respond by pulling apart.

Neutrophils also migrate through endothelial cells by **transcellular diapedesis**. Instead of inducing endothelial cell retraction, PMNs may squeeze through small circular pores in the endothelial cell cytoplasm. In tissues that contain fenestrated microvessels, such as the gastrointestinal mucosa and secretory glands, PMNs may traverse thin regions of endothelium, called **fenestrae**, without damaging endothelial cells. In nonfenestrated microvessels, PMNs may cross the endothelium using endothelial cell caveolae or pinocytotic vesicles, which form small, membrane-bound passageways across the cell.

Leukocyte Functions in Acute Inflammation

Leukocytes Phagocytose Microorganisms and Tissue Debris

Many inflammatory cells (including monocytes, tissue macrophages, dendritic cells, and neutrophils) recognize, internalize, and digest foreign material, microorganisms, or cellular debris by a process termed **phagocytosis**. This is now defined as ingestion by eukaryotic cells of large (usually > 0.5 μm) insoluble particles and microorganisms. The effector cells are **phagocytes**. The complex process involves a sequence of transmembrane and intracellular signaling events.

1. **Recognition:** Phagocytosis is initiated by the recognition of particles by specific receptors on the surface of phagocytic cells (Fig. 2-14). Phagocytosis of most biological agents is enhanced by, if not dependent on, their coating (opsonization) with plasma components (opsonins), particularly immunoglobulins or C3b. Phagocytic cells possess specific opsonic receptors, including those for immunoglobulin Fcγ and complement components. Many pathogens, however, have evolved mechanisms to evade phagocytosis by leukocytes. Polysaccharide capsules, protein A, protein M, or peptidoglycans around bacteria can prevent complement deposition or antigen recognition and receptor binding.

2. **Signaling:** Clumping of opsonins on bacterial surfaces causes Fcγ receptors on phagocytes to cluster. Subsequent phosphorylation of immunoreceptor tyrosine-based activation motifs, located in the cytosolic domain or γ subunit of the receptor, triggers intracellular signaling events. Tyrosine kinases that associate with the Fcγ receptor are required for signaling during phagocytosis.

3. **Internalization:** In the case of phagocytosis initiated via the Fcγ receptor or CR3 (CD11b/CD18 receptor), actin assembly occurs directly under the phagocytosed target. Polymerized actin filaments push the plasma membrane forward. The plasma membrane remodels to increase surface area and to form pseudopods surrounding the foreign material. The resulting phagocytic cup engulfs the foreign agent. The membrane then "zippers" around the opsonized particle to enclose it in a cytoplasmic vacuole called a **phagosome** (see Fig. 2-14).

4. **Digestion:** The phagosome that contains the foreign material fuses with cytoplasmic lysosomes to form a **phagolysosome**, into which lysosomal enzymes are released. The acid pH within the phagolysosome activates these hydrolytic enzymes, which then degrade the phagocytosed material. Some microorganisms have evolved mechanisms for evading killing by neutrophils by preventing lysosomal degranulation or inhibiting neutrophil enzymes.

Neutrophil Enzymes are Required for Antimicrobial Defense and Debridement

Although PMNs are critical for degrading microbes and cell debris, they also contribute to tissue injury. The release of PMN granules at sites of injury is a double-edged sword. On the one hand, debridement of damaged tissue by proteolytic breakdown is beneficial. On the other hand, degradative enzymes can damage endothelial and epithelial cells, as well as degrade connective tissue.

Neutrophil Granules

The armamentarium of enzymes required for degradation of microbes and tissue is generated and contained within PMN cytoplasmic granules. Primary, secondary, and tertiary granules in neutrophils are differentiated morphologically and biochemically; each granule has a unique spectrum of enzymes (see Fig. 2-11A).

Inflammatory Cells Have Oxidative and Nonoxidative Bactericidal Activity

The bactericidal activity of PMNs and macrophages is mediated in part by production of ROS and in part by oxygen-independent mechanisms.

Bacterial Killing by Oxygen Species

Phagocytosis is accompanied by metabolic reactions in inflammatory cells that lead to the production of several oxygen metabolites

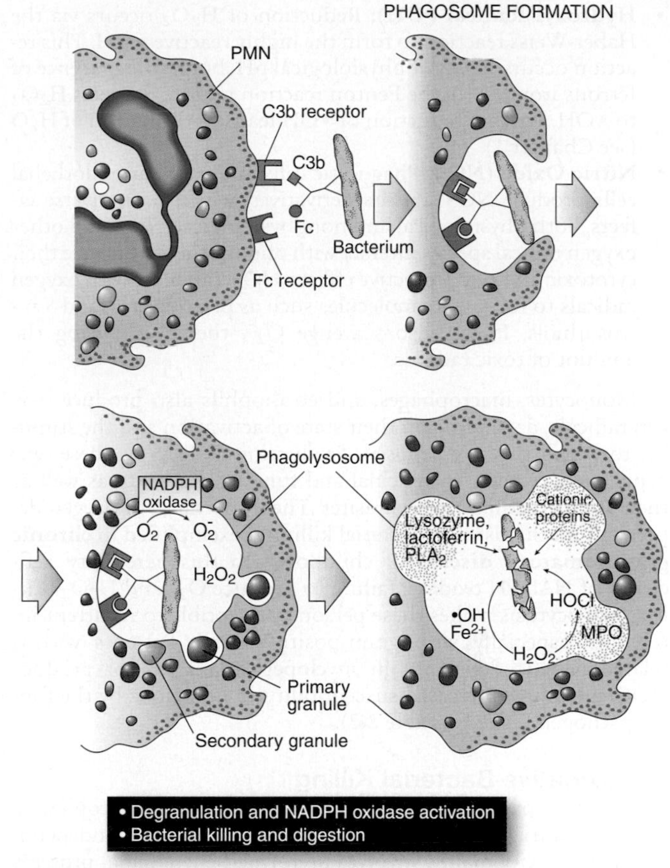

FIGURE 2-14. **Mechanisms of neutrophil bacterial phagocytosis and cell killing.** Opsonins such as C3b coat the surface of microbes, allowing recognition by the neutrophil C3b receptor. Receptor clustering triggers intracellular signalling and actin assembly within the neutrophil. Pseudopods form around the microbe to enclose it within a phagosome. Lysosomal granules fuse with the phagosome to form a phagolysosome into which the lysosomal enzymes and oxygen radicals are released to kill and degrade the microbe. Fe^{2+}, ferrous iron; HOCl, hypochlorous acid; MPO, myeloperoxidase; PLA_2, phospholipase A_2; PMN, polymorphonuclear neutrophil.

(see Chapter 1). These products are more reactive than oxygen itself and contribute to the killing of ingested bacteria (see Fig. 2-14).

- **Superoxide Anion (O_2^-):** Phagocytosis activates a nicotinamide adenine dinucleotide phosphate (NADPH) oxidase in PMN cell membranes. NADPH oxidase is a multicomponent electron transport complex that reduces molecular oxygen to O_2^-. Activation of this enzyme is enhanced by prior exposure of cells to a chemotactic stimulus or LPS. NADPH oxidase activation increases oxygen consumption and stimulates the hexose monophosphate shunt. Together, these cell responses are referred to as the **respiratory burst.**

- **Hydrogen Peroxide (H_2O_2):** O_2^- is rapidly converted to H_2O_2 by superoxide dismutase at the cell surface and in phagolysosomes. H_2O_2 is stable and serves as a substrate for generating additional reactive oxidants.

- **Hypochlorous Acid (HOCl):** Myeloperoxidase (MPO), a neutrophil product with a strong cationic charge, is secreted from granules during exocytosis. In the presence of a halide, usually chlorine, MPO catalyzes the conversion of H_2O_2 to HOCl. This powerful oxidant is a major bactericidal agent produced by phagocytic cells. HOCl also participates in activating neutrophil-derived collagenase and gelatinase, both of which are secreted as latent enzymes. At the same time, HOCl inactivates α_1-antitrypsin.

- **Hydroxyl Radical ($\cdot$OH):** Reduction of H_2O_2 occurs via the Haber-Weiss reaction to form the highly reactive $\cdot$OH. This reaction occurs slowly at physiological pH, but in the presence of ferrous iron (Fe^{2+}), the Fenton reaction rapidly converts H_2O_2 to $\cdot$OH. Further reduction of $\cdot$OH leads to formation of H_2O (see Chapter 1).
- **Nitric Oxide ($NO\cdot$):** Phagocytic cells and vascular endothelial cells produce $NO\cdot$ and its derivatives, which have diverse effects, both physiological and nonphysiological. $NO\cdot$ and other oxygen radical species interact with one another to balance their cytotoxic and cytoprotective effects. $NO\cdot$ can react with oxygen radicals to form toxic molecules such as peroxynitrite and S-nitrosothiols. It can also scavenge O_2^-, thereby reducing the amount of toxic radicals.

Monocytes, macrophages, and eosinophils also produce oxygen radicals, depending on their state of activation and the stimulus to which they are exposed. Production of ROS by these cells contributes to their bactericidal and fungicidal activity as well as their ability to kill certain parasites. The importance of oxygen-dependent mechanisms in bacterial killing is exemplified in **chronic granulomatous disease** of childhood. In this hereditary deficiency of NADPH oxidase, failure to produce O_2^- and H_2O_2 during phagocytosis makes these persons susceptible to recurrent infections, especially with gram-positive cocci. Patients with a related genetic deficiency in myeloperoxidase cannot produce HOCl and show increased susceptibility to infections by the fungal pathogen *Candida* (Table 2-2).

Nonoxidative Bacterial Killing

Phagocytes, particularly PMNs and monocytes/macrophages, have substantial antimicrobial activity, which is oxygen independent. This activity mainly involves preformed bactericidal proteins in cytoplasmic granules. These include lysosomal acid hydrolases and specialized noncatalytic proteins unique to inflammatory cells.

- **Lysosomal hydrolases:** Neutrophil primary and secondary granules and lysosomes of mononuclear phagocytes contain hydrolases, including sulfatases, phosphatases, and other enzymes capable of digesting polysaccharides and DNA.
- **Bactericidal/permeability-increasing protein:** This cationic protein in PMN primary granules can kill many gram-negative bacteria but is not toxic to gram-positive bacteria or to eukaryotic cells.
- **Defensins:** Primary granules of PMNs and lysosomes of some mononuclear phagocytes contain this family of cationic proteins, which kill an extensive variety of gram-positive and gram-negative bacteria, fungi, and some enveloped viruses.
- **Lactoferrin:** Lactoferrin is an iron-binding glycoprotein in the secondary granules of neutrophils and in most body secretory fluids. Its iron-chelating capacity allows it to compete with bacteria for iron. It may also facilitate oxidative killing of bacteria by enhancing $\cdot$OH formation.
- **Lysozyme:** This bactericidal enzyme is found in many tissues and body fluids, in primary and secondary granules of neutrophils, and in lysosomes of mononuclear phagocytes. Peptidoglycans of gram-positive bacterial cell walls are exquisitely sensitive to degradation by lysozyme; gram-negative bacteria are usually resistant to it.
- **Bactericidal Proteins of Eosinophils:** Eosinophils contain several granule-bound cationic proteins, the most important of which are major basic protein and eosinophilic cationic protein. Major basic protein accounts for about half of the total protein of the eosinophil granule. Both proteins are ineffective against bacteria but are potent cytotoxic agents for many parasites.

Defects in Leukocyte Function

The importance of protection afforded by acute inflammatory cells is emphasized by the frequency and severity of infections

TABLE 2-2

Congenital Diseases of Defective Phagocytic Cell Function Characterized by Recurrent Bacterial Infections

Disease	Defect
LAD	LAD-1 defective β_2-integrin expression or function (CD11/CD18) LAD-2 (defective fucosylation, selectin binding)
Hyper-IgE-recurrent infection, (Job) syndrome	Poor chemotaxis
Chediak-Higashi syndrome	Defective lysosomal granules, poor chemotaxis
Neutrophil-specific granule deficiency	Absent neutrophil granules
Chronic granulomatous disease	Deficient NADPH oxidase, with absent H_2O_2 production
Myeloperoxidase deficiency	Deficient HOCl production

H_2O_2, hydrogen peroxide; HOCl, hypochlorous acid; Ig, immunoglobulin, LAD, leukocyte adhesion deficiency; NADPH, nicotinamide adenine dinucleotide phosphate.

when PMNs are greatly decreased or defective. *The most common such deficit is iatrogenic neutropenia resulting from cancer chemotherapy.* Functional impairment of phagocytes may occur at any step in the sequence: adherence, emigration, chemotaxis, or phagocytosis. These disorders may be acquired or congenital. Acquired diseases, such as leukemia, diabetes mellitus, malnutrition, viral infections, and sepsis are often accompanied by defects in inflammatory cell function. Table 2-2 shows representative examples of congenital diseases linked to defective phagocytic function.

Outcomes of Acute Inflammation

As a result of regulatory components and the short life span of neutrophils, acute inflammatory reactions are usually self-limited and are followed by restoration of normal tissue architecture and physiological function (**resolution**). Resolution involves removal of dead cells, clearance of acute response cells, and re-establishment of the stroma. However, inflammatory responses can lead to other outcomes:

- **Scar:** If a tissue is irreversibly injured, the normal architecture is often replaced by a scar, despite elimination of the initial pathological insult (see Chapter 3).
- **Abscess:** If the area of acute inflammation is walled off by inflammatory cells and fibrosis, PMN products destroy the tissue, forming an abscess.
- **Lymphadenitis:** Localized acute inflammation and chronic inflammation may cause secondary inflammation of lymphatic channels (**lymphangitis**) and lymph nodes (**lymphadenitis**). The inflamed lymphatic channels in the skin appear as red streaks, and the lymph nodes are enlarged and painful. Microscopically, the lymph nodes show hyperplasia of lymphoid follicles and proliferation of mononuclear phagocytes in the sinuses (**sinus histiocytosis**).
- **Persistent inflammation:** Failure to eliminate a pathological insult or inability to trigger resolution results in a persistent inflammatory reaction. This may be evident as a prolonged acute response, with continued influx of neutrophils and tissue destruction, or more commonly as chronic inflammation.

Chronic Inflammation

When acute inflammation does not resolve or becomes disordered, chronic inflammation occurs. Inflammatory cells persist, stroma responds by becoming hyperplastic, and tissue destruction and scarring lead to organ dysfunction. This process may be localized but more commonly progresses to disabling diseases such as chronic lung disease, rheumatoid arthritis, asthma, ulcerative colitis, granulomatous diseases, autoimmune diseases, and chronic dermatitis. Acute and chronic inflammation are ends of a dynamic continuum with overlapping morphological features: (1) Inflammation with continued recruitment of chronic inflammatory cells is followed by (2) tissue injury due to prolongation of the inflammatory response, and (3) an often-disordered attempt to restore tissue integrity. The events leading to an amplified inflammatory response resemble those of acute inflammation in a number of aspects:

- **Specific triggers**, microbial products or injury, initiate the response.
- **Chemical mediators** direct recruitment, activation, and interaction of inflammatory cells. Activation of coagulation and complement cascades generates small peptides that function to prolong the inflammatory response. Cytokines, specifically IL-6 and RANTES, regulate a switch in chemokines, such that mononuclear cells are directed to the site. Other cytokines (e.g., IFN-γ) then promote macrophage proliferation and activation.
- **Inflammatory cells** are recruited from the blood. Interactions between lymphocytes, macrophages, dendritic cells, and fibroblasts generate antigen-specific responses.
- **Stromal cell activation and extracellular matrix** remodeling occur, both of which affect the cellular immune response. Varying degrees of fibrosis may result, depending on the extent of tissue injury and persistence of the pathological stimulus and inflammatory response.

Chronic inflammation is not synonymous with chronic infection, but if the inflammatory response to infectious agents, including bacteria, viruses, and notably parasites, cannot eliminate the organism, infection may persist. Chronic inflammation may also be associated with a variety of noninfectious disease states including:

- **Trauma:** Extensive tissue damage releases mediators capable of inducing an extended inflammatory response.
- **Cancer:** Chronic inflammatory cells, especially macrophages and T lymphocytes, may be the morphological expression of an immune response to malignant cells. Chemotherapy may suppress normal inflammatory responses, thereby increasing susceptibility to infection.
- **Immune factors:** Many autoimmune diseases, including rheumatoid arthritis, chronic thyroiditis, and primary biliary cirrhosis, are characterized by chronic inflammatory responses in affected tissues. This may be associated with activation of antibody-dependent and cell-mediated immune mechanisms (see Chapter 4). Such autoimmune responses may account for injury in affected organs.

Cells from Both the Circulation and Affected Tissue Play a Role in Chronic Inflammation

Monocyte/macrophages, lymphocytes, and plasma cells (see Chapter 4), and cells discussed previously under Acute Inflammation play an active role in chronic inflammation. The latter are recruited from the circulation, as well as cells from the affected tissue including fibroblasts and vascular endothelial cells (see Chapter 3).

Monocyte/Macrophages

Activated macrophages and their cytokines are central to initiating inflammation and prolonging responses that lead to chronic

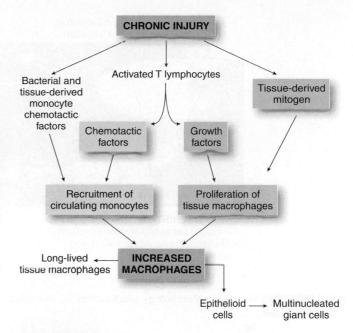

FIGURE 2-15. Accumulation of macrophages in chronic inflammation.

inflammation. (see Fig. 2-11C). Macrophages produce inflammatory and immunological mediators and regulate reactions leading to chronic inflammation. They also control lymphocyte responses to antigens and secrete other mediators that modulate the proliferation and activities of fibroblasts and endothelial cells.

The **mononuclear phagocyte system** includes blood monocytes and different types of tissue macrophages, particularly Kupffer cells of the liver. Under the influence of chemotactic stimuli, IFN-γ and bacterial endotoxins, resident tissue macrophages are activated and proliferate, while circulating monocytes are recruited and differentiate into tissue macrophages (Fig. 2-15).

Within different tissues, resident macrophages differ in their armamentarium of enzymes and can respond to local inflammatory signals. The activity of these enzymes is central to the tissue destruction in chronic inflammation. In emphysema, for example, resident macrophages generate proteinases, particularly matrix metalloproteinases (MMPs) with elastolytic activity, which destroy alveolar walls and recruit blood monocytes into the lung. Other macrophage products include oxygen metabolites, chemotactic factors, cytokines, and growth factors.

Lymphocytes and Plasma Cells

Lymphocytes and plasma cells play a central role in the adaptive immune response to pathogens and foreign agents in damaged tissue and are discussed in detail in Chapter 4.

Fibroblasts

Fibroblasts are long-lived, ubiquitous cells whose chief function is to produce components of the extracellular matrix (ECM) (Fig. 2-16). They can also differentiate into other connective tissue cells, including chondrocytes, adipocytes, osteocytes, and smooth muscle cells. Fibroblasts are the construction workers of the tissue, rebuilding the scaffold of the ECM upon which tissue is re-established.

Fibroblasts not only respond to immune signals that induce their proliferation and activation but are also active players in the immune response. They interact with inflammatory cells, particularly lymphocytes, via surface molecules and receptors on both cells. For example, when CD40 on fibroblasts binds its ligand on lymphocytes, both cells are activated. Activated fibroblasts pro-

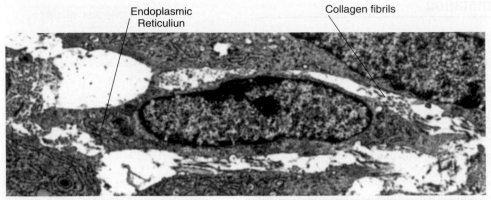

Endoplasmic Reticuliun

Collagen fibrils

CHARACTERISTICS AND FUNCTIONS
- Produce extracellular matrix proteins
- Mediate chronic inflammation and wound healing

PRIMARY INFLAMMATORY MEDIATORS
- IL-6
- IL-8
- Cyclooxygenase-2
- Hyaluronan
- PGE$_2$
- CD40 expression
- Matricellular proteins
- Extracellular proteins

FIGURE 2-16. Fibroblast: Morphology and function. IL, interleukin.

duce cytokines, chemokines, and prostanoids, creating a tissue microenvironment that further regulates the behavior of inflammatory cells in the damaged tissue. Fibroblasts function in wound healing in combination with regenerating vascular endothelial cells. Both are discussed more fully in Chapter 3.

Injury and Repair in Chronic Inflammation

Chronic inflammation is mediated by both immunological and nonimmunological mechanisms and is frequently observed in conjunction with reparative responses, namely, granulation tissue and fibrosis. Neutrophil products, such as proteases and ROS, protect the host by participating in antimicrobial defense and debridement of damaged tissue. However, these same products may prolong tissue damage and promote chronic inflammation if not appropriately regulated. Persistent tissue injury produced by inflammatory cells is important in the pathogenesis of several diseases, for instance, pulmonary emphysema, rheumatoid arthritis, certain immune complex diseases, gout, and adult respiratory distress syndrome.

Granulomatous Inflammation

Granuloma formation is a protective response to chronic infection (fungal infections, tuberculosis, leprosy, schistosomiasis) or the presence of foreign material (e.g., suture or talc). It prevents dissemination and restricts inflammation due to exogenous substances that are not effectively digested during the acute response, thereby protecting the host tissues. Some autoimmune diseases (e.g., rheumatoid arthritis, Crohn disease, and sarcoidosis [a mysterious disease of unknown etiology]) are also associated with granulomas.

The principal cells involved in granulomatous inflammation are macrophages and lymphocytes. Macrophages are mobile cells that continuously migrate through the extravascular connective tissues. After amassing substances that they cannot digest, macrophages lose their motility, accumulate at the site of injury, and undergo transformation into nodular collections of pale, epithelioid cells, creating a **granuloma** (Fig. 2-17A,B). Multinucleated giant cells are formed by the cytoplasmic fusion of

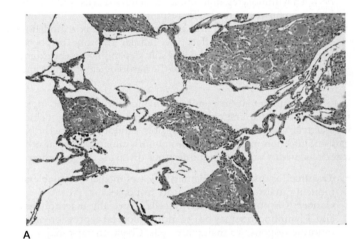

A

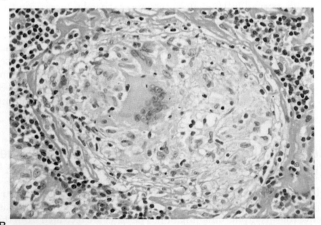

B

FIGURE 2-17. Granulomatous inflammation. **A.** Section of lung from a patient with sarcoidosis reveals numerous discrete granulomas. **B.** A higher-power photomicrograph of a single granuloma in a lymph node from the same patient depicts a multinucleated giant cell amid numerous pale epithelioid cells. A thin rim of fibrosis separates the granuloma from the lymphoid cells of the node.

macrophages. When the nuclei of such giant cells are arranged around the periphery of the cell in a horseshoe pattern, the cell is called a **Langhans giant cell**. If a foreign agent (e.g., silica or a *Histoplasma spore*) or other indigestible material is identified within the cytoplasm of a multinucleated giant cell, it is termed a **foreign body giant cell**. Granulomas are further classified histopathologically by the presence or absence of necrosis. Certain infectious agents such as *Mycobacterium tuberculosis* characteristically produce **caseating granulomas**, the necrotic centers of which are filled with an amorphous mixture of debris and dead microorganisms and cells. Other diseases, such as sarcoidosis, are characterized by granulomas that lack necrosis.

Systemic Manifestations of Inflammation

Under certain conditions, local injury may result in prominent systemic effects that can themselves be debilitating. For example, systemic effects are likely to result when a pathogen enters the bloodstream, a condition known as **sepsis**. The systemic symptoms associated with inflammation, e.g. fever, myalgia, arthralgia, anorexia and somnolence, are attributable to cytokines, including IL-1α, IL-1β, TNF-α, IL-6, and interferons. The most prominent systemic manifestations of inflammation, termed the **systemic inflammatory response syndrome**, are leukocytosis and the acute phase response, fever and shock.

The Acute Phase Response is a Systemic Response to Elevated Levels of IL-1, IL-6, and TNF-α

The acute phase response is a regulated physiological reaction that occurs in inflammatory conditions in response to elevated levels of IL-1, IL-6, and TNF-α. It is characterized clinically by fever, leukocytosis, decreased appetite, and altered sleep patterns and notably by changes in plasma levels of certain *acute phase proteins*. These proteins (Table 2-3) are synthesized primarily by the liver and released in elevated amounts into the circulation, where they may serve as markers for ongoing inflammation. For example, increases in acute phase proteins lead to the accelerated erythrocyte sedimentation rate, a qualitative index used clinically to monitor the activity of many inflammatory diseases.

Fever is a Clinical Hallmark of Inflammation

Fever is a clinical hallmark of inflammation. Release of **pyrogens** (molecules that cause fever) by bacteria, viruses, or injured cells may directly affect hypothalamic thermoregulation. More impor-

TABLE 2-3

Acute Phase Proteins

Protein	Function
Mannose binding protein	Opsonization/complement activation
C-reactive protein	Opsonization
α_1-Antitrypsin	Serine protease inhibitor
Haptoglobin	Binds hemoglobin
Ceruloplasmin	Antioxidant, binds copper
Fibrinogen	Coagulation
Serum amyloid A protein	Apolipoprotein
α_2-Macroglobulin	Antiprotease
Cysteine protease inhibitor	Antiprotease

tantly, they stimulate the production of **endogenous pyrogens**, namely cytokines—including IL-1α, IL-1β, TNF-α, IL-6—and interferons, which produce local and systemic effects. IL-1 stimulates prostaglandin synthesis in hypothalamic thermoregulatory centers, thereby altering the "thermostat" that controls body temperature. Inhibitors of cyclooxygenase (e.g., aspirin) block the fever response by inhibiting IL-1–stimulated synthesis of PGE_2. Chills (the sensation of cold), rigor (profound chills with shivering and piloerection), and sweats (to allow heat dissipation) are symptoms associated with fever.

Shock is Characterized by Cardiac Decompensation

Under conditions of massive tissue injury or infection that spreads to the blood (sepsis), significant quantities of cytokines, especially TNF-α and other chemical mediators of inflammation, may be generated in the circulation. The sustained presence of these mediators induces cardiovascular decompensation through its effects on the heart and on the peripheral vascular system, a process termed **shock**. Systemic effects include generalized vasodilation, increased vascular permeability, intravascular volume loss, myocardial depression with decreased cardiac output, and potentially death (see Chapter 7). In severe cases, activation of coagulation pathways may generate microthrombi throughout the body, with consumption of clotting components and subsequent predisposition to bleeding, a condition defined as **disseminated intravascular coagulation** (see Chapter 20). The net result is **multisystem organ dysfunction** and death.

3 Repair, Regeneration, and Fibrosis

Gregory C. Sephel
Stephen C. Woodward

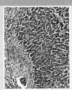

*The study of wound healing involves a complex interaction among many cell types, matrix proteins, growth factors, and cytokines, which regulate and modulate the repair process. Successful healing maintains tissue function and repairs tissue barriers, preventing blood loss and infection. Optimally, repair is accomplished by regeneration—restoration of the original tissue matrix and architecture. More often, healing proceeds through collagen deposition or **scarring (fibrosis)**.*

*Successful repair relies upon a balance between matrix deposition and matrix degradation. **Tissue regeneration is favored when the matrix composition and architecture are unaltered.** Thus, wounds that do not heal may reflect damage to the tissue architecture by excess proteinase activity, decreased matrix accumulation, or altered matrix assembly. By contrast, fibrosis and scarring may result either from reduced proteinase activity or increased matrix accumulation. The formation of new collagen during repair is required for increased strength of the healing site. However, excess col-*

lagen formation (chronic fibrosis) is a major component of diseases that involve chronic injury.

The Basic Processes of Healing

Three key cellular mechanisms are necessary for wound healing:

- **Cellular migration**
- **Extracellular matrix organization, reorganization, and remodeling**
- **Cell proliferation**

Migration of Cells Initiates Repair

Cells at the Site of Injury
The entry of cells into a wound and the activation of local cells is initiated by mediators that are (1) released from reserves stored in the granules of **platelets** and **basophils** at the site of injury or (2) synthesized de novo by tissue resident cell**s**. These mediators (1) control vascular permeability to fluid and cells, (2) degrade damaged tissue, and (3) initiate the repair cascade (see also Chapter 2).

- **Platelets** are activated when bound to collagen exposed by endothelial damage, after which they aggregate and, with fibrin, form a thrombus that limits blood loss. They release platelet-derived growth factor (PDGF) and other molecules that facilitate repair (see Fig. 2-12B).
- **Mast cell** granules release heparin and other contents, many of which promote blood vessel formation (angiogenesis). They reside next to small blood vessels (see Fig. 2-11D).

- **Resident macrophages** in connective tissue secrete mediators that not only contribute to the early response but also perpetuate it. Their numbers are increased through proliferation and recruitment to the site of injury (see Fig. 2-11C).

Cells that Migrate to the Wound

Inflammatory stimuli (see also Chapter 2) and cells activated at the site of injury produce mediators that initiate the migration of the following cells to the site of injury (Fig. 3-1):

- **Polymorphonuclear leukocytes** are rapidly recruited from the bone marrow and invade the wound site within the first day. They degrade and destroy nonviable tissue by releasing their granular contents (see Fig. 2-11A).
- **Macrophages** arrive shortly after neutrophils but persist for days or longer. They phagocytose debris and orchestrate the development of reparative tissue (granulation tissue) by the release of cytokines and chemoattractants.
- **Fibroblasts, myofibroblasts, pericytes, and smooth muscle cells** are recruited by growth factors and matrix degradation products, arriving in a skin wound by day 3 or 4. These cells are responsible for increased collagen synthesis (fibroplasia), synthesis of connective tissue matrix, tissue remodeling, wound contraction, and (indirectly) wound strength.
- **Endothelial cells** form nascent capillaries by responding to growth factors and are visible in a skin wound beyond day 3. The development of capillaries is necessary for the exchange of gases, the delivery of nutrients, and the influx of inflammatory cells (see Fig. 2-11B).
- **Epithelial cells** in the epidermis move across the surface of a skin wound, penetrate the provisional matrix (see below), and migrate upon stromal collagen.
- **Stem cells** from the bone marrow, the bulb of the hair follicle, and the basal layer of the epidermis provide a renewable source of epidermal and dermal cells, which are capable of differentiation, proliferation, and migration. Under appropriate conditions, these cells form new blood vessels and epithelium and regenerate skin structures, such as hair follicles and sebaceous glands.

Mechanisms of Cell Migration

Cell migration depends on the response of cells to chemical signals (**cytokines**) and insoluble substrates of the extracellular matrix. Locomotion of the rapidly migrating leukocytes is powered by broad, wavelike, membrane extensions called **lamellipodia**. Slower moving cells, such as fibroblasts, extend narrower, finger-like, membrane protrusions labeled **filopodia**. Cell polarization and membrane extensions are initiated by growth factors or chemokines, which trigger a response by binding to their specific receptors on the cell surface. **Actin fibrils** polymerize and form a network at the membrane's leading edge, thereby propelling lamellipodia and filopodia forward, with traction provided via attachments to the extracellular matrix substrate. Actin-related proteins stimulate actin assembly, and numerous actin-binding proteins act like molecular tinker toys, rapidly constructing, stabilizing, and destabilizing actin networks.

The leading edge of the cell membrane impinges upon the extracellular matrix and adheres to it through transmembrane adhesion receptors, termed **integrins,** which recognize matrix components such as collagen, laminin, and fibronectin. Such adhesive interactions between cell body and matrix are critical for cell migration. Integrins also transmit intracellular signals to cells that regulate cellular survival, proliferation, and differentiation. Cytoskeletal connections are involved in cell–cell and cell–matrix connections and determine the shape and differentiation of epithelial, endothelial, and other cells.

The Organization of Extracellular Matrix Sustains the Repair Process

Two types of extracellular matrix contribute to the organization, physical properties, and function of both normal and injured tissue, namely connective tissue (interstitial matrix or stroma) and basement membranes.

Connective Tissue (Matrix)

Connective tissue forms an interconnected matrix between tissue elements, such as epithelia, muscles, nerves, and blood vessels. This stromal matrix consists of both cells and an extracellular compartment, the latter including structural elements and a proteinaceous ground substance. Connective tissue provides physical protection by conferring resistance to compression or stretching. The stroma also acts as a storage medium for bioactive proteins.

The cells in connective tissue are primarily of mesenchymal origin and include fibroblasts, myofibroblasts, adipocytes, chondrocytes, osteocytes, and endothelial cells. Bone marrow–derived cells (e.g., mast cells, macrophages, and transient leukocytes) also populate connective tissue (see above).

The extracellular matrix of connective tissue is defined by the type of collagen fibers, selected from a large family of collagen molecules (Table 3-1). Another important structural component of the stroma is elastic fibers, which impart elasticity principally to skin, large blood vessels, and lungs. The fibers are composed of an elastin core, surrounded by microfibrillar proteins, such as fibrillin. The so-called **ground substance** of the interstitium represents a number of molecules, including glycosaminoglycans (GAGs), proteoglycans, and fibronectin, which provide for many important biological functions of connective tissue, in addition to the support and modulation of cell attachment.

Collagens

Collagen is the most abundant protein in the animal kingdom; it is essential for the structural integrity of tissues and organs. When collagen synthesis is reduced, delayed, or abnormal, the result is failed wound healing, as seen in scurvy. Mutational alterations of fibrillar collagen are responsible for diseases of bone (osteogenesis imperfecta), cartilage (chondroplasias), skin, joints, and blood vessels (Ehlers-Danlos syndrome) (see Chapters 6 and 26). Excess collagen deposition leads to **fibrosis,** the basis of several connective tissue diseases and the loss of function that accompanies chronic damage to many organs, including kidneys, lungs, and the liver. Collagens are divided into three types (see Table 3-1):

- **Fibrillar collagens.** Of the fibrillar collagens, type I collagen is the major constituent of bone. Type I and type III collagens are prominent in skin; type II collagen is the predominant form in cartilege. Fibrillar collagens turn over slowly and are generally resistant to proteinase digestion.
- **Nonfibrillar** collagens contain globular domains that prevent fibril formation. They act as **transmembrane** proteins (type XVII) in the hemidesmosome that attaches epidermal cells to the basement membrane and as **fibrillar anchors** (type VII) connecting the hemidesmosome and basement membrane to the underlying stroma in the skin.
- **Network-forming collagens** facilitate the formation of flexible "chicken wire"–like networks of basement membrane collagen (type IV).

Noncollagenous Matrix Constituents of Stroma

Noncollagenous matrix components of stroma include a complex variety of proteins, glycoproteins, elastic fibers, and proteoglycans (Table 3-2):

- **Elastin** is a secreted matrix protein that allows deformable tissues, such as skin, uterus, ligament, lung, elastic cartilage, and

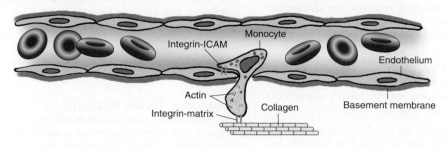

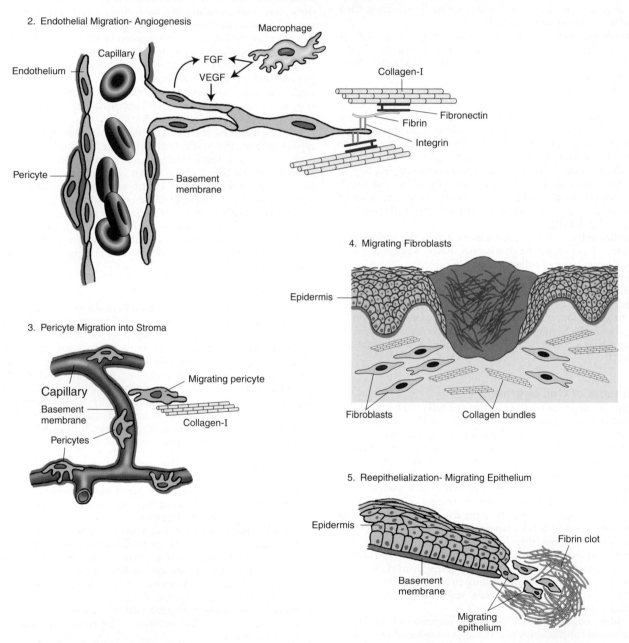

1. Leukocyte Migration

Integrin-ICAM
Monocyte
Endothelium
Actin
Integrin-matrix
Collagen
Basement membrane

2. Endothelial Migration- Angiogenesis

Macrophage
Capillary
Endothelium
FGF
VEGF
Collagen-I
Fibronectin
Fibrin
Integrin
Pericyte
Basement membrane

3. Pericyte Migration into Stroma

Capillary
Migrating pericyte
Basement membrane
Collagen-I
Pericytes

4. Migrating Fibroblasts

Epidermis
Fibroblasts
Collagen bundles

5. Reepithelialization- Migrating Epithelium

Epidermis
Fibrin clot
Basement membrane
Migrating epithelium

FIGURE 3-1. **Cell migrations during repair.** *(1)* Leukocytes attach to, and migrate between, capillary endothelial cells, penetrate the basement membrane, and enter the matrix. *(2)* Capillary endothelial cells, released from the basement membrane, migrate through the matrix to form new capillaries. *(3)* Pericytes detach from endothelial cells and their basement membranes to migrate into the matrix. *(4)* Fibroblasts become bipolar and migrate through the matrix to the site of injury. *(5)* Epithelial keratinocytes detach from neighboring cells and basement membranes and migrate between the scab and the wound along the provisional matrix of the dermis. FGF, fibroblast growth factor; VEGF, vascular endothelial growth factor.

TABLE 3–1

Collagen Molecular Composition and Structure

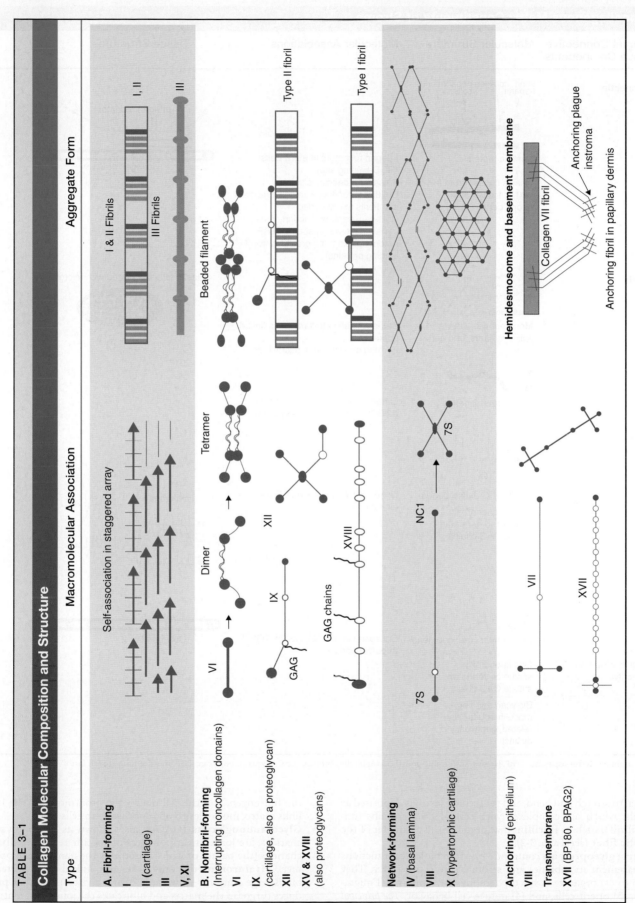

Type	Macromolecular Association	Aggregate Form
A. Fibril-forming	Self-association in staggered array	I & II Fibrils
I		III Fibrils
II (cartilage)		
III		
V, XI		
B. Nonfibril-forming (Interrupting noncollagen domains)	Dimer Tetramer	Beaded filament
VI		
IX (cartilage, also a proteoglycan)	GAG IX	Type II fibril
XII		XII
XV & XVIII (also proteoglycans)	GAG chains XVIII	Type I fibril
Network-forming	7S NC1 7S	Hemidesmosome and basement membrane
IV (basal lamina)		
VIII		
X (hypertorphic cartilage)		
Anchoring (epithelium)	VII	Collagen VII fibril
VIII		Anchoring plaque instroma
Transmembrane	XVII	Anchoring fibril in papillary dermis
XVII (BP180, BPAG2)		

GAG, glycosaminoglycan.

TABLE 3-2

Noncollagenous Matrix Constituents of Stroma

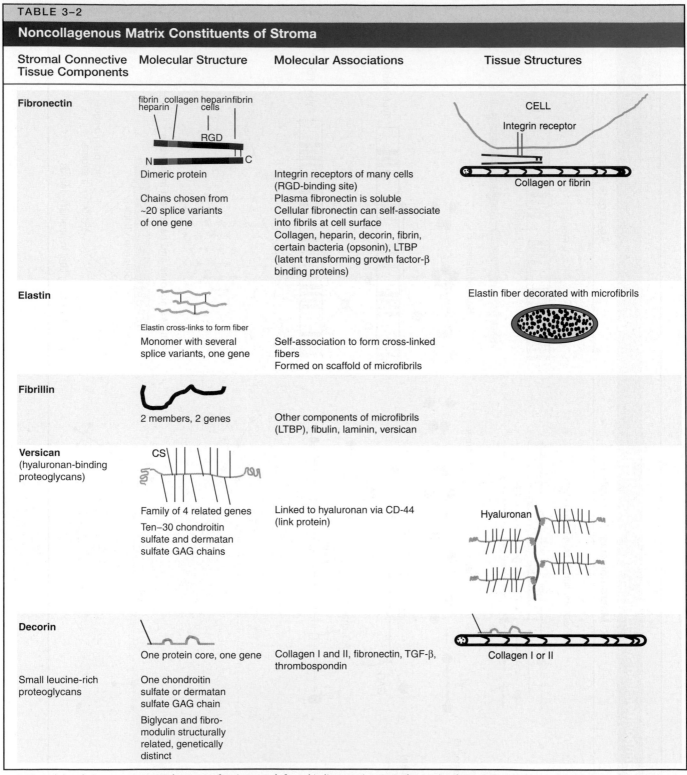

Stromal Connective Tissue Components	Molecular Structure	Molecular Associations	Tissue Structures
Fibronectin	Dimeric protein Chains chosen from ~20 splice variants of one gene	Integrin receptors of many cells (RGD-binding site) Plasma fibronectin is soluble Cellular fibronectin can self-associate into fibrils at cell surface Collagen, heparin, decorin, fibrin, certain bacteria (opsonin), LTBP (latent transforming growth factor-β binding proteins)	CELL Integrin receptor Collagen or fibrin
Elastin	Elastin cross-links to form fiber Monomer with several splice variants, one gene	Self-association to form cross-linked fibers Formed on scaffold of microfibrils	Elastin fiber decorated with microfibrils
Fibrillin	2 members, 2 genes	Other components of microfibrils (LTBP), fibulin, laminin, versican	
Versican (hyaluronan-binding proteoglycans)	Family of 4 related genes Ten–30 chondroitin sulfate and dermatan sulfate GAG chains	Linked to hyaluronan via CD-44 (link protein)	Hyaluronan
Decorin Small leucine-rich proteoglycans	One protein core, one gene One chondroitin sulfate or dermatan sulfate GAG chain Biglycan and fibromodulin structurally related, genetically distinct	Collagen I and II, fibronectin, TGF-β, thrombospondin	Collagen I or II

RGD, arginine-glycine-aspartate; LTBP, latent transforming growth factor binding proteins; GAG, glycosaminoglycan; TGF, transforming growth factor.

aorta, to stretch and bend, and yet recoil. Elastin is deposited as fibrils, which are complexed with several glycoproteins (microfibrils), such as **fibrillin**, that decorate the perimeter of the **elastic fiber** (see Table 3-2).

- **Matrix glycoproteins** contribute essential biological functions to basement membranes and stromal connective tissue. They help to (1) organize tissue topography, (2) support cell migration, (3) orient cells, and (4) induce cell behavior. *The principal matrix glycoprotein of stromal connective tissue is **fibronectin**.* Specific domains within fibronectin bind bacteria, collagen, heparin, fib-

rin, fibrinogen, and the cell matrix receptor, integrin. The last links matrix molecules to one another or to cells.
- **Glycosaminoglycans** (**GAGs**), also known as mucopolysaccharides, are long, linear polymers of specific repeating disaccharides (the names of which determine the name of the polymer). **Hyaluronin** (the only GAG not linked to a protein) binds large amounts of water, creating a viscous gel that produces turgor in the matrix and lubricates the joints and matrix.
- **Proteoglycans** consist of varying numbers of GAGs, heparan, chondroitin sulfate, and keratan sulfate, linked to specific core

TABLE 3-3

Basement Membrane Constituents and Organization

Basement Membrane Components	Molecular Structure	Molecular Associations	Basement Membrane Aggregate Form
Perlecan (heparan sulfate proteoglycan)	GAG chains	Laminin, collagen IV, fibronectin, growth factors (VEGF, FGF), chemokines	
Laminin	α β γ	Integrin and dystroglycan receptors on variety of cells (epithelium, endothelium, muscle, Schwann cells, adipocytes)	
		Forms self-associated noncovalent network assisted by perlecan	
		Laminin, nidogen/entactin, perlecan, agrin, fibulin	
Nidogen/Entactin		Collagen IV, laminin, perlecan, fibulin	
		Stabilizes basement membrane through association of laminin and collagen IV networks	
Collagen IV		Integrin receptors on many cells	
		Forms covalent self-associated network	
		Collagen IV, perlecan nidogen/entactin, SPARC	
Minor Collagens VIII, XV, XVIII			

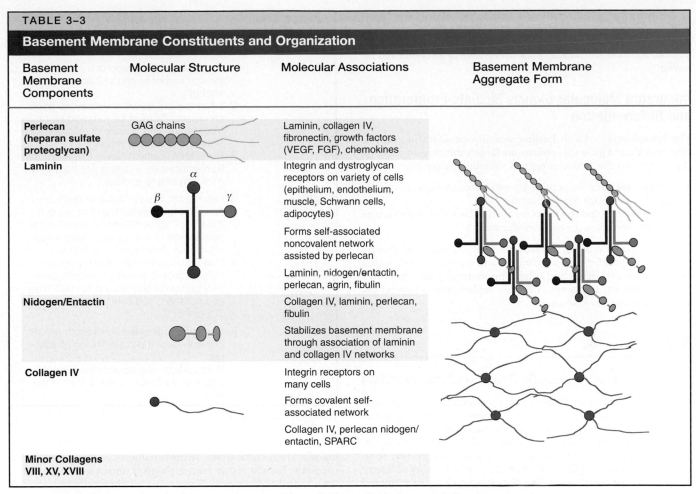

FGF, fibroblast growth factor; SPARC, secreted protein acidic and rich in cysteine; VEGF, vascular endothelial growth factor.

proteins. They participate in matrix organization, structural integrity, and cell attachment.

Basement Membranes

Basement membranes, also called **basal lamina**, are thin, well-defined layers of specialized extracellular matrix that separate the cells that synthesize it from connective tissue. Epithelium, adipocytes, muscle cells, Schwann cells, and capillary endothelium produce basement membranes (Table 3-3).

- Basement membranes are constructed from extracellular matrix molecules. They self-assemble into a sandwich-like structure composed of two interacting networks.
- Within different tissues and during development, the expression of unique members of the collagen IV and laminin families imparts diversity to the basement membrane and the many structures and functions it supports.
- Basement membranes act as filters, cellular anchors, and a surface for migrating epidermal cells after injury. Basement membranes also determine cell shape and provide a repository for growth factors and chemotactic peptides.
- Lamins are a biologically versatile family of basement membrane glycoproteins that contribute to the heterogeneity of tissue morphology and function, in part, by supporting cell attachment. Laminin is key for both normal epidermal function and re-epithelialization of wounds.

Stromal Reorganization is Critical to Repair

The matrix metalloproteins (MMPs) are crucial components in wound healing. They enable cells to migrate through the stroma by degrading matrix proteins at the site of injury, thereby allowing re-

organization of the tissue. MMPs are also involved in cell–cell communication and the activation or inactivation of bioactive molecules (e.g., matrix fragments and growth factors), in addition to influencing cell growth and apoptosis. MMPs can disrupt cell–cell adhesions and release, activate, or inactivate bioactive molecules stored in the matrix. In the later stages of the repair process, inflammatory cells diminish in number, and capillary formation is completed. Remodeling of the injury site into a mechanically strong, mature scar indicates that the equilibrium between collagen deposition and degradation has been restored. In this context, MMPs are the main digestive enzymes in remodeling, although neutrophil and serine proteases are also present.

Once secreted, MMP activity can be inactivated by binding to specific proteinase inhibitors. In addition to the important plasma-derived proteinase inhibitor, α_2-macroglobulin, there is a family of endogenous tissue inhibitors of metalloproteinases.

Cell Proliferation is Evoked by Cytokines and Matrix

A prominent early feature in injured tissue is a transient increase in cellularity, which serves to replace damaged cells. Cell proliferation also initiates and perpetuates the formation of granulation tissue, which is a specialized vascular tissue that is formed transiently during repair (discussed below). Cells of granulation tissue accumulate from labile cell populations, including circulating leukocytes and basal epithelial cells, and from stable cells, such as capillary endothelia and resident mesenchymal cells (fibroblasts, myofibroblasts, pericytes, and smooth muscle cells). Local and marrow-derived stem cells or committed progenitor cells may also populate wounds, differentiating into endothelial and fibroblast populations. Cells that are terminally differentiated (e.g., cardiac myocytes, neurons) do not contribute to repair or regeneration.

Growth factors and small chemotactic peptides (chemokines) provide soluble autocrine and paracrine signals for cell proliferation, differentiation, and migration. Signals from soluble factors and extracellular matrix also work collectively to influence cell behavior.

Integrated Molecular Signals Mediate Proliferation and Differentiation

The behaviors of cells in healing wounds—proliferation, migration, and altered gene expression—are largely initiated by three receptor systems that share integrated signaling pathways.

- Protein receptors for peptide growth factors, which contain cytoplasmic tyrosine kinase domains
- G protein-coupled receptors for chemokines and other factors
- Integrin receptors for extracellular matrix

The myriad signaling mechanisms that regulate cell growth, survival, and proliferation are complex and involve the integration of numerous activating and inhibiting molecules and cross-talk between different pathways. A further explanation is beyond the scope of the current discussion.

Repair

Outcomes of Injury Include Repair and Regeneration

Repair and regeneration develop with the waning of inflammatory responses, as inflammation itself is the primary response to tissue injury (see Chapter 2). *Transient* acute inflammation may resolve completely, with locally injured parenchymal elements being regenerated without significant scarring. For example, in recovery from moderate sunburn, small numbers of acute inflammatory cells temporarily accompany transient vasodilation beneath the solar-injured epidermis. By contrast, *sustained* acute inflammation, with emergence of macrophage-predominant inflammation, is a precursor to the sequence of collagen elaboration and repair associated with scar formation and fibrosis.

Wound Healing Exhibits a Defined Sequence

Wound healing that results in scar formation remains the predominant mode of repair. Given that wounds in the skin and the extremities are easily accessible, they have been extensively used as models. Although more difficult to study, healing within hollow viscera and body cavities generally parallels the repair sequence in skin (Table 3-4 and Fig. 3-2).

Hemostasis

A thrombus is formed at the site of injury primarily by the conversion of plasma fibrinogen to fibrin. The thrombus is also rich in fibronectin. Fibrin and fibronectin are soon cross-linked by transglutaminase to provide local tensile strength and maintain closure. The thrombus also contains contracting platelets, an initial source of growth factors. In the skin, a **scab** or **eschar** results from the drying of the exposed surface of the thrombus and forms a barrier to invading microorganisms. With time, the thrombus undergoes proteolysis, after which it is penetrated by regenerating epithelium. The scab then detaches.

Inflammation

Repair sites vary in the amount of local tissue destruction. For example, the surgical excision of a minor skin lesion leaves little or no devitalized tissue. Demarcated, localized necrosis accompanies medium-sized myocardial infarcts. By contrast, widespread, irregularly defined necrosis is a feature of a large third-degree burn. Initially, an acute, neutrophil-dominated, inflammatory response

TABLE 3-4	
Repair in Skin	
EARLY	1. Thrombosis: Formation of a growth factor-rich barrier having significant tensile strength
	2. Inflammation: Necrotic debris and microorganisms must be removed by neutrophils; the appearance of macrophages signals and initiates repair
	3. Re-epithelialization: Newly formed epithelium establishes a permanent barrier to microorganisms and fluid
MID	4. Granulation tissue formation and function: This specialized organ of repair is the site of extracellular matrix and collagen secretion; it is vascular, edematous, insensitive, and resistant to infection
	5. Contraction: Fibroblasts and possibly other cells also transform to actin-containing myofibroblasts, link to each other and collagen, and contract, stimulated by TGF-ß1 or ß2
LATE	6. Accretion of final tensile strength results primarily from the cross-linking of collagen
	7. Remodeling: The wound site devascularizes and conforms to stress lines in the skin

TGF, transforming growth factor.

liquefies the necrotic tissue. Acute inflammation persists as long as necessary, because repair cannot progress until necrotic structures are liquefied and removed. Plasma-derived fibronectin binds to collagen and cell membranes to facilitate phagocytosis. Fibronectin and cellular debris are chemotactic for macrophages and fibroblasts (see Fig. 3-2 parts 4 and 5). The appearance of macrophages as the predominant cell at the site of injury signals the onset of the repair process. Macrophages ingest proteolytic products of neutrophils and secrete collagenase, thereby promoting further liquefaction. They also provide growth factors that stimulate fibroblast proliferation, collagen secretion, and neovascularization.

Fibroblasts are also early responders to injury. These collagen-secreting cells are involved in inflammatory, proliferative, and remodeling phases of wound repair. Fibroblasts are capable of further differentiation to contractile myofibroblasts.

Provisional Matrix

Provisional matrix is a term that describes the temporary extracellular organization of plasma-derived matrix proteins and tissue-derived components that accumulate at sites of injury. These molecules are associated with the pre-existing stromal matrix and serve to stop blood or fluid loss. They also support the migration of monocytes, endothelial cells, epidermal cells, and fibroblasts to the wound site. *Plasma-derived provisional matrix proteins include fibrinogen, fibronectin, and vitronectin.* These proteins become insoluble by binding to the stromal matrix and by forming cross-links via the action of tissue- and plasma-derived transglutaminases.

Granulation Tissue

Granulation tissue is the transient, specialized tissue of repair, which replaces the provisional matrix. On gross examination, it is deceptively simple, with a glistening and pebbled appearance (Fig. 3-3). Microscopically, a mixture of fibroblasts and red blood cells first appears, followed by the development of provisional matrix and patent single cell-lined capillaries, which are surrounded by fibroblasts and inflammatory cells.

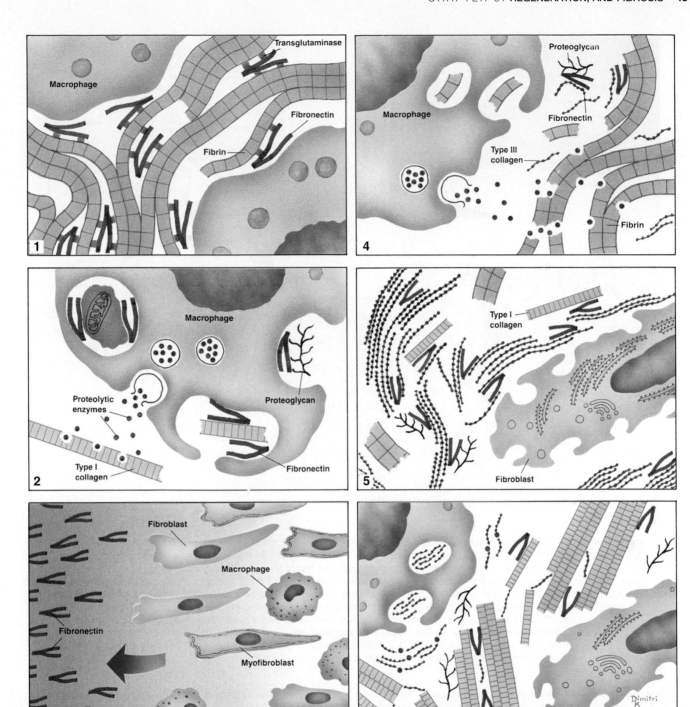

FIGURE 3-2. **Summary of the healing process.** The initial phase of the repair reaction, which typically begins with hemorrhage into the tissues. *(1)* A fibrin clot forms and fills the gap created by the wound. Fibronectin in the extravasated plasma is cross-linked to fibrin, collagen, and other extracellular matrix components by the action of transglutaminases. This cross-linking provides a provisional mechanical stabilization of the wound (0 to 4 hours). *(2)* Macrophages recruited to the wound area process cell remnants and damaged extracellular matrix. The binding of fibronectin to cell membranes, collagens, proteoglycans, DNA, and bacteria (opsonization) facilitates phagocytosis by these macrophages and contributes to the removal of debris (1 to 3 days). *(3)* Fibronectin, cell debris, and bacterial products are chemoattractants for a variety of cells that are recruited to the wound site (2 to 4 days). The intermediate phase of the repair reaction. *(4)* As a new extracellular matrix is deposited at the wound site, the initial fibrin clot is lysed by a combination of extracellular proteolytic enzymes and phagocytosis (2 to 4 days). *(5)* Concurrent with fibrin removal, there is deposition of a temporary matrix formed by proteoglycans, glycoproteins, and type III collagen (2 to 5 days). *(6)* Final phase of the repair reaction. Eventually, the temporary matrix is removed by a combination of extracellular and intracellular digestion, and the definitive matrix, rich in type I collagen, is deposited (5 days to weeks).

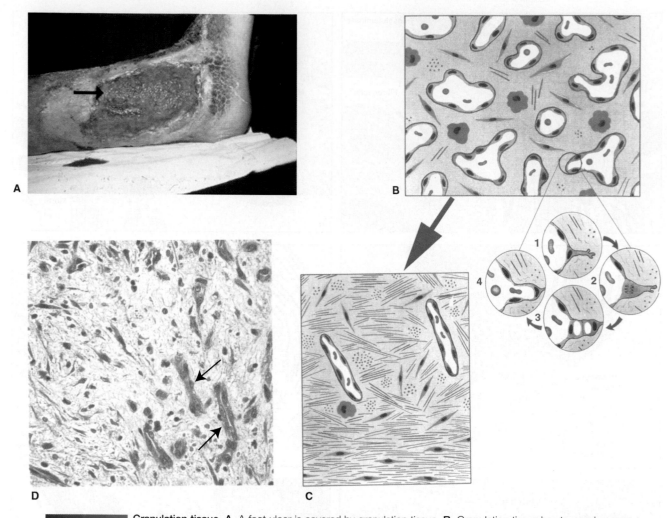

FIGURE 3-3. **Granulation tissue. A.** A foot ulcer is covered by granulation tissue. **B.** Granulation tissue has two major components: cells and proliferating capillaries. The cells are mostly fibroblasts, myofibroblasts, and macrophages. The macrophages are derived from monocytes and macrophages. The fibroblasts and myofibroblasts derive from mesenchymal stem cells, and the capillaries arise from adjacent vessels by division of the lining endothelial cells *(detail),* in a process termed *angiogenesis.* Endothelial cells put out cell extensions, called pseudopodia that grow toward the wound site. Cytoplasmic growth enlarges the *pseudopodia,* and eventually, the cells divide. Vacuoles formed in the daughter cells eventually fuse to create a new lumen. The entire process continues until the sprout encounters another capillary, with which it will connect. At its peak, granulation tissue is the most richly vascularized tissue in the body. **C.** Once repair has been achieved, most of the newly formed capillaries are obliterated and then reabsorbed, leaving a pale avascular scar. **D.** A photomicrograph of granulation tissue shows thin-walled vessels embedded in a loose connective tissue matrix containing mesenchymal cells and occasional inflammatory cells.

A key step in the development of granulation tissue is the recruitment of monocytes to the site of injury by chemokines and fragments of damaged matrix. Later, plasma cells are conspicuous, even predominant. Activated macrophages coordinate the development of granulation tissue through the release of growth factors and cytokines, which (1) direct angiogenesis (see angiogenesis below), (2) activate fibroblasts to form new stroma, and (3) continue the degradation and removal of the provisional matrix. However, recent studies challenge established concepts regarding the central role of the macrophage in wound repair. Granulation tissue is fluid-laden, and its cellular constituents supply antibacterial antibodies and growth factors. It is highly resistant to bacterial infection, allowing the surgeon to create anastomoses at such nonsterile sites as the colon.

Fibroblast Proliferation and Matrix Accumulation

The temporary early matrix of granulation tissue contains proteoglycans, glycoproteins, and type III collagen (see Fig. 3-2). The release of cytokines from fixed cells in the damaged tissue causes hemorrhage and attracts inflammatory cells to the site. About 2 to 3 days

after injury, activated fibroblasts and capillary sprouts are detected. The shape of fibroblasts in the wound changes from oval to bipolar, as they begin to form collagen and synthesize other matrix proteins, such as fibronectin. Extracellular cross-linking of newly synthesized collagen progressively increases wound strength.

Growth Factors and Fibroplasia

The initial discovery of epidermal growth factor and the subsequent identification of at least 20 other growth factors have provided explanations for many of the rapidly changing events in repair and regeneration. Interactions among growth factors, other cytokines, and MMPs are illustrated in Figures 3-4 and 3-5. Each has a predominant function in repair. Growth factors that are expressed as an early wound response support migration, recruitment, and proliferation of cells involved in fibroplasia, re-epithelialization, and angiogenesis. Growth factors that peak later sustain the maturation phase and remodeling of granulation tissue.

Although the roles of growth factors in the initiation and progression of repair are reasonably well understood, the limiting and

2–4 Days

Thrombus

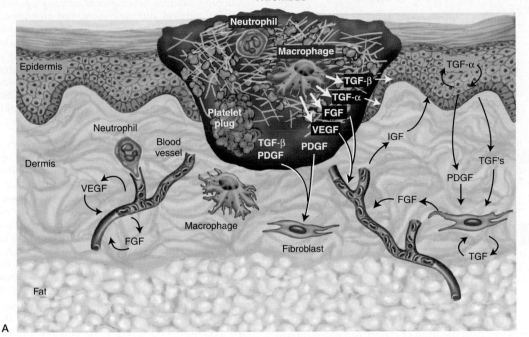

4–8 Days

Thrombus

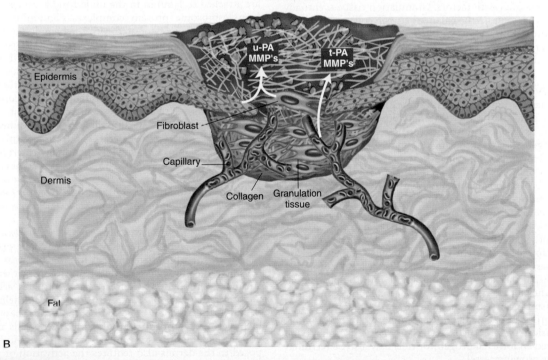

FIGURE 3-4.   **Cutaneous wound. A.** At 2 to 4 days, growth factors controlling migration of cells are illustrated. Extensive redundancy is present, and no growth factor is rate limiting. **B.** At 4 to 8 days, the blood vessels are proliferating, and the epidermis is penetrating the thrombus, but not at its surface. The upper portion will become an eschar or scab. FGF, fibroblast growth factor; IGF, insulin-like growth factor; TGF, transforming growth factor; PDGF, platelet-derived growth factor; VEGF, vascular endothelial growth factor; MMPs, matrix metalloproteinases; t-PA, tissue plasminogen activator; u-PA, urokinase-type plasminogen activator.

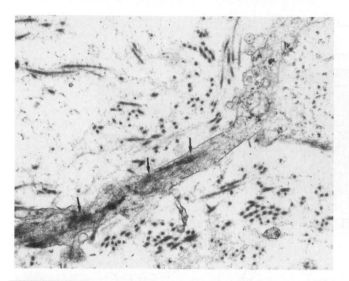

FIGURE 3-5. **Myofibroblast viewed by electron microscopy.** Myofibroblasts have an important role in the repair reaction. These cells, with features intermediate between those of smooth muscle cells and fibroblasts, are characterized by the presence of discrete bundles of myofilaments in the cytoplasm (*arrows*).

terminating events are not well defined. Diminishing anoxia as repair progresses may be key to the arrest of the repair process. Repair may also cease because of reduced turnover of extracellular matrix. Finally, increased storage and decreased availability of growth factors may stabilize the matrix, which may then transmit signals that reduce the effects of growth factors. Granulation tissue eventually transitions to scar tissue, as the balance between collagen synthesis and collagen breakdown begins within weeks of injury. Fibroblasts remain active at the wound site, much increasing the density of the scar over several years.

Angiogenesis

At its peak, granulation tissue has more capillaries per unit volume than any other tissue. New capillary growth is essential for the delivery of oxygen and nutrients to the cells. New capillaries form by angiogenesis (i.e., sprouting of endothelial cells from pre-existing capillary venules) (see Fig. 3-3) and create the granular appearance for which granulation tissue is named. Less often, new blood vessels form de novo from angioblasts. The latter process is known as **vasculogenesis** and is primarily associated with developmental processes.

Angiogenesis in wound repair is tightly regulated. Quiescent capillary endothelial cells are activated by the local release of cytokines and growth factors. The endothelial cells and pericytes are bordered by basement membranes, which must be locally degraded before endothelial cells and pericytes migrate into the provisional matrix. Endothelial passage through the matrix requires the cooperation of plasminogen activators, matrix MMPs, and integrin receptors. The growth of new capillaries is supported by the proliferation and fusion of endothelial cells (see Fig. 3-3), and bone marrow-derived endothelial progenitor cells may also be recruited to support the growing vessel.

Migration of cells into the wound site is directed by soluble ligands (**chemotaxis**) and proceeds along adhesive matrix substrates (**haptotaxis**). Once capillary endothelial cells are immobilized, cell–cell contacts form, and an organized basement membrane develops on the exterior of the nascent capillary. The association with pericytes and signals from angiopoietin, TGF-β, and PDGF establish a mature vessel phenotype and help form nonleaky capillaries.

In vivo angiogenesis is initiated by hypoxia and a redundance of cytokines, growth factors, and various lipids, which stimulate or regulate vascular endothelial growth factor (VEGF). Activated granulation tissue macrophages and endothelial cells produce

FGF and VEGF, and epidermal cells in the wound release VEGF in response to keratinocyte growth factor. Because the chief target of VEGF is the endothelial cell, this molecule is a critical regulator of embryonic vascular development and angiogenesis, regulating endothelial survival, differentiation, and migration. The binding of angiogenic growth factors to heparan sulfate-containing GAG chains is a crucial feature of angiogenesis. The association with heparan sulfate chains affects the availability and action of growth factors and vessel formation by (1) creating a storage reservoir of VEGF and βFGF in capillary basement membranes and (2) using cell surface proteoglycan receptors to regulate VEGF and βFGF receptor congregation, as well as signal delivery and intensity.

Re-Epithelialization

Skin provides the best-studied example of epithelial repair. Epidermis constantly renews itself via mitosis of keratinocytes at the basal layer. The squamous cells then cornify or keratinize as they mature, move toward the surface, and are shed. *Maturation requires an intact layer of basal cells that are in direct contact with one another and the basement membrane.* If cell–cell contact is disrupted, basal epithelial cells re-establish contact with other basal cells through mitosis. Epithelial regeneration is illustrated in Figures 3-5 and 3-6. Once re-established, the epithelial barrier demarcates the scab from the newly covered wound, providing a protective barrier against infection and fluid loss. When epithelial continuity is re-established, the epidermis resumes its normal cycle of maturation and shedding.

During the process of re-epithelialization in the skin, the basal layer of epithelial cells contributes important cytokines (interleukin [IL]-1, VEGF, TGF-α, TGF-β, PDGF) for the initiation of healing. To begin migration, keratinocytes must undergo cellular differentiation before forming a new covering over the wound. Normally, these cells are attached to laminin in the underlying basement membrane by hemidesmosome protein complexes containing $\alpha_6\beta_4$ integrin. Collagen fibers are associated with the hemidesmosome, including types XVII and VII, also termed **anchoring fibril** (see Table 3-1). The anchoring fibril connects the hemidesmosome–basement membrane complex to the dermal connective tissue collagen fibers.

Epithelial cells are connected to each other at their lateral edges by **tight junctions** and by **adherens junctions** composed of cadherin receptors. Cadherins are calcium-dependent, integral membrane proteins that form extracellular cell–cell connections and anchor intracellular cytoskeletal connections. In the adherens junctions, cadherins bind stable actin bundles to a cytoplasmic complex of α-, β-, and γ-catenins. The layer of actin that encircles the epithelial cytoplasm creates lateral tension and strength and is referred to as the **adhesion belt**. *The shape and the strength of connected epithelial sheets result from tension created by cytoskeletal connections to basement membrane and cell-to-cell connections.*

Cellular migration is the predominant means by which the wound surface is re-epithelialized. Migrating epidermal cells originate at the margin of the wound and in hair follicles or sweat glands. If the basement membrane is lost, cells come in contact with unfamiliar stromal components, an effect that stimulates cell locomotion and proteinase expression. Activation of epithelial motility is driven by the assembly of actin fibers at focal adhesions organized by integrin receptors, directing the migrating cells along the margin of viable dermis. Movement through cross-linked fibrin apposed to the dermis also requires the activation of plasmin from plasminogen to degrade fibrin. Plasmin also aids in the activation of specific MMPs. Proteolytic cleavage of stromal collagens I and III and laminin at focal adhesion contacts can release adhesion or enable keratinocyte migration. Migrating keratinocytes eventually resume their normal phenotype after reforming a confluent layer and attaching to their newly formed basement membranes.

Wound Contraction

As they heal, open wounds contract and deform in a process mediated by a specialized cell of granulation tissue, the **myofibroblast**. This modified fibroblast cannot be distinguished from the collagen-

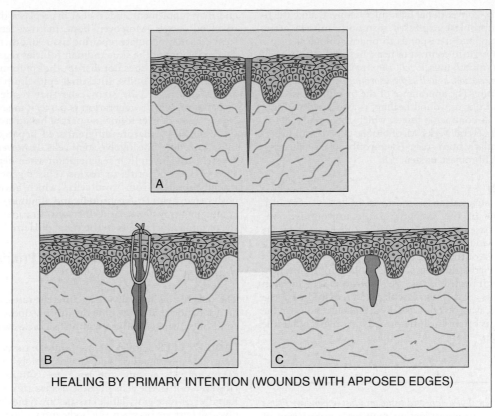

HEALING BY PRIMARY INTENTION (WOUNDS WITH APPOSED EDGES)

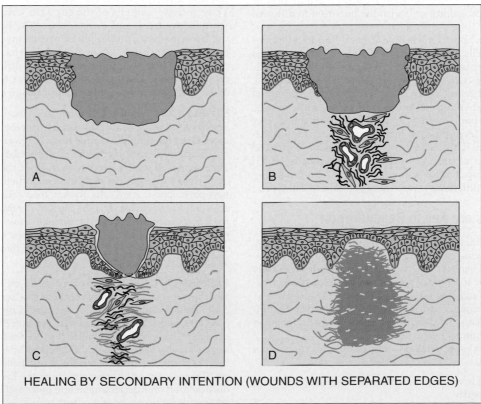

HEALING BY SECONDARY INTENTION (WOUNDS WITH SEPARATED EDGES)

FIGURE 3-6.   **Top: Healing by primary intention. A.** A wound with closely apposed edges and minimal tissue loss. **B.** Such a wound requires only minimal cell proliferation and neovascularization to heal. **C.** The result is a small scar.
Bottom: Healing by secondary intention. A. A gouged wound, in which the edges are far apart and in which there is substantial tissue loss. **B.** This wound requires wound contraction, extensive cell proliferation, and neovascularization (granulation tissue) to heal. **C.** The wound is re-epithelialized from the margins, and collagen fibers are deposited in the granulation tissue. **D.** Granulation tissue is eventually resorbed and replaced by a large scar that is functionally and esthetically unsatisfactory.

secreting fibroblast by conventional light microscopy. Unlike the fibroblast, the myofibroblast expresses α-smooth muscle actin, desmin, and vimentin, and it responds to pharmacological agents that cause smooth muscle to contract or relax. In short, it is a fibroblast that reacts like a smooth muscle cell. *The myofib-roblast is the cell responsible for wound contraction, as well as the deforming pathological process termed wound contracture.* The appearance of the myofibroblast, usually around the third day of wound healing, is associated with the sudden appearance of contractile forces, which then gradually diminish over the next several weeks. Myofibroblasts persist in hypertrophic scars, particularly burn scars. The myofibroblast may originate from a pericyte, fibroblast, or stem cell.

Wound Strength

Skin incisions and surgical anastomoses in hollow viscera ultimately develop 75% of the strength of the unwounded site. Despite a rapid increase in tensile strength at 7 to 14 days, by the end of 2 weeks, the wound has acquired only about 20% of its ultimate strength. Most of the strength of the healed wound results from intermolecular cross-linking of type I collagen. A 2-month-old incision, although healed, is still visibly obvious. The incision line and suture marks are distinct, vascular, and red. By 1 year, the incision is white and avascular but usually still identifiable. As the scar fades further, it is often slowly deformed into an irregular line by stresses in the skin.

Regeneration

Regeneration is the renewal of a damaged tissue or a lost appendage that is identical to the original one. Regeneration requires a population of stem or committed progenitor cells with the potential to differentiate and replicate.

The adult human body is made up of several hundred types of well-differentiated cells, yet it maintains the remarkable potential to rebuild itself by replenishing dying cells and to heal itself by recruiting or activating cells that repair or regenerate injured tissue. Tissues are adept at healing injury, but their regenerative potential is unfortunately restricted to a limited number of adult tissues. Unique cells within bone marrow, epidermis, intestine, and liver maintain sufficient developmental memory to orchestrate tissue-specific regeneration. The power to regenerate tissue is derived from a small number of unspecialized cells, or **stem cells**, which are unique in their capacity for self-renewal while also producing clonal progeny that differentiate into more specialized cell types.

Adult Stem Cells are Key to Regeneration

Cells able to divide indefinitely, without terminally differentiating, continue to inhabit many adult tissues and have even been identified in tissues not observed to regenerate. These **adult stem cells** may exist in a specific tissue or be seeded in that tissue from circulating cells of bone marrow origin. Either way, the presence of stem cells within a broader variety of tissues underscores the importance of a permissive and supportive environment for stem cell-driven regeneration.

Stem cells may be more generally defined by certain common properties including:

- The ability to divide without limit, avoid senescence, and maintain genomic integrity
- The ability to undergo division intermittently or to remain quiescent
- The ability to propagate by self-renewal and differentiation
- The absence of lineage markers

Bone marrow contains hematopoietic, mesenchymal, and endothelial stem cells, providing a multifaceted regenerative capacity. Bone marrow stem cells, which are set aside during embryonic development, replenish the hematopoietic population. Endothelial stem cells from bone marrow have been implicated in tissue angiogenesis

and may supplement endothelial hyperplasia during regeneration of blood vessels. Moreover, bone marrow-derived mesenchymal stem cells may populate repairing tissue in other parts of the body.

Epithelium of the skin and hair follicles regenerates from stem cells if the wound does not disrupt the epidermal basement membrane or the hair bulbs. Intestinal epithelium turns over rapidly and is replenished by stem cells that reside in the crypts of Lieberkuhn. Liver regeneration is partly a misnomer, because the regeneration of liver following partial hepatectomy is a hyperplastic response by mature differentiated hepatocytes and, for the most part, does not involve stem cells. However, there is evidence for stem cell-driven liver regeneration when hepatocytes are damaged by viral hepatitis or toxins. This regenerative potential is thought to arise from "oval cells," which have characteristics of both hepatocytes (α-fetoprotein and albumin) and bile duct cells (γ-glutamyl transferase and duct cytokeratins) and may reside in the terminal ductal cells in the canal of Hering.

Cells Can be Classified by their Proliferative Potential

The cells of the body divide at different rates. Some mature cells do not divide at all and some divide only under certain permissive conditions, whereas others complete a cycle every 16 to 24 hours.

LABILE CELLS: Labile cells are found in tissues that are in a constant state of renewal. Tissues in which more than 1.5% of the cells are in mitosis at any one time are composed of labile cells. However, not all the cells in these tissues are continuously cycling. Rapidly self-renewing (labile) tissues are typically tissues that form physical barriers between the body and the external environment. These include epithelia of the gut, skin, cornea, respiratory tract, reproductive tract, and urinary tract. The hematopoietic cells of the bone marrow and lymphoid organs involved in immune defense also constitute labile tissues. Polymor-phonuclear leukocytes are the best example of a terminally differentiated cell that is rapidly renewed. *Under appropriate conditions, tissues composed of labile cells regenerate after injury, provided that enough stem cells remain.*

STABLE CELLS: Stable cells populate tissues that normally are renewed very slowly but are populated with progenitor cells capable of more rapid renewal after tissue loss. The liver and the proximal renal tubules are examples of stable cell populations. Stable cells populate tissues in which fewer than 1.5% of the cells are in mitosis. Such tissues (e.g., endocrine glands, endothelium, and liver) do not have conspicuous stem cells. Rather, their cells require an appropriate stimulus to divide. *It is the potential to replicate and not the actual number of steady state mitoses that determines the ability of an organ to regenerate.* For example, the liver, a stable tissue with less than one mitosis for every 15,000 cells, regenerates rapidly after a loss of as much as 75% of its mass.

PERMANENT CELLS: Permanent cells are terminally differentiated, have lost all capacity for regeneration, and do not enter the cell cycle. Traditionally, neurons of the central nervous system, cardiac myocytes, and cells of the lens were considered permanent cells, although recent studies are challenging previous dogma. *If lost, permanent cells cannot be replaced.* Although permanent cells do not divide, most of them do renew their cellular organelles. The extreme example of permanent cells is the lens of the eye. Every lens cell generated during embryonic development and postnatal life is preserved in the adult without turnover of its constituents.

Conditions that Modify Repair

Local Factors May Influence Healing

Location of the Wound

In addition to the size and shape of the wound, its location also affects healing. Sites in which skin covers bone with little intervening tissue, such as skin over the anterior tibia, are locations where skin cannot contract. Skin lesions in such areas, particularly burns, often require skin grafts because their edges cannot be apposed. Complications or other treatments, such as infection or ionizing radiation, also slow the repair process.

Blood Supply

Lower-extremity wounds of diabetics who suffer from disease-related vasculopathies often heal poorly or even require amputation. In such cases, advanced atherosclerosis in the legs compromises blood supply and impedes repair. Varicose veins of the legs slow the venous return and can also cause ulceration and nonhealing. Bedsores (decubitus ulcers) result from prolonged, localized, dependent pressure, which diminishes both arterial and venous blood flow. Joint (articular) cartilage is largely avascular and has limited diffusion capacity; often, it cannot mount a vigorous inflammatory response. As a result, articular cartilage repairs poorly, a condition (osteoarthritis) that usually worsens with age.

Systemic Factors

No specific effect of age alone on repair has been found. Although the skin of a 90-year-old person—which exhibits reduced collagen and elastin—may heal slowly, the same person's cataract extraction or colon resection heals normally because the bowel and the eye are practically unaffected by age. Iatrogenic factors such as therapeutic corticosteroids retard wound repair by inhibiting collagen and protein synthesis as well as by exerting anti-inflammatory effects.

Fibrosis and Scarring Contrasted

Successful wound repair that leads to localized scarring is a transient, not chronic, process that leads to resolution of local injury. By contrast, many chronic diseases involve persistent, unresolved inflammation, with progression of the repair response culminating in diffuse fibrosis in affected tissues. For example, inhaled smoke or silica particles induce persistent inflammation in the lung, ultimately leading to pulmonary fibrosis. Continuing insult or inflammation, mediated through the interplay of monocytes and lymphocytes, results in persistent high levels of cytokines, growth factors, and locally destructive enzymes such as collagenases. Whatever the cause, long-standing fibrosis of parenchymal organs such as the lung, kidney, or liver, disrupts the normal architecture and reduces function. Chronic fibrosis is generally irreversible, calling for measures to prevent exposure to the cause, or therapeutic measures to limit the inflammatory process. Fibrosis should be viewed as the pathological end result of persistent injury. Scarring, however, is often beneficial—the scar resulting from a surgical incision in skin, although cosmetically unattractive, holds the skin together.

Specific Sites Exhibit Different Repair Patterns

Skin

Healing in the skin involves both repair (primarily dermal scarring) and regeneration (principally of the epidermis and vasculature). The salient features of primary and secondary healing are provided in Figure 3-6.

Healing by primary intention occurs when the surgeon closely approximates the edges of a wound. The actions of myofibroblasts are minimized, and regeneration of the epidermis is optimal, because epidermal cells need migrate only a minimal distance.

Healing by secondary intention proceeds when a large area of hemorrhage and necrosis cannot be completely corrected surgically. In this situation, myofibroblasts contract the wound, and subsequent scarring repairs the defect.

The success and method of healing following a burn wound depends on the depth of the burn injury. If the burn is superficial or does not extend beyond the upper dermis, stem cells from the sweat glands and hair follicles will regenerate the epidermis. If the deep dermis is involved, the regenerative elements are destroyed,

and surgery and engraftment are necessary to cover or heal the wound site and reduce scarring and contractures.

Liver

Acute chemical injury or fulminant viral hepatitis causes widespread necrosis of hepatocytes. However, if liver failure is not quickly fatal, the parenchyma regenerates and normal form and function are restored. In addition to mitosis of hepatocytes, small cells at the canal of Hering, termed oval cells, are thought to be the stem cell responsible for liver regeneration under these conditions. By contrast, chronic injury in viral hepatitis or alcoholism is associated with the development of broad collagenous scars within the hepatic parenchyma, termed **cirrhosis** of the liver (Fig. 3-7). The hepatocytes form regenerative nodules that lack central veins and expand to obstruct blood vessels and bile flow. Portal hypertension and jaundice ensue despite adequate numbers of regenerated but disconnected hepatocytes.

Kidney

Although the kidney has limited regenerative capacity, the removal of one kidney (nephrectomy) is followed by compensatory hypertrophy of the remaining kidney. If renal injury is not extensive and the extracellular matrix framework is not destroyed, the tubular epithelium regenerates. In most renal diseases, however, there is some destruction of the framework. Regeneration is then incomplete, and scar formation is the usual outcome. The regenerative capacity of renal tissue is maximal in cortical tubules, less in medullary tubules, and nonexistent in glomeruli. Recent data suggest tubule repair occurs by proliferation of endogenous renal progenitor cells.

Lung

The epithelium lining the respiratory tract has an effective regenerative capacity, provided that the underlying extracellular matrix framework is not destroyed. Superficial injuries to tracheal and bronchial epithelia heal by regeneration from the adjacent epithelium. The outcome of alveolar injury ranges from complete regeneration of structure and function to incapacitating fibrosis (Fig. 3-8).

Alveolar injury that does not result in damage to the basement membrane is followed by healing by regeneration. Alveolar type II pneumocytes (the alveolar reserve cells) migrate to denuded areas and undergo mitosis to form cells with features intermediate between those of type I and type II pneumocytes. As these cells cover

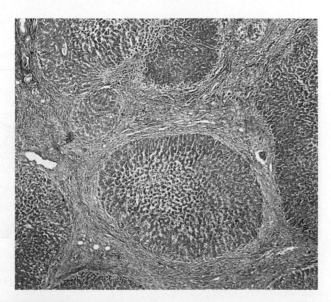

FIGURE 3-7. **Cirrhosis of the liver.** The consequences of chronic hepatic injury are the formation of regenerating nodules separated by fibrous bands. A microscopic section shows regenerating nodules (*red*) surrounded by bands of connective tissue (*blue*).

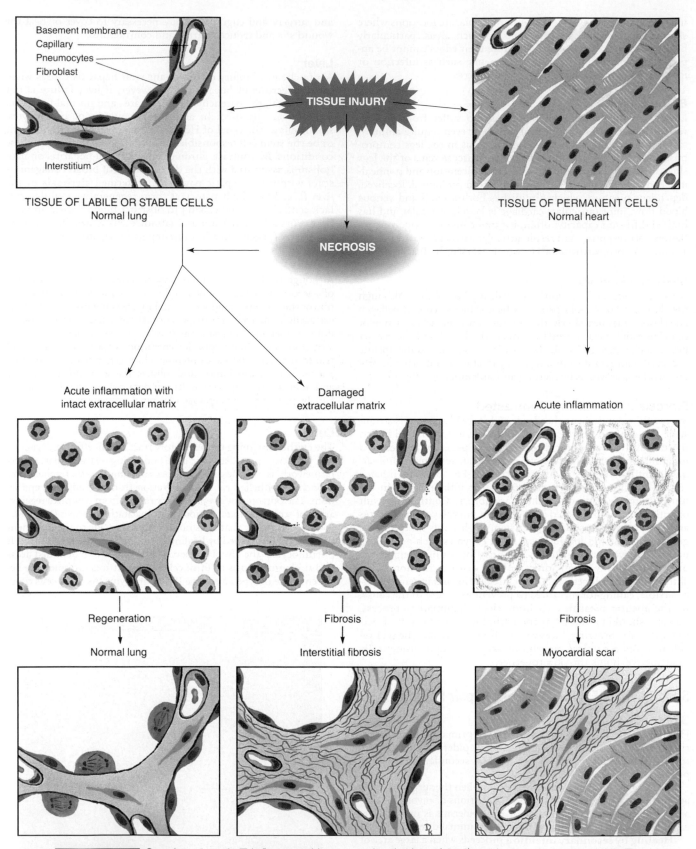

FIGURE 3-8. **Overview of repair.** This figure provides an overview that interrelates the early dynamic events in repair. The time scale in this figure is not linear; initial tensile strength, the first phase, develops almost immediately. Remodeling is ill defined, extending from its early beginning in repair for weeks or months.

the alveolar surface, they establish contact with other epithelial cells. Mitosis then stops, and the cells differentiate into type I pneumocytes. If there is extensive disruption to the basement membrane of the alveolus, scarring and fibrosis result. Stimulated by macrophage products, mesenchymal cells from the alveolar septa proliferate and differentiate into fibroblasts and myofibroblasts. These cells migrate into the alveolar space, where they secrete type 1 collagen and proteoglycans, leading to pulmonary fibrosis. The most common chronic pulmonary disease is emphysema, which involves airspace enlargement, the destruction of alveolar walls, and ineffective replacement of elastin. This process results in irreversible loss of tissue resiliency and function.

Heart

Cardiac myocytes are permanent, nondividing, terminally differentiated cells. Recent studies, however, have provided evidence for minimal regeneration of cardiac myocytes from previously unrecognized stem or committed progenitor cells. The origin of these cells, whether they reside in the myocardium or migrate there following injury from sites unknown, is not resolved. For practical purposes, myocardial necrosis, from whatever cause, heals by the formation of granulation tissue and eventual scarring (Fig. 3-9). Not only does myocardial scarring result in the loss of contractile elements, but the fibrotic tissue also decreases the effectiveness of contraction in the surviving myocardium.

Nervous System

Mature neurons have been described as permanent and postmitotic cells, and recent studies suggesting possible regenerative capacity have not altered well-established observations about injury in the nervous system. Following trauma, only regrowth and reorganization of the surviving neuronal cell processes can re-establish neural connections. Although the peripheral nervous system has the capacity for axonal regeneration, the central nervous system lacks this ability. Any damage to the brain or spinal cord is followed by the growth of capillaries and gliosis (i.e., the proliferation of astrocytes and microglia). Gliosis in the central nervous system is the equivalent of scar formation elsewhere; once established, it remains permanently.

Neurons in the peripheral nervous system can regenerate their axons, and under ideal circumstances, interruption in the continuity of a peripheral nerve results in complete functional recovery. However, if the cut ends are not in perfect alignment or are prevented from establishing continuity by inflammation or a scar, a traumatic neuroma results (Fig. 3-10). This bulbous lesion consists of disorganized axons and proliferating Schwann cells, as well as fibroblasts.

Effects of Scarring

Although scarring is essential to the repair of most injuries, scarring in parenchymal organs modifies their complex structure and never improves their function. For example, in the heart, the scar of a myocardial infarction serves to prevent rupture of the weakened wall of the heart but reduces the amount of contractile tissue. If extensive enough, it may be associated with congestive heart failure or the formation of a ventricular aneurysm. Persistent inflammation within the pericardium may result in organization of the inflammatory exudate and conversion of the deposited fibrin into collagen. This is likely to produce fibrous adhesions, which result in constrictive pericarditis and heart failure (Fig. 3-11).

Alveolar fibrosis in the lung causes respiratory failure. Infection within the peritoneum or even surgical exploration may lead to adhesions and intestinal obstruction. Immunological injury to the renal glomerulus eventuates in its replacement by a collagenous scar and, if this process is extensive, renal failure. Scarring in the skin following burns or surgical excision of lesions may produce unsatisfactory cosmetic results or worse, deficits in limb function because of wound contractions.

Wound Repair is Often Suboptimal

Abnormalities in any of three healing processes—repair, contraction, and regeneration—result in unsuccessful or prolonged wound healing. The skill of the surgeon is often of critical importance.

Deficient Scar Formation

Inadequate formation of granulation tissue or an inability to form a suitable extracellular matrix leads to deficient scar formation and its complications, such as wound dehiscence (splitting upon increased stress) and incisional hernias at prior surgical sites. Systemic factors predisposing to such defects include metabolic deficiency, hypoproteinemia, and the general inanition that often accompanies metastatic cancer.

Ulceration

Wounds can ulcerate when there is an inadequate intrinsic blood supply or insufficient vascularization during healing. For example, leg wounds in persons with varicose veins or severe atherosclerosis often ulcerate. Nonhealing wounds also develop in areas

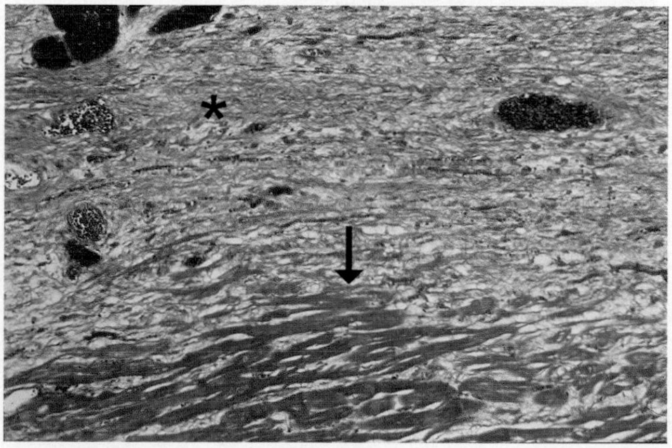

FIGURE 3-9. **Myocardial infarction.** A section through a healed myocardial infarct shows mature fibrosis (*) and disrupted myocardial fibers (*arrow*).

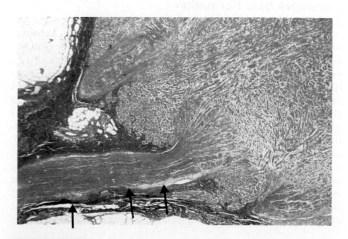

FIGURE 3-10. **Traumatic neuroma.** In this photomicrograph, the original nerve (*arrows*) enters the neuroma. The nerve is surrounded by dense collagenous tissue, which appears dark blue with this trichrome stain.

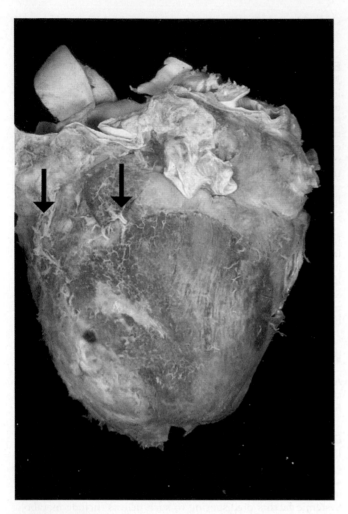

FIGURE 3-11. **Organized strands of collagen** in constrictive pericarditis (*arrows*).

ture and results in severe deformity of the wound and surrounding tissues. Interestingly, the regions that normally show minimal wound contraction (e.g., the palms, the soles, and the anterior aspect of the thorax) are the ones prone to contractures. Contractures are particularly conspicuous in the healing of serious burns and can be severe enough to compromise the movement of joints. In the alimentary tract, a contracture (stricture) can result in obstruction to the passage of food in the esophagus or a block in the flow of intestinal contents.

Excessive Regeneration and Repair

In addition to the many responses to injury described thus far, an additional lesion merits consideration, namely **pyogenic granuloma**. This lesion is a localized, persistent, exuberant overgrowth of granulation tissue, most commonly seen in gum tissue in pregnant women. It also develops in the squamocolumnar junction of the uterine cervix and at other sites. An injury preceding the development of pyogenic granuloma cannot usually be found. Like injury-induced granulation tissue, it lacks nerves and can be surgically trimmed without anesthesia. Conceptually, pyogenic granuloma is a transitional lesion, resembling granulation tissue but behaving almost as an autonomous benign neoplasm.

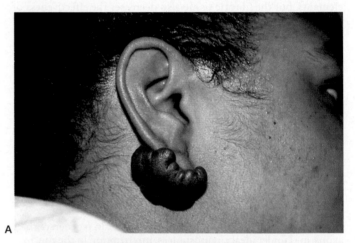

A

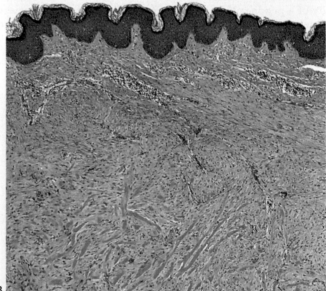

B

FIGURE 3-12. **Keloid. A.** A light-skinned black woman developed a keloid as a reaction to having her earlobe pierced. **B.** Microscopically, the dermis is markedly thickened by the presence of collagen bundles with random orientation and abundant cells.

devoid of sensation because of persistent trauma. Such **trophic** or **neuropathic** ulcers are commonly seen in diabetic peripheral neuropathy.

Excessive Scar Formation

Inordinate deposition of extracellular matrix, mostly excessive collagen, at the wound site results in a hypertrophic scar. **A keloid** is an exuberant hypertrophic scar that tends to progress beyond the site of initial injury and recurs after excision (Fig. 3-12). Histologically, both of these types of scars exhibit broad and irregular collagen bundles, with more capillaries and fibroblasts than expected for a scar of the same age. More clearly defined in keloids than in hypertrophic scars, the rate of collagen synthesis, the ratio of type III to type I collagen, and the number of reducible cross-links, remain high. This situation indicates a "maturation arrest," or block, in the process of wound maturation. Keloids are unsightly, and attempts at surgical repair are always problematic—the outcome likely being a still-larger keloid. Dark-skinned individuals are more frequently affected by keloids than light-skinned ones, and the tendency is sometimes hereditary. By contrast, the occurrence of **hypertrophic scars** is not associated with skin color or heredity.

Excessive Contraction

A decrease in the size of a wound depends on the presence of myofibroblasts, development of cell–cell contacts, and sustained cell contraction. An exaggeration of these processes is termed **contrac-**

4 Immunopathology

Jeffrey S. Warren
Douglas P. Bartlett
Roger J. Pomerantz

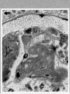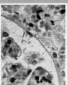

*The immune system protects the host from invasion by foreign and potentially harmful agents. As components of host defense, immune responses are characterized by their ability to (1) distinguish self from nonself, (2) discriminate among potential invaders (specificity), (3) maintain the presence of immune memory (anamnesis), and (4) recall previous exposures and mount an amplified response to them. Immune responses can be elicited by a wide range of agents (termed **antigens**) including parasites, bacteria, viruses, chemicals, toxins, drugs, and transplanted tissues. Immune responses that show antigen specificity and immune memory are termed **adaptive immunity**. **Innate immunity** (discussed in part in Chapter 2) does not demonstrate immune memory and lacks the exacting specificity of adaptive immunity (although patterns and classes of harmful agents such as* bacterial cell wall components are recognized). The host defense systems that constitute the acute inflammatory response, including cell surface-associated and soluble mediator systems (e.g., complement and coagulation systems) and phagocytes (most important being tissue resident macrophages), are integral to innate immunity.

The adaptive immune response is critical to host survival, and failure is associated with overwhelming infectious disease. One need only consider the ravages of AIDS. Adaptive immune responses can be appropriate in terms of defense, but nevertheless may lead to host injury (such as the immune rejection of a transplanted organ). The diseases associated with either the lack of appropriate adaptive immunity or injury produced by inappropriate or excessive adaptive immunity constitute the study of immunopathology.

Biology of the Immune System

The Cells that Comprise the Immune System Derive from Hematopoietic Stem Cells

The antigen-specific or "adaptive" immune system encompasses lymphocytes, plasma cells, antigen-presenting cells (APCs), spe-cific effector molecules (e.g., immunoglobulins), and a vast array of regulatory mediators.

The cellular components of the immune system are derived from pluripotent hematopoietic stem cells (Fig. 4-1). By 8 weeks of gestation, lymphoid stem cells derived from hematopoietic stem cells and fated to become T cells circulate to the thymus, where they differentiate into mature T lymphocytes. Lymphoid stem cells destined to become B cells differentiate first within fetal liver

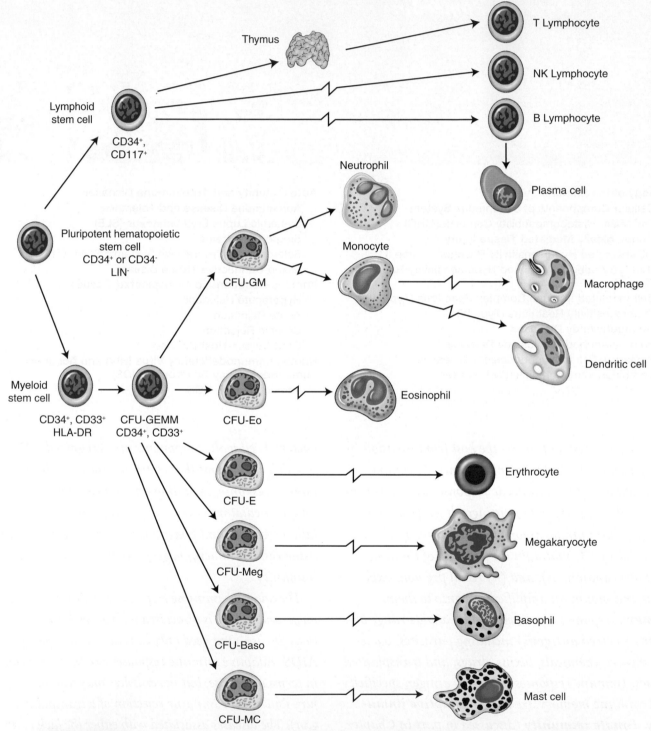

FIGURE 4-1. Pluripotent hematopoietic stem cells differentiate into either lymphoid or myeloid stem cells and, in the case of myeloid stem cells, into lineage-specific colony-forming units (CFUs). Under the influence of an appropriate microenvironment, CFUs give rise to definitive cell types. Lymphoid stem cells are precursors of natural killer (NK) cells, T lymphocytes, and B lymphocytes. B lymphocytes give rise to plasma cells. CD, cluster designation; CFU-GEMM, granu-locytic, erythroid, monocytic–dendritic, and megakaryocytic colony-forming units; HLA, human leukocyte antigen.

(8 weeks) and later within bone marrow (12 weeks). The primary branch point in differentiation is between lymphoid progenitors and myeloid progenitors. The former ultimately give rise to T lymphocytes, B lymphocytes, and natural killer (NK) cells, whereas the latter develop into granulocytic, erythroid, monocytic–dendritic, and megakaryocytic cells. The definition of developing and mature cells of the immune and hematopoietic systems depends in large part on cell surface markers, which are designated by cluster designation (CD) numbers.

Lymphocytes

There are three major types of lymphocytes—T cells, B cells, and NK cells—which account for 25% of peripheral blood leukocytes. Some 80% of blood lymphocytes are T cells, 10% B cells, and 10% are NK cells. The relative proportions of lymphocytes in the peripheral blood and central and peripheral lymphoid tissues vary. In contrast to the blood, only 30% to 40% of splenic and bone marrow lymphocytes are T cells.

T lymphocytes can be subdivided into subpopulations by virtue of their specialized functions, by surface CD molecules, and in some cases, by morphologic features. Lymphoid progenitor cells destined to become T cells exit the bone marrow and migrate to the thymus, where they undergo a complex multistep maturation process that accomplishes three goals:

1. Recombination of dispersed gene segments that encode the antigen-binding regions of the heterodimeric α/β or γ/δ T-cell receptor (TCR)
2. Formation of functionally distinct helper (CD4$^+$) and cytotoxic/suppressor (CD8$^+$) T-cell populations
3. Positive, followed by negative, thymic selection to produce a T-cell population that recognizes self-peptides plus major histocompatibility antigens, but **not** with sufficient avidity to result in autoimmunity

During this process, the developing T lymphocytes transit from the subcapsular zone of the thymus (containing the least mature T cells) to the medullary region, from which the mature naive T cells are released into the peripheral circulation. During this process, immature T cells interact with thymic epithelial cells (in the cortex) and dendritic cells (in the medulla) and undergo the following maturational events.

- Subcapsular zone of thymus: T cells are CD4$^-$, CD8$^-$ (double negative). TCR gene arrangements commence.
- Cortical zone of thymus: T cells are CD4$^+$, CD8$^+$ (double positive). **Positive selection** of cells interacting with self-major histocompatibility (MHC) molecules and self-peptides that are displayed by cortical epithelial cells
- Cortical zone of thymus: T cells are CD4$^+$ **or** CD8$^+$ (single positive), depending on preferential binding to MHC class II or MHC class I molecules, respectively.
- Medullary zone of thymus: T cells that react strongly with MHC and self-peptide displayed by medullary dendritic cells are **negatively selected** and undergo apoptosis to eliminate self-reactivity.
- Mature single-positive naive T cells enter the circulation.

T lymphocytes exit the thymus and populate peripheral lymphoid tissues. In the thymus, antigen-specific TCRs are formed and are expressed in conjunction with CD3, an essential accessory molecule. Nearly 95% of circulating T lymphocytes express α/β TCRs. In turn, circulating α/β T cells also express either CD4 or CD8. A smaller population (5%) of T cells expresses γ/δ TCRs and CD3, but neither CD4 nor CD8.

T lymphocytes recognize specific antigens, usually proteins or haptens bound to proteins. CD4$^+$ and CD8$^+$ T-cell subsets possess a variety of effector and regulatory functions. Effector functions include secretion of proinflammatory cytokines and killing of cells that express foreign or altered membrane antigens. Regulatory functions comprise augmenting and suppressing immune responses, usually by secreting specific helper or suppressor cytokines.

In general, CD4$^+$ T cells promote antibody and inflammatory responses. Such cells recognize antigen in the context of self-MHC class II molecules on APCs. CD4$^+$ T cells can be further distinguished by the types of cytokines produced. Helper type 1, or Th1, cells produce interferon (IFN)-γ and interleukin (IL)-2, whereas helper type 2, or Th2, cells secrete IL-4, IL-5, and IL-10. Th1 lymphocytes have been associated with cell-mediated phenomena and Th2 cells with B-cell activation and allergic responses. By contrast, CD8$^+$ cells, for the most part, exert suppressor and cytotoxic functions. CD8$^+$ cells recognize antigen in the context of self-MHC class I molecules present on many cells. Suppressor cells inhibit the activation phase of immune responses; cytotoxic cells can kill target cells that express specific antigens (see Fig. 4-2).

Foreign class I and class II molecules, which are not histocompatible with the host (e.g., transplanted histocompatibility antigens), are themselves potent immunogens and can be recognized by host T cells. This is why human tissue transplantation requires that donor and recipient be HLA-matched. In addition to the binding of foreign peptides presented by MHC molecules to the TCR complex, a number of other receptor–ligand interactions must occur to maximally activate lymphocytes. See Figure 4-2, which summarizes some of the key interactions that occur between CD4$^+$ T-helper cells and APCs.

B lymphocytes pass through a series of carefully regulated developmental pathways in a manner analogous to those of T cells. Initially, pro-B cells are produced in the fetal liver and continue to differentiate in the bone marrow after birth. The microenvironment of the bone marrow is critical to B-lymphocyte development; Pro-B cells traverse radially from the marrow nearest to the bone toward the central sinus of the marrow as they mature. They are released to the periphery as immature B cells. Only B lymphocytes that pass through the many ordered stages of DNA recombination necessary to produce surface immunoglobulins survive and exit to the periphery. Immature B cells upregulate the expression of surface immunoglobulins (the B-cell receptor) and undergo a process of negative selection by self-antigens they encounter, resulting in mature B cells. Developing B cells in which surface immunoglobulin binds too avidly to self-antigens are negatively selected and eliminated. B cells express a surface antigen-binding receptor, the membrane-bound immunoglobulin B-cell receptor, which bears the same antigen-binding specificity as the soluble immunoglobulin that will ultimately be secreted by the corresponding terminally differentiated B cell, termed a **plasma cell.**

Mature B lymphocytes exist primarily in a resting state, awaiting activation by foreign antigens. Activation requires (1) cross-linking of membrane immunoglobulin receptors by antigens presented by accessory cells or (2) interactions with membrane molecules of helper T cells via a mechanism called **cognate T-cell—B-cell help** (see Fig. 4-2). The initial stimulus leads to B-cell proliferation and clonal expansion, a process amplified by cytokines from both accessory cells and T cells. If no additional signal is provided, proliferating B cells return to a resting state and enter the memory cell pool. These events occur largely in lymphoid tissues and can be seen as germinal centers. Within germinal centers, B cells also undergo further somatic gene rearrangements, leading to generation of cells that produce the various immunoglobulin isotypes and subclasses.

An **isotype** is the class of the defining heavy chain of an immunoglobulin molecule. In turn, each immunoglobulin subtype exhibits a different array of biological activities. In the presence of antigen, T cells produce helper cytokines that stimulate isotype switching or induce proliferation of previously committed isotype populations. For example, IL-4 induces switching to the IgE isotype. The final stage of B-cell differentiation into antibody-synthesizing

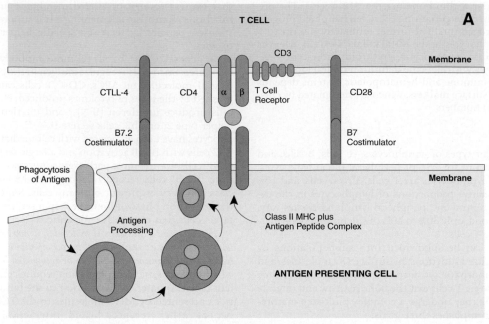

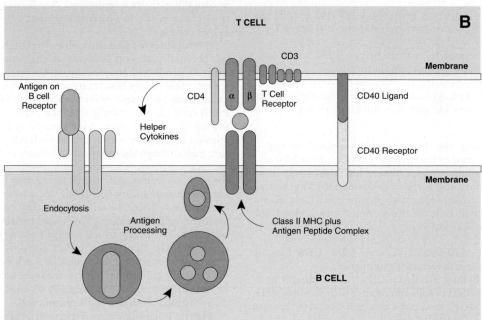

FIGURE 4-2. **A. T-lymphocyte activation (by the T-cell receptor [TCR]) occurs via peptides cleaved from the phago-cytized antigen** (antigen processing) and presented to the TCR in the context of a histocompatible class II major histocompatibility complex (MHC) molecule. T-cell activation also requires accessory or costimulatory signals from cytotoxic lymphoid line (CTLL)-4 or CD28. **B. A similar process applies to B-cell–T-cell interactions.** The B-lymphocyte antigen recep-tor is membrane immunoglobulin.

plasma cells requires exposure to additional products of T lym-phocytes (e.g., IL-5, IL-6), especially in the case of protein anti-gens. The predominant type of immunoglobulin produced dur-ing an immune response changes with age. Newborns tend to produce predominantly IgM. By contrast, older children and adults initially produce IgM following an antigenic challenge, but rapidly shift toward IgG synthesis.

NK cells, which are believed to form in both the thymus and bone marrow, recognize target cells via an antigen-independent mechanism. NK cells do not express either a functional TCR or sur-face immunoglobulin. They bear several types of class I MHC mol-ecule receptors, which when engaged, **inhibit** the NK cell's capacity

to secrete cytolytic products. Certain tumor cells and virus-infected cells bear reduced numbers of MHC class I molecules and thus do not inhibit NK cells. NK cells that engage virus-infected or tumor cells secrete complement-like cytolytic proteins (perforin), granzymes A and B, and other lytic factors. NK cells also secrete granulysin, a cationic protein that induces target cell apoptosis.

Mononuclear Phagocytes, Antigen-Presenting Cells, and Dendritic Cells

Mononuclear phagocyte is a general term applied to phagocytic cell populations in virtually all organs and connective tissues. Among these cells are macrophages, monocytes, Kupffer cells of the liver, and lung alveolar macrophages. Precursor cells (monoblasts and promonocytes) arise in the bone marrow, enter the circulation as monocytes, and then migrate into tissues, where they take up residence as tissue macrophages. In the lung, liver, and spleen, numerous macrophages populate sinuses and pericapillary zones to form an effective filtering system, which removes effete cells and foreign particulate material from blood.

Macrophages are important accessory cells by virtue of their expression of class II histocompatibility antigens. They ingest and process antigens for presentation to T cells in conjunction with class II MHC molecules. The subsequent T-cell responses are further amplified by macrophage-derived cytokines. One of the best-characterized cytokines is IL-1, which promotes expression of the IL-2 receptor on T cells, augmenting T-cell proliferation that is driven by IL-2. Among many effects of IL-1 on other tissues is preparation of the body to combat infection. For example, IL-1 induces fever and promotes catabolic metabolism (see Chapter 2).

The functional activities of macrophages and the spectrum of molecules that they produce are regulated by external factors, such as T-cell–derived cytokines. Macrophages exposed to such factors become "activated," after which they produce a variety of reactive oxygen metabolites, cytokines, and soluble mediators of host defense (e.g., IFN-γ, IL-1β, tumor necrosis factor-α, and complement components), and are a critical part of innate, as well as adaptive, immunity.

Antigen-presenting cells (APCs) acquire the capacity to present antigen to T-helper lymphocytes in the context of histocompatibility, after cytokine-driven upregulation of MHC class II molecules (Fig. 4-2). Monocytes, macrophages, dendritic cells and, under certain conditions, B lymphocytes, endothelial cells and epithelial cells, can act as APCs. In some locations, APCs are highly specialized for this function. For instance, in B-cell-rich follicles of lymph nodes and spleen, antigen presentation by follicular dendritic cells leads to generation of memory B lymphocytes, which are important in anamnesis (immune memory) (Fig. 4-3).

Dendritic cells are specialized APCs that are termed "dendritic" by virtue of their spider-like morphologic appearance. They are found in B-lymphocyte-rich lymphoid follicles, in thymic medulla, and in many peripheral sites, including intestinal lamina propria, lung, genitourinary tract, and skin. An example of a peripheral APC is the **epidermal Langerhans cell**. Upon exposure, the Langerhans cell engulfs antigen, migrates to a regional lymph node through an afferent lymphatic, and differentiates into a more mature dendritic cell. Langerhans cell-derived dendritic cells express high densities of MHC class I and II molecules and present antigen efficiently to T lymphocytes (see Fig. 4-3).

The MHC Coordinates Interactions Among Immune Cells

The MHC, in humans termed the HLA complex, orchestrates many of the cell–cell interactions fundamental to the immune response. These antigens are major immunogens and were first recognized as targets in transplant rejection. The MHC includes class I, II, and III antigens. (Class III antigens represent certain complement components and are not histocompatibility antigens *per se*; Fig. 4-4).

Class I MHC molecules are encoded by highly polymorphic genes in the A, B, and C regions of the MHC (see Fig. 4-4). These loci encode similarly structured molecules that are expressed in virtually all tissues. Because the alleles are expressed codominantly, tissues bear class I antigens inherited from each parent. These antigens are recognized by cytotoxic T cells during graft rejection or T-lymphocyte-mediated killing of virus-infected cells.

Class II MHC molecules are encoded by multiple loci in the D region. The D region loci encode structurally similar molecules that are expressed primarily on antigen-presenting cells, including monocytes, macrophages, dendritic cells, and B lymphocytes. Class II antigens have also been referred to as "Ia" (immunity-associated) antigens. As with class I antigens, D region alleles are expressed codominantly, and tissues bear antigens from each parent.

Immunologically Mediated Tissue Injury

Immune responses not only protect against invasion by foreign organisms but may also themselves cause tissue damage. Thus, many inflammatory diseases are examples of "friendly fire" in which the immune system attacks the body's own tissues. An immune response that leads to tissue injury or disease is broadly called a **hypersensitivity** reaction. Immune, or hypersensitivity-mediated, diseases are common and include such entities as hives (urticaria), asthma, hay fever, hepatitis, glomerulonephritis, and arthritis.

Hypersensitivity reactions are classified according to the type of immune mechanism (Table 4-1). Type I, II, and III hypersensitivity reactions all require formation of a specific antibody against an exogenous (foreign) or an endogenous (self) antigen. The antibody class is a critical determinant of the mechanism by which tissue injury occurs.

In most **type I**, or **immediate-type hypersensitivity reactions**, IgE antibody is formed and binds to high-affinity receptors on mast cells and/or basophils via its Fc domain. Subsequent binding of antigen and cross-linking of IgE trigger rapid (immediate) release of products from these cells, leading to the characteristic symptoms of such diseases as urticaria, asthma, and anaphylaxis.

In type II hypersensitivity reactions, IgG or IgM antibody is formed against an antigen, usually a protein on a cell surface. Less commonly, the antigen is an intrinsic structural component of the extracellular matrix (e.g., part of the basement membrane). Such antigen–antibody binding activates complement, which in turn lyses the cell (cytotoxicity) or damages the extracellular matrix. In some type II reactions, other antibody-mediated effects are operative.

In type III hypersensitivity reactions, the antibody responsible for tissue injury is also usually IgM or IgG, but the mechanism of tissue injury differs. The antigen circulates in the vascular compartment until it is bound by antibody. The resulting immune complex is deposited in tissues. Complement activation at sites of antigen–antibody deposition leads to leukocyte recruitment, which is responsible for the subsequent tissue injury. In some type III reactions, antigen is bound by antibody in situ.

Type IV reactions, also known as **cell-mediated**, or **delayed-type hypersensitivity reactions**, do not involve antibodies. Rather, antigen activation of T lymphocytes, usually with the help of macrophages, causes release of products by these cells, thereby leading to tissue injury.

Many immunologic diseases are mediated by more than one type of hypersensitivity reaction. Thus, in hypersensitivity pneumonitis, lung injury results from hypersensitivity to inhaled fungal antigens. Types I, III, and IV hypersensitivity reactions all appear to be operative in this disease.

Type I or Immediate Hypersensitivity Reactions are Triggered by IgE Bound to Mast Cells

Immediate-type hypersensitivity is manifested by a localized or generalized reaction that occurs within minutes of exposure to an antigen or "allergen" to which the person has previously been sensitized. The clinical manifes-

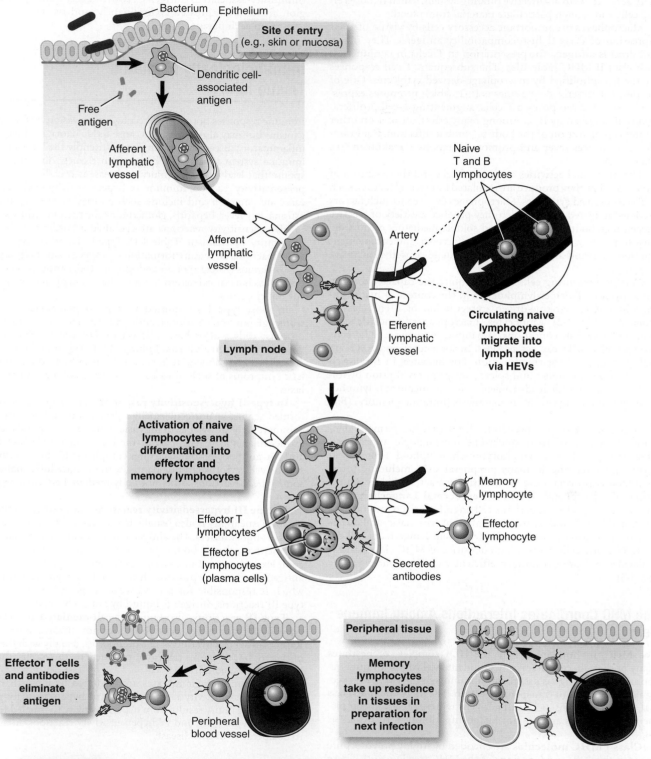

In an integrated immune response, antigen is processed and presented by a dendritic cell, which migrates via the afferent lymphatics to a regional lymph node. Within the regional lymph node, antigen is presented to lymphocytes, which in turn are activated and may migrate (via homing mechanism) to specific peripheral sites. HEVs, high endothelial venules.

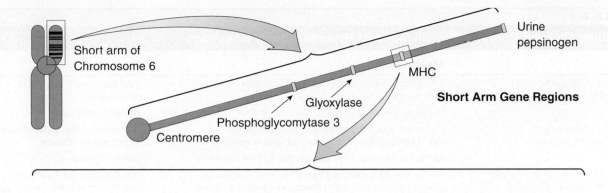

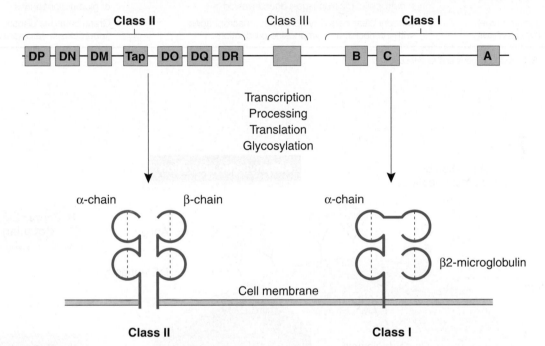

FIGURE 4-4. **The highly polymorphic loci that encode major histocompatibility antigens are located on the short arm of chromosome 6.** Class I and class II molecules exhibit different structures, but each participates in fundamentally important T-cell—cell interactions.

tations of a reaction depend on the site of antigen exposure and extent of sensitization. For example, when a reaction involves the skin, the characteristic local reaction is a "wheal and flare," or **urticaria (hives)**. When the localized manifestations of immediate hypersensitivity involve the upper respiratory tract and conjunctiva, causing sneezing and conjunctivitis, we speak of **hay fever** (allergic rhinitis). In its generalized and most severe form, immediate hypersensitivity reactions are associated with bronchoconstriction, airway obstruction, and circulatory collapse, as seen in **anaphylactic shock**. There is a high degree of variability in susceptibility to type I hypersensitivity reactions, which is genetically determined.

Type I hypersensitivity reactions usually feature IgE antibodies, which are formed by a CD4+, Th2, T-cell–dependent mechanism and which bind avidly to Fcε receptors on mast cells and basophils. The high avidity of binding of IgE accounts for the term **cytophilic** antibody. Once exposed to a specific allergen that elicits IgE, a person is sensitized, and subsequent exposures to that allergen induce immediate hypersensitivity reactions. After IgE is elicited, repeat exposure to antigens typically induces additional IgE antibodies, rather than antibodies of other classes, such as IgM or IgG.

IgE can persist for years bound to Fcε receptors on mast cells and basophils, a feature unique to these cells. Upon subsequent re-exposure, the soluble antigen or allergen binds the IgE coupled to its surface Fcε receptor and activates the mast cell or basophil. This event releases the potent inflammatory mediators that are responsible for the manifestations of this type I hypersensitivity reaction. As shown in Figure 4-5, the antigen (allergen) binds to the IgE antibody through its Fab sites. Cross-linking of the antigen to more than one IgE antibody molecule is required to activate the cell. Figure 4-5 shows that the complement-derived anaphylatoxic peptides, C3a and C5a, can directly stimulate mast cells by a different receptor-mediated process. These cell-activating events trigger the release of stored granule constituents and rapid synthesis as well as release of other mediators.

A number of potent mediators are preformed and released from granules within minutes, after which they exert immediate biological effects (see Fig. 4-5).

• Histamine induces (1) constriction of vascular and nonvascular smooth muscle, (2) microvascular dilation, and (3) an increase in venule permeability, mediated largely through H_1 receptors.

TABLE 4–1

Modified Cell and Coombs Classification of Hypersensitivity Reactions

Type	Mechanism	Examples
Type I (anaphylactic type): Immediate hypersensitivity	IgE antibody-mediated mast cell activation and degranulation	Hay fever, asthma, hives, anaphylaxis
	Non–Ige-mediated	Physical urticarias
Type II (cytotoxic type): Cytotoxic antibodies	Cytotoxic (IgG, IgM) antibodies formed against cell-surface antigens; complement usually involved	Autoimmune hemolytic anemias, Goodpasture disease
	Noncytotoxic antibodies against cell surface receptors	Graves disease
Type III (immune complex type): Immune complex disease	Antibodies (IgG, IgM, IgA) formed against exogenous or endogenous antigens; complement and leukocytes (neutrophils, macrophages) often involved	Autoimmune diseases (SLE, rheumatoid arthritis), many types of glomerulonephritis
Type IV (cell-mediated type): Delayed-type hypersensitivity	Mononuclear cells (T lymphocytes, macrophages) with interleukin and lymphokine production	Granulomatous disease (tuberculosis, sarcoidosis)

Ig, immunoglobulin; SLE, systemic lupus erythematosus.

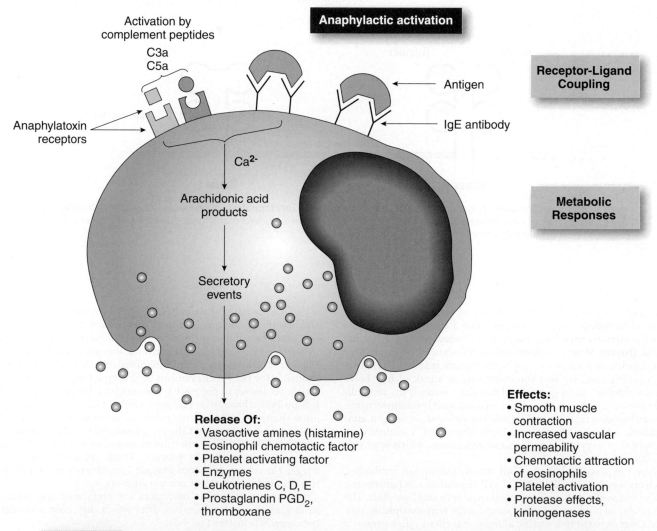

FIGURE 4-5. In a type I hypersensitivity reaction, allergen binds to cytophilic surface IgE antibody on a mast cell or basophil and triggers cell activation and the release of a cascade of proinflammatory mediators. These mediators are responsible for smooth muscle contraction, edema formation, and the recruitment of eosinophils. Ca^{2+}, calcium ion; Ig, immunoglobulin; PGD_2, prostaglandin D_2.

The biologic effects include urticaria in the skin and bron-chospasm, vascular congestion, and edema in the lung.
• Chemotactic factors for neutrophils and eosinophils (the later is the hallmark cell of immediate hypersensitivity)

Activation of macrophages also results in the synthesis of many other potent inflammatory mediators that are important in the late phase response of immediate hypersensitivity reactions.

• Cytokines that are responsible in part for the development of a mixed inflammatory infiltrate
• Products of arachidonic acid metabolism, including prostaglandins and leukotrienes (C_4, D_4, and E_4), the "slow-reacting substances of anaphylaxis," which are responsible for the delayed bronchoconstriction phase of anaphylaxis, and leukotriene B_4, a potent chemotactic factor for neutrophils, macrophages, and eosinophils
• **Platelet-activating factor (PAF)**, a powerful inducer of platelet activation, neutrophil chemotaxis, and activation of many phagocytic cells

Activated T cells, specifically the Th2 type, produce cytokines that have important roles in allergic responses. Activated Th2 T-cell subsets produce IL-4, IL-5, and IL-13, leading to IgE production and increased numbers of mast cells and eosinophils. Allergy-prone persons have reduced levels of IFN-γ, which suppresses development of Th2 clones and subsequent production of IgE. The factors responsible for human susceptibility to immediate hypersensitive reactions (allergy) are complex and involve the interaction of environment and multiple genetic loci.

Type II Hypersensitivity Reactions are Mediated by Antibodies Against Fixed Cellular or Extracellular Antigens

IgG and IgM typically mediate type II reactions. An important characteristic of these antibodies is their ability to activate complement through the immunoglobulin Fc domain. This occurs when IgM or IgG antibody binds an antigen on the surface of the erythrocyte membrane. At sufficient density, bound immunoglobulin leads to complement fixation via C1q and the classic pathway (see Chapter 2). Once activated, complement can destroy target cells by several methods.

• Insertion of the membrane attack complex into the red cell plasma membrane, thereby inducing lysis.
• Opsonization, the coating of target cells with immunoglobulin or C3b and subsequent phagocytosis by cells having receptors for these molecules (including neutrophils and macrophages) (Fig. 4-6).

Such complement-dependent mechanisms are responsible for transfusion reactions related to major blood group incompatibilities and some autoimmune hemolytic anemias.

There is another type of antibody-mediated cytotoxicity that does not require complement. Antibody-dependent cell-mediated cytotoxicity (**ADCC**) involves cytolytic leukocytes that attack antibody-coated target cells after binding via Fc receptors. Phagocytic cells and NK cells can function as effector cells in ADCC. The mechanisms by which target cells are destroyed in these reactions are not entirely understood. ADCC may also be involved in the pathogenesis of some autoimmune diseases (e.g., autoimmune thyroiditis).

In some type II reactions, antibody binding to a specific target cell receptor does not lead to cell death but rather to a change in function. Autoimmune diseases such as Graves disease and myasthenia gravis feature autoantibodies against cell-surface hormone receptors. In Graves disease, autoantibody directed against the thyroid-stimulating hormone (TSH) receptor on thyrocytes mimics the effect of TSH, stimulating thyroxine production and leading to hyperthyroidism (see Chapter 21). By contrast, in myasthenia gravis, autoantibodies to acetylcholine receptors in neuromuscular endplates either block acetylcholine binding or mediate internalization or destruction of receptors, thereby inhibiting efficient synaptic transmission (see Chapter 27). Patients with myasthenia gravis thus suffer from muscle weakness. Modulatory autoantibodies against receptors for insulin, prolactin, growth hormone, and other messengers are reported.

Some type II hypersensitivity reactions result from antibody directed against a structural connective tissue component. A classic example is Goodpasture syndrome, in which antibodies bind the noncollagenous domain of type IV collagen, which is a major structural component of pulmonary and glomerular basement membranes. Local complement activation recruits neutrophils to the site, resulting in tissue injury, pulmonary hemorrhage, and glomerulonephritis. Direct complement-mediated damage to the basement membranes of the glomeruli and the lung alveoli through formation of membrane attack complexes may also be involved.

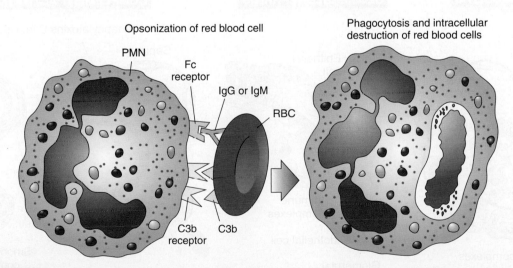

FIGURE 4-6. In a type II hypersensitivity reaction, opsonization by antibody or complement leads to phagocytosis via either Fc or C3b receptors, respectively. Ig, immunoglobulin; PMN, polymorphonuclear neutrophil; RBC, red blood cell.

In Type III Hypersensitivity Reactions, Immune Complex Deposition or Formation In Situ Leads to Complement Fixation and Inflammation

IgG, IgM, and occasionally IgA antibody against either a circulating antigen or an antigen that is deposited or "planted" in a tissue can cause a type III response. Physicochemical characteristics of the immune complexes, such as size, charge, and solubility, in addition to immunoglobulin isotype, determine whether an immune complex can deposit in tissue or fix complement. Immune complexes elicit inflammatory responses by activating complement, leading to chemotactic recruitment of neutrophils and monocytes to the site. Activated phagocytes release tissue-damaging mediators, such as proteases and reactive oxygen intermediates.

Immune complexes have been implicated in many human diseases (Fig. 4-7). The most compelling cases are those in which the demonstration of immune complexes in injured tissue correlates with the development of injury, because in some diseases immune complexes can be detected in plasma without concomitant evidence of tissue injury. Diseases that seem to be most clearly attributable to immune complex deposition are collagen-vascular autoimmune diseases, such as systemic lupus erythematosus (SLE)

and rheumatoid arthritis, some types of vasculitis, and many varieties of glomerulonephritis.

Once immune complexes are deposited in tissues, they may trigger an inflammatory response. Local activation of complement by immune complexes results in the formation of C5a, which is a potent neutrophil chemoattractant. Inflammation proceeds much as described for nonimmune-mediated acute inflammation (see Chapter 2). Once neutrophils arrive, they are activated through contact with, and ingestion of, immune complexes. Activated leukocytes release many inflammatory mediators, including proteases, reactive oxygen intermediates, and arachidonic acid products, which collectively produce tissue injury.

Type IV, or Cell-Mediated, Hypersensitivity Reactions are Cellular Immune Responses that Do Not Involve Antibodies

Included among these reactions are delayed-type cellular inflammatory responses and cell-mediated cytotoxic effects. Type IV reactions often occur together with antibody-dependent reactions, which can make it difficult to distinguish these processes. Both clinical obser-

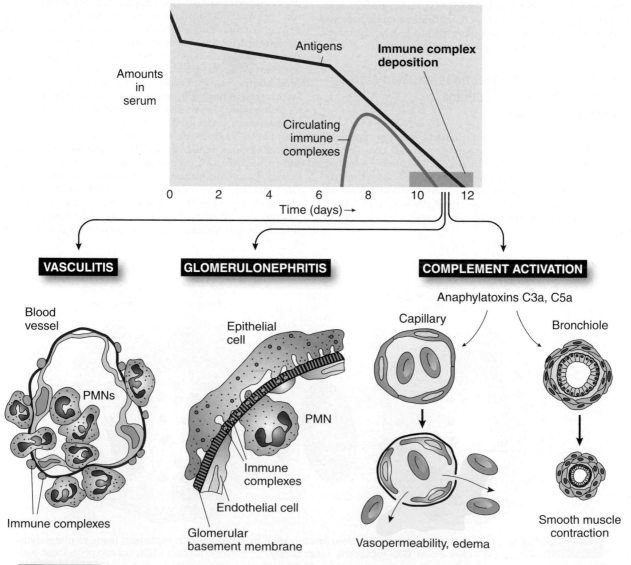

FIGURE 4-7. In type III hypersensitivity, immune complexes are deposited and can lead to complement activation and the recruitment of tissue-damaging inflammatory cells. The ability of immune complexes to mediate tissue injury depends on size, solubility, net charge, and ability to fix complement. PMN, polymorphonuclear neutrophil.

vations and experimental studies suggest that the type of tissue response is largely determined by the nature of the inciting agent.

Classically, delayed-type hypersensitivity is a tissue reaction, primarily involving lymphocytes and mononuclear phagocytes, which occurs in response to a soluble protein antigen and reaches greatest intensity 24 to 48 hours after initiation. A classic example of a type IV reaction is the contact sensitivity response to poison ivy. Although chemical ligands in poison ivy are not proteins, they bind covalently to cell proteins, after which the compound molecules are recognized by antigen-specific lymphocytes.

Figure 4-8 summarizes the stages of a delayed-type hypersensitivity reaction. In the initial phase, foreign protein antigens or chemical ligands interact with accessory cells that express class II human leukocyte antigen (HLA) molecules (Fig. 4-8A). Such accessory cells (macrophages, dendritic cells) secrete IL-12, which along with processed and presented antigen, activates CD4$^+$ T cells. In turn, activated CD4$^+$ T cells secrete IFN-γ and IL-2, which activate more macrophages and trigger T-lymphocyte proliferation, respectively (Fig. 4-8B). The protein antigens are actively processed into short peptides within phagolysosomes of macrophages and then presented on the cell surface in conjunction with class II MHC molecules. Processed and presented antigens are recognized by MHC-restricted, antigen-specific CD4$^+$ T cells, which become activated and synthesize an array of cytokines (Fig. 4-8C). Such activated CD4 cells are referred to as T$_H$1 cells. In turn, the cytokines recruit and activate lymphocytes, monocytes, fibroblasts, and other inflammatory cells. If the antigenic stimulus is eliminated, the reaction spontaneously resolves after about 48 hours. If the stimulus persists (e.g., poorly biodegradable mycobacterial cell wall components), an attempt to sequester the inciting agent may result in a granulomatous reaction.

Other mechanisms by which T cells (especially CD8$^+$) mediate tissue damage is direct cytolysis of target cells (Fig. 4-9). These immune mechanisms are important in destroying and eliminating cells infected by viruses and possibly tumor cells that express neoantigens. Cytotoxic T cells also play an important role in transplant graft rejection. Figure 4-9 summarizes the events in T-cell-mediated cytotoxicity. In contrast to delayed-type hypersensitivity reactions, cytotoxic CD8$^+$ T cells specifically recognize target antigens in the context of class I MHC molecules. In the case of virus-infected cells and tumor cells, foreign antigens are actively presented together with self-MHC antigens (Fig. 4-9A,B). In graft rejection, foreign MHC antigens are themselves potent activators of CD8$^+$ T cells. Once activated by antigen, proliferation of cytotoxic cells is promoted by helper cells and mediated by soluble growth factors, such as IL-2 (Fig. 4-9C). An expanded population of antigen-specific cytotoxic cells is thus generated. Actual cell killing involves several mechanisms (Fig. 4-9D). Cytolytic T cells (CTLs) secrete perforins that form pores in target cell membranes, through which they introduce granzymes that activate intracellular caspases, leading to apoptosis. CTLs can also kill targets via engagement of the Fas ligand (by the CTL) and Fas (on the target cell). The Fas ligand-Fas interaction triggers apoptosis of the Fas-bearing cell (see Chapter 2). The chronic inflammation in many autoimmune diseases—including type 1 diabetes, chronic thyroiditis, Sjögren syndrome (SS), and primary biliary cirrhosis—is the result of type IV hypersensitivity.

Immunodeficiency Diseases

Immunodeficiency diseases are classified according to two characteristics: (1) whether the defect is congenital (primary) or acquired (secondary) and (2) whether the specific host defense system is defective. The great majority of primary immunodeficiency disorders are genetically determined and uncommon. Disorders of the complement system and primary defects of phagocytes are discussed elsewhere (see Chapters 2 and 20). In contrast to the low prevalence of congenital immunodeficiency disorders, acquired immune deficiencies, like that caused by HIV-1 infection (AIDS), are common.

Functional defects in lymphocytes can be localized to particular maturational stages in the ontogeny of the immune system or

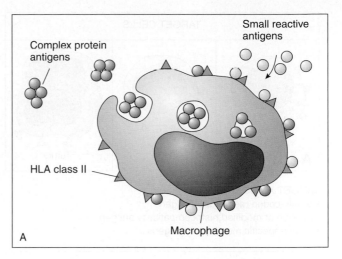

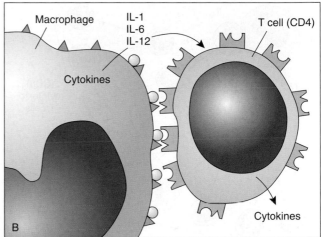

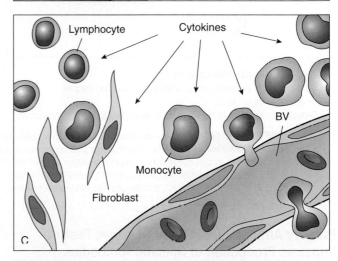

FIGURE 4-8. In a type IV (delayed type) hypersensitivity reaction, complex antigens are phagocytized, processed, and presented on macrophage cell membranes in conjunction with class II major histocompatibility complex (MHC) antigens. Antigen-specific, histocompatible, cytotoxic T lymphocytes bind the presented antigens and are activated. Activated cytotoxic T cells secrete cytokines that amplify the response. BV, blood vessel.

to interruption of discrete immune activation events. The explosive growth of knowledge regarding molecular mechanisms of immunodeficiency disorders has led to improved diagnosis, clinical management, and therapeutic strategies.

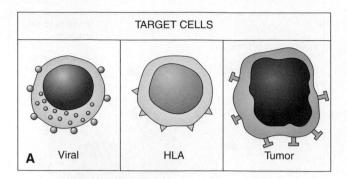

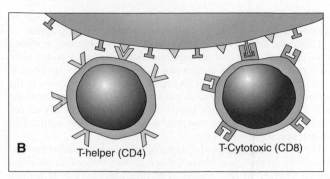

TARGET ANTIGENS
- Virally-coded membrane antigen
- Foreign or modified histocompatibility antigen
- Tumor-specific membrane antigens

RECOGNITION OF ANTIGEN BY T CELLS
- T-helper cells recognize antigen plus class II molecules
- T-cytotoxic/killer cells recognize antigen plus class I molecules

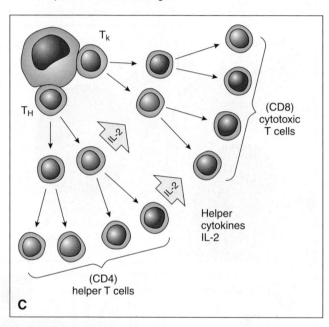

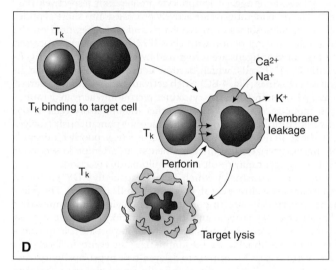

ACTIVATION AND AMPLIFICATION
- T-helper cells activate and proliferate, releasing helper molecules (e.g., IL-2)
- T-cytotoxic/killer cells proliferate in response to helper molecules

TARGET CELL KILLING
- T-cytotoxic/killer cells bind to target cell
- Killing signals perforin release and target cell loses membrane integrity
- Target cell undergoes lysis

FIGURE 4-9. In T-cell—mediated cytotoxicity, potential target cells include (A) virus-infected host cells, malignant host cells, and foreign (histoincompatible transplanted) cells. **B.** Cytotoxic T lymphocytes recognize foreign antigens in the context of human leukocyte antigen (HLA) class I molecules. **C.** Activated T cells secrete lytic compounds (e.g., perforin and other mediators) and cytokines that amplify the response, which is apoptosis (target cell killing). **D.** Ca^{2+}, calcium ion; IL, interleukin; K$^+$, potassium ion; Na$^+$, sodium ion.

Primary Antibody Deficiency Diseases Feature Impaired Production of Specific Antibodies

Bruton X-Linked Agammaglobulinemia
The congenital disorder, Bruton X-linked agammaglobulinemia, typically presents in male infants at 5 to 8 months old, the period during which maternal antibody levels have declined. The infant suffers from recurrent pyogenic infections and severe hypogammaglobulinemia involving all immunoglobulin isotypes. Occasional patients develop chronic enterovirus infections of the central nervous system (CNS). Immunization with live attenuated poliovirus can lead to paralytic poliomyelitis. Approximately one third of Bruton patients have a poorly understood form of arthritis, believed in some cases to be caused by *Mycoplasma*. There are no mature B cells in peripheral blood or plasma cells in lymphoid tissues. Pre-B cells, however, can be detected. The genetic defect, on the long arm of the X chromosome (Xq21.22), inactivates the gene that encodes a B-cell tyrosine kinase (Bruton tyrosine kinase), an enzyme critical to B-lymphocyte maturation.

Selective IgA Deficiency
Characterized by low serum and secretory concentrations of IgA, selective IgA deficiency is the most common primary immunodeficiency syndrome. Its incidence is 1:700 among Europeans, but is less frequently seen in Japan (1:18,000). Although patients are often asymptomatic, they occasionally present with respiratory or GI infections of varying severity. They display a strong predilection for allergies and collagen vascular diseases. They are also at high risk of anaphylactic reactions to IgA in transfused blood products. Patients with IgA deficiency have normal numbers of IgA-bearing B cells; their varied defects result in an inability to synthesize and secrete IgA.

Common Variable Immunodeficiency (CVID)

CVID is a heterogenous group of disorders characterized by pronounced hypogammaglobulinemia. A variety of defects in either B-lymphocyte maturation or T- lymphocyte-mediated B-lymphocyte maturation appear to be operative. Many relatives of patients with CVID have selective IgA deficiency. Affected patients present with recurrent severe pyogenic infections, especially pneumonia and diarrhea, the latter often due to infestation with *Giardia lamblia*. Recurrent attacks of herpes simplex are common; herpes zoster develops in one fifth of patients. The disease appears years to decades after birth, with a mean age at onset of 30 years. The incidence is estimated to be between 1:50,000 and 1:200,000. The inheritance pattern is variable, and the malady features a variety of maturational and regulatory defects of the immune system. A high incidence of malignant disease is seen in CVID, including a 50-fold increase in stomach cancer. Interestingly, lymphoma is 300 times more frequent in women with this immunodeficiency than in affected men. Malabsorption secondary to lymphoid hyperplasia and inflammatory bowel diseases is more frequent than in the general population. CVID patients are also susceptible to other autoimmune disorders, including hemolytic anemia, neutropenia, thrombocytopenia, and pernicious anemia.

Primary T-Cell Immunodeficiency Diseases Typically Result in Recurrent or Protracted Viral and Fungal Infections

DiGeorge Syndrome

In its complete form, DiGeorge syndrome is one of the most severe T-lymphocyte immunodeficiency disorders. Infants who survive the neonatal period are subject to recurrent or chronic viral, bacterial, fungal, and protozoal infections. The syndrome is caused by defective embryologic development of the third and fourth pharyngeal pouches, which give rise to the thymus and parathyroid glands and influence conotruncal cardiac development, all of which may be abnormal. Most patients have a point deletion in the long arm of chromosome 22. In the absence of a thymus, T-cell maturation is interrupted at the pre–T-cell stage. The disease has been corrected by transplanting thymic tissue. Most patients have partial DiGeorge syndrome, in which a small remnant of thymus is present. With time, these persons recover T-cell function without treatment.

Chronic Mucocutaneous Candidiasis

The yeast infection, chronic mucocutaneous candidiasis, is the result of a congenital defect in T-cell function. It is characterized by susceptibility to candidal infections and is associated with an endocrinopathy (hypoparathyroidism, Addison disease, diabetes mellitus). Although most T-cell functions are intact, there is an impaired response to *Candida* antigens, the precise cause of which is unknown, although it could occur at any of several points during T-cell development. Recent studies suggest that persons with this disorder react to *Candida* antigens differently than do healthy individuals. In particular, they mount a type 2 (IL-4/IL-6) helper T-cell response, which is ineffective in resisting the organism. By contrast, the normal response features type 1 (IL-2/IFN-γ) T cells, which effectively control candidal infections.

Combined Immunodeficiency Diseases Exhibit Reduced Immunoglobulins and Defects in T-Lymphocyte Function

Severe combined immunodeficiencies are conspicuously heterogenous and represent life-threatening disorders.

Severe Combined Immunodeficiency (SCID)

SCID is a group of disorders that ultimately affect both T and B lymphocytes. It is characterized by severe, recurrent, viral, bacterial, fungal, and protozoal infections. A virtually complete absence of T cells is associated with severe hypogammaglobulinemia. Many of these infants have a severely reduced mass of lymphoid tissue and an immature thymus that lacks lymphocytes. In some patients, lymphocytes fail to develop beyond pre-B cells and pre-T cells. Because patients with SCID have profound T- and B-lymphocyte dysfunction, they are susceptible to many pathogens, including cytomegalovirus (CMV), varicella, Pneumocystis, *Candida,* and many different bacteria.

SCID occurs in both X-linked and autosomal recessive forms and typically appears before 6 months of age. In some patients with the autosomal recessive form, B lymphocytes are present but do not function, possibly because of a lack of helper cell activity. In the X-linked form, the most common defect is due to a mutation of the common γ-chain of the IL-2 receptor, which is also used by receptors for other cytokines, namely IL-4, IL-7, IL-9, IL-11, and IL-15.

Adenosine Deaminase (ADA) Deficiency

ADA deficiency is an autosomal recessive form of combined immunodeficiency with mutations in the adenosine deaminase gene. The clinical manifestations range from mild to severe dysfunction of T cells and B cells and include characteristic developmental abnormalities of cartilage.

Wiskott-Aldrich Syndrome (WAS)

This rare syndrome is characterized by (1) recurrent infections, (2) hemorrhages secondary to thrombocytopenia, and (3) eczema. It typically manifests in boys within the first few months of life as petechiae and recurrent infections. WAS is caused by numerous distinct mutations in a gene on the X chromosome that encodes a protein called WASP (Wiskott-Aldrich syndrome protein), which is expressed at high levels in lymphocytes and megakaryocytes. Cellular and humoral immunity are both impaired in WAS. Boys with WAS have selective deficiencies in cell-mediated immunity. The numbers of CD4+ and CD8+ T cells are normal, but these children are largely lacking cutaneous delayed hypersensitivity. Virus-specific cytotoxic T-cell immunity is usually absent, although virus-specific antibody responses appear to be normal. Although levels of most immunoglobulins are normal or elevated, however, IgM is only about half of normal. Antibody responses to some antigens are normal, but responses to others may be absent. As many polysaccharide antigens, particularly some bacterial polysaccharides, elicit mainly IgM antibody responses, patients with WAS are susceptible to infection with encapsulated organisms, e.g. *Streptococcus pneumoniae, Haemophilus influenzae* and such opportunistic pathogens as *Pneumocystis jiroveci*. They are also prone to viral infections such as CMV, and may die of disseminated herpes simplex or varicella infections and a variety of autoimmune disorders. Thrombo-cytopenia may be severe (<30,000/μL), and the platelets are generally small. One third of these patients typically die of hemorrhage. Rarely, thrombocytopenia alone may be the sole manifestation of mutation in WAS.

Autoimmunity and Autoimmune Diseases

Autoimmune Disease Involves an Immune Response Against Self-Antigens

Autoimmunity implies that the immune system can no longer differentiate between self- and non–self-antigens effectively. It was classically interpreted as an abnormal immune response that invariably caused disease, but it is now clear that autoimmune responses are common and are necessary in order to regulate the immune system. When these regulatory mechanisms are in some way disrupted, uncontrolled production of autoantibodies or abnormal cell–cell recognition leads to tissue injury, and autoimmune disease results. To define an autoimmune etiology, one must demonstrate that the autoimmune reaction (whether cellular or humoral) is directly related to the disease process. Auto-immune diseases may be organ-specific or generalized.

At present, only a few diseases (e.g., Hashimoto thyroiditis, type 1 diabetes, SLE) fit this rigorous criterion.

Theories of Autoimmunity

An abnormal autoimmune response to self-antigens implies a loss of **immune tolerance,** a situation in which there is no measurable (or clinically consequential) immune response to specific (usually self) antigens. The reasons for loss of tolerance in autoimmune diseases are not well understood. There is extensive evidence that induction and maintenance of tolerance are active and ongoing immune activities, which can be produced through a variety of mechanisms. Thus, tolerance is an active state in which an immune response is blocked or prevented. Induction of tolerance to an antigen is partly related to the dose of antigen to which cells are exposed. Several theories have been suggested to explain the loss of tolerance in autoimmune disease.

Inaccessible Self-Antigens

The simplest hypothesis to explain the loss of tolerance in autoimmune disease states that an immune reaction develops to a self-antigen not normally "accessible" to the immune system. Intracellular antigens are not exposed or released until some type of tissue injury releases them. At that time, an immune response develops. Examples of this type of response are antibody formation against spermatozoa, lens tissue, and myelin after injury to target organs. Although autoantibodies may form against normally "sequestered" antigens, there is little evidence that they are pathogenic.

Abnormal T-Cell Function

Autoimmune reactions have been suggested to develop as a result of abnormalities in the T-lymphocyte system. Most immune responses require T-cell participation to activate antigen-specific B cells. Thus, alterations in the number or functional activities of helper or, more significantly, suppressor T cells would be expected to influence the ability to mount an immune response. Abnormalities in suppressor cell function have been reported in many autoimmune diseases, including SLE, primary biliary cirrhosis, thyroiditis, multiple sclerosis, myasthenia gravis, rheumatoid arthritis, and scleroderma, and have been described in persons with no evidence of disease. Therefore, the question is whether these alterations in suppressor cell function cause these diseases or whether they merely represent an epiphenomenon.

Molecular Mimicry

Another mechanism by which the helper T-cell tolerance is overcome involves antibodies against foreign antigens that cross-react with self-antigens. Here helper T cells function "correctly" and do not induce autoantibody formation. Rather, the efferent limb of the immune response is abnormal. Thus, in rheumatic heart disease, antibodies against streptococcal bacterial antigens cross-react with antigens from cardiac muscle—a phenomenon known as molecular mimicry.

Polyclonal B-Cell Activation

Loss of tolerance may also involve polyclonal B-cell activation, in which B lymphocytes are directly activated by complex substances that contain many antigenic sites (e.g., bacterial cell walls and viruses). Rheumatoid factor (a complex group of IgM autoantibodies reactive with IgG) in rheumatoid arthritis, anti-DNA antibodies in lupus erythematosus, and other autoantibodies have been described after bacterial, viral, and parasitic infections. They may represent the loss of active tolerance to common self-antigens as an inadvertent result of polyclonal B-cell activation.

Tissue Injury in Autoimmune Diseases

Autoimmune diseases have traditionally been considered to be prototypic of immune complex disease, which involves complexes that form either in the circulation or in tissues. Thus, type II (cytotoxic) and type III (immune complex) hypersensitivity reactions are implicated as the cause of tissue injury in most types of autoimmune diseases. Although it is probably true that these hypersensitivity reactions explain most autoimmune tissue injury, the story is more complicated. In some types of autoimmune diseases, T cells sensitized to self-antigens (such as thyroglobulin) may directly cause tissue injury (type IV reaction), but it is not clear to what extent.

Type III hypersensitivity reactions (immune complex disease) explain tissue injury in some types of autoimmune diseases. The prototypical disease in this category is SLE. In this disorder, DNA–anti-DNA complexes formed in the circulation (or at local sites) are deposited in tissues, where they induce inflammation and injury, such as occurs in vasculitis and glomerulonephritis. Other examples are rheumatoid arthritis, scleroderma, polymyositis/dermatomyositis, and Sjögren syndrome. All of these disorders are characterized by immune phenomena and are classified under the rubric collagen vascular diseases. The clinical manifestations are systemic, and many organs and tissues are typically involved. By contrast, cytotoxic (type II-mediated) autoimmune reactions are, for the most part, organ specific.

Systemic Lupus Erythematous is a Prototypical Systemic Immune Complex Disease

SLE is a chronic, autoimmune, multisystem, inflammatory disease that may involve almost any organ but characteristically affects kidneys, joints, serous membranes, and skin. Autoantibodies are formed against a variety of self-antigens, including plasma proteins (complement components, clotting factors) and protein-phospholipid complexes, cell-surface antigens (lymphocytes, neutrophils, platelets, erythrocytes), intracellular cytoplasmic components (microfilaments, microtubules, lysosomes, ribosomes, RNA), and nuclear factors (DNA, ribonucleoproteins, and histones). The most important diagnostic disease-associated autoantibodies are those against nuclear antigens—in particular, antibody to double-stranded DNA and to a soluble nuclear antigen complex that is part of the spliceosome, termed Sm (Smith) antigen. High titers of these two **antinuclear antibodies** (ANAs) are nearly pathognomonic of SLE but are not directly cytotoxic. Antigen–antibody complexes deposit in tissues, leading to the characteristic vasculitis, synovitis, and glomerulonephritis. For this reason, SLE is a prototype of type III hypersensitivity reactions. Occasionally, directly cytotoxic antibodies are present, particularly antibodies against cell-surface antigens of leukocytes and erythrocytes.

The prevalence of SLE varies worldwide, and in North America and northern Europe is 40 out of 100,000. In the United States, it appears to be more common and severe in blacks and Hispanics. More than 80% of cases occur in women of childbearing age, and SLE may strike as many as 1 in 700 women in this age group.

 Pathogenesis: The etiology of SLE is unknown. The presence of numerous autoantibodies, particularly against nuclear components (ANAs), suggests a breakdown in immune surveillance mechanisms that leads to a loss of tolerance. Many manifestations of SLE result from tissue injury caused by immune complex-mediated vasculitis. The presence of immune complexes containing nuclear antigen in injured tissues lends strong support to the concept that the bulk of the injury in lupus is due to the deposition of circulating immune complexes against self-antigens, particularly against DNA. Other clinical manifestations (e.g., thrombocytopenia or the secondary antiphospholipid syndrome) are caused by autoantibodies against serum components or molecules on cell membranes. However, the diagnostically helpful ANAs are not incriminated in the pathogenesis of SLE.

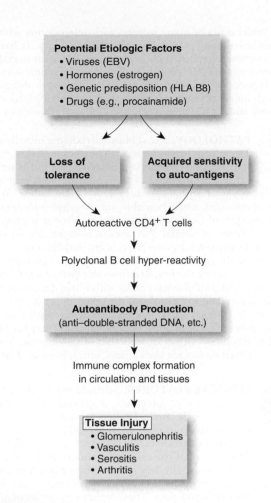

Potential Etiologic Factors
- Viruses (EBV)
- Hormones (estrogen)
- Genetic predisposition (HLA B8)
- Drugs (e.g., procainamide)

Loss of tolerance **Acquired sensitivity to auto-antigens**

Autoreactive CD4$^+$ T cells

Polyclonal B cell hyper-reactivity

Autoantibody Production
(anti–double-stranded DNA, etc.)

Immune complex formation in circulation and tissues

Tissue Injury
- Glomerulonephritis
- Vasculitis
- Serositis
- Arthritis

FIGURE 4-10. The pathogenesis of systemic lupus erythematosus is multifactorial. EBV, Epstein-Barr virus; HLA, human leukocyte antigen.

There appear to be many factors that predispose to the development of SLE, although there is no general agreement as to which play a significant role (Fig. 4-10). Some of the more likely factors are as follows:

- Endocrine factors are suggested by the clear female predominance and ability of estrogens to promote disease.
- Genetic factors are supported by increased concordant disease rates (of about 20% to 30%) in monozygotic twins (also suggesting the importance of nongenetic, environmental factors).
- MHC class II (HLA DR and DQ) antigens appear critical. The incidence of SLE (and other autoimmune diseases) is higher among persons who express certain sets of HLA class II antigens.
- Deficiencies in certain complement components, particularly C2, C4, and C1q, are associated with an increased incidence of the disease. The genes that encode these early complement components are within the HLA region, close to the D/DR locus.

PATHOLOGY AND CLINICAL FEATURES: Because circulating immune complexes deposit in almost all tissues, virtually every organ in the body can be involved.

Skin involvement (see Chapter 24) is common and is manifested by an erythematous rash in sun-exposed sites, a malar "butterfly" rash being the most characteristic. Microscopically, the skin exhibits a perivascular lymphoid infiltrate and liquefactive degeneration of the basal cells. Immunofluorescence studies reveal immunoglobulin and complement deposition at the dermal–epidermal junction ("lupus band").

Joint disease is the most common manifestation of SLE; more than 90% of patients have polyarthralgia. An inflammatory synovitis occurs, but unlike rheumatoid arthritis, joint destruction is unusual.

Renal disease, in particular glomerulonephritis, afflicts three fourths of patients with SLE. Immune complexes between DNA and IgG antibodies to double-stranded DNA deposit in glomeruli and lead to glomerulonephritis (see Chapter 16).

Serous membranes are commonly involved in SLE. More than one third of patients have pleuritis and pleural effusion. Pericarditis and peritonitis occur, but less frequently.

Respiratory disorders in SLE occur frequently. The clinical manifestations are diverse, ranging from pleural disease to upper airway involvement and pulmonary parenchymal disease.

Cardiac involvement (see Chapter 11) is often encountered in SLE, although congestive heart failure is rare and is usually associated with myocarditis. All layers of the heart may be involved, with pericarditis being the most common finding. **Libman-Sacks endocarditis**, which is usually not clinically significant, is characterized by small nonbacterial vegetations on valve leaflets.

Disease of the CNS is a life-threatening complication of lupus. Vasculitis is the common underlying lesion, leading to hemorrhage and infarction of the brain, which are often lethal.

Antiphospholipid antibodies are encountered in one third of patients with SLE. This autoimmune phenomenon predisposes patients to thromboembolic complications, including stroke, pulmonary embolism, deep venous thrombosis, portal vein thrombosis, and spontaneous abortions.

The clinical course of SLE is highly variable, typically with exacerbations and remissions. Because of immunosuppressive therapies, better recognition of mild forms of the disease, and improved antihypertensive medications, the overall 10-year survival rate approaches 90%. The worst prognosis is in patients with severe renal or CNS disease and those with systolic hypertension.

Sjögren Syndrome Targets the Salivary and Lacrimal Glands

Sjögren syndrome (SS) is an autoimmune disorder characterized by keratoconjunctivitis sicca (dry eyes) and xerostomia (dry mouth) in the absence of other connective tissue disease. This definition separates primary SS from secondary types that are occasionally associated with other autoimmune conditions, such as SLE, rheumatoid arthritis, scleroderma, and polymyositis. SS is also frequently associated with involvement of other organs, including the thyroid, lung, and kidney.

Primary SS is the second most common connective tissue disorder after SLE and affects up to 3% of the population. Like most autoimmune diseases, it occurs mostly in women, 30 to 65 years old. There are strong associations between primary SS and certain MHC (HLA) types. Familial clustering occurs, and these families also exhibit a high prevalence of other autoimmune diseases.

The cause of SS is unknown. The production of autoantibodies, particularly ANAs against DNA or nonhistone proteins, typically occurs in patients with SS. Autoantibodies to soluble nuclear nonhistone proteins, especially antigens SS-A (Ro) and SS-B (La), are found in half of patients with primary SS and are associated with more severe glandular and extraglandular manifestations. Autoantibodies to DNA or histones are rare, and their presence suggests secondary SS associated with lupus. Organ-specific autoantibodies (e.g., against salivary gland antigens) are distinctly uncommon. As in SLE, it remains controversial whether the autoantibodies in SS mainly reflect polyclonal B-cell activation or are essentially antigen-driven.

SS has become the prototype for investigation of a viral etiology for autoimmune disease. Particular attention has been paid to possible roles of Epstein-Barr virus (EBV) and human T-cell leukemia virus-1 (HTLV-1). Although it is still difficult to assign a role for EBV in the pathogenesis of SS, there is evidence that reactivation of this virus may be involved in perpetuating the disease, polyclonal B-cell activation, and the development of lymphoma.

In Japan, the seroprevalence of HTLV-1 among patients with SS is 23%, compared with 3.4% among unselected blood donors. Conversely, among HTLV-1 seropositive persons, more than three-quarters demonstrated evidence of SS.

 PATHOLOGY AND CLINICAL FEATURES: SS is characterized by an intense lymphocytic infiltrate in the salivary and lacrimal glands, composed predominantly of CD4⁺ T cells, and a few B cells. The lymphoid infiltrates destroy acini and ducts, and in the late stage of the disease, the glands atrophy and may be replaced by hyalinized tissue and fibrosis. Owing due to the absence of tears, the corneas become dry and fissured and may ulcerate. The lack of saliva causes atrophy, inflammation, and cracking of the oral mucosa. The pathology of the salivary and lacrimal glands is described in greater detail in Chapter 25. Involvement of extraglandular sites is also common in SS. Pulmonary disease occurs in most patients, particularly bronchial gland atrophy in association with lymphoid infiltration. This causes thick tenacious secretions, focal atelectasis, recurrent infections, and bronchiectasis. The GI tract is also affected, and many patients have difficulty swallowing (dysphagia). Esophageal submucosal glands are infiltrated by lymphocytes. In addition, atrophic gastritis occurs secondary to lymphoid infiltration of the gastric mucosa. Liver disease, especially primary biliary cirrhosis, is present in 5% to 10% of patients with SS and is associated with destruction of intrahepatic bile ducts and nodular lymphoid infiltrates. Interstitial nephritis and chronic thyroiditis occasionally accompany the disorder. SS is associated with a 40-fold increased risk of malignant lymphoma, probably through B-cell clonal expansion.

Scleroderma (Progressive Systemic Sclerosis) is an Autoimmune Disease of Connective Tissue

 PATHOGENESIS: Scleroderma is characterized by vasculopathy and excessive collagen deposition in the skin and internal organs, such as the lungs, GI tract, heart, and kidneys. It is four times as common in women as in men, mostly in persons 25 to 50 years of age. An increased familial incidence has been reported. There is an association between HLA-DQB1 and the formation of the autoantibodies characteristic of this disease.

Patients with scleroderma exhibit abnormalities of the humoral and cellular immune systems. The number of circulating B lymphocytes is normal, but there is evidence of hyperactivity, as manifested by hypergammaglobulinemia and cryoglobulinemia. ANAs are common but are usually at lower titers than in SLE. Antibodies commonly found in scleroderma include nucleolar autoantibodies (primarily against RNA polymerase); antibodies to Scl-70, a nonhistone nuclear protein topoisomerase; and anticentromere antibodies, which are associated with the "CREST" variant of the disease (see below). Rheumatoid factor is commonly present in scleroderma, and autoantibodies are occasionally directed against other issues, such as smooth muscle, thyroid gland, and salivary glands. Antibodies against collagen types I and IV have also been described.

Cellular immune derangements are also seen in patients with progressive systemic sclerosis. Reduced circulating CD8⁺ T-suppressor cells, evidence of T-cell activation, alterations in functions mediated by IL-1, IL-2, and soluble IL-2 receptor occur in active disease. Increased levels of IL-4 and IL-6 have also been described. Tissues exhibit active mononuclear inflammation, which precedes the development of the vasculopathy and fibrosis characteristic of this disease. The incidence of other autoimmune disorders, such as thyroiditis and primary biliary cirrhosis, is increased in patients with progressive systemic sclerosis. Circulating male fetal cells have been demonstrated in blood and

blood vessel walls of many women with scleroderma who bore male children many years before the disease began. It has been suggested that scleroderma in these patients is similar to graft-versus-host disease (GVHD see below). Progressive systemic sclerosis is characterized by widespread excessive collagen deposition. Although the cause remains unclear, there is emerging evidence for expansion and activation of fibrogenic clones of fibroblasts.

 PATHOLOGY: The skin in scleroderma initially shows edema and then induration. The thickened skin exhibits (1) a striking increase in collagen fibers in the reticular dermis, (2) thinning of the epidermis with loss of rete pegs, (3) atrophy of dermal appendages, (4) hyalinization, (5) obliteration of arterioles, and (6) variable mononuclear infiltrates, consisting primarily of T cells. The stage of induration may progress to atrophy or revert to normal. Increases in collagen deposition can also occur in synovia, lungs, GI tract, heart, and kidneys.

Lesions in the arteries, arterioles, and capillaries are typical, and in some cases may be the first demonstrable pathologic finding in the disease. Initial subintimal edema with fibrin deposition is followed by thickening and fibrosis of the vessel and reduplication or fraying of the internal elastic lamina. The involved vessels can become severely restricted in terms of blood flow and may become occluded by thrombus. Organ systems that display fibrosis, vascular injury, and necrosis include the kidneys, lungs, heart, and GI tract.

 CLINICAL FEATURES: Scleroderma presents as two distinct clinical categories, a generalized (progressive systemic) form and a limited variant. Progressive systemic sclerosis (diffuse scleroderma) is characterized by severe and worsening disease of the skin and early onset and progression of most or all of the associated abnormalities of visceral organs. Symptoms usually begin with Raynaud phenomenon, namely, intermittent episodes of ischemia of fingers, marked by pallor, paresthesias, and pain. These symptoms are accompanied or followed by edema of fingers and hands, tightening and thickening of skin, polyarthralgia, and complaints referable to involvement of specific internal organs. The typical patient with generalized scleroderma exhibits "stone facies," due to tightening of facial skin and restricted motion of the mouth.

The so-called limited form of scleroderma is a milder disease than generalized scleroderma. Typically, such patients exhibit skin involvement, particularly of the face and fingers. A variant within the spectrum of limited scleroderma is CREST syndrome. CREST is characterized by calcinosis, Raynaud phenomenon, esophageal dysmotility, sclerodactyly, and telangiectasia. The limited variant usually does not entail severe systemic involvement early in disease but later can progress, primarily in the form of diffuse interstitial pulmonary fibrosis. Patients with limited scleroderma often posses circulating anticentromere antibodies.

Mixed Connective Tissue Disease Combines Features of SLE, Scleroderma, and Dermatomyositis

The incidence of mixed connective tissue disease (MCTD) is unknown. Between 80% and 90% of patients are female, and most are adults (mean age, 37 years). Those symptoms that are characteristic of SLE include rash, Raynaud phenomenon, arthritis, and arthralgia. The characteristics of scleroderma are swollen hands, esophageal hypomotility, and pulmonary interstitial disease. Some patients also develop symptoms suggestive of rheumatoid arthritis. Patients with MCTD have been reported to respond well to corticosteroid therapy, although some studies have challenged this assertion.

The etiology and pathogenesis of MCTD are unknown. Patients often have evidence of B-cell activation, with hypergammaglobulinemia and a positive rheumatoid factor assay. ANAs are present but, unlike in SLE, they are usually not directed against double-stranded DNA. The most distinctive ANA is directed against an extractable nuclear antigen, uridine-rich ribonucleoprotein (anti-U1-RNP).

The cause of the formation and maintenance of the high titer of anti-RNP antibody is unclear. However, there is an association with HLA-DR4 and HLA-DR2 genotypes, suggesting a role for T cells in autoantibody production. There is no direct evidence that these antibodies induce the characteristic involvement of the various organ systems. At this time, it is unclear whether MCTD is a distinct entity or simply an overlap of symptoms in patients with other types of collagen vascular diseases.

Immune Reactions to Transplanted Tissues

Antigens encoded by the MHC on chromosome 6 are critical immunogenic molecules that can stimulate rejection of transplanted tissues. Thus, optimal graft survival occurs when recipient and donor are closely matched (most similar) with regard to histocompatibility antigens. In practice, an exact HLA match is obtained infrequently, except in the case of transplantation between monozygotic twins and in 25% of siblings. Vigilant monitoring of the functional status of the graft and immunosuppressive therapy are thus required after transplantation. In recent years, therapeutic advances (immunosuppressives such as cyclosporine and tacrolimus) have greatly improved transplant success rates, even when there is a degree of histoincompatibility. When host-versus-graft immune reactions (rejection) occur, any combination of immune responses may injure the graft.

Both T-cell–mediated and antibody-mediated reactions are important in the pathophysiology of transplant rejection. **Donor** APCs, bearing foreign MHC molecules within the graft, are recognized by **host** CD8$^+$ cytotoxic T lymphocytes that mediate tissue injury. In addition, host CD4$^+$ T-helper cells augment antibody production, induce IFN-γ production, and activate macrophages. Induction of IFN-γ leads to enhanced MHC expression and amplification of tissue injury. **Host** APCs also process foreign donor antigens, leading to CD4$^+$-mediated delayed type hypersensitivity.

Transplant rejection reactions have been traditionally categorized as "hyperacute, acute, and chronic" rejection, based on the clinical tempo of the response and on the pathophysiologic mechanisms

involved. However, in practice, there can be overlap of features and ambiguity in diagnosis. The diagnosis of transplant rejection is further complicated by the toxic effects of immunosuppressive drugs and by the potential for either mechanical problems (e.g., vascular thrombosis) or recurrence of the disease that necessitated transplantation (e.g., some types of glomerulonephritis). The next sections illustrate rejection in the context of renal transplantation. Similar responses occur in other transplanted tissues, although each transplanted tissue type exhibits its own unique problems.

Hyperacute Rejection Occurs Within Minutes to Hours after Transplantation

Hyperacute rejection of the kidney is manifested clinically as a sudden cessation of urine output, along with fever and pain in the area of the graft site. This immediate rejection is catastrophic and necessitates prompt surgical removal of the kidney. The histologic features of hyperacute rejection within the transplanted kidney are vascular congestion, fibrin–platelet thrombi within capillaries, neutrophilic vasculitis with fibrinoid necrosis, prominent interstitial edema, and neutrophilic infiltrates (Fig. 4-11A). This form of rejection is mediated by preformed host anti-HLA antibodies that react with donor tissue. This process leads to the formation of complement activation products, including chemotactic and other inflammatory mediators. Fortunately, hyperacute rejection is not common when appropriate pretransplantation antibody screening is performed.

Acute Rejection is Seen Within the First Few Weeks or Months after Transplantation

Acute renal rejection is characterized by the abrupt onset of azotemia and oliguria, which may be associated with fever and graft tenderness. A needle biopsy is often used to differentiate between acute rejection and acute tubular necrosis or toxicity from immunosuppressive agents. Findings vary depending on whether the rejection is primarily cellular or humoral. In the former case, microscopic find-

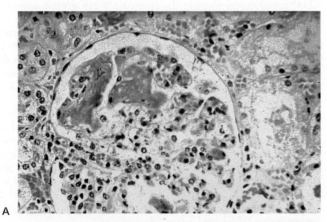

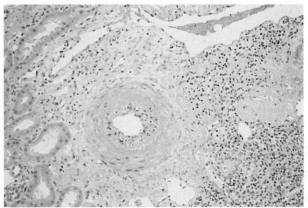

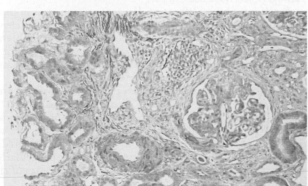

FIGURE 4-11. **There are three major forms of renal transplant rejection. A.** Hyperacute rejection occurs within minutes to hours after transplantation and is characterized by intravascular fibrin–platelet thrombi. **B.** Acute cellular rejection occurs within weeks to months after transplantation and is characterized by tubular damage and mononuclear leukocyte infiltration. In this example, the small artery *(in the center of the frame)* exhibits vasculitis. **C.** Chronic rejection is observed months to years after transplantation and is characterized by tubular atrophy, patchy interstitial mononuclear cell infiltrates, and fibrosis. In this example, glomeruli capillary walls are focally thickened.

ings include interstitial infiltrates of lymphocytes and macrophages, edema, lymphocytic tubulitis, and tubular necrosis (see Fig. 4-11B). The acute humoral form, sometimes called rejection vasculitis, shows vascular damage, manifested as arteritis, fibrinoid necrosis, and thrombosis. Vascular involvement is an ominous sign because it usually means that the rejection episode will be refractory to therapy. Acute rejection most typically involves both cell-mediated and humoral mechanisms of tissue damage. If detected in its early stages, acute rejection can be reversed with immunosuppressive therapy.

Chronic Rejection Appears Months to Years after Transplantation

In chronic rejection of the transplanted kidney, the patient typically develops progressive azotemia, oliguria, hypertension, and weight gain over a period of months. The dominant histologic features are arterial and arteriolar intimal thickening, causing vascular stenosis or obstruction, thickened glomerular capillary walls, tubular atrophy, and interstitial fibrosis (see Fig. 4-11C). The interstitium often exhibits scattered mononuclear infiltrates, and tubules contain proteinaceous casts. Chronic rejection may be the end result of repeated episodes of cellular rejection, either asymptomatic or clinically apparent. This advanced state of damage does not respond to therapy. As in the clinical diagnosis, histologic features of acute and chronic rejection may overlap and vary in degree, so that a clear distinction may not be possible on renal biopsy.

Graft Versus Host Disease (GVHD) Occurs When Donor Lymphocytes React to the Recipient Tissues

The advent of transplantation of allogeneic (donor) bone marrow into patients with hematogenous malignancies or other disorders, has allowed treatment of conditions that were refractory to previous therapies. Immunocompetent lymphocytes in the grafted marrow may "reject" host tissues, leading to GVHD. GVHD can also occur when a profoundly immunodeficient patient is transfused with blood products containing HLA-incompatible lymphocytes.

The major organs affected in GVHD are skin, GI tract, and liver. The skin and intestine exhibit mononuclear cell infiltrates and epithelial cell necrosis. The liver displays periportal inflammation, damaged bile ducts, and liver cell injury. Clinically, acute GVHD manifests as rash, diarrhea, abdominal cramps, anemia, and liver dysfunction. The chronic form of GVHD is characterized by dermal sclerosis, sicca syndrome (dry eyes and mouth due to chronic inflammation of lacrimal and salivary glands), and immunodeficiency. Treatment of GVHD requires immunosuppressive therapy to modulate donor cell immunoreactivity. Patients, especially those with chronic GVHD, may be at a higher risk for opportunistic infections. In some cases, mild GVHD may be beneficial, as it may aid in suppressing residual host neoplastic cells.

Human Immunodeficiency Virus (HIV) and Acquired Immunodeficiency Syndrome (AIDS)

AIDS is the most common immunodeficiency state worldwide. It is mainly caused by HIV-1, although a small minority of patients are infected with HIV-2, primarily in western Africa. Persons infected with HIV-1 exhibit a variety of immunologic defects, the most devastating of which is a loss of cellular immunity. The disease is progressive if not treated with appropriate antiretroviral therapy. Catastrophic opportunistic infections are virtually inevitable if the patient is left untreated. The relentless progression of HIV infection is now recognized as a continuum that extends from an initial asymptomatic state to the immune depletion that characterizes patients with overt AIDS, and the continuum is often referred to as HIV/AIDS. The basic lesion is infection of $CD4^+$ (helper) T lymphocytes by HIV, which leads to depletion of this cell population and consequent impaired immune function and dys-

regulation. As a result, rather than dying of HIV infection itself, patients with AIDS usually die of opportunistic infections. There is also a high incidence of malignant tumors, principally B-cell lymphomas and Kaposi sarcoma. Finally, infection of the CNS with HIV often leads to an array of syndromes, ranging from minor cognitive or motor neuron disorders to dementia.

Immunology of AIDS

The destruction of $CD4^+$ T cells by HIV-1 can essentially disable the entire immune system because this subset of lymphocytes exerts critical regulatory and effector functions that involve both cellular and humoral immunity. Thus, in typical AIDS patients, all elements of the immune system are eventually perturbed, including T cells, B cells, NK cells, and monocyte/macrophages.

Of the two functional types of $CD4^+$ T lymphocytes, that is helper and amplifier (or inducer) cells, those affected first in HIV infection are the amplifier subset. Eventually, total $CD4^+$ lymphocyte counts fall to less than 500 cells/μL, and helper-to-suppressor T-cell ratios decline from a normal value of 2.0 to as little as 0.5. The numbers of $CD8^+$ (cytotoxic/suppressor) cells are variable, although in AIDS, most of these cells seem to be of the cytotoxic variety.

Defects in T-cell function are manifested by defective responses to skin testing with a variety of antigens (delayed hypersensitivity) and impaired proliferative responses to mitogens and antigens in vitro. Moreover, the deficiency of $CD4^+$ cells reduces the levels of IL-2, the cytokine produced in response to antigens that stimulate cytotoxic T-cell killing. Thus, patients with AIDS cannot generate the antigen-specific cytotoxic T cells that are required to clear viruses and other infectious agents.

Humoral immunity is also abnormal. Production of antibodies in response to specific antigenic stimulation is markedly decreased, often to under 10% of normal. B cells also show poor proliferative responses in vitro to mitogens and antigens. Yet, sera of patients with AIDS usually show high levels of polyclonal immunoglobulins, autoantibodies, and immune complexes. This apparent paradox is probably explained by the concurrent infection with polyclonal B-cell-activating viruses (e.g., EBV or CMV), which constantly stimulate B cells nonspecifically to produce immunoglobulins. Lack of $CD4^+$ lymphocytes impairs the cytotoxic T-cell proliferation that normally would eliminate B cells infected with EBV.

NK-cell activity is severely decreased in AIDS as well. Because these cells kill both virus-infected cells and tumor cells, this defect may contribute to the malignant tumors and viral infections that plague these patients. Suppression of NK-cell activity is related both to a decrease in NK-cell number and to reduction in IL-2 levels, owing to a loss of $CD4^+$ cells.

HIV-1 tends to target monocyte/macrophages, and infected macrophages may serve as reservoirs for dissemination of the virus. Interestingly, some macrophages express CD4 on their surfaces. Unlike T lymphocytes, which are killed by HIV, infected macrophages generally survive. Macrophages from patients with AIDS display impaired phagocytosis of immune complexes and opsonized particles, decreased chemotaxis, and impaired responses to antigenic challenges. For details on the pathology and pathogenesis HIV-1 see Chapter 9.

B-cell lymphoproliferative diseases are common in patients with AIDS. The lymphomas in chronically immunodeficient patients may manifest as an invasive polyclonal B-cell proliferation or as a monoclonal B-cell lymphoma. Many patients exhibit serologic evidence of infection with EBV, and the EBV genome has been demonstrated in the lymphoma cells.

B-cell hyperplasia and generalized lymphadenopathy precede malignant lymphoproliferative disease. HIV-associated lymphomas are usually of the large cell variety, as in other immunodeficiency conditions, although small cell lymphomas are sometimes seen. A conspicuous feature of lymphomas associated with AIDS is their predilection for extranodal disease, particularly primary lymphomas of the brain. In addition, lymphomas of the GI tract, liver, and bone marrow are frequent.

5 Neoplasia

Antonio Giordano
Giulia De Falco
Emanuel Rubin
Raphael Rubin

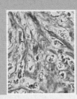

A **neoplasm** (Greek, neo, new + plasma, thing formed) is the autonomous growth of tissues that have escaped normal restraints on cell proliferation and exhibit varying degrees of fidelity to their precursors. The structural resemblance of the neoplastic cell to its cell of origin usually enables conclusions about its source and potential behavior. In view of their space-occupying properties, solid neoplasms are termed **tumors** (Greek, swelling). Tumors that remain localized are considered **benign**, whereas those that spread to distant sites are termed **malignant**, or **cancer**. The neoplastic process entails not only cellular proliferation but also altered differentiation of the tumor cell and, in some cases, an aberration of programmed cell death (apoptosis).

The incidence of cancer increases with age, and the greater longevity in modern times necessarily enlarges the population at risk. If all deaths from cancers caused by tobacco smoke are removed from the statistics, there has been no increase in the overall age-adjusted cancer death rate in men in the past half-century, and there has been a continually decreasing rate in women. However, the age-adjusted incidence of specific cancers has fluctuated over this time period.

In general, neoplasms are irreversible, and their growth is, for the most part, autonomous. Several observations are important:

- Neoplasms are derived from cells that normally maintain a proliferative capacity. Thus, mature neurons and cardiac myocytes do not give rise to tumors.
- A tumor may express varying degrees of differentiation, from relatively mature structures that mimic normal tissues to a collection of cells so primitive in appearance that the cell of origin cannot be identified.
- The exact stimulus responsible for the uncontrolled proliferation may not be identifiable; in fact, it is not known for most human neoplasms.
- Neoplasia arises from mutations in genes that regulate cell growth, apoptosis, or DNA repair.

Benign Versus Malignant Tumors

By definition, benign tumors do not penetrate (invade) adjacent tissue borders, nor do they spread (metastasize) to distant sites. They remain as localized overgrowths in the area in which they arise. As a rule, benign tumors are more differentiated than malignant ones—that is, they more closely resemble their tissue of origin. *By contrast, malignant tumors, or cancers, have the added property of invading contiguous tissues and metastasizing to distant sites, where subpopulations of malignant cells take up residence, grow anew, and again invade.*

In common usage, the terms **benign** and **malignant** refer to the overall biological behavior of a tumor rather than to its morphologic characteristics. In most circumstances, malignant tumors kill, whereas benign ones spare the host. However, so-called benign tumors in critical locations can be deadly. For example, a benign intracranial tumor of the meninges (meningioma) can kill by exerting pressure on the brain. A benign mesenchymal tumor of the left atrium (myxoma) may kill suddenly by blocking the mitral valve orifice. In certain locations, the erosion of a benign tumor of smooth muscle can lead to serious hemorrhage—witness the peptic ulceration of a stromal tumor in the gastric wall. On rare occasions, a functioning, benign endocrine adenoma can be life-threatening, as in the case of sudden hypoglycemia associated with an insulinoma of the pancreas or a hypertensive crisis produced by a pheochromocytoma of the adrenal medulla. Conversely, certain types of malignant tumors are so indolent that they are curable by surgical resection. In this category are many cancers of breast and some malignant tumors of connective tissue (e.g., fibrosarcoma).

A number of tumors are difficult to classify because they do not fit all the criteria for either benign or malignant neoplasms. The best-known example is basal cell carcinoma of the skin, which is histologically malignant (i.e., it invades aggressively) but only rarely has been reported to metastasize to distant sites. Similarly, the local growth of a pleomorphic adenoma of a salivary gland, which is classified as benign, may be so aggressive that it defies surgical cure.

Classification of Neoplasms

The classification of tumors reflects historical concepts, technical jargon, location, origin, descriptive modifiers, and predictors of biological behavior. Although the language of tumor classification is neither rigidly logical nor consistent, it still serves as a reasonable mode of communication.

Benign Tumors Carry the Suffix "oma"

The primary descriptor of any tumor, benign or malignant, is its cell or tissue of origin. The classification of benign tumors is the basis for the names of their malignant variants. *The suffix "oma" for benign tumors is preceded by reference to the cell or tissue of origin.* For example, a benign tumor that resembles chondrocytes is called a **chondroma** (Fig. 5-1). If the tumor resembles the precursor of the chondrocyte, it is labeled **chondroblastoma**.

Tumors of epithelial origin are given a variety of names based on what is believed to be their outstanding characteristic. Thus, a benign tumor of the squamous epithelium may be called simply **epithelioma** or, when branched and exophytic, may be termed **papilloma**. Benign tumors arising from glandular epithelium, such as in the colon or the endocrine glands, are named **adenoma**. Accordingly, we refer to a **thyroid adenoma** or a **pancreatic islet cell adenoma**. In some instances, the predominating feature is the gross appearance, in which case we speak, for example, of an **adenomatous polyp** of the colon.

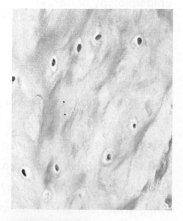
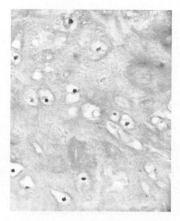

A
B

FIGURE 5-1. **Benign chondroma. A.** Normal cartilage. **B.** A benign chondroma closely resembles normal cartilage.

Benign tumors that arise from germ cells and contain derivatives of different germ layers are labeled **teratoma**. These tumors occur principally in the gonads and occasionally in the mediastinum and may contain a variety of structures, such as skin, neurons and glial cells, thyroid, intestinal epithelium, and cartilage. Localized, disordered differentiation during embryonic development results in a **hamartoma**, a disorganized caricature of normal tissue components. Such tumors, which are not strictly neoplasms, contain varying combinations of cartilage, ducts or bronchi, connective tissue, blood vessels, and lymphoid tissue. Ectopic islands of normal tissue, called **choristoma**, may also be mistaken for true neoplasms. These small lesions are represented by pancreatic tissue in the wall of the stomach or intestine, adrenal rests under the renal capsule, and nodules of splenic tissue in the peritoneal cavity. Certain benign growths, recognized clinically as tumors, are not truly neoplastic but rather represent overgrowth of normal tissue elements. Examples are vocal cord polyps, skin tags, and hyperplastic polyps of the colon.

Malignant Tumors are Mostly Carcinomas or Sarcomas

In general, the malignant counterparts of benign tumors usually carry the same name, except that the suffix "carcinoma" is applied to epithelial cancers and "sarcoma" to those of mesenchymal origin. For instance, a malignant tumor of the stomach is a **gastric adenocarcinoma** or **adenocarcinoma of the stomach** (Fig. 5-2). **Squamous cell carcinoma** is an invasive tumor of the skin or other organs lined by a squamous epithelium (e.g., the esophagus). Squamous cell carcinomas also arise in the metaplastic squamous epithelium of the bronchus or endocervix. **Transitional cell carcinoma** is a malignant neoplasm of the bladder or ureters. By contrast, we speak of **chondrosarcoma** (Fig. 5-3) or **fibrosarcoma**. Sometimes the name of the tumor suggests the tissue type of origin, as in **osteogenic sarcoma** or **bronchogenic carcinoma**. Some tumors display neoplastic elements of different cell types but are not germ cell tumors. For example, **fibroadenoma** of the breast, composed of epithelial and stromal elements, is benign, whereas, as the name implies, **adenosquamous carcinoma** of the uterus or the lung is malignant. A rare malignant tumor that contains intermingled carcinomatous and sarcomatous elements is known as **carcinosarcoma**.

The persistence of certain historical terms adds a note of confusion. **Hepatoma** of the liver, **melanoma** of the skin, **seminoma** of the testis, and the lymphoproliferative tumor, **lymphoma**, are all highly malignant. Tumors of the hematopoietic system are a special case in which the relationship to the blood is indicated by the suffix "emia." Thus, **leukemia** refers to a malignant proliferation of leukocytes.

Secondary descriptors (again, with some inconsistencies) refer to a tumor's morphologic and functional characteristics. For example, the term **papillary** describes a frond-like structure (Fig. 5-4). **Medullary** signifies a soft, cellular tumor with little connective tissue stroma, whereas **scirrhous** or **desmoplastic** implies a dense fibrous stroma (Fig. 5-5). **Colloid** carcinomas secrete abundant mucus, in which float islands of tumor cells. **Comedocarcinoma** is an intraductal neoplasm in which necrotic material can be expressed from the ducts. Certain visible secretions of the tumor cells lend their characteristics to the classification—for example, production of mucin or serous fluid. A further designation describes the gross appearance of a cystic mass. From all these considerations, we derive such common terms as **papillary serous cystadenocarcinoma** of the ovary, **comedocarcinoma** of the breast, **adenoid cystic carcinoma** of the salivary glands, **polypoid adenocarcinoma** of the stomach, and **medullary carcinoma** of the thyroid. Finally, tumors in which the histogenesis is poorly understood are often given an eponym—for example, Hodgkin disease, Ewing sarcoma of bone, or Brenner tumor of the ovary.

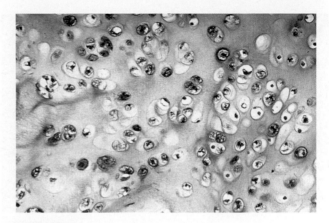

FIGURE 5-3. **Chondrosarcoma of bone.** The tumor is composed of malignant chondrocytes, which have bizarre shapes and irregular hyperchromatic nuclei, embedded in a cartilaginous matrix. Compare with Figure 5-1.

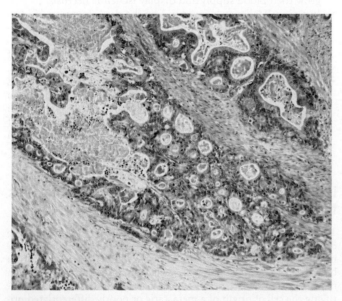

FIGURE 5-2. **Adenocarcinoma of the stomach.** Irregular neoplastic glands infiltrate the gastric wall.

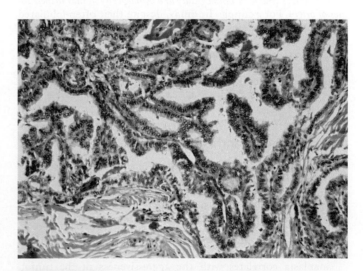

FIGURE 5-4. **Papillary adenocarcinoma of the thyroid.** The tumor exhibits numerous fronds lined by malignant epithelial cells.

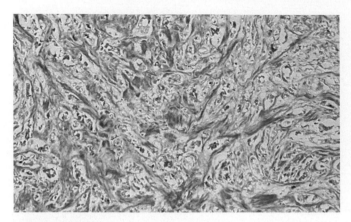

FIGURE 5-5. **Scirrhous adenocarcinoma of the breast.** A trichrome stain shows nests of cancer cells (*red*) embedded in a dense fibrous stroma (*blue*).

Histologic Diagnosis of Malignancy

There are no reliable molecular indicators of malignancy, and the "gold standard" for diagnosis of cancer remains routine microscopy. The distinction between benign and malignant tumors is, from a practical point of view, the most important diagnostic challenge faced by the pathologist. In most cases, the differentiation poses few problems; in a few, careful study is required before an accurate diagnosis is secure. However, there remain tumors that defy the diagnostic skills and experience of any pathologist. In these cases, the correct diagnosis must await the clinical outcome. In effect, the criteria used to assess the true biological nature of any tumor are based not on scientific principles but rather on a historical correlation of histologic and cytologic patterns with clinical outcomes. Although general criteria for malignancy are recognized, they must be used with caution in specific cases. For example, a reactive proliferation of connective cells termed **nodular fasciitis** has a more alarming histologic appearance than many fibrosarcomas, and misdiagnosis can lead to unnecessary surgery. Conversely, many well-differentiated endocrine adenocarcinomas are histologically indistinguishable from benign adenomas.

Benign Tumors Resemble Their Parent Tissue

Benign tumors tend to be histologically and cytologically similar to their tissues of origin. For example, **lipomas**, despite their often-lobulated gross appearance, seem to be composed of normal adipocytes (Fig. 5-6). **Fibromas** are composed of mature fibroblasts and a collagenous stroma. **Chondromas** exhibit chondrocytes dispersed in a cartilaginous matrix. **Thyroid adenomas** form acini and produce thyroglobulin. *Remember that the definition of a benign tumor resides above all in its inability to invade adjacent tissue and to metastasize.*

Malignant Tumors Depart from the Parent Tissue Morphologically and Functionally

Despite the histologic divergence of malignant tumors from their tissue of origin, an accurate identification of their source depends not only on the location but also on a morphologic resemblance to a normal tissue. Some of the histologic features that favor malignancy include the following:

- **Anaplasia or cellular atypia:** These terms refer to the lack of differentiated features in a cancer cell. In general, the degree of anaplasia correlates with the aggressiveness of the tumor. Cytologic evidence of anaplasia includes (1) variation in the size and shape of cells and cell nuclei **(pleomorphism)**, (2) enlarged and hyperchromatic nuclei with coarsely clumped chro-

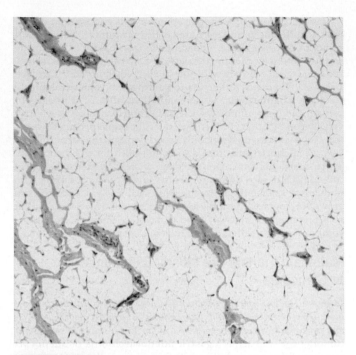

FIGURE 5-6. **Lipoma.** This subcutaneous, nodular tumor of adipocytes is grossly and microscopically indistinguishable from normal fat.

matin and prominent nucleoli, (3) atypical mitoses, and (4) bizarre cells, including tumor giant cells (Fig. 5-7). Many of these features are preceded by a preneoplastic dysplastic epithelium, which may lead to carcinoma in situ (see Chapter 1).

- **Mitotic activity:** Abundant mitoses are characteristic of many malignant tumors but are not a necessary criterion. However, in some cases (e.g., leiomyosarcomas), the diagnosis of malignancy is based on the finding of even a few mitoses.
- **Growth pattern:** In common with many benign tumors, malignant neoplasms often exhibit a disorganized and random growth pattern, which may be expressed as uniform sheets of cells, arrangements around blood vessels, papillary structures, whorls, rosettes, and so forth. Malignant tumors often outgrow their blood supply and display ischemic necrosis.
- **Invasion:** Malignancy is proved by the demonstration of invasion, particularly of blood vessels and lymphatics. In some circumstances (e.g., squamous carcinoma of the cervix or carcinoma arising in an adenomatous polyp), the diagnosis of malignant transformation is made on the basis of local invasion.
- **Metastases:** The presence of metastases identifies a tumor as malignant. In metastatic disease that was not preceded by a clinically diagnosed primary tumor, the site of origin is often not readily apparent from the morphologic characteristics of the tumor. In such cases, electron microscopic examination and the demonstration of specific tumor markers may establish the correct origin.

Immunohistochemical Tumor Markers are Antigens that Point to the Origin of Neoplasms

Tumor markers are products of malignant neoplasms that can be detected in the cells themselves or in body fluids. The ultimate tumor marker would be one that allows the unequivocal distinction between benign and malignant cells, but unfortunately no such marker exists. Nevertheless, some markers are often useful in identifying the cell of origin of a metastatic or poorly differentiated primary tumor. Metastatic tumors may be so undifferentiated microscopically as to preclude even the distinction between an epithelial

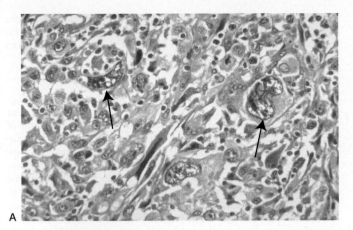
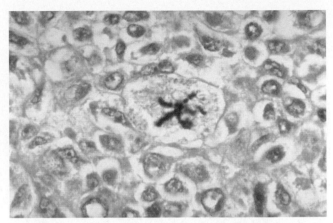

FIGURE 5-7. **Anaplastic features of malignant tumors. A.** The cells of this anaplastic carcinoma are highly pleomorphic (i.e., they vary in size and shape). The nuclei are hyperchromatic and are large relative to the cytoplasm. Multinucleated tumor giant cells are present (*arrows*). **B.** A malignant cell in metaphase exhibits an abnormal mitotic figure.

and a mesenchymal origin. Tumor markers rely on the preservation of characteristics of the progenitor cell or the synthesis of specialized proteins by the neoplastic cell to make this distinction. The determination of cell lineage of undifferentiated tumors is more than an academic exercise, because therapeutic decisions may be based on their appropriate identification. For example, the treatment of carcinomas usually involves surgery, whereas malignant lymphomas are treated with radiation therapy and chemotherapy. Among these diagnostically useful markers are such diverse products as immunoglobulins, fetal proteins, enzymes, hormones, and cytoskeletal and junctional proteins.

- **Carcinomas** uniformly express **cytokeratins**, which are intermediate filaments belonging to a multigene family of proteins. Lineage-associated markers are often useful in establishing the origin of a poorly differentiated carcinoma. For example, prostatic carcinomas consistently express the glycoprotein **prostate-specific antigen** and **prostate-specific acid phosphatase**. By contrast, colon cancers are negative for these markers, but most of them express **carcinoembryonic antigen** (CEA).
- **Neuroendocrine tumors** share the positivity for cytokeratins with other carcinomas. However, they can be identified by their content of **chromogranins**, a family of proteins found in neurosecretory granules, or **synaptophysins**.
- **Malignant melanomas** may be unpigmented and appear similar to other poorly differentiated carcinomas. They can often be distinguished by immunohistochemical studies. Melanomas express HMB-45 and S-100 protein, but unlike most carcinomas, they are not positive for cytokeratins.
- **Soft tissue sarcomas** express the intermediate filament **vimentin**. Because this marker is also present in numerous non-mesenchymal tumors, its expression is meaningful only in concert with other markers and morphologic criteria.
- **Malignant lymphomas** are generally positive for **leukocyte common antigen** (CD45). Markers for lymphomas and leukemias are grouped by so-called cluster designations (CDs), at present numbering over 200. Markers for CD antigens help to discriminate between T and B lymphocytes, monocytes, and granulocytes, as well as the mature and immature variants of these cells.
- **Vascular tumors** derived from endothelial cells, including hemangiomas and hemangiosarcomas, are identified by antibodies against **factor VIII-related antigen** or by the binding of certain lectins.
- **Proliferating cells** display **Ki-67** and **proliferating cell nuclear antigen**. Although the presence of proliferating cells alone does not establish a diagnosis of malignancy, the presence of cycling cells at sites in which cell growth is normally absent frequently suggests a cancer.

Serum tumor markers are not disease-specific, but they allow monitoring of tumor recurrence after surgery. For example, high serum levels of carcinoembryonic antigen (CEA) are associated with carcinomas of the gastrointestinal tract and some carcinomas of the breast. Increased levels of **serum α-fetoprotein** suggest liver cancer or a yolk sac tumor. **Human chorionic gonadotropin (hCG)** is used for monitoring the recurrence of malignant trophoblastic tumors. Increased serum levels of prostate-specific antigen accompany prostatic cancers.

Invasion and Metastasis

The two properties that are unique to cancer cells are the ability to invade locally and the capacity to metastasize to distant sites. These characteristics are responsible for the vast majority of deaths from cancer; the primary tumor itself is generally amenable to surgical extirpation.

Direct Extension Damages the Involved Organ and Adjacent Tissues

Most carcinomas begin as localized growths confined to the epithelium in which they arise. As long as these early cancers do not penetrate the basement membrane on which the epithelium rests, such tumors are termed carcinoma in situ (Fig. 5-8). In this stage, it is unfortunate that in situ tumors are asymptomatic, because they are invariably curable. When the in situ tumor acquires invasive potential and extends directly through the underlying basement membrane, it can compromise neighboring tissues and metastasize. In situations in which cancer arises from cells that are not confined by a basement membrane—such as connective tissue cells, lymphoid elements, and hepatocytes—an in situ stage is not defined.

Malignant tumors characteristically grow within the tissue of origin, where they enlarge and infiltrate normal structures. They may also extend directly beyond the confines of that organ to involve adjacent tissues. The growth of the cancer is occasionally so extensive that replacement of the normal tissue results in functional insufficiency of the organ. Such a situation is not uncommon in primary liver cancer. Brain tumors, such as astrocytomas, infiltrate the brain until they compromise vital regions. The direct extension of malignant tumors within an organ may also be life-threatening because of their location. A common example is the intestinal obstruction produced by cancer of the colon.

The invasive growth pattern of cancers often leads to their direct extension outside the tissue of origin, in which case the tumor may secondarily impair the function of an adjacent organ. Squamous carcinoma of the cervix frequently grows beyond the genital tract to produce vesicovaginal fistulas and to obstruct the ureters. Neglected

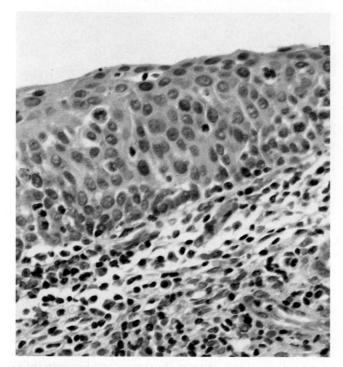

FIGURE 5-8. **Carcinoma in situ.** A section of the uterine cervix shows neoplastic squamous cells occupying the full thickness of the epithelium and confined to the mucosa by the underlying basement membrane.

cases of breast cancer are often complicated by extensive skin ulceration. Even small tumors can produce severe consequences when they invade vital structures. A small lung cancer can cause exsanguinating hemorrhage when it erodes a blood vessel. The agonizing pain of pancreatic carcinoma results from direct extension of the tumor to the celiac nerve plexus. Tumor cells that reach serous cavities (e.g., those of the peritoneum or pleura) spread easily by direct extension or can be carried by the fluid to new locations on the serous membranes. The most common example is the seeding of the peritoneal cavity by certain types of ovarian cancer.

Metastatic Spread is the Most Common Cause of Cancer Death

Metastasis refers to the transfer of malignant cells from one site to another not directly connected with it. The invasive properties of malignant tumors bring them into contact with blood and lymphatic vessels. *In the same way that they can invade parenchymal tissue, neoplastic cells can also penetrate vascular and lymphatic channels, through which they are disseminated to distant sites.* In general, metastases resemble the primary tumor histologically, although they are occasionally so anaplastic that their cell of origin is obscure.

Hematogenous Metastases

Cancer cells commonly invade capillaries and venules, whereas thicker-walled arterioles and arteries are relatively resistant. Before they can form viable metastases, circulating tumor cells must lodge in the vascular bed of the metastatic site (Fig. 5-9). Here, they presumably attach to the walls of blood vessels, either to endothelial cells or to naked basement membranes. For many tumors, this sequence of events explains why the liver and the lung are so frequently the sites of metastases. Because abdominal tumors seed the portal system, they lead to hepatic metastases; other tumors penetrate systemic veins that eventually drain into the vena cava and hence to the lungs. Some tumor cells released into the venous system survive passage through the microcirculation and are thus transported to more distant organs. For instance, tumor cells may survive passage through the pulmonary microcirculation to reach

the brain, bones, and other organs through arterial dissemination. Neoplastic cells arrested in the microcirculation penetrate the vessel walls at the site of metastasis by use of the same mechanisms by which the primary tumor invades.

Lymphatic Metastases

Tumors arising in tissues that have a rich lymphatic network (e.g., the breast) often metastasize by this route, although the particular properties of specific neoplasms may play a role in the route of spread. Basement membranes envelop only large lymphatic channels; they are lacking in lymphatic capillaries. Thus, invasive tumor cells may penetrate lymphatic channels more readily than blood vessels. Once in lymphatic vessels, the cells are carried to the regional draining lymph nodes, where they initially lodge in the marginal sinus and then extend throughout the node. Lymph nodes bearing metastatic deposits may be enlarged to many times their normal size, often exceeding the diameter of the primary lesion. The cut surface of the lymph node usually resembles that of the primary tumor in color and consistency and may also exhibit the necrosis and hemorrhage commonly seen in primary cancers (Fig. 5-10).

The regional lymphatic pattern of metastatic spread is most prominently exemplified by breast cancer. The initial metastases are almost always lymphatic, and these regional lymphatic metastases have considerable prognostic significance. Cancers that arise in the lateral aspect of the breast characteristically spread to axillary lymph nodes; those arising in the medial portion drain to the internal mammary thoracic lymph nodes. Identification of the specific **sentinel nodes** that drain the site of a breast cancer is an important aid in attempting to assess whether a tumor has metastasized via the lymphatic system.

Seeding of Body Cavities

Malignant tumors that arise in organs adjacent to body cavities (e.g., ovaries, gastrointestinal tract, and lung) may shed malignant cells into these spaces. Such body cavities principally include the peritoneal and pleural cavities, although occasional seeding of the pericardial cavity, joint space, and subarachnoid space are observed. Similar to tissue culture, tumors in these sites grow in masses and may provoke the formation of fluid (e.g., ascites, pleural fluid), sometimes in very large quantities. Mucinous adenocarcinoma may also secrete copious amounts of mucin in these locations.

Invasion and Metastasis are Multistep Events

Several steps are required for malignant cells to establish a metastasis (Fig. 5-11):

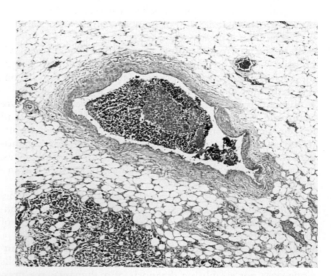

FIGURE 5-9. **Hematogenous spread of cancer.** A malignant tumor (*bottom*) has invaded adipose tissue and penetrated into a small vein.

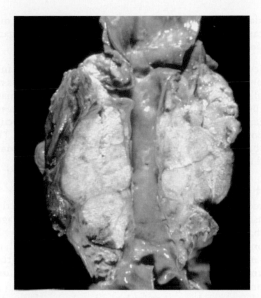

FIGURE 5-10. Metastatic carcinoma in periaortic lymph nodes. The aorta has been opened and the nodes bisected.

1. Invasion of the basement membrane underlying the tumor
2. Movement through extracellular matrix
3. Penetration of vascular or lymphatic channels
4. Survival and arrest within circulating blood or lymph nodes
5. Exit from the circulation into a new tissue site
6. Survival and growth as a metastasis, a process that involves angiogenesis.

Most cancers originate from the malignant transformation of a single cell (**monoclonal origin of tumors**). Nevertheless, the inherent genetic instability of the malignant phenotype leads to the appearance of subpopulations with diverse biological characteristics and profound variations in their metastatic potential (**tumor heterogeneity**). The demonstration of tumor heterogeneity has led to the concept that at each step of the metastatic cascade, only the fittest cells survive. Thus, the metastatic process can be viewed as a competition in which a subpopulation of cells within the primary cancer ultimately prevails as a metastasis.

Invasion

Inherent in the definition of a malignant cell is the capacity to invade surrounding tissue. In epithelial tumors, invasion requires disruption of, and penetration through, the underlying basement membrane and passage through the extracellular matrix. Similarly, circulating cells destined to establish metastases must reproduce these same events to exit from the vascular or lymphatic compartment and establish residence at a distant site.

Adhesion Molecules

The entire metastatic sequence, from the initial binding of the tumor cell to the underlying extracellular matrix, to its growth in a distant location, depends on the expression of numerous adhesion molecules by the malignant cells. The display of such surface molecules varies with (1) the type of tumor, (2) the individual clone (tumor heterogeneity), (3) the stage of the malignant progression, and (4) the specific step in the metastatic process. Among some of the most important cell adhesion molecules active in the process of invasion are the following:

- **Integrins** directly mediate cell-cell and cell-matrix interactions and indirectly act to promote cell division and migration. They bind to and target matrix metalloproteins (MMPs) such as collagenase, so as to pave the way for metastatic cells (see below).
- **Immunoglobulin supergene family** such as ICAM-1, correlates positively with the aggressiveness of a number of tumor types.

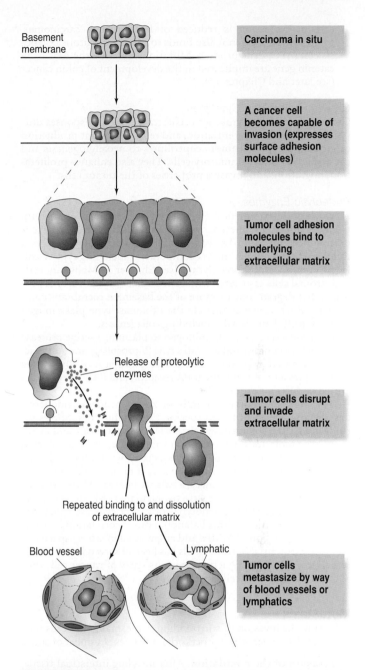

FIGURE 5-11. Mechanisms of tumor invasion and metastasis. The mechanism by which a malignant tumor initially penetrates a confining basement membrane and then invades the surrounding extracellular environment involves several steps. The tumor first acquires the ability to bind components of the extracellular matrix. These interactions are mediated by the expression of a number of adhesion molecules. Proteolytic enzymes are then released from the tumor cells, and the extracellular matrix is degraded. After moving through the extracellular environment, the invading cancer penetrates blood vessels and lymphatics by the same mechanisms.

- **Cadherins** are a family of calcium (Ca^{2+})-dependent, transmembrane, cell–cell adhesion molecules. E-cadherin, is expressed on the surface of all epithelia and mediates cell–cell adhesion by mutual **zipper** interactions. It appears to suppress metastasis, as its expression is lost in most carcinomas, thereby permitting malignant cells to leave the tumor mass.
- **Catenins** are proteins that interact with the intracellular domain of E-cadherin and create a mechanical linkage between that molecule and the cytoskeleton, which is essential for effective epithelial cell interactions Like E-cadherin (above),

catenin expression is reduced or lost in most carcinomas. Interestingly, β-catenin also binds to the adenomatous polyposis coli (APC) gene product. Mutations in either the APC or β-catenin gene are implicated in the development of colon cancer (see later and Chapter 13).

Growth Factors and Cytokines

Growth factors and cytokines orchestrate cellular responses during development, differentiation, and repair. Aberrant production of growth factors by tumors contributes to neoangiogenesis and the attraction of inflammatory cells. They also enhance proliferation, migration, and invasive properties of the tumor cells.

Proteolytic Enzymes

A breach of the basement membrane that separates an epithelium from the underlying mesenchymal compartment is the first event in tumor cell invasion. The basement membrane is composed of a number of extracellular matrix components, including type IV collagen, laminin, and proteoglycans (see Chapter 3). Malignant cells and stromal cells associated with cancers elaborate a variety of proteases that degrade one or more of the basement membrane components. Such enzymes include the urokinase-type plasminogen activator (u-PA) and MMPs, including collagenases.

u-PA converts serum plasminogen to plasmin, a serine protease that degrades laminin and activates type IV procollagenase. u-PA activity is balanced by plasminogen activator inhibitor (PAI); changes in the expression of u-PA, the u-PA receptor, and PAI have been reported in different cancers.

The MMPs comprise a family of zinc-dependent endopeptidases that are susceptible to specific tissue inhibitors. MMPs include interstitial collagenases, stromelysins, gelatinases, and membrane-type molecules. These enzymes are synthesized and secreted by normal cells under conditions associated with physiologic tissue remodeling, such as wound healing and placental implantation. Under these circumstances, a balance between MMPs and tissue inhibitors of MMPs is strictly regulated. By contrast, the invasive and metastatic phenotypes of cancer cells are characterized by dysregulation of this balance. A direct correlation between increased expression of MMPs and augmented invasive capacity or metastatic potential of tumor cells has been observed in many cancers. Deregulated MMP activity permits entry of cancer cells into and through the extracellular matrix.

Metastasis

Following the invasion of surrounding tissue, malignant cells may spread to distant sites by a process that includes a number of steps:

1. **Invasion of the circulation:** After invading interstitial tissue, malignant cells penetrate lymphatic or vascular channels. In lymph nodes, communications between lymphatics and venous tributaries allow the cells access to the systemic circulation. Most tumor cells do not survive their journey in the bloodstream, and less than 0.1% remain to establish a new colony.
2. **Escape from the circulation:** Circulating tumor cells may arrest mechanically in capillaries and venules, where they attach to endothelial cells. This adherence causes retraction of the endothelium, thereby exposing the underlying basement membrane to which tumor cells now bind. Clumps of circulating tumor cells may also arrest in arterioles, where they grow within vascular lumens. In both situations, tumor cells eventually extravasate by mechanisms similar to those responsible for local invasion.
3. **Local growth:** In a hospitable site, the extravasated cancer cells grow in response to autocrine and possibly local growth factors produced by the host tissue. However, a new vascular supply is necessary for the tumor to grow to a diameter greater than 0.5 mm. Thus, many tumors secrete polypeptides (e.g., FGF, VEGF, TGF ß and PDGF), which together trigger and

regulate the process of **angiogenesis** (see below). The metastasis can metastasize again, either within the same organ or to distant sites.

The establishment of a metastatic colony does not mean that it inevitably enlarges. It is well known clinically that tumors may recur locally or at metastatic sites many years after the primary cancer has been surgically removed. For example, patients treated for breast cancer or malignant melanoma may be apparently cured for 20 or more years, only to have the tumor suddenly recur. The molecular basis for this phenomenon, termed **tumor dormancy**, is not well understood.

Target Organs in Metastatic Disease

It was recognized more than a century ago that the distribution of metastases in breast cancer is not random. In 1889, Paget proposed that the spread of tumor cells to specific secondary sites depends on compatibility between the tumor cells (the seed) and favorable microenvironment factors in the secondary site (the soil). By contrast, others have argued that metastatic spread depends solely on anatomical factors and the blood flow to an organ. Today, there is evidence that both mechanisms operate, depending on the tumor. For example, cancers of the breast, prostate, and thyroid metastasize to bone, a tropism that suggests a favored "soil." Conversely, despite their size and abundant blood flow, neither the spleen nor skeletal muscle is a common site of metastases. Yet for many cancers, the vascular anatomy unquestionably influences the pattern of metastatic spread. Malignant tumors of the gastrointestinal tract commonly metastasize to the first capillary bed they encounter, namely the liver. Similarly, lung cancers often spread to the brain. An additional factor that regulates homing of malignant cells may be the expression of complementary adhesion molecules, either by the cancer cells or those of the organ to which they home.

The Grading and Staging of Cancers

In an attempt to predict the clinical behavior of a malignant tumor and to establish criteria for therapy, many cancers are classified according to cytologic and histologic grading schemes or by staging protocols that describe the extent of spread.

Cancer Grading Reflects Cellular Characteristics

Low-grade tumors are **well differentiated**; high-grade ones tend to be **anaplastic** (that is, they lack those differentiated features that indicate the tissue of origin). Cytologic and histologic grading, which are necessarily subjective and at best semiquantitative, are based on the degree of anaplasia and on the number of proliferating cells. The degree of anaplasia is determined from the shape and regularity of the cells and from the presence of distinct differentiated features, such as functioning glandlike structures in adenocarcinomas or epithelial pearls in squamous carcinomas. The presence of such characteristics identify a tumor as well differentiated. By contrast, the cells of "poorly differentiated" malignancies bear little resemblance to their normal counterparts. Evidence of rapid or abnormal growth is provided by (1) large numbers of mitoses, (2) atypical mitoses, (3) nuclear pleomorphism, and (4) tumor giant cells. Most grading schemes classify tumors into three or four grades of increasing malignancy. The general correlation between the cytologic grade and the biological behavior of a neoplasm is not invariable: There are many examples of tumors of low cytologic grades that exhibit substantial malignant properties.

Cancer Staging Refers to the Extent of Spread

The choice of a surgical approach or the selection of treatment modalities is influenced more by the stage of a cancer than by its cytologic grade. Moreover, most statistical data related to cancer survival are based on the stage rather than the cytologic grade of the tumor. Clinical staging is independent of cytologic grading. The significant criteria used for staging vary with different organs. Commonly used criteria include:

- Tumor size
- Extent of local growth, whether within or without the organ
- Presence of lymph node metastases
- Presence of distant metastases

These criteria have been codified in the international **TNM cancer staging system**, in which "T" refers to the size of the primary tumor, "N" to regional node metastases, and "M" to the presence and extent of distant metastases. The definitions of numerical scores for T, N, and M (e.g., T1–T4, N1–N3) vary according to specific tumor types.

Tumor size and degree of local spread influence prognosis and therapy. For instance, a primary breast cancer smaller than 2 cm in diameter can be treated with local excision and radiation therapy; larger masses often necessitate mastectomy. The Duke's classification of colorectal cancer penetration of the tumor into the muscularis and serosa of the bowel is associated with a poorer prognosis than that of a more superficial tumor. Clearly, the presence of lymph node metastases mandates more aggressive treatment than does their absence, whereas the presence of distant metastases is generally a contraindication to surgical intervention other than for palliation.

The Clonal Origin of Cancer

Studies of human and experimental tumors have provided strong evidence that most cancers arise from a single transformed cell. This theory has been most thoroughly examined in connection with proliferative disorders of the hematopoietic system. Cell surface markers have been used to establish a monoclonal origin for many hematopoietic malignant disorders. For example, B-cell lymphomas are composed of cells that exclusively display either κ or λ light chains on their surface, whereas polyclonal lymphoid proliferations exhibit both types of cells. Monoclonality has also been demonstrated in the individual metastases of a number of solid tumors. An early observation in regard to the monoclonal origin of cancer was derived from the study of glucose-6-phosphate dehydrogenase in women who were heterozygous for its two isozymes, A and B (Fig. 5-12). These isozymes are encoded by genes located on the X chromosome. Because one X chromosome is randomly inactivated, only one of these genes is expressed in any given cell. Thus, although the genotypes of all cells are the same, their phenotypes vary with regard to the expression of isozyme A or B. An examination of benign uterine smooth muscle tumors (leiomyomas, or "fibroids") revealed that all the cells in an individual tumor expressed either A or B but not both, indicating that each tumor was derived from a single progenitor cell.

The Growth of Cancers

Historically, cancer was considered to result from a totally unregulated growth of cells, and a logical corollary was that neoplastic cells divide at a faster rate than normal ones. *It is now clear that tumor cells do not necessarily proliferate more rapidly than their normal counterparts.* Tumor growth depends on other factors, such as the growth fraction (proportion of cycling cells) and the rate of cell death. In normal proliferating tissues (e.g., intestine and bone marrow), an exquisite balance between cell renewal and cell death is strictly maintained. *By contrast, the major determinant of tumor growth is clearly the fact that more cells are produced than die in a given time.* Such an effect can reflect either an excess of cell proliferation

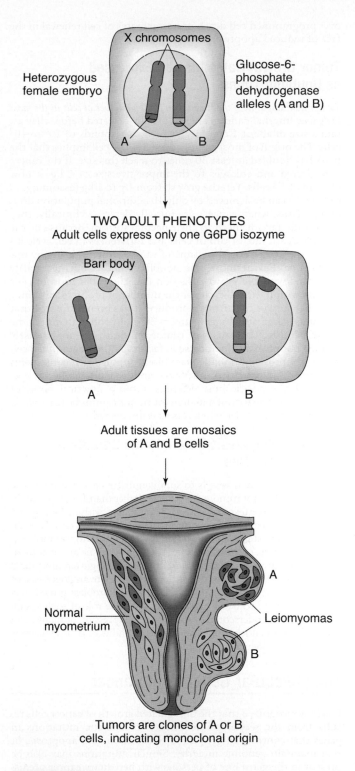

FIGURE 5-12. **Monoclonal origin of human tumors.** Some females are heterozygous for the two alleles of glucose-6-phosphate dehydrogenase (G6PD) on the long arm of the X chromosome. Early in embryogenesis, one of the X chromosomes is randomly inactivated in every somatic cell and appears cytologically as a Barr body attached to the nuclear membrane. As a result, the tissues are a mosaic of cells that express either the A or the B isozyme of G6PD. Leiomyomas of the uterus have been shown to contain one or the other isozyme (A or B) but not both, a finding that demonstrates the monoclonal origin of the tumors.

over programmed cell death or normal rates of cell renewal in the face of reduced apoptosis.

Tumor Growth Rates May be Expressed as Doubling Times

Tumor doubling time is the time taken for the number of cells in the mass to double. Internal cancers are not usually detected before they attain a size of about 1 cm³ (1 g), which corresponds to 10^8 to 10^9 cells. The origin of most tumors from a single cell implies that the mass has doubled at least 30 times to reach this size. If the cancer is neglected and enlarges to the impressive size of 1 kg, it now contains 10^{12} cells. Yet, the growth from 1 g to 1 kg (assuming no cell death) can be achieved by only 10 additional population doublings. Thus, when cancers are initially detected clinically, they are already far advanced in their natural history. Because of the variable death rate of tumor cells and differences in cell cycle kinetics, the actual doubling time of human tumors is highly unpredictable. Furthermore, the doubling time is not necessarily correlated with the growth fraction (i.e., the proportion of cells that are within the cell cycle) or the number of proliferated tumor cells that survive to further reproduce. It has been estimated that in human skin tumors, as many as 97% of proliferated cells die spontaneously. The causes of tumor cell death are not precisely defined but probably include such factors as (1) programmed cell death (apoptosis), (2) inadequate blood supply, with consequent ischemia, (3) a paucity of nutrients, and (4) vulnerability to specific and nonspecific host defenses. From a practical point of view, the prior history of a malignant tumor cannot be reasonably estimated from its size when it is first discovered.

Tumor Angiogenesis Refers to the Sprouting of New Capillaries

In the absence of new vessels to supply nutrients and remove waste products, malignant tumors do not grow larger than 1 to 2 mm in diameter. In this context, the density of capillaries within the primary tumor (e.g., cancers of the breast, prostate, and colon) correlates directly with metastases and decreased host survival. Importantly, tumor angiogenesis occurs in non-neoplastic host tissue and is comparable to that in wound healing and other physiologic circumstances (see Chapter 3). A number of factors can stimulate angiogenesis, of which vascular endothelial growth factor and fibroblast growth factor-2 are thought to be the most important. The role of such angiogenic factors is underscored by the growth suppression of many solid tumors by both endogenous and synthetic inhibitors of angiogenesis factors, some of which are in clinical use.

The Molecular Genetics of Cancer

It is now recognized that the unregulated growth of cancer cells results from the sequential acquisition of somatic mutations in genes that control cell growth, differentiation, and apoptosis, or that maintain genomic integrity. Similar mutations may also be present in the germ line of persons with hereditary cancer predispositions. Mutations can be produced by environmental mutagens such as chemical carcinogens or radiation (see below). They can also arise during normal cellular metabolism, particularly from the formation of activated oxygen species (see Chapter 1).

It is likely that the most common mechanism of mutagenesis relates to spontaneous errors in DNA replication and repair. Assuming a mutation rate of about 2.5×10^{-8} per nucleotide, it has been estimated that humans acquire about 175 mutations per generation. Thus, it is inevitable that everyone is a somatic mosaic at many genetic loci. If the mutation involves genes that control growth or stabilize the genome, it may give rise to a clone of cells that possess a growth advantage over their normal neighbors. Successive mutations in similar genes result in increasingly aberrant clones until a malignant phenotype eventually emerges.

In a sense, the emergence of malignancy may be viewed as an evolutionary process wherein we see only the surviving clones.

Transformed Cells Share Common Attributes

Cancer cells are remarkably heterogeneous in appearance, growth rate, invasiveness, and metastatic potential, presumably due to the interplay between diverse acquired mutations and the inherent gene expression of specific cell lineages. Nevertheless, transformed cells share certain biological features. The disruption of a limited number of regulatory pathways (involving about 4 to 7 mutated genes, or more) leads to deregulation of cell proliferation and suppression of apoptosis, and confers a neoplastic phenotype to diverse cell types This **is a multistep** process, which takes place over a period of years. The process involves:

- Autonomous generation of mitogenic signals
- Insensitivity to exogenous antigrowth signals
- Resistance to apoptosis
- Limitless replicative potential (immortalization)
- Blocked differentiation
- Ability to sustain angiogenesis
- Capacity to invade surrounding tissues
- Potential to metastasize

The normal genes that are mutated in various cancers, include cell cycle regulators, signal transduction factors, transcriptional factors, DNA-binding proteins, growth factor receptors, adhesion molecules, effectors of apoptosis, and telomerase. Such "transforming genes" can be grouped into three categories:

- **Oncogenes** are altered versions of normal genes, termed **protooncogenes**, which regulate normal cell growth, differentiation, and survival. Gain-of-function (dominant) mutations **activate** protooncogenes to become oncogenes. Such mutated genes are **positive effectors** of the neoplastic phenotype.
- **Tumor suppressor genes** are normal genes with products that inhibit cellular proliferation. Loss-of-function (recessive) mutations **inactivate** the normal inhibitory activities of tumor suppressor genes. By permitting unregulated cell growth, tumor suppressor genes serve as **negative effectors** of the neoplastic phenotype.
- **Mutator genes (DNA mismatch repair genes)** normally maintain the integrity of the genome and the fidelity of DNA replication. Inactivating mutations of these genes allows the successive accumulation of further mutations.

Oncogenes are Counterparts of Normal Genes

The transfer of specific genes (**oncogenes**) from human tumor cells into rodent cells by viral vectors in vitro can transform the recipient cells. The transforming genes were discovered to be mutant versions of normal genes involved in growth regulation and were termed **protooncogenes**. Transforming viral oncogenes were termed v-*onc* genes, and their cellular counterparts (c-) were individual normal genes (e.g., c-*myc*, c-*jun*, c-*src*).

Mechanisms of Activation of Cellular Oncogenes

There are three general mechanisms by which protooncogene activation is accomplished:

- An activating mutation of a protooncogene leads to the **constitutive** (dysregulated) production of an abnormal protein. The mutations may involve (1) point mutations, (2) deletions, or (3) chromosomal translocations.
- An increase in the expression of the protooncogene may cause overproduction of a normal gene product.
- The activation of protooncogenes is regulated by numerous autoinhibitory mechanisms, which operate as a safeguard against inappropriate activity. Thus, many mutations in protooncogenes lead to **resistance** to normal autoinhibitory and regulatory constraints.

Activation by Mutation

Activating, or gain-of-function, mutations in protooncogenes are usually somatic rather than germline alterations. Germline mutations in protooncogenes, which are known to be important regulators of growth during development, are ordinarily lethal in utero. There are several exceptions to this rule. For example, c-ret is incriminated in the pathogenesis of certain heritable endocrine cancers, and c-met, which encodes the receptor for hepatocyte growth factor, is associated with a hereditary form of renal cancer.

Activation by Chromosomal Translocation

Chromosomal translocations (i.e., the transfer of a portion of one chromosome to another) have been implicated in the pathogenesis of several human leukemias and lymphomas (See Chapter 20). The first and still the best-known example of an acquired chromosomal translocation in a human cancer is the **Philadelphia chromosome**, which is found in 95% of patients with chronic myelogenous leukemia (Fig. 5-13A,B). The translocation activates the c-abl protooncogene (a nonreceptor protein kinase) by the formation of an aberrant fusion protein. The resultant BCR/ABL oncogene has very high tyrosine kinase activity, which generates mitogenic and antiapoptotic signals. In Burkitt lymphoma (Fig. 5-13C) the c-myc protooncogene involved in cell cycle progression is translocated next to genes that control transcription of immunoglobulin light or heavy chains, thereby leading to the overproduction of a normal product. The excessive amount of the normal c-myc product, probably in association with other genetic alterations, promotes the emergence of a dominant clone of B cells, driven relentlessly to proliferate as a monoclonal neoplasm. Although the above malignant conditions are **initiated** by chromosomal translocations, during the **progression** of many cancers, myriad chromosomal abnormalities take place (translocations, breaks, aneuploidy, etc.).

Activation by Gene Amplification

Chromosomal alterations that result in an increased number of gene copies (i.e., gene amplification) have been found primarily in human solid tumors. The erb B protooncogene is amplified in up to one third of breast and ovarian cancers. The erb B2 gene (also designated HER2/neu) encodes a receptor-type tyrosine kinase that shows close structural similarity to the EGF receptor. Amplification of erb B2 in breast and ovarian cancer may be associated with poor overall survival and decreased time to relapse. In this context, an antibody targeted against HER2/neu (trastuzumab) is now used as adjunctive therapy for breast cancers that overexpress this protein.

Mechanisms of Oncogene Action

Oncogenes can be classified according to the roles of their normal counterparts (protooncogenes) in the biochemical pathways that regulate growth and differentiation. These include the following (Fig. 5-14):

- Growth factors
- Cell surface receptors
- Intracellular signal transduction pathways
- DNA-binding nuclear proteins (transcription factors)
- Cell cycle proteins (cyclins and cyclin-dependent protein kinases)
- Inhibitors of apoptosis (bcl-2)

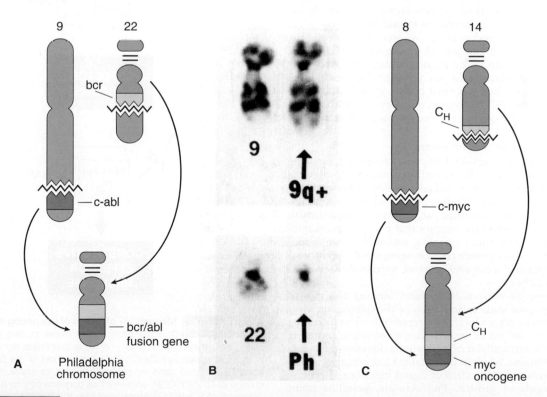

FIGURE 5-13. **Oncogene activation by chromosomal translocation. A.** Chronic myelogenous leukemia. Breaks at the ends of the long arms of chromosomes 9 and 22 allow reciprocal translocations to occur. The c-abl protooncogene on chromosome 9 is translocated to the breakpoint region (bcr) of chromosome 22. The result is the Philadelphia chromosome (Ph¹), which contains a new fusion gene coding for a hybrid oncogenic protein (bcr-abl), presumably involved in the pathogenesis of chronic myelogenous leukemia. **B.** Karyotypes of a patient with chronic myelogenous leukemia showing the results of reciprocal translocations between chromosomes 9 and 22. The Philadelphia chromosome is recognized by a smaller-than-normal chromosome 22 (22q–). One chromosome 9 (9q+) is larger than its normal counterpart. **C.** Burkitt lymphoma. In this disorder, chromosomal breaks involve the long arms of chromosomes 8 and 14. The c-myc gene on chromosome 8 is translocated to a region on chromosome 14 adjacent to the gene coding for the constant region of an immunoglobulin heavy chain (C_H). The expression of c-myc is enhanced by its association with the promoter/enhancer regions of the actively transcribed immunoglobulin genes.

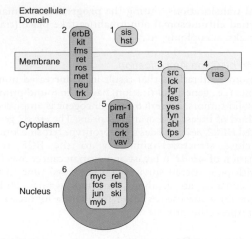

FIGURE 5-14. Cellular compartments in which oncogene or protooncogene products reside. *(1)* Growth factors, *(2)* transmembrane growth factor receptors (tyrosine kinase), *(3)* membrane-associated kinases, *(4) ras* GTPase family, *(5)* cytoplasmic kinases, *(6)* nuclear transcriptional regulators. GTP, guanosine triphosphate.

Oncogenes and Growth Factors

The binding of soluble extracellular growth factors to their specific surface receptors initiates signaling cascades that eventuate in entry of the cell into the mitotic cycle. A few protooncogenes encode growth factors that stimulate tumor cell growth. In some instances, a growth factor acts upon the same cell that produces it (**autocrine stimulation**). Other growth factors act upon the receptors of neighboring cells (**paracrine stimulation**).

PDGF is the protein product of the *c-sis* protooncogene and is a potent mitogen for fibroblasts, smooth muscle cells, and glial cells. Cells derived from human sarcomas and glioblastomas (malignant glial cell tumors) produce PDGF-like polypeptides; their normal counterparts do not. Thus, a normal human gene (*c-sis*) that encodes a growth factor (PDGF) acquires transforming capacity when it is constitutively expressed in a cell that responds to this signal.

Oncogenes and Growth Factor Receptors

The regulation of the functional responses to growth factors—including cell proliferation, differentiation, and survival—depends principally on the expression of, and relative balance between, various growth factor receptors. Binding of a ligand to the extracellular domain of its receptor stimulates an intrinsic kinase activity in the cytoplasmic domain of the receptor that phosphorylates tyrosine residues on intracellular signaling molecules. *Thus, because growth factor receptors can generate potent mitogenic signals, they harbor a latent oncogenic potential, which when activated, overrides the normal controls of signaling pathways.*

Under normal circumstances, transient binding of a growth factor to its receptor leads to activation of the cytoplasmic tyrosine kinase domain, after which the receptor reverts to its resting state. Certain mutations of growth factor receptors, including truncation of the extracellular or intracellular domains, point mutations, and deletions, result in unrestrained (constitutive) activation of the receptor, independent of ligand binding and promotion of dysregulated growth. For example, germline point mutations in *c-ret* lead to constitutive activation of the receptor and are associated with multiple endocrine neoplasia syndromes and familial medullary thyroid carcinoma (see Chapter 21).

Ras Oncogenes

Activation of ras genes (Ha-ras, Ki-ras, or N-ras) is the most frequent dominant mutation in human cancers. Ras is an effector molecule in the signal transduction cascade that couples the activation of growth factor receptors to changes in nuclear gene transcription. The *ras*

protooncogene codes for a product, p21, that belongs to a family of small cytoplasmic proteins (G proteins) that bind guanosine triphosphate (GTP) and guanosine diphosphate (GDP) (Fig. 5-15). The protein p21 is active when it binds GTP. Bound GTP is converted to GDP by the intrinsic GTPase of p21, an activity that is stimulated by a GTPase-activating protein (GAP). The intrinsic GTPase activity is the "off" switch for the molecule. Point mutations of ras, which either directly reduce p21 GTPase activity or render it resistant to GAP, result in uncontrolled stimulation of *ras*-related functions, because p21 is locked in the "on" position.

Oncogenes and Nuclear Regulatory Proteins

A number of nuclear proteins encoded by protooncogenes are intimately involved in the sequential expression of genes that regulate cellular proliferation and differentiation. Many of these proteins can bind to DNA, where they regulate the expression of other

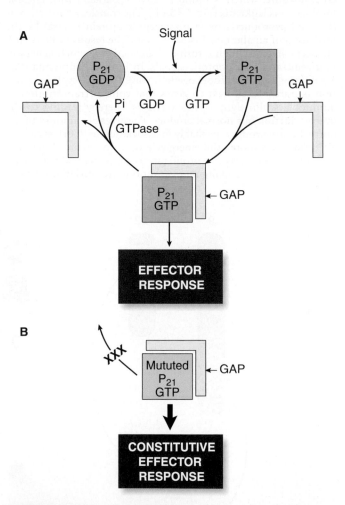

FIGURE 5-15. Mechanism of action of ras oncogene. **A.** Normal. The ras protein p21 exists in two conformational states, determined by the binding of either guanosine diphosphate (GDP) or guanosine triphosphate (GTP). Normally, most of the p21 is in the inactive GDP-bound state. An external stimulus, or signal, triggers the exchange of GTP for GDP, an event that converts p21 to the active state. Activated p21, which is associated with the plasma membrane, binds GTPase-activating protein (GAP) from the cytosol. The binding of GAP has two consequences. In association with other plasma membrane constituents, it initiates the effector response. At the same time, the binding of GAP to p21 GTP stimulates by about 100-fold the intrinsic GTPase activity of p21, thereby promoting the hydrolysis of GTP to GDP and the return of p21 to its inactive state. **B.** Mutated ras protein is locked into the active GTP-bound state because of an insensitivity of its intrinsic GTPase to GAP or because of a lack of the GTPase activity itself. As a result, the effector response is exaggerated, and the cell is transformed.

genes. The transitory expression of several protooncogenes is necessary for the cells to pass through specific points in the cell cycle. Protooncogenes that are expressed early in the cell cycle (such as c-myc, c-fos and c-jun) render the cells competent to receive the final signals for mitosis and are, therefore, termed **competence genes**. In general, competence genes play a role in (1) progression from the G_1 to the S phase in the cell cycle, (2) stability of the genome, (3) apoptosis, and (4) positive or negative effects on cellular maturation. However, the cells are not yet fully programmed to divide after the expression of these genes and will enter the S phase and mitosis only after further stimulation by other factors, such as EGF or IGF-I (**progression factors**).

Bcl-2 and Apoptosis

Normal tissue requires an exquisite balance between cell proliferation and cell death mediated by apoptosis (see Chapter 1). The most prominent example of suppression of apoptosis in a tumor cell is the upregulation of the antiapoptotic protein bcl-2 in B-cell neoplasia. Bcl-2 and its family regulate the permeability of mitochondrial membranes. Bcl-2 itself exerts an antiapoptotic effect by preventing the release of cytochrome c, thereby protecting the cell from the mitochondrial apoptotic pathway. Follicular B-cell lymphomas (see Chapter 20) display a characteristic chromosomal translocation, t(14;18), in which the *bcl*-2 gene on chromosome 18 is brought under the transcriptional control of the immunoglobulin light-chain gene promoter, thereby causing overexpression of *bcl*-2. As a result of the antiapoptotic properties of bcl-2, the neoplastic clone accumulates in the affected lymph nodes.

Tumor Suppressor Genes Negatively Regulate Cell Growth

A second general mechanism by which a genetic alteration contributes to carcinogenesis is a mutation that creates a deficiency of a normal gene product (**tumor suppressors** or **"gate keepers"**) that exerts a negative regulatory control of cell growth and thereby suppresses tumor formation (**"loss of function mutations"**). Such genes encode *negative* transcriptional regulators of the cell cycle, signal-transducing molecules, and cell surface receptors.

Because both alleles of tumor suppressor genes must be inactivated to produce the deficit that allows the development of a tumor, the normal suppressor gene is functionally dominant. In this circumstance, the heterozygous state is sufficient to protect against cancer. **Loss of heterozygosity** in a tumor suppressor gene by deletion or somatic mutation of the remaining normal allele predisposes to tumor development.

The Role of Tumor Suppressor Genes in Carcinogenesis

Tumor suppressor genes are increasingly being incriminated in the pathogenesis of both hereditary and spontaneous cancers in humans. Two such genes have been particularly well studied. The Rb and p53 gene products serve to restrain cell division in many tissues, and their absence or inactivation is linked to the development of malignant tumors. In this context, oncogenic DNA viruses encode products that interact with these suppressor proteins, thereby inactivating their functions. *Thus, the mechanisms underlying the development of some tumors associated with germline and somatic mutations and infections with DNA viruses involve the same cellular gene products.*

Retinoblastoma Gene

Retinoblastoma, a rare childhood cancer, is the prototype of a human tumor in which the origin is attributed to the inactivation of a specific tumor suppressor gene (the Rb gene) located on the long arm of chromosome 13. About 40% of cases are associated with a germline mutation; the remainder are sporadic. In sporadic cases of retinoblastoma, the child begins life with two normal *Rb* alleles in all somatic cells, but both are inactivated by somatic mutations

in the retina. Because somatic mutations in the *Rb* gene are uncommon, the incidence of sporadic retinoblastoma is very low (1/30,000).

In patients with *hereditary* retinoblastoma, all somatic cells carry one missing or mutated allele of the *Rb* gene. This heterozygous state is not associated with any observable changes in the retina, presumably because 50% of the *Rb* gene product is sufficient to prevent the development of disease. If the remaining normal *Rb* allele is inactivated by deletion or mutation (loss of heterozygosity), the absence of the Rb gene product allows the appearance of a retinoblastoma, in which both alleles of the *Rb* gene are inactive in all tumor cells. Thus, the *Rb* gene exerts a tumor suppressor function, and the development of hereditary retinoblastoma is associated with two genetic events (Knudson's "two-hit" hypothesis) (Fig. 5-16). Children who inherit a mutant *Rb* gene also suffer a 200-fold increased risk of developing mesenchymal tumors in early adult life. More than 20 different cancers have been described, with osteosarcoma being by far the most common. Chromosomal analysis has demonstrated abnormalities of the *Rb* locus in 70% of cases of osteosarcoma and in many instances of small cell lung cancer, carcinomas of the breast, bladder, pancreas, and other human tumors.

The function of Rb genes is at the most critical checkpoint in the cell cycle, and **inactivating** mutations in Rb genes permits unregulated cell proliferation by allowing cells to escape the G_1 restriction (R) checkpoint and proceed to G_1–S phase transition. In addition, certain products of human DNA viruses (e.g., human papillomavirus [HPV]) inactivate Rb by binding to it, thereby leading to dysregulated cell growth.

The p53 Gene Family

The *p53* tumor suppressor gene is a principal mediator of growth arrest, senescence, and apoptosis. Therefore, loss of p53 function is, not unexpectedly, associated with cancer. In response to DNA damage, oncogenic activation of other proteins, and other stresses (e.g., hypoxia), p53 levels rise. Increased p53 levels enhance the synthesis of cyclin–dependent kinase inhibitors and the inactivation of cyclin-dependent kinase (CDK) complexes, thereby leading to cell arrest at the G_1/S checkpoint. Hence, cells are prevented from entering the S phase of the cell cycle. Such arrested cells may repair DNA damage or undergo apoptosis. In this manner, p53 acts as a "guardian of the genome" by restricting uncontrolled cellular proliferation under circumstances in which cells with abnormal DNA might propagate.

The *p53* gene is located on the small arm of chromosome 17, and its protein product is present in virtually all normal tissues. This gene is deleted or mutated in 75% of cases of colorectal cancer and frequently in breast cancer, small cell carcinoma of the lung, hepatocellular carcinoma, astrocytoma, and numerous other tumors. *In fact, mutations of p53 seem to be the most common genetic change in human cancer.* Many human cancers exhibit deletion of both *p53* alleles, in which case the cell contains no *p53* gene product. By contrast, in some cancers, the malignant cells express one normal *p53* allele and one mutant version. In these cases, the mutant p53 protein forms complexes with the normal p53 protein and inactivates the function of the normal suppressor gene. When a mutant allele inactivates the normal one, the mutant allele is said be a **dominant negative** gene. Theoretically, a cell containing one mutant *p53* allele (i.e., a heterozygote) might have a growth advantage over normal cells, a situation that would increase the number of cells at risk for a second mutation (loss of heterozygosity) and the development of cancer.

Li-Fraumeni syndrome refers to an inherited predisposition to develop cancers in many organs due to germline mutations of p53. Persons with this condition carry germline mutations in one *p53* allele, but their tumors display mutations at both alleles. This situation is similar to that determining inherited retinoblastoma and is another example of the two-hit hypothesis (see Fig. 5-16) and loss of heterozygosity.

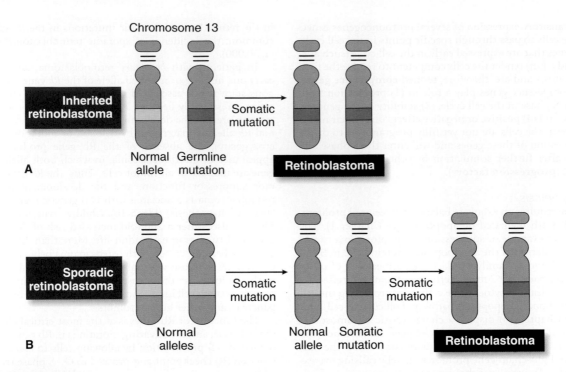

FIGURE 5-16. **The "two-hit" origin of retinoblastoma. A.** A child with the inherited form of retinoblastoma is born with a germline mutation in one allele of the retinoblastoma gene located on the long arm of chromosome 13. A second somatic mutation in the retina leads to the inactivation of the functioning *Rb* allele and the subsequent development of a retinoblastoma. **B.** In sporadic cases of retinoblastoma, the child is born with two normal *Rb* alleles. It requires two independent somatic mutations to inactivate *Rb* gene function and allow the appearance of a neoplastic clone.

Other Tumor Suppressor Genes

A number of unrelated syndromes have now been shown to result from germline mutations in various tumor suppressor genes. For example, the APC gene is implicated in the pathogenesis of familial adenomatous polyposis coli and most sporadic colorectal cancers (see Chapter 13). The *APC* gene product binds to and inhibits the function of β-catenin (see above), Mutations in both *APC* and β-catenin genes have also been described in other malignant tumors, including malignant melanoma and ovarian cancer. Hereditary Wilms tumor, neurofibromatosis type 1, von Hippel-Lindau syndrome (associated with renal cell carcinoma), hemangioblastoma of the brain, and pheochromocytoma are all associated with germline mutations of genes with tumor suppressor functions.

Tumor Suppressor Genes and Oncogenic DNA Viruses

Unlike RNA tumor viruses whose oncogenes have normal cellular counterparts, the transforming genes of DNA viruses are not homologous with any cellular genes. *The gene products of oncogenic DNA viruses lead to the inactivation of tumor suppressor proteins.* This phenomenon is analogous to the ability of mutant tumor suppressor proteins to inhibit their normal counterparts. For example, the binding of an HPV protein to p53 accelerates the degradation of the latter protein. The transforming proteins of polyoma viruses (including SV40), adenoviruses, HPVs, and human herpes virus (HHV)-8 also bind and inactivate Rb. These observations indicate that oncogenic DNA viruses use common mechanisms for altering growth regulation and, thereby, transforming cells.

DNA Repair Genes Protect the Integrity of the Genome

The third class of genes in which mutations contribute to the pathogenesis of cancer are those involved in DNA mismatch repair, so-called **mutator genes** or **caretaker genes**. The loss of these gene functions renders the DNA susceptible to the progres-sive accumulation of mutations; when these affect protoonco-genes or tumor suppressor genes, cancer may result. A number of syndromes demonstrating a familial predisposition to cancer have been associated with mutations in genes involved in DNA repair. For example, hereditary nonpolyposis colon cancer (or Lynch syndrome) reflects a familial predisposition to the development of colorectal cancer (not associated with APC), which accounts for about 5% of the disease (see Chapter 13). Patients are heterozygous for one of five genes involved in DNA mismatch repair. Tumors have lost the function of both alleles and demonstrate microsatel-lite instability associated with uncorrected nucleotide mispairing. Several other syndromes with cancer susceptibility, including ataxia telangiectasia, xeroderma pigmentosum, and Bloom syndrome, all demonstrate an increased risk of cancer related to mutations in genes involved in DNA repair.

Telomerase is Activated in Most Cancers

As cells in tissue culture continue to divide, the tips of the chromosomes, termed **telomeres**, progressively shorten (see Chapter 1). Somatic cells do not normally express telomerase, an enzyme that recognizes the end of a chromosome and adds repetitive telomeric sequences to maintain telomere length. Most human cancers show activation of the gene for the catalytic subunit of telomerase, namely human telomerase reverse transcriptase. Telomerase is not classified as an oncogene because it does not lead to growth deregulation. Many immortalized cell lines that express telomerase show no evidence of neoplastic capacity. Thus, despite extensive research in the field, the role of telomerase in oncogenesis remains controversial.

Viruses and Human Cancer

Despite the existence of viral oncogenes, the number of human cancers definitely associated with viral infections is limited.

Nevertheless, it is estimated that viral infections are responsible for some 15% of all human cancers. The strongest associations between the presence of viruses and the development of cancer in humans are:

- Human T-cell leukemia virus type I (HTLV-I) (RNA retrovirus) and T-cell leukemia/lymphoma
- HPV (**DNA virus**) and carcinoma of the cervix
- Hepatitis B virus (HBV) (**DNA virus**) and hepatitis C virus (**RNA**) and primary hepatocellular carcinoma
- Epstein-Barr virus (EBV) (**DNA virus**) and certain forms of lymphoma and nasopharyngeal carcinoma
- HHV 8 (DNA virus) and Kaposi sarcoma.

Worldwide, infections with hepatitis B and C viruses and HPVs alone account for 80% of all virus-associated cancers.

Human T-Cell Leukemia Virus-I (HTLV-I) is a Lymphotropic Agent

The one human cancer that has been firmly linked to infection with an RNA retrovirus is adult T-cell leukemia, which is endemic in southern Japan as well as the Caribbean basin and occurs sporadically in other parts of the world. The etiological agent, HTLV-I, is tropic for CD4$^+$ T lymphocytes and has also been incriminated in the pathogenesis of a number of neurologic disorders. It is estimated that leukemia develops in less than 5% of persons infected with HTLV-I and exhibits a latency period on the order of 40 years for its development. Oncogenic stimulation by HTLV-I is mediated principally by the viral transcriptional activation protein *tax*. Tax protein not only increases the transcription from its own viral genome, but it also promotes the activity of other genes involved in host cell proliferation.

DNA Viruses Encode Proteins that Bind Regulatory Proteins

Four DNA viruses (HPV, EBV, HBV, and HHV 8) are incriminated in the development of human cancers. The transforming genes of oncogenic DNA viruses exhibit virtually no homology with cellular genes, whereas those of RNA retroviruses (oncogenes) are derived from, and are homologous with, their cellular counterparts (protooncogenes). As discussed above, oncogenic DNA viruses have genes that encode protein products that bind to, and inactivate, specific host proteins (the products of tumor suppressor genes, e.g., *Rb, p53*) involved in the regulation of cell proliferation and apoptosis.

Human Papilloma Viruses (HPVs)

HPVs induce lesions in humans that progress to squamous cell carcinoma. Papillomaviruses manifest a pronounced tropism for epithelial tissues, and their full productive life cycle occurs only in squamous cells. At least 20 HPV types are associated with cancer of the uterine cervix, especially HPV 16 and 18 (see Chapter 18).The major oncoproteins encoded by HPV are E6 and E7. E6 binds to p53 and targets it for degradation. E7 binds to Rb, thereby releasing its inhibitory effect on cell cycle progression.

Epstein-Barr Virus (EBV)

EBV is a human herpesvirus that is so widely disseminated that 95% of adults in the world have antibodies against it. EBV infects B lymphocytes, transforming them into lymphoblasts with an indefinite lifespan. In a small proportion of primary infections with EBV, this lymphoblastoid transformation is manifested as infectious mononucleosis (see Chapter 9), a short-lived lymphoproliferative disease. However, EBV is also intimately associated with the development of certain human cancers.

When B lymphocytes are infected with EBV, they acquire the ability to proliferate indefinitely in vitro. A number of EBV genes are implicated in this lymphocyte immortalization, including Epstein-Barr nuclear antigens (EBNAs) and latent-infection—associated membrane proteins (LMPs). The EBNAs maintain the EBV genome in its episomal state and activate the transcription of viral and cellular genes. LMP1 interacts with cellular proteins that normally transduce signals from the TNF receptor, a critical pathway in lymphocyte activation and proliferation. *Both EBNAs and LMPs can be demonstrated in most EBV-associated cancers. These include the following:*

Burkitt Lymphoma

African Burkitt lymphoma is a B-cell tumor, in which the neoplastic lymphocytes invariably contain EBV in their DNA and manifest EBV-related antigens (see Chapter 20). The tumor has also been recognized in non-African populations, but in those cases, only about 20% contain the EBV genome. The localization of Burkitt lymphoma to equatorial Africa is not understood, but it has been suggested that prolonged stimulation of the immune system by endemic malaria may be important. As discussed above, lymphoma production in African Burkitt lymphoma is associated with a chromosomal translocation, in which the c-*myc* protooncogene is deregulated by being brought into proximity with an immunoglobulin promoter region. Ultimately, this leads to uncontrolled proliferation of a malignant clone of B lymphocytes.

Polyclonal Lymphoproliferation in Immunodeficient States

Congenital or acquired immunodeficiency states can be complicated by the development of EBV-induced, B-cell proliferative disorders. These lesions may be clinically and pathologically indistinguishable from true malignant lymphomas, but they differ in that most of them are polyclonal. The incidence of lymphoid neoplasia in immunosuppressed renal transplant recipients is 30 to 50 times that of the general population. In virtually all cases of lymphoproliferations associated with organ transplantation, EBNA or EBV genomic material is present in the neoplastic tissue. Similar B-cell lymphoproliferative disorders are seen in a number of other acquired immunodeficiencies, notably, AIDS.

Nasopharyngeal Carcinoma

Nasopharyngeal carcinoma is a variant of squamous cell carcinoma that has a worldwide distribution and is particularly common in certain parts of Africa and Asia. EBV DNA and EBNA are present in virtually all of these cancers. The pathogenesis of nasopharyngeal carcinoma may be related to infection with EBV in early childhood, with reactivation at 40 to 50 years of age and the appearance of tumors 1 to 2 years thereafter. Fortunately, 70% of patients with this disease are cured by radiation therapy alone.

Hepatitis B and C Viruses

Epidemiologic studies have established a strong association between chronic infection with HBV and hepatitis C virus (chronic hepatitis and cirrhosis) and the development of primary hepatocellular carcinoma (see Chapter 14). Two mechanisms have been invoked to explain the mechanism of carcinogenesis in virus-related liver cancer. One theory holds that the continued liver cell proliferation that accompanies chronic liver injury eventually leads to malignant transformation.. A second theory implicates a virally encoded protein (the HBx gene product, which inactivates p53) in the pathogenesis of HBV-induced liver cancer. The underlying mechanisms in HBV-induced carcinogenesis are still controversial and require further investigation.

HHV 8

Kaposi sarcoma is a vascular neoplasm that was originally described in eastern European elderly men and later in central African blacks (see Chapter 10). Kaposi sarcoma is today the most common neoplasm associated with AIDS. The neoplastic cells contain sequences of a novel herpesvirus, HHV 8. Interestingly, HHV 8 has also been demonstrated in specimens of Kaposi sarcoma from HIV-negative patients. Like other DNA viruses, the viral genome encodes proteins that interfere with the p53 and Rb tumor suppressor pathways.

Chemical Carcinogenesis

The field of chemical carcinogenesis originated about two centuries ago in descriptions of an occupational disease. The English physician Sir Percival Pott gets credit for relating cancer of the scrotum in chimney sweeps to a specific chemical exposure, namely, soot. Today, we realize that other products of the combustion of organic materials are responsible for a man-made epidemic of cancer, namely, lung cancer in cigarette smokers.

The experimental production of cancer by chemicals dates to 1915, when Japanese investigators produced skin cancers in rabbits with coal tar. Since that time, the list of organic and inorganic carcinogens has grown exponentially. Yet a curious paradox existed for many years. Many compounds known to be potent carcinogens are relatively inert in terms of chemical reactivity. *The solution to this riddle became apparent in the early 1960s, when it was shown that most, although not all, chemical carcinogens require metabolic activation before they can react with cell constituents.* On the basis of those observations and the close correlation between mutagenicity and carcinogenicity, an in vitro assay using *Salmonella* organisms for screening potential chemical carcinogens—the Ames test—was developed a decade later. Subsequently, a variety of genotoxicity assays have been developed and are still used to screen chemicals and new drugs for potential carcinogenicity.

Chemical Carcinogens are Mostly Mutagens

A *mutagen* is an agent that can permanently alter the genetic constitution of a cell. About 90% of known carcinogens are mutagenic in a variety of *in vitro* systems, which detect mutations in bacteria and in cultured animal and human cells. Moreover, most, but not all, mutagens are carcinogenic. This close correlation between carcinogenicity and mutagenicity presumably occurs because both reflect damage to DNA. Although not infallible, in vitro mutagenicity assays have proved to be valuable tools in screening for the carcinogenic potential of chemicals.

Chemical Carcinogenesis is a Multistep Process

Chemical carcinogenesis is best understood as a multistep process that involves numerous mutations. Four stages of chemical carcinogenesis summarize this process:

1. **Initiation** likely represents a mutation in a single cell.
2. **Promotion** reflects the clonal expansion of the initiated cell, in which the mutation has conferred a growth advantage. During promotion, the altered cells remain dependent on the continued presence of the promoting stimulus. This stimulus may be an exogenous chemical or physical agent or may reflect an endogenous mechanism (e.g., hormonal stimulation in the breast and prostate).
3. **Progression** is the stage in which growth becomes autonomous (i.e., independent of the carcinogen or the promoter). By this time, sufficient mutations have accumulated to immortalize cells.
4. **Cancer**, the end result of the entire sequence, is established when the cells acquire the capacity to invade and metastasize.

The morphologic changes that reflect multistep carcinogenesis in humans are best exemplified in epithelia, such as those of the skin, cervix, and colon. Although initiation has no visible counterpart, *promotion and progression are represented by the sequence of hyperplasia, dysplasia, and carcinoma in situ.*

Chemical Carcinogens Usually Undergo Metabolic Activation

About 75 chemicals are recognized as human carcinogens. Chemicals cause cancer either directly or, more often, after metabolic activation. The direct-acting carcinogens are inherently reactive enough to bind covalently to cellular macromolecules. Most organic carcinogens, however, require conversion to an ultimate, more reactive compound. This conversion is enzymatic and, for the most part, is effected by the cellular systems involved in drug metabolism and detoxification. Many cells in the body, particularly liver cells, possess enzyme systems that can convert procarcinogens to their active forms. Yet each carcinogen has its own spectrum of target tissues, often limited to a single organ. The basis for organ specificity in chemical carcinogenesis is not well understood.

POLYCYCLIC AROMATIC HYDROCARBONS: The polycyclic aromatic hydrocarbons are among the most extensively studied carcinogens. Found in cigarette smoke, they may well be involved in the production of lung cancer. These compounds have a broad range of target organs and, in experimental models, generally produce cancers at the site of application including the skin, soft tissues, and breast.

Polycyclic hydrocarbons are metabolized by cytochrome P450-dependent mixed-function oxidases to electrophilic epoxides, which in turn react with proteins and nucleic acids. For example, vinyl chloride, the simple two-carbon molecule from which the widely used plastic polyvinyl chloride is synthesized, is metabolized to an epoxide, which is responsible for its carcinogenic properties. Workers exposed to the vinyl chloride monomer in the ambient atmosphere later developed hepatic angiosarcomas.

ALKYLATING AGENTS: Many chemotherapeutic drugs (e.g., cyclophosphamide, cisplatin, busulfan) are alkylating agents that transfer alkyl groups (methyl, ethyl, etc.) to macromolecules, including guanines within DNA. Although such drugs destroy cancer cells by damaging DNA, they also injure normal cells. Thus, alkylating chemotherapy carries a significant risk of solid and hematological malignancies at a later time.

AFLATOXIN: Aflatoxin B_1, a natural product of the fungus *Aspergillus flavus*, is among the most potent liver carcinogens recognized. Like the polycyclic aromatic hydrocarbons, aflatoxin B_1 is metabolized to an epoxide, which can bind covalently to DNA. Because *Aspergillus* species are ubiquitous, contamination of peanuts and grains exposed to warm moist conditions may result in the formation of significant amounts of aflatoxin B_1. It has been suggested that in addition to hepatitis B and C, aflatoxin-rich foods may contribute to the high incidence of cancer of the liver in parts of Africa and Asia. Interestingly, human liver cancers in areas of high dietary concentrations of aflatoxin carry a specific inactivating mutation in the *p53* gene (G:C→T:A transversion at codon 249) as do aflatoxin-dosed rodents.

AROMATIC AMINES AND AZO DYES: Aromatic amines and azo (aniline) dyes, in contrast to the polycyclic aromatic hydrocarbons, are not ordinarily carcinogenic at the point of application. However, occupational exposure to aniline dyes has resulted in bladder cancer. Both aromatic amines and azo dyes are primarily metabolized in the liver to form the hydroxylamine derivatives, which are then detoxified by conjugation with glucuronic acid. In the bladder, hydrolysis of the glucuronide releases the reactive hydroxylamine.

NITROSAMINES: Carcinogenic nitrosamines are a subject of considerable study because it is suspected that they may play a role in human gastrointestinal neoplasms and possibly other cancers. Nitrosamines are potent carcinogens in primates, although unambiguous evidence of cancer induction in humans is lacking.

However, the extremely high incidence of esophageal carcinoma in the Hunan province of China (100 times higher than in other areas) has been correlated with the high nitrosamine content of the diet. Nitrosamines may also be implicated in other gastrointestinal cancers because nitrites, commonly added to preserve processed meats and other foods, may react with other dietary components to form nitrosamines. Nitrosamines are activated by hydroxylation, followed by the formation of a reactive alkyl carbonium ion.

METALS: A number of metals or metal compounds can induce cancer, but the carcinogenic mechanisms are unknown. Divalent metal cations, such as nickel (Ni^{2+}), lead (Pb^{2+}), cadmium (Cd^{2+}), cobalt (Co^{2+}), and beryllium (Be^{2+}) are electrophilic and can, therefore, react with macromolecules. Most metal-induced cancers occur in an occupational setting (see Chapter 9).

Endogenous and Environmental Factors Influence Chemical Carcinogenesis

Chemical carcinogenesis in experimental animals involves consideration of genetic aspects, species and strain, age and gender of the animal, hormonal status, diet, and the presence or absence of inducers of drug-metabolizing systems and tumor promoters. A similar role for such factors in humans has been postulated on the basis of epidemiologic studies, but details remain unclear.

Physical Carcinogenesis

The physical agents of carcinogenesis discussed here are ultraviolet (UV) light, asbestos, and foreign bodies. Radiation carcinogenesis is discussed in Chapter 9.

UV Radiation Causes Skin Cancers

The current fad for a tanned complexion has been accompanied not only by cosmetic deterioration of facial skin but also by an increased incidence of the major skin cancers. *Cancers attributed to sun exposure, namely, basal cell carcinoma, squamous carcinoma, and melanoma occur predominantly in the white population.* The skin of persons of the darker races is protected by the increased concentration of melanin pigment, which absorbs UV radiation. In fair-skinned people, the areas exposed to the sun are most prone to develop skin cancer. Moreover, there is a direct correlation between total exposure to sunlight and the incidence of skin cancer.

Only certain portions of the UV spectrum are associated with tissue damage, and a carcinogenic effect occurs at wavelengths between 290 and 320 nm. *The effects of UV radiation on cells include enzyme inactivation, inhibition of cell division, mutagenesis, cell death, and cancer.* The most important biochemical effect of UV radiation is the formation of **pyrimidine dimers** in DNA, a type of DNA damage that is not seen with any other carcinogen. Dimer formation leads to a cyclobutane ring, which distorts the phosphodiester backbone of the double helix in the region of each dimer. Unless efficiently eliminated by the nucleotide excision repair pathway, genomic injury produced by UV radiation is mutagenic and carcinogenic.

Xeroderma pigmentosum, an autosomal recessive disease, exemplifies the importance of DNA repair in protecting against the harmful effects of UV radiation. In this rare disorder, sensitivity to sunlight is accompanied by a high incidence of skin cancers, including basal cell carcinoma, squamous cell carcinoma, and melanoma. Both the neoplastic and non-neoplastic disorders of the skin in xeroderma pigmentosum are attributed to an impairment in the excision of UV-damaged DNA.

Asbestos Causes Mesothelioma

Pulmonary asbestosis and asbestosis-associated neoplasms are discussed in Chapter 12. Asbestos, a material widely used in construction, insulation, and manufacturing, is a family of related fibrous silicates that occur in several different physical forms.

*The characteristic tumor associated with asbestos exposure is **malignant mesothelioma** of the pleural and peritoneal cavities.* This cancer, which is exceedingly rare in the general population, has been reported to occur in 2% to 3% (in some studies even more) of heavily exposed workers. The latent period (i.e., the interval between exposure and the appearance of a tumor) is usually about 20 years but may be twice that figure. It is reasonable to surmise that mesotheliomas of both pleura and peritoneum reflect the close contact of these membranes with asbestos fibers transported to them by lymphatic channels. Although the pathogenesis of asbestos-associated mesotheliomas is obscure, the significant public health risk is well recognized and has led to great care in the use of the material.

Tumor Immunology: Immunologic Defenses Against Cancer in Animals and Humans

It has long been recognized that malignant tumors elicit a chronic inflammatory response that is unrelated to necrosis or infection of the tumor. This observation led early investigators to postulate a host immune reaction to the neoplastic cells. The inflammatory reaction is correlated with a better prognosis in some tumors, such as medullary carcinoma of the breast and seminoma, but in general, no clear correlation exists. Although the infiltrate is composed principally of T cells and macrophages, suggesting a cell-mediated immune response, the antigens to which the cells respond have not been identified. Despite the paucity of direct evidence in human cancers, it is clear from animal experiments that immune defenses against malignant tumors exist.

To invoke a role for an immune defense against cancer, it is necessary to postulate that tumor cells express antigens that differ from those of normal cells and that are recognized as foreign by the host. Such a condition has been indirectly demonstrated in experiments with inbred mice. When cells from a chemically induced or virally induced tumor are transplanted into a syngeneic mouse, the cells form a tumor. *If the transplanted tumor is removed before it metastasizes (i.e., the mouse is cured of its tumor), reinjection of the tumor cells back into the cured mouse will not produce a tumor (although the cells remain capable of forming a tumor in a second naive mouse).* The transplanted tumor is **rejected** because of immunity acquired as a result of the initial tumor transplant. Why the original tumor is not destroyed by the immunologic reaction remains unexplained.

An important observation is that tumors induced by the same chemical in different mice are antigenically distinct, whereas those induced by the same virus express the same virally determined antigens. Accordingly, mice sensitized to one chemically induced tumor do not reject a second tumor induced by the same chemical. By contrast, mice that have received a virus-induced tumor reject another similar tumor. These experiments provide compelling evidence that immunologic mechanisms can play a role in host defenses against tumors, at least against experimental tumors in animals.

Tumor Antigens are Potential Targets for the Immune Response

The immune response to experimental tumors must necessarily be directed against tumor antigens on the surface of malignant cells. Such antigens can be tumor-specific; that is, they are uniquely expressed by the cancer cells but not by their normal cellular counterparts. Alternatively, other tumor antigens represent proteins that are expressed by some normal cells, such as those in developing embryos. Such antigens are tumor-associated, rather than tumor-specific.

As noted above, tumor-specific antigens have been demonstrated in animal models. It is much more difficult to document the presence of tumor-specific antigens in human cancers because of technical and ethical limitations. Nevertheless, candidate human tumor-specific antigens have begun to emerge, for example, virally encoded antigens in tumors with a pathogenesis that is linked to viruses (e.g., HPV). In this context, an anti-HPV vaccine is now used to prevent the development of cancer of the uterine cervix. The tumor-specific antigens identified to date are peptides complexed to human leukocyte antigen (HLA) molecules on tumor cell surfaces.

There has been even more progress in identifying tumor-associated antigens, which correspond to proteins that are present in small amounts in the adult but are abundant during development. Such tumor-associated oncodevelopmental antigens are not specific for a given patient's tumor per se but instead are shared by cancers in different people and sometimes of varying histologic type. Although there is no reason to believe that immune responses to these fetal antigens play any role in the host defense against cancer, their presence in the blood or the tumor (e.g., CEA, serum α-fetoprotein) is useful in clinical diagnosis and monitoring efficacy of treatment.

Inroads into the identification of tumor antigens have created new opportunities for developing immunotherapies against human cancers, at least in theory. Passive immunotherapies can draw upon tumor-infiltrating lymphocytes with specificity for HLA-associated tumor peptide antigens and antibodies directed against various tumor surface proteins. Alternatively, as noted above, active immunotherapeutic strategies can invoke tumor antigens as vaccines to elicit systemic antitumor immune responses.

Mechanisms of Immunologic Response to Tumors

Although some circumstantial evidence exists for the participation of immunologic defenses in the resistance to cancer in humans, conclusive proof that immunologic tumor surveillance is an ongoing process is lacking. Perhaps the strongest argument for immunologic tumor rejection in humans is the observation that immunodeficiency, whether acquired or congenital, is associated with an increased incidence of cancers, almost all of which are B-cell lymphomas. The potential contribution of any specific immunologic mechanism to tumor cell destruction in vivo has not been clearly defined. A number of possible mechanisms are recognized.

- **T-cell-mediated cytotoxicity:** The capacity of cytotoxic T cells to mediate the specific rejection of transplanted tumors is evidenced by the demonstration that lymphocytes from tumor-bearing hosts can transfer tumor immunity when injected into healthy animals. Moreover, the transferred immunity is eliminated by the administration of antibodies directed against T-cell antigens. The mechanisms of T-cell-mediated immunological cell killing are discussed in Chapter 4.
- **Natural killer (NK) cell-mediated cytotoxicity:** Another set of lymphocytes, the NK cells, have tumoricidal activity that does not depend on prior sensitization. Tumor cells that are resistant to the action of NK cells may be lysed by NK cells that have been activated by IL-2. Such activated NK cells are referred to as **lymphokine-activated killer cells**.
- **Macrophage-mediated cytotoxicity:** Macrophages are capable of killing tumor cells in a nonspecific manner. However, their role in the control of malignant tumors is far from clear, because under some circumstances, in vitro factors derived from macrophages can actually stimulate the proliferation of tumor cells.

- **Antibody-dependent cell-mediated cytotoxicity:** Tumor-associated antigens can elicit a humoral antibody response, but these immunoglobulins by themselves do not kill tumor cells. However, as discussed in Chapter 4, such antibodies can participate in antibody-dependent cell-mediated cytotoxicity. The antibody binds both to the tumor antigen and to the Fc receptor of the effector cell, thereby bringing the effector cell into direct contact with its target. Depending on the conditions, the effector cells may be a lymphocyte killer cell (null cell), macrophage, or neutrophil.
- **Complement-mediated cytotoxicity:** Tumor cells that have been coated with specific antibodies may be lysed by the activation of complement.

Evasion of Immunologic Responses by Tumors

The fact that cancer is alive and well despite the presence of potential immunologic defenses implies that such mechanisms are either ineffective or that tumor cells can evade immunologic destruction. A number of factors have been proposed to account for the failure of immune responses to limit tumor growth. These explanations remain theoretical and even controversial. These include:

- Absence or paucity of tumor-specific antigens on the neoplastic cell
- Absence or paucity of cell surface molecules necessary for antigenic recognition (such as HLA) on the tumor cell
- Tumor heterogeneity leading to the selection of resistant tumor clones (as described above)
- Expression of immunosuppressive molecules by tumor cells

Defining and tackling these immune evasion mechanisms will be essential for developing effective immunotherapies for cancer.

Systemic Effects of Cancer on the Host

The symptoms of cancer are, for the most part, referable to the local effects of either the primary tumor or its metastases. However, in a minority of patients, cancer produces remote effects that are not attributable to tumor invasion or to metastasis but may be related to the synthesis of bioactive compounds by the tumor. Such effects are collectively termed **paraneoplastic syndromes**. Although such effects are rarely lethal, in some cases, they dominate the clinical course. Paraneoplastic syndromes are also of diagnostic and therapeutic significance.

Common systemic effects include:

- **Fever:** It is not uncommon for cancer patients to present initially with fever of unknown origin that cannot be explained by an infectious disease. Fever attributed to cancer (1) correlates with tumor growth, (2) disappears after treatment, and (3) reappears on recurrence. This is likely related to the release of pyrogens by the tumor or associated stromal inflammatory cells.
- **Anorexia and weight loss:** A paraneoplastic syndrome of anorexia, weight loss, and cachexia is very common in patients with cancer, often appearing before its malignant cause becomes apparent. The mechanisms responsible for this phenomenon are poorly understood but may be related to the production of a variety of cytokines, including TNF-α, interferons, and IL-6.
- **Endocrine syndromes:** Malignant tumors may produce a number of peptide hormones with secretion that is not under normal regulatory control. Most of these hormones are usually present in the brain, gastrointestinal tract, or endocrine organs. Their inappropriate secretion can cause a variety of effects. Cushing syndrome (see Chapter 21), inappropriate an-

tidiuresis, hyper- and hypocalcemia, gonadotropic syndromes, and hypoglycemia may all result from inappropriate hormone secretion by tumors.

Organ-Specific Effects of Cancer on the Host

Cancer may have specific effects on different host organ systems that may result from mechanical, metabolic, or other poorly defined causes related to the growth of the tumor.

Neurologic Syndromes are Common in Cancer Patients

Neurologic disorders usually result from metastases or from endocrine or electrolyte disturbances. Vascular, hemorrhagic, and infectious conditions affecting the nervous system are also common. However, there remains a small group of cancer patients who suffer from a variety of neurologic complaints without any demonstrable cause. Most of these cases reflect an autoimmune etiology mediated by circulating antibodies directed against neural antigens or by reactive T cells. Cerebral complications include dementia, subacute cerebellar degeneration, limbic encephalitis, and optic neuritis.

Spinal Cord
Subacute motor neuropathy, a disorder of the spinal cord, is characterized by slowly developing lower motor neuron weakness without sensory changes. It is so strongly associated with cancer that an intensive search for an occult neoplasm, often a lymphoma, should be made in patients who present with these symptoms.

Amyotrophic lateral sclerosis is well described among cancer patients. Conversely, as many as 10% of patients with this neurologic disease are found to have cancer.

Peripheral Nerves
Sensorimotor peripheral neuropathy, characterized by distal weakness, wasting, and sensory loss, is common in cancer patients and when not associated with an overt neoplasm suggests the possibility of an occult tumor. Interestingly, the removal of the primary tumor usually does not reverse the neuropathy.

Purely sensory neuropathy, resulting from degenerative changes in the dorsal root ganglia, may also develop in persons with cancer.

Autonomic and gastrointestinal neuropathies, manifested as orthostatic hypotension, neurogenic bladder, and intestinal pseudoobstruction, are associated with small cell carcinoma of the lung.

Skeletal Muscle Syndromes Can be Strongly Associated with Cancer

Patients with dermatomyositis or polymyositis have an incidence of cancer five to seven times higher than that in the general population. The association is most conspicuous in affected men older than 50 years; in this group, more than 70% have cancer. In most cases, the muscle disorder and cancer present within a year of each other.

Hematologic Syndromes Commonly Relate to Marrow Infiltration

The most common hematologic complications of neoplastic diseases result either from direct infiltration of the marrow or from treatment. However, hematologic paraneoplastic syndromes, which antedate the modern era of chemotherapy and radiation therapy, are well described. Erythrocytosis (polycythemia), ane-

mias, and defects of leukocytes and platelets may have a paraneoplastic (or possibly autoimmune) etiology. Treatment-related hematologic defects are, of course, also common.

A Hypercoagulable State is Often Associated with Cancer

The association between cancer and venous thrombosis was noted more than a century ago. Since then, other abnormalities resulting from a hypercoagulable state (e.g., disseminated intravascular coagulation and nonbacterial thrombotic endocarditis) have been recognized. The cause of this hypercoagulable state is still debated.

VENOUS THROMBOSIS: This condition is most distinctly associated with carcinoma of the pancreas, in which there is a 50-fold increased incidence of this complication. Venous thrombosis, normally in the deep veins of the legs, is also particularly common in association with other mucin-secreting adenocarcinomas of the gastrointestinal tract and with lung cancer.

DISSEMINATED INTRAVASCULAR COAGULATION: This complication is most commonly found with acute promyelocytic leukemia and adenocarcinomas.

NONBACTERIAL THROMBOTIC ENDOCARDITIS: The presence of noninfected verrucous deposits of fibrin and platelets on the left-sided heart valves occurs in cancer patients, particularly in those who are debilitated (see Chapter 11). Although the effects on the heart are not of clinical importance, emboli to the brain and rarely the coronary arteries present a great danger. This cardiac complication is most common with solid tumors but may occasionally be noted with leukemias and lymphomas.

Cancer also Affects a Number of Other Organ Systems

Cancer may affect a variety of other organ systems either as a direct consequence of tumor growth or as a paraneoplastic effect. Some of the more common organ systems affected include the following:

GASTROINTESTINAL SYSTEM: Malabsorption of a variety of dietary components is an occasional paraneoplastic symptom, and half of cancer patients develop some histologic abnormalities of the small intestine, even though the tumor may not directly involve the bowel.

KIDNEY: Nephrotic syndrome, as a consequence of renal vein thrombosis or amyloidosis, is a well-known complication of cancer. The nephrotic syndrome may also represent a paraneoplastic complication in the form of minimal-change disease (lipoid nephrosis) or glomerulonephritis produced by the deposition of immune complexes.

SKIN: A number of pigmented lesions and keratoses are well-recognized paraneoplastic effects. Acanthosis nigricans is a cutaneous disorder marked by hyperkeratosis and pigmentation of the axilla, neck, flexures, and anogenital region. *It is of particular interest because more than half of patients with acanthosis nigricans have cancer.* The development of the disease may precede, accompany, or follow, the detection of the cancer. More than 90% of cases occur in association with gastrointestinal carcinomas, with tumors of the stomach accounting for one-half to two-thirds. Exfoliative dermatitis occasionally complicates certain lymphomas and Hodgkin disease without any cutaneous involvement by tumor.

Amyloidosis May be a Systemic Effect of Cancer

About 15% of cases of amyloidosis occur in association with cancers, particularly with multiple myeloma and renal cell carcinoma but also with other solid tumors and lymphomas (see Chapter 23). The presence of amyloidosis implies a poor prognosis; in patients with myeloma, amyloidosis is associated with a median survival of 14 months or less.

Epidemiology of Cancer

Cancer accounts for one fifth of the total mortality in the United States and is the second leading cause of death after cardiovascular diseases and stroke. For most cancers, death rates in the United States have largely remained flat for more than half a century, with some notable exceptions (Fig. 5-17). The death rate from lung cancer among men has risen dramatically from 1930, when it was an uncommon tumor, to the present, when it is by far the most common cause of death from cancer in men. As discussed in Chapter 8, the entire epidemic of lung cancer deaths is attributable to smoking. Among women, smoking did not become fashionable until World War II. Considering the time lag needed between starting to smoke and the development of lung cancer, it is not surprising that the increased death rate from lung cancer in women did not become significant until after 1965. In the United States, the death rate from lung cancer in women now exceeds that for breast cancer, and it is now, as in men, the most common fatal cancer. By contrast, for reasons difficult to fathom, cancer of the stomach, which in 1930 was by far the most common cancer in men and was more common than breast cancer in women, has shown a remarkable and sustained decline in frequency. Similarly, there has been a conspicuous decline in the death rate from cancer of the uterus corpus and cervix, possibly explained by better screening, diagnostic techniques, and therapeutic methods. Overall, after decades of steady increases, the age-adjusted mortality rate due to all cancers has now reached a plateau. The ranking of the incidence of tumors in men and women in the United States is shown in Table 5-1.

Individual cancers have their own age-related profiles, but for most, increased age is associated with an increased incidence. The most striking example of the dependency on age is carcinoma of the prostate, in which the incidence increases 30-fold in men between the ages of 50 and 85. Certain neoplastic diseases, such as acute lymphoblastic leukemia in children and testicular cancer in young adults, show different age-related peaks of incidence.

Geographic and Ethnic Differences Influence Cancer Incidence

It is difficult to find a cancer that does **not** show signif-icant differences in incidence in different ethnic groups or geographical regions. It is equally difficult to find an explanation for such differences. This in part relates to the complexity in undertaking human population-based studies, the plethora of potential genetic and environmental variables between populations, and the uncertainty involved in translating animal experimental data to humans. Hypotheses attempting to explain population-based differences in frequency for some types of cancer have achieved some level of acceptance. These include:

LIVER CANCER: There is a strong correlation between the incidence of primary hepatocellular carcinoma and the prevalence of hepatitis B and C. Endemic regions for both diseases include large parts of sub-Saharan Africa and most of Asia, Indonesia, and the Philippines. It must be remembered that levels of aflatoxin B_1 are high in the staple diets of many of the high-risk areas.

SKIN CANCER: The rates for skin cancers vary with skin color and exposure to the sun. Thus, particularly high rates have been reported in northern Australia, where sun exposure is intense and much of the current population is derived from the British Isles (and fair skinned). Although the data are scanty, darker aboriginal

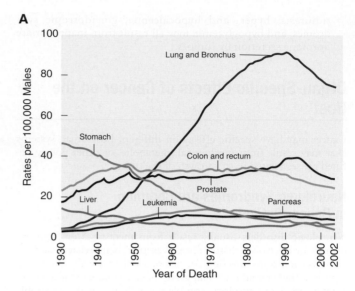

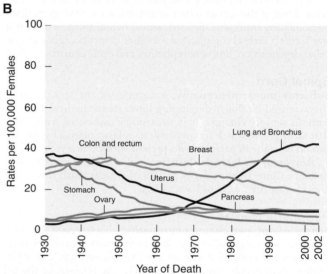

FIGURE 5-17. Cancer death rates in the United States, 1930 to 2002, among men **(A)** and women **(B)**.

Australians appear to have lower rates of skin cancer. Increased rates of skin cancer have also been noted among the white population of the American Southwest. The lowest rates are found among those with pigmented skin (e.g., Japanese, Chinese, and Indians). The rates for African blacks, despite their heavily pigmented skin, are occasionally higher than those for Asians because of the higher incidence of melanomas of the soles and palms in blacks.

CERVICAL CARCINOMA: Striking differences in the incidence of squamous carcinoma of the cervix exist between ethnic groups and different socioeconomic levels. For instance, the very low rate in Ashkenazi Jews of Israel contrasts with a 25 times greater rate in the Hispanic population of Texas. In general, groups of low socioeconomic status have a higher incidence of cervical cancer than the more prosperous and better educated. This cancer is also directly correlated with early sexual activity and multiparity and is rare among women who are not sexually active, such as nuns. It is also uncommon among women whose husbands are circumcised. A strong association with infection by HPVs has been

TABLE 5–1

Most Common Tumor Types in Men and Women

Tumor Type	%
Men	
Prostate	33
Lung and bronchus	14
Colon and rectum	11
Urinary bladder	6
Melanoma	4
Non-Hodgkin lymphoma	4
Kidney	3
Oral cavity	3
Leukemia	3
Pancreas	2
All other sites	17
Women	
Breast	32
Lung and bronchus	12
Colon and rectum	11
Uterine corpus	6
Ovary	4
Non-Hodgkin lymphoma	4
Melanoma	3
Thyroid	3
Pancreas	2
Urinary bladder	2
All other sites	20

demonstrated, and cervical cancer should be classed as a venereal disease. Hence, differences in frequency correlate with sexual practices and the use of condoms.

BURKITT LYMPHOMA: Burkitt lymphoma, a disease of children, was first described in Uganda, where it accounts for half of all childhood tumors. Since then, a high frequency has been observed in other African countries, particularly in hot, humid lowlands. It has been noted that these are areas where malaria is also endemic. High rates have been recorded in other tropical areas, such as Malaysia and New Guinea, but European and American cases are encountered only sporadically. An interaction between chronic malarial infection and EBV virus appears likely (see above).

Studies of Migrant Populations Give Clues to Cancer Development

Although planned experiments on the etiology of human cancer are rarely feasible, certain populations have unwittingly performed such experiments by migrating from one environment to another. Initially at least, the genetic characteristics of such persons remained the same, but the new environment differed in climate, diet, infectious agents, occupations, and so on. *Consequently, epidemiologic studies of migrant populations have provided many intriguing clues to the factors that may influence the pathogenesis of cancer.* The United States, which has been the destination of one of the greatest population movements of all time, is the source of most of the important data in this field.

CANCER OF THE STOMACH: A study of Japanese residents of Hawaii found that emigrants from Japanese regions with the highest risk of stomach cancer continued to exhibit an excess risk in Hawaii. By contrast, their offspring who were born in Hawaii had the same incidence of this cancer as American whites. Although dietary factors, such as pickled vegetables and salted fish, have been postulated to account for the higher incidence in Japan and the lower incidence in Hawaii, no firm evidence has been adduced to support this contention. More recently, it has been shown in Japan that the population in regions at high risk for stomach cancer also displays a high prevalence of chronic atrophic gastritis with intestinal metaplasia, lesions that are considered precursors of gastric cancer. Interestingly, when people from these regions move to low-risk areas, they carry the high prevalence of intestinal metaplasia with them. Thus, the environmental factors associated with stomach cancer may not be directly carcinogenic but rather may be related to atrophic gastritis and intestinal metaplasia.

COLORECTAL, BREAST, ENDOMETRIAL, OVARIAN, AND PROSTATIC CANCERS: Emigrant studies of the incidence of colorectal cancer show opposite trends to those of stomach cancer. Emigrants from low-risk areas in Europe and Japan exhibit an increased risk of colorectal cancer in the United States. Moreover, their offspring continue at a higher risk and reach the incidence levels of the general American population. This rule for colorectal cancer also prevails for cancers of the breast, endometrium, ovary, and prostate.

CANCER OF THE LIVER: As noted above, primary hepatocellular carcinoma is common in Asia and Africa, where it has been associated with hepatitis B and C. In American blacks and Asians, however, the neoplasm is no more common than in American whites, a situation that presumably reflects the relatively low prevalence of chronic viral hepatitis in the United States.

HODGKIN DISEASE: In poorly developed countries, the childhood form of Hodgkin disease is the type reported most often. In developed Western countries, by contrast, the disease is most common among young adults. Such a pattern is characteristic of certain viral infections, although there is no evidence for an infectious etiology of Hodgkin disease. An exception to this generalization is noted in Japan, a developed country where young adult disease is distinctly uncommon. Further evidence for an environmental influence is the higher incidence of Hodgkin disease in Americans of Japanese descent than that in Japan.

6 Developmental and Genetic Diseases

Anthony A. Killeen
Emanuel Rubin
David S. Strayer

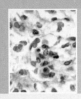
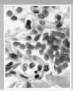
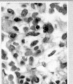
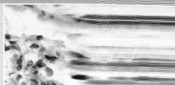

Diseases that present during the perinatal period may be caused (1) by factors in the fetal environment, (2) genomic abnormalities, or (3) interaction between genetic defects and environmental influences. An example of the last is phenylketonuria, in which a genetic deficiency of phenylalanine hydroxylase causes mental retardation only if an infant is exposed to dietary phenylalanine.

Developmental and genetic disorders are classified as follows:

- Errors of morphogenesis
- Chromosomal abnormalities
- Single-gene defects
- Polygenic inherited diseases

The fetus may also be injured by adverse transplacental influences or by intrauterine trauma or during parturition. After birth, acquired diseases of infancy and childhood are also important causes of morbidity and mortality.

Principles of Teratology

Teratology is the study of developmental anomalies (Greek, *ton,* monster). **Teratogens** are chemical, physical, and biolog agents that cause developmental anomalies. The list of proven atogens is long and includes most cytotoxic drugs, alcohol, s antiepileptic drugs, heavy metals, and thalidomide.

Malformations are morphologic defects or abnormalities of an or part of an organ, or anatomical region due to perturbed morphoge Exposure to a teratogen may result in a malformation, but th not invariably the case. Such observations have led to the form tion of general principles of teratology:

- **Susceptibility to teratogens is variable.** Presumably, principal determinants of this variability are the genotyp the fetus and the mother.
- **Susceptibility to teratogens is specific for each embryol stage.** Most agents are teratogenic only at particular tim development (Fig. 6-1). For example, maternal rubella i tion only causes fetal abnormalities if it occurs during the trimester of pregnancy.

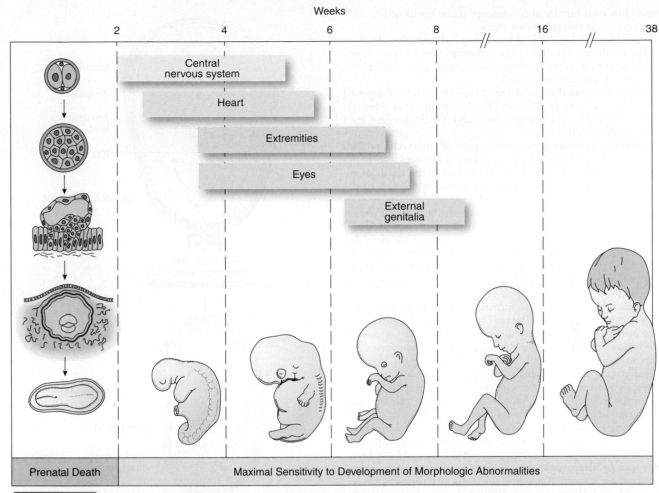

FIGURE 6-1. **Sensitivity of specific organs to teratogenic agents at critical stages of human embryogenesis.** Exposure to adverse influences in the preimplantation and early postimplantation stages of development (*far left*) leads to prenatal death. Periods of maximal sensitivity to teratogens (*horizontal bars*) vary for different organ systems but overall are limited to the first 8 weeks of pregnancy.

- **The mechanism of teratogenesis is specific for each teratogen.** Teratogenic drugs inhibit metabolic steps critical for normal morphogenesis. Many drugs and viruses affect specific tissues (e.g., neurotropism, cardiotropism) and so damage some developing organs more than others.
- **Teratogenesis is dose dependent.** Because of the multiple determinants of teratogenesis, all established teratogens should be avoided during pregnancy; an absolutely safe dose cannot be predicted for every woman.
- **Teratogens produce death, growth retardation, malformation, or functional impairment.** The outcome depends on the interaction between the teratogenic influences, the maternal organism, and the fetal–placental unit.

Errors of Morphogenesis

As a rule, exogenous toxins acting on preimplantation-stage embryos do not produce errors of morphogenesis and do not cause malformations (see Fig. 6-1). The most common consequence of toxic exposure at the preimplantation stage is death of the embryo, which often passes unnoticed or is perceived as heavy, albeit delayed, menstrual bleeding. Injury during the first 8 to 10 days after fertilization usually causes incomplete separation of blastomeres, which leads to conjoined twins ("Siamese twins") joined at the head (craniopagus), thorax (thoracopagus), or rump (ischiopagus).

Most complex developmental abnormalities affecting several organ systems are due to injuries that occur between implantation of the blastocyst and early organogenesis. *Formation of primordial organ systems is the stage of embryonic development most susceptible to teratogenesis, and many major developmental abnormalities are probably due to faulty gene activity or the effects of exogenous toxins (see Fig. 6-1).* Disorganized or disrupted morphogenesis may have minor or major consequences at the level of (1) cells and tissues, (2) organs or organ systems, and (3) anatomical regions.

After the third month of pregnancy, exposure of the human fetus to teratogenic influences rarely results in major errors of morphogenesis. However, morphologic and, especially, functional consequences may still occur in children exposed to exogenous teratogens during the second and third trimesters. Although organs are already formed by the end of the third month of pregnancy, most still undergo the restructuring and maturation required for extrauterine life. Functional maturation proceeds at different rates in different organs; the central nervous system (CNS) requires several years after birth to attain functional maturity and so is still susceptible to adverse exogenous influences for some time after birth.

- **Agenesis** is the complete absence of an organ primordium. It may manifest as (1) total lack of an organ, as in renal agenesis; (2) absence of part of an organ, for example, agenesis of the corpus callosum of the brain; or (3) lack of tissue or cells within an organ.
- **Aplasia** is the persistence of an organ anlage or rudiment, without the mature organ. Thus, in aplasia of the lung, the main

bronchus ends blindly in nondescript tissue composed of rudimentary ducts and connective tissue.

- **Hypoplasia** means reduced size owing to incomplete development of all or part of an organ. Examples include microphthalmia (small eyes), micrognathia (small jaw), and microcephaly (small brain and head).
- **Dysraphic anomalies** are defects caused by failure of apposed structures to fuse. In spina bifida, the spinal canal does not close completely, and overlying bone and skin do not fuse, leaving a midline defect.
- **Involution failures** denote persistence of embryonic or fetal structures that should have disappeared at certain stages of development. A persistent thyroglossal duct is the result of incomplete involution of the tract that connects the base of the tongue with the developing thyroid.
- **Division failures** are caused by incomplete cleavage of embryonic tissues, when that process depends on programmed cell death. For example, fingers and toes are formed at the distal end of the limb bud through the loss of cells located between the primordia that contain the cartilage. If these cells do not undergo apoptosis, the fingers will be conjoined or incompletely separated (syndactyly).
- **Atresia** reflects incomplete formation of a lumen. Many hollow organs originate as cell strands and cords with centers that are programmed to die, producing a central cavity or lumen. Esophageal atresia is characterized by partial occlusion of the lumen, which was not fully established in embryogenesis.
- **Dysplasia** is caused by abnormal organization of cells into tissues, a situation that results in abnormal histogenesis. (This is different from the use of "dysplasia" to describe precancerous epithelial lesions [see Chapters 1 and 5].) Tuberous sclerosis is a striking example of dysplasia, being characterized by abnormal development of the brain, which contains aggregates of normally developed cells arranged into grossly visible "tubers."
- **Ectopia, or heterotopia,** is an anomaly in which an organ is situated outside its normal anatomic site. Thus, an ectopic heart is not in the thorax. Heterotopic parathyroid glands can be within the thymus in the anterior mediastinum.
- **Dystopia** refers to inadequate migration of an organ that remains where it was during development, rather than migrating to its proper site. For example, the kidneys are first located in the pelvis and then move cephalad out of the pelvis. Dystopic kidneys remain in the pelvis. Dystopic testes are retained in the inguinal canal and do not descend into the scrotum (cryptorchidism).

Clinically Important Malformations

- *A developmental sequence anomaly (anomalad or complex anomaly) is a pattern of defects related to a single anomaly or pathogenetic mechanics*—different factors lead to the same consequences through a common pathway. In the Potter complex (Fig. 6-2), pulmonary hypoplasia, external signs of intrauterine fetal compression, and morphologic changes of the amnion are all related to oligohydramnios (a severely reduced amount of amniotic fluid). A fetus in an amniotic sac with insufficient fluid develops the distinctive features of Potter complex regardless of the cause of oligohydramnios.
- *A **developmental syndrome** refers to multiple anomalies that are pathogenetically related.* The term **syndrome** implies a single cause for anomalies in diverse organs that have been damaged by the same effect during a critical developmental period.
- *A **deformation** is defined as an abnormality of form, shape, or position of a part of the body that is caused by mechanical forces.* Most anatomic defects caused by adverse influences in the last two trimesters of pregnancy fall into this category. The responsible forces may be external (e.g., amniotic bands in the uterus) or intrinsic (e.g., fetal hypomobility caused by CNS injury).

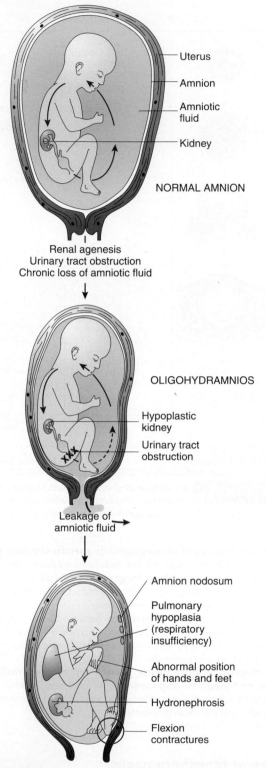

FIGURE 6-2. **Potter complex.** The fetus normally swallows amniotic fluid and, in turn, excretes urine, thereby maintaining its normal volume of amniotic fluid. In the face of urinary tract disease (e.g., renal agenesis or urinary tract obstruction) or leakage of amniotic fluid, the volume of amniotic fluid decreases, a situation termed **oligohydramnios**. Oligohydramnios results in a number of congenital abnormalities termed **Potter complex**, which includes pulmonary hypoplasia and contractures of the limbs. The amnion has a nodular appearance. In cases of urinary tract obstruction, congenital hydronephrosis is also seen, although this abnormality is not considered part of Potter complex.

Fetal Alcohol Syndrome Demonstrates the Teratogenic Potential of Common Chemicals

Fetal alcohol syndrome is caused by maternal consumption of alcoholic beverages during pregnancy. It is a complex of abnormalities including (1) growth retardation, (2) CNS dysfunction, and (3) characteristic facial dysmorphology. Because not all children adversely affected by maternal alcohol abuse show all these abnormalities, the term **fetal alcohol effect** is also used.

 EPIDEMIOLOGY AND PATHOGENESIS: The prevalence of fetal alcohol syndrome in the United States and Europe is 1 to 3 per 1,000 live births. However, in populations with extremely high rates of alcoholism, the prevalence may reach 20 to 150 per 1,000. *It is thought that abnormalities related to fetal alcohol effect, particularly mild mental deficiency and emotional disorders, are far more common than the full-blown fetal alcohol syndrome.*

The minimum amount of alcohol that results in fetal injury is not well established, but children with the entire spectrum of fetal alcohol syndrome are usually born to mothers who are chronic alcoholics. Heavy alcohol consumption during the first trimester of pregnancy is particularly dangerous. The mechanism by which alcohol damages the developing fetus remains unknown despite a large body of research.

 PATHOLOGY AND CLINICAL FEATURES: Infants born to alcoholic mothers often show prenatal growth retardation, which continues after birth. These infants may also display microcephaly, epicanthal folds, short palpebral fissures, maxillary hypoplasia, a thin upper lip, a small jaw (micrognathia), and a poorly developed philtrum. Cardiac septal defects may affect up to one third of patients, although these often close spontaneously. Minor abnormalities of joints and limbs may occur.

Fetal alcohol syndrome is a common cause of acquired mental retardation. One fifth of children with fetal alcohol syndrome have intelligence quotients (IQs) below 70, and 40% are between 70 and 85. Even if their IQ is normal, these children tend to have short memory spans and to exhibit impulsive behavior and emotional instability (see Chapter 8).

Anencephaly and Related Neural Tube Defects are Malformations that are Related in Part to Nutritional Deficiency

Anencephaly is the congenital absence of the cranial vault. The cerebral hemispheres are completely missing or are reduced to small masses at the base of the skull. The disorder is a dysraphic defect of neural tube closure. The neural tube closes sequentially in a craniocaudal direction, so a defect in this process causes abnormalities of the vertebral column. **Spina bifida** is incomplete closure of the spinal cord or vertebral column or both. Hernial protrusion of the meninges through a defect in the vertebral column is termed **meningocele**. **Myelomeningocele** is the same condition as meningocele but complicated by herniation of the spinal cord itself.

Folic acid supplementation during pregnancy lowers the incidence of neural tube defects. Mandatory food supplementation with folate since 1998 has resulted in a significant decrease in the incidence of neural tube defects, although other factors, some genetic in origin, play a significant role in formation of the defects. Neural tube defects are discussed in detail in Chapter 28.

Malformations May be Produced by Fetal or Neonatal Infections

TORCH Complex

The acronym, TORCH, refers to a complex of similar signs and symptoms produced by fetal or neonatal infection with Toxoplasma *(T), rubella (R), cytomegalovirus (C), and herpes simplex virus (H). In the acronym TORCH, the letter "O" represents "others"* (Fig. 6-3), including syphilis, tuberculosis, listeriosis, leptospirosis, varicella-zoster virus infection, and Epstein-Barr virus infection. Human immunodeficiency virus and human parvovirus (B19) have been suggested as additions to the list.

Infections with TORCH agents occur in 1% to 5% of all liveborn infants in the United States and are major causes of neonatal morbidity and mortality. The severe damage inflicted by these organisms is mostly irreparable, and prevention (if possible) is the only alternative. Unfortunately, titers of serum antibodies against TORCH agents in infants or mothers are usually not diagnostic, and the precise etiology is often unclear.

- **Toxoplasmosis:** Asymptomatic toxoplasmosis is common, and 25% of women in their reproductive years have antibodies to this organism. However, intrauterine *Toxoplasma* infection occurs in only 0.1% of all pregnancies.
- **Rubella:** Vaccination against rubella in the United States has virtually eliminated congenital rubella. Fewer than 10 cases are reported each year.
- **Cytomegalovirus (CMV):** In the United States, two thirds of women of childbearing age have antibodies to CMV, and up to 2% of newborns are congenitally infected. Because most normal infants have maternally derived antibodies, CMV is diagnosed by urine culture.
- **Herpesvirus:** Intrauterine infection with herpes simplex virus type 2 is uncommon. The neonatal infection is usually acquired during passage through the birth canal of a mother with active genital herpes. Clinical examination of the mother, the appearance of typical skin lesions in the newborn, and serologic testing and culture for herpes simplex virus type 2 establish the diagnosis. Congenital herpes infection can be pre-

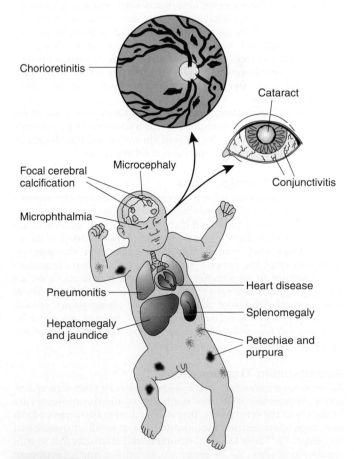

FIGURE 6-3. **TORCH complex.** Children infected in utero with *Toxoplasma*, rubella virus, cytomegalovirus, or herpes simplex virus show remarkably similar effects.

vented by cesarean section of mothers who have active genital lesions or by antenatal treatment of the mother with antiviral drugs.

The specific organisms of the TORCH complex are discussed in detail in Chapter 9.

 PATHOLOGY: The clinical and pathologic findings in the symptomatic newborn vary. Only a minority present with multisystem disease and the entire spectrum of abnormalities. Growth retardation and abnormalities of the brain, eyes, liver, hematopoietic system, and heart are seen in TORCH syndrome (Fig. 6-3).

Chromosomal Abnormalities

Cytogenetics is the study of chromosomes and their abnormalities. The current system of classification is the International System for Human Cytogenetic Nomenclature.

Structural Chromosomal Abnormalities May Arise During Somatic Cell Division (Mitosis) or During Gametogenesis (Meiosis)

Changes in chromosome structure that occur in somatic cells during mitosis may (1) not affect a cell's basic functions and thus be silent, (2) interfere with one or more key cellular activities and lead to cell death, or (3) change a key cell function (e.g., increased mitotic activity) that has effects on cell function but does not cause cell death. Such changes may be associated with neoplastic transformation (see Chapter 5).

The structural chromosomal abnormalities that arise during gametogenesis are important in a different context, because they are transmitted to all somatic cells of the offspring and may result in heritable diseases. During normal meiosis, homologous chromosomes (e.g., two chromosomes 1) form pairs, termed **bivalents**. A normal process, known as **crossing-over**, results in exchange of parts of these chromosomes and a rearrangement of the genetic constituents of each chromosome.

An abnormal process, termed **translocation,** can result in exchanges between nonhomologous chromosomes (e.g., chromosomes 3 and 21). Two major types of chromosomal translocations are recognized, namely, reciprocal and robertsonian.

Reciprocal Translocations

Reciprocal translocation refers to the exchange of acentric chromosomal segments between different (nonhomologous) chromosomes. A reciprocal translocation is **balanced** if there is no loss of genetic material, so that each chromosomal segment is translocated in its entirety. When such translocations are present in the gametes (sperm or ova), the progeny maintain the abnormal chromosomal structure in all somatic cells. *Balanced translocations are not generally associated with loss of genes or disruption of vital gene loci, so most carriers of balanced translocations are phenotypically normal. Offspring of carriers of balanced translocations, however, are at risk because they will have unbalanced karyotypes and may show severe phenotypic abnormalities.*

Robertsonian Translocations

Robertsonian translocation (centric fusion) involves the centromere of acrocentric chromosomes. When two nonhomologous chromosomes are broken near the centromere, they may exchange two arms to form one large metacentric chromosome and a small chromosomal fragment. The latter lacks a centromere and is usually lost in subsequent divisions. As in reciprocal translocation, robertsonian translocation is balanced if there is no significant loss of genetic material. The carrier is also usually phenotypically normal, but may be infertile. *If the carrier is fertile, however, his or her gametes may produce unbalanced translocations, in which case the offspring may have congenital malformations.*

Chromosomal Deletions

A deletion is loss of a portion of a chromosome and involves either a terminal or an intercalary (middle) segment. Disturbances during meiosis in germ cells or breaks of chromatids during mitosis in somatic cells may result in formation of chromosomal fragments that are not incorporated into any chromosome and are thus lost in subsequent cell divisions (Fig. 6-4).

Gametic deletion can be associated with either normal or abnormal development. An example of the latter is the **cri du chat syndrome**, in which the short arm of chromosome 5 is deleted. Deletions may be related to several human cancers, including some hereditary forms of cancer. For example, some familial **retinoblastomas** are associated with deletions in the long arm of chromosome 13 (see Chapter 5).

Chromosomal Inversions

Chromosomal inversion refers to a process in which a chromosome breaks at two points, the affected segment inverts and then reattaches. **Pericentric inversions** result from breaks on opposite sides of the centromere, whereas **paracentric inversions** involve breaks on the same arm of the chromosome (see Fig. 6-4). During meiosis, homologous chromosomes that carry inversions do not exchange segments of chromatids by crossing over as readily as do normal chromosomes, because of interference with pairing. Although this is of little consequence for the phenotype of the offspring, it may be important in evolutionary terms, because it may lead to clustering of certain hereditary features.

Ring Chromosomes

Ring chromosomes are formed by a break involving both telomeric ends of a chromosome, deletion of the acentric fragments, and end-to-end fusion of the remaining centric portion of the chromosome (see Fig. 6-4). The consequences depend primarily on the amount of genetic material lost because of the break. The abnormally shaped chromosome may impede normal meiotic division, but in most instances, this chromosomal abnormality is of no consequence.

Isochromosomes

Isochromosomes are formed by faulty centromere division. Normally, centromeres divide in a plane parallel to a chromosome's long axis, to give two identical hemichromosomes. If a centromere divides in a plane transverse to the long axis, pairs of isochromosomes are formed. One pair corresponds to the short arms attached to the upper portion of the centromere and the other to the long arms attached to the lower segment (see Fig. 6-4).

The most important clinical condition involving isochromosomes is **Turner syndrome**, in which 15% of those affected have an isochromosome of the X chromosome.

The Causes of Abnormal Chromosome Numbers are Largely Unknown

A number of terms are important in understanding developmental defects associated with abnormal chromosome numbers.

- **Haploid:** A single set of each chromosome (23 in humans). Only germ cells have a haploid number (n) of chromosomes.
- **Diploid:** A double set (2n) of each of the chromosomes (46 in humans). Most somatic cells are diploid.
- **Euploid:** Any multiple (from n to 8n) of the haploid number of chromosomes. For example, many normal liver cells have twice (4n) the diploid DNA of somatic cells and are, therefore, euploid or, more specifically, tetraploid. If the multiple is greater than 2 (i.e., greater than diploid), the karyotype is **polyploid**.
- **Aneuploid:** Karyotypes that are not exact multiples of the haploid number. Many cancer cells are aneuploid, a characteristic often associated with aggressive behavior.

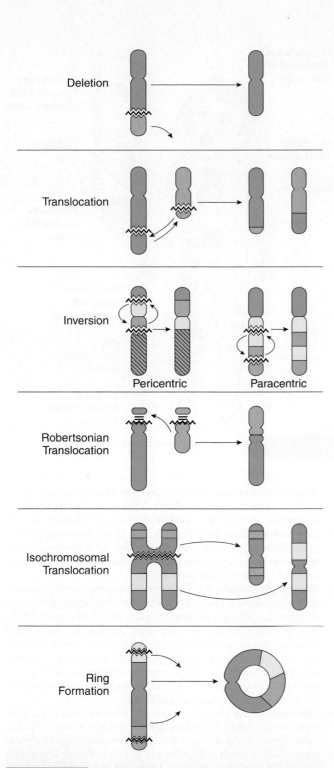

FIGURE 6-4. **Structural abnormalities of human chromosomes.** The deletion of a portion of a chromosome leads to the loss of genetic material and a shortened chromosome. A reciprocal translocation involves breaks on two nonhomologous chromosomes, with exchange of the acentric segments. An inversion requires two breaks in a single chromosome. If the breaks are on opposite sides of the centromere, the inversion is **pericentric**; it is **paracentric** if the breaks are on the same arm. A robertsonian translocation occurs when two nonhomologous acrocentric chromosomes break near their centromeres, after which the long arms fuse to form one large metacentric chromosome. Isochromosomes arise from faulty centromere division, which leads to duplication of the long arm (iso q) and deletion of the short arm or the reverse (iso p). Ring chromosomes involve breaks of both telomeric portions of a chromosome, deletion of the acentric fragments, and fusion of the remaining centric portion.

- **Monosomy:** The absence in a somatic cell of one chromosome of a homologous pair. For example, Turner syndrome is characterized by a single X chromosome.
- **Trisomy:** The presence of an extra copy of a normally paired chromosome. For example, Down syndrome is caused by the presence of three copies of chromosome 21.

Nondisjunction

*Nondisjunction is a failure of paired chromosomes or chromatids to separate and move to opposite poles of the spindle at anaphase, during mitosis or meiosis. **Numerical chromosomal abnormalities arise primarily from nondisjunction**.* Nondisjunction leads to aneuploidy if only one pair of chromosomes fails to separate. It results in polyploidy if the entire set does not divide and all the chromosomes are segregated into a single daughter cell.

Nomenclature of Chromosomal Aberrations

Structural or numerical chromosomal aberrations are seen in 5 to 7 per 1,000 liveborn infants, although most are balanced translocations and are asymptomatic. A schema for describing chromosomal aberrations is detailed in Table 6-1.

Numerical Autosomal Aberrations in Liveborn Infants are Virtually all Trisomies

Structural aberrations that may result in clinical disorders include translocations, deletions, and chromosomal breakage.

Trisomy 21 (Down Syndrome)

Trisomy 21 is the most common cause of congenital mental retardation. Furthermore, liveborn infants are only a fraction of all conceptuses with this defect. Two-thirds abort spontaneously or die in utero. Life expectancy is also reduced. Advances in treating infections, congenital heart defects, and leukemia—the leading causes of death in patients with Down syndrome—have increased life expectancy.

TABLE 6–1	
Chromosomal Nomenclature	
Numerical designation of autosomes	1–22
Sex chromosomes	X, Y
Addition of a whole or part of a chromosome	+
Loss of a whole or part of a chromosome	−
Numerical mosaicism (e.g., 46/47)	/
Short arm of chromosome (petite)	p
Long arm of chromosome	q
Isochromosome	i
Ring chromosome	r
Deletion	del
Insertion	ins
Translocation	t
Derivative chromosome (carrying translocation)	der
Terminal	ter
Representative karyotypes	
Male with trisomy 21 (Down syndrome)	47, XY, +21
Female carrier of fusion-type translocation between chromosomes 14 and 21	45, XX, −14, −21, + t(14q21q)
Cri-du-chat syndrome (male) with deletion of a portion of the short arm of chromosome 5	46, XY, del(5p)
Male with ring chromosome 19	46, XY, r(19)
Turner syndrome with monosomy X	45, X
Mosaic Klinefelter syndrome	46, XY/47, XXY

PATHOGENESIS: There are three mechanisms by which three copies of the genes on chromosome 21 that cause Down syndrome may be present in somatic cells:

- **Nondisjunction** in the first meiotic division of gametogenesis accounts for most (92% to 95%) patients with trisomy 21. The extra chromosome 21 is of maternal origin in about 95% of Down syndrome children. Virtually all maternal nondisjunction seems to result from events in the first meiotic division (meiosis I).
- **Translocation** of an extra long arm of chromosome 21 to another acrocentric chromosome causes about 5% of cases of Down syndrome.
- **Mosaicism** for trisomy 21 is caused by nondisjunction during mitosis of a somatic cell early in embryogenesis and accounts for 2% of children born with Down syndrome.

Down syndrome caused by translocation of an extra portion of chromosome 21 occurs in two situations. Either parent may be a phenotypically normal carrier of a balanced translocation, or a translocation may arise de novo during gametogenesis. If the translocation is inherited from a parent, a balanced translocation has been converted to an unbalanced one.

The incidence of trisomy 21 correlates strongly with increasing maternal age; children of older mothers have a much greater risk of having Down syndrome. Up to their mid-30s, women have a constant risk of giving birth to a trisomic child of about 1 per 1,000 liveborn infants. The incidence then increases sharply to 1 in 30 at age 45 years. The risk of a mother having a second child with Down syndrome is 1%, regardless of maternal age, unless the syndrome is associated with translocation of chromosome 21.

The mechanism by which increasing maternal age increases the risk of bearing a child with trisomy 21 is poorly understood. Molecular studies have shown that the maternal age effect is related to maternal nondisjunction events, which implies that the defect lies in meiosis in oocytes. Down syndrome associated with translocation or mosaicism is not related to maternal age.

 PATHOLOGY AND CLINICAL FEATURES: The diagnosis of Down syndrome is ordinarily made at the time of birth by virtue of the infant's flaccid state and characteristic appearance. The diagnosis is then confirmed by cytogenetic analysis. As the child develops, a typical constellation of abnormalities appears (Fig. 6-5).

- **Mental status:** Children with Down syndrome are invariably mentally retarded. Their IQs decline relentlessly and progressively with age. Mean IQs are 70 below the age of 1 year, declining during the first decade of life to a mean of 30.
- **Craniofacial features:** Face and occiput tend to be flat, with a low-bridged nose, reduced interpupillary distance, and oblique palpebral fissures. Epicanthal folds of the eyes impart an Oriental appearance, which accounts for the obsolete term **mongolism**. A speckled appearance of the iris is referred to as **Brushfield spots.** Ears are enlarged and malformed. A prominent tongue, which typically lacks a central fissure, protrudes through an open mouth.
- **Heart:** One third of children with Down syndrome have cardiac malformations.
- **Skeleton:** These children tend to be small, owing to shorter than normal bones of the ribs, pelvis, and extremities. The hands are broad and short and exhibit a "simian crease," that is, a single transverse crease across the palm. The middle phalanx of the fifth finger is hypoplastic, an abnormality that leads to inward curvature of this digit.

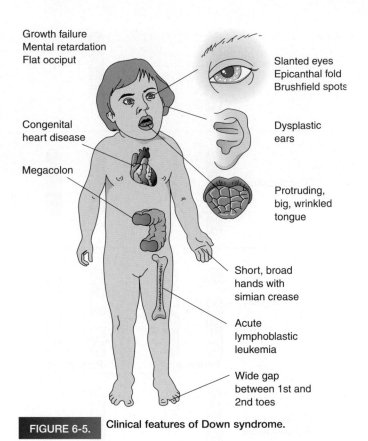

Growth failure
Mental retardation
Flat occiput

Slanted eyes
Epicanthal fold
Brushfield spots

Congenital
heart disease

Dysplastic
ears

Megacolon

Protruding,
big, wrinkled
tongue

Short, broad
hands with
simian crease

Acute
lymphoblastic
leukemia

Wide gap
between 1st and
2nd toes

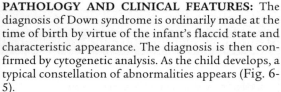 **FIGURE 6-5.** Clinical features of Down syndrome.

- **Reproductive system:** Men with trisomy 21 are invariably sterile, owing to arrested spermatogenesis. A few women with Down syndrome have given birth to children, 40% of whom had trisomy 21.
- **Hematologic disorders:** Persons with Down syndrome are at a particularly high risk of developing leukemia at all ages. *The risk of leukemia in Down syndrome children younger than the age of 15 years is about 15-fold greater than normal.*
- **Neurologic disorders:** *One of the most intriguing neurologic features of Down syndrome is its association with Alzheimer disease,* a relationship that has been appreciated for more than half a century. The lesions characteristic of Alzheimer disease are universally demonstrable by age 35, including (1) granulovacuolar degeneration, (2) neurofibrillary tangles, (3) senile plaques, and (4) loss of neurons (see Chapter 28). Dementia appears in one-fourth to one-half of older patients with Down syndrome, with a progressive loss of many intellectual functions.
- **Life expectancy:** Only about 5% of Down syndrome patients with normal hearts die before age 10, whereas about 25% with heart disease die by that age. For those who reach age 10, the estimated age at death is 55, which is 20 years or more lower than that of the general population. Only 10% reach age 70.

Additional Sex Chromosomes Produce less Severe Disease than do Extra Autosomes

The reasons are not entirely clear, but additional sex chromosomes produce less severe clinical manifestations than do extra autosomes and are less likely to disturb critical stages of development. In the case of additional X chromosomes, the reason that the phenotype tends to be less severely affected is probably related to *lyonization*, a normal process in which each cell has only one active X chromosome (see below).

The contrast between the X and Y chromosomes is striking. Whereas the X chromosome is one of the larger chromosomes, with 6% of all DNA, the Y chromosome is very small. More than 1,300 genes have been identified on the X chromosome. By contrast, the Y chromosome has fewer than 400 genes, one of which is the testis-determining gene (*SRY*, also known as *TDF*).

The Y Chromosome

In humans, it appears that genes on the Y chromosome are the key determinants of gender phenotype. Thus, the phenotype of people who are XXY (Klinefelter syndrome; see below) is male, and those who are XO (Turner syndrome) are female. The testis-determining gene (*SRY*, sex-determining region, Y) is an intron-less gene near the end of the short arm of the Y chromosome, which encodes a small nuclear protein with a DNA-binding domain. This protein binds another protein (SIP-1) to form a complex that is a transcriptional activator of autosomal genes that control development of a male phenotype. Mutations in this gene lead to XY females, whereas translocations that introduce this gene into an X chromosome produce XX males.

The X Chromosome

Males carry only one X chromosome but produce the same amounts of X chromosome gene products as do females. This seeming discrepancy is explained by the **Lyon effect:**

- In females, one X chromosome is irreversibly inactivated at random early in embryogenesis. The inactivated X chromosome is detectable in interphase nuclei as a heterochromatic clump of chromatin attached to the inner nuclear membrane, termed the **Barr body**.
- Inactivation of the X chromosome is virtually complete. However, a significant minority of X-linked genes escapes inactivation and continues to be expressed by both X chromosomes (see below).
- Inactivation of the X chromosome is permanent and is transmitted to progeny cells. Thus, paternally or maternally derived X chromosomes are propagated clonally. *All females are therefore mosaic for paternally and maternally derived X chromosomes.*
- A part of the short arm of the X chromosome (the **pseudoautosomal region**) is known to escape X-inactivation. This region is homologous with a region of the short arm of the Y chromosome. Genes in this location are present in two functional copies in both males and females.

Klinefelter Syndrome (47, XXY)

In Klinefelter syndrome, or testicular dysgenesis, there are one or more X chromosomes beyond the normal male XY complement. This is the most important clinical condition involving trisomy of sex chromosomes (Fig. 6-6). This syndrome is a prominent cause of male hypogonadism and infertility.

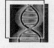 **PATHOGENESIS:** Most people (80%) with Klinefelter syndrome have a single extra X chromosome, that is, a 47, XXY karyotype. A minority are mosaics (e.g., 46, XY/47, XXY) or have more than two X chromosomes (e.g., 48, XXXY). *Interestingly, regardless of the number of supernumerary X chromosomes, the Y chromosome ensures a male phenotype.* The number of additional X chromosomes correlates with a more abnormal phenotype, despite the inactivation of the extra X chromosomes. Presumably, the same genes that escape inactivation in healthy females are still functional in Klinefelter syndrome.

Klinefelter syndrome occurs in 1 per 1,000 male newborns, roughly comparable to the incidence of Down syndrome. Interestingly, half of all 47, XXY conceptuses are lost by spontaneous abortion. In half of the cases, nondisjunction occurs during

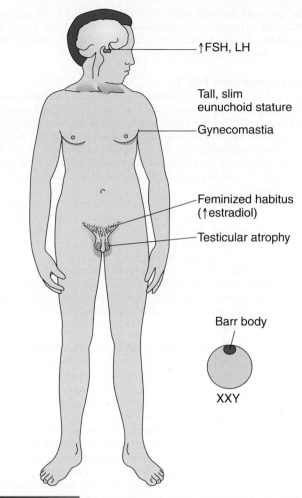

FIGURE 6-6. Clinical features of Klinefelter syndrome. FSH, follicle-stimulating hormone; LH, leuteinizing hormone.

paternal meiosis I, leading to a sperm that contains both an X and a Y chromosome. Fertilization of a normal oocyte by such a sperm produces a 47, XXY karyotype.

 PATHOLOGY: After puberty, the intrinsically abnormal testes do not respond to gonadotropin stimulation and show sequentially regressive alterations. Seminiferous tubules display atrophy, hyalinization, and peritubular fibrosis. Germ cells and Sertoli cells are usually absent, and eventually the tubules become dense cords of collagen. Leydig cells are increased in number, but their function is impaired, as evidenced by low testosterone levels in the face of elevated luteinizing hormone levels.

 CLINICAL FEATURES: The diagnosis of Klinefelter syndrome is ordinarily made after puberty. Gross mental retardation is uncommon, although average IQ is probably somewhat reduced.

Children with Klinefelter syndrome tend to be tall and thin, with relatively long legs (eunuchoid body habitus). Normal testicular growth and masculinization do not occur at puberty, and the testes and penis remain small. Feminine characteristics include a high-pitched voice, gynecomastia, and a female pattern of pubic hair (female escutcheon). Azoospermia results in infertility. All of these changes are due to hypogonadism and a resulting lack of androgens. Serum testosterone is low to normal, but luteinizing hormone and follicle-stimulating hormone are remarkably high, indicating normal pituitary function. High circulating estradiol levels increase the estradiol-to-testosterone ratio, which determines the degree of feminization. Although treatment with testosterone virilizes these patients, it does not restore fertility.

Turner Syndrome (45, X)

Turner syndrome refers to the spectrum of abnormalities that results from complete or partial X chromosome monosomy in a phenotypic female. It occurs in about 1 liveborn female infant in 5,000. In three fourths of cases, the single X chromosome of Turner syndrome is of maternal origin, suggesting that the meiotic error tends to be paternal. The incidence of the syndrome does not correlate with maternal age, and the risk of producing a second affected female infant is not increased.

The 45, X karyotype is actually one of the most common aneuploid abnormalities in human conceptuses, but almost all are aborted spontaneously. In fact, up to 2% of abortuses show this aberration. Only about half of women with Turner syndrome lack an entire X chromosome (monosomy X). The rest of these women are mosaics or have structural X chromosome aberrations, such as isochromosome of the long arm, translocations, and deletions. Mosaics with a 45, X/46, XX karyotype (15%) tend to have milder phenotypic manifestations of Turner syndrome and may even be fertile.

 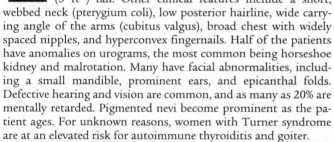 **PATHOLOGY AND CLINICAL FEATURES:** The clinical hallmark of Turner syndrome is sexual infantilism, with primary amenorrhea and sterility (Fig. 6-7). In most cases, the disorder is not discovered until the absence of menarche brings the child to medical attention. Virtually all of these women are less than 152 cm (5 ft) tall. Other clinical features include a short, webbed neck (pterygium coli), low posterior hairline, wide carrying angle of the arms (cubitus valgus), broad chest with widely spaced nipples, and hyperconvex fingernails. Half of the patients have anomalies on urograms, the most common being horseshoe kidney and malrotation. Many have facial abnormalities, including a small mandible, prominent ears, and epicanthal folds. Defective hearing and vision are common, and as many as 20% are mentally retarded. Pigmented nevi become prominent as the patient ages. For unknown reasons, women with Turner syndrome are at an elevated risk for autoimmune thyroiditis and goiter.

Cardiovascular anomalies occur in almost half the patients with Turner syndrome. Coarctation of the aorta is seen in 15%, and a bicuspid aortic valve is seen in as many as one third. Essential hypertension occurs in some patients, and dissecting aneurysm of the aorta is occasionally a cause of death.

Ovaries of fetuses with Turner syndrome contain oocytes at first, but they lose them rapidly, so that none remain by 2 years of age. The ovaries are converted to fibrous streaks, whereas the uterus, fallopian tubes, and vagina develop normally. It may be said that the child with Turner syndrome has undergone menopause long before normal females reach menarche.

Single Gene Abnormalities Result in Traits that Segregate Within Families

Familial traits that are inherited in a Mendelian fashion are characterized as having the following patterns of inheritances:

1. **Autosomal dominant** traits require the presence of only one allele of a homologous gene pair located on an autosomal chromosome, provided that the person is heterozygous for the trait.
2. **Autosomal recessive** traits are expressed only if both alleles of a homologous autosomal gene are defective (i.e., the individual is homozygous for the trait).
3. **Sex-linked dominant** traits require the presence of only one allele of a homologous gene pair located on the X chromosome.
4. **Sex-linked recessive** traits are expressed only if both alleles of a homologous gene on the X chromosome are defective in the

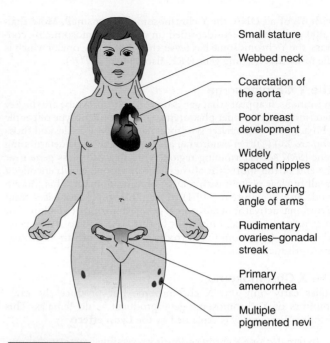

Small stature
Webbed neck
Coarctation of the aorta
Poor breast development
Widely spaced nipples
Wide carrying angle of arms
Rudimentary ovaries–gonadal streak
Primary amenorrhea
Multiple pigmented nevi

FIGURE 6-7. Clinical features of Turner syndrome.

female (i.e., the individual is homozygous for the trait). Sex-linked recessive traits (such as hemophilia) are expressed in a male who carries a single X chromosome.
5. **Codominance** refers to a situation in which both alleles in a heterozygous gene pair are fully expressed (e.g., the AB blood group genes).

Diseases due to sex-linked dominant genes are rare and of little practical importance.

Mutations

A mutation is a stable heritable change in DNA. The consequences of mutations are highly variable. Some have no functional consequences, whereas others are lethal and cannot be transmitted from one generation to another. An exhaustive reference to mutations causing human disease is available from Online Mendelian Inheritance in Man™ (http://www.ncbi.nlm.nih.gov/entrez/query.fcgi?db=OMIM). Certain regions of the genome mutate at a much higher rate than average. The best-characterized hotspot is the dinucleotide pair CG, which is prone to undergo mutation to form TG. Several additional types of mutations are also known to be associated with human disease:

- **Large deletions:** When a large segment of DNA is deleted, the coding region of a gene may be entirely removed, in which case the protein product is absent. On the other hand, a large deletion may result in the apposition of coding regions of nearby genes, giving rise to a fused gene that codes for a hybrid protein, one in which part or all of one protein is followed by part or all of another.
- **Expansion of unstable trinucleotide repeat sequences:** The human genome contains frequent tandem trinucleotide repeat sequences. The number of repeats within such repetitive trinucleotide sequences varies among individuals. In general, the number of repeats below a particular threshold does not change during mitosis or meiosis, whereas above this threshold, the number of repeats can expand or contract, expansion being far more common. A number of distinct trinucleotide expansions have been identified in human diseases, including Huntington disease, fragile X syndrome (see below), and myotonic dystrophy, the most common form of autosomal muscular dystrophy (see Chapter 27).

Autosomal Dominant Disorders are Expressed in Heterozygotes

An autosomal dominant disease occurs when only one defective gene (i.e., mutant allele) is present, whereas its paired allele on the homologous chromosome is normal (Fig. 6-8).

- Males and females are equally affected, because by definition, the mutant gene resides on one of the 22 autosomal chromosomes.
- The trait encoded by the mutant gene can be transmitted to successive generations (unless the disease interferes with reproductive capacity).
- Unaffected family members do not transmit the trait to their offspring. Unless the disease represents a new mutation, everyone with the disease has an affected parent.
- The proportions of normal and diseased offspring of patients with the disorder are on average equal, because most affected individuals are heterozygous, whereas their normal siblings do not harbor the defective gene.
- In many human pedigrees, the picture is far more complex. Autosomal dominant traits often vary in **penetrance** (whether an inherited mutant allele results in detectable disease) and **expressivity** (the degree to which a trait is expressed, i.e., the severity of disease) even within a single pedigree.

More than 1,000 human diseases are inherited as autosomal dominant traits, although most are rare. Examples of human autosomal dominant diseases are given in Table 6-2.

Heritable Diseases of Connective Tissue are Heterogeneous and Often Inherited as Autosomal Dominant Traits

This discussion is limited to two of the most common and best-studied entities: Marfan syndrome and Ehlers-Danlos syndrome. Even in these well-delineated disorders, clinical symptomatology often overlaps.

Marfan Syndrome

Marfan syndrome is an autosomal dominant, inherited disorder of connective tissue characterized by a variety of abnormalities in many organs, including the heart, aorta, skeleton, eyes, and skin. One third of cases represent sporadic mutations. The incidence in the United States is 1 per 10,000.

Autosomal Dominant

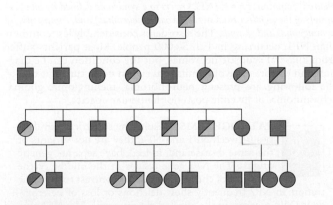

☑⊘ Heterozygote with disease

FIGURE 6-8. **Autosomal dominant inheritance.** Only symptomatic individuals transmit the trait to the next generation, and heterozygotes are symptomatic. Both males and females are affected.

 PATHOGENESIS: The cause of Marfan syndrome is a missense mutation in the gene for *fibrillin-1(FBN1)* on the long arm of chromosome 15. Fibrillin is a family of connective tissue proteins analogous to the collagens, of which there are now about a dozen genetically distinct forms. It is widely distributed in many tissues in the form of a fiber system termed **microfibrils**, which are organized into rods, sheets, and interlaced networks. **Such microfibrillar fibers** are scaffolds for elastin deposition during embryonic development, after which they constitute part of elastic tissues. Abnormal microfibrillar fibers have been visualized in all the tissues affected in Marfan syndrome.

 PATHOLOGY AND CLINICAL FEATURES: People with Marfan syndrome are usually (but not invariably) tall, and the lower body segment (pubis-to-sole) is longer than the upper body segment. A slender habitus, which reflects a paucity of subcutaneous fat, is complemented by long, thin extremities and fingers, which accounts for the term **arachnodactyly** (spider fingers). Other defects include:

- **Skeletal system:** The skull in Marfan syndrome is characteristically long (dolichocephalic) with prominent frontal eminences. Disorders of the ribs are conspicuous and produce pectus excavatum (concave sternum) and pectus carinatum (pigeon breast). The tendons, ligaments, and joint capsules are weak, a condition that leads to hyperextensibility of the joints (double-jointedness), dislocations, hernias, and kyphoscoliosis; the last is often severe.
- **Cardiovascular system:** *The most important vascular defect is in the aorta, in which the principal lesion is a weak tunica media.* Weakness of the media leads to variable dilation of the ascending aorta and a high incidence of dissecting aneurysms. The aneurysm, usually of the ascending aorta, may rupture into the pericardial cavity or make its way down the aorta and rupture into the retroperitoneal space. Cardiovascular disorders are the most common causes of death in Marfan syndrome.
- **Eyes:** Ocular changes are common in Marfan syndrome and reflect the intrinsic lesion in connective tissue. These include dislocation of the lens (ectopia lentis), severe myopia due to elongation of the eye, and retinal detachment.

Untreated men with Marfan syndrome usually die in their 30s, and untreated women often die in their 40s. However, with antihy-

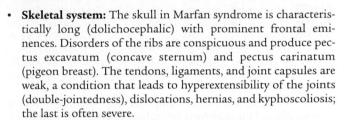

TABLE 6–2

Representative Autosomal Dominant Disorders

Disease	Frequency	Chromosome
Familial hypercholesterolemia	1/500	19p
von Willebrand disease	1/8,000	12p
Hereditary spherocytosis (major forms)	1/5,000	14,8
Hereditary elliptocytosis (all forms)	1/2,500	1, 1p, 2q, 14
Osteogenosis imperfecta (types I–IV)	1/10,000	17q, 7q
Ehlers-Danlos syndrome, type III	1/5,000	?
Marfan syndrome	1/10,000	15q
Neurofibromatosis type 1	1/3,500	17q
Huntington chorea	1/15,000	4p
Retinoblastoma	1/14,000	13q
Wilms' tumor	1/10,000	11p
Familial adenomatous polyposis	1/10,000	5q
Acute intermittent porphyria	1/15,000	11q
Hereditary amyloidosis	1/100,000	18q
Adult polycystic kidney disease	1/1,000	16p

pertensive therapy and replacement of the aorta with prosthetic grafts, life expectancy approaches normal.

Ehlers-Danlos Syndromes

The Ehlers-Danlos syndromes (EDS) are rare, autosomal dominant, inherited disorders of connective tissue that feature remarkable hyperelasticity and fragility of the skin, joint hypermobility, and often a bleeding diathesis. The disorder is clinically and genetically heterogeneous, and more than 10 varieties of EDS have been distinguished.

 PATHOGENESIS: The genetic and biochemical lesions in 7 of the 10 types of EDS have been established. *The common feature of all is a generalized defect in collagen, including abnormalities in its molecular structure, synthesis, secretion, and degradation.* Depending on the type of EDS, these molecular lesions are associated with conspicuous weakness of the supporting structures of the skin, joints, arteries, and visceral organs.

 PATHOLOGY AND CLINICAL FEATURES: All types of EDS are characterized by soft, fragile, hyperextensible skin. Patients typically can stretch their skin many centimeters, and trivial injuries can lead to serious wounds. Sutures do not hold well, so dehiscence of surgical incisions is common. Hypermobility of the joints allows unusual extension and flexion. **EDS VI** is the most dangerous variety, owing to a tendency to spontaneous rupture of the large arteries, bowel, and gravid uterus. Death from such complications is common in the third and fourth decades of life.

EDS VI also has major complications, including severe kyphoscoliosis, blindness from retinal hemorrhage (or rupture of the globe), and death from aortic rupture. Severe periodontal disease, with loss of teeth by the third decade, characterizes EDS VIII. EDS IX features the development of bladder diverticula during childhood, with a danger of bladder rupture and skeletal deformities.

Many people who exhibit clinical abnormalities suggesting EDS do not conform to any of the documented types of this disorder. Further genetic and biochemical characterization of such cases is likely to expand the classification of EDS.

Neurofibromatosis Includes Two Distinct Autosomal Dominant Disorders that Feature Benign Tumors of Peripheral Nerves

Neurofibromatosis Type I (von Recklinghausen Disease)

Neurofibromatosis type I (NF1) is characterized by (1) disfiguring neurofibromas, (2) areas of dark pigmentation of the skin (café-au-lait spots), and (3) pigmented lesions of the iris (Lisch nodules). It is one of the more common autosomal dominant disorders, affecting 1 in 3,500 persons of all races. The *NF1* gene has an unusually high rate of mutation, and half of the cases are sporadic rather than familial.

 PATHOGENESIS: Germline mutations in the NF1 gene, on the long arm of chromosome 17, include deletions, missense mutations, and nonsense mutations. The gene product, *neurofibromin*, belongs to a family of GTPase-activating proteins (GAP), which inactivate the ras protein (see Chapter 5). In this sense, NF1 is a classic tumor suppressor. The loss of GTPase-activating protein activity permits uncontrolled ras activation, which presumably predisposes to the formation of neurofibromas.

 PATHOLOGY AND CLINICAL FEATURES: The clinical manifestations of NF1 are highly variable and difficult to explain entirely on the basis of a single gene defect. The typical features of NF1 include:

- **Neurofibromas:** More than 90% of patients with NF1 develop cutaneous and subcutaneous neurofibromas in late childhood or adolescence. These cutaneous tumors, which may total more than 500, appear as soft, pedunculated masses, usually about 1 cm in diameter. However, on occasion, they may reach alarming proportions and dominate the physical appearance of a patient, attaining 25 cm in diameter. Subcutaneous neurofibromas present as soft nodules along the course of peripheral nerves. **Plexiform neurofibromas** occur only within the context of NF1 and are diagnostic of that condition. Although these tumors usually involve the larger peripheral nerves, they sometimes may arise from cranial or intraspinal nerves. Plexiform neurofibromas are often large, infiltrative tumors that cause severe disfigurement of the face or an extremity. The microscopic appearance of neurofibromas is discussed in Chapter 28. *A major complication of NF1, occurring in 3% to 5% of patients, is the appearance of a neurofibrosarcoma in a neurofibroma, usually a larger one of the plexiform type.* NF1 is also associated with an increased incidence of other neurogenic tumors, including meningioma, optic glioma, and pheochromocytoma.
- **Café-au-lait spots:** Although normal individuals may exhibit occasional light brown patches on the skin, more than 95% of persons affected by NF1 display six or more such lesions. These are larger than 5 mm before puberty and greater than 1.5 cm thereafter.
- **Lisch nodules:** More than 90% of patients with NF1 have pigmented nodules of the iris, which are masses of melanocytes. These lesions are thought to be hamartomas.
- **Skeletal lesions:** A number of bone lesions occur frequently in NF1. These include malformations of the sphenoid bone and thinning of the cortex of the long bones, with bowing and pseudarthrosis of the tibia, bone cysts, and scoliosis.
- **Mental status:** Mild intellectual impairment is frequent in patients with NF1, but severe retardation is not part of the syndrome.
- **Leukemia:** The risk of malignant myeloid disorders in children with NF1 is 200 to 500 times the normal risk. In some patients, both alleles of the NF1 gene are inactivated in leukemic cells.

Neurofibromatosis Type II (Central Neurofibromatosis)

Neurofibromatosis type II (NF2) refers to a syndrome defined by bilateral tumors of the eighth cranial nerve (acoustic neuromas) and, commonly, by meningiomas and gliomas. The disorder is considerably less common than NF1, occurring in 1 in 50,000 people. Most patients suffer from bilateral acoustic neuromas, but the condition can be diagnosed in the presence of a unilateral eighth nerve tumor if two of the following are present: neurofibroma, meningioma, glioma, schwannoma, or juvenile posterior lenticular opacity.

 PATHOGENESIS: Despite the superficial similarities between NF1 and NF2, they are not variants of the same disease and, indeed, have separate genetic origins. The *NF2* gene resides in the middle of the long arm of chromosome 22. In contrast to NF1, the tumors in NF2 frequently show deletions or loss of heterozygous DNA markers in the affected chromosome. The *NF2* gene encodes a tumor-suppressor protein termed **merlin**, or **schwannomin**, which is a member of a superfamily of proteins that link the cytoskeleton to the cell membrane. Merlin is detectable in most differentiated tissues, including Schwann cells.

Familial Hypercholesterolemia is One of the Most Common Autosomal Dominant Disorders

Familial hypercholesterolemia is an autosomal dominant disorder characterized by high levels of low-density lipoproteins (LDLs) in the blood and deposition of cholesterol in arteries, tendons, and skin. It is one of the most common autosomal dominant disorders, affecting 1 in 500 adults in the United States in its heterozygous form. Only 1 person in 1 million is homozygous for the disease. *Interest in this disease stems from the striking acceleration of atherosclerosis and its complications* (see Chapter 10).

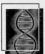 **PATHOGENESIS:** Familial hypercholesterolemia results from abnormalities in the low-density-lipoprotein receptor gene (19p13) that codes for the cell surface receptor that removes LDL from the blood. More than 750 different mutations in the low-density-lipoprotein receptor gene are known. The LDL receptor is (1) synthesized in the endoplasmic reticulum, (2) transferred to the Golgi complex, (3) transported to the cell surface, and (4) internalized by receptor-mediated endocytosis in coated pits after binding LDL. Genetic defects in each of these steps have been described.

Hepatocytes are the main cell type expressing the LDL receptor. After LDL binds the receptors, they are internalized and degraded in lysosomes, freeing cholesterol for further metabolism. Lacking LDL receptor function, high levels of LDL circulate, are taken up by tissue macrophages, and accumulate to form occlusive arterial plaques (atheromas) and papules or nodules of lipid-laden macrophages (xanthomas) (see Chapter 10).

 CLINICAL FEATURES: Heterozygous and homozygous familial hypercholesterolemia are two distinct clinical syndromes, reflecting a clear **gene-dosage effect**. In heterozygotes, elevated blood cholesterol (mean, 350 mg/dL; normal, <200 mg/dL) is seen at birth. Tendon xanthomas develop in half of the patients before the age of 30, and symptoms of coronary heart disease often occur before age 40. In homozygotes, blood cholesterol content reaches astronomic levels (600 to 1,200 mg/dL), and virtually all patients have tendon xanthomas as well as generalized atherosclerosis in childhood. Untreated homozygotes typically die of myocardial infarction before they reach 30 years of age.

Autosomal Recessive Disorders Cause Symptoms in People Who Have Defective Alleles on Both Homologous Chromosomes

Most genetic metabolic diseases exhibit an autosomal recessive mode of inheritance (Fig. 6-9; Table 6-3). Some of the salient features of such disorders are:

- The more infrequent the mutant gene in the general population, the higher the chance that parents of an affected individual are related. *Rare autosomal recessive disorders often derive from consanguineous marriages.*
- Both parents are usually heterozygous for the trait and are clinically normal.
- Symptoms appear on average in one of four of their offspring. Half of all offspring are heterozygous for the trait and are asymptomatic. Thus, two thirds of unaffected offspring are heterozygous carriers.
- As in autosomal dominant disorders, autosomal recessive traits are transmitted equally to males and females.
- Symptomatology of autosomal recessive disorders is ordinarily less variable than with dominant diseases.
- The variability in clinical expression of many autosomal recessive diseases is often a function of the residual functionality of the affected enzyme.

Autosomal Recessive

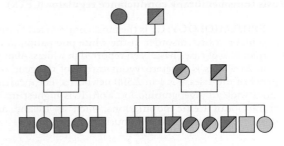

☐○ Homozygote with disease

◪◐ Heterozygote without disease (silent carrier)

FIGURE 6-9. **Autosomal recessive inheritance.** Symptoms of the disease appear only in homozygotes, male or female. Heterozygotes are asymptomatic carriers. Symptomatic homozygotes result from the mating of asymptomatic heterozygotes.

Many mutant genes responsible for autosomal recessive disorders are rare in the general population. Paradoxically, a few lethal autosomal recessive diseases are common. For example, sickle cell anemia may confer a biological advantage by increasing the resistance of heterozygotes to malarial parasitization and thus compensating for the loss of homozygotes.

Autosomal recessive diseases characteristically are caused by deficiencies in enzymes rather than in structural proteins. A mutation that inactivates an enzyme does not usually cause an abnormal phenotype in heterozygotes because most cellular enzymes operate at substrate concentrations well below saturation. An enzyme deficiency is easily corrected simply by increasing the amount of substrate. By contrast, loss of both alleles in a homozygote results in complete loss of enzyme activity, a situation that cannot be corrected by such mechanisms.

Cystic Fibrosis (CF) is the Most Common Lethal Autosomal Recessive Disease in Whites

CF is characterized by (1) chronic pulmonary disease; (2) deficient exocrine pancreatic function; and (3) other complications of inspissated mucus in several organs, including the small intestine, liver, and reproductive

TABLE 6–3		
Representative Autosomal Recessive Disorders		
Disease	**Frequency**	**Chromosome**
Cystic fibrosis	1/2,500	7q
α-Thalassemia	High	16p
β-Thalassemia	High	11p
Sickle cell anemia	High	11p
Myeloperoxidase deficiency	1/2,000	17q
Phenylketonuria	1/10,000	12q
Gaucher disease	1/1,000	1q
Tay-Sachs disease	1/4,000	15q
Hurler syndrome	1/100,000	22p
Glycogen storage disease Ia (von Gierke disease)	1/100,000	17
Wilson disease	1/50,000	13q
Hereditary hemochromatosis	1/1,000	6p
α₁-Antitrypsin deficiency	1/7,000	14q
Oculocutaneous albinism	1/20,000	11q
Alkaptonuria	<1/100,000	3q
Metachromatic leukodystrophy	1/100,000	22q

tract. The disease results from a defective chloride channel, the **cystic fibrosis transmembrane conductance regulator** (CFTR).

 EPIDEMIOLOGY: CF is the most common lethal autosomal recessive disorder in the white population. More than 95% of cases have been reported in whites. About 1 in 25 whites is a heterozygous carrier of the gene, and the incidence of the disease is 1 in 2,500 newborns. The incidence of CF varies widely by geographic location. It is highest in the northern European Celtic populations, such as Ireland and Scotland, and is much lower among southern Europeans.

 PATHOGENESIS: The CFTR gene is on the long arm of chromosome 7 and encodes a protein that is a member of the ATP-binding family of membrane transporter proteins. It is a chloride channel in most epithelia, with two membrane-spanning domains, two domains that bind ATP, and an "R" domain that contains phosphorylation sites.

Secretion of chloride anions by mucus-secreting epithelial cells controls the parallel secretion of fluid and, consequently, the viscosity of the mucus. In normal mucus-secreting epithelia, cAMP activates protein kinase A, which phosphorylates the regulatory domain of CFTR and permits channel opening. The most common (70%) mutation in the white population is a deletion of three base pairs that deletes a phenylalanine residue (ΔF_{508}). The next most common mutation accounts for only 2% of all mutations.

All pathologic consequences of CF can be attributed to the abnormally thick mucus that obstructs the lumina of airways, pancreatic and biliary ducts, as well as the fetal intestine, and impairs airway mucociliary function.

 PATHOLOGY: CF affects many organs that produce exocrine secretions.

RESPIRATORY TRACT: *Pulmonary disease is responsible for most of the morbidity and mortality associated with CF.* The earliest lesion is obstruction of bronchioles by mucus, with secondary infection and inflammation of bronchiolar walls. Recurrent cycles of obstruction and infection result in **chronic bronchiolitis** and **bronchitis**, which increase in severity as the disease progresses. Bronchial mucous glands undergo hypertrophy and hyperplasia, and airways are distended by thick and tenacious secretions. Widespread **bronchiectasis** becomes apparent by age 10 and often earlier. In late stages of the disease, large bronchiectatic cysts and lung abscesses are common. Secondary pulmonary hypertension may complicate the chronic bronchitis.

PANCREAS: Most (85%) patients with CF have a form of **chronic pancreatitis**, and in long-standing cases, little or no functional exocrine pancreas remains. Inspissated secretions in the pancreatic ducts produce secondary dilation and cystic change of the distal ducts (Fig. 6-10). Recurrent pancreatitis leads to loss of acinar cells and extensive fibrosis. At autopsy, the pancreas is often simply cystic fibroadipose tissue containing islets of Langerhans.

LIVER: Inspissated mucous secretions in the intrahepatic biliary system obstruct the flow of bile in the drainage areas of the affected ducts and lead to focal **secondary biliary cirrhosis**, which is seen in one fourth of patients at autopsy. Microscopically, the liver shows inspissated concretions in bile ducts and ductules, chronic portal inflammation, and septal fibrosis. On occasion, the hepatic lesions are sufficiently widespread to lead to the clinical manifestations of biliary cirrhosis.

GASTROINTESTINAL TRACT: Shortly after birth, a normal newborn passes the intestinal contents that have accumulated in utero (meconium). The most important lesion of the gut in CF is

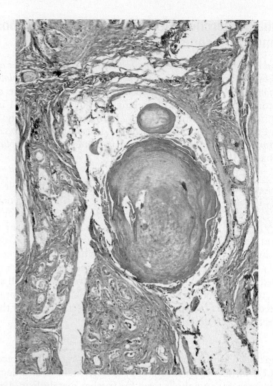

FIGURE 6-10. Intraductal concretion and atrophy of the acini in the pancreas of a patient with cystic fibrosis.

small-bowel obstruction in 5% to 10% of newborns, termed **meconium ileus**, which is caused by failure to pass meconium in the immediate postpartum period. This complication has been attributed to the failure of pancreatic secretions to digest meconium, possibly augmented by the greater viscosity of small-bowel secretions.

REPRODUCTIVE TRACT: Almost all boys with CF have atrophy or fibrosis of the reproductive duct system, including the vas deferens, epididymis, and seminal vesicles. The pathogenesis of these lesions relates to obstruction of the lumen by inspissated secretions early in life and even in utero. As a result, only 2% to 3% of males become fertile, most demonstrating an absence of spermatozoa in the semen.

Only a minority of women with CF are fertile, and many of them suffer from anovulatory cycles as a result of poor nutrition and chronic infections. Moreover, the cervical mucous plug is abnormally thick and tenacious.

 CLINICAL FEATURES: *The diagnosis of CF is most reliably made by detecting increased concentrations of electrolytes in the sweat and by genetic studies that demonstrate the disease-causing mutations.* The decreased chloride conductance characteristic of CF results in a failure of chloride reabsorption by the cells of the sweat gland ducts and hence to the accumulation of sodium chloride in the sweat (Fig. 6-11). Children with CF have been described as "tasting salty" and may even display salt crystals on their skin after vigorous sweating.

The clinical course of CF is highly variable. At one extreme, death may result from meconium ileus in the neonatal period, whereas some patients have reportedly survived to age 50. Improved medical care and recognition of milder cases of CF have served to prolong the average life span to about 30 years of age.

The most common organisms that infect the respiratory tract in CF are *Staphylococcus* and *Pseudomonas* species. As the disease advances, *Pseudomonas* may be the only organism cultured from the lung. *In fact, the recovery of* Pseudomonas *species, particularly the mucoid variety, from the lungs of a child with chronic pulmonary disease is virtually diagnostic of CF.* Infection with *Burkholderia cepacia* is associated with **cepacia syndrome**, a severe pulmonary infection that is highly resistant to treatment with antibiotics and is commonly fatal.

Postural drainage of the airways, antibiotic therapy, and pancreatic enzyme supplementation are the mainstays of treatment. Molecular prenatal diagnosis of CF is now accurate in 95% of cases. Lung transplantation may also be successful in cases of terminal lung disease.

Lysosomal Storage Diseases are Characterized by the Accumulation of Unmetabolized Normal Substrates

Extracellular macromolecules that are incorporated by endocytosis or phagocytosis and intracellular constituents that are subjected to autophagy are digested in lysosomes to their basic components. End products may be transported across the lysosomal membrane into the cytosol, where they are reused in the synthesis of new macromolecules.

Virtually all lysosomal storage diseases result from mutations in genes that encode lysosomal hydrolases. A deficiency in one of the more than 40 acid hydrolases can result in an inability to catabolize the normal macromolecular substrate of that enzyme. As a result, undigested substrate accumulates in and engorges lysosomes, expanding the lysosomal compartment of the cell. The resulting lysosomal distention is often at the expense of other critical cellular components, particularly in the brain and heart, and can lead to a failure of cell function.

Lysosomal storage diseases are classified according to the material retained within the lysosomes. Thus, when the substrates that accumulate are sphingolipid, they are **sphingolipidoses**. Storage of mucopolysaccharides (glycosaminoglycans) leads to the **mucopolysaccharidoses**. More than 30 distinct lysosomal storage diseases are known, but we restrict our discussion to the more important examples.

Gaucher Disease

Gaucher disease is characterized by the accumulation of glucosylceramide, primarily in macrophage lysosomes.

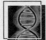 **PATHOGENESIS:** The abnormality in Gaucher disease is a deficiency in glucocerebrosidase, a lysosomal acid β-glucosidase. The enzyme deficiency can be traced to a variety of single-base mutations in the β-glucosidase gene, on the long arm of chromosome 1. Each of the three clinical types of the disease exhibits heterogeneous mutations in the β-glucosidase gene, although the molecular basis for the phenotypic differences remains to be firmly established.

The glucosylceramide that accumulates in Gaucher cells of the spleen, liver, bone marrow, and lymph nodes derives principally from the catabolism of senescent leukocytes. The membranes of these cells are rich in cerebrosides, and when their degradation is blocked by the deficiency of glucocerebrosidase, the intermediate metabolite, glucosylceramide, accumulates. The glucosylceramide of Gaucher cells in the brain is believed to originate from turnover of plasma membrane gangliosides of cells in the CNS.

 PATHOLOGY: The hallmark of this disorder is the presence of **Gaucher cells**, which are lipid-laden macrophages characteristically present in the red pulp of the spleen, liver sinusoids, lymph nodes, lungs, and bone marrow, although they may be found in virtually any organ. These cells are derived from resident macrophages in the respective organs, for example, Kupffer cells in the liver and alveolar macrophages in the lung.

Gaucher cells are large (20 to 100 µm) with clear cytoplasm and eccentric nuclei (Fig. 6-12). By light microscopy, the cytoplasm has a characteristic fibrillar appearance, which has been likened to wrinkled tissue paper and is intensely positive with the periodic acid-Schiff stain.

Enlargement of the spleen is virtually universal in Gaucher disease. In the adult form of the disorder, splenomegaly may be massive, with spleen weights up to 10 kg. The liver is usually enlarged by Gaucher cells within sinusoids, but hepatocytes are unaffected. In severe cases, hepatic fibrosis and even cirrhosis may ensue. The extent of bone marrow involvement is variable but leads to radiological abnormalities in 50% to 75% of cases.

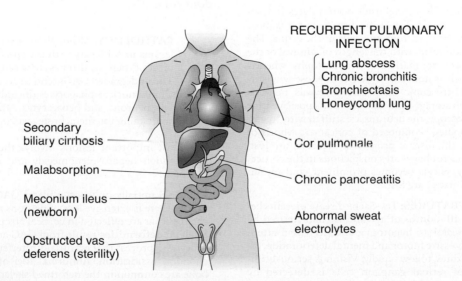

FIGURE 6-11. Clinical features of of cystic fibrosis.

RECURRENT PULMONARY INFECTION

Lung abscess
Chronic bronchitis
Bronchiectasis
Honeycomb lung

Cor pulmonale

Chronic pancreatitis

Abnormal sweat electrolytes

Secondary biliary cirrhosis

Malabsorption

Meconium ileus (newborn)

Obstructed vas deferens (sterility)

CLINICAL FEATURES: Gaucher disease is the most common of all lysosomal storage diseases. It is subclassified into three distinct forms, based on the age at onset and degree of neurologic involvement. The most common form is type 1 and is found principally in adult Ashkenazi Jews, among whom the incidence is 1 in 600 to 1 in 2,500. The age at onset and disease severity is highly variable—some cases are diagnosed in infants and others in individuals 70 years old. The disease usually presents initially as painless splenomegaly and the complications of hypersplenism (i.e., anemia, leukopenia, and thrombocytopenia). Bone involvement, in the form of pain and pathologic fractures, is the leading cause of disability. The life expectancy of most persons with type 1 Gaucher disease is normal. This type of Gaucher disease is now successfully treated by intravenous administration of modified acid glucose cerebrosidase. Other rare variants of the disease present in infants and are associated with neurological degeneration and early death.

Tay-Sachs Disease (GM$_2$ Gangliosidosis, Type 1)

Tay-Sachs disease is the catastrophic infantile form of a class of lysosomal storage diseases known as the GM$_2$ gangliosidoses, in which this ganglioside is deposited in neurons of the CNS, owing to a failure of lysosomal degradation. Tay-Sachs disease is inherited as an autosomal recessive trait and is predominantly a disorder of Ashkenazi Jews, in whom the carrier rate is 1 in 30, and the natural incidence of homozygotes is 1 in 4,000 live newborns. By contrast, the incidence of Tay-Sachs disease in non-Jewish American populations is less than 1 in 100,000 live births. The other GM$_2$ gangliosidoses are exceedingly rare.

 PATHOGENESIS: Gangliosides are glycosphingolipids consisting of a ceramide and an oligosaccharide chain that contains *N*-acetylneuraminic acid. They are present in the outer leaflet of the plasma membrane of animal cells, particularly in brain neurons.

Tay-Sachs disease (also known as hexosaminidase α-subunit deficiency) results from about 50 different mutations in the gene that codes for the α subunit of hexosaminidase A, with a resulting defect in the synthesis of this enzyme.

 PATHOLOGY: GM$_2$ ganglioside accumulates in lysosomes of all organs in Tay-Sachs disease, but it is most prominent in brain neurons and cells of the retina. The size of the brain varies with the length of survival of the affected infant. Early cases are marked by brain atrophy, whereas the brain may be as much as doubled in weight in those who survive beyond a year. Microscopic examination reveals neurons markedly distended with storage material that stains positively for lipids. By electron microscopy, the neurons are stuffed with "membranous cytoplasmic bodies," composed of concentric whorls of lamellar structures. As the disease progresses, neurons are lost, and many lipid-laden macrophages are conspicuous in the cortical gray matter. Eventually, gliosis becomes prominent, and myelin and axons in the white matter are lost.

 CLINICAL FEATURES: Tay-Sachs disease presents between 6 and 10 months of age and is characterized by progressive weakness, hypotonia, and decreased attentiveness. Progressive motor and mental deterioration, often with generalized seizures, follow rapidly. Vision is seriously impaired. Involvement of retinal ganglion cells is detected by ophthalmoscopy as a **cherry-red spot** in the macula. This feature reflects the pallor of the affected cells, which enhances the prominence of blood vessels underlying the central fovea. Most children with Tay-Sachs disease die before 4 years of age.

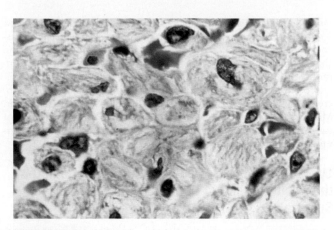

FIGURE 6-12. **The spleen in Gaucher disease.** Typical Gaucher cells have foamy cytoplasm and eccentrically located nuclei.

Mucopolysaccharidoses

The mucopolysaccharidoses (MPS) are an assortment of lysosomal storage diseases characterized by the accumulation of glycosaminoglycans (mucopolysaccharides) in many organs. All types of MPS are inherited as autosomal recessive traits, except for Hunter syndrome, which is X-linked. These rare diseases are caused by deficiencies in any one of the 10 lysosomal enzymes that catabolize glycosaminoglycans. Six abnormal phenotypes are described, and each varies with the specific enzyme deficiency.

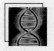 **PATHOGENESIS:** Glycosaminoglycans (GAGs) are large polymers of repeating disaccharide units containing *N*-acetylhexosamine and a hexose or hexuronic acid. Either disaccharide may be sulfated. The accumulated GAGs (dermatan sulfate, heparan sulfate, keratan sulfate, and chondroitin sulfates) in MPS are all derived from the cleavage of proteoglycans, which are important extracellular matrix constituents. GAGs are degraded stepwise by removing sugar residues or sulfate groups. Thus, a deficiency in any one of the glycosidases or sulfatases results in the accumulation of undegraded GAGs.

 PATHOLOGY: Although the severity and location of the lesions in MPS vary with the specific enzyme deficiency, most of these syndromes share certain common features. The undegraded GAGs tend to accumulate in connective tissue cells, mononuclear phagocytes (including Kupffer cells), endothelial cells, neurons, and hepatocytes. Affected cells are swollen and clear, and stains for metachromasia confirm the presence of GAGs.

The most important lesions involve the CNS, skeleton, and heart, although hepatosplenomegaly and corneal clouding are common.

- **The CNS** initially only accumulates GAGs, but as disease advances, there is extensive loss of neurons and increasing gliosis, changes that are reflected in cortical atrophy.
- **Skeletal deformities** result from GAG accumulation in chondrocytes, a process that eventually interferes with normal endochondral ossification. Abnormal foci of osteoid and woven bone are common in the deformed skeleton.
- **Cardiac lesions** are often severe, with thickening and distortion of valves, chordae tendineae, and endocardium. The coronary arteries are frequently narrowed by intimal thickening caused by GAG deposits in smooth muscle cells.

- **Hepatosplenomegaly** is secondary to distention of Kupffer cells and hepatocytes in the liver and accumulation of GAG-filled macrophages in the spleen.

 CLINICAL FEATURES: Hurler syndrome (MPS IH), the most severe clinical form of MPS, remains the prototype of these syndromes. The symptoms of Hurler syndrome are apparent between the ages of 6 months and 2 years. These children typically show skeletal deformities, enlarged livers and spleens, a characteristic facies, and joint stiffness.

Children with Hurler syndrome suffer developmental delay, hearing loss, corneal clouding, and progressive mental deterioration. Most patients die from recurrent pulmonary infections and cardiac complications before they reach 10 years.

Glycogenoses (Glycogen Storage Diseases)

The glycogenoses are a group of at least 10 distinct inherited disorders characterized by glycogen accumulation, principally in the liver, skeletal muscle, and heart. Each entity reflects a deficiency of one of the specific enzymes involved in glycogen metabolism. With one rare exception (X-linked phosphorylase kinase deficiency), all types of glycogen storage disease are autosomal recessive traits. The glycogenoses are rare, varying in frequency from 1 in 100,000 to 1 in 1 million.

Glycogen is a large glucose polymer (20,000 to 30,000 glucose units per molecule), which is stored in most cells to provide a ready source of energy during the fasting state. Liver and muscle are particularly rich in glycogen, although its function is different in each organ. Glycogen is synthesized and degraded sequentially by a number of enzymes, a deficiency in any of which leads to the accumulation of glycogen.

Although each of the glycogen storage diseases causes glycogen accumulation, the significant organ involvement varies with the specific enzyme defect. Some mainly affect the liver, whereas others principally cause cardiac or skeletal muscle dysfunction. *Importantly, the symptoms of a glycogenosis can reflect either accumulation of glycogen itself (Pompe disease, Andersen disease) or the lack of the glucose that is normally derived from glycogen degradation (von Gierke disease, McArdle disease).* We discuss only several representative examples of the known glycogenoses.

VON **GIERKE DISEASE (TYPE IA GLYCOGENOSIS):** *von Gierke disease results from a deficiency in glucose-6-phosphatase and is characterized by the accumulation of glycogen in the liver.* Symptoms reflect the inability of the liver to convert glycogen to glucose, a defect that results in hepatomegaly and hypoglycemia. The disorder is usually evident in infancy or early childhood. Growth is commonly stunted, but with treatment, the prognosis for normal mental development and longevity is generally good.

POMPE DISEASE (TYPE II GLYCOGENOSIS): Pompe disease is a lysosomal storage disease that involves virtually all organs and results in death from heart failure before the age of 2. The juvenile and adult variants are less common and have a better prognosis. Normally, a small proportion of cytoplasmic glycogen is degraded within lysosomes after an autophagic sequence. Type II glycogenosis is caused by a deficiency in the lysosomal enzyme acid α-glucosidase, which leads to inexorable accumulation of undegraded glycogen in lysosomes of many different cells. Interestingly, patients do not suffer from hypoglycemia, because the major metabolic pathways of glycogen synthesis and degradation in the cytoplasm are intact.

MCARDLE DISEASE (TYPE V GLYCOGENOSIS): McArdle disease is characterized by the accumulation of glycogen in skeletal muscles, owing to a deficiency of muscle phosphorylase, the enzyme that releases glucose-1-phosphate from glycogen. Symptoms usually appear in adolescence or early adulthood and consist of muscle cramps and spasms during exercise and sometimes myocytolysis and resulting myoglobinuria. Avoidance of exercise prevents the symptoms.

Inborn Errors of Amino Acid Metabolism Manifest with Variably Severe Symptomatology

Heritable disorders involving the metabolism of many amino acids have been described. Some are lethal in early childhood; others are asymptomatic biochemical defects that have no clinical significance. Some of these are treated in chapters dealing with specific organs. Here we restrict our discussion to the examples provided by two defects in the metabolism of phenylalanine.

Phenylketonuria

Phenylketonuria (PKU, hyperphenylalaninemia) is an autosomal recessive deficiency of the hepatic enzyme phenylalanine hydroxylase. The disorder features high levels of circulating phenylalanine, which leads to progressive mental deterioration in the first few years of life. The overall incidence of PKU is 1 per 10,000 in white and Asian populations, but it varies widely across different geographic areas (Fig. 6-13).

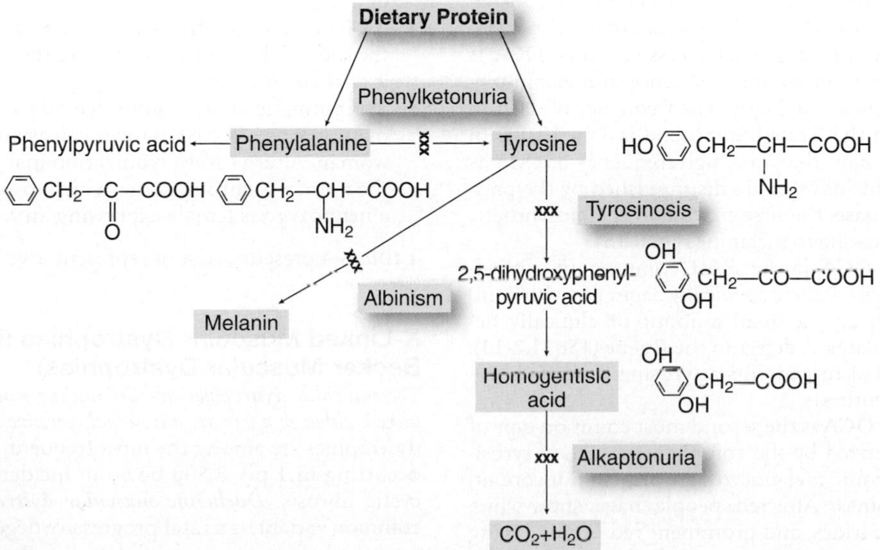

FIGURE 6-13. Diseases caused by disturbances of phenylalanine and tyrosine metabolism. CO_2, carbon dioxide; H_2O, water.

PATHOGENESIS: Phenylalanine is an essential amino acid derived exclusively from the diet. It is oxidized in the liver to tyrosine by phenylalanine hydroxylase (PAH), the product of the *PAH* gene on the long arm of chromosome 12. Deficiency in PAH results in both hyperphenylalaninemia and the formation of phenylketones from transamination of phenylalanine. Phenylpyruvic acid and its derivatives are excreted in the urine, but phenylalanine itself, rather than its metabolites, causes the neurologic damage central to this disease. *Thus, the term* **hyperphenylalaninemia** *is actually a more appropriate designation than PKU.*

The mechanism of the neurotoxicity associated with hyperphenylalaninemia during infancy has not been precisely established, but several processes have been implicated: (1) competitive interference with amino acid transport systems in the brain; (2) inhibition of the synthesis of neurotransmitters; and (3) disturbance of other metabolic processes. These effects presumably lead to inadequate development of neurons and defective synthesis of myelin.

CLINICAL FEATURES: Phenylketonuria illustrates the interaction between "nature and nurture" in the pathogenesis of disease. The disorder is based on a genetic defect, but its expression depends on the ingestion of phenylalanine, a dietary constituent. *The affected infant appears normal at birth, but mental retardation is evident within a few months.* By the age of 12 months, the untreated infant has suffered severe retardation. Infants with PKU tend to have fair skin, blond hair, and blue eyes, because the inability to convert phenylalanine to tyrosine leads to reduced melanin synthesis. They exude a "mousy" odor, which reflects the presence of phenylacetic acid.

Treatment of PKU involves restriction of dietary phenylalanine to 250 to 500 mg per day, which usually requires a semisynthetic formula. How long phenylalanine restriction should be maintained is controversial. Nevertheless, the success of newborn screening programs in detecting PKU and the prompt institution of a low-phenylalanine diet allows many PKU homozygotes to live a normal life.

Albinism

Albinism refers to a heterogeneous group of at least 10 inherited disorders in which absent or reduced biosynthesis of melanin causes hypopigmentation. This condition is found throughout the animal kingdom (from insects to humans). The most common type is oculocutaneous albinism (OCA), a family of closely related diseases that (with a single rare exception) represent autosomal recessive traits. OCA is characterized by a deficiency or complete absence of melanin pigment in the skin, hair follicles, and eyes. The frequency of OCA in whites is 1 per 18,000 in the United States and is 1 in 10,000 in Ireland. American blacks have the same high frequency of OCA as the Irish. Two major forms of OCA are distinguished by the presence or absence of tyrosinase, the first enzyme in the biosynthetic pathway that converts tyrosine to melanin (Fig. 6-13).

Tyrosinase-positive OCA is the most common type of albinism in whites and blacks. Patients typically begin life with complete albinism, but with age, a small amount of clinically detectable pigment accumulates. A defect in the *P* gene (15q11.2-13), which has been postulated to code for a tyrosine-transport protein, prevents melanin synthesis.

Tyrosinase-negative OCA is the second most common type of albinism and is characterized by the complete absence of tyrosinase (11q14-21) and melanin: melanocytes are present but contain unpigmented melanosomes. Affected people have snow-white hair, pale pink skin, blue irides, and prominent red pupils, owing to an absence of retinal pigment. They typically have severe ophthalmic problems, including photophobia, strabismus, nystagmus, and decreased visual acuity.

The skin of all types of albinos is strikingly sensitive to sunlight. Exposed skin areas require strong sunscreen lotions. These patients are at a greatly increased risk for squamous cell carcinomas of sun-exposed skin.

An X-Linked Disorder Features an Abnormal Gene on the X Chromosome

Expression of an X-linked disorder is different in males and females. Females, having two X chromosomes, may be homozygous or heterozygous for a given trait. It follows that clinical expression of the trait in a female is variable, depending on whether it is dominant or recessive. By contrast, males have only one X chromosome and are said to be **hemizygous** for the same trait. *Thus in the male, regardless of whether the trait is dominant or recessive, it is invariably expressed.*

A cardinal attribute of all X-linked inheritance is lack of transmission from father to son. A symptomatic father donates only a normal Y chromosome to his male offspring. By contrast, he always donates his abnormal X chromosome to his daughters, who are therefore obligate carriers of the trait. As a consequence, the disease classically skips a generation in the male, as the female carrier transmits it to grandsons of the original symptomatic male.

X-Linked Dominant Traits

- X-linked dominance refers to expression of a trait only in the female, as the hemizygous state in the male precludes a distinction between dominant and recessive inheritance. Only a few X-linked dominant disorders are described, among which are familial hypophosphatemic rickets and ornithine transcarbamylase deficiency. In such diseases, variations in the phenotype of the trait in the female may be explained, at least in part, by the Lyon effect (i.e., inactivation of one X chromosome). This random inactivation results in mosaicism for the mutant allele, leading to inconstant expression of the trait.

X-Linked Recessive Traits

Most X-linked traits are recessive; that is, heterozygous females do not have clinical disease (Fig. 6-14). The characteristics of this mode of inheritance are:

- Sons of women who are carriers have a 50% chance of inheriting the disease; daughters are not symptomatic. However, 50% of daughters will also be carriers.
- All daughters of affected men are asymptomatic carriers, but the sons of these men do not have the trait and cannot transmit it to their children.
- Symptomatic homozygous females can result from the rare mating of an affected man and an asymptomatic, heterozygous woman. Alternatively, lyonization may preferentially inactivate the normal X chromosome, which in extreme cases may lead to a heterozygous female expressing an X-linked recessive trait.

Table 6-4 presents a list of representative X-linked recessive disorders.

X-Linked Muscular Dystrophies (Duchenne and Becker Muscular Dystrophies)

The muscular dystrophies are devastating muscle diseases. Most are X-linked, although a few are autosomal recessive. The X-linked muscular dystrophies are among the most frequent human genetic diseases, occurring in 1 per 3,500 boys, an incidence approaching that of cystic fibrosis. **Duchenne muscular dystrophy (DMD)**, the most common variant, is a fatal progressive degeneration of muscle that appears before the age of 4 years. **Becker muscular dystrophy (BMD)** is allelic with DMD but is less common and milder. Muscular dystrophy is discussed in Chapter 27.

X-LINKED RECESSIVE

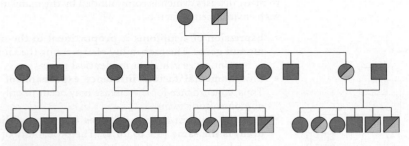

☑ Affected male

◍ Heterozygous female
without disease
(silent carrier)

FIGURE 6-14.   **X-linked recessive inheritance.** Only males are affected; daughters of affected men are all asymptomatic carriers. Asymptomatic men do not transmit the trait. Clinical expression of the disease skips a generation.

Hemophilia A (Factor VIII Deficiency)

Hemophilia A is an X-linked recessive disorder of blood clotting that results in spontaneous bleeding, particularly into joints, muscles, and internal organs. The disease is discussed in Chapter 20.

Fragile X Syndrome

Fragile X syndrome is the most common form of inherited mental retardation and is caused by the expansion of a CGG repeat at the Xq27 fragile site. It is second in frequency only to Down syndrome as an identifiable cause of mental retardation. The disease afflicts 1 in 1,250 males and 1 in 2,500 females.

  PATHOGENESIS: About 20% of all cases of heritable mental retardation are X-linked disorders, and one fifth of these are associated with a single genetic defect, namely, a fragile site on the X chromosome (Xq27). A **fragile site** represents a specific locus, or band, on a chromosome that breaks easily. The fragile site at Xq27 is a distinct kind of mutation characterized by amplification of a CGG repeat.

Within fragile X families, the probability of being affected is related to position in the pedigree; that is, later generations are more likely than earlier ones to be affected **(Sherman paradox or genetic anticipation)**. Chromosomes with more than about 52 repeats can increase the number of repeats—so-called expansion. Small expansions, which tend to be asymptomatic, can enlarge, particularly during meiosis in females, leading to larger expansions

in successive generations. Such small expansions are known as **premutations**. Expansions with more than 200 repeats are associated with mental retardation and represent full mutations. Expansion of a premutation to a full mutation during gametogenesis only occurs in females. As fragile X syndrome is recessive, most daughters of carrier males transmit mental retardation to 50% of their sons. These considerations explain the greater risk of the disorder in succeeding generations of fragile X families (Fig. 6-15).

  CLINICAL FEATURES: A male newborn with fragile X syndrome appears normal, but during childhood, typical features appear, including increased head circumference, facial coarsening, joint hyperextensibility, enlarged testes, and heart valve abnormalities. Mental retardation is profound: IQ scores vary from 20 to 60. *Interestingly, a significant proportion of autistic male children carry a fragile X chromosome.* Among female carriers who are mentally handicapped, the severity of the impairment varies from a learning disability with normal IQ to serious retardation.

Some Diseases are Associated with Non-Mendelian Patterns of Inheritance

MITOCHONDRIAL DISEASES: Most inherited defects in mitochondrial function result from maternally inherited mutations in the mitochondrial genome itself. All vertebrate mitochondria are inherited exclusively from the female via the ovum. Because any given cell has many mitochondria with multiple copies of mtDNA and thus hundreds or thousands of mtDNA copies, mutations in mtDNA lead to mixed populations of mutant and normal mitochondrial genomes. The phenotype associated with mtDNA mutations reflects the severity of the mutation, the proportion of mutant genomes, and the demand of the tissue for ATP. Diseases caused by mutations in the mitochondrial genome are rare and principally affect the nervous system, heart, and skeletal muscle. The functional deficits in all of these disorders can be traced to inadequate oxidative phosphorylation. The first human mitochondrial disease characterized was **Leber hereditary optic neuropathy**, which is associated with progressive loss of vision. Various mitochondrial myopathies, hypertrophic cardiomyopathy, and encephalomyopathies are known (see Chapter 27).

GENETIC IMPRINTING: Genetic imprinting refers to the observation that the phenotype associated with some genes differs, depending on whether the allele is inherited from the mother or the father. Either the maternal or paternal allele is maintained in an inactive state (is imprinted). If the nonimprinted allele is disrupted through mutation, the imprinted allele cannot compensate and disease results. Imprinting can result in hereditary diseases that have phenotypes determined by the parental source of the mutant allele. Deletion of the 15q11-13 locus results in

TABLE 6–4

Representative X-Linked Recessive Diseases

Disease	Frequency in Males
Fragile X syndrome	1/2,000
Hemophilia A (factor VIII deficiency)	1/10,000
Hemophilia B (factor IX deficiency)	1/70,000
Duchenne-Becker muscular dystrophy	1/3,500
Glucose-6-phosphate dehydrogenase deficiency	Up to 30%
Lesch-Nyhan syndrome (HPRT deficiency)	1/10,000
Chronic granulomatous disease	Not rare
X-linked agammaglobulinemia	Not rare
X-linked severe combined immunodeficiency	Rare
Fabry disease	1/40,000
Hunter syndrome	1/70,000
Adrenoleukodystrophy	1/100,000
Menke disease	1/100,000

HPRT, hypoxanthine-guanine phosphoribosyltransferase.

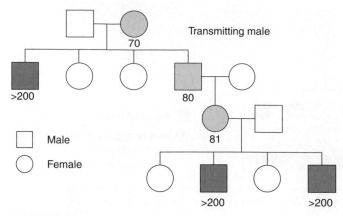

Transmitting male

FIGURE 6-15. Inheritance pattern of fragile X syndrome. The number of copies of the trinucleotide repeat (CGG) is shown below selected members in this pedigree. Expansion occurs primarily during meiosis in females. When the number of repeats exceeds ~200, the clinical syndrome is manifested. Individuals shaded pink carry a premutation and are asymptomatic.

Prader-Willi syndrome when the affected chromosome is inherited from the father and in **Angelman syndrome** when the mutated chromosome is of maternal origin. The phenotypes of these disorders are remarkably different. Prader-Willi syndrome features hypotonia, obesity, hypogonadism, mental retardation, and a specific facies. By contrast, patients with Angelman syndrome are hyperactive, display inappropriate laughter, and have a facies different from that of Prader-Willi syndrome.

UNIPARENTAL INHERITANCE: Uniparental disomy results when both members of a single chromosome pair are inherited from the same parent. Uniparental disomy is rare but has been implicated in unexpected patterns of inheritance of genetic traits. For instance, a child with uniparental disomy may manifest a recessive disease when only one parent carries the trait, as has been observed in a few cases of cystic fibrosis and hemophilia A. About 30% of Prader-Willi disease results from maternal uniparental disomy. Such affected persons have two identical inactivated regions of chromosome 15 and no active paternal contribution.

Multifactorial Inheritance

Multifactorial inheritance *describes a process by which a disease results from the effects of a number of abnormal genes and environmental factors.* Most normal human traits reflect such complexities and are not inherited as simple dominant or as recessive Mendelian attributes. For example, multifactorial inheritance determines height, skin color, and body habitus. Similarly, most of the common chronic disorders of adults—diabetes, atherosclerosis, and many forms of cancer, arthritis, and hypertension—represent multifactorial genetic diseases and are well known to "run in families." The inheritance of many birth defects is also multifactorial (e.g., cleft lip and palate, pyloric stenosis, and congenital heart disease).

The concept of multifactorial inheritance is based on the notion that multiple genes interact with each other and with environmental factors to produce disease in an individual patient. Such inheritance leads to familial aggregation that does not obey simple Mendelian rules.

The Biological Basis of Polygenic Inheritance Resides in Genetic Polymorphism

*The biological basis of polygenic inheritance rests on the evidence that more than one fourth of all genetic loci in normal humans contain polymor-*phic alleles (i.e., alleles that show genetic variation). Such genetic heterogeneity provides a background for wide variability in susceptibility to many diseases, which is compounded by the many interactions with environmental factors.

- **Expression of symptoms is proportional to the number of mutant genes.** The probability of expressing the same number of mutant genes is highest in identical twins.
- **Environmental factors influence expression of the trait.** Thus, concordance for the disease may occur in only one third of monozygotic twins.
- **The risk in first-degree relatives (parents, siblings, children) is the same (5% to 10%).** The probability of disease is much lower in second-degree relatives.
- **The probability of a trait's expression in later offspring is influenced by its expression in earlier siblings.** If one or more children are born with a multifactorial defect, the chance of its recurrence in later offspring is doubled. For simple Mendelian traits, in contrast, the probability is independent of the number of affected siblings.
- **The more severe a defect, the greater the risk of transmitting it to offspring.** Patients with more severe polygenic defects presumably have more mutant genes, and their children thus have a greater chance of inheriting the abnormal genes than do the offspring of less severely affected persons.
- **Some abnormalities characterized by multifactorial inheritance show a sex predilection.** Such differential susceptibility is believed to represent a difference in the threshold for expression of mutant genes in the two sexes.

Cleft Lip and Cleft Palate Exemplify Multifactorial Inheritance

At the 35th day of gestation, the frontal prominence fuses with the maxillary process to form the upper lip. This process is under the control of many genes, and disturbances in gene expression (hereditary or environmental) at this time lead to interference with proper fusion and result in cleft lip, with or without cleft palate (Fig. 6-16).

The incidence of cleft lip, with or without cleft palate, is 1 in 1,000, and the incidence of cleft palate alone is 1 in 2,500. If one child is born with a cleft lip, the chances are 4% that the second child will exhibit the same defect. If the first two children are affected, the risk of cleft lip increases to 9% for the third child. The more severe the anatomical defect, the greater is the probability of transmitting cleft lip. Whereas 75% of cases of cleft lip occur in boys, the sons of women with cleft lip have a four times higher risk of acquiring the defect than do the sons of affected fathers.

Diseases of Infancy and Childhood

Morbidity and mortality rates in the neonatal period differ considerably from those in infancy and childhood. Infants and children are not simply "small adults," and they may be afflicted by diseases unique to their particular age group.

Prematurity and Intrauterine Growth Retardation

Human pregnancy normally lasts 40 ± 2 weeks, and most newborns weigh $3,300 \pm 600$ g. The World Health Organization defines prematurity as a gestational age of less than 37 weeks (timed from the first day of the last menstrual period). **Low-birth-weight**

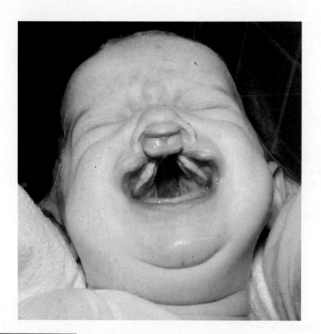

FIGURE 6-16. Cleft lip and palate in an infant.

infants (<2,500 g) are termed (1) appropriate for gestational age (AGA) or (2) small for gestational age (SGA).

About 1% of all infants born in the United States weigh less than 1,500 g and are classified as **very-low-birth-weight infants**. Such babies account for half of neonatal deaths, and their survival is determined by their birth weight. If premature newborns are cared for in neonatal intensive care units, 90% of infants over 750 g survive. Between 500 g and 750 g, 45% survive, of whom more than half develop normally.

The factors that predispose to the premature birth of an infant (AGA) are (1) maternal illness, (2) uterine incompetence, (3) fetal disorders, and (4) placental abnormalities. In a substantial proportion of AGA infants, the cause of premature birth is unknown. Intrauterine growth retardation and the resulting birth of SGA infants are associated with disorders that (1) impair maternal health and nutrition, (2) interfere with placental circulation or function, or (3) disturb the growth or development of the fetus.

CLINICAL FEATURES: There is a substantial overlap between the complications of prematurity itself (AGA) and intrauterine growth retardation (SGA). However, certain general principles apply. Prematurity is often associated with severe respiratory distress, metabolic disturbances (e.g., hyperbilirubinemia, hypoglycemia, hypocalcemia), circulatory problems (anemia, hypothermia, hypotension), and bacterial sepsis. By contrast, SGA infants are a much more heterogeneous group and include many infants with congenital anomalies and infections acquired in utero. In addition to the many problems associated with prematurity, SGA infants often suffer from perinatal asphyxia, meconium aspiration, necrotizing enterocolitis, pulmonary hemorrhage, and disorders related to birth defects or inherited metabolic diseases.

Organ Immaturity is a Cause of Neonatal Disease

Maturing organs in infants born prematurely differ from those in term infants, although complete maturation of many organs may require days (lungs) to years (brain) after birth.

LUNGS: Pulmonary immaturity is a common and immediate threat to the viability of low-birth-weight infants. The lining cells of the fetal alveoli do not differentiate into type I and type II pneumocytes until late pregnancy. Amniotic fluid fills the fetal alveoli and drains from the lungs at birth. Sometimes immature infants show sluggish respiratory movements that do not fully expel the amniotic fluid from the lungs. Sometimes termed amniotic fluid aspiration syndrome, this actually represents retained amniotic fluid. Air passages contain desquamated squamous cells (squames) and lanugo hair from the fetal skin and protein-rich amniotic fluid.

Neonatal respiratory distress syndrome resulting from insufficient pulmonary surfactant in the immature lung is discussed below.

LIVER: The liver of premature infants is morphologically similar to that of the adult organ, with the exception of conspicuous extramedullary hematopoiesis. However, the hepatocytes tend to be functionally immature. The fetal liver is deficient in glucuronyl transferase, and the resulting inability of the organ to conjugate bilirubin often leads to neonatal jaundice. This enzyme deficiency is aggravated by the rapid destruction of fetal erythrocytes, a process that results in an increased supply of bilirubin.

BRAIN: Although the brain of the immature newborn differs from that of the adult, both morphologically and functionally, this difference is rarely fatal. On the other hand, the incomplete development of the CNS is often reflected in poor vasomotor control, hypothermia, feeding difficulties, and recurrent apnea.

Neonatal Respiratory Distress Syndrome (RDS) is due to Deficiency of Surfactant

Neonatal RDS is the leading cause of morbidity and mortality among premature infants, accounting for half of all neonatal deaths in the United States. Its incidence varies inversely with gestational age and birth weight. Thus, more than half of newborns younger than 28 weeks gestational age have RDS, compared with only one fifth of infants between 32 and 36 weeks.

PATHOGENESIS: *The pathogenesis of RDS of the newborn is intimately linked to a deficiency of surfactant* (Fig. 6-17). When a newborn starts breathing, type II cells release their surfactant stores. The presence of surfactant reduces surface tension, that is, it decreases the affinity of alveolar surfaces for each other. When the alveoli remain open, the baby exhales and reduces resistance to reinflating the lungs with the second breath. If surfactant function is inadequate, the alveoli collapse when the baby exhales and resist expansion when the child tries to take its second breath, resulting in alveolar damage. The injured alveoli leak plasma into air spaces. Plasma constituents, including fibrinogen and albumin, bind surfactant and impair its function, thus further exacerbating the respiratory insufficiency. Many alveoli are perfused with blood, but not ventilated by air, an effect that leads to hypoxia as well as acidosis and further compromises the ability of type II pneumocytes to produce surfactant. Moreover, hypoxia produces pulmonary arterial vasoconstriction, thereby increasing right-to-left shunting through the ductus arteriosus and foramen ovale and within the lung itself. The resulting pulmonary ischemia further aggravates alveolar epithelial damage and injures the endothelium of the pulmonary capillaries.

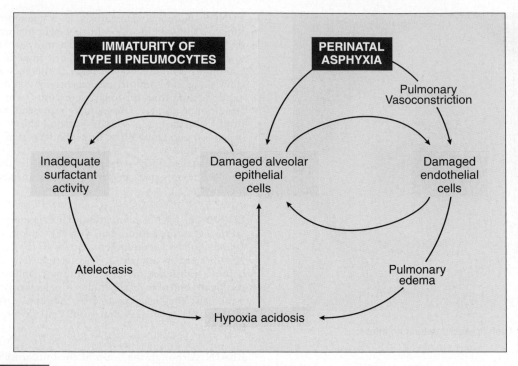

FIGURE 6-17. **Pathogenesis of the respiratory distress syndrome of the neonate.** Immaturity of the lungs and perinatal asphyxia are the major pathogenetic factors.

 PATHOLOGY: On gross examination, the lungs are dark red and airless. The alveoli are collapsed, and alveolar ducts and respiratory bronchioles are dilated and contain cellular debris, proteinaceous edema fluid, and erythrocytes. The alveolar ducts are lined by conspicuous, eosinophilic, fibrin-rich, amorphous structures, called **hyaline membranes**, hence the original term for neonatal RDS, **hyaline membrane disease** (Fig. 6-18). Walls of collapsed alveoli are thick, capillaries are congested, and lymphatics are filled with proteinaceous material.

CLINICAL FEATURES: Most newborns destined to develop RDS appear normal at birth. The first symptom, usually appearing within an hour of birth, is increased respiratory effort, with forceful intercostal retraction and the use of accessory neck muscles. The respiratory rate increases to more than 100 breaths per minute, and the baby becomes cyanotic. In severe cases, the infant becomes progressively obtunded and flaccid. Long periods of apnea ensue, and the infant eventually dies of asphyxia. Despite advances in neonatal intensive care, the overall mortality rate of RDS is about 15%, and one third of infants born before 30 weeks of gestational age die of this disorder. In milder cases, the symptoms peak within 3 days, after which gradual improvement takes place. The major complications of RDS relate to anoxia and acidosis.

Fetal lung maturity can be ascertained by a variety of tests. Pulmonary surfactant is released into the amniotic fluid, which can be sampled by amniocentesis to assess the maturity of the fetal lung. A lecithin-to-sphingomyelin ratio above 2:1 implies that the fetus will survive without developing RDS. After the 35th week, the appearance of phosphatidylglycerol in the amniotic fluid is the best proof of the maturity of the fetal lungs.

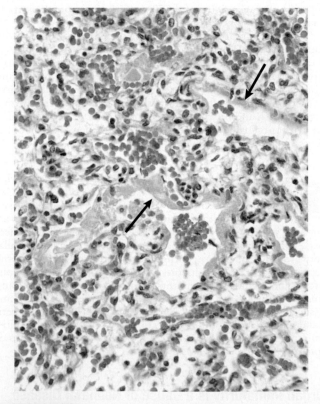

FIGURE 6-18. **The lung in respiratory distress syndrome of the neonate.** The alveoli are atelectatic, and a dilated alveolar duct is lined by a fibrin-rich hyaline membrane *(arrows)*.

Erythroblastosis Fetalis is a Hemolytic Disease caused by Maternal Antibodies against Fetal Erythrocytes

Erythroblastosis fetalis is a hemolytic disease of the fetus or newborn caused by the transplacental passage of maternal antibodies against fetal erythrocyte antigens. Only antibodies against Rh D antigen, Kell$_1$ antigen, the Rh c antigen, and the ABO system cause a significant incidence of hemolytic disease, with anti-Rh D being the most common by far. The distribution of Rh antigens among ethnic groups varies. In American whites, 15% are Rh-negative (Rh D–), whereas only 8% of blacks are Rh D–. Japanese, Chinese, and Native American Indian populations contain essentially no Rh D– individuals.

PATHOGENESIS: Among infants with erythroblastosis fetalis caused by Rh incompatibility, 90% of cases are due to antibodies against fetal D antigen. Rh-positive fetal erythrocytes (>1 mL) enter the circulation of an Rh-negative mother at the time of delivery, eliciting maternal antibodies to the D antigen (Fig. 6-19). Because the quantity of fetal blood necessary to sensitize the mother is introduced into her circulation only at the time of delivery, erythroblastosis fetalis does not ordinarily affect the first baby. However, when a sensitized mother again carries an Rh-positive fetus, much smaller quantities of fetal D antigen elicit an increase in antibody titer. In contrast to IgM, IgG antibodies are small enough to cross the placenta and thus produce hemolysis in the fetus. This cycle is exaggerated in multiparous women, and the severity of erythroblastosis tends to increase progressively with each succeeding pregnancy.

Even in those Rh-negative women who are exposed to significant amounts of fetal Rh-positive blood, many do not mount a substantial immune response. In fact, after multiple pregnancies, only 5% of Rh-negative women deliver infants with erythroblastosis fetalis. A second potential source of maternal sensitization is blood transfusions.

PATHOLOGY AND CLINICAL FEATURES: The severity of erythroblastosis fetalis varies from mild hemolysis to fatal anemia, and the pathologic findings are determined by the extent of the hemolytic disease.

- **Death in utero** occurs in the most extreme form of the disease, in which case severe maceration is evident on delivery. Numerous erythroblasts are demonstrable in visceral organs that are not extensively autolyzed.
- *Hydrops fetalis is the most serious form of erythroblastosis fetalis in liveborn infants. It is characterized by severe edema secondary to congestive heart failure caused by severe anemia.* Affected infants generally die, unless adequate exchange transfusions with Rh-negative cells correct the anemia and ameliorate the hemolytic disease.
- *Kernicterus, also termed* **bilirubin encephalopathy,** *is defined as a neurologic condition associated with severe jaundice and is characterized by bile staining of the brain, particularly of the basal ganglia, pontine nuclei, and dentate nuclei in the cerebellum.* Kernicterus (from the German, *kern*, nucleus) is essentially confined to newborns with severe unconjugated hyperbilirubinemia, usually related to erythroblastosis. The bilirubin derived from the destruction of erythrocytes and the catabolism of the released heme is not easily conjugated by the immature liver, which is deficient in glucuronyl transferase.

- **Bilirubin** is thought to injure the cells of the brain by interfering with mitochondrial function. Severe kernicterus leads initially to loss of the startle reflex and athetoid movements, which in 75% of newborns progresses to lethargy and death. Most surviving infants have severe choreoathetosis and mental retardation; a minority display varying degrees of intellectual and motor retardation.

The incidence of erythroblastosis fetalis secondary to Rh incompatibility has been greatly reduced (to <1% of women at risk) by the use of human anti-D globulin (RhoGAM) within 72 hours of delivery. The quantity of RhoGAM administered to the mother suffices to neutralize 10 mL of antigenic fetal cells that may have entered the maternal circulation during delivery.

Birth Injury Spans the Spectrum from Mechanical Trauma to Anoxic Damage

Some birth injuries relate to poor obstetric manipulation, whereas many are unavoidable sequelae of routine delivery. Birth injuries occur in about 5 per 1,000 live births. Factors that predispose to birth injury include cephalopelvic disproportion, dystocia (difficult labor), prematurity, and breech presentation.

Cranial Injury

Cranial injuries range from the minor scalp edema (caput succedaneum) caused by passage through the birth canal to potentially serious skull fractures that result from head impact on the pelvis or instrumentation. **Intracranial hemorrhage** is one of the most dangerous birth injuries and may be traumatic, secondary to asphyxia, or a result of an underlying bleeding diathesis. Traumatic intracranial hemorrhage occurs in the setting of (1) significant cephalopelvic disproportion, (2) precipitous delivery, (3) breech presentation, (4) prolonged labor, or (5) the inappropriate use of forceps. These traumas can result in **subdural or subarachnoid hemorrhage.** The prognosis for newborns with intracranial hemorrhage depends on its extent. Massive hemorrhage is often rapidly fatal. A surviving infant may recover completely or may have long-term impairment.

Peripheral Nerve Injury

Brachial palsy, with varying degrees of paralysis of the upper extremity, is caused by excessive traction on the head and neck or shoulders during delivery. The injury may be permanent if the nerves are severed. Function may return within a few months if the palsy results from edema and hemorrhage. **Phrenic nerve paralysis** and associated paralysis of a hemidiaphragm may be associated with brachial palsy and result in breathing difficulties. The condition generally resolves spontaneously within a few months.

Facial nerve palsy usually presents as a unilateral flaccid paralysis of the face caused by injury to the seventh cranial nerve during labor or delivery, especially with forceps. When severe, the entire affected side of the face is paralyzed, and even the eyelid cannot be closed. The prognosis again depends on whether the nerve was lacerated or simply injured by pressure.

Sudden Infant Death Syndrome (SIDS) Does Not Have a Known Cause

The sudden infant death syndrome (SIDS), also known as "crib death," is defined as "the sudden death of an infant or young child which is unexpected by history and in which a thorough postmortem examination fails to demonstrate an adequate cause of death." Although the diagnosis of SIDS is arrived at solely by excluding other specific causes of sud-

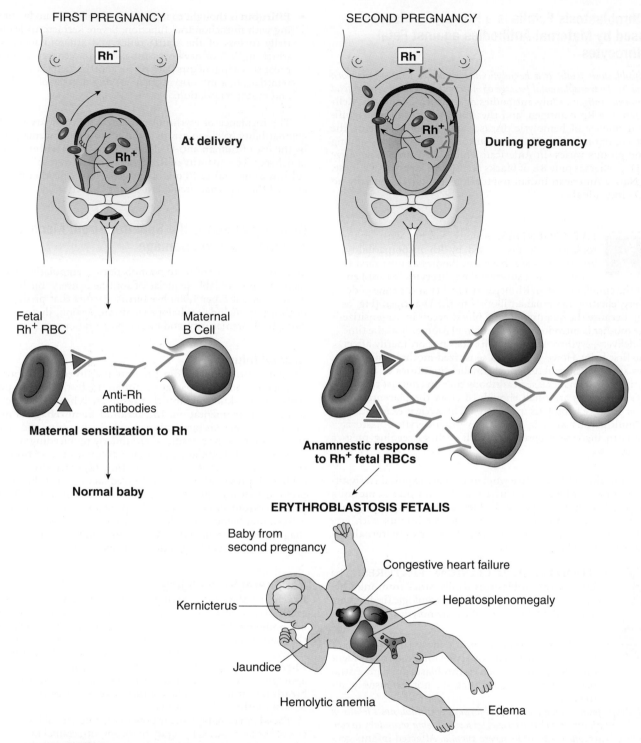

FIRST PREGNANCY

Rh⁻

At delivery

SECOND PREGNANCY

Rh⁻

Rh⁺

During pregnancy

Fetal
Rh⁺ RBC

Maternal
B Cell

Anti-Rh
antibodies

Maternal sensitization to Rh

Normal baby

**Anamnestic response
to Rh⁺ fetal RBCs**

ERYTHROBLASTOSIS FETALIS

Baby from
second pregnancy

Congestive heart failure

Hepatosplenomegaly

Kernicterus

Jaundice

Hemolytic anemia

Edema

FIGURE 6-19. **Pathogenesis of erythroblastosis fetalis due to maternal–fetal Rh incompatibility.** Immunization of the Rh-negative mother with Rh-positive erythrocytes in the first pregnancy leads to the formation of anti-Rh antibodies of the immunoglobulin (Ig)G type. These antibodies cross the placenta and damage the Rh-positive fetus in subsequent pregnancies.

den death, this catastrophe is nevertheless considered a distinct clinicopathologic entity.

Typically, the victim of SIDS is an apparently healthy young infant who has been asleep without any hint of illness. Clinically, the infant does not awaken from an otherwise normal sleep period. Postmortem examination does not identify a cause of death, such as pneumonia, food aspiration, sepsis, or cerebral hemorrhage. This tragic sequence has aroused great public concern, because it

must be separated from homicide, which has been demonstrated in a number of cases to be the true cause of mysterious death in children.

 EPIDEMIOLOGY: After the neonatal period, SIDS is the leading cause of death in the first year of life, accounting for more than one third of all deaths in this period. The incidence in the United States is 2 per 1,000

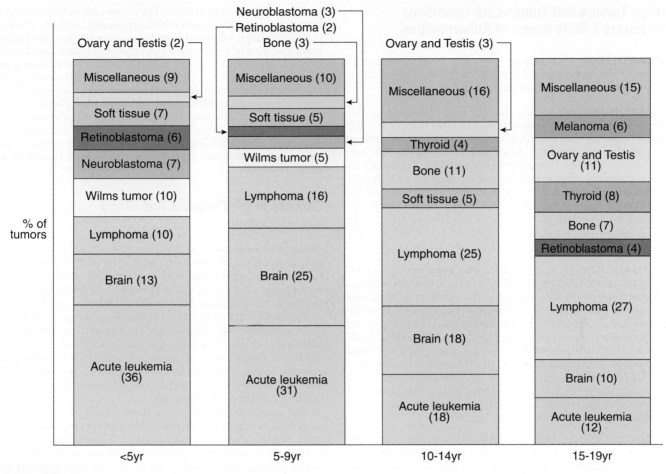

FIGURE 6-20. Distribution of childhood tumors according to age and primary site.

live births. The large majority of cases (90%) occur before 6 months of age. Most deaths from SIDS present during the winter months, but no association between particular respiratory infections and infant death has been established. Deaths typically occur at night or during periods associated with sleep. The reported death rates for SIDS have declined dramatically. This has been attributed to "Back to Sleep" campaigns that encourage parents to place infants on their backs for sleeping.

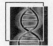

PATHOGENESIS: The pathogenesis of SIDS is elusive and controversial and no clear answers are available at this time. It is also unclear whether SIDS is a single entity or the common end point of several different conditions. The most popular hypothesis relates SIDS to a prolonged spell of apnea, followed by cardiac arrhythmia or shock. However, fewer than 10% of parents of SIDS victims report episodes of apnea or an apparent life-threatening event at any time prior to the fatal event. *Thus, sleep apnea may contribute to the sequence of events leading to SIDS, but available data do not support a strong and predictable relationship between the two conditions.*

PATHOLOGY: At autopsy, several morphologic alterations are described in victims of SIDS, but their relevance to the etiology and pathogenesis of this disorder remains unclear. Chronic hypoxia may be evidenced by brainstem gliosis, which occurs with some regularity. Petechiae on

the surfaces of the lungs, heart, pleura, and thymus, which have been reported in most infants dying of SIDS, are probably terminal events and have been attributed to negative intrathoracic pressure produced by respiratory efforts.

Neoplasms of Infancy and Childhood

Malignant tumors between the ages of 1 and 15 years are distinctly uncommon, but cancer remains the leading cause of death from disease in this age group. In children, 10% of all deaths are due to malignancies, and only accidental trauma kills a larger number. **Unlike adults, in whom most cancers are of epithelial origin (e.g., carcinomas of the lung, breast, and gastrointestinal tract), most malignant tumors in children arise from hematopoietic, nervous and soft tissues** (Fig. 6-20). Another feature that distinguishes childhood tumors from those of adults is the fact that many childhood tumors are part of developmental complexes. Examples include Wilms tumor associated with aniridia, genitourinary malformations, and mental retardation (WAGR complex); hemihypertrophy of the body associated with Wilms tumor, hepatoblastoma, and adrenal carcinoma; and tuberous sclerosis in association with renal tumors and rhabdomyomas of the heart. Some neoplasms are apparent at birth and are obviously developmental tumors that have evolved in utero. In addition, abnormally developed organs, persistent organ primordia, and displaced organ rests are all vulnerable to neoplastic transformation.

Benign Tumors and Tumor-Like Conditions Encompass a Wide Range of Abnormalities

HAMARTOMAS: These lesions represent focal, benign overgrowths of one or more of the mature cellular elements of a normal tissue, often with one element predominating.

HEMANGIOMAS: Of varying size and in diverse locations, hemangiomas are the most frequently encountered tumors in childhood. Whether they are true neoplasms or hamartomas is unclear, although half are present at birth and most regress with age. Large, rapidly growing hemangiomas occasionally can be serious lesions, especially when they occur on the head or neck. A **port wine stain** is a congenital capillary hemangioma that involves the skin of the face and scalp and is often large enough to be disfiguring, imparting a dark purple color to the affected area. Unlike many small hemangiomas, they persist for life and are not easily treated.

LYMPHANGIOMAS: Also termed **cystic hygromas**, lymphangiomas are poorly demarcated swellings that are usually present at birth and thereafter rapidly increase in size. Most lymphangiomas occur on the head and neck, but the floor of the mouth, mediastinum, and buttocks are not uncommon sites. The classification of these tumors is imprecise; some researchers consider them developmental malformations or hamartomas, and others call them neoplasms. Lymphangiomas appear as unilocular or multilocular cysts with thin, transparent walls and straw-colored fluid. Microscopically, myriad dilated lymphatic channels are separated by fibrous septa. Unlike hemangiomas, these lesions do not regress spontaneously and should be resected.

SACROCOCCYGEAL TERATOMAS: Although rare, these germ cell neoplasms are the most common solid tumors in the newborn, with an incidence of 1 in 40,000 live births. At least 75% of sacrococcygeal teratomas occur in girls, and a substantial number have been encountered in twins. The tumors are usually noticed at birth as a mass in the region of the sacrum and buttocks. They are commonly large, lobulated masses, often as large as the infant's head. One half of these tumors grow externally and may be connected to the body by a small stalk. Some have both external and intrapelvic components, whereas a few grow entirely in the pelvis. Microscopically, sacrococcygeal teratomas are composed of numerous tissues, particularly of neural origin. Most (90%) sacrococcygeal teratomas detected before the age of 2 months are benign, but up to half of those diagnosed later in life are malignant. Associated congenital anomalies of the vertebrae, genitourinary system, and anorectum are common. The lesion should be resected promptly.

Cancers in the Pediatric Age Group are Uncommon

The incidence of childhood malignancies is 1.3 per 10,000 per year in children under the age of 15 years. The mortality rate clearly varies with the intrinsic behavior of the tumor and the response to therapy, but as an overall figure, the death rate for childhood cancer is only about one-third the incidence. Almost half of all malignant diseases in patients under 15 years of age are acute leukemias and lymphomas (see Chapter 20). Leukemias alone, particularly acute lymphoblastic leukemia, account for one third of all cases of childhood cancer. Most of the other malignant neoplasms are neuroblastomas, brain tumors, Wilms tumors, retinoblastomas, bone cancers, and various soft tissue sarcomas and are discussed in detail in appropriate chapters.

The genetic influences in the development of childhood tumors have been particularly well studied in the case of retinoblastoma, Wilms tumor, and osteosarcoma. The issues relating to the interaction of inherited mutations and environmental influences in the pathogenesis of malignant tumors in both children and adults are discussed in Chapter 5.

7 Hemodynamic Disorders

Bruce M. McManus
Michael F. Allard
Bobby Yanagawa

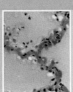

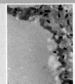

Hemodynamic disorders are characterized by disturbed perfusion that may result in organ and cellular injury. The metabolism of organs and cells depends on an intact circulation, both for the continuous delivery of oxygen, nutrients, hormones, electrolytes, and water and also for the removal of metabolic waste and carbon dioxide. Delivery and elimination at the cellular level are controlled by exchanges between the intravascular, interstitial, cellular, and lymphatic spaces.

Disorders of Perfusion

Hyperemia is an Excess of Blood in an Organ

Hyperemia may be caused either by an increased supply of blood from the arterial system (**active hyperemia**) or by impaired exit of blood through venous pathways (**passive hyperemia** or **congestion**).

Active Hyperemia

Active hyperemia is an augmented supply of blood to an organ. It is usually a physiologic response to increased functional demand, as in the heart and skeletal muscle during exercise. Neurogenic and hormonal influences play a role in active hyperemia. Cutaneous hyperemia in febrile states serves to dissipate heat. Skeletal muscle may increase its blood flow (and thus oxygen delivery) 20-fold during exercise. The increased blood supply occurs by arteriolar dilation and recruitment of unperfused capillaries.

The most striking active hyperemia occurs in association with inflammation (see Chapter 2). Because inflammation can also damage endothelial cells and increase capillary permeability, inflammatory hyperemia is often accompanied by edema and local extravasation of erythrocytes.

Passive Hyperemia (Congestion)

Passive hyperemia, or congestion, is engorgement of an organ with venous blood. Acute passive congestion is clinically a consequence of acute left or right ventricular failure. A generalized increase in venous pressure, typically from chronic heart failure, results in slower blood flow and a consequent increase in blood volume in many organs, including the liver, spleen, and kidneys. Congestive heart failure secondary to coronary artery disease and hypertension and right-sided failure due to pulmonary disease are common causes of passive congestion (see below).

Passive congestion may also be confined to a limb or an organ as a result of more localized obstruction to venous drainage. Examples include deep venous thrombosis of the leg veins, with resulting edema of the lower extremity and thrombosis of hepatic veins (Budd-Chiari syndrome), with secondary chronic passive congestion of the liver.

LUNGS: Chronic left ventricular failure impedes venous blood flow out of the lungs and leads to chronic passive pulmonary congestion. As a result, pressure in the alveolar capillaries increases as these vessels become engorged with blood. Increased pressure in the alveolar capillaries has four major consequences:

- **Microhemorrhages** release erythrocytes into alveolar spaces, where they are phagocytosed and degraded by alveolar macrophages. The released iron, in the form of hemosiderin, remains in the macrophages, which are then called "heart failure cells."
- **Fluid** is forced from the blood into the alveolar spaces, resulting in pulmonary edema, which interferes with gas exchange in the lung (Fig. 7-1).
- **Fibrosis** increases in the interstitium of the lung. The presence of fibrosis and iron is viewed grossly as a firm brown lung (**brown induration**).
- **Pulmonary hypertension** occurs when the pressure is transmitted to the pulmonary arterial system. This may lead to right-sided heart failure and consequent generalized systemic venous congestion.

LIVER: Because the hepatic veins empty into the vena cava immediately inferior to the heart, it is particularly vulnerable to acute or chronic passive congestion (see Chapter 14). The central veins of hepatic lobules become dilated. The increased venous pressure is transmitted to the sinusoids, which dilate, and centrilobular hepatocytes undergo pressure atrophy. Grossly, the cut surface of the chronically congested liver exhibits dark foci of centrilobular congestion surrounded by paler zones of unaffected peripheral portions of the lobules. The result is a reticulated appearance that resembles a cross-section of a nutmeg ("nutmeg liver") (Fig. 7-2).

SPLEEN: Increased intravascular pressure in the liver, from cardiac failure or an intrahepatic obstruction to blood flow (e.g., cirrhosis), leads to higher pressure in the splenic vein and congestion of the spleen. The organ becomes enlarged and tense, and the cut section oozes dark blood. In long-standing congestion, diffuse splenic fibrosis develops, and iron-containing, fibrotic, and calcified foci of old hemorrhage (Gamna-Gandy bodies) appear. Such a spleen may weigh 250 to 750 g, compared with a normal weight of 150 g. The enlarged spleen sometimes displays excessive functional activity—termed **hypersplenism**—which leads to hematologic abnormalities (e.g., anemia, leukopenia, thrombocytopenia).

EDEMA AND ASCITES: Venous congestion impedes blood flow through the capillaries, thereby increasing hydrostatic pressure and promoting edema formation (see below for a discussion of the mechanisms of edema formation). Accumulation of edema fluid in heart failure is particularly noticeable in dependent tissues—the legs

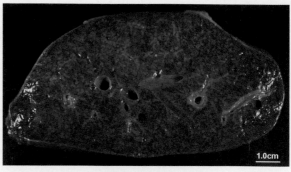

A

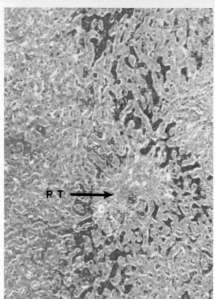

B

FIGURE 7-2. **Passive congestion of liver. A.** A gross photograph of liver shows nutmeg appearance, reflecting congestive failure of the right ventricle. **B.** A photomicrograph of liver shows centrilobular sinusoids dilated with blood. The intervening plates of hepatocytes exhibit pressure atrophy. PT, portal tract.

and feet in ambulatory patients and the back in those who are bedridden. **Ascites** is an accumulation of fluid in the peritoneal space and reflects (among other factors) lack of tissue rigor, a condition in which there is no countervailing external pressure to oppose hydrostatic pressure within the blood vessels.

Hemorrhage is a Discharge of Blood Out of the Vascular Compartment

Blood can be released from the circulation to the exterior of the body or into nonvascular body spaces. The most common and obvious cause is trauma. Severe atherosclerosis may so weaken the wall of the abdominal aorta that it balloons to form an aneurysm, which then may rupture and bleed into the retroperitoneal space (see Chapter 10). Congenital berry aneurysms at the branch points of the carotid system in the brain may give way and cause subarachnoid hemorrhage (see Chapter 28). Certain infections (e.g., pulmonary tuberculosis) and invasive neoplasms may erode blood vessels and lead to hemorrhage.

Hemorrhage also results from damage to capillaries. For instance, rupture of capillaries by blunt trauma leads to a bruise. Increased venous pressure also causes extravasation of blood from pulmonary capillaries. Vitamin C deficiency is associated with capillary fragility and bleeding, owing to a defect in the supporting connective tissue structures. The minor trauma imposed on small vessels and capillaries by normal movement requires an intact co-

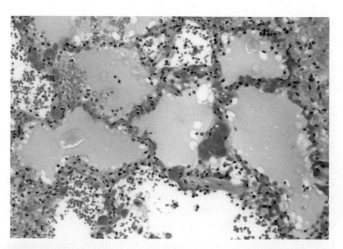

FIGURE 7-1. **Pulmonary edema.** A patient with congestive heart failure shows pink-staining fluid in the alveoli.

agulation system to prevent hemorrhage. Thus, a severe decrease in the number of platelets (thrombocytopenia) or a deficiency of a coagulation factor (e.g., factor VIII in hemophilia A) is associated with spontaneous hemorrhage into joints without apparent trauma (see Chapter 10).

A person may exsanguinate into an internal cavity, as in gastrointestinal hemorrhage from a peptic ulcer (arterial hemorrhage) or esophageal varices (venous hemorrhage). In such cases, fresh blood may fill the entire gastrointestinal tract. Bleeding into a serous cavity can result in accumulation of a large amount of blood, even to the point of exsanguination.

A few definitions are in order:

- **Hematoma:** Hemorrhage into soft tissue. Such collections of blood can be merely painful, as in a muscle bruise, or fatal, if located in the brain.
- **Hemothorax:** Hemorrhage into the pleural cavity.
- **Hemopericardium:** Hemorrhage into the pericardial space.
- **Hemoperitoneum:** Bleeding into the peritoneal cavity.
- **Hemarthrosis:** Bleeding into a joint space.
- **Purpura:** Diffuse superficial hemorrhages in the skin, up to 1 cm in diameter.
- **Ecchymosis:** A larger superficial hemorrhage in the skin.
- **Petechiae:** Pinpoint hemorrhages, usually in the skin or conjunctiva. This lesion represents the rupture of a capillary or arteriole and occurs in conjunction with coagulopathies or vasculitis.

Thrombosis

Thrombosis refers to the formation of a thrombus, defined as an aggregate of coagulated blood containing platelets, fibrin, and entrapped cellular elements, within a vascular lumen. A **thrombus** by definition adheres to vascular endothelium and should be distinguished from a simple blood clot, which reflects only activation of the coagulation cascade and can form in vitro or even postmortem. Similarly, a thrombus differs from a hematoma, which results from hemorrhage and subsequent clotting outside the vascular system. Thrombus formation and the coagulation cascade are discussed in more detail in Chapters 10 and 20.

Thrombosis in the Arterial System is Usually due to Atherosclerosis

 PATHOGENESIS: The vessels most commonly involved in arterial thrombosis due to atherosclerosis are the coronary, cerebral, mesenteric, renal arteries, and arteries of the lower extremities. Less commonly, arterial thrombosis occurs in other disorders, including inflammation of arteries (arteritis), trauma, and blood diseases.

A major risk factor for thrombosis is immobilization after surgery or after leg casting. Other risk factors include obesity, advanced age, previous thrombosis, and cancer. The pathogenesis of arterial thrombosis involves principally three factors:

- **Damage to endothelium**, almost always a result of atherosclerosis, disturbs the anticoagulant properties of the vessel wall and serves as a nidus for platelet aggregation and fibrin formation.
- **Alterations in blood flow**, whether from turbulence in an aneurysm or at sites of arterial bifurcation, is conducive to thrombosis. Slowing of blood flow in narrowed arteries favors thrombosis.

 PATHOLOGY: An arterial thrombus attached to a vessel wall is initially soft, friable, and dark red, with fine alternating bands of yellowish platelets and fibrin, the lines of Zahn (Fig. 7-3). Once formed, arterial thrombi have several possible outcomes.

- **Lysis**, owing to the potent thrombolytic activity of the blood.
- **Propagation** (i.e., an increase in its size), because a thrombus serves as a focus for further thrombosis.
- **Organization**, the eventual invasion of connective tissue elements involved in repair (see Chapter 3), which causes a thrombus to become firm and grayish white.
- **Canalization**, by which new lumina lined by endothelial cells form in an organized thrombus (Fig. 7-4).
- **Embolization**, when part or all of the thrombus becomes dislodged, travels through the circulation, and lodges in a blood vessel some distance from the site of thrombus formation (see below for further discussion).

 CLINICAL FEATURES: *Arterial thrombosis due to atherosclerosis is the most common cause of death in Western industrialized countries.* Because most arterial thrombi occlude the vessel, they often lead to ischemic necrosis of tissue supplied by that artery (i.e., an **infarct**). Thus, thrombosis of a coronary or cerebral artery results in **myocardial infarct** (heart attack) or **cerebral infarct** (stroke), respectively. Other end-arteries that are affected by atherosclerosis and often suffer thrombosis include mesenteric arteries (intestinal infarction), renal arteries (kidney infarcts), and arteries of the leg (gangrene).

Thrombosis in the Heart Develops on the Endocardium

As in the arterial system, endocardial injury and changes in blood flow in the heart may lead to mural thrombosis (i.e., a thrombus adhering to the underlying wall of the heart). Myocardial infarction is often associated with mural thrombi adherent to the left ventricle resulting from damage to the endocardium and altered blood flow. Mural thrombi also occur in association with atrial fibrillation, cardiomyopathies, and endocarditis—the last produc-

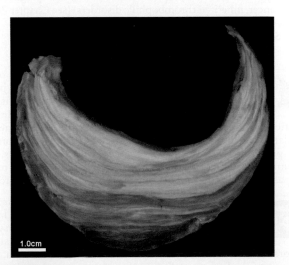

1.0cm

FIGURE 7-3. **Arterial thrombus.** Gross photograph of a thrombus from an aortic aneurysm shows the laminations of fibrin and platelets known as the lines of Zahn.

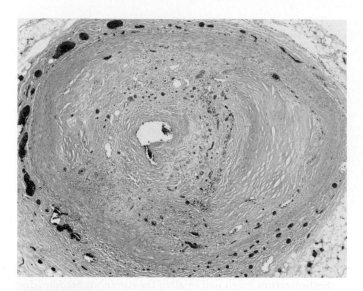

FIGURE 7-4. **Canalization of thrombus.** Photomicrograph of the left anterior descending coronary artery shows severe atherosclerosis and canalization.

ing small thrombi (vegetations) on cardiac valves (see Chapter 11 for additional detail). The major complication of thrombi in any location in the heart is detachment of fragments and their lodgement in blood vessels at distant sites (**embolization**).

Thrombosis in the Venous System is Multifactorial

The most common manifestation of thrombosis in the venous system is thrombosis of the deep venous system of the legs (**deep venous thrombosis or DVT**).

PATHOGENESIS: DVT is caused by the same factors that favor arterial and cardiac thrombosis: endothelial injury, stasis, and a hypercoagulable state. Conditions that favor the development of DVT include:

- **Stasis** (heart failure, chronic venous insufficiency, postoperative immobilization, prolonged bed rest).
- **Injury** (trauma, surgery, childbirth).
- **Hypercoagulability** (oral contraceptives, late pregnancy, cancer, inherited thrombophilic disorders) (see Chapter 20).
- **Advanced age** (venous varicosities, phlebosclerosis).
- **Sickle cell disease** (see Chapter 20).

PATHOLOGY: Most (>90%) venous thromboses occur in deep veins of the legs; the rest usually involve pelvic veins. Most venous thrombi begin in the calf veins, frequently in the sinuses above the venous valves. In this location, venous thrombi have several potential fates, generally similar to those discussed above for arterial thrombi. A thrombus may propagate so as to involve the larger iliofemoral veins. The thrombus may then dislodge (embolization) and be carried to the lung as a pulmonary embolus, which is a significant hazard to life.

CLINICAL FEATURES: Small thrombi in the calf veins are ordinarily asymptomatic, and even larger thrombi in the iliofemoral system may cause no symptoms or calf tenderness. Occlusive thrombosis of femoral or iliac veins leads to severe congestion, edema, and cyanosis of the lower extremity.

The function of venous valves is always impaired in a vein subjected to thrombosis and organization. As a result, chronic deep venous insufficiency (i.e., impaired venous drainage) is virtually inevitable. If a lesion is restricted to a small segment of the deep venous system, the condition may remain asymptomatic. However, more extensive involvement leads to pigmentation, edema, and induration of leg skin. Ulceration above the medial malleolus can occur and is often difficult to treat.

Venous thrombi elsewhere may also be dangerous. Thrombosis of mesenteric veins can cause hemorrhagic small bowel infarction, thrombosis of cerebral veins may be fatal, and hepatic vein thrombosis (Budd-Chiari syndrome) may destroy the liver.

Embolism

An embolism is the sudden blockage of the venous or arterial circulations by any material that can lodge in a blood vessel and obstruct its lumen. The most common embolus is a thromboembolus—that is, a thrombus formed in one location that detaches from a vessel wall at its point of origin and travels to a distant site.

Pulmonary Arterial Embolism is Potentially Fatal

Most pulmonary emboli (90%) arise from deep veins of the lower extremities, and fatal emboli tend to form in iliofemoral veins (Fig. 7-5). The clinical features of pulmonary embolism are determined by the size of the embolus and the patient's health. Acute pulmonary embolism is divided into the following syndromes:

- Asymptomatic small pulmonary emboli
- Transient dyspnea and tachypnea without other symptoms
- Pulmonary infarction with pleuritic chest pain, hemoptysis, and pleural effusion
- Cardiovascular collapse with sudden death.

Massive Pulmonary Embolism

One of the most dramatic calamities complicating hospitalization is the sudden collapse and death of a patient who appeared to be well on the way to an uneventful recovery. The cause of this catastrophe is often massive pulmonary embolism due to the release of a large deep venous thrombus from a lower extremity. Classically, a postoperative patient succumbs upon getting out of bed for the first time. The muscular activity dislodges a thrombus that formed as a result of the stasis from prolonged bed rest. Excluding deaths related to surgery itself, pulmonary embolism is the most common cause of death after major orthopedic surgery and is the most frequent nonobstetric cause of postpartum death. It also is an especially common factor in deaths of patients who suffer from chronic heart and lung diseases and in those who are subjected to prolonged immobilization for any reason. Prolonged immobilization associated with air travel can also lead to venous thrombosis ("economy class syndrome") and, occasionally, sudden death from a pulmonary embolus.

A large pulmonary embolus often lodges at the bifurcation of the main pulmonary artery (**saddle embolus**), obstructing blood flow to both lungs (Fig. 7-6). Large lethal emboli may also be found in the first branching of the right or left pulmonary arteries. Multiple smaller emboli may obstruct secondary branches and prove fatal. With acute obstruction of more than half of the pulmonary arterial tree, the patient often experiences immediate severe hypotension (or shock) and may die within minutes.

The hemodynamic consequences of such massive pulmonary embolism are acute right ventricular failure from sudden obstruction of outflow and pronounced reduction in left ventricular cardiac output, secondary to the loss of right ventricular function. The low cardiac output is responsible for the sudden appearance of severe hypotension.

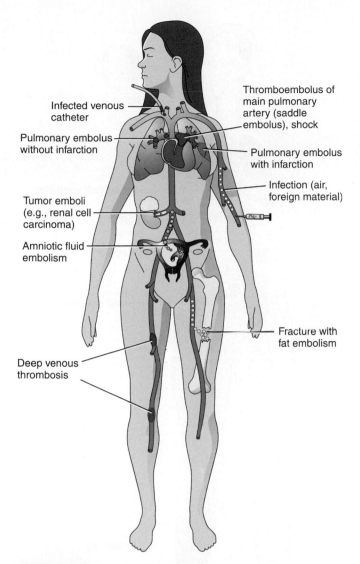

Infected venous catheter

Pulmonary embolus without infarction

Tumor emboli (e.g., renal cell carcinoma)

Amniotic fluid embolism

Deep venous thrombosis

Thromboembolus of main pulmonary artery (saddle embolus), shock

Pulmonary embolus with infarction

Infection (air, foreign material)

Fracture with fat embolism

FIGURE 7-5. Sources and effects of venous emboli.

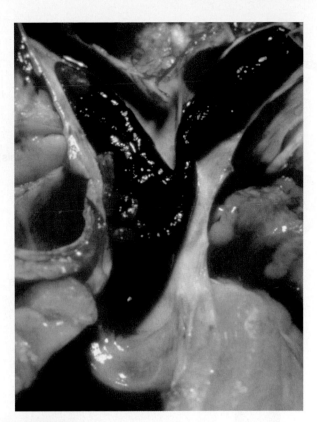

FIGURE 7-6. **Pulmonary embolism.** The main pulmonary artery and its bifurcation have been opened to reveal a large saddle embolus.

Pulmonary Infarction

Small pulmonary emboli tend to locate in peripheral pulmonary arteries and are not ordinarily lethal. Clinically, pulmonary infarction is usually seen in the context of congestive heart failure or chronic lung disease, because the normal dual circulation of the lung ordinarily protects against ischemic necrosis. When pulmonary infarcts do occur, they tend to be hemorrhagic, as the bronchial artery pumps blood into the necrotic area. The infarcts are generally pyramidal, with the base of the pyramid on the pleural surface. Patients experience cough, stabbing pleuritic pain, shortness of breath, and occasional hemoptysis. Pleural effusion is common and often bloody. With time, the blood in the infarct is resorbed, and the center of the infarct becomes pale. Granulation tissue forms on the edge of the infarct, after which it is organized to form a fibrous scar. Half of all pulmonary thromboemboli are resorbed and organized within 8 weeks, with little narrowing of the vessels.

Systemic Arterial Embolism Often Causes Infarcts

Thromboembolism

The heart is the most common source of arterial thromboemboli (Fig. 7-7), which usually arise from mural thrombi or diseased valves (see above). These emboli tend to lodge at points where the vessel lumen narrows abruptly (e.g., at bifurcations or in the area of an atheroscle-

rotic plaque). Organs that suffer the most from arterial thromboembolism include:

- **Brain:** Arterial emboli to the brain cause ischemic necrosis (strokes).
- **Intestine:** In the mesenteric circulation, emboli result in bowel infarction, which manifests as an acute abdomen and requires immediate surgery.
- **Lower extremity:** Embolism to an artery of the leg leads to sudden pain, absence of pulses, and a cold limb. In some cases, the limb must be amputated.
- **Kidney:** Renal artery embolism may infarct an entire kidney but more commonly causes small peripheral infarcts.
- **Heart:** Coronary artery embolism and resulting myocardial infarcts occur but are rare.

The more common sites of infarction from arterial emboli are summarized in Figure 7-8.

Air/Gas Embolism

Air may enter the venous circulation through neck wounds, thoracocentesis, or punctures of the great veins during invasive procedures or hemodialysis. Small amounts of circulating air in the form of bubbles are of little consequence, but quantities of 100 mL or more can lead to sudden death. Air bubbles tend to coalesce and physically obstruct blood flow in the right side of the heart, the pulmonary circulation, and the brain. Histologically, air bubbles appear as empty spaces in capillaries and small vessels of the lung.

Persons exposed to increased atmospheric pressure, such as scuba divers and workers in underwater occupations (e.g., tunnels, drilling platform construction), are subject to **decompression sickness**, a unique form of gas embolism. During descent, large amounts of inert gas (nitrogen or helium) are dissolved in bodily fluids. When the diver ascends, the gas is released from solution

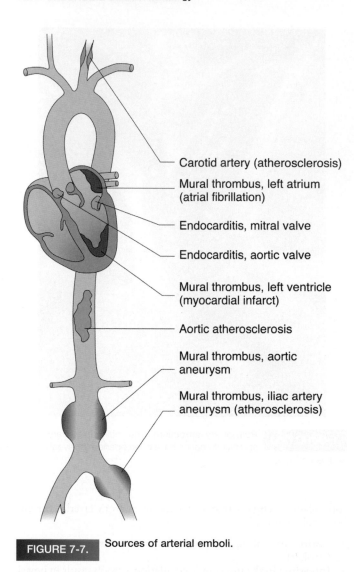

FIGURE 7-7. Sources of arterial emboli.

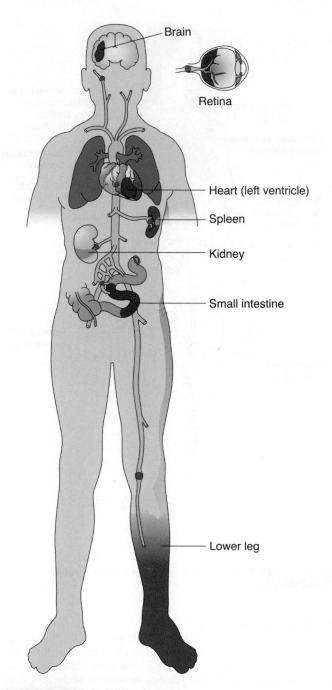

FIGURE 7-8. Common sites of infarction from arterial emboli.

and exhaled. However, if ascent is too rapid, gas bubbles form in the circulation and within tissues, obstructing blood flow and directly injuring cells. Air embolism is the second most common cause of death in sport diving (drowning is the first). **Acute decompression sickness**, "the bends," is characterized by temporary muscular and joint pain, as a result of small vessel obstruction in these tissues. However, severe involvement of cerebral blood vessels may cause coma or even death.

Amniotic Fluid Embolism

In amniotic fluid embolism, amniotic fluid containing fetal cells and debris enter the maternal circulation through open uterine and cervical veins. It is a rare maternal complication of childbirth but can be catastrophic when it occurs. This disorder usually occurs at the end of labor when the pulmonary emboli are composed of the solid epithelial constituents (squames) contained in the amniotic fluid. Of greater importance is the initiation of potentially fatal disseminated intravascular coagulation caused by the high thromboplastin activity of amniotic fluid.

Fat Embolism

Fat embolism refers to the release of emboli of fatty marrow into damaged blood vessels following severe trauma to fat-containing tissue, particularly accompanying bone fractures. In most instances, fat embolism is clinically inapparent. However, when severe it leads to **fat embolism syndrome** 1 to 3 days after the injury. In its most severe form, which may be fatal, this syndrome is characterized by respiratory

failure, mental changes, thrombocytopenia, and widespread petechiae. At autopsy, innumerable fat globules are seen in the microvasculature of the lungs and brain and sometimes other organs. The lungs typically exhibit the changes of acute respiratory distress syndrome (ARDS) (see Chapter 12). The lesions in the brain include cerebral edema, small hemorrhages, and occasionally microinfarcts.

Infarction

Infarction is the process by which coagulative necrosis develops in an area distal to the occlusion of an end artery. The necrotic zone is an **infarct**. Infarcts of vital organs such as the heart, brain, and intestine are serious medical conditions and are major causes of morbidity and mortality. If the victim survives, the infarct heals with a scar.

PATHOLOGY: The gross and microscopic appearance of an infarct depends on its location and age. Upon arterial occlusion, the area supplied by the vessel rapidly becomes swollen and deep red. Microscopically, vascular dilation and congestion and occasionally interstitial hemorrhage are noted. Subsequently, several types of infarcts are distinguishable by gross examination.

Pale infarcts are typical in the heart, kidneys, and spleen (Fig. 7-9). On gross examination, 1 or 2 days after the initial hyperemia, the infarct becomes soft, sharply delineated, and light yellow (Fig. 7-10). The border tends to be dark red, reflecting hemorrhage into surrounding viable tissue. Microscopically, a pale infarct exhibits uniform coagulative necrosis.

Red infarcts may result from either arterial or venous occlusion and are also characterized by coagulative necrosis. However, they are distinguished by bleeding into the necrotic area from adjacent arteries and veins. *Red infarcts occur principally in organs with a dual blood supply,* such as the lung, or those with extensive collateral circulation, such as the small intestine and brain. In the heart, a red infarct occurs when the infarcted area is reperfused, as may occur following spontaneous or therapeutically induced lysis of the occluding thrombus. Grossly, red infarcts are sharply circumscribed, firm, and dark red to purple (Fig. 7-11). Over a period of several days, acute inflammatory cells infiltrate the necrotic area from the viable border, followed by granulation tissue, healing, and scar formation (see Chapter 3). In the brain, an infarct typically undergoes liquefactive necrosis and may become a fluid-filled cyst, which is referred to as a **cystic infarct** (Fig. 7-12).

Infarcts of the lung (pulmonary infarct, see above), heart (myocardial infarcts, see Chapter 11), brain (cerebral infarcts, see Chapter 28), and intestine (see Chapter 13) are medical emergencies responsible for significant morbidity and mortality in the population. Details of the pathogenesis and clinical features of infarctions occurring in specific organs are found in the appropriate chapter references.

Edema

Edema is excess fluid in interstitial spaces of the body and may be local or generalized. Edema fluid may accumulate in body spaces, such as the pleural cavity (**hydrothorax**), peritoneal cavity (**ascites**), or pericardial cavity (**hydropericardium**).

LOCAL EDEMA in many instances occurs as a result of the vascular effects of inflammation (see Chapter 2). Local edema of a limb, usually the leg, results from venous or lymphatic obstruction.

GENERALIZED EDEMA, affecting visceral organs and the skin of the trunk and lower extremities reflects a global disorder of fluid and electrolyte metabolism, most often occasioned by heart failure. Generalized edema is also seen in certain renal diseases as-

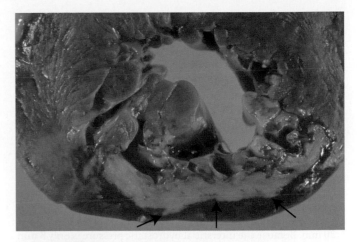

FIGURE 7-10. **Acute myocardial infarct.** A cross-section of the left ventricle reveals a sharply circumscribed, soft, yellow area of necrosis in the posterior free wall (*arrows*).

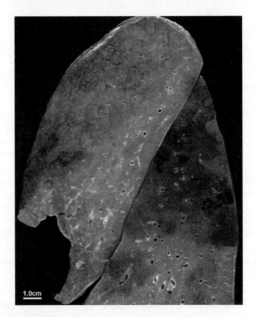

FIGURE 7-11. **Red infarct.** A sagittal slice of lung shows a hemorrhagic infarct in upper segments of the lower lobe.

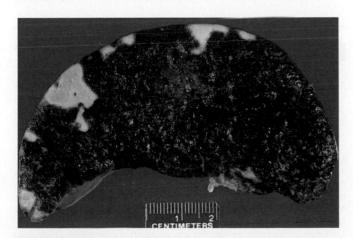

FIGURE 7-9. **Spleen infarcts.** A cut section of spleen displays multiple pale, wedge-shaped infarcts beneath the capsule.

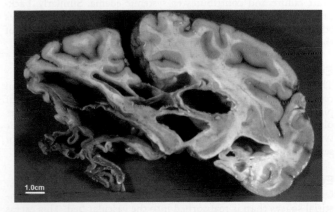

FIGURE 7-12. **Cystic infarct.** A cross-section of brain in the frontal plane shows a healed cystic infarct.

sociated with loss of serum proteins into the urine (nephrotic syndrome) and in cirrhosis of the liver.

ANASARCA is extreme generalized edema, a condition evidenced by conspicuous fluid accumulation in subcutaneous tissues, visceral organs, and body cavities.

The Mechanisms of Edema Formation Alter the Equilibrium of Fluid Between the Vasculature and Interstitium

Normal Capillary Filtration
Normal formation and retention of interstitial fluid depends on filtration and reabsorption at the level of the capillaries (Starling forces). The internal or hydrostatic pressure in the arteriolar segment of the capillary is 32 mm Hg. At the middle of the capillary, it is 20 mm. Because the interstitial hydrostatic pressure is only 3 mm Hg, there is an outward fluid filtration of 14 mL/min. Hydrostatic pressure is opposed by plasma oncotic pressure (26 mm Hg), which results in osmotic reabsorption of 12 mL/min at the venous end of the capillary. Thus, interstitial fluid is formed at the rate of 2 mL/min and is reabsorbed by the lymphatics, so that in equilibrium, there is no net fluid gain or loss in the interstitium.

Sodium and Water Metabolism
Water represents 50% to 70% of body weight and is divided between the extracellular and the intracellular fluid spaces. Extracellular fluid is further divided into interstitial and vascular compartments. Interstitial fluid constitutes about 75% of the extracellular compartment.

Total body sodium is the principal determinant of extracellular fluid volume because it is the major cation in the extracellular fluid. In other words, increased total body sodium must be balanced by more extracellular water to maintain constant osmolality. Control of extracellular fluid volume depends to a large extent on regulation of renal sodium excretion, which is influenced by (1) atrial natriuretic factor, (2) the renin–angiotensin system of the juxtaglomerular apparatus, and (3) sympathetic nervous system activity (see Chapter 10). Generalized edema and ascites invariably reflect increased total body sodium, as a consequence of renal sodium retention. The most common conditions in which generalized edema is found include congestive heart failure, cirrhosis of the liver, nephrotic syndrome, and some cases of chronic renal insufficiency.

Edema Produced by Increased Hydrostatic Pressure
Unopposed increases in hydrostatic pressure result in greater filtration of fluid into the interstitial space and its retention as edema. Such a situation is particularly prominent in decompensated heart disease, in which back-pressure in the lungs secondary to left ventricular failure leads to acute pulmonary edema and right-sided heart failure and contributes to systemic edema. Similarly, back-pressure caused by venous obstruction in the lower extremity causes edema of the leg. Obstruction to portal blood flow in cirrhosis of the liver contributes to the formation of abdominal fluid (ascites).

Edema Caused by Decreased Oncotic Pressure
The difference in pressure between intravascular and interstitial compartments is largely determined by the concentration of plasma proteins, especially albumin. Any condition that lowers plasma albumin levels, whether it is albuminuria in the nephrotic syndrome or reduced albumin synthesis in chronic liver disease or severe malnutrition, tends to promote generalized edema.

Edema Secondary to Lymphatic Obstruction
Under normal circumstances, more fluid is filtered into the interstitial spaces than is reabsorbed into the vascular bed. This excess interstitial fluid is removed by lymphatics. Thus, obstruction to lymphatic flow leads to localized edema. Lymphatic channels can be obstructed by (1) malignant neoplasms, (2) fibrosis resulting from inflammation or irradiation, and (3) surgical ablation. Lymphedema of the arm sometimes complicates radical mastectomies for breast cancer, owing to the removal of axillary lymph nodes and lymphatics.

The mechanisms of edema formation and disorders associated with them are summarized in Figure 7-13 and Table 7-1.

Congestive Heart Failure is the Consequence of Inadequate Cardiac Output

Congestive heart failure occurs when cardiac compensatory mechanisms fail to provide an adequate supply of blood to peripheral tissues. In the United States, this disorder is most commonly associated with ischemic heart disease, although virtually any chronic cardiac disorder may ultimately result in congestive heart failure. The pathogenesis of congestive heart failure is complex (see Chapter 11 for detailed discussion).

Concentrating on the role of cardiac failure in sodium/water balance, inadequate cardiac output in congestive heart failure leads to decreased glomerular filtration and increased renin secretion. The latter activates angiotensin, leading to the release of aldosterone, subsequent sodium reabsorption, and fluid retention. Furthermore, reduced hepatic blood flow impairs catabolism of aldosterone, thereby further raising its concentration in the blood. Distention of the atria by the increased blood volume promotes release of atrial natriuretic peptide, which stimulates renal sodium excretion.

When compensatory mechanisms fail, the further expansion of plasma volume leads to increased pulmonary and systemic venous pressure, which produces greater hydrostatic pressure in the respective capillary beds. The increased capillary pressure, together with decreased plasma oncotic pressure, results in the edema of congestive heart failure.

 PATHOLOGY: Failure of the left ventricle is associated principally with passive congestion of the lungs and pulmonary edema (Fig. 7-14). When chronic, these conditions lead to pulmonary hypertension and eventual failure of the right ventricle. Right ventricular failure is characterized by generalized subcutaneous edema (most prominent in the dependent portions of the body), ascites, and pleural effusions. The liver, spleen, and other splanchnic organs are typically congested. At autopsy, the heart is enlarged and its chambers dilated.

 CLINICAL FEATURES: Patients may complain of shortness of breath (**dyspnea**) on exertion and when recumbent (**orthopnea**). They may be awakened from sleep by sudden episodes of shortness of breath (**paroxysmal nocturnal dyspnea**). Physical examination usually reveals distended jugular veins, pitting edema of the legs, and an

---

FIGURE 7-13. The capillary system and mechanisms of edema formation. **A.** Normal. The differential between the hydrostatic and oncotic pressures at the arterial end of the capillary system is responsible for the filtration into the interstitial space of approximately 14 mL of fluid per minute. This fluid is reabsorbed at the venous end at the rate of 12 mL/min. It is also drained through the lymphatic capillaries at a rate of 2 mL/min. Proteins are removed by the lymphatics from the interstitial space. **B.** Hydrostatic edema. If the hydrostatic pressure at the venous end of the capillary system is elevated, reabsorption decreases. As long as the lymphatics can drain the surplus fluid, no edema results. If their capacity is exceeded, however, edema fluid accumulates. **C.** Oncotic edema. Edema fluid also accumulates if reabsorption is diminished by decreased oncotic pressure of the vascular bed, due to a loss of albumin. **D.** Inflammatory and traumatic edema. Edema, either local or systemic, results if the vascular bed becomes leaky following injury to the endothelium. **E.** Lymphedema. Lymphatic obstruction causes the accumulation of interstitial fluid because of insufficient reabsorption and deficient removal of proteins, the latter increasing the oncotic pressure of the fluid in the interstitial space.

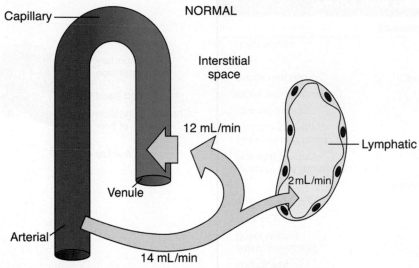

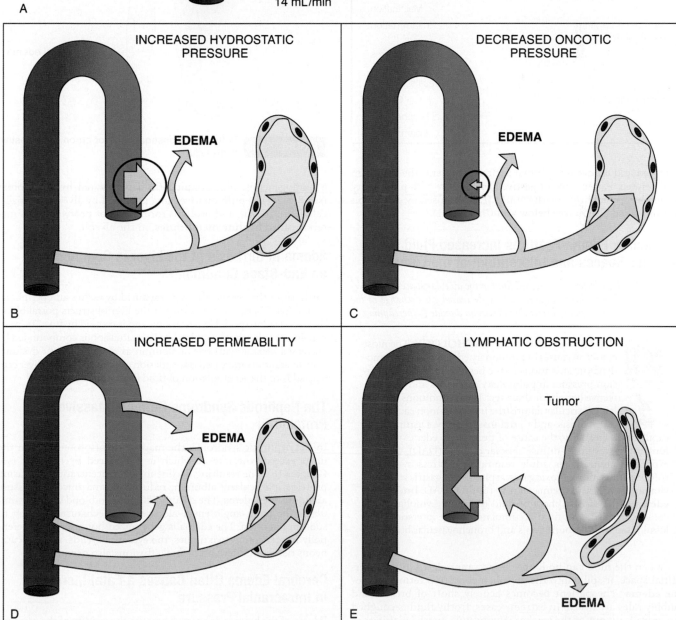

TABLE 7–1

Disorders Associated With Edema

Increased hydrostatic pressure	
Arteriolar dilation	Inflammation
	Heat
Increased venous pressure	Venous thrombosis
	Congestive heart failure
	Cirrhosis (ascites)
	Postural inactivity (e.g., prolonged standing)
Hypervolemia	Sodium retention (e.g., decreased renal function)
Decreased oncotic pressure	
Hypoproteinemia	Nephrotic syndrome
	Cirrhosis
	Protein-losing gastroenteropathy
	Malnutrition
Increased capillary permeability	Inflammation
	Burns
	Acute respiratory distress syndrome
Lymphatic obstruction	Cancer
	Postsurgical lymphedema
	Inflammation

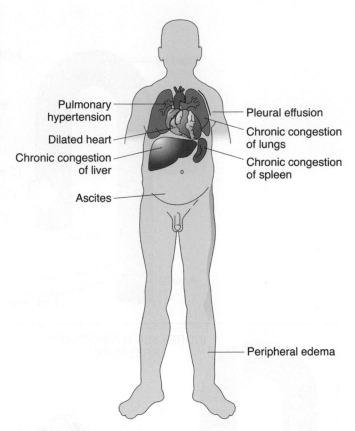

FIGURE 7-14. Pathologic consequences of chronic congestive heart failure.

enlarged and tender liver. When ascites is present, the abdomen is distended. Patients in congestive heart failure with pulmonary edema have crackling breath sounds (**rales**) caused by expansion of fluid-filled alveoli (see below and Chapter 11).

Pulmonary Edema Features Increased Fluid in the Alveolar Spaces and Interstitium of the Lung

Pulmonary edema refers to increased fluid in the alveolar spaces and interstitium of the lung. This condition leads to decreased gas exchange in the lung and causes hypoxia and retention of carbon dioxide (hypercapnia).

 PATHOGENESIS AND PATHOLOGY: The most common causes of pulmonary edema relate to hemodynamic alterations in the heart that increase perfusion pressure in pulmonary capillaries and block effective lymphatic drainage. These conditions include left ventricular failure (the most common cause), mitral stenosis, and mitral insufficiency. Disruption of capillary permeability, the cause of pulmonary edema in acute lung injury, results in diffuse alveolar damage (DAD), which is expressed clinically as adult respiratory distress syndrome (ARDS). Inhalation of toxic gases, aspiration of gastric contents, viral infections, and uremia all may result in DAD. **Interstitial edema** is the earliest phase of fluid filtration. Lymphatics become distended, and fluid accumulates in the interstitium of lobular septa and around veins and bronchovascular bundles.

When the fluid can no longer be accommodated in the interstitial space, it spills into the alveoli, a condition termed **alveolar edema**. The patient becomes acutely short of breath, and bubbly rales are heard. In extreme cases, frothy fluid is coughed up or wells up out of the trachea. Hypoxemia may be manifest as cyanosis. Microscopic examination of the edematous lung reveals severely congested alveolar capillaries and alveoli filled with

a homogeneous, pink-staining fluid permeated by air bubbles (see Fig. 7-1). If pulmonary edema is caused by alveolar damage, cell debris, fibrin, and proteins form films of proteinaceous material, called **hyaline membranes**, in the alveoli.

Edema in Cirrhosis of the Liver is Commonly an End-Stage Condition

Cirrhosis of the liver is often accompanied by ascites and peripheral edema (see Chapter 14). Scarring of the liver obstructs portal blood flow and leads to portal hypertension and increased hydrostatic pressure in the splanchnic circulation. This situation is compounded by decreased hepatic synthesis of albumin as a result of liver dysfunction. In addition, increased transudation of lymph from the liver capsule adds to the accumulation of fluid in the abdomen.

The Nephrotic Syndrome Reflects Massive Proteinuria

In the nephrotic syndrome, the magnitude of protein loss in the urine exceeds the rate at which it is replaced by the liver (see Chapter 16). The resulting decline in the concentration of plasma proteins, particularly albumin, reduces plasma oncotic pressure and promotes edema. The ensuing decrease in blood volume stimulates the renin–angiotensin–aldosterone mechanism, leading to sodium retention. The edema is generalized but appears preferentially in soft connective tissues, the eyes, the eyelids, and subcutaneous tissues. Ascites and pleural effusions also occur.

Cerebral Edema Often Causes a Fatal Increase in Intracranial Pressure

Edema of the brain is dangerous because the rigidity of the cranium allows little room for expansion. Increased intracranial pressure from edema compromises cerebral blood supply, distorts the gross structure of the brain, and interferes with central nervous system function. At autopsy, an edematous brain is soft and heavy. Gyri are flattened and sulci narrowed. Because of alterations in brain function, patients with cerebral edema suffer vomiting, disorientation, and convulsions. Severe cerebral edema causes herniation of the cerebral tonsils, a lethal event.

Fluid Accumulates in Body Cavities as Extensions of the Interstitial Space

The Pleural Space

Pleural effusion (fluid in the pleural space) is a straw-colored transudate of low specific gravity that contains few cells (mainly exfoliated mesothelial cells). Fluid commonly accumulates as an expression of a generalized tendency to form edema in diseases such as the nephrotic syndrome, cirrhosis of the liver, and congestive heart failure. Pleural effusion is also a frequent response to an inflammatory process or tumor in the lung or on the pleural surface.

The Pericardium

Fluid in the pericardial sac may result from either hemorrhage (**hemopericardium**) or injury to the pericardium (**pericardial effusion**). Pericardial effusions occur with pericardial infections, metastatic neoplasms to the pericardium, uremia, and systemic lupus erythematosus. They are also occasionally encountered after cardiac operations (**postpericardiotomy syndrome**) or radiation therapy for cancer.

Pericardial fluid may accumulate rapidly, for example, with hemorrhage from a ruptured myocardial infarct, dissecting aortic aneurysm, or trauma. In these cases, the pressure in the pericardial cavity rises to exceed the filling pressure of the heart, a condition termed **cardiac tamponade**. The resulting precipitous decline in cardiac output is often fatal. If pericardial fluid accumulates rapidly, the tolerable limit may be only 90 to 120 mL, but a liter or more of fluid can be accommodated if the process is gradual.

Peritoneum

Peritoneal effusion, also called **ascites**, is caused mainly by cirrhosis of the liver, abdominal neoplasms, pancreatitis, cardiac failure, the nephrotic syndrome, and hepatic venous obstruction (Budd-Chiari syndrome). Obstruction of the thoracic duct by cancer may lead to **chylous ascites**, in which the fluid has a milky appearance and a high fat content. The pathogenesis of ascites in cirrhosis of the liver is discussed above.

Patients with severe ascites accumulate many liters of fluid and have hugely distended abdomens. The complications of ascites derive from increased abdominal pressure and include anorexia and vomiting, reflux esophagitis, dyspnea, ventral hernia, and leakage of fluid into the pleural space.

Shock

Shock is a condition of profound hemodynamic and metabolic disturbance characterized by failure of the circulatory system to maintain an appropriate blood supply to the microcirculation, with consequent inadequate perfusion of vital organs. The term **shock** encompasses all the reactions that occur in response to such disturbances. In the course of uncompensated shock, a rapid circulatory collapse leads to impaired cellular metabolism and death. However, in many cases, compensatory mechanisms sustain the patient, at least for a while. When these adaptations fail, shock becomes irreversible.

 PATHOGENESIS: Decreased perfusion in shock most commonly results from decreased cardiac output, either due to the inability of the heart to pump the normal venous return or to decreased effective blood volume that leads to decreased venous return. These two

mechanisms underlie two of the major types of shock: **cardiogenic** and **hypovolemic** shock. Systemic vasodilation, with or without increases in vascular permeability, is responsible for the other categories of shock: septic shock, anaphylactic shock, and neurogenic shock (Fig. 7-15).

- **Cardiogenic shock** is caused by myocardial pump failure. It usually arises after massive myocardial infarction, but myocarditis may also be responsible. "Obstructive" shock may result from pulmonary embolism, cardiac tamponade, and (rarely) atrial myxoma.
- **Hypovolemic shock** is secondary to a pronounced decrease in blood or plasma volume, caused by loss of fluid from the vascular compartment. Hemorrhage, fluid loss from severe burns, diarrhea, excessive urine formation, perspiration, and trauma are the major mechanisms of fluid loss that can produce hypovolemic shock. In the case of burns or trauma, direct damage to the microcirculation increases vascular permeability.
- **Septic shock** is caused by severe systemic microbial infections. The pathogenesis of septic shock is complex and is discussed in detail below.
- **Anaphylactic shock** is a consequence of a systemic type I hypersensitivity reaction, which causes widespread vasodilation and increased vascular permeability (see Chapter 4).
- **Neurogenic shock** can follow acute injury to the brain or spinal cord, which impairs the neural control of vasomotor tone, causing generalized vasodilation. In the case of both anaphylactic and neurogenic shock, the subsequent redistribution of blood to the periphery, with or without increased vascular permeability, reduces the effective circulating blood and plasma volume. This effect ultimately leads to the same consequences as does hypovolemic shock.

In hypovolemic and cardiogenic shock, lower cardiac output and resultant decreased tissue perfusion are the key steps in the progression from reversible to irreversible shock. Cellular hypoxia is the common consequence of the initial decrease in tissue perfusion. Although such changes do not initially result in irreversible injury, a vicious circle of decreasing tissue perfusion and further hypoxic injury to endothelial cells, cardiac myocytes, and other organs may lead to death.

Systemic Inflammatory Response Syndrome (SIRS) Characterizes Septic Shock

Systemic inflammatory response syndrome (SIRS) is an exaggerated and generalized manifestation of a local immune or inflammatory reaction, which is often fatal. SIRS is a hypermetabolic state that features two or more signs of systemic inflammation—such as fever, tachycardia, tachypnea, leukocytosis, or leukopenia—in the setting of a known cause of inflammation. **Septic shock** (see above) is defined as clinical SIRS so severe that it leads to organ dysfunction and hypotension. The mechanisms responsible for the development of septic shock are illustrated in Figure 7-16. These processes often progress to **multiple organ dysfunction syndrome** (MODS), a term used to describe otherwise unexplained abnormalities of organ function in critically ill patients (see below).

The massive inflammatory reaction defined by SIRS results from systemic release of cytokines, the most important being tumor necrosis factor (TNF), interleukin-1 (IL-1), IL-6, and platelet-activating factor (PAF). More than 30 endogenous mediators are described in this condition, and their interactions may be important in the pathogenesis of SIRS.

Septicemia with gram-negative organisms is the most common cause of septic shock. The invading bacteria release **endotoxin**, a lipopolysaccharide (LPS), with toxic activity that resides in the lipid A component. The binding of LPS to CD14 and to toll-like receptor-4, both primary sensors of monocytes/ macrophages for innate immune responses, leads to (1) the upregulation of TNF expression and (2) the secretion

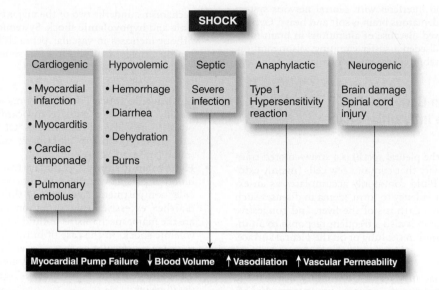

FIGURE 7-15. **Classification of shock.** Shock results from (1) an inability of the heart to pump adequately (cardiogenic shock), (2) decreased effective blood volume as a consequence of severely reduced blood or plasma volume (hypovolemic shock), or (3) widespread vasodilation (septic, anaphylactic, or neurogenic shock). Increased vascular permeability may complicate vasodilation by contributing to reduced effective blood volume.

of large quantities of cytokines, such as IL-1, IL-6, IL-8, IL-12, and others, which mediate a variety of responses. These cytokines, as well as subsequent production of nitric oxide and procoagulant proteins, ultimately cause the overwhelming cardiovascular collapse characteristic of septic shock.

Multiple Organ Dysfunction Syndrome (MODS) is the End-Result of Shock

Multiple organ dysfunction occurs in one third of patients with septic shock, trauma, or burns and in one quarter of those with acute pancreatitis. Whatever the cause, the clinical deterioration of MODS results from the common mechanisms of tissue injury defined as SIRS. Mortality of SIRS/MODS exceeds 50%, making it responsible for most deaths in noncoronary intensive care units in the United States.

It is now thought that following bacterial infection, there is an initial response of excessive inflammation and septic shock characteristic of SIRS. However, such uncontrolled cytokine induction is preceded by a stage of anergy and immune repression, termed **compensated anti-inflammatory response syndrome**. Septic patients may cycle between SIRS and compensated anti-inflammatory response syndrome, in which case they tend to exhibit increased mortality rates.

Vascular Compensatory Mechanisms

Compensatory mechanisms in shock shift blood flow away from the periphery, so as to maintain flow to the heart and the brain. These responses involve the sympathetic nervous system, release of endogenous vasoconstrictors and hormonal substances, and local vasoregulation. The result is increased cardiac output achieved by increasing heart rate and myocardial contractility, while constricting arteries and arterioles.

 PATHOLOGY: Shock is associated with specific changes in a number of organs (Fig. 7-17), including failure of the heart, liver, and kidneys, ARDS, and depression of host defense mechanisms.

Heart

The heart shows petechial hemorrhages of the epicardium and endocardium. Microscopically, prominent contraction bands and necrotic foci in the myocardium range from loss of single fibers to large areas of necrosis.

Kidney

Acute tubular necrosis known clinically as acute renal failure, is a major complication of shock. During acute renal failure, the kidney is large, swollen, and congested, although the cortex may be pale. A cross-section reveals blood pooling in the outer stripe of the medulla. Microscopically, fully developed acute tubular necrosis is evidenced by dilation of the proximal tubules and focal necrosis of cells. Frequently, pigmented casts in tubular lumina indicate leakage of hemoglobin or myoglobin. Coarse "ropy" casts are seen in the distal nephron and distal convoluted tubules. Interstitial edema is prominent in the cortex, and mononuclear cells accumulate within tubules and surrounding interstitium. Acute tubular necrosis is discussed in more detail in Chapter 16.

Lung

After the onset of severe and prolonged shock, injury to alveolar walls can result in **shock lung**, a cause of **ARDS**. The sequence of changes is mediated by polymorphonuclear leukocytes and includes interstitial edema, necrosis of endothelial and alveolar epithelial cells, and formation of intravascular microthrombi and hyaline membranes lining the alveolar surface. This process (DAD) is more fully discussed in Chapter 12.

Gastrointestinal Tract

Shock often results in diffuse gastrointestinal hemorrhage. Erosions of the gastric mucosa and superficial ischemic necrosis in the intestines are the usual sources of this bleeding. Interruption of the barrier function of the intestine may promote septicemia. More severe necrotizing lesions contribute to deterioration in the final phase of shock (see Chapter 13).

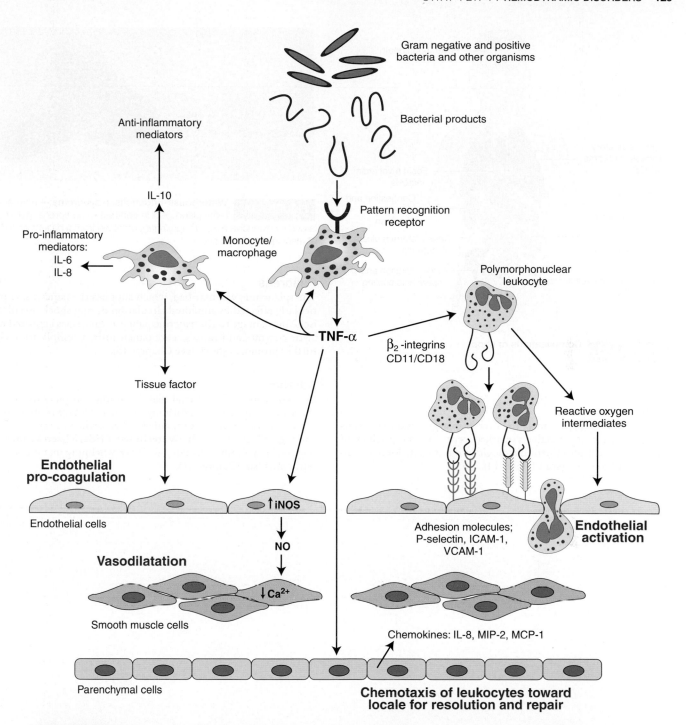

FIGURE 7-16. **Pathogenesis of endotoxic shock.** Sepsis is caused primarily by gram-negative bacteria and bacterial products such as endotoxin (lipopolysaccharide [LPS]), which is released into the circulation, where it binds to a pattern recognition receptor on the surface of monocyte/macrophages. Such binding stimulates the secretion of substantial quantities of tumor necrosis factor-alpha (TNF-α). TNF-α mediates septic shock by a number of mechanisms: (1) stimulation of the release of various pro- and anti-inflammatory mediators; (2) induction of endothelial procoagulation by tissue factor, thereby leading to thrombosis and local ischemia; (3) direct cytotoxic damage to endothelial cells; (4) endothelial activation, which enhances the adherence of polymorphonuclear leukocytes; (5) stimulation of endothelial cell nitric oxide production and vasodilation; and (6) release of chemokines to attract leukocytes for resolution and repair of tissue injury. Ca²⁺, calcium ion; ICAM, intercellular adhesion molecule; IL, interleukin; iNOS, inducible nitric oxide synthetase; MCP-1, monocyte chemotactic protein-1; MIP-2, macrophage-inflammatory protein-2; NO, nitric oxide; VCAM-1, vascular cell adhesion molecule-1.

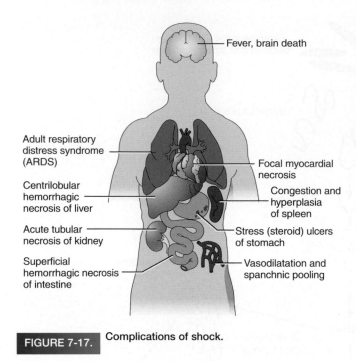

Fever, brain death

Adult respiratory distress syndrome (ARDS)

Centrilobular hemorrhagic necrosis of liver

Acute tubular necrosis of kidney

Superficial hemorrhagic necrosis of intestine

Focal myocardial necrosis

Congestion and hyperplasia of spleen

Stress (steroid) ulcers of stomach

Vasodilatation and spanchnic pooling

FIGURE 7-17. Complications of shock.

Liver

In patients who die in shock, the liver is enlarged and has a mottled cut surface that reflects marked centrilobular pooling of blood. The most prominent histologic lesion is centrilobular congestion and necrosis (see Chapter 14).

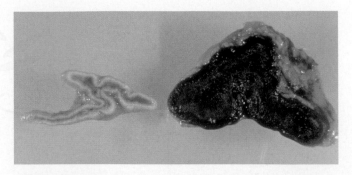

FIGURE 7-18. **Waterhouse-Friderichsen syndrome.** A normal adrenal gland *(left)* in contrast to an adrenal gland enlarged by extensive hemorrhage *(right)*, obtained from a patient who died of meningococcemic shock.

Pancreas

The splanchnic vascular bed, which supplies the pancreas, is particularly affected by impaired circulation during shock. Resulting ischemic damage to the exocrine pancreas unleashes activated catalytic enzymes and causes acute pancreatitis, a complication that further promotes shock (see Chapter 15).

Adrenals

In severe shock, the adrenal glands exhibit conspicuous hemorrhage in the inner cortex. Although the hemorrhage is often focal, it can be massive and accompanied by hemorrhagic necrosis of the entire gland, as seen in the **Waterhouse-Friderichsen syndrome** (Fig. 7-18), typically associated with overwhelming meningococcal septicemia (see Chapter 21).

8 Environmental and Nutritional Pathology

David S. Strayer
Emanuel Rubin

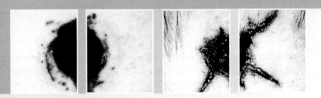

Environmental pathology is the study of diseases caused by exposure to harmful external agents and deficiencies of substances vital to life. In this chapter, we concentrate on diseases caused by (1) exposure to toxic agents, (2) physical damage, and (3) nutritional deficiencies.

Smoking

The use of tobacco is the single largest preventable cause of death in the United States, *with more than 400,000 deaths per year—about one sixth of the total deaths in the United States—occurring prematurely because of smoking. The major diseases responsible for excess mortality reported in cigarette smokers are, in order of frequency, coronary heart disease, lung cancer, and chronic obstructive pulmonary disease.* Life expectancy is shortened, and overall mortality is proportional to the amount and duration of cigarette smoking, commonly quantitated as "pack-years" (Fig. 8-1). Mortality from lung cancer, almost all of which is related to cigarette smoking, exceeds that from cancers of the colon, breast, pancreas, and prostate, the four next most common

causes of cancer-related death in the United States. After 15 years of abstinence from cigarettes, the mortality rate of ex-smokers approaches that of people who have never smoked.

Cardiovascular Disease is a Major Complication of Smoking

Cigarette smoking is a major independent risk factor for myocardial infarction and acts synergistically with other risk factors, such as elevated blood pressure and blood cholesterol levels (Fig. 8-2). Smoking precipitates initial myocardial infarction, increases the risk for second heart attacks, and diminishes survival after a heart attack. Smoking also increases the incidence of sudden cardiac death: It contributes to instability and erosion of atherosclerotic plaques and may lead to ischemia, arrhythmias, and ischemic stroke as well. The combination of smoking and oral contraceptive use in women older than 30 years of age further increases the likelihood of myocardial infarction and stroke in an age-dependent manner.

Atherosclerosis of the coronary arteries and aorta is more severe and extensive among cigarette smokers than among nonsmokers, and the effect is dose related. As a consequence, cigarette smoking is a strong risk factor for atherosclerotic aortic aneurysms and peripheral vascular disease. The pharmacologic actions of nicotine itself, carbon

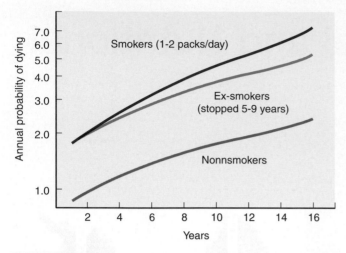

FIGURE 8-1. The risk of dying in smokers and nonsmokers. Note that the annual probability of an individual dying, indicated on the ordinate, is a logarithmic scale. Individuals who have smoked for 1 year have a twofold greater probability of dying than a nonsmoker, whereas those who have smoked for more than 15 years have more than a threefold greater probability of dying.

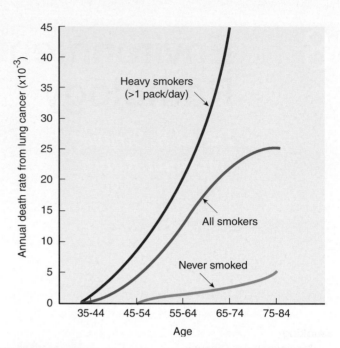

FIGURE 8-3. Death rate from lung cancer among smokers and nonsmokers. Nonsmokers exhibit a small, linear rise in the death rate from lung cancer from the age of 50 onward. By contrast, those who smoke more than one pack per day show an exponential rise in the annual death rate from lung cancer starting at about age 35. By age 70, heavy smokers have about a 20-fold greater death rate from lung cancer than nonsmokers.

monoxide (CO) inhalation, reduced plasma high-density lipoprotein levels, increased plasma fibrinogen levels, and higher leukocyte counts are all consequences of smoking that may predispose to myocardial infarction and stroke. **Buerger disease**, a now uncommon peculiar inflammatory and occlusive disease of the lower leg vasculature, occurs almost only in heavy smokers, mainly Eastern European Jews (see Chapter 10).

Cancer of the Lung is Largely a Disease of Cigarette Smokers

More than 85% of deaths from lung cancer, the single most common cancer death in both men and women in the United States today, are attributed to cigarette smoking (Fig. 8-3). Cigarette smoke is toxic and carcinogenic to the bronchial mucosa. The particulate tars, and to a lesser

extent, the gas phase of cigarette smoke contain thousands of substances that have been identified as carcinogens, tumor promoters, and ciliotoxic agents.

- **Cancers of the lip, tongue, and buccal mucosa** occur principally (>90%) in tobacco users. All forms of tobacco smoke—cigarette, cigar and pipe smoking—expose the oral cavity to toxic compounds.

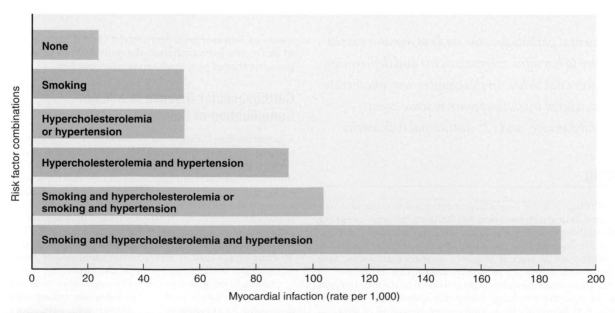

FIGURE 8-2. The risk of myocardial infarction in cigarette smokers. Smoking is an independent risk factor and increases the risk of a myocardial infarction to about the same extent as does hypertension or hypercholesterolemia alone. The effects of smoking are additive to those of these other two risk factors.

- **Cancer of the larynx** is similarly related to cigarette smoking. In some large studies, white male smokers are 6 to 13 times more likely to die from laryngeal cancer as nonsmokers.
- **Cancer of the esophagus** is estimated to result from smoking in 80% of cases in the United States and Great Britain.
- **Cancer of the bladder** is attributable to smoking in 30% to 40% of all cases.
- **Adenocarcinoma of the kidney** is increased 50% to 100% among smokers. A modest increase in cancer of the renal pelvis has also been documented.
- **Cancer of the pancreas** has shown a dramatic increase in incidence, which is, at least in part, related to cigarette smoking. The risk for adenocarcinoma of the pancreas in male smokers is two- to threefold greater than in nonsmokers, and a dose-response relationship exists.
- **Cancer of the uterine cervix** is significantly increased (about 30%) in female smokers.

Smokers are at Higher Risk for Certain Non-Neoplastic Diseases

- **Chronic bronchitis and emphysema** occur primarily in cigarette smokers. The incidence of these diseases is a function of the amount of cigarettes smoked (Fig. 8-4; see Chapter 12).
- **Peptic ulcer disease** is 70% more common in male cigarette smokers than in nonsmokers.
- **Ocular diseases**, particularly macular degeneration and cataracts, are reportedly more frequent in smokers.

Of particular concern to women:

- **Osteoporosis** in women is exacerbated by tobacco use. Women who smoke have a diminution of bone density sufficient to increase the risk of bone fractures.
- **Thyroid diseases** are linked to cigarette smoking. The most conspicuous association is with Graves disease, especially when hyperthyroidism is complicated by exophthalmos.
- **Earlier menopause** is experienced by female smokers, possibly because of the effects of tobacco on estrogen metabolism.

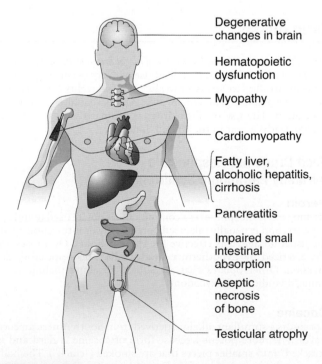

Complications of chronic alcohol abuse.

Degenerative changes in brain

Hematopoietic dysfunction

Myopathy

Cardiomyopathy

Fatty liver, alcoholic hepatitis, cirrhosis

Pancreatitis

Impaired small intestinal absorption

Aseptic necrosis of bone

Testicular atrophy

Fetal Tobacco Syndrome Produces Infants Who are Small for Gestational Age

Maternal cigarette smoking impairs the development of the fetus. These infants are not born preterm but rather are small for gestational age at every stage of pregnancy. In fact, 20% to 40% of the incidence of low birth weight can be attributed to maternal cigarette smoking. Perinatal mortality is higher among offspring of smokers, reaching almost 40% among children of those who smoke more than one pack per day. *Incidences of abruptio placentae, placenta previa, uterine bleeding, and premature rupture of membranes are all increased.* These complications of smoking tend to occur at times when the fetus is not viable or is at great risk, (i.e., from 20 to 32 weeks of gestation). Children born of cigarette-smoking mothers have been reported to be more susceptible to several respiratory diseases, including respiratory infections and otitis media. Substantial evidence indicates that maternal cigarette smoking inflicts lasting harm on children, impairing physical, cognitive, and emotional development.

Environmental Tobacco Smoke May Produce a Variety of Diseases in Nonsmokers

Environmental tobacco smoke representing involuntary exposure to tobacco smoke in the environment is a risk factor for some diseases in nonsmokers, although the relative risks are not great and deserve further study. For example:

- **Lung cancer** is reported to be increased 20% to 30% in nonsmoking spouses of smokers.
- **Respiratory illnesses and hospitalizations** are increased among infants whose parents smoke.
- **Coronary artery disease and sudden cardiac death** are linked to environmental tobacco smoke. The magnitude of the risk is dose dependent and disproportionately increased for the level of smoke exposure as compared to smokers.

Alcoholism

Alcoholism is addiction to ethanol that features dependence and withdrawal symptoms, resulting in acute and chronic toxic effects of alcohol on the body. It is estimated that there are about 15 million alcoholics in the United States (about 5.5% of the population). The proportion has been estimated to be even higher in other countries. Certain ethnic groups, such as Native Americans and Eskimos, have high rates of alcoholism, whereas others, such as Chinese and Jewish individuals, are less afflicted. Although alcoholism is more common in males, the number of female alcoholics has been increasing.

Chronic alcoholism has been defined as the regular intake of sufficient alcohol to injure a person socially, psychologically, or physically. Although there are no firm rules, for most people, daily consumption of more than 45 g alcohol should probably be discouraged, and 100 g or more a day may be dangerous (10 g alcohol = 1 oz, or 30 mL, of 86 proof [43%] spirits).

Acute alcohol intoxication is hardly a benign condition. Approximately 40% of all fatalities from motor vehicle accidents involve alcohol—more than 16,000 deaths in 2004 in the United States. Alcoholism is also a major contributor to fatal home accidents, deaths in fires, and suicides.

Alcohol Ingestion Affects Organs and Tissues

The pathogenesis of ethanol-induced organ damage remains obscure. Acetaldehyde is the highly toxic product of alcohol metabolism. However, circulating levels of acetaldehyde are extremely low, and it is difficult to attribute all of the changes associated with alcoholism solely to this metabolite (Fig. 8-4).

Liver

Alcoholic liver disease, the most common medical complication of alcoholism, has been known for thousands of years and accounts for a large proportion of cases of cirrhosis of the liver in industrialized countries. The nature of the alcoholic beverage is largely irrelevant; consumed in excess, beer, wine, whiskey, hard cider, and so on all produce cirrhosis. Only the total dose of alcohol itself is relevant (see Chapter 14).

Pancreas

Both acute and chronic pancreatitis are complications of alcoholism (see Chapter 15). *Chronic calcifying pancreatitis is an unquestioned result of alcoholism and an important cause of incapacitating pain, pancreatic insufficiency, and pancreatic stones.*

Heart

"Beer-drinker's heart" is a form of dilated cardiomyopathy, termed **alcoholic cardiomyopathy**, which leads to low-output congestive heart failure (see Chapter 11). Alcoholics' hearts seem also to be more susceptible to arrhythmias, and many cases of sudden death in alcoholics are probably caused by sudden, fatal arrhythmias. Ironically, moderate alcohol consumption, or "social drinking" (one to two drinks a day), provides significant protection against coronary artery disease (atherosclerosis) and its consequence, myocardial infarction. Similarly, compared with abstainers, social drinkers have a lower incidence of ischemic stroke.

Skeletal Muscle

Muscle weakness, particularly of the proximal muscles, is common in alcoholics. A wide range of changes in skeletal muscle occurs in chronic alcoholics, varying from mild weakness to severe, debilitating chronic myopathy, with degeneration of muscle fibers and diffuse fibrosis. **Acute alcoholic rhabdomyolysis** (necrosis of muscle fibers and release of myoglobin into the circulation) rarely occurs. This sudden event can be fatal because of renal failure secondary to myoglobinuria.

Endocrine System

Feminization of male alcoholics, plus loss of libido and potency, is common. Breasts become enlarged (gynecomastia), body hair is lost, and a female distribution of pubic hair (female escutcheon) develops. Some of these changes can be attributed to impaired estrogen metabolism due to chronic liver disease, but many of the changes—particularly atrophy of the testes—occur even its absence. This may result from lower levels of circulating testosterone because of interference with the pituitary–gonadal axis, possibly complicated by accelerated hepatic metabolism of the hormone. Alcohol also has a direct toxic effect on the testes.

Gastrointestinal Tract

Alcohol is directly toxic to the mucosa of the esophagus and stomach. Such injury is potentiated by hypersecretion of gastric hydrochloric acid stimulated by ethanol. **Reflux esophagitis** may be particularly painful, and peptic ulcers are also more common in alcoholics. Violent retching may lead to tears at the esophageal-gastric junction (**Mallory-Weiss syndrome**), sometimes severe enough to cause exsanguinating hemorrhage.

Blood

Megaloblastic anemia is common in alcoholics and reflects a combination of dietary deficiency of folic acid and the fact that alcohol is a weak folic acid antagonist in humans. Moreover, folate absorption by the small intestine may be decreased in alcoholics. Acute transient **thrombocytopenia** is common after acute alcohol intoxication and may result in bleeding. Alcohol also interferes with platelet aggregation, thereby contributing to bleeding.

Bone

Chronic alcoholics, particularly postmenopausal women, are at increased risk for **osteoporosis**, although the precise mechanism responsible for accelerated bone loss is not understood. Interestingly, moderate alcohol intake seems to exert a protective effect against osteoporosis.

Nervous System

General cortical atrophy of the brain is common in alcoholics and may reflect a toxic effect of alcohol (see Chapter 28). By contrast, most of the characteristic brain diseases in alcoholics are probably a result of nutritional deficiency.

- **Wernicke encephalopathy** is caused by thiamine deficiency and is characterized by mental confusion, ataxia, abnormal ocular motility, and polyneuropathy, reflecting pathologic changes in the diencephalon and brainstem.
- **Korsakoff psychosis** is characterized by retrograde amnesia and confabulatory symptoms. It was once believed to be pathognomonic of chronic alcoholism, but it has also been seen in several organic mental syndromes and is considered nonspecific.
- **Alcoholic cerebellar degeneration** is differentiated from other acquired or familial cerebellar degeneration by the uniformity of its manifestations. Progressive unsteadiness of gait, ataxia, incoordination, and reduced deep tendon reflex activity are present.
- **Central pontine myelinolysis** is another characteristic change in the brain of alcoholics, apparently caused by electrolyte imbalance. In this complication, a progressive weakness of bulbar muscles terminates in respiratory paralysis.
- **Polyneuropathy** is common in chronic alcoholics. It is usually associated with deficiencies of thiamine and other B vitamins, but a direct neurotoxic effect of ethanol may play a role. The most common complaints include numbness, paresthesias, pain, weakness, and ataxia.

Fetal Alcohol Syndrome Results from Alcohol Abuse in Pregnancy

Infants born to mothers who consume excess alcohol during pregnancy may show a cluster of abnormalities that together constitute the fetal alcohol syndrome. This disorder is discussed in detail in Chapter 6.

Drug Abuse

Drug abuse has been defined as the use of illegal drugs or the inappropriate use of legal drugs. The repeated illicit use of drugs occurs to produce pleasure, to alleviate stress, or to alter or avoid reality (or all three). Hence, drug abuse generally involves agents that alter mood and perception. The use of illicit drugs is estimated to cause about 17,000 deaths a year in the United States.

Illicit Drugs are Responsible for Many Pathologic Syndromes

Heroin

Heroin (acetyl morphine) is a common illicit opiate used to induce euphoria and is usually taken subcutaneously or intravenously. In the usual dosage, it is effective for about 5 hours. Overdoses are characterized by hypothermia, bradycardia, and respiratory depression. Other opiates that are subject to abuse include morphine, dilaudid, and oxycodone.

Cocaine

Cocaine is a stimulant alkaloid derived from South American coca leaves. The more potent freebase form of cocaine is hard and is "cracked" into smaller pieces that are smoked ("crack"). The half-life of cocaine in the blood is about 1 hour. Cocaine users report extreme euphoria and heightened sensitivity to a variety of stimuli. However, with addiction, paranoid states and conspicuous emotional lability occur. Cocaine's mechanism of action is related to its interference with the reuptake of the neurotransmitter dopamine, thereby increasing the synaptic concentration.

Cocaine overdose leads to anxiety and delirium and occasionally to seizures. Cardiac arrhythmias and other effects on the heart may cause sudden death in otherwise apparently healthy individuals. Chronic abuse of cocaine is associated with the occasional development of a characteristic dilated cardiomyopathy, which may be fatal. "Snorted" cocaine produces destructive midline lesions in the nasal passage and septal perforation.

Amphetamines

Amphetamines, mainly methamphetamine, are sympathomimetic and resemble cocaine in their effects, although they have a longer duration of action. The most serious complications of amphetamine abuse are seizures, cardiac arrhythmias, and hyperthermia. Amphetamine use has been reported to lead to vasculitis of the brain, and both subarachnoid and intracerebral hemorrhages have been described.

Hallucinogens

Hallucinogens are a group of chemically unrelated drugs that alter perception and sensory experience.

Phencyclidine (PCP) is an anesthetic agent that has psychedelic or hallucinogenic effects. As a recreational drug, it is known as "angel dust" and is taken orally, intranasally, or by smoking. The anesthetic properties of PCP lead to a diminished capacity to perceive pain and, therefore, to self-injury and trauma. Other than the behavioral effects, PCP commonly produces tachycardia and hypertension. High doses result in deep coma, seizures, and even decerebrate posturing.

Lysergic acid diethylamide (LSD) is a hallucinogenic drug. Its popularity peaked in the late 1960s, and it is little used today. LSD causes perceptual distortion of the senses, interference with logical thought, alteration of time perception, and a sense of depersonalization. "Bad trips" are characterized by anxiety and panic and objectively by sympathomimetic effects that include tachycardia, hypertension, and hyperthermia. Large overdoses cause coma, convulsions, and respiratory arrest.

Marijuana is the most commonly used illicit drug. Its effect is mediated by the active agent delta-9-tetrahydrocannabinol. It binds to brain cannabinoid receptors and produces perceptual changes, loss of coordination, and other psychotropic effects. Chronic use is associated with a variety of pulmonary problems similar to those seen in cigarette users, which are most likely related to smoke-derived tars. Effects on learning and social behavior are also common with prolonged use.

Organic Solvents

The recreational inhalation of organic solvents is widespread, particularly among adolescents. Various commercial preparations such as fingernail polish, glues, plastic cements, and lighter fluid are all sniffed. Among the active ingredients are benzene, carbon tetrachloride, acetone, xylene, and toluene. These compounds are all central nervous system (CNS) depressants, although early effects (e.g., with xylene) may be excitatory. Acute intoxication with organic solvents resembles inebriation with alcohol. Large doses produce nausea and vomiting, hallucinations, and eventually coma. Respiratory depression and death may follow. Chronic exposure to, or abuse of, organic solvents may result in damage to the brain, kidneys, liver, lungs, and hematopoietic system.

Intravenous Drug Abuse Has Many Medical Complications

Apart from reactions related to pharmacologic or physiological effects of the abused substance, the most common complications (15% of directly drug-related deaths) are caused by introducing infectious organisms by a parenteral route. Most occur at the site of

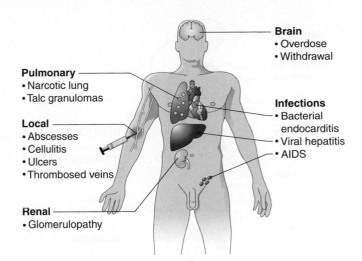

FIGURE 8-5. Complications of intravenous drug abuse. AIDS, acquired immunodeficiency syndrome.

injection, including cutaneous abscesses, cellulitis, and ulcers (Fig. 8-5). Intravenous introduction of bacteria may lead to septic complications in internal organs, such as bacterial endocarditis. Intravenous drug abusers are at very high risk for AIDS, as well as hepatitis B and C and their many complications.

Oral Contraceptives

Orally administered hormonal contraceptives (OCs) are now the most commonly used method of birth control in industrialized countries. Current formulations are combinations of synthetic estrogens and steroids with progesterone-like activity. They act either by inhibiting the gonadotropin surge at midcycle, thereby preventing ovulation, or by preventing implantation by altering the phase of the endometrium. Data available to date include studies focusing on second- and third-generation OCs, which contain lower doses of both estrogens and progestogens than did earlier oral contraceptives. Most complications of oral contraceptives involve either the vasculature or reproductive organs (Fig. 8-6).

- **Deep vein thrombosis** and the potential for thromboembolism has an increased risk of three to four times, even in users of "third-generation" OCs. The risk is much higher in women who also have thrombophilia (see Chapter 20).
- **Myocardial infarctions and ischemic stroke do not** appear to be at increased risk in otherwise normal users of modern formulations of OCs in most studies. It must be emphasized that smoking, hypertension, and other risk factors for arterial thrombosis act synergistically with OC use to elevate the risk (see above).
- **Tumors of several of the female reproductive organs** and possibly colon cancer are **reduced** in risk in OC users. **Benign liver adenomas** are rare hepatic neoplasms that are significantly increased in incidence among women who use OCs.
- **Breast cancer** risk with OC use remains controversial. A small increase in relative risk (to 1.24) has been reported, although other studies report no increase in risk.

In considering the potential side effects of the use of OCs, it is important to recognize that certain benefits accrue. In addition to a significant reduction in the risk of ovarian and endometrial cancers, the use of these agents decreases the risk of pelvic inflammatory disease, uterine leiomyomas, endometriosis, and fibrocystic disease of the breast, and substantially reduces the severity of acne.

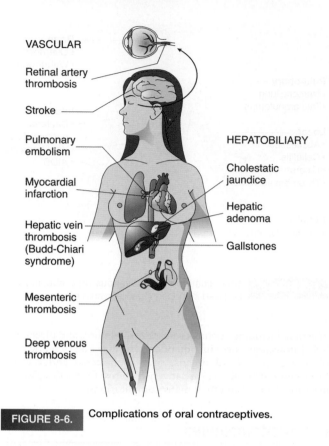

VASCULAR

Retinal artery
thrombosis

Stroke

Pulmonary
embolism

HEPATOBILIARY

Myocardial
infarction

Cholestatic
jaundice

Hepatic
adenoma

Hepatic vein
thrombosis
(Budd-Chiari
syndrome)

Gallstones

Mesenteric
thrombosis

Deep venous
thrombosis

FIGURE 8-6.   Complications of oral contraceptives.

Postmenopausal Hormone Replacement Therapy Increases the Risk of Some Cancers

Hormone replacement preparations containing either estrogen or estrogen plus progestin are given to postmenopausal women in an effort to alleviate menopausal symptoms and decrease the risk of myocardial infarction and osteoporosis. These agents have proved effective in the treatment of postmenopausal symptoms. However, recent studies have cast doubt on their effectiveness in preventing myocardial infarction and osteoporosis.

Women who take these preparations have an increased risk for cancers of the breast and endometrium. Hormone replacement regimens involving estrogens with or without added progestins increase the risk of both cancers. However, an increased breast cancer incidence is somewhat greater for hormone replacements that contain both progestin and estrogen, compared to estrogen only but is significant for both types of formulation.

Environmental Chemicals

Humans are surrounded by chemicals that are added to, or appear as contaminants in, foods, water, and air. Several important mechanisms govern the effect of toxic agents, including the toxin's absorption, distribution, metabolism, and excretion. Among the most important chemical hazards to which humans are exposed are environmental dusts and carcinogens. Inhalation of mineral and organic dusts occurs primarily in occupational settings (e.g., mining, industrial manufacturing, farming) and occasionally as a result of unusual situations (e.g., bird fanciers). Inhaling mineral dusts leads to pulmonary diseases known as pneumoconioses, whereas organic dusts may produce hypersensitivity pneumonitis. Pneumoconioses were formerly common, but control of dust exposure in the workplace by modifying manufacturing techniques, improvements in air handling, and the use of masks has substantially reduced the incidence of these diseases. Because of their im-

portance, pneumoconioses and hypersensitivity pneumonitis are discussed in detail in Chapter 12.

Chemical carcinogens are ubiquitous in the environment, and their potential for causing disease has elicited widespread concern. In particular, exposure to carcinogens in the workplace has been associated epidemiologically with a number of cancers (Table 8-1), which are reviewed in Chapter 5.

Toxic Effects Differ from Hypersensitivity Responses

Many substances elicit disease in a variety of animal species in a dose-dependent manner, with a regular time delay and a predictable target organ response. Furthermore, the morphologic changes in injured tissues are constant and reproducible. By contrast, other agents show great variability in their ability to produce disease—irregular lag times before injury are apparent, no dose dependency, and lack of reproducibility. Generally, predictable dose-response reactions reflect direct actions of a compound or its metabolite on a tissue (i.e., a "toxic" effect). The second, unpredictable type of reaction is believed to reflect "hypersensitivity," probably an immunologic response or idiosyncratic side effect. Scorecard.org (http://www.scorecard.org/chemical-profiles/index.tcl) provides a helpful summary of uses and toxicity of more than 10,000 industrial chemicals.

Volatile Organic Solvents and Vapors

Volatile organic solvents and vapors are widely used in industry in many capacities. With few exceptions, exposures to these compounds are industrial or accidental and represent short-term dangers rather than long-term toxicity. For the most part, exposure to solvents is by inhalation rather than by ingestion, although exceptions occur.

- **Chloroform ($CHCl_3$) and carbon tetrachloride (CCl_4):** These solvents exert anesthetic (depressant) effects on the CNS and on the heart and blood vessels but are better known as hepatotoxins. Large doses lead to acute hepatic necrosis, fatty liver, and liver failure.
- **Trichloroethylene (C_2HCl_3):** A ubiquitous industrial solvent, trichloroethylene in high concentrations depresses the CNS,

TABLE 8–1	
Cancers Associated with Exposure to Occupational Carcinogens	
Agent or Occupation	**Site of Cancer**
Arsenic	Lung cancer
Asbestos	Mesothelioma (pleura and peritoneum) Lung cancer (in smokers)
Aromatic amines	Bladder cancer
Benzene	Leukemia, multiple myeloma
bis-(chloromethyl)ether	Lung cancer
Chromium	Lung cancer
Furniture and shoe manufacturing	Nasal carcinoma
Hematite mining	Lung cancer
Nickel	Lung cancer, paranasal sinus cancer
Tars and oils	Cancers of lung, gastrointestinal tract, bladder, and skin
Vinyl chloride	Angiosarcoma of liver

but hepatotoxicity is minimal. It is listed as a possible carcinogen by several groups but more study is needed.

- **Methanol (CH₃OH):** Because methanol, unlike ethanol, is not taxed, it is used by some impoverished alcoholics as a substitute for ethanol. It produces inebriation similar to that produced by ethanol but is succeeded by gastrointestinal symptoms, visual dysfunction, seizures, coma, and death. The major toxicity of methanol is believed to arise from its metabolism, first to formaldehyde and then to formic acid. Metabolic acidosis is common after methanol ingestion. The most characteristic lesion of methanol toxicity is necrosis of retinal ganglion cells and subsequent degeneration of the optic nerve. Severe poisoning may lead to lesions in the putamen and globus pallidus.
- **Ethylene glycol (HOCH₂CH₂OH):** Because of its low vapor pressure, the toxicity of ethylene glycol chiefly results from ingestion. It is commonly used in antifreeze, and has been drunk by chronic alcoholics as a substitute for ethanol for many years. Accidental ingestion by children and animals occurs because of its sweet taste, although the product is now deliberately made bitter by additives. The toxicity of ethylene glycol is chiefly due to its metabolites, particularly oxalic acid, and occurs within minutes of ingestion. Metabolic acidosis, CNS depression, nausea and vomiting, and hypocalcemia-related cardiotoxicity are seen. Oxalate crystals in the tubules and oxaluria are often noted and may cause renal failure.
- **Gasoline and kerosene:** These fuels are mixtures of aliphatic hydrocarbons and branched, unsaturated, and aromatic hydrocarbons. Chronic exposure is by inhalation. Despite prolonged exposure to gasoline by gas station attendants and auto mechanics, there is no evidence that inhalation of gasoline over the long term is particularly injurious.
- **Benzene (C₆H₆):** The prototypic aromatic hydrocarbon is benzene, which must be distinguished from benzine, a mixture of aliphatic hydrocarbons. Benzene is one of the most widely used chemicals in industrial processes, as it is a starting point for innumerable syntheses and a solvent. It is also a constituent of fuels, accounting for as much as 3% of gasoline. Virtually all cases of acute and chronic benzene toxicity have occurred as industrial exposures. Acute benzene poisoning primarily affects the CNS, and death results from respiratory failure. However, with chronic exposure, the bone marrow is the principal target. Patients who develop hematologic abnormalities characteristically exhibit **hypoplasia or aplasia of the bone marrow and pancytopenia**. With higher exposure, aplastic anemia and subsequent development of acute myeloid leukemia are significant consequences (see Chapter 20). Overall, the risk of leukemia is increased 60-fold in workers exposed to the highest atmospheric concentrations of benzene. The closely related compound toluene is occasionally abused as an inhalent. Although it has not been incriminated as a cause of hematologic abnormalities, it is suspected to produce developmental abnormalities.

Agricultural Chemicals

Pesticides, fungicides, herbicides, fumigants, and organic fertilizers are central to the success of modern agriculture. However, many of these chemicals persist in soil and water and may pose potential long-term hazards. Acute exposure to industrial concentrations or inadvertently contaminated food can cause severe acute illness. Children are particularly susceptible and may ingest home gardening preparations.

Symptoms of acute toxicity are often related to the toxin's mode of action. For example, organophosphate insecticides are acetylcholinesterase inhibitors that are readily absorbed through the skin. Thus, acute toxicity in humans mainly involves neuromuscular disorders, such as visual disturbances, dyspnea, mucous hypersecretion, and bronchoconstriction. Death may come from respiratory failure. Each year, in the United States, 30 to 40 people die of acute pesticide poisoning. Long-term exposure produces symptoms similar to acute exposure. Organochlorine pesticides,

such as DDT (dichlorodiphenyltrichloroethane), chlordane, and others, have caused concern because they accumulate in soils and in human tissues, break down very slowly, and have harmful environmental effects. High levels of any such pesticide can be harmful to humans in acute exposures, but the side effects of chronic contact with the materials and their buildup are of greatest interest. Many of these compounds function as weak estrogens, but no harmful effects related to this activity have been documented. There is equivocal evidence suggesting DDT may be a carcinogen. Some compounds, such as aldrin and dieldrin, have been associated with tumor development, but the toxicity of most organochlorine insecticides relates to effects on the CNS.

Human exposure to herbicides is not infrequent. Among the best known of these is the highly toxic agent paraquat. Occupational paraquat exposure is usually via the skin, although toxicity from ingestion and inhalation are documented. The compound is very corrosive and causes burns or ulcers on whatever it contacts. It is transported actively to the lung, where it can damage the pulmonary epithelium, causing edema and even respiratory failure. Pulmonary fibrosis may ultimately lead to death. Pulmonary toxicity is likely related to redox cycling and peroxidation.

Aromatic Halogenated Hydrocarbons

The halogenated aromatic hydrocarbons that have received considerable attention include (1) the polychlorinated biphenyls (PCBs); (2) chlorophenols (pentachlorophenol, used as a wood preservative); (3) hexachlorophene, used as an antibacterial agent in soaps; and (4) the dioxin TCDD (2,3,7,8-tetrachlorodibenzo-p-dioxin), a byproduct of the synthesis of herbicides and hexachlorophene and, therefore, a potential contaminant of these preparations. Chronic exposure to TCDD does not appear to produce demonstrable toxicity. Serious questions have been raised regarding the danger of long-term exposure to dioxin, particularly its carcinogenic potential. The compound is, however, classified as carcinogenic to humans by the WHO. The problem of the presence of PCBs in the environment resembles that of agricultural chemicals: long-term animal toxicity is well documented, but there are no significant increases in the incidence of cancer or other diseases in workers exposed to PCBs. The same situation pertains to hexachlorophene and pentachlorophenol.

Air Pollutants

A precise definition of air pollution is elusive, because the meaning of "pure air" is not established. However, for the purposes of this discussion, the most important pollutants are those generated by the combustion of fossil fuels, industrial and agricultural processes, and so forth. The most important air pollutants that are implicated as factors in human disease are the irritants sulfur dioxide (SO₂), oxides of nitrogen, carbon monoxide (CO), and ozone, as well as suspended particulates and acid aerosols. All of the gaseous pollutants are capable of causing toxicity with either acute or high-dose chronic experimental exposure. For example, **CO** is a colorless, odorless gas that has a very high affinity for hemoglobin. It may be deadly when produced by indoor combustion (see below). The effects of chronic environmental exposure via smog remain unclear. Exposure to atmospheric ozone is reported to lead to deterioration in pulmonary function and may be associated with a slight but significant increase in mortality.

Most studies of the effects of air pollution on health have focused on particulates. Many large short-term and long-term epidemiologic studies have shown that particulate air pollution is associated with increased mortality, both overall and from cardiovascular disease and cancer. Shorter-term studies suggested significant increases in acute myocardial infarction as a consequence of exposure to higher levels of fine particulates. It has been proposed that residence within 100 meters of a freeway greatly increases the likelihood of cardiovascular death. Furthermore, experimental studies have demonstrated that particulate exposure may increase atherosclerosis, blood pressure, heart rate, coagulability, and levels of inflammatory mediators. There is experimental evidence to support a suggestion that inflammation and oxidative stress are responsible for at least part of the harmful effects of pollutants. Thus, the frequency of exacerbations of asthma is related to levels of fine particulates, especially derived from diesel exhaust and ozone in the air.

Carbon Monoxide

CO is an odorless and nonirritating gas that results from the incomplete combustion of organic substances. It combines with hemoglobin with an affinity 240 times greater than that of oxygen to form carboxyhemoglobin. CO binding to hemoglobin also increases the affinity of the remaining heme moieties for oxygen, inhibiting its dissociation into tissues. As a consequence, the hypoxia that results from CO poisoning is far greater than can be attributed to loss of oxygen-carrying capacity alone.

Atmospheric CO is derived principally from automobile exhaust and does not pose a health problem. Carboxyhemoglobin concentrations under 10% are found in some smokers and may accelerate the onset of exertional angina and cause changes in electrocardiograms in smokers with ischemic heart disease. Indoor combustion, particularly from space heaters, however, can generate much higher concentrations of CO, which can be hazardous. Concentrations up to 30% usually cause only headache and mild exertional dyspnea. Higher levels of carboxyhemoglobin lead to confusion and lethargy. Above 50%, coma and convulsions ensue. Levels greater than 60% are usually fatal. In fatal CO poisoning, a characteristic cherry-red color is imparted to the skin by the carboxyhemoglobin in the superficial capillaries. Recovery from severe CO poisoning may be associated with brain damage, which may be manifested as subtle intellectual deficits, memory loss, or extrapyramidal symptoms (e.g., parkinsonism). Treatment of acute CO poisoning, as in those who attempt suicide or are trapped in fires, consists principally of administering 100% oxygen.

Metals

Metals are an important group of environmental chemicals that have caused disease in humans from ancient times to the present.

Lead

Lead is a ubiquitous heavy metal that is common in the environment of industrialized countries. Before widespread awareness of chronic exposure to lead in the 1950s and 1960s, the classic symptoms of lead poisoning were commonly encountered in children and adults. In the United States, lead poisoning was primarily a pediatric problem related to pica—the habit of chewing on cribs, toys, furniture, and woodwork—and eating painted plaster and fallen paint flakes. To these sources of lead was added a heavy burden of atmospheric lead in the form of dust derived from the combustion of lead-containing gasoline. Children and adults living near point sources of environmental lead contamination, such as smelters, were exposed to even higher levels of lead.

In adults, occupational exposure to lead occurred primarily among those engaged in lead smelting and in the production and recycling of automobile batteries. Accidental poisonings occasionally occur from the use of pottery with lead-based glaze, renovation of old residences heavily coated with lead paint, and recently in children who play with inexpensive novelty jewelry and other items manufactured from lead.

METABOLISM: Lead is absorbed through the lungs or, less often, the gastrointestinal tract. It crosses the blood-brain barrier readily and concentrations in the brain, liver, kidneys, and bone marrow are directly related to its toxic effects. Lead binds sulfhydryl groups and interferes with the activities of zinc-dependent enzymes and with enzymes involved in synthesis of steroids and cell membranes.

TOXICITY: Classic lead overexposure, which is rarely seen in the United States today, affects many organs, but its major toxicity involves dysfunction in (1) the nervous system, (2) the kidneys, and (3) hematopoiesis (Fig. 8-7). *The brain is the target of lead toxicity in children; adults usually present with manifestation of peripheral neuropathy.* Children with lead encephalopathy (lead levels of 120 mg/mL) are typically irritable and ataxic. They may convulse or display altered states of consciousness, from drowsiness to frank coma. Children with lower blood lead levels exhibit mild CNS symptoms, such as clumsiness, irritability, and hyperactivity.

Lead encephalopathy is a condition in which the brain is edematous and displays flattened gyri and compressed ventricles. There may be herniation of the uncus and cerebellar tonsils. Microscopically, congestion, petechial hemorrhages, and foci of

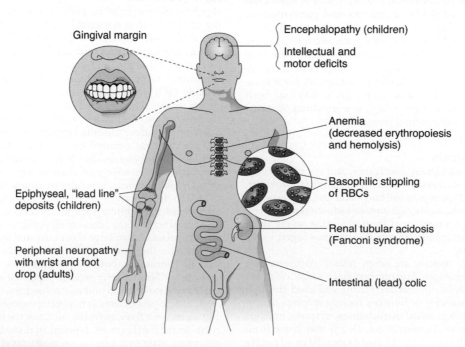

FIGURE 8-7.   Complications of lead intoxication. RBCs, red blood cells.

neuronal necrosis are seen. A diffuse astrocytic proliferation in both the gray and white matter may accompany these changes. Vascular lesions in the brain are particularly prominent, with capillary dilation and proliferation.

Peripheral motor neuropathy is the most common manifestation of lead neurotoxicity in the adult, typically affecting the radial and peroneal nerves and resulting in **wristdrop** and **footdrop**, respectively. Lead-induced neuropathy is probably also the basis of the paroxysms of gastrointestinal pain known as lead colic.

Anemia is a cardinal sign of lead intoxication. Lead disrupts heme synthesis in bone marrow erythroblasts and is expressed as a microcytic and hypochromic anemia resembling that seen in iron deficiency. The anemia of lead intoxication is also characterized by prominent basophilic stippling of erythrocytes, related to clustering of ribosomes. Erythrocyte life span is decreased; thus, the anemia of lead intoxication is due to both ineffective hematopoiesis and accelerated erythrocyte turnover.

Lead nephropathy reflects the toxic effect of the metal on the proximal tubular cells of the kidney. The resulting dysfunction is characterized by aminoaciduria, glycosuria, and hyperphosphaturia (Fanconi syndrome).

Lead poisoning is treated with chelating agents such as calcium ethylene diamine tetra-acetic acid (EDTA), either alone or in combination with dimercaprol (BAL). Both the hematologic and renal manifestations of lead intoxication are usually reversible, but alterations in the CNS are generally irreversible.

EFFECTS OF CHRONIC EXPOSURE TO LOW LEAD LEVELS: Due to the removal of lead from gasoline, improvements in housing and paint reformulation, ambient levels of lead have fallen significantly: blood levels in the general population of the United States have decreased dramatically, resulting in the near elimination of lead-related childhood fatalities and encephalopathy. However, low lead exposure in children, although not producing recognizable symptoms, may permanently decrease cognitive performance. The regulatory safe threshold for blood levels of lead in children has been progressively reduced and is now thought to be below 10 μg/dL. High blood lead concentrations remain a problem among poor, mainly urban children, and more vigorous campaigns to address this situation are justified.

Mercury

Inorganic mercury has been used since prehistoric times and has been known to be an occupation-related hazard, at least since the Middle Ages. Although mercury poisoning still occurs in some occupations, there has been increasing concern over the potential health hazards brought about by the contamination of many ecosystems following several well-known outbreaks of methylmercury poisoning. Mercury released into the environment may be bioconcentrated and enter the food chain. Bacteria in bays and oceans can convert inorganic mercury compounds from industrial wastes into highly neurotoxic organomercurials. These compounds are then transferred up the food chain and are eventually concentrated in the large predatory fish (e.g., tuna, pike), which make up a substantial part of the diet in many countries.

Although inorganic mercury is not efficiently absorbed in the gastrointestinal tract, organic mercurial compounds are readily absorbed because of their lipid solubility. Both inorganic and organic mercury are preferentially concentrated in the kidney, and methylmercury also distributes to the brain. *The kidney is the principal target of the toxicity of inorganic mercury, but the brain is damaged by organic mercurials.*

NEPHROTOXICITY: At one time, mercuric chloride was widely used as an antiseptic, and acute mercuric chloride poisoning was much more common. Today, most cases are industrial accidents. Under such circumstances, **proximal tubular necrosis** is accompanied by oliguric renal failure. Proteinuria is common in chronic mercurial nephrotoxicity, and there may be a nephrotic syndrome with more severe intoxication. Pathologically, there is a membranous glomerulonephritis with subepithelial electron-dense deposits, suggesting immune complex deposition.

NEUROTOXICITY: The neurologic effects of mercury are manifested as a constriction of visual fields, paresthesias, ataxia, dysarthria, and hearing loss. Pathologically, there is cerebral and cerebellar atrophy. Microscopically, the cerebellum exhibits atrophy of the granular layer, without loss of Purkinje cells and spongy softening in the visual cortex and other cortical regions.

Arsenic

The toxic properties of arsenic have been known for centuries. Arsenic-containing compounds have been widely used as insecticides, weed killers, wood preservatives, and pigments. Arsenicals may also contaminate soil and leach into ground water as a result of naturally occurring arsenic-rich rock formations or from soil contaminants. As with mercury, there is evidence for the bioaccumulation of arsenic along the food chain.

Acute arsenic poisoning is almost always the result of accidental or homicidal ingestion. Death is due to **CNS toxicity**. Chronic arsenic intoxication affects many organ systems. It is characterized initially by such nonspecific symptoms as malaise and fatigue, followed by gastrointestinal, cardiovascular, and hematologic dysfunction. Both encephalopathy and peripheral neuropathy develop. The latter is characterized by paresthesias, motor palsies, and painful neuritis. On epidemiological grounds, **cancers of the skin, respiratory tract, and gastrointestinal tract** have been attributed to industrial and agricultural exposure to arsenic. In some parts of the world, notably areas of Bangladesh that use deep tube wells as a water source, chronic exposure of workers in rice paddies to arsenic in the ground water has been associated with keratotic skin disorders and cancer.

Nickel

Nickel is a widely used metal in electronics, coins, steel alloys, batteries, and food processing. Dermatitis ("nickel itch"), the most frequent effect of exposure to nickel, may occur from direct contact with metals containing nickel, such as coins and costume jewelry. The dermatitis is a sensitization reaction; the body reacts to nickel-conjugated proteins formed following the penetration of the epidermis by nickel ions. Exposure to nickel, as to arsenic, increases the risk of development of specific cancer types. Epidemiologic studies have demonstrated that workers who were occupationally exposed to nickel compounds have an increased incidence of lung cancer and cancer of the nasal cavities.

Thermal Regulatory Dysfunction

Hypothermia is a Decrease in Body Temperature Below 35°C (95°F)

Hypothermia can result in systemic or focal injury. In localized hypothermia, actual tissue freezing does not occur. **Frostbite**, by contrast, involves the crystallization of tissue water.

Generalized Hypothermia

Acute immersion in water at 4°C to 10°C (39.2° to 50°F) reduces central blood flow. Coupled with decreased core body temperature and cooling of the blood perfusing the brain, this results in mental confusion. Tetany makes swimming impossible. Increased vagal discharge leads to premature ventricular contractions, ventricular arrhythmias, and even fibrillation. Within 30 minutes, heat loss exceeds heat production, and core temperature then begins to fall. Below 35°C, respiratory rate, heart rate, and blood pressure decline. If hypothermia is prolonged, decreased body temperature alters cerebrovascular function. When body core temperature reaches

32°C (89.6°F), the person becomes lethargic, apathetic, and withdrawn. When it falls below 28°C (82.4°F), pulse and breathing weaken and coma supervenes. The most important factor in causing death is a cardiac arrhythmia or sudden cardiac arrest. These observations have been confirmed and extended, largely due to the indication of hypothermia in some patients undergoing open heart surgery. In fact, with careful pharmacologic control, prolonged periods of lower body temperature can be achieved with no residual harm.

Focal Hypothermia

Local reduction in tissue temperature, particularly in the skin, is associated with local vasoconstriction. Tissue water crystallizes if blood circulation is insufficient to counter persistent thermal loss. When freezing occurs slowly, ice crystals form within tissue cells and in the interstitial space. Denaturation of macromolecules and physical disruption of cellular membranes by the ice ensue.

The most biologically significant cell injury appears in the endothelial lining of the capillaries and venules, which alters small-vessel permeability. This injury initiates extravasation of plasma, formation of localized edema and blisters, and an inflammatory reaction. **Immersion foot** (trench foot) is caused by a prolonged reduction in tissue temperature to a point not low enough to freeze tissue. This cooling causes cellular disruption, and endothelial cell damage leads to local thrombosis and changes caused by altered permeability. Vascular occlusion often produces gangrene.

Hyperthermia Means an Increase in Body Temperature

Tissue responses to hyperthermia are similar in some respects to those caused by freezing injuries. In both instances, injury to the vascular endothelium results in altered vascular permeability, edema, and blisters. The degree of injury depends on the extent of temperature elevation and how quickly it is reached. Small increases in body temperature increase the metabolic rate. However, above a certain limit, enzymes denature, other proteins precipitate, and "melting" of lipid bilayers of cell membranes takes place.

Systemic Hyperthermia

Fever is an elevation of body core temperature resulting from a change in the thermoregulatory center. It occurs because of (1) increased heat production, (2) decreased elimination of heat from the body (when reflecting an aberrant response of the thermal regulatory center), or (3) a disturbance of the thermal regulatory center itself. In a strict sense, **systemic hyperthermia** is an elevation of core temperature above the thermal set point, as a result of insufficient dissipation of heat. A body temperature above 42.5°C (108.5°F) leads to profound functional disturbances, including general vasodilation, inefficient cardiac function, altered respiration, and ultimately, death. Few, if any, defined pathologic changes are associated with fever alone.

Malignant hyperthermia is a thermal alteration, accompanied by a hypermetabolic state and often by rhabdomyolysis (muscle necrosis), which occurs after gaseous anesthesia in susceptible individuals. This autosomal dominant disorder is associated with mutations in the gene for the sarcoplasmic reticulum ryanodine receptor.

Heat stroke is a form of hyperthermia that occurs under conditions of very high ambient temperatures and is not mediated by endogenous pyrogens. It reflects impaired thermal regulatory cooling responses and characteristically occurs in infants, young children, and the very aged. The disorder is often associated with an underlying chronic illness and the use of diuretics, tranquilizers that may affect the hypothalamic thermal regulatory center, or drugs that inhibit perspiration. Another form of heatstroke is seen in healthy men during unusually vigorous exercise. Lactic acidosis, hypocalcemia, and rhabdomyolysis may be severe problems, and almost one third of patients with exertional heatstroke develop myoglobinuric acute renal failure. Heatstroke is not amenable to treatment with standard antipyretics, and only external cooling and fluid and electrolyte replacement are effective therapy.

Local Hyperthermia: Burns

Cutaneous burns are the most common form of localized hyperthermia. Both the degree and rate of temperature elevation determine the tissue response. A temperature of 50°C (120°F) may be sustained for 10 minutes or more without cell death, whereas a temperature of 70°C (158°F) or higher for even several seconds causes necrosis of the entire epidermis. Cutaneous burns have been separated into three categories of severity: first-, second-, and third-degree burns (Fig. 8-8).

- **First-degree burns**, such as mild sunburn, are recognized by congestion and pain but are not associated with necrosis. Mild endothelial injury produces vasodilation, increased vascular permeability, and slight edema.
- **Second-degree burns** cause epidermal necrosis but spare the dermis. Clinically, these burns are recognized by blisters, in which the epithelium separates from the dermis.
- **Third-degree burns** char both epidermis and dermis. Histologically, tissue is carbonized and cellular structure is lost.

Among the most important functions of the skin are fluid retention and protection from infectious agents. Not surprisingly, one of the most serious systemic disturbances caused by extensive cutaneous burns is fluid loss. Many severely burned persons, particularly those with more than 70% of their body surface involved

FIRST DEGREE

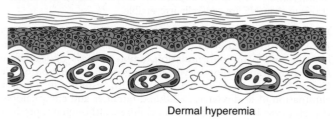

Dermal hyperemia

SECOND DEGREE

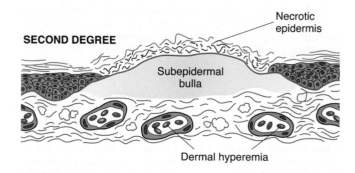

Necrotic epidermis

Subepidermal bulla

Dermal hyperemia

THIRD DEGREE

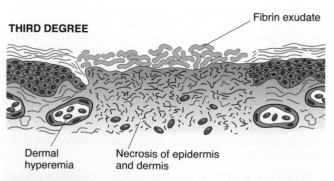

Fibrin exudate

Dermal hyperemia

Necrosis of epidermis and dermis

FIGURE 8-8. **The pathology of cutaneous burns.** A first-degree skin burn exhibits only dilation of the dermal blood vessels. In a second-degree burn, there is necrosis of the epidermis, and subepidermal edema collects under the necrotic epidermis to form a bulla. In a third-degree burn, both the epidermis and dermis are necrotic.

with third-degree burns, develop shock as well as acute tubular necrosis of the kidneys, and mortality is very high. Severely burned patients who survive longer are at great risk of lethal surface infections and sepsis. Even normal skin saprophytes may cause infection of charred tissue and pose another difficulty for healing.

Healing of cutaneous burns is related to the extent of tissue destruction. First-degree burns, by definition, have little if any cell loss, and healing requires only repair or replacement of injured endothelial cells. Second-degree burns also heal without a scar because epidermal basal cells remain and are a source of regenerating cells for the epithelium. Third-degree burns, in which the entire thickness of the epidermis is destroyed, pose a separate set of problems. If the skin appendages are spared, re-epithelialization can arise from them. Deeper burns that destroy the skin appendages require new epidermis or cultured autologous keratinocytes to be grafted to the débrided area to establish a functional covering. Burned skin that is not replaced by a graft heals with dense scarring. Because this scar tissue lacks the elasticity of normal skin, contractures that limit motion may eventually result.

Inhalation burns result from exposure to air and aerosolized flammable materials heated to very high temperatures. Inhalation of these noxious fumes injures or destroys respiratory tract epithelium from the oral cavity to the alveoli. If a patient survives the acute episode, potentially fatal acute respiratory distress syndrome/diffuse alveolar damage may develop (see Chapter 12).

Electrical burns are produced by conversion of electrical energy to heat energy when the current encounters the resistance of the tissues. *Because electrical energy can potentially disrupt the electrical system within the heart, it frequently causes death through ventricular fibrillation.* Electrical burns of the skin reflect the voltage, the area of electrical conductance, and the duration of current flow. Very high-voltage current chars tissue and produces a third-degree burn. Larger areas exposed suffer less injury than small areas exposed under equal conditions.

Physical Injuries

The effect of mechanical trauma is related to (1) the force transmitted to the tissue, (2) the rate at which the transfer occurs, (3) the surface area to which the force is transferred, and (4) the area of the body involved. Blows over a hollow viscus can rupture the organ because of compression of the fluid or gas the space contains; organs nestled beneath the skin, such as the liver, can be easily ruptured. An impact directly over the heart can even disturb its electrical systems. The injury may be **patterned**, giving evidence of the causative agent. Reproducible sets of injuries (**injury patterns**) may be characteristic of particular injurious circumstances. These findings are of particular interest to the forensic pathologist who must determine both the cause and the **manner** of death—for example, is the death natural, accidental, suicidal, or homicidal?

A Contusion (Bruise) is a Localized Mechanical Injury with Focal Hemorrhage

A force with sufficient energy may disrupt capillaries and venules within an organ by physical means alone. The result may be so limited that the only histologic change is hemorrhage in tissue spaces outside the vascular compartment. A discrete extravascular blood pool within the tissue is called a **hematoma or bruise**. Initially, the deoxygenated blood renders the area blue to blue-black, as in the classic "black eye." Macrophages ingest the erythrocytes, convert their hemoglobin to bilirubin and so change the color from blue to yellow. Both mobilization of the pigment by macrophages and further metabolism of bilirubin cause the yellow to fade to yellowish-green and then to disappear.

An Abrasion (Scrape) is a Skin Defect Caused by the Application of Tangential Force

The disruptive force may provide a portal of entry for microorganisms because it leads to damage or loss of the superficial (and sometimes deeper) epithelial layers.

A Laceration is a Split or Tear of the Skin Caused by Crushing or Twisting Force

Lacerations are more common over bone prominences and have irregular margins. When they have crushed margins, they are termed abraded lacerations. Lacerations are generally **not** produced by sharp objects.

Wounds are Mechanical Disruptions of Tissue Integrity

An **incision** is a deliberate opening in the skin by a cutting instrument such as a surgeon's scalpel. Incisions have sharp edges and, importantly, tissues are cleanly separated through the wound's extent. **Deep penetrating wounds** made by high-velocity projectiles, such as bullets, are often deceptive, because the energy of the missile as it passes through the body may be released at sites distant from the entrance itself. Bullets rotate axially and do not tumble, producing a well-defined and usually round entrance wound. Once the projectile enters the flesh, however, it may fragment, tumble, or actually explode, resulting in considerable tissue damage and a large, ragged exit wound (Fig. 8-9).

Radiation

Radiation is the transmission of energy by electromagnetic waves and by certain charged particles (alpha and beta particles and neutrons) emitted by radioactive elements. High-energy radiation, in the form of gamma or x-rays, mediates most of the biological effects discussed here. We do not consider the effects of ultraviolet radiation here; they are discussed in Chapters 5 and 24.

Radiation is quantitated in a number of ways:

- **A rad** defines the energy, expressed as ergs, absorbed by a tissue. One rad equals 100 ergs per gram of tissue.
- **A gray** (Gy) corresponds to 100 rads (1 joule/kg of tissue), and a centigray (cGy) is equivalent to 1 rad.
- **A sievert** (Sv) is the dose in grays multiplied by an appropriate quality factor Q, so that 1 Sv of radiation is roughly equivalent in biological effectiveness to 1 Gy of gamma rays.

Sieverts measure radiation effects in tissue, whereas grays measure absorption in tissue. For example, background radiation averages about 3 milliSv, and 3 Sv will lead to the death of half of exposed people.

For the purposes of this discussion of radiation-induced pathology, the rad, gray, and sievert are considered comparable, with 1 Sv being equal to 100 rads.

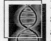 **PATHOGENESIS:** At the cellular level, radiation essentially has two effects: (1) a somatic effect, associated with acute cell killing and (2) genetic damage. Radiation-induced cell death is believed to be caused by the acute effects of the radiolysis of water and the production of activated oxygen species (see Chapter 1). Genetic damage to the cell (whether caused by direct absorption of energy by DNA or indirectly by a reaction of DNA with oxygen radicals) is expressed either as a mutation or as reproductive failure. Both mutations and reproductive failure may lead to delayed cell death, and mutation is incriminated in the development of radiation-induced neoplasia (see Chapter 5).

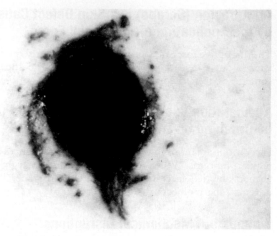
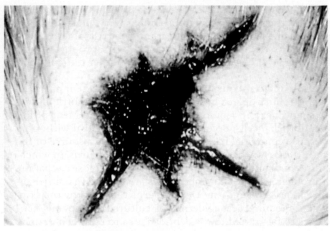

A   B

FIGURE 8-9.   **Bullet wounds. A.** The entrance wound is sharply punched out. **B.** The exit wound is irregular with characteristic stellate lacerations.

Different tissues vary in their sensitivity to radiation. The vulnerability of a tissue to radiation-induced damage depends on its proliferative rate, which in turn, correlates with the natural life span of the constituent cells. For example, the intestine and hematopoietic bone marrow are far more vulnerable to radiation than are tissues such as bone and brain. Damage to the DNA of a long-lived, nonproliferating cell does not necessarily impair its function or viability. By contrast, a short-lived, proliferating cell, such as an intestinal crypt cell or a hematopoietic precursor, must be rapidly replaced by division of precursor cells. If radiation-induced DNA damage precludes mitosis of these cells, the mature elements are not replaced, and the tissue can no longer function. Rapid somatic cell death occurs only with extremely high doses of radiation, well in excess of 1,000 cGy. By contrast, irreversible damage to the replicative capacity of cells requires far lower doses, possibly as few as 50 cGy.

Whole-body Irradiation Injures Many Organs

Most of our information about whole-body irradiation has been derived from studies of Japanese atom bomb survivors and persons exposed during the Chernobyl nuclear power plant accident (Fig. 8-10).

- **300 cGy:** At this dose, a syndrome characterized by **hematopoietic failure** develops within 2 weeks, leading to bleeding, anemia, and infection. The last is often the cause of death, which occurs in about half of the people exposed.
- **10 Gy:** In the vicinity of this dose, the main cause of death is related to the **gastrointestinal system**. At this dose, the entire epithelium of the gastrointestinal tract is destroyed within 3 days, which is the time of the normal life span of villous and crypt cells. As a result, fluid homeostasis of the bowel is disrupted, and severe diarrhea and dehydration ensue. Moreover, the epithelial barrier to intestinal bacteria is breached; gut organisms invade and disseminate throughout the body. Septicemia and shock kill the victim.
- **20 Gy:** With whole-body doses of 20 Gy and above, CNS damage causes death within hours. In most cases, cerebral edema and loss of the integrity of the blood–brain barrier, owing to endothelial injury, predominate. With extreme doses, radiation necrosis of neurons can be expected. Convulsions, coma, and death follow.

FETAL EFFECTS: The effects of whole-body irradiation on the human fetus have been documented in studies of Hiroshima nuclear bomb survivors. Pregnant women exposed to 25 cGy or more gave birth to infants with reduced head size, diminished overall growth, and mental retardation. Other effects of irradiation in utero include hydrocephaly, microphthalmia, chorioretinitis, blindness, spina bifida, cleft palate, clubfeet, and genital abnormalities. Data from experimental and human studies strongly suggest that major congenital malformations are highly unlikely at doses below 20 cGy after day 14 of pregnancy. However, lower doses may produce more subtle effects, such as a decrease in mental capacity.

GENETIC EFFECTS: Most data on which predictions of human genetic effects are based are derived from experimental data and analysis of nuclear bomb survivors. *After long-term follow-up, even survivors of Hiroshima and Nagasaki have shown no evidence of genetic damage in the form of either congenital abnormalities or heritable diseases in subsequent offspring or their descendants.* Consequently, the risk of heritable genetic damage from radiation appears to be small.

Localized Radiation Injury Complicates Radiation Therapy for Tumors

During radiation therapy for malignant neoplasms, some normal tissue is inevitably irradiated. Although almost any organ can be damaged by radiation, the skin, lungs, heart, kidney, bladder, and intestine are all susceptible and difficult to shield (Fig. 8-11). Localized damage to the bone marrow is clearly of little functional consequence because of the immense reserve capacity of the hematopoietic system.

 PATHOLOGY: Persistent damage to radiation-exposed tissue can be attributed to: (1) compromise of the vascular supply and (2) a fibrotic repair reaction to acute necrosis and chronic ischemia. Radiation-induced tissue injury predominantly affects small arteries and arterioles. The endothelial cells are the most sensitive elements in the blood vessels, and in the short term, exhibit swelling and necrosis. With time, vascular walls become thickened by endothelial cell proliferation, and subintimal deposition of collagen and other connective tissue elements occurs. Vacuolization of intimal cells, so called foam cells, is typical. Fragmentation of the internal elastic lamina, loss of smooth muscle cells, scarring in the media, and fibrosis of the adventitia are seen in the small arteries. Bizarre fibroblasts with large hyperchromatic nuclei are common and probably reflect radiation-induced DNA damage.

 CLINICAL FEATURES: Acute necrosis from radiation is represented by such disorders as **radiation pneumonitis**, **cystitis**, **dermatitis**, and diarrhea from **enteritis**. Chronic disease is characterized by **interstitial fibrosis** in the heart and lungs, strictures in the esophagus and small intestine, and **constrictive pericarditis**. Chronic **radiation nephritis**, which simulates malignant nephrosclerosis, is

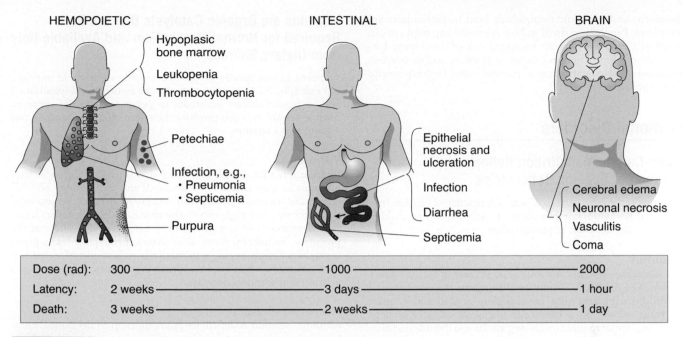

FIGURE 8-10. **Acute radiation syndromes.** At a dose of approximately 300 rads of whole body radiation, a syndrome characterized by hematopoietic failure develops within 2 weeks. In the vicinity of 1,000 rads, a gastrointestinal syndrome with a latency of only 3 days is seen. With doses of 2,000 rads or more, disease of the central nervous system appears within 1 hour, and death ensues rapidly.

primarily a vascular disease that leads to severe hypertension and progressive renal insufficiency. Additional sites affected by local radiation include:

- **Skin:** Radiation dermatitis may occur where the therapeutic radiation traverses the skin. Poorly healed or dehisced wounds or persistent ulcers may occur at such sites and often require full-thickness skin grafts.
- **Gonads:** The combination of radiation-induced vascular injury and direct damage to the continuously dividing germ cells leads to progressive atrophy and loss of reproductive function, with persistence of normal hormonal status.
- **Other sites:** Cataracts (lenticular opacities) may be produced if the eye lies in the path of the radiation beam. Transverse myelitis and paraplegia occur with spinal cord irradiation as a result of vascular damage and local ischemia.

High Doses of Radiation Cause Cancer

The evidence that radiation can lead to cancer is incontrovertible and comes from many sources. The survivors of the nuclear bomb explosions in Japan suffered from a number of cancers. They exhibited more than a 10-fold increase in the incidence of leukemia, which had peaked by 5 years after exposure, then declined over the next 3 decades to near-background rates, although significant excess risk was detectable 30 years after exposure. The frequency of solid tumors, although not as great as that for leukemia, was clearly increased for the breast, lung, thyroid, gastrointestinal tract, and urinary tract. A striking increase in the incidence of thyroid cancer, resulting in at least 1,000 additional cases among children, occurred in geographical areas contaminated by the nuclear catastrophe at Chernobyl in Ukraine in 1986. The increase has been linked to release of radioactive iodine isotopes in that incident.

LOW-LEVEL RADIATION AND CANCER: *The key question that needs to be answered is whether there is a threshold dose of radiation below which there is no increase in the incidence of cancer or whether any exposure carries a significant risk.* Data currently available show that the estimates of cancer risk at low radiation doses is very low, although they do not demonstrate that the risk is zero. *When data from atomic bomb survivors are subjected to a conservative analysis, the lifetime risk from 1 cGy of whole-body x- or gamma irradiation is 1 excess cancer death per 10,000 persons.*

RADON: The finding that some homes in the United States contain radon formed from the decay of naturally occurring uranium 238 (^{238}U), which is found in some soil and rock formations, has raised concern. Although radon is itself inert, its radioactive decay products are chemically active α alpha particle emitting isotopes

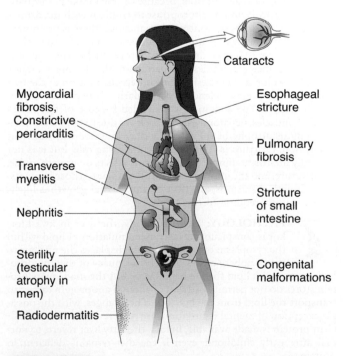

FIGURE 8-11. The nonneoplastic complications of radiation.

of bismuth, lead, and polonium, which bind to particulates and lung tissues. People who dwell in homes containing high concentrations of radon gas have an increased risk of developing lung cancer, although it may be restricted to smokers and ex-smokers. Ventilation of basement spaces to prevent radon buildup ameliorates the problem.

Nutritional Disorders

Protein-Calorie Malnutrition Reflects Starvation or Specific Deficiencies

Marasmus is the term used to denote a deficiency of calories from all sources. **Kwashiorkor** is a form of malnutrition in children caused by a diet deficient in protein alone.

Marasmus

Global starvation—that is, a deficiency of all elements of the diet—leads to marasmus. The condition is common throughout the nonindustrialized world, particularly when breast-feeding is unavailable, and a child must subsist on a calorically inadequate diet. Pathologic changes are similar to those in starving adults and include decreased body weight, diminished subcutaneous fat, a protuberant abdomen, muscle wasting, and a wrinkled face. Wasting and increased lipofuscin pigment are seen in most visceral organs, especially the heart and the liver. Pulse, blood pressure, and temperature are low, and diarrhea is common. Because immune responses are impaired, the child suffers from numerous infections. An important consequence of marasmus is growth failure and the inability to reach full potential adult stature. Although still controversial, marasmus also appears to reduce cognitive ability during development.

Kwashiorkor

Kwashiorkor (Fig. 8-12) results from a deficiency of protein in diets relatively high in carbohydrates. It is one of the most common diseases of infancy and childhood in the nonindustrialized world. Like marasmus, it usually occurs after an infant is weaned to a protein-poor diet, consisting principally of staple carbohydrates. There is generalized growth failure and muscle wasting, as in marasmus, but subcutaneous fat is normal, because caloric intake is adequate. Extreme apathy is notable, in contrast to children with marasmus, who may be alert. Also in contrast to marasmus, there is prominent edema, hepatomegaly, and depigmentation of the skin. Dermatoses consisting of dry, hyperkeratotic "flaky paint" lesions occur on the face, extremities, and perineum. Hair becomes a sandy or reddish color; a characteristic linear depigmentation of the hair ("flag sign") provides evidence of particularly severe periods of protein deficiency. The abdomen is distended because of flaccid abdominal muscles, hepatomegaly, and ascites due to hypoalbuminemia. Villous atrophy of the intestine may interfere with nutrient absorption. Diarrhea is common. Anemia is the rule, but it is not generally life-threatening. The nonspecific effects on growth, pulse, temperature, and the immune system are similar to those in marasmus. As with marasmus, an effect on intellectual growth is likely, but the subject requires further study.

 PATHOLOGY: Microscopically, the liver in kwashiorkor is conspicuously fatty. Accumulation of lipid within the cytoplasm of the hepatocyte displaces the nucleus to the periphery of the cell. The adequacy of dietary carbohydrate provides lipid for the hepatocyte, but the inadequate protein stores do not permit synthesis of enough apoprotein carrier to transport the lipid from the liver cell. The changes, with the possible exception of mental retardation, are fully reversible when sufficient protein is made available. In fact, the fatty liver reverts to normal after early childhood, even if the diet remains deficient in protein.

Vitamins are Organic Catalysts that are Both Required for Normal Metabolism and Available Only from Dietary Sources

Vitamins in one species are not necessarily vitamins in another. For example, humans cannot synthesize ascorbic acid (vitamin C) and so require dietary ascorbate to prevent scurvy. By contrast, most lower animals can produce their own vitamin C and do not require it as a vitamin.

Vitamin A

Vitamin A is a fat-soluble substance that is important for skeletal maturation, maintenance of specialized epithelial linings, and cell membrane structure. In addition, it is an important constituent of the photosensitive pigments in the retina. Vitamin A occurs naturally as retinoids or as a precursor, β-carotene. The source of the precursor, namely carotene, is in plants, principally leafy, green vegetables. Fish livers are a particularly rich source of vitamin A itself. At times when fat absorption is impaired (e.g., diarrhea), vitamin A absorption decreases.

Vitamin A Deficiency

Although vitamin A deficiency is uncommon in developed countries, it is a significant health problem in poorer regions of the world, including much of Africa, China, and Southeast Asia.

 PATHOLOGY: *Deficiency of vitamin A results principally in squamous metaplasia, especially in glandular epithelium* (Fig. 8-13). Thus, keratin debris blocks sweat and tear glands (**follicular hyperkeratosis**). Squamous metaplasia is

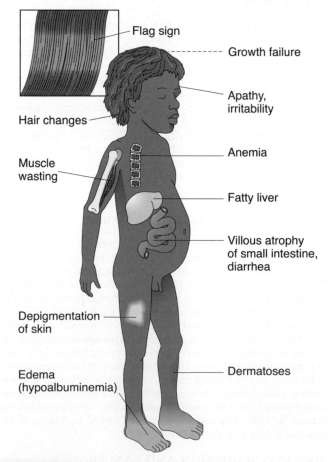

FIGURE 8-12. Complications of kwashiorkor.

common in the trachea and bronchi, and bronchopneumonia is a frequent cause of death. With further diminution of vitamin A stores, squamous metaplasia of conjunctival and tear duct epithelial cells occurs, which leads to **xerophthalmia** (dryness of the cornea and conjunctiva). The cornea becomes softened (**keratomalacia**) and vulnerable to ulceration and bacterial infection, which may lead to blindness.

Excess vitamin A is toxic. Poisoning may be caused by overenthusiastic administration of vitamin supplements to children. Enlargement of the liver and spleen are common; microscopically, these organs show lipid-laden macrophages. Discontinuing the excess vitamin A consumption reverses all or most of the lesions. Both retinoic acid derivatives (used to alleviate severe acne) and a high dietary intake of preformed vitamin A are particularly dangerous in pregnancy because they are potent teratogens. Excessive carotene intake is benign and simply stains the skin yellow, which may be mistaken for jaundice.

 CLINICAL FEATURES: The earliest sign of vitamin A deficiency is often diminished vision in dim light. Vitamin A is a continuously necessary component in retinal rod pigment and is active in light transduction. Vitamin A deficiency is a leading cause of preventable childhood blindness in the developing world.

Vitamin B Complex

Vitamins in the B group of water-soluble vitamins are numbered 1 through 12, but most are not distinct vitamins. The members of the complex currently recognized as true vitamins are vitamins B_1 (thiamine), B_3 (niacin), B_2 (riboflavin), B_6 (pyridoxine), and B_{12} (cyanocobalamin). With the exception of vitamin B_{12}, which is derived only from animal sources, B complex vitamins are found principally in leafy green vegetables, milk, and liver.

Thiamine

Thiamine was the active ingredient in the original description of vitamin B, which was defined as a water-soluble extract in rice polishings that cured beriberi (clinical thiamine deficiency). This disease was classically seen in Asia, where the staple food was polished rice that had been deprived of its thiamine content by processing. In Western countries, the disease occurs in alcoholics, neglected persons with poor overall nutrition, and food faddists. *The cardinal symptoms of thiamine deficiency are polyneuropathy, edema, and cardiac failure.* The deficiency syndrome is classically divided into **dry beriberi**, with symptoms referable to the neuromuscular system, and **wet beriberi**, in which manifestations of cardiac failure predominate.

 PATHOGENESIS: Patients with dry beriberi present with paresthesias, depressed reflexes and weakness, and muscle atrophy in the extremities. Wet beriberi is characterized by generalized edema, a reflection of severe congestive failure. The basic lesion is uncontrolled, generalized vasodilation and significant peripheral arteriovenous shunting. This combination leads to compensatory increases in cardiac output, and eventually to a large dilated heart and congestive heart failure.

 PATHOLOGY: Thiamine deficiency in chronic alcoholics may be manifested by CNS involvement, in the form of Wernicke syndrome, in which progressive **dementia, ataxia, and ophthalmoplegia** (paralysis of the extraocular muscles) are prominent. A characteristic alteration is myelin sheath degeneration, which often begins in the sciatic nerve and then involves other peripheral nerves and sometimes the spinal cord itself. The most striking lesions in Wernicke encephalopathy comprise atrophy in the mamillary bodies and surrounding areas that abut on the third ventricle. Microscopically, degeneration and loss of ganglion cells, rupture of small blood vessels, and ring hemorrhages are seen in the brain.

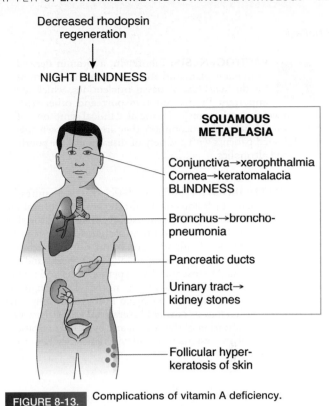

FIGURE 8-13. Complications of vitamin A deficiency.

Decreased rhodopsin regeneration → NIGHT BLINDNESS

SQUAMOUS METAPLASIA

Conjunctiva→xerophthalmia
Cornea→keratomalacia
BLINDNESS

Bronchus→bronchopneumonia

Pancreatic ducts

Urinary tract→ kidney stones

Follicular hyperkeratosis of skin

The changes in the heart are also nonspecific. Grossly, the heart is flabby, dilated, and increased in weight. The process may affect either the right or the left side of the heart, or both. The microscopic changes are nondescript and include edema, inconsistent fiber hypertrophy, and occasional foci of fiber degeneration.

Niacin

Niacin refers to two chemically distinct compounds: nicotinic acid and nicotinamide. These components are derived from dietary niacin or are biosynthesized from tryptophan. Niacin plays a major role in formation of nicotinamide adenine dinucleotide (NAD) and its phosphate (NADP). Animal protein, as found in meat, eggs, and milk, is high in tryptophan and is, therefore, a good source of endogenously synthesized niacin. Niacin itself is available in many types of grain. **Pellagra** is the term for clinical niacin deficiency. It is uncommon today and is seen principally in patients who have been weakened by other diseases and also in malnourished alcoholics.

 PATHOLOGY: Pellagra is particularly prevalent in areas where corn (maize) is the staple food, because the niacin in corn is chemically bound and is thus poorly available. Corn is also a poor source of tryptophan. The disease is characterized by the three "Ds" of niacin deficiency: **dermatitis, diarrhea, and dementia**. Areas exposed to light, such as the face and the hands, and those subjected to pressure, such as the knees and the elbows, exhibit a rough, scaly dermatitis. The involvement of the hands leads to so-called glove dermatitis. Microscopically, hyperkeratosis, vascularization, and chronic inflammation of the skin are characteristic. Subcutaneous fibrosis and scarring may be seen in late stages. Similar lesions are found in the mucous membranes of the mouth and vagina. In the mouth, chronic inflammation and edema lead to a large, red fissured tongue. Chronic, watery diarrhea is typical for the disease, presumably due to mucosal atrophy and ulceration in the entire gastrointestinal tract, particularly in the colon. The dementia, characterized by aberrant ideation bordering on psychosis, is represented in the brain by degeneration of ganglion cells in the cortex. Myelin degeneration of tracts in the spinal cord resembles the subacute combined degeneration of vitamin B_{12} deficiency (see below).

Riboflavin

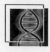

PATHOGENESIS: Riboflavin, a vitamin derived from many plant and animal sources, is important for the synthesis of flavin nucleotides, which are important in electron transport and other reactions in which energy transfer is crucial. Clinical symptoms of riboflavin deficiency are uncommon; they are usually seen only in debilitated patients with a variety of diseases and in poorly nourished alcoholics.

PATHOLOGY: Riboflavin deficiency is manifested principally by lesions of the facial skin and corneal epithelium. **Cheilosis**, a term used for fissures in the skin at the angles of the mouth, is a characteristic feature. **Seborrheic dermatitis**, an inflammation of the skin that exhibits a greasy, scaling appearance, typically involves the cheeks and the areas behind the ears. Microscopically, hyperkeratosis and a mild mononuclear infiltrate of the skin are noted. The tongue is smooth and purplish (magenta), owing to mucosal atrophy. The most troubling lesion may be **corneal interstitial keratitis**, which is followed by opacification of the cornea and eventual ulceration. The localization of the lesions in riboflavin deficiency is not explained biochemically.

Pyridoxine

Vitamin B_6 activity is found in three related, naturally occurring compounds: pyridoxine, pyridoxal, and pyridoxamine. For convenience, they are grouped under the heading pyridoxine. These compounds are widely distributed in vegetable and animal foods.

PATHOGENESIS: Pyridoxine is converted to pyridoxal phosphate, a coenzyme for many enzymes, including transaminases and carboxylases. Pyridoxine deficiency is rarely caused by an inadequate diet. Of particular concern is the deficiency of pyridoxine that follows prolonged medication with a number of drugs, particularly isoniazid, cycloserine, and penicillamine. A deficiency state is also occasionally reported in alcoholics.

CLINICAL FEATURES: There are no clinical manifestations of pyridoxine deficiency that can be considered characteristic or pathognomonic. The usual dermatologic complications of other B vitamin deficiencies occur with pyridoxine deficiency. *The primary expression of the disease is in the CNS, a feature consistent with the role of this vitamin in the formation of pyridoxal-dependent decarboxylase of the neurotransmitter GABA.* In infants and children, diarrhea, anemia, and seizures have occurred. Pyridoxine-responsive anemia is hypochromic and microcytic and therefore can be confused with iron-deficiency anemia. By definition, the anemia responds well to massive doses of pyridoxine.

Vitamin B_{12} and Folic Acid Deficiencies

Comprehensive discussions of **vitamin B_{12} and folic acid deficiencies** are found in Chapters 20 and 28. In pregnant women, deficiency of folate may lead to spina bifida and other dysraphic anomalies in the fetus, which are in turn prevented by folate supplementation (see Chapter 6).

Vitamin C (Ascorbic Acid)

PATHOGENESIS: Ascorbic acid is a powerful biological reducing agent involved in many oxidation–reduction reactions and in proton transfer. This vitamin is important for chondroitin sulfate synthesis and for proline hydroxylation to form the hydrox-

yproline of collagen. Wound healing and immune functions also involve ascorbic acid. The best dietary sources of vitamin C are citrus fruits, green vegetables, and tomatoes. *Scurvy is the clinical vitamin C deficiency state.* Scurvy is now a disease of persons afflicted with chronic diseases who do not eat well, the neglected aged, and malnourished alcoholics. The stress of cold, heat, fever, or trauma (accidental or surgical) leads to an increased requirement for vitamin C. Children who are fed only milk for the first year of life tend to develop scurvy.

PATHOLOGY: Most of the events associated with vitamin C deficiency are caused by the formation of abnormal collagen that lacks tensile strength (Fig. 8-14). Within 1 to 3 months, subperiosteal hemorrhages produce pain in the bones and joints. Petechial hemorrhages, ecchymoses, and purpura are common, particularly after mild trauma or at pressure points. Perifollicular hemorrhages in the skin are particularly typical of scurvy. In advanced cases, swollen, bleeding gums are a classic finding. Alveolar bone resorption results in loss of teeth. Wound healing is poor, and dehiscence of previously healed wounds occurs. Anemia may result from prolonged bleeding, impaired iron absorption, or associated folic acid deficiency. In children, vitamin C deficiency leads to growth failure, and collagen-rich structures, such as teeth, bones, and blood vessels, develop abnormally. Although the claims that ascorbic acid may help to prevent upper respiratory infections lack substantiation, ingestion of large amounts of vitamin C is not known to be harmful.

Vitamin D

Vitamin D is a fat-soluble steroid hormone found in two forms: vitamin D_3 (cholecalciferol) and vitamin D_2 (ergocalciferol), both of which have equal biological potency in humans. Vitamin D_3 is produced in the skin, and D_2 is derived from plant ergosterol. The vitamin is absorbed in the jejunum along with fats and is transported in the blood bound to an α-globulin (vitamin D-binding protein). *To achieve biological potency, vitamin D must be hydroxylated to active metabolites in the liver and kidney. The active form of the vitamin promotes calcium and phosphate absorption from the small intestine and may directly influence mineralization of bone.*

Vitamin D Deficiency

PATHOGENESIS: *In children, vitamin D deficiency causes rickets; in adults, osteomalacia occurs.* Vitamin D deficiency results from (1) insufficient dietary vitamin D, (2) insufficient production of vitamin D in the skin because of limited sunlight exposure, (3) inadequate absorption of vitamin D from the diet (as in the fat malabsorption syndromes), or (4) abnormal conversion of vitamin D to its bioactive metabolites. The last occurs in liver disease and chronic renal failure.

CLINICAL FEATURES: The bone lesions of vitamin D deficiency in children (rickets) have been recognized for centuries and were common in the Western industrialized world until recently. Addition of vitamin D to milk and many processed foods, administration of vitamin preparations to young children, and generally improved levels of nutrition have made rickets a curiosity in industrialized countries (See Chapter 26).

Excess vitamin D may be harmful and result in **hypercalcemia**, which leads to nonspecific symptoms such as weakness and headaches and ultimately to **nephrolithiasis** or **nephrocalcinosis. Ectopic calcification** in other organs may be seen. Infants are particularly susceptible to excess vitamin D and may develop premature arteriosclerosis, supravalvular aortic stenosis, and renal acidosis.

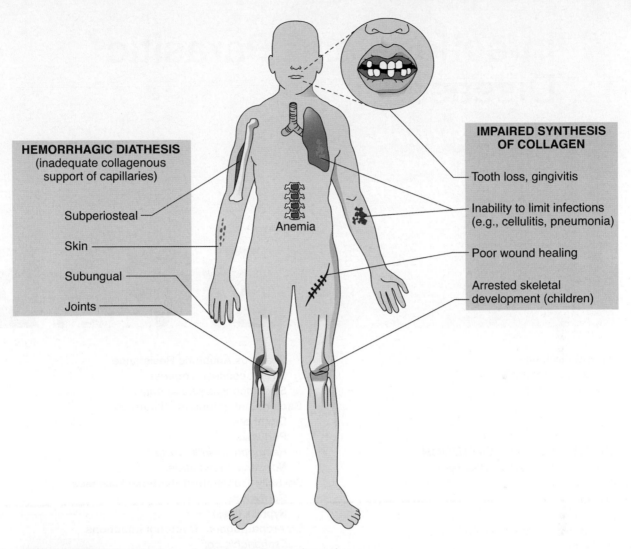

FIGURE 8-14. Complications of vitamin C deficiency (scurvy).

Vitamin E

Vitamin E is an antioxidant that (experimentally at least) protects membrane phospholipids against lipid peroxidation by free radicals formed by cellular metabolism. The activity of this fat-soluble vitamin is found in a number of dietary constituents, principally in α-tocopherol. Corn and soy beans are particularly rich in vitamin E. Dietary deficiency of vitamin E is rare, and no clearly definable syndrome is associated with it. In premature infants, hemolytic anemia, thrombocytosis, and edema have been reported with vitamin E deficiency. Claims for a variety of beneficial effects of vitamin E abound, but the evidence for efficacy is unsubstantiated.

Vitamin K

Vitamin K, a fat-soluble material, occurs in two forms: vitamin K_1, from plants and vitamin K_2, which is principally synthesized by the normal intestinal bacteria. Green leafy vegetables are rich in vitamin K, and liver and dairy products contain smaller amounts. Dietary deficiency is very uncommon in the United States; most cases are associated with other disorders. However, newborn infants may exhibit vitamin K deficiency because the vitamin is not transported well across the placenta, and the sterile gut of the newborn does not have bacteria to produce it. Vitamin K confers calcium-binding properties to certain proteins and is important for the activity of several clotting factors. For this reason, a deficiency of this vitamin can lead to catastrophic bleeding (see Chapter 20). Parenteral vitamin K therapy is rapidly effective.

Essential Trace Minerals are Mostly Components of Enzymes and Cofactors

Essential trace minerals include iron, copper, iodine, zinc, cobalt, selenium, manganese, nickel, chromium, tin, molybdenum, vanadium, silicon, and fluorine. Dietary deficiencies of these minerals are clinically important in the case of iron and iodine. These are discussed in Chapters 20 and 21, which deal with blood and endocrine diseases, respectively.

9 Infectious and Parasitic Diseases

David A. Schwartz
Robert M. Genta
Douglas P. Bennett
Roger J. Pomerantz

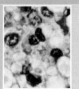

SPIROCHETAL INFECTIONS
Syphilis
  Primary Syphilis
  Secondary Syphilis
  Tertiary Syphilis
  Congenital Syphilis
Lyme Disease
CHLAMYDIAL INFECTIONS
Chlamydia Trachomatis Infection
Psittacosis (Ornithosis)
RICKETTSIAL INFECTIONS
Rocky Mountain Spotted Fever
Epidemic (Louse-Borne) Typhus
MYCOPLASMAL INFECTIONS: MYCOPLASMA PNEUMONIA
MYCOBACTERIAL INFECTIONS
Tuberculosis
  Primary Tuberculosis
  Secondary (Cavitary) Tuberculosis
Leprosy
FUNGAL INFECTIONS
Pneumocystis Jiroveci Pneumonia
Candida
Aspergillosis
Cryptococcosis
Histoplasmosis
Coccidioidomycosis
Blastomycosis
Dermatophyte Infections

PROTOZOAL INFECTIONS
Malaria
Toxoplasmosis
  Congenital *Toxoplasma* Infections
  Toxoplasmosis in Immunocompromised Hosts
Amebiasis
Cryptosporidiosis
Giardiasis
Leishmaniasis
  Localized and Diffuse Cutaneous Leishmaniasis
  Mucocutaneous Leishmaniasis
  Viscaral Leishmaniasis (Kala Azar)
Chagas Disease (American Trypanosomiasis)
African Trypanosomiasis
HELMINTHIC INFECTION
Filarial Nematodes
  Lymphatic Filariasis
  Onchocerciasis
Intestinal Nematodes
  Ascariasis
  Trichuriasis
  Hookworms
  Strongyloidiasis
Tissue Nematodes: Trichinellosis
Trematodes (Flukes)
  Schistosomiasis
  Clonorchiasis
Cestodes: Intestinal Tapeworms
Echinococcosis

Bacterial and viral diarrheas and pneumonias, tuberculosis, measles, malaria, hepatitis B, pertussis, as well as tetanus kill more people each year than do all cancers and cardiovascular diseases. The impact of infectious diseases is greatest in less-developed countries, where millions of people, mostly children younger than 5 years of age, die of treatable or preventable infectious diseases. Even in the industrialized countries of Europe and North America, the mortality, morbidity, and loss of economic productivity from infectious diseases is enormous. In the United States each year, infectious diseases cause more than 200,000 deaths and more than 50 million days of hospitalization.

Infectivity and Virulence

Infectious organisms cause diseases in which tissue dysfunction results from an invading transmissible agent. Virulence refers to the complex of properties that allows that agent to achieve infection and cause diseases of different degrees of severity. The organism must (1) gain access to the body, (2) avoid multiple host defenses, (3) accommodate to growth in the human milieu, and (4) parasitize human resources. Virulence reflects both the structures inherent to the offending microbe and the interplay of those factors with host defense mechanisms.

Host Defense Mechanisms

The means by which the body prevents or contains infections are known as host defense mechanisms. There are major anatomical barriers to infection—mainly the skin and the aerodynamic filtration system of the upper airway—that prevent most organisms from ever penetrating the body. The mucociliary blanket of the airways is also an essential defense, providing a means of expelling organisms that gain access to the respiratory system. The microbial flora normally resident in the gastrointestinal tract and in various body orifices compete with outside organisms, preventing them from gaining sufficient nutrients or binding sites in the host. The body's orifices are also protected by secretions that possess antimicrobial properties, both nonspecific (e.g., lysozyme and interferon) and specific (IgA). In addition, gastric acid and bile chemically destroy many ingested organisms.

Heritable Differences in the Host Influence Organism Virulence

The first step in infection is often a specific interaction of a binding molecule on the infecting organism with a receptor molecule on the host. If the host lacks a suitable receptor, the organism cannot attach to the target. An example is *Plasmodium vivax,* one of the parasites that causes malaria. It infects human erythrocytes by using Duffy blood group determinants on the cell surface as receptors. Many individuals, particularly blacks, lack these determinants and are not susceptible to infection with *P. vivax*. As a result, *P. vivax* malaria is absent from much of Africa.

Age Influences the Outcome of Infection

The effect of age on the outcome of exposure to many infectious agents is illustrated by fetal infections. Some organisms produce more severe disease in utero than in children or adults. Infections of the fetus with cytomegalovirus (CMV), rubellavirus, parvovirus B19, and *Toxoplasma gondii* interfere with fetal development. Fetal protection is dependent on the presence of maternal IgG antibodies, which cross the placenta. An acute infection in a nonimmune pregnant woman may allow the organism to infect the fetus. These infections are usually subclinical or produce minimal disease in the mother but may lead to major congenital abnormalities or death in the fetus.

Age also affects the course of common illnesses, such as the diverse viral and bacterial diarrheas. In older children and adults, these infections cause discomfort and inconvenience, but rarely severe disease. The outcome can be different in children under 3 years, who cannot compensate for the rapid volume loss that results from profuse diarrhea. In 2000, the World Health Organization estimated that acute diarrheal diseases kill 2.2 million children yearly.

The elderly fare more poorly with almost all infections than younger persons. Common respiratory illnesses such as influenza and pneumococcal pneumonia are more often fatal in those older than 65 years of age.

Human Behavior Plays a Large Role in Exposure to Infectious Agents

The link between behavior and infection is probably most obvious for sexually transmitted diseases, in which the type and number of sexual encounters profoundly influence the risk of acquiring disease.

Other aspects of behavior also influence the risk of acquiring infections. Humans contract brucellosis and Q fever, which are primarily bacterial diseases transmitted by close contact with domesticated farm animals or their secretions. These infections occur in farmers, herders, meat processors, and, in the case of brucellosis, in persons who drink unpasteurized milk. Transmission of a number of parasitic diseases is strongly affected by behavior. Schistosomiasis, acquired when water-borne parasite larvae penetrate the skin of a susceptible host, is primarily a disease of farmers who work in fields irrigated by infected water. The larvae of hookworm and *Strongyloides stercoralis* live in humid soil and make their way through the skin of the lower extremities in people who walk barefoot. The introduction of shoes has probably been the single most important factor in reducing the prevalence of infection with soil-transmitted nematodes. Botulism is contracted by (1) ingestion of improperly canned food that contains the toxin; (2) ingestion of clostridia spores, often via honey, by infants; or (3) from inoculation of wounds by spores, which then germinate in devitalized tissue.

People with Compromised Defenses are More Likely to Contract Infections and to Have More Severe Infections

Disruption or absence of any host defense mechanism results in increased numbers and severity of infections. Disruption of epithelial surfaces by trauma or burns frequently leads to invasive bacterial or fungal infections. Injury to the mucociliary apparatus of the airways, as in smoking or influenza, impairs clearance of inhaled microorganisms and leads to an increased incidence of bacterial pneumonia. Congenital absence of complement components C5, C6, C7, and C8 prevents formation of a fully functional membrane attack complex and permits disseminated, and often recurrent, *Neisseria* infections (see Chapter 2). Diseases such as diabetes mellitus and chemotherapeutic drugs that interfere with the production

or function of neutrophils increase the likelihood of bacterial infections or invasive fungal infections (see Chapter 20).

Organisms that cause disease *mainly* in hosts with impaired immunity are termed **opportunistic pathogens**. These organisms, many of which are part of the normal endogenous human or environmental microbial flora, take advantage of a host's inadequate defenses to stage a more violent and sustained attack.

VIRAL INFECTIONS

Viruses range from 20 to 300 nm and consist of RNA or DNA contained in a protein shell. Some are also enveloped in lipid membranes. *Viruses do not engage in metabolism or reproduction independently, and thus are obligate intracellular parasites that require living cells in order to replicate.* After invading cells, they divert the cells' biosynthetic and metabolic capacities toward the synthesis of virus-encoded nucleic acids and proteins.

Viruses often cause disease by killing infected cells, but many do not. For example, rotavirus, a common cause of diarrhea, interferes with the function of infected enterocytes without immediately killing them. It prevents enterocytes from synthesizing proteins that transport molecules from the intestinal lumen and thereby causes diarrhea.

Viruses may also promote the release of chemical mediators that elicit inflammatory or immunologic responses. The symptoms of the common cold are due to the release of bradykinin from infected cells. Other viruses cause cells to proliferate and form tumors. Human papillomaviruses (HPVs), for instance, cause squamous cell proliferative lesions, which range from common warts to cervical cancer.

Some viruses infect and persist in cells without interfering with cellular functions, a process known as **latency**. Latent viruses can emerge to produce disease years after the primary infection. Opportunistic infections are frequently caused by viruses that have established latent infections. CMV and herpes simplex viruses are among the most frequent opportunistic pathogens because they are commonly present as latent agents and emerge in persons with impaired cell-mediated immunity.

Finally, some viruses may reside within cells, either by integrating into their genomes or by remaining episomal, and cause those cells to generate tumors. Examples of this are Epstein-Barr virus (EBV), which causes endemic Burkitt lymphoma in Africa, and other tumors in different settings, and human T-cell leukemia virus-1 (see Chapter 5), which causes a form of T-cell lymphoma.

In the following section, viruses with highly organ-specific tropisms are not described in detail, but are addressed in those chapters that deal with the organs that are principally affected (e.g., hepatitis B and C) (see Chapter 14).

RNA VIRUSES

A number of important pathogenic RNA viruses (e.g., human immunodeficiency virus [HIV]-1, hepatitis C virus) differ from many DNA viruses in that the RNA viral polymerases do not proofread the RNA strand being synthesized. This has two important consequences. First, the mutation rate—and therefore the plasticity of these viruses in circumventing therapies—is very high. Second, a greater percentage of daughter virions are inactive.

Respiratory Viruses

The Common Cold is the Most Common Viral Disease

The common cold (coryza) is an acute, self-limited upper respiratory tract disorder caused by infection with a variety of RNA viruses, including more than 100 distinct rhinoviruses and several coronaviruses. Colds are frequent and worldwide in distribution, spreading from person to person by contact with infected secretions. Infection is more likely during the winter months in temperate areas and during the rainy seasons in the tropics, when spread is facilitated by indoor crowding. In the United States, children usually suffer six to eight colds per year and adults two to three.

 PATHOGENESIS: The viruses infect the nasal respiratory epithelial cells, causing increased mucus production and edema. Rhinoviruses and coronaviruses have a tropism for respiratory epithelium and optimally reproduce at temperatures well below 37°C (98.6°F). Thus, infection remains confined to the cooler passages of the upper airway. Infected cells release chemical mediators, such as bradykinin, which produce most of the symptoms associated with the common cold, namely increased mucus production, nasal congestion, and eustachian tube obstruction. The resulting stasis of secretions may predispose to secondary bacterial infection and lead to bacterial sinusitis and otitis media. Rhinoviruses and coronaviruses do not destroy the respiratory epithelium and produce no visible alterations. Clinically, the common cold is characterized by rhinorrhea, pharyngitis, cough, low-grade fever. and malaise.

Influenza Virus is a Highly Contagious Epidemic Disease

Influenza is an acute, usually self-limited, infection of upper and lower airways caused by influenza virus. These viruses are enveloped and contain single-stranded RNA.

  PATHOGENESIS AND PATHOLOGY: Influenza spreads from person to person by virus-containing respiratory droplets and secretions. Upon reaching the respiratory epithelial cell surface, the virus binds and enters the cell by fusion with the cell membrane, a process mediated by a viral glycoprotein (hemagglutinin) that binds to sialic acid residues on human respiratory epithelium. Once inside, the virus directs the cell to produce progeny viruses and causes cell death. The infection usually involves both the upper and lower airways. Influenza virus causes necrosis and desquamation of the ciliated respiratory tract epithelium and is associated with a predominantly lymphocytic inflammatory infiltrate. Extension of the infection to the lungs leads to necrosis and sloughing of alveolar lining cells and the histologic appearance of viral pneumonitis. Destruction of the ciliated epithelium cripples the mucociliary blanket, predisposing to bacterial pneumonia, especially with *Staphylococcus aureus* and *Streptococcus pneumoniae.*

 CLINICAL FEATURES: Influenza manifests with a rapid onset of fever, chills, myalgia, headaches, weakness, and nonproductive cough. Symptoms may be primarily those of an upper respiratory infection or those of tracheitis, bronchitis, and pneumonia. Epidemics are accompanied by deaths from both the disease and its complications, particularly in the elderly and in persons with underlying cardiopulmonary disease. Killed viral vaccines specific to epidemic strains are 75% effective in preventing influenza.

Respiratory Syncytial Virus (RSV) Causes Bronchiolitis in Infants

RSV is a major cause of bronchiolitis and pneumonia in children under 1 year of age with most children having been infected by school age. It is spread by respiratory aerosols and secretions, often in the setting of hospitals or daycare centers.

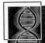 **PATHOGENESIS AND PATHOLOGY:** Viral surface proteins bind to specific receptors on host respiratory epithelium and then fuse with the cell membrane. RSV produces necrosis and sloughing of bronchial, bronchiolar, and alveolar epithelium, which are associated with a predominantly lymphocytic inflammatory infiltrate. Multinucleated syncytial cells are sometimes seen in infected tissues.

 CLINICAL FEATURES: Infants and young children with RSV bronchiolitis or pneumonitis present with wheezing, cough, and respiratory distress, sometimes accompanied by fever. The illness is usually self-limited, resolving in 1 to 2 weeks. In older children and adults, RSV produces much milder disease. Among otherwise healthy young children, the mortality rate from RSV infection is very low, but it rises dramatically to 20% to 40% among children with congenital heart disease or immunosuppression.

Viral Exanthems

Measles (Rubeola) is a Highly Contagious Virus that May Cause Fatal Infection

Measles virus is an enveloped, single-stranded RNA virus that causes an acute illness, characterized by upper respiratory tract symptoms, fever, and rash. The virus is transmitted in respiratory aerosols and secretions. In nonimmunized populations, measles is primarily a disease of children.

 PATHOGENESIS AND PATHOLOGY: The initial site of infection is the mucous membranes of the nasopharynx and bronchi, where the virus produces necrosis of respiratory epithelium and is associated with a predominantly lymphocytic inflammatory infiltrate. The virus extends to the regional lymph nodes and then to the bloodstream, leading to widespread dissemination and prominent involvement of the skin and lymphoid tissues. Lymphoid hyperplasia is often prominent in the cervical and mesenteric lymph nodes, spleen, and appendix. In lymphoid tissues, the virus sometimes causes fusion of infected cells, producing multinucleated giant cells containing up to 100 nuclei, with both intracytoplasmic and intranuclear inclusions. These cells, named **Warthin-Finkeldey giant cells**, are pathognomonic for measles. The virus produces a T-cell-mediated vasculitis of small blood vessels in the skin and a resultant rash.

 CLINICAL FEATURES: Measles first manifests with fever, rhinorrhea, cough, and conjunctivitis and progresses to the characteristic mucosal and skin lesions. The mucosal lesions, known as "Koplik spots," appear on the posterior buccal mucosa and consist of minute gray-white dots on a red base. The skin lesions begin on the face as an erythematous maculopapular rash, which usually spreads to involve the trunk and extremities. The rash fades in 3 to 5 days, and the symptoms gradually resolve. Measles often leads to secondary bacterial infections, especially otitis media and pneumonia. Measles is a particularly severe disease in the very young, the sick, or the malnourished. In impoverished countries, the disease has a high mortality rate (10% to 25%). Uncommonly, patients can develop subacute sclerosing panencephalitis (SSPE), a slow, chronic neurodegenerative disorder that occurs years after a measles infection. The exact pathophysiology of SSPE is unclear. Live attenuated vaccines are highly effective in preventing measles and in eliminating the spread of the virus and have also greatly reduced the incidence of SSPE.

Rubella Infection in Utero is Associated with Congenital Anomalies

Rubellavirus is an enveloped, single-stranded RNA virus that causes a mild, self-limited systemic disease, usually associated with a rash, which is spread primarily by the respiratory route. Many infections are so mild that they go unnoticed. However, in pregnant women, rubella (part of the TORCH complex) is a destructive fetal pathogen (see Chapter 5). Infection early in gestation can produce fetal death, premature delivery, and congenital anomalies, including deafness, cataracts, glaucoma, heart defects, and mental retardation. The live attenuated vaccine currently available prevents rubella and has largely eliminated the disease from developed countries.

 PATHOGENESIS: Rubella infects respiratory epithelium and then disseminates to various organs through the bloodstream and lymphatics. The rubella rash is believed to result from an immunologic response to the disseminated virus. Fetal infection occurs through the placenta during the viremic phase of maternal illness. A congenitally infected fetus remains persistently infected and sheds large amounts of virus in body fluids, even after birth. Maternal infection after 20 weeks' gestation usually does not cause significant fetal disease.

Mumps

Mumps virus is an enveloped, single-stranded highly contagious RNA virus that causes an acute, self-limited systemic illness, characterized by parotid gland swelling and meningoencephalitis.

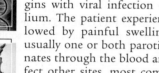 **PATHOGENESIS AND PATHOLOGY:** Mumps begins with viral infection of respiratory tract epithelium. The patient experiences fever and malaise, followed by painful swelling of the salivary glands, usually one or both parotids. The virus then disseminates through the blood and lymphatic systems to infect other sites, most commonly the salivary glands, CNS, pancreas, and testes. The virus causes necrosis of infected cells and a predominantly lymphocytic inflammatory infiltrate. The affected salivary glands are swollen, the ducts lined by necrotic epithelium, and the interstitium infiltrated with lymphocytes. The CNS is involved in more than half of cases, producing symptomatic disease in 10%. Epididymoorchitis occurs in 30% of males infected after puberty. The swelling of testicular parenchyma, confined within the tunica albuginea, produces focal infarcts. Mumps orchitis is usually unilateral and, thus, rarely causes sterility. A live attenuated vaccine prevents mumps, and the disease has been largely eliminated from most developed countries.

Intestinal Virus Infections: Rotavirus

Rotavirus infection is the most common cause of severe diarrhea worldwide. The organism produces profuse watery diarrhea that can lead to dehydration and death if untreated. This double-stranded RNA virus usually infects young children. Rotavirus infection spreads from person to person by the oral–fecal route.

 PATHOGENESIS AND PATHOLOGY: Rotavirus infects the enterocytes of the upper small intestine, disrupting the absorption of sugars, fats, and various ions. The resulting osmotic load causes a net loss of fluid into the bowel lumen, producing profuse watery diarrhea and dehydration. Infected cells are shed from intestinal villi, and the regenerating epithelium initially lacks full absorptive capabilities. Pathologic changes in rotavirus infection are largely confined to the duodenum and jejunum, where there is shortening of the intestinal villi, associated with a mild infiltrate of neutrophils and lymphocytes.

Viral Hemorrhagic Fevers

Viral hemorrhagic fevers are a group of at least 20 distinct viral infections that cause varying degrees of hemorrhage and shock and often death. There are many similar viral hemorrhagic fevers in different parts of the world, for the most part named for the area where they were first described. The viral hemorrhagic fevers encompass members of four virus families—the *Bunyaviridae, Flaviviridae, Arenaviridae,* and *Filoviridae*. On the basis of differences in routes of transmission, vectors, and other epidemiologic characteristics, the viral hemorrhagic fevers have been divided into four groups (Table 9-1): mosquito-borne; tick-borne; zoonotic; and the filoviruses, Marburg and Ebola virus, in which the route of transmission is unknown.

Yellow Fever May Lead to Fulminant Hepatic Failure

Yellow fever is an acute hemorrhagic fever, sometimes associated with extensive hepatic necrosis and jaundice. The illness is caused by an insect-borne flavivirus, an enveloped, single-stranded RNA virus. The usual reservoir for the virus is tree-dwelling monkeys, and the agent is passed among them in the forest canopy by mosquitoes. These monkeys serve as a reservoir because the virus does not makes them ill. Humans acquire jungle yellow fever by entering the forest and being bitten by infected *Aedes* mosquitoes. On returning to the village or city, the human victim becomes the reservoir for epidemic yellow fever in the urban setting in Africa or South America, where *Aedes aegypti* is the vector.

 PATHOGENESIS AND PATHOLOGY: On inoculation by the mosquito, the virus multiplies within tissue and vascular endothelium and then disseminates through the bloodstream. The virus has a tropism for liver cells, where it causes coagulative necrosis of hepatocytes, which begins among cells in the middle of hepatic lobules and spreads toward the central veins and portal tracts. In the most severe cases, the entire lobule may be necrotic. Some necrotic hepatocytes lose their nuclei and become intensely eosinophilic Councilman bodies (recognized today as apoptotic bodies). The jaundice in yellow fever results from the hepatic damage. Extensive damage to the endothelium of small blood vessels may lead to a loss of vascular integrity, hemorrhages, and shock, hallmarks of the hemorrhagic fevers.

Ebola and Marburg Hemorrhagic Fevers are Fatal African Diseases

Ebola and Marburg hemorrhagic fevers are severe viral diseases caused by the Ebola and Marburg RNA filoviruses. Both diseases continue to cause sporadic outbreaks in sub-Saharan Africa. Infections with Ebola (Zaire strain) and Marburg viruses have case fatality rates of 80% to 90% in major occurrences. Ebola (Sudan strain) has a somewhat lower fatality rate of about 50%. In the wild, the Ebola virus infects humans, gorillas, chimpanzees, and monkeys. Recent field evidence has implicated several species of fruit bats as the natural reservoir of the Ebola virus. The natural reservoir for Marburg virus remains unknown. Healthcare workers and family members have become infected while treating patients with Ebola and Marburg hemorrhagic fever or during funerary preparation of the bodies of deceased victims. The virus can be transmitted via bodily secretions, blood, and used needles.

 PATHOGENESIS AND PATHOLOGY: *Ebola and Marburg viruses result in the most widespread destructive tissue lesions of all viral hemorrhagic fever agents.* The viruses undergo massive replication in endothelial cells, mononuclear phagocytes, and hepatocytes. Necrosis is most severe in the liver, kidneys, gonads, spleen, and lymph nodes. Characteristic findings in the liver include hepatocellular necrosis, Kupffer cell hyperplasia, Councilman

TABLE 9-1	
Viral Hemorrhagic Fevers	
Vector	Viral Fever
Mosquitoes	Yellow fever Rift Valley fever Dengue hemorrhagic fever Chikungunya hemorrhagic fever
Ticks	Omsk hemorrhagic fever Crimean hemorrhagic fever Kyasanur forest disease
Rodents	Lassa fever Bolivian hemorrhagic fever Argentine hemorrhagic fever Korean hemorrhagic fever
Undefined	Ebola virus disease Marburg virus disease

(acidophilic, apoptotic) bodies, and microsteatosis. The lungs are usually hemorrhagic, and petechial hemorrhages are present in the skin, mucous membranes, and internal organs. Injury to the microvasculature and increased endothelial permeability are important causes of shock. Multiorgan dysfunction syndrome is common and results in death (see Chapter 7).

Human Immunodeficiency Virus (HIV) and Acquired Immunodeficiency Syndrome (AIDS)

AIDS is a widespread disease caused principally by the enveloped RNA retrovirus HIV-1, a member of the lentivirus subfamily. A small minority of patients, primarily in western Africa, are infected with HIV-2, a very similar virus. Persons infected with HIV-1 exhibit a variety of immunologic defects, the most devastating of which is a progressive loss of cellular immunity. Immunosuppression is progressive and may become complete if not treated with appropriate drugs (see Chapter 4 for details on immune aspects and pathology of infection). As a result, rather than dying of HIV infection itself, patients with AIDS usually die of opportunistic infections. There is also a high incidence of malignant tumors, principally B-cell lymphomas and Kaposi sarcoma (KS). Finally, infection of the CNS with HIV often leads to an array of syndromes, ranging from minor cognitive or motor neuron disorders to frank dementia.

HIV is Transmitted by Contact with Blood and Certain Body Fluids

With the exception of intravenous drug users and transfusion recipients, AIDS is transmitted principally as a venereal disease, in both homosexuals and heterosexuals. Transmission to newborns via breast milk is a concern in the developing world. Significant amounts of HIV have been isolated from blood, semen, vaginal secretions, breast milk, and cerebrospinal fluid. Except for the last, HIV in these fluids is both present in lymphocytes and as free virus.

The receptive partner in unprotected anal intercourse is at particularly high risk of becoming infected with HIV. The virus is transmitted via semen through tears in the rectal mucosa, where it can directly infect epithelial cells. In heterosexual contact, transmission from male to female is more likely than the reverse, perhaps reflecting the greater concentration of HIV in semen than in vaginal fluids. Genital lesions, usually caused by other sexually transmitted diseases such as syphilis and HPV, facilitate entry of the virus and lead to a particularly high risk of contracting AIDS.

AIDS is not transmissible by nonsexual, casual exposure to infected persons. In prospective studies of hundreds of health care workers who sustained "needle sticks" or other accidental exposures to

blood from patients with AIDS, fewer than 1% actually seroconverted and became infected with HIV-1. Immediate postexposure prophylaxis with antiretroviral therapy is indicated in such accidental exposures, with the goal of preventing HIV-1 infection. (Specific recommendations are available online at the Centers for Disease Control and Prevention [CDC]. See www.cdc.gov/mmwr/preview/ mmwrhtml/rr5409a1.htm.)

 PATHOGENESIS: Specific target cells for HIV-1 are CD4+ helper T lymphocytes and mononuclear phagocytes, although infection of other cells can occur, such as in B lymphocytes, glial cells, and intestinal epithelial cells. Free HIV or an infected lymphocyte can transmit the virus to an uninfected cell. The HIV envelope glycoprotein, gp120, either on the free virus or on the surface of an infected cell, binds the CD4 molecule on the surface of helper T lymphocytes and other cells, as well as one of a family of β–chemokine receptors. The most important of these chemokine receptors are CXCR4 (on T lymphocytes) and CCR-5 (on many phagocytic cells). Binding of both receptors is necessary for HIV entry. Virus cDNA integrates into the host genome using a viral integrase protein, generating the latent proviral form of HIV-1. Viral genes are replicated along with host DNA and therefore persist for the life of the cell. As memory T cells have long life spans, some experts estimate that even if total suppression of HIV-1 replication were achieved, more than 60 years would be needed for infected T cells to die off. To complete its cycle, nascent virus is assembled in the cytoplasm just beneath the cell membrane and disseminated to other target cells. This is accomplished either by fusion of an infected cell with an uninfected one or by the budding of virions from the plasma membrane of the infected cell (see Fig. 9-1 for details).

The long interval between HIV-1 infection and the appearance of clinical symptoms of AIDS is related to the small number of infected T lymphocytes and viral latency. Only 10^5 to 10^{-4} circulating mononuclear cells display detectable viral messenger RNA, but about 1% of circulating T cells contain proviral DNA. Initiation of viral replication in latent HIV-1 infection depends on the induction of host proteins during T-cell activation. Viral transcription may be activated by many T-cell mitogens and cytokines produced by monocyte/macrophages including tumor necrosis factor (TNF)-α and IL-1, and in addition, by proteins produced by other viruses that infect patients with AIDS, such as herpes virus, EBV, adenovirus, and CMV. *Thus, immune system activation by a variety of infectious agents may promote HIV replication. Active HIV replication and increasing viral loads render such individuals more likely to transmit disease.*

 PATHOLOGY AND CLINICAL FEATURES: Patients recently infected with HIV-1 may have an acute, usually self-limited, infectious mononucleosis-like illness called the **acute retroviral syndrome**, which is associated with intense viremia and a drop in CD4+ T cells. This occurs 2 to 3 weeks after exposure to HIV, before the appearance of antibodies against the virus. Fever, myalgia, lymphadenopathy, sore throat, and a macular rash are common. Most of these symptoms usually resolve within 2 to 3 weeks. Seroconversion occurs 1 to 10 weeks after the onset of this illness. *Thus, the standard HIV-1 enzyme immunoassay and Western blot testing, which depend on the presence of anti–HIV-1 antibodies, are negative during the initial stage of the infection.*

As a patient's immune system begins to recognize the new infection, the viral load drops, and the CD4+ T-cell count begins to climb as a result of a vigorous cytotoxic T-cell response, although a small percentage of persons progress to frank AIDS. After the initial acute syndrome, most newly infected individuals enter a period of latency and slow immune system decline, which averages approximately 10 years before they reach a state of serious immune compromise.

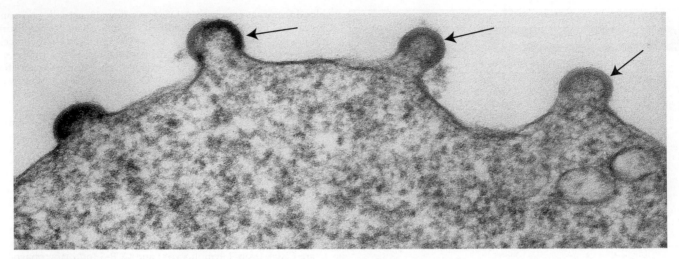

FIGURE 9-1.   Human immunodeficiency virus-1 (HIV-1) virions can be seen budding from infected cells (*arrows*).

During this period, viral replication continues but is constrained by the immune response. However, viral replication virtually always begins to increase, with a concomitant decrease in CD4$^+$ T cells. Nonspecific constitutional symptoms and opportunistic infections begin to appear when CD4$^+$ lymphocyte counts fall below 500/μL. If unrecognized or untreated, the outcome is fulminant immunodeficiency and its fatal complications (Fig. 9-2). As CD4$^+$ T cells fall below 350/μL, patients become much more susceptible to primary or reactivation *Mycobacterium tuberculosis,* which may progress rapidly to severe disease or death. Once CD4$^+$ levels are under 150/μL and CD4:CD8 ratios are less than 0.8, the disease progresses rapidly. A variety of bacteria, viruses, fungi, and protozoa attack the immunocompromised patient. Kaposi sarcoma (KS) and lymphoproliferative disorders may appear, and neurologic disease is common.

Discussion of the diversity of infectious agents that ravage patients with AIDS is beyond the scope of this discussion, and only a few representative examples are mentioned (see Fig. 9-2). It is important to recognize that although most persons with normal immune function will suffer only one infection at a time, HIV-1-infected patients can develop multiple severe infections simultaneously.

Opportunistic Infections, Particularly Polymicrobial Infections, are Common in Patients with AIDS

The majority of patients with HIV-1/AIDS suffer from opportunistic pulmonary infections, although this complication has been greatly reduced through the use of prophylactic antibiotics. *Pneumocystis jiroveci* pneumonia may occur in patients with advanced HIV-1 disease. Lung infection with CMV, *Mycobacterium avium-intracellulare,* and Legionella are less common.

Diarrhea occurs in more than 75% of AIDS patients, often representing simultaneous infections with more than one organism. The most frequent pathogens are protozoans, including *Cryptosporidium, Isospora belli,* and *Giardia lamblia. M. avium-intracellulare* and *Salmonella* species are the most common bacterial cause. CMV infection of the gastrointestinal tract can manifest as a colitis associated with watery diarrhea in patients whose CD4 counts are under 50 cells/μL.

Cryptococcal meningitis is a devastating complication and represents 5% to 8% of all opportunistic infections in patients with AIDS. CNS complications include cerebral toxoplasmosis; primary CNS lymphoma; encephalitis caused by herpes simplex, varicella, or CMV; and progressive multifocal leukoencephalopathy, which is produced by the JC virus.

Virtually all patients with AIDS develop some form of skin disease, infections being the most prominent. *Staphylococcus aureus* is the most common, causing bullous impetigo, deeper purulent le-

sions (ecthyma), and folliculitis. Chronic mucocutaneous herpes simplex infection is so characteristic of AIDS that it is considered an index infection in establishing the diagnosis. Among the most common causes of death in patients with HIV/AIDS is hepatitis C (see Chapter 14). Patients with AIDS, especially homosexual men, are at very high risk for Kaposi sarcoma (KS) (see Chapter 24). In fact, the occurrence of KS in an otherwise healthy person under 60 years is strong evidence of AIDS. KS in AIDS is usually aggressive, often involving viscera such as the gastrointestinal tract or lungs. Lung involvement frequently leads to death. A strain of herpesvirus, namely human herpesvirus 8 (HHV8), is implicated in all forms of KS, including that associated with AIDS.

DNA VIRUSES

Herpes Viruses

The virus family Herpesviridae includes a large number of enveloped, DNA viruses, many of which infect humans. Almost all herpes viruses express some common antigenic determinants, and many produce type A nuclear inclusions (acidophilic bodies surrounded by a halo). The most important human pathogens among the herpes viruses are varicella-zoster, herpes simplex, EBV, human herpesvirus 6 (HHV6, the cause of roseola), and CMV. Recently, HHV8 was implicated in the pathogenesis of KS in HIV-infected patients. These viruses are also distinguished by their capacity to remain latent for long periods of time.

Varicella-Zoster Infection Causes Chickenpox and Herpes Zoster

The first exposure to varicella-zoster virus (VZV) produces chickenpox, an acute systemic illness, which has a dominant feature of generalized vesicular skin eruption (Fig. 9-3). The virus then becomes latent, and its reactivation in ganglion cells later in life causes herpes zoster ("shingles"). The virus travels down the sensory nerve for a single dermatome. It then infects the corresponding epidermis, producing a localized, painful vesicular eruption.

VZV is restricted to human hosts and spreads from person to person primarily by the respiratory route. It can also be spread by contact with secretions from skin lesions. The virus is present worldwide and is highly contagious. Most children in the United States are infected by early school age, but an effective vaccine has reduced this incidence. An adult VZV vaccine has recently proved effective in reducing the incidence of herpes zoster.

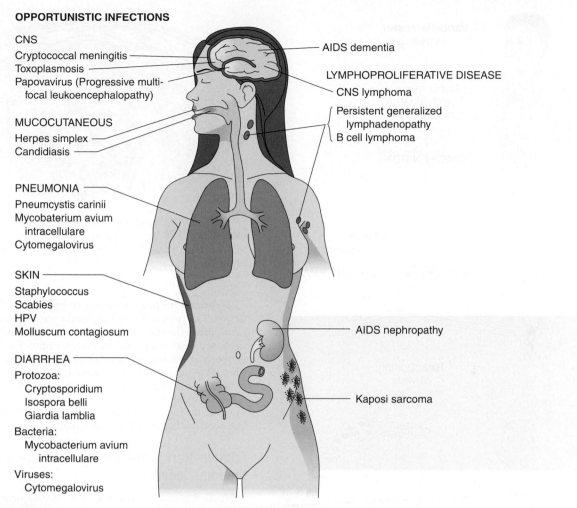

OPPORTUNISTIC INFECTIONS

CNS
Cryptococcal meningitis
Toxoplasmosis
Papovavirus (Progressive multi-
  focal leukoencephalopathy)

MUCOCUTANEOUS
Herpes simplex
Candidiasis

PNEUMONIA
Pneumcystis carinii
Mycobaterium avium
  intracellulare
Cytomegalovirus

SKIN
Staphylococcus
Scabies
HPV
Molluscum contagiosum

DIARRHEA
Protozoa:
  Cryptosporidium
  Isospora belli
  Giardia lamblia
Bacteria:
  Mycobacterium avium
    intracellulare
Viruses:
  Cytomegalovirus

AIDS dementia

LYMPHOPROLIFERATIVE DISEASE
CNS lymphoma
Persistent generalized
  lymphadenopathy
B cell lymphoma

AIDS nephropathy

Kaposi sarcoma

FIGURE 9-2. **Human immunodeficiency virus-1 (HIV-1)–mediated destruction of the cellular immune system results in acquired immunodeficiency syndrome (AIDS).** The infectious and neoplastic complications of AIDS can affect practically every organ system. CNS, central nervous system; HPV, human papilloma virus.

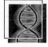**PATHOGENESIS AND PATHOLOGY:** VZV initially infects cells of the respiratory tract or conjunctival epithelium. There it reproduces and spreads through the blood and lymphatic systems. Many organs are infected during this viremic stage, but skin involvement usually dominates the clinical picture. Skin lesions begin as maculopapules that rapidly evolve into vesicles and then pustules that soon ulcerate and crust. The virus spreads from the capillary endothelium to the epidermis, where its replication destroys the basal cells. As a result, the upper layers of the epidermis separate from the basal layer to form vesicles that fill with neutrophils and soon erode to become shallow ulcers. In infected cells, VZV produces a characteristic cytopathic effect, consisting of nuclear homogenization and intranuclear inclusions (Cowdry type A). The inclusion is large and eosinophilic and is separated from the nuclear membrane by a clear zone (halo). Multinucleated cells are common (Fig. 9-4). During primary infection, VZV establishes latent infection in perineuronal satellite cells of the dorsal nerve root ganglia. Transcription of viral genes continues during latency, and viral DNA can be demonstrated years after the initial infection. The skin lesions of chickenpox and shingles are identical and are also similar to the lesions of herpes simplex virus (HSV) (see below).

Herpesvirus (HSV) Produces Necrotizing Infections at Diverse Body Sites

HSVs are common human viral pathogens, which most frequently produce recurrent painful vesicular eruptions of the skin and mucous membranes (Table 9-2). HSV spreads from person to person, primarily through direct contact with infected secretions or open lesions. Two antigenically and epidemiologically distinct HSVs cause human disease (Fig. 9-5). Clusters of painful, ulcerating, vesicular lesions on the skin or mucous membranes are the most frequent manifestation of HSV infection. These lesions persist for 1 to 2 weeks and then resolve.

- **HSV-1** is transmitted in oral secretions and typically causes disease "above the waist," including oral, facial, and ocular lesions.
- **HSV-2** is transmitted in genital secretions and typically produces disease "below the waist," including genital ulcers and neonatal herpes infection acquired by passage through the infected birth canal.

PATHOGENESIS AND PATHOLOGY: Primary HSV disease occurs at a site of initial viral inoculation, such as the oropharynx, genital mucosa, or skin. The virus infects epithelial cells, producing progeny viruses and destroying basal cells in the squamous epithelium, with resulting formation of vesicles. Cell necrosis also elicits an inflammatory response, initially dominated by neutrophils and then followed by lymphocytes. The cellular alterations are similar to those produced by VZV (see Fig. 9-4). Primary infection resolves with the development of humoral- and cell-mediated immunity to the virus. Latent infection is established in a manner analogous to that of VZV. Upon reactivation, HSV travels back down the nerve to the epithelial site served by the ganglion, where it again infects epithelial cells. Sometimes, this

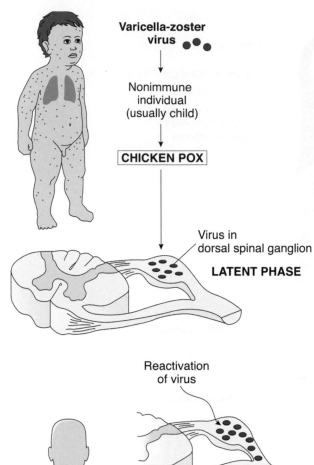

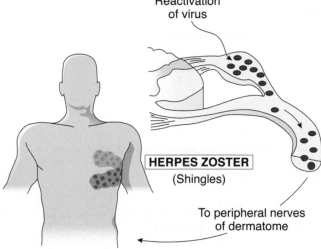

FIGURE 9-3. **Varicella (chickenpox) and herpes zoster (shingles).** Varicella-zoster virus (VZV) in droplets is inhaled by a nonimmune person (usually a child) and initially causes a "silent" infection of the nasopharynx. This progresses to viremia, seeding of fixed macrophages and dissemination of VZV to skin (chickenpox) and viscera. VZV resides in a dorsal spinal ganglion, where it remains dormant for many years. Latent VZV is reactivated and spreads from ganglia along the sensory nerves to the peripheral nerves of sensory dermatomes, causing shingles.

secondary infection produces ulcerating vesicular lesions. At other times, the secondary infection does not cause visible tissue destruction, but contagious progeny viruses are shed from the site of infection. Both HSV-1 and HSV-2 can cause severe protracted and disseminated disease in immunocompromised persons.

Herpes encephalitis is a rare (1 in 100,000 HSV infections), but devastating manifestation of HSV-1 infection. In some instances, it occurs when a virus that is latent in the trigeminal ganglion is reactivated and travels retrograde to the brain. However, herpes encephalitis also occurs in people who have no history of "cold sores" (see Chapter 28). Equally rare is **herpes hepatitis**, which may occur in immunocompromised patients but has also been reported in young, previously healthy, pregnant women.

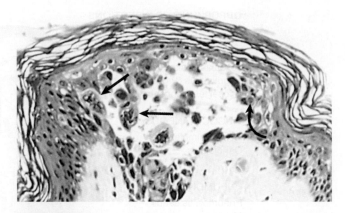

FIGURE 9-4. **Varicella.** Photomicrograph of the skin from a patient with chickenpox shows an intraepidermal vesicle. Multinucleated giant cells (*straight arrows*) and nuclear inclusions (*curved arrow*) are present.

Neonatal herpes is a serious complication of maternal genital herpes. The virus is transmitted to the fetus from the infected birth canal, often the uterine cervix, and readily disseminates in the unprotected newborn child. The disease begins 5 to 7 days after delivery, with irritability, lethargy, and a mucocutaneous vesicular eruption. The infection rapidly spreads to involve multiple organs, including the brain. The infected newborn develops jaundice, bleeding problems, respiratory distress, seizures, and coma. Treatment of severe HSV infections with acyclovir is often effective, but neonatal herpes still carries a high mortality rate.

Epstein-Barr Virus (EBV) is the Cause of Infectious Mononucleosis

Infectious mononucleosis is a viral disease characterized by fever, pharyngitis, lymphadenopathy, and increased circulating lymphocytes. By adulthood, most persons have been infected with EBV. Infection in early childhood is usually asymptomatic, but two thirds of individuals with primary infections occurring in adolescence or early adulthood develop infectious mononucleosis. EBV has also been associated with several cancers, including African Burkitt lymphoma, B-cell lymphoma in immunosuppressed persons, and nasopharyngeal carcinoma. These neoplastic complications are discussed in Chapters 5, 20, and 25.

EBV spreads from person to person primarily through contact with infected oral secretions. Once it enters the body, EBV remains for life, analogous to latent infections with other herpesviruses. A few people (10% to 20%) intermittently shed the virus. Transmission requires close contact with infected persons. Thus, EBV spreads readily among young children in crowded conditions, where there is considerable "sharing" of oral secretions.

TABLE 9-2		
Herpes Simplex Viral Diseases		
Viral Type	Common Presentations	Infrequent Presentations
HSV-1	Oral-labial herpes	Conjunctivitis, keratitis Encephalitis Herpetic whitlow Esophagitis* Pneumonia* Disseminated infection*
HSV-2	Genital herpes	Perinatal infection Disseminated infection*

*These conditions usually occur in immunocompromised hosts.

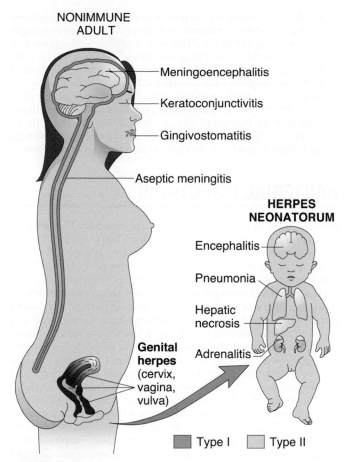

NONIMMUNE ADULT

- Meningoencephalitis
- Keratoconjunctivitis
- Gingivostomatitis
- Aseptic meningitis

Genital herpes (cervix, vagina, vulva)

HERPES NEONATORUM

- Encephalitis
- Pneumonia
- Hepatic necrosis
- Adrenalitis

Type I ▮ Type II ▯

FIGURE 9-5. **Herpesvirus infections.** HSV-1 infects a nonimmune adult, causing gingivostomatitis ("fever blister" or "cold sore"), keratoconjunctivitis, meningoencephalitis, and aseptic spinal meningitis. HSV-2 infects the genitalia of a nonimmune adult, involving the cervix, vagina, and vulva. HSV-2 infects the fetus as it passes through the birth canal of an infected mother. The infant's lack of a mature immune system results in disseminated infection with HSV-1. The infection is often fatal, involving the lung, liver, adrenal glands, and central nervous system.

PATHOGENESIS AND PATHOLOGY: The virus first binds to and infects nasopharyngeal cells and then B lymphocytes, which carry the virus throughout the body, producing a generalized infection of lymphoid tissues and spleen. The resultant asymmetric lymphadenopathy is most striking in the neck. Microscopically, the general nodal architecture is preserved. The germinal centers are enlarged and have indistinct margins because of a proliferation of immunoblasts. The nodes contain occasional large hyperchromatic cells with polylobular nuclei that resemble Reed-Sternberg cells. In fact, the appearance of the lymph nodes histology may be difficult to distinguish from that of Hodgkin disease or other lymphomas (see Chapter 20). The liver is almost always involved, and the sinusoids and portal tracts contain atypical lymphocytes.

A distinguishing feature of infectious mononucleosis is a lymphocytosis with atypical lymphocytes. The atypical cells (characterized by lobulated, eccentric nuclei and vacuolated cytoplasm) are activated T cells, which are involved in the suppression and killing of polyclonally stimulated EBV-infected B lymphocytes.

Cytomegalovirus (CMV) Infects Many Persons but Rarely Produces Disease

CMV is a congenital and opportunistic pathogen that usually produces an asymptomatic infection. However, the fetus and immunocompro-

mised persons are particularly vulnerable to the destructive effects of the virus. CMV (a member of the TORCH complex) crosses the placenta, infects 0.5% to 2.0% of all fetuses, and injures 10% to 20% of those infected, making it the most common congenital pathogen. The brain, inner ears, eyes, liver, and bone marrow are the most common fetal organ systems affected (see Chapter 6).

PATHOGENESIS AND PATHOLOGY: CMV infects various human cells, including epithelial cells, lymphocytes, and monocytes, and establishes latency in white blood cells. The normal immune response rapidly controls CMV infection; infected persons rarely show ill effects, although they shed the virus periodically in body secretions. Like other herpes viruses, CMV may remain latent for life. Microscopically, the lesions of fetal CMV disease show cellular necrosis and a characteristic cytopathic effect, consisting of marked cellular and nuclear enlargement, with nuclear and cytoplasmic inclusions. The giant nucleus, which is usually solitary, contains a large central inclusion surrounded by a clear zone (Fig. 9-6). The cytoplasmic inclusions are less prominent.

CLINICAL FEATURES: When an infected pregnant woman passes CMV to her fetus, the fetus is not protected by maternally derived antibodies, and the virus invades fetal cells with little initial immunologic response, causing widespread necrosis and inflammation. CMV disease in immunosuppressed patients has diverse clinical manifestations. It can manifest as decreased visual acuity (chorioretinitis), diarrhea or gastrointestinal hemorrhage (colonic ulcerations), change in mental status (encephalitis), shortness of breath (pneumonitis), or a wide range of other symptoms.

Human Papillomavirus (HPV)

HPVs cause proliferative lesions of squamous epithelium, including common warts, flat warts, plantar warts, anogenital warts (condyloma acuminatum), and laryngeal papillomatosis. Some HPV serotypes cause squamous cell dysplasia and squamous cell carcinomas of the female genital tract (see Chapter 18).

HPVs are nonenveloped, double-stranded DNA viruses. More than 100 types of HPV are known, and different types are associated with different lesions. Thus, HPV types 1, 2, and 4 produce common warts and plantar warts. Types 6, 10, 11, and 40 through 45 cause anogenital warts. Types 16, 18, and 31 are associated with

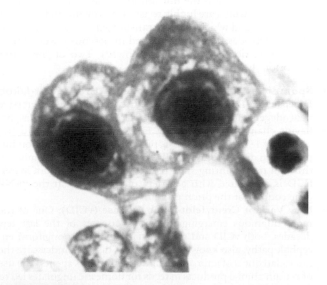

FIGURE 9-6. **Cytomegalovirus pneumonitis.** Type II pneumocytes display enlarged nuclei containing solitary inclusions surrounded by a clear zone.

squamous carcinoma of the female genital tract. HPV infection is widespread and is transmitted from person to person by direct contact. The viruses that cause genital lesions are transmitted sexually.

PATHOGENESIS AND PATHOLOGY: HPV infection begins with viral inoculation into a stratified squamous epithelium where the virus enters the nuclei of basal cells. Some infected cells display a characteristic cytopathic effect, termed **koilocytosis**, which features large squamous cells with shrunken nuclei enveloped in large cytoplasmic vacuoles (koilocytes). Infection stimulates replication of the squamous epithelium, producing the various HPV-associated proliferative lesions. The rapidly growing squamous epithelium replicates innumerable progeny viruses, which are shed in the degenerating superficial cells. Many HPV lesions resolve spontaneously, although depressed cell-mediated immunity is associated with the persistence and spread of HPV lesions. The mechanism by which HPV infections participate in malignant change is discussed in Chapter 5.

Common warts (verruca vulgaris) are firm, circumscribed, raised, rough-surfaced lesions, which usually appear on surfaces subject to trauma, especially the hands. **Plantar warts** are similar squamous proliferative lesions on the soles of the feet but are compressed inward by standing and walking.

Anogenital warts (condyloma acuminatum) are soft, raised, fleshy lesions found on the penis, vulva, vaginal wall, cervix, or perianal region. When caused by certain HPV types, flat warts can develop into malignant squamous cell proliferations. The relationship between HPV, cervical intraepithelial neoplasia, and invasive squamous carcinoma of the cervix is discussed in Chapter 18.

PRIONS: A NEW DISEASE PARADIGM

In the last several decades, it has become clear that infection can be transmitted and propagated solely by proteins without the participation of nucleic acids. These protein aggregates, termed **prions**, are only known to cause CNS disease, the prototype being Kuru, a now-extinct disease of the Fore people of New Guinea transmitted by cannibalism. Prions are essentially misfolded proteins that aggregate in the CNS and cause progressive neurodegeneration that leads to death. The prion protein (PrP) exists in a normal isoform and in a pathogenic form that can transmit the disease. These pathogenic isoforms aggregate into prion rods, which are a diagnostic characteristic of these rare disorders. Of particular importance is the uncommon persistence of these infectious agents, which are highly resistant to the normal methods of sterilization and which may be transmitted via surgical instruments or electrodes that are implanted in nervous tissue (unless special sterilization protocols are followed). Two of the better known prion diseases are:

- **Sporadic, Familial, and Iatrogenic Creutzfeldt-Jakob Disease (sCJD, fCJD, and iCJD):** CJD is a rapidly progressive neurodegenerative disorder characterized by myoclonus, behavior changes, and dementia (see Chapter 28). With a frequency of 1/1,000,000, sCJD is probably the most common human prion disease. Rarely, iCJD has resulted from transmission through transplanting such tissues as cornea and dura mater. fCJD is associated with a variety of mutations in the PRNP gene coding for the prion protein.
- **New Variant Creutzfeldt-Jakob Disease (vCJD):** One of the more infamous emerging infectious diseases of the last few decades, both vCJD and the associated bovine spongiform encephalopathy, also known as "mad cow" disease, underscore the interrelatedness of animal and human infectious agents. The use of certain animal products in feeds for domestic ungulates led to a prion disease epidemic, initially in cattle herds in the United Kingdom and subsequently found in many other countries. Nearly 150 persons have been infected with this relentless termi-

nal disease, presumably contracted by eating the meat of infected animals. To date, all patients have been homozygous for methionine at codon 129 of the PRNP gene that encodes the prion protein, a condition found in about 40% of Europeans. The same homozygous residue is also found in most (but not all) cases of sCJD. Although the mean onset of sCJD has been 65 years of age, vCJD has mainly occurred in young adults, with a mean age of 26 years. Psychiatric signs and symptoms have also been predominant in vCJD. Pathologic changes in vCJD are strikingly similar to those seen in bovine spongiform encephalopathy, although they differ somewhat from changes seen in the sporadic form.

BACTERIAL INFECTIONS

Bacteria, at 0.1 to 10 μm, are the smallest living cells. They are classified according to the structural features of their envelope. The simplest envelope found in mycoplasmas is only a phospholipid–protein bilayer membrane. Most bacteria, however, have a rigid cell wall that surrounds the cell membrane. Two types of bacterial cell walls are identified by their Gram-stain properties. Gram-positive bacteria stain dark blue and have cell walls containing teichoic acids and a thick peptidoglycan layer. Gram-negative bacteria stain red and have an outer membrane containing a lipopolysaccharide component known as endotoxin, a potent mediator of shock (see Chapter 7). Both classes of bacteria may be surrounded by an additional layer of polysaccharide or protein gel (a capsule), which contributes to the virulence of the organism; hence, bacteria may also be classified as **encapsulated** or **unencapsulated**. The cell wall confers rigidity to bacteria and allows them to be distinguished on the basis of shape and pattern of growth in cultures. Round or oval bacteria are **cocci**. Those that grow in clusters are called **staphylococci**, whereas those that grow in chains are called **streptococci**. Elongate bacteria are **rods** or **bacilli**, and curved ones are **vibrios**. Some spiral-shaped bacteria are called **spirochetes**.

Pyogenic Gram-Positive Cocci

Staphylococcus aureus Produces Suppurative Infections

S. aureus *is a gram-positive coccus that typically grows in clusters and is one of the most common bacterial pathogens.* It normally resides on the skin, is spread by direct contact, and is readily inoculated into deeper tissues. *It is the most common cause of suppurative infections of the skin, joints, and bones, and is a leading cause of infective endocarditis.* S. aureus is commonly distinguished from other, less virulent staphylococci by the coagulase test. *S. aureus* is coagulase-positive; the other staphylococci are coagulase-negative.

PATHOGENESIS: Many *S. aureus* infections begin as localized infections of the skin and skin appendages, producing cellulitis and abscesses filled with pus and bacteria. The organism, equipped with destructive enzymes and toxins, sometimes invades beyond the initial site, spreading by the blood or lymphatics to almost any location in the body. The bones, joints, and heart valves are the most common sites of metastatic *S. aureus* infections. The organism also causes several distinct diseases by elaborating toxins that are carried to distant sites.

CLINICAL FEATURES: The clinical manifestations of *S. aureus* disease vary according to the sites and types of infection.

- **Furuncles (boils) and carbuncles:** Deep-seated *S. aureus* infections occur in and around hair follicles, often in a nasal carrier.

The boil begins as a nodule at the base of a hair follicle, followed by a pimple that remains painful and red for a few days. A yellow apex forms, and the central core becomes pus-filled, soft, and necrotic. Rupture or incision of the boil relieves the pain. Carbuncles result from coalescent furuncles and produce draining sinuses.

- **Scalded skin syndrome:** This disease affects infants and children under 3 years of age, who present with a sunburn-like rash that begins on the face and spreads over the body. Bullae begin to form, and even gentle rubbing causes the skin to desquamate. The disease begins to resolve in 1 to 2 weeks, as the skin regenerates. Desquamation is due to systemic effects of a specific exotoxin, often from an unknown site of infection.
- **Osteomyelitis:** Acute staphylococcal osteomyelitis, usually in the bones of the legs, most commonly afflicts boys between 3 and 10 years old, most of whom have a history of infection or trauma. Osteomyelitis may become chronic if not properly treated. Adults older than 50 are more frequently afflicted with vertebral osteomyelitis, which may follow staphylococcal infections of the skin or urinary tract, prostatic surgery, or pinning of a fracture.
- **Respiratory tract infections:** Staphylococcal respiratory tract infections are most common in infants under 2 years of age and especially under 2 months. The infection is characterized by ulcers of the upper airway, scattered foci of pneumonia, pleural effusions, empyema, and pneumothorax. In adults, staphylococcal pneumonia may follow viral influenza, which destroys the ciliated surface epithelium and leaves the bronchial surface vulnerable to secondary infection.
- **Bacterial arthritis:** *S. aureus* is the causative organism in half of all cases of septic arthritis, mostly in patients 50 to 70 years old. Rheumatoid arthritis and corticosteroid therapy are common predisposing conditions.
- **Septicemia:** Septicemia with *S. aureus* afflicts patients with lowered resistance who are in the hospital for other diseases. Miliary abscesses and endocarditis are serious complications.
- **Bacterial endocarditis:** Bacterial endocarditis is a common serious complication of *S. aureus* septicemia (see Chapter 11).
- **Toxic shock syndrome:** This disorder most commonly afflicts menstruating women who present with high fever, nausea, vomiting, diarrhea, and myalgias. Subsequently, they develop shock and within several days, a sunburn-like rash. The disease is associated with use of tampons, which provide a site for replication and toxin elaboration by *S. aureus* but can occur in nontampon users. Toxic shock syndrome occurs rarely in children and men and when it does, it is usually associated with an occult *S. aureus* infection.
- **Staphylococcal food poisoning:** Staphylococcal food poisoning typically begins less than 6 hours after a meal. Nausea and vomiting begin abruptly and usually resolve within 12 hours. This disease is caused by preformed toxin, rather than by secretion of toxin by ingested bacteria.

Antibiotic-Resistant *S. aureus* Presents an Increasing Clinical Challenge

One of the most important clinical issues concerning S. aureus is the relentless increase in antibiotic resistance that has occurred over the last 6 decades. Today, methicillin-resistant *S. aureus* (MRSA) infections represent one of the most dreaded of nosocomial infections. According to the CDC, between 1995 and 2004, the percentage of MRSA infections in patients in intensive care units almost doubled, from slightly over one-third to almost two-thirds. The recent increase in **community-acquired** MRSA raises concerns of dissemination of antibiotic resistance among *Staphylococcus* and other bacteria.

Streptococcus pyogenes Causes Suppurative, Toxin-Related, and Immunologic Reactions

S. pyogenes, also known as group A streptococcus, is one of the most common human bacterial pathogens, causing many diseases of diverse organ systems, from acute self-limited pharyngitis to major illnesses such as rheumatic fever (Fig. 9-7). *S. pyogenes* is a gram-positive coccus that is frequently part of the endogenous flora of the skin and oropharynx.

Diseases caused by *S. pyogenes* fall into two categories, namely suppurative and nonsuppurative. Suppurative diseases occur at sites where the bacteria invade and cause tissue necrosis, usually inducing an acute inflammatory response. Suppurative *S. pyogenes* infections include pharyngitis, impetigo, cellulitis, myositis, pneumonia, and puerperal sepsis. By contrast, nonsuppurative diseases occur at locations remote from the site of bacterial invasion. *S. pyogenes* causes two major nonsuppurative complications: rheumatic fever and acute poststreptococcal glomerulonephritis. Rheumatic fever is discussed in Chapter 11 and poststreptococcal glomerulonephritis in Chapter 16.

Streptococcal Pharyngitis ("Strep Throat")

S. pyogenes is the common bacterial cause of pharyngitis with associated fever, malaise, headache, and elevated leukocyte count. It spreads from person to person by direct contact with oral or respiratory secretions. "Strep throat" occurs worldwide, predominantly affecting children and adolescents. *Streptococcal pharyngitis may lead to rheumatic fever or acute poststreptococcal glomerulonephritis if not promptly treated with penicillin.*

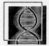 **PATHOGENESIS:** *S. pyogenes* attaches to epithelial cells by binding to fibronectin on their surface. The bacterium produces hemolysins, DNAase, hyaluronidase, and streptokinase, which allow it to damage and invade human tissues. A bacterial cell wall component, designated **M protein**, is associated with virulence and prevents complement deposition, thereby protecting bacteria from phagocytosis. The invading organism elicits an acute inflammatory response, often producing an exudate of neutrophils in the tonsillar fossae.

Scarlet Fever

Scarlet fever describes a punctate red rash on skin and mucous membranes seen in some cases of Streptococcal pharyngitis and occasionally other S. pyogenes infections. The rash is associated with production of a bacterial erythrogenic toxin.

Erysipelas

Erysipelas is an erythematous swelling of the skin caused chiefly by S. pyogenes. The rash usually begins on the face and spreads rapidly. A diffuse, edematous, acute inflammatory reaction in the epidermis and dermis extends into subcutaneous tissues. The inflammatory infiltrate is principally composed of neutrophils and is most intense around vessels and adnexa of the skin. Cutaneous microabscesses and small foci of necrosis are common.

Impetigo

Impetigo (pyoderma) is a localized, intraepidermal infection of the skin that is caused by S. pyogenes or S. aureus and most commonly seen in children. The strains of *S. pyogenes* that cause impetigo are antigenically and epidemiologically distinct from those that cause pharyngitis. Minor trauma or an insect bite inoculates the bacteria into the skin, where they form an intraepidermal pustule, which ruptures and leaks a purulent exudate.

Streptococcal Cellulitis

S. pyogenes causes an acute spreading infection of the loose connective tissue of the deeper layers of the dermis. This suppurative infection results from traumatic inoculation of microorganisms into the skin and frequently occurs on the extremities in the context of impaired lymphatic drainage.

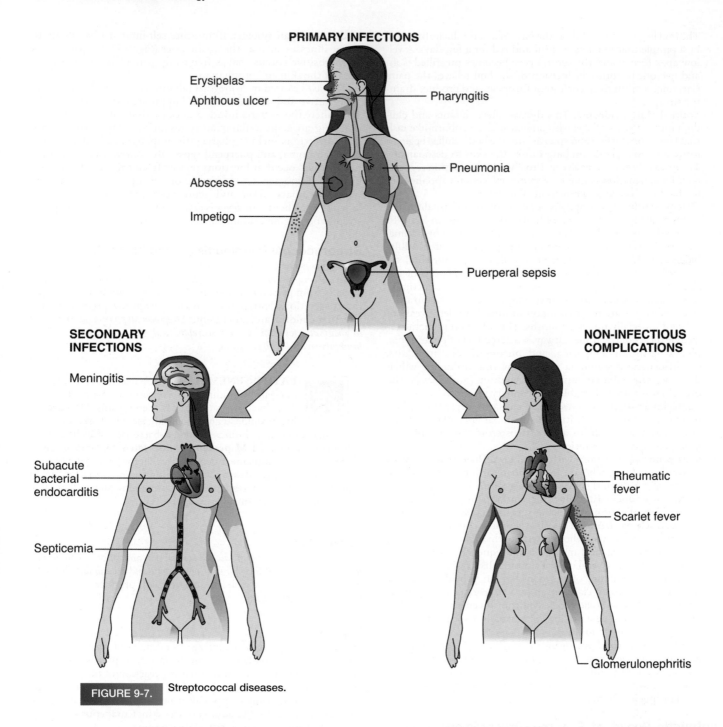

FIGURE 9-7. Streptococcal diseases.

Streptococcus pneumoniae Infection is a Major Cause of Lobar Pneumonia

Streptococcus pneumoniae is an aerobic, gram-positive diplococcus, often simply called **pneumococcus**, which causes pyogenic infections, primarily involving the lungs (pneumonia), middle ear (otitis media), sinuses (sinusitis), and meninges (meningitis). *It is one of the most common bacterial pathogens of humans, and by age 5, most children in the world have suffered from at least one episode of pneumococcal disease (usually otitis media).* S. pneumoniae is a commensal organism in the oropharynx, and virtually all persons are colonized at some time.

 PATHOGENESIS: Pneumococcal pneumonia commonly arises in the wake of viral, smoking, or alcohol-related injury to the mucociliary blanket and cough response that allows *S. pneumoniae* access to the lower airway. Once in the alveoli, the organisms proliferate and elicit

an acute inflammatory response. Unlike pneumonia caused by *Staphylococcus aureus,* which can cause permanent lung damage, pneumonia caused by *S. pneumoniae* often resolves completely. Invasive disease generally occurs in the setting of an illness that compromises the host's ability to opsonize the bacteria. Splenectomized patients have a high risk of fulminant disease and septic shock. The pathogenesis and clinical features of pneumococcal infections are discussed further in Chapter 12.

Bacterial Infections of Childhood

Diphtheria is a Necrotizing Upper Respiratory Tract Infection

Infection with *Corynebacterium diphtheriae,* an aerobic, pleomorphic, gram-positive rod may lead to cardiac and neurologic disturbances via toxin production. Humans are the only known reservoir for *C. diphtheria,* which spreads from person to person in respiratory droplets or oral secretions. Immunization has largely eliminated the disease in developed countries, but it persists in areas lacking aggressive vaccination programs.

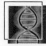 **PATHOGENESIS AND PATHOLOGY:** *C. diphtheriae* enters the pharynx and proliferates, often on the tonsils, producing a characteristic *pseudomembrane.* This lesion is composed of sloughed epithelium, necrotic debris, neutrophils, fibrin, and bacteria that line affected respiratory passages. The inflammatory process in the mucosal epithelium below the membrane often produces swelling in the surrounding soft tissues, which can be severe enough to cause respiratory compromise. Diphtheria toxin produced by some bacterial strains is absorbed systemically and acts on tissues throughout the body; the heart, nerves, and kidneys are most susceptible to damage. When the heart is affected, the myocardium displays fat droplets in the myocytes and focal necrosis. In the case of neural involvement, the affected peripheral nerves exhibit demyelination.

Pertussis is Characterized by Debilitating Paroxysmal Coughing

Pertussis infection, commonly called whooping cough, is a prolonged upper respiratory tract illness, which lasts 4 to 5 weeks. It is characterized by paroxysmal coughing, followed by a long, high-pitched inspiration, the "whoop," which gives the disease its common name. The causative organism is *Bordetella pertussis,* a small, gram-negative coccobacillus, which is highly contagious and spreads from person to person, primarily by infected respiratory aerosols. Pertussis is primarily a disease of children younger than the age of 5 years, although the incidence is increasing among adults.

 PATHOGENESIS: *B. pertussis* initiates infection by attaching to the cilia of respiratory epithelial cells. The organism then elaborates a cytotoxin that results in necrosis of the ciliated respiratory epithelium and an acute inflammatory response, thereby producing an extensive tracheobronchitis. Vaccination protects against *B. pertussis,* but worldwide, there are approximately 50 million cases of pertussis each year, resulting in almost 1 million deaths, particularly in infants, who often die from secondary pneumonia.

Haemophilus influenzae Causes Pyogenic Infections in Young Children

Haemophilus influenzae *infections involve the middle ear, sinuses, facial skin, epiglottis, meninges, lungs, and joints and are the most common cause of meningitis in children younger than 2 years of age.* The organism is a major pediatric bacterial pathogen with the incidence of serious disease peaking at 6 to 18 months of age. The bacteria is an aerobic, pleomorphic, gram-negative coccobacillus, which spreads from person to person in respiratory droplets and secretions. Nonencapsulated strains (type a) usually produce localized infections; encapsulated strains, designated type b, are more virulent and cause more than 95% of the invasive bacteremic infections. Inoculating infants with a specific vaccine has greatly reduced H. influenzae type b disease, particularly meningitis, in children.

PATHOGENESIS: *H. influenzae* type b is capable of invading tissue and eliciting a strong acute inflammatory response. The capsular polysaccharide of type b organisms allows them to evade phagocytosis, and bacteremic infections are common. Epiglottitis, facial cellulitis, septic arthritis, and meningitis result from invasive bacteremic infections. *H. influenzae* type b also elaborates an IgA protease, which facilitates local survival of the organism in the respiratory tract.

 CLINICAL FEATURES

- *H. influenzae* **meningitis** is characterized by predominantly acute, inflammatory, leptomeningeal infiltrates, sometimes involving the subarachnoid space.
- *H. influenzae* **pneumonia** usually complicates chronic lung disease. In half of patients, it follows a viral infection of the respiratory tract. The alveoli are filled with neutrophils, macrophages containing bacilli, and fibrin. The bronchiolar epithelium is necrotic and infiltrated by macrophages.
- *H. influenzae* **epiglottitis** is characterized by swelling and acute inflammation of the epiglottis, aryepiglottic folds, and pyriform sinuses. It may sometimes completely obstruct the upper airway.

Neisseria meningitidis Causes Pyogenic Meningitis and Overwhelming Shock

Neisseria meningitidis, *commonly termed* **meningococcus**, *produces disseminated blood-borne infections, often accompanied by shock and profound disturbances in coagulation.* The organism is aerobic, appears as paired, bean-shaped, gram-negative cocci and is spread from person to person, primarily by respiratory droplets. Meningococcal diseases appear as sporadic cases, clusters of cases, and epidemics (the last seen most frequently in crowded quarters). Most infections in industrialized countries are sporadic and afflict children under the age of 5.

 PATHOGENESIS AND PATHOLOGY: On colonizing the upper respiratory tract, *N. meningitidis* attaches to nonciliated respiratory epithelium by means of its pili. If the organism spreads to the bloodstream before the development of protective immunity, it can proliferate rapidly in unprotected human tissue, resulting in fulminant meningococcal disease. Meningococcal disease can be confined to the CNS, with the leptomeninges and subarachnoid space infiltrated with neutrophils and the underlying brain parenchyma swollen and congested. The organism may also be disseminated throughout the body (septicemia), resulting in diffuse damage to the endothelium of small blood vessels, with widespread petechiae and purpura in the skin and viscera.

Many of the systemic effects of meningococcal disease are due to the endotoxin of the outer membrane lipopolysaccharide, which promotes an increase in production of TNF by macrophages and the simultaneous activation of the complement and coagulation cascades. Disseminated intravascular coagulation, fibrinolysis, and shock follow abruptly. Vasculitis and thrombosis rarely (3% to 4% of all cases) produce hemorrhagic necrosis of both adrenals, called the **Waterhouse-Friderichsen syndrome**. Meningococcal disease was once almost invariably fatal, but antibiotic treatment has reduced the mortality rate to less than 15%.

Sexually Transmitted Bacterial Diseases

Gonorrhea Remains a Common Infection that Causes Sterility

Neisseria gonorrhoeae, *also termed* **gonococcus**, *causes gonorrhea, an acute suppurative genital tract infection, which is reflected in urethritis in men and endocervicitis in women. It may ascend the female genital tract to produce endometritis, salpingitis, and pelvic inflammatory disease.* N. gonorrhoeae is an aerobic, bean-shaped, gram-negative diplococcus. Neonatal infections derived from the birth canal of a mother with gonorrhea usually manifest as conjunctivitis, although disseminated infections are occasionally seen. Except for perinatal transmission, spread is almost always by sexual intercourse.

PATHOGENESIS AND PATHOLOGY: Gonorrhea is a suppurative infection, which begins in the mucous membranes of the urogenital tract (Fig. 9-8). Bacteria attach to surface cells using hair-like extensions, termed "pili," which project from the gonococcal cell wall. The pili contain a protease that digests IgA on the mucous membrane, thereby facilitating the attachment of the bacterium to the columnar and transitional epithelium of the urogenital tract. After attachment, the bacteria invade superficially, provoking acute inflammation and the formation of copious pus and often-submucosal abscesses. Men present with purulent urethral discharge and dysuria, which, if left untreated, may lead to stricture and extension of the infection in the genitourinary tract. In about one half of infected women, gonorrhea remains asymptomatic. Symptomatic women initially exhibit endocervicitis, with a vaginal discharge or bleeding and dysuria. Infection often extends to produce acute and chronic salpingitis and eventually pelvic inflammatory disease. The fallopian tubes swell with pus, causing acute abdominal pain. Infertility occurs when inflammatory adhesions block the tubes.

Syphilis (lues)

Syphilis (lues) is a chronic, sexually transmitted, systemic infection caused by *Treponema pallidum*. The disease is discussed below under Diseases Caused by Spirochetes.

Enteropathogenic Bacterial Infections

Escherichia coli is a Common Cause of Diarrhea and Urinary Tract Infections

E. coli *is among the most common and important human bacterial pathogens, causing more than 90% of all urinary tract infections and many cases of diarrheal illness worldwide.* It is also a major opportunistic pathogen and frequently causes pneumonia and sepsis in immunocompromised hosts and meningitis and sepsis in newborns.

E. coli comprises a group of diverse, aerobic (facultatively anaerobic), gram-negative bacteria. Most strains are intestinal commensals, well adapted to grow in the human colon without harming the host. However, *E. coli* can be aggressive when it gains access to usually sterile body sites, such as the urinary tract, meninges, or peritoneum. Strains of *E. coli* that produce diarrhea possess specialized virulence properties, usually plasmid-borne, which confer the capacity to cause intestinal disease.

E. coli Diarrhea

Of the four distinct strains of *E. coli* that cause diarrhea, two are associated with serious illness in developed countries.

- **ENTEROHEMORRHAGIC E. coli:** Enterohemorrhagic E. coli *(serotype O157:H7)* causes a bloody diarrhea, which occasionally is followed by the hemolytic–uremic syndrome (see Chapter 16). The source of infection is usually the ingestion of contaminated meat, milk, vegetables or other food products contaminated with bovine feces, a common source for the serotype. *Enterohemorrhagic E. coli* adheres to the colonic mucosa and elaborates an enterotoxin, virtually identical to Shigatoxin (see below), which destroys the epithelial cells. Patients infected with *E. coli* O157:H7 present with cramping abdominal pain, low-grade fever, and sometimes bloody diarrhea. Occasional fatalities occur in the very young and elderly, often associated with hemolytic–uremic syndrome.
- **ENTEROINVASIVE E. coli** causes food-borne dysentery that is clinically and pathologically indistinguishable from that caused by Shigella. It invades and destroys mucosal cells of the distal ileum and colon. As in shigellosis, the mucosa of the distal ileum and colon are acutely inflamed and focally eroded and are some-

times covered by an inflammatory pseudomembrane. Patients exhibit abdominal pain, fever, tenesmus, and bloody diarrhea.

E. coli Urinary Tract Infection

Urinary tract infections with *E. coli* are most common in sexually active women and in persons of both sexes who have structural or functional abnormalities of the urinary tract. Such infections are extremely common, afflicting more than 10% of the human population, often repeatedly.

PATHOGENESIS: E. coli gains access to the sterile proximal urinary tract by ascending from the distal urethra. Because the shorter female urethra provides a less effective mechanical barrier to infection, women are much more prone to urinary tract infections. Uropathogenic *E. coli* have specialized adherence factors on the pili, which enable them to bind the uroepithelium. Urinary tract infections initially produce an acute inflammatory infiltrate at the site of infection, usually the bladder mucosa, which may ascend to the kidney to produce **pyelonephritis** (see Chapter 16).

E. coli Sepsis (Gram-Negative Sepsis)

E. coli is the most common cause of enteric gram-negative sepsis, but other gram-negative rods, including *Pseudomonas*, *Klebsiella*, and *Enterobacter* species, produce identical disease. *This discussion relates to gram-negative sepsis in general.*

PATHOGENESIS: E. coli sepsis is usually an opportunistic infection, occurring in persons with predisposing conditions, such as neutropenia, pyelonephritis, or cirrhosis, and in hospitalized patients. The microbe occasionally seeds the bloodstream. Patients with neutropenia or cirrhosis develop *E. coli* sepsis because of an impaired capacity to eliminate even low-level bacteremias. Persons with ruptured abdominal organs or acute pyelonephritis suffer gram-negative sepsis because the large numbers of organisms that gain access to the circulation overwhelm the normal defenses. The presence of *E. coli* in the bloodstream causes septic shock through the effects of TNF, whose release from macrophages is stimulated by bacterial endotoxin. Septic shock is discussed in Chapters 7 and 20.

Salmonella Enterocolitis and Typhoid Fever are Both Intestinal Infections

The bacterial genus *Salmonella* comprises more than 1,500 antigenically distinct but biochemically and genetically related gram-negative rods, which cause two important human diseases: *Salmonella* enterocolitis and typhoid fever.

SALMONELLA ENTEROCOLITIS: Salmonella enterocolitis is an acute, self-limited (1 to 3 days), gastrointestinal illness that manifests as *nausea, vomiting, diarrhea, and fever.* Infection is typically acquired by eating food contaminated with nontyphoidal *Salmonella* strains and is commonly called *Salmonella food poisoning.* The organisms proliferate in the small intestine and invade enterocytes in the distal small bowel and colon. The nontyphoidal *Salmonella* species elaborate several toxins that contribute to the dysfunction of intestinal cells. The mucosa of the ileum and colon is acutely inflamed and sometimes superficially ulcerated.

TYPHOID FEVER: Typhoid fever is an acute systemic illness caused by infection with Salmonella typhi. The disease is acquired from infected patients or chronic carriers and is spread primarily by ingestion of contaminated water and food. *S. typhi* attaches to and invades the ileum in areas overlying Peyer patches, which become hypertrophic. In some cases, concomitant capillary thrombosis causes necrosis of overlying mucosa and characteristic ulcers ori-

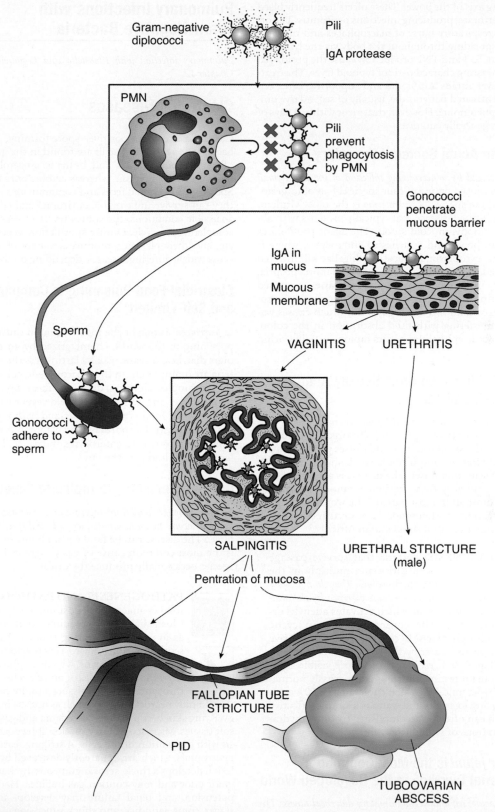

FIGURE 9-8. **Pathogenesis of gonococcal infections.** *Neisseria gonorrhoeae* is a gram-negative diplococcus with surface pili that form a barrier against phagocytosis by neutrophils. The pili contain an IgA protease that digests IgA on the luminal surface of the mucous membranes of the urethra, endocervix, and fallopian tube, thereby facilitating attachment of gonococci. Gonococci cause endocervicitis, vaginitis, and salpingitis. In men, gonococci attached to the mucous membrane of the urethra cause urethritis and, sometimes, urethral stricture. Gonococci may also attach to sperm heads and be carried into the fallopian tube. Penetration of the mucous membrane by gonococci leads to stricture of the fallopian tube, pelvic inflammatory disease (PID), or tuboovarian abscess. IgA, immunoglobulin A; PMN, polymorphonuclear neutrophil.

ented along the long axis of the bowel. These ulcers frequently bleed and occasionally perforate, producing infectious peritonitis. The organisms block the respiratory burst of macrophages and multiply within these cells, spreading throughout the body via the lymphatics and bloodstream. IL-1 and TNF production cause the prolonged fever, malaise, and wasting characteristic of typhoid fever. The treatment of typhoid fever entails antibiotics and supportive care. Ten percent to 20% of untreated patients die, usually of secondary complications, such as pneumonia. However, treatment within 3 days of the onset of fever is generally curative.

Shigellosis is an Acute Bacterial Dysentery

Shigellosis is characterized by a necrotizing infection of the distal small bowel and colon. It is caused by any of four species of aerobic, gram-negative rods. Of these species, *S. dysenteriae* is the most virulent. Shigellosis is a self-limited disease that typically presents with abdominal pain and bloody, mucoid stools. The agent proliferates rapidly in the small bowel and attaches to enterocytes, where it replicates within the cytoplasm. Replicating shigellae kill infected cells and then spread to adjacent cells and into the lamina propria, producing a patchy inflammatory **pseudomembrane**, composed of neutrophils, fibrin, and necrotic epithelium. Shigellae also produce a potent exotoxin, known as **Shiga toxin**, which causes watery diarrhea, by interfering with fluid absorption in the colon. Regeneration of colonic epithelium occurs rapidly, usually within 10 to 14 days.

Cholera is an Epidemic Enteritis Usually Acquired from Contaminated Water

Cholera is a severe diarrheal illness caused by the enterotoxin of Vibrio cholerae, *an aerobic, curved gram-negative rod.* The organism proliferates in the lumen of the small intestine and causes profuse watery diarrhea, rapid dehydration, and if not treated, shock and death within 24 hours of symptom onset. The disease is acquired by ingesting *V. cholerae,* primarily from fecally contaminated food or water. Cholera is common in most parts of the world, and major epidemics affecting tens of thousands have occurred in South America and currently in central sub-Saharan Africa.

 PATHOGENESIS: Bacteria that survive passage through the stomach thrive and multiply in the mucous layer of the small bowel. *They do not themselves invade the mucosa but cause diarrhea by elaborating a potent exotoxin,* **cholera toxin,** which activates adenylyl cyclase of the enterocyte. The consequent rise in cyclic adenosine monophosphate (cAMP content results in massive secretion of sodium and water by the enterocyte into the intestinal lumen (Fig. 9-9). *V. cholerae* causes little visible alteration in the affected intestine, which appears grossly normal or only slightly hyperemic. Untreated cholera has a 50% mortality rate. Replacing lost salts and water is a simple, effective treatment, which can often be accomplished by oral rehydration with preparations of salt, glucose, and water.

Campylobacter jejuni is the Most Common Cause of Bacterial Diarrhea in the Developed World

C. jejuni *causes an acute, self-limited inflammatory diarrheal illness.* The bacterium is a microaerophilic, curved gram-negative rod, morphologically similar to the vibrios.

C. jejuni infection is acquired through food or water contaminated by animal waste. Raw milk and inadequately cooked poultry and meat are frequent sources of disease. *C. jejuni* can also spread from person to person by fecal–oral contact. Ingested *C. jejuni* multiply in the alkaline environment of the upper small intestine. The organisms produce a superficial enterocolitis of the terminal ileum and colon and secrete several toxic proteins.

Pulmonary Infections with Gram-Negative Bacteria

Pulmonary infection with Klebsiella and Legionellosis are discussed in Chapter 12.

Clostridial Diseases

Clostridia are gram-positive, spore-forming, obligate anaerobic bacilli. The vegetative bacilli are found in the gastrointestinal tract of herbivorous animals and humans. Anaerobic conditions promote vegetative division, whereas aerobic ones lead to sporulation. Spores pass in animal feces and contaminate soil and plants, where they can survive unfavorable environmental circumstances. Under anaerobic conditions, the spores revert to vegetative cells, thereby completing the cycle. During sporulation, vegetative cells degenerate, and their plasmids produce a variety of specific toxins that cause widely differing diseases, depending on the species (Fig. 9-10).

Clostridial Food Poisoning is Common and Self-Limited

C. perfringens is one of the most common causes of bacterial food poisoning in the world, characterized by an acute, generally benign, diarrheal disease, usually lasting less than 24 hours. The bacteria are omnipresent in the environment, contaminating soil, water, air samples, clothing, dust, and meat. Spores survive cooking temperatures and germinate to yield vegetative forms, which proliferate when food is allowed to stand without refrigeration. The vegetative clostridia sporulate and elaborate a variety of exotoxins, which are cytotoxic to enterocytes and cause the loss of intracellular ions and fluid into the gut.

Gas Gangrene May Complicate Penetrating Wounds

Gas gangrene (clostridial myonecrosis) is a necrotizing, gas-forming infection that begins in contaminated wounds and spreads rapidly to adjacent tissues. The disease can be fatal within hours of onset. *C. perfringens* is the most common cause of gas gangrene, but other clostridial species occasionally produce the disease.

  PATHOGENESIS AND PATHOLOGY: Gas gangrene follows anaerobic deposition of *C. perfringens* into tissue. Clostridial growth requires extensive devitalized tissue, as in severe penetrating trauma, wartime injuries, and septic abortions. Necrosis of previously healthy muscle is caused by myotoxins, which are phospholipases that destroy the membranes of muscle cells, leukocytes, and erythrocytes. Affected tissues rapidly become mottled and then frankly necrotic. Tissues such as muscle may even liquefy. The overlying skin becomes tense, as edema and gas expand underlying soft tissues. Microscopic examination shows extensive tissue necrosis with dissolution of the cells. A striking feature is the paucity of neutrophils, which are apparently destroyed by the myotoxin. The lesion develops a thick, serosanguineous discharge, which has a fragrant odor and may contain gas bubbles. Hemolytic anemia, hypotension, and renal failure may develop, and in the terminal stages, coma, jaundice, and shock supervene.

Tetanus is a Disease Characterized by Spastic Skeletal Muscle Contractions Caused by *C. tetani* Neurotoxin

Tetanus occurs when *C. tetani* contaminates wounds and proliferates in tissue, releasing its exotoxin. Immunization programs using inactivated tetanus toxin have largely eliminated the disease

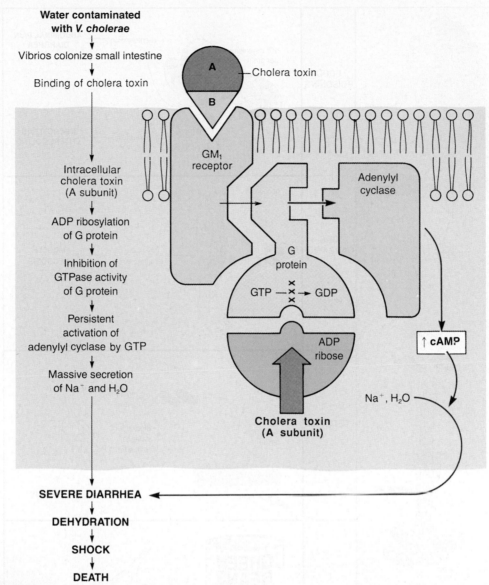

**Water contaminated
with *V. cholerae***
↓
Vibrios colonize small intestine
↓
Binding of cholera toxin

A — Cholera toxin
B

GM₁
receptor

Intracellular
cholera toxin
(A subunit)
↓
ADP ribosylation
of G protein
↓
Inhibition of
GTPase activity
of G protein
↓
Persistent
activation of
adenylyl cyclase by GTP
↓
Massive secretion
of Na⁺ and H₂O

Adenylyl
cyclase

G
protein

GTP ⟶ ✕✕✕ ⟶ GDP

ADP
ribose

↑ cAMP

Na⁺, H₂O

**Cholera toxin
(A subunit)**

SEVERE DIARRHEA
↓
DEHYDRATION
↓
SHOCK
↓
DEATH

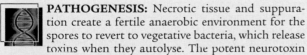 **FIGURE 9-9.**   **Cholera.** Infection comes from water contaminated with *Vibrio cholerae* or food prepared with contaminated water. Vibrios traverse the stomach, enter the small intestine, and propagate. Although they do not invade the intestinal mucosa, vibrios elaborate a potent toxin that induces a massive outpouring of water and electrolytes. Severe diarrhea ("ricewater stool") leads to dehydration and hypovolemic shock.

from developed countries. Nonetheless, tetanus remains a frequent and lethal disease in developing countries.

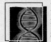 **PATHOGENESIS:** Necrotic tissue and suppuration create a fertile anaerobic environment for the spores to revert to vegetative bacteria, which release toxins when they autolyse. The potent neurotoxin *(tetanospasmin)* undergoes retrograde transport through the ventral roots of peripheral nerves to the anterior horn cells of the spinal cord, where it binds to receptors on inhibitory motor neurons in the ventral horns. The release of inhibitory neurotransmitters is blocked, permitting unopposed neural stimulation and sustained contraction of skeletal muscles **(tetany)**. Spastic rigidity often begins in the muscles of the face, giving rise to "lockjaw," which extends to several facial muscles, causing a fixed grin *(risus sardonicus)*. Rigidity of the muscles of the back produces a backward arching *(opisthotonos)*. Prolonged spasm of respiratory and laryngeal musculature may lead to death.

Botulism is a Paralyzing Disease due to *C. botulinum* Neurotoxin

C. botulinum spores are widely distributed and are especially resistant to drying and boiling. *In the United States, the toxin is most often present in foods that have been improperly home canned and stored without refrigeration. These circumstances provide suitable anaerobic conditions for growth of the vegetative cells that elaborate the neurotoxin.* Botulism can also be contracted from home-cured ham, other meats, and nonacidic vegetable products, such as carrot juice that has been left unrefrigerated for several days.

PATHOGENESIS: Ingested botulinum neurotoxin is readily absorbed into the blood from the proximal small intestine. When it reaches cholinergic nerve endings at the myoneural junction, it inhibits acetylcholine (ACh) release. Ultimately, untreated botulism can progress to respiratory weakness, respiratory arrest, and death. Treatment with antitoxin reduces the mortality rate to 25%.

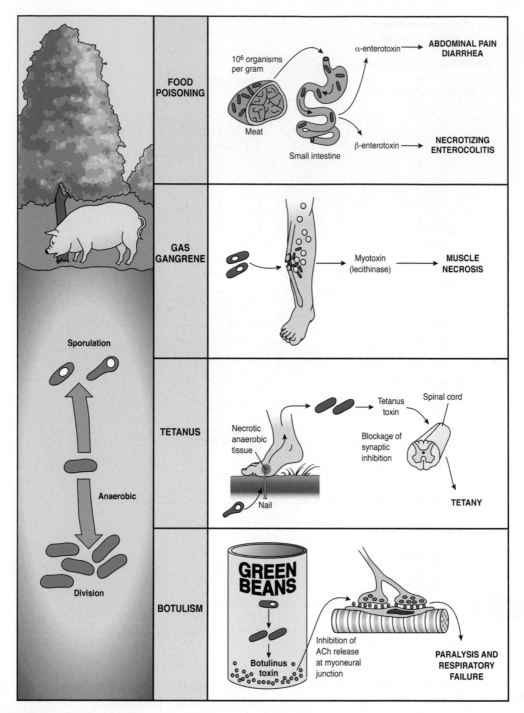

FIGURE 9-10. **Clostridial diseases.** Clostridia in the vegetative form (bacilli) inhabit the gastrointestinal tract of humans and animals. Spores pass in the feces, contaminate soil and plant materials, and are ingested or enter sites of penetrating wounds. Under anaerobic conditions, they revert to vegetative forms. Plasmids in the vegetative forms elaborate toxins that cause several clostridial diseases. **Food poisoning and necrotizing enteritis.** Meat dishes left to cool at room temperature grow large numbers of clostridia (>10^6 organisms per gram). When contaminated meat is ingested, *Clostridium perfringens* types A and C produce α enterotoxin in the small intestine during sporulation, causing abdominal pain and diarrhea. Type C also produces ß enterotoxin. **Gas gangrene.** Clostridia are widespread and may contaminate a traumatic wound or surgical operation. *C. perfringens* type A elaborates a myotoxin (α toxin), a lecithinase that destroys cell membranes, alters capillary permeability, and causes severe hemolysis following intravenous injection. The toxin causes necrosis of previously healthy skeletal muscle.
Tetanus. Spores of *Clostridium tetani* are in soil and enter the site of an accidental wound. Necrotic tissue at the wound site causes spores to revert to the vegetative form (bacilli). Autolysis of vegetative forms releases tetanus toxin. The toxin is transported in peripheral nerves and (retrograde) through axons to the anterior horn cells of the spinal cord. The toxin blocks synaptic inhibition, and the accumulation of ACh in damaged synapses leads to rigidity and spasms of the skeletal musculature (tetany).
Botulism. Improperly canned food is contaminated by the vegetative form of *Clostridium botulinum,* which proliferates under aerobic conditions and elaborates a neurotoxin. After the food is ingested, the neurotoxin is absorbed from the small intestine and eventually reaches the myoneural junction, where it inhibits the release of ACh. The result is a symmetric descending paralysis of cranial nerves, trunk and limbs, with eventual respiratory paralysis and death.

Clostridium difficile Colitis Follows Antibiotic Treatment

C. difficile colitis is an acute necrotizing infection of the terminal small bowel and colon. It is responsible for a large fraction (25% to 50%) of antibiotic-associated diarrheas and is potentially lethal. *C. difficile* colitis is often called **pseudomembranous colitis**, although that condition may have many etiologies (see Chapter 13).

Bacterial Infections with Animal Reservoirs or Insect Vectors

Brucellosis is a Chronic Febrile Disease Acquired from Domestic Animals

Brucellosis is a zoonotic disease caused by one of four Brucella *species. Human brucellosis may manifest as an acute systemic disease or as a chronic infection and is characterized by waxing and waning febrile episodes, weight loss, and fatigue.* Brucella *species are small, aerobic, gram-negative rods that in humans primarily infect monocytes/macrophages.* Each species of *Brucella* has its own animal reservoir:

- *Brucella melitensis:* sheep and goats
- *Brucella abortus:* cattle
- *Brucella suis:* swine
- *Brucella canis:* dogs (human infections are very uncommon)

Humans acquire the bacteria by several mechanisms including (1) contact with infected blood or tissue, (2) ingestion of contaminated meat or milk, or (3) inhalation of contaminated aerosols. Brucellosis is an occupational hazard among ranchers, herders, veterinarians, and slaughterhouse workers. Elimination of infected animals and vaccination of herds have reduced the incidence of brucellosis in many countries, including the United States, where only about 100 cases are reported annually. However, the disease remains common in many parts of the world.

  PATHOGENESIS AND PATHOLOGY: Brucellosis is a systemic infection that can involve any organ or organ system of the body. Bacteria enter the circulation through skin abrasions, the conjunctiva, oropharynx, or lungs. They then spread in the bloodstream to the liver, spleen, lymph nodes, and bone marrow, where they multiply in macrophages. Generalized hyperplasia of these cells may ensue.

CLINICAL FEATURES: Patients infected with *B.abortus* develop conspicuous noncaseating granulomas in the liver, spleen, lymph nodes, and bone marrow. Periodic release of organisms from infected phagocytic cells may be responsible for the febrile episodes of the illness, which wax and wane (hence the term **undulant fever**). The most common complications of brucellosis involve the bones and joints and include spondylitis of the lumbar spine and suppuration in large joints. Endocarditis, although uncommon, can be lethal. Treatment with doxycycline and rifampin is usually effective.

Yersinia pestis Causes Bubonic Plague, the Medieval "Black Death"

Plague is a bacteremic, often fatal, infection that is usually accompanied by enlarged, painful regional lymph nodes (buboes). Historically, plague caused massive epidemics that killed a substantial portion of the population affected. *Y. pestis* is a short gram-negative rod that stains more heavily at the ends (i.e., bipolar staining). *Y. pestis* infection is an endemic zoonosis in many parts of the world, including the Americas, Africa, and Asia. The organisms are found in wild rodents, such as rats, squirrels, and prairie dogs. Fleas transmit it from animal to animal,

and most human infections result from bites of infected fleas. Some infected humans develop plague pneumonia and shed large numbers of organisms in aerosolized respiratory secretions, which allow disease transmission from person to person. In the United States, 30 to 40 cases of plague occur annually, mostly in the four corners region of the Southwest and South-Central California.

 PATHOGENESIS: After inoculation into the skin, *Y. pestis* is phagocytosed by neutrophils and macrophages. Organisms ingested by neutrophils are killed, but those engulfed by macrophages survive and replicate intracellularly. The bacteria are carried to regional lymph nodes, where they continue to multiply, producing extensive hemorrhagic necrosis. Affected lymph nodes, known as "buboes," are enlarged and fluctuant. From the regional lymph nodes, the bacteria disseminate through the bloodstream and lymphatics, producing septic shock and death (bubonic plague). In the lungs, *Y. pestis* produces a necrotizing pneumonitis that releases organisms into the alveoli and airways. These are expelled by coughing, enabling pneumonic spread of the disease (pneumonic plague). Septicemic plague occurs when bacteria are inoculated directly into the blood and do not produce buboes.

All types of plague carry a high mortality rate (50% to 75%) if untreated. Streptomycin or gentamicin is the recommended therapy.

Tularemia is an Acute Febrile Disease Usually Acquired from Rabbits

Tularemia is caused by Francisella tularensis, *a small, gram-negative coccobacillus.* The most important reservoirs of this zoonosis are rabbits and rodents. Human infection results from contact with infected animals (generally rabbits) or from the bites of infected insects, most commonly ticks. The incidence of the infection has fallen to about 200 cases annually, presumably related to a decline in hunting and trapping, formerly major sources of infection. There is renewed awareness of the organism because of its potential as a bioterrorism agent.

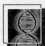 **PATHOGENESIS:** *F. tularensis* multiplies at the site of inoculation, where it initially produces an exudative pyogenic ulcer. The bacteria then spread to regional lymph nodes. Dissemination in the bloodstream leads to metastatic infections that involve the monocyte/macrophage system and sometimes the lungs, heart, and kidneys. *F. tularensis* survives within macrophages until these cells are activated by a cell-mediated immune response to the infection. Disseminated lesions undergo central necrosis and are surrounded by a perimeter of granulomatous reaction resembling the lesions of tuberculosis. The most serious infections are complicated by secondary pneumonia and endotoxic shock, in which case the prognosis is grave.

Anthrax is Rapidly Fatal When it Disseminates

Anthrax is a necrotizing disease caused by Bacillus anthracis, *a large spore-forming, gram-positive rod.* Anthrax is a zoonosis with major reservoirs in goats, sheep, cattle, horses, pigs, and dogs. Spores form in the soil and dead animals, resisting heat, desiccation, and chemical disinfection for years. Humans are infected when spores enter the body through breaks in the skin, by inhalation, or by ingestion. Human disease may also result from exposure to contaminated animal byproducts, such as hides, wool, brushes, or bone meal. In North America, human infection is extremely rare (one case per year for the past few years) and usually results from exposure to imported animal products. However, increased vigilance for anthrax has emerged following a recent act of bioterrorism that used spores delivered in mail and resulted in 11 cases of pulmonary disease.

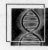

PATHOGENESIS: The spores of *B. anthracis* germinate in the human body to yield vegetative bacteria that multiply and release a potent necrotizing toxin. In 80% of cutaneous anthrax cases, the infection remains localized, and the host immunologic response eventually eliminates the organism. Cutaneous lesions are ulcerated, contain numerous organisms, and are covered by a black scab. Extensive tissue necrosis occurs at the sites of infection and is associated with only a mild infiltrate of neutrophils. Pulmonary infection produces a necrotizing, hemorrhagic pneumonia, associated with hemorrhagic necrosis of mediastinal lymph nodes and widespread dissemination of the organism.

Listeriosis is a Systemic Multiorgan Infection that Carries a High Mortality Rate

Listeriosis is caused by Listeria monocytogenes, *a small, motile, gram-positive coccobacillus with a widespread distribution in the environment. L. monocytogenes* grows at refrigerator temperatures, and outbreaks have been traced to unpasteurized milk, cheese, and dairy products.

PATHOGENESIS: *L. monocytogenes* has an unusual life cycle, which accounts for its ability to evade intracellular and extracellular antibacterial defense mechanisms. After phagocytosis by host cells, the organism enters a phagolysosome, where the acidic pH activates *listeriolysin O*, an exotoxin that disrupts the vesicular membrane and permits the bacterium to escape into the cytoplasm. After replicating, bacteria usurp the contractile elements of the host cytoskeleton to form elongated protrusions that are engulfed by adjacent cells. Thus, *Listeria* spread from one cell to another without exposure to the extracellular environment.

PATHOLOGY AND CLINICAL FEATURES: **Listeriosis of pregnancy** includes prenatal and postnatal infections. Maternal infection early in pregnancy may lead to abortion or premature delivery. Infected infants rapidly develop respiratory distress, hepatosplenomegaly, cutaneous and mucosal papules, leukopenia, and thrombocytopenia. Intrauterine infections involve many organs and tissues, including amniotic fluid, placenta, and the umbilical cord. Abscesses are found in many organs. Microscopically, foci of necrosis and suppuration contain many bacteria. Older lesions tend to be granulomatous. Neurologic sequelae are common, and the mortality rate of neonatal listeriosis is high even with prompt antibiotic therapy.

Chronic alcoholics, patients with cancer, those receiving immunosuppressive therapy, and patients with AIDS are far more susceptible to infection than is the general population. Meningitis is the most common form of the disease in adults. **Septicemic listeriosis** is a severe febrile illness most common in immunodeficient patients. It may lead to shock and disseminated intravascular coagulation, a situation that may be misdiagnosed as gram-negative sepsis. The mortality rate from systemic listeriosis remains at 25%.

Infections Caused by Branching Filamentous Organisms

Actinomycosis is Characterized by Abscesses and Sinus Tracts

Actinomycosis is a slowly progressive, suppurative, fibrosing infection involving the jaw, thorax, or abdomen. The disease is caused by a number of anaerobic and microaerophilic bacteria termed *Actinomyces,*

and the most common is *Actinomyces israelii.* These organisms are branching, filamentous, gram-positive rods that normally reside as saprophytes in the oropharynx, gastrointestinal tract, and vagina without producing disease.

PATHOGENESIS AND PATHOLOGY: Actino-myces can cause disease only if inoculated into anaerobic deep tissues. Trauma can produce tissue necrosis, providing an excellent anaerobic medium for growth of Actinomyces and can inoculate the organism into normally sterile tissue. Actinomycosis occurs at four distinct sites:

- **Cervicofacial actinomycosis** results from jaw injury, dental extraction, or dental manipulation.
- **Thoracic actinomycosis** is caused by the aspiration of organisms contaminating dental debris.
- **Abdominal actinomycosis** follows traumatic or surgical disruption of the bowel, especially the appendix.
- **Pelvic actinomycosis** is associated with the prolonged use of intrauterine devices.

Actinomycosis begins as a nidus of proliferating organisms that attract an acute inflammatory infiltrate. The small abscess grows slowly, becoming a series of abscesses connected by sinus tracts that burrow across normal tissue boundaries and into adjacent organs. Eventually, a tract may penetrate onto an external surface or mucosal membrane, producing a draining sinus. Within the abscesses and sinuses are pus and colonies of organisms that appear as hard, yellow grains, known as **sulfur granules,** because of their resemblance to elemental sulfur. Histologically, the colonies appear as rounded, basophilic grains with scalloped eosinophilic borders (Fig. 9-11A,B).

Nocardiosis is a Suppurative Respiratory Infection in Immunocompromised Hosts

Nocardia are aerobic, gram-positive filamentous, branching bacteria that are widely distributed in soil. Human disease is caused by inhaling or inoculating soil-borne organisms. From the lung, the infection often spreads to the brain and skin. Nocardiosis is most common in persons with impaired immunity, particularly cell-mediated immunity. Organ transplantation, long-term corticosteroid therapy, lymphomas, leukemias, and other debilitating diseases predispose to *Nocardia* infections.

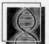

PATHOGENESIS: The respiratory tract is the usual portal of entry for *Nocardia.* The organism elicits a brisk infiltrate of neutrophils, and disease begins as a slowly progressive, pyogenic pneumonia. In immunocompromised persons, *Nocardia* produces pulmonary abscesses, which are frequently multiple and confluent. Direct extension to the pleura, trachea, and heart, and metastases to the brain or skin through the circulation, carry a grave prognosis. Untreated nocardiosis is usually fatal. Sulfonamides or related antibiotics for several months are often effective therapy.

SPIROCHETAL INFECTIONS

Spirochetes are long, slender, helical bacteria with specialized cell envelopes that permit them to move by flexion and rotation. Although spirochetes have the basic cell wall structure of gram-negative bacteria, they stain poorly with the Gram stain.

Three genera of spirochetes, *Treponema, Borrelia,* and *Leptospira* cause human disease (Table 9-3). They are adept at evading host inflammatory and immunological defenses, and diseases caused by these organisms are all chronic or relapsing.

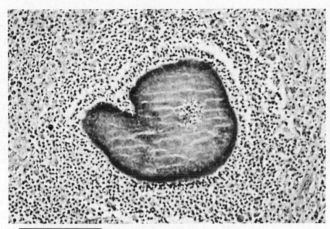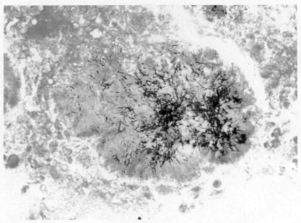

FIGURE 9-11. **Actinomycosis. A.** A typical sulfur granule lies within an abscess. **B.** The individual filaments of *Actinomyces israeli* are readily visible with the silver impregnation technique.

Syphilis

Syphilis (lues) is a chronic systemic infection that is transmitted almost exclusively by sexual contact or from an infected mother to her fetus (**congenital syphilis**). *Infection is caused by* Treponema pallidum, a thin, long spirochete (Fig. 9-12).

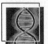 **PATHOGENESIS AND PATHOLOGY:** Person-to-person transmission requires direct contact between a rich source of spirochetes (e.g., an open lesion) and mucous membranes or abraded skin of the genital organs, rectum, mouth, fingers, or nipples. The organisms reproduce at the site of inoculation, pass to regional lymph nodes, gain access to systemic circulation, and disseminate throughout the body. Although *T. pallidum* induces an inflammatory response and is taken up by phagocytic cells, it persists and proliferates. Chronic infection and inflammation cause tissue destruction, sometimes for decades. The course of syphilis is classically divided into three stages (Fig. 9-13).

Primary Syphilis is Characterized by the Chancre

The classic lesion of primary syphilis is the **chancre** (Fig. 9-14), a characteristic ulcer at the site of *T. pallidum* entry. It appears 1 week to 3 months after exposure and tends to be solitary. Spirochetes tend to concentrate in vessel walls and in the epidermis around the ulcer. The vessels display a characteristic "luetic vasculitis," in which endothelial cells proliferate and swell, and vessel walls become thickened by lymphocytes and fibrous tissue. Chancres are painless and heal without scarring.

Secondary Syphilis Features the Systemic Spread of the Organism

In secondary syphilis, *T. pallidum* spreads systemically and proliferates to cause lesions in the skin, mucous membranes, lymph nodes, meninges, stomach, and liver. Lesions show perivascular lymphocytic infiltration and endarteritis obliterans. The most common presentation of secondary syphilis is an erythematous

TABLE 9–3				
Spirochete Infections				
Disease	**Organism**	**Clinical Manifestation**	**Distribution**	**Mode of Transmission**
	Treponemes			
Syphilis	*Treponema pallidum*	See text	Common worldwide	Sexual contact, congenital
Bejel	*Treponema endenicum (Treponema pallidum,* subspecies *endenicum)*	Mucosal, skin, and bone lesions	Middle East	Mouth-to-mouth contact
Yaws	*Treponema pertenue (Treponema pallidum* subspecies *pertenue)*	Skin and bone	Tropics	Skin-to-skin contact
Pinta	Treponem acarateum	Skin lesions	Latin America	Skin-to-skin contact
	Borrelia			
Lyme disease	*Borrelia burgdorferi*	See text	North America, Europe, Russia, Asia, Africa, Australia	Tick bite
Relapsing fever	*Borrelia recurrentis* and related species	Relapsing flu-like illness	Worldwide	Tick bite, louse bite
	Leptospira			
Leptospirosis	*Leptospira interrogans*	Flu-like illness, meningitis	Worldwide	Contact with animal urine

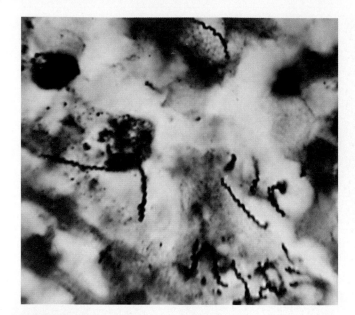

FIGURE 9-12. **Syphilis.** Spirochetes of *Treponema pallidum,* visualized by silver impregnation, in the eye of a child with congenital syphilis.

and maculopapular rash, involving the trunk and extremities and often includes the palms and soles. The rash appears 2 weeks to 3 months after the chancre heals. Lesions on mucosal surfaces of the mouth and genital organs, called **mucous patches**, teem with organisms and are highly infectious.

The Gumma is the Hallmark Lesion of Tertiary Syphilis

Following secondary syphilis, an asymptomatic period lasts for years. However, spirochetes continue to multiply, and the deep-seated lesions of tertiary syphilis gradually develop in one third of untreated patients. The appearance of a **gumma** in any organ or tissue is the hallmark of tertiary syphilis. Gummas are most commonly found in the skin, bone, and joints, although they can occur anywhere. These granulomatous lesions are composed of a central area of coagulative necrosis, epithelioid macrophages, occasional giant cells, and peripheral fibrous tissue. Gummas are usually localized lesions and generally do not contribute to the disease process. Rather, the underlying mechanism for much of the damage associated with tertiary syphilis is focal ischemic necrosis secondary to obliterative endarteritis. *T. pallidum* induces a mononuclear inflammatory infiltrate composed predominantly of lymphocytes and plasma cells. These cells infiltrate small arteries and arterioles, producing a characteristic obstructive vascular lesion (**endarteritis obliterans**). The small arteries are inflamed, and their endothelial cells are swollen. They are surrounded by concentric layers of proliferating fibroblasts, which confer an "onion skin" appearance to the vascular lesions. **Syphilitic aortitis** results from destruction of the vasa vasorum, eventually leading to necrosis of the aortic media, gradual weakening and stretching of the aortic wall, aortic aneurysm, and ultimately rupture, causing sudden death. Syphilitic aneurysms are saccular and involve the ascending aorta. On gross examination, the aortic intima is rough and pitted (**tree-bark appearance**). Damage to, and scarring of, the ascending aorta also commonly lead to dilation of the aortic ring, separation of the valve cusps, and regurgitation of blood through the aortic valve (aortic insufficiency) (see Chapter 10). **Neurosyphilis** results from the slowly progressive infection and damages the meninges, cerebral cortex, spinal cord, cranial nerves, or eyes.

Congenital Syphilis Affects the Fetus

In this setting, the organism disseminates in fetal tissues, which are injured by the proliferating organisms and accompanying inflammatory response. Fetal infection produces stillbirth, neonatal illness or death, or progressive postnatal disease. Histopathologically, the lesions of congenital syphilis are identical to those of adult disease.

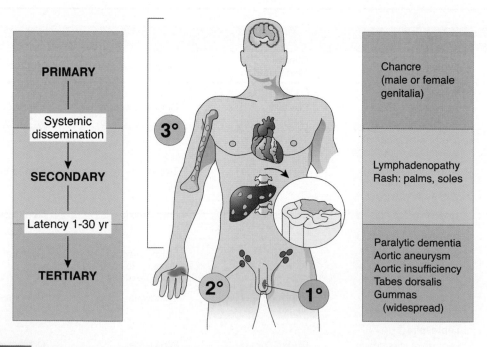

FIGURE 9-13. Clinical characteristics of the various stages of syphilis.

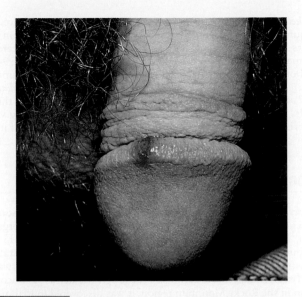

FIGURE 9-14. **Syphilitic chancre.** A patient with primary syphilis displays a raised, erythematous penile lesion.

Lyme Disease

Lyme disease is a chronic systemic infection, which begins with a characteristic skin lesion and later manifests as cardiac, neurologic, or joint disturbances. The causative agent is *Borrelia burgdorferi,* a large, microaerophilic spirochete transmitted from its animal reservoir to humans by the bite of the minute *Ixodes* tick, which usually feeds on mice and deer. Lyme disease has become the most common tick-borne illness in the United States, causing an estimated 20,000 to 25,000 cases annually.

PATHOGENESIS, PATHOLOGY, AND CLINICAL FEATURES: *B. burgdorferi* reproduces locally at the site of inoculation, spreads to regional lymph nodes, and is disseminated throughout the body in the bloodstream. Like other spirochetal diseases, Lyme disease is chronic, occurring in stages, with remissions and exacerbations. *B. burgdorferi* elicits a chronic inflammatory infiltrate composed of lymphocytes and plasma cells. Three clinical stages are recognized in Lyme disease:

- **Stage 1:** The characteristic skin lesion, **erythema chronicum migrans**, appears at the site of the tick bite. It begins as an erythematous macule or papule, which grows into an erythematous patch. The last often is intensely red at its periphery and pale in the center, imparting an annular appearance. Secondary annular skin lesions develop in about half of patients and may persist for long periods. During this phase, patients experience constant malaise, fatigue, headache, and fever. Intermittent manifestations may also include meningeal irritation, migratory myalgia, cough, generalized lymphadenopathy, and testicular swelling.
- **Stage 2:** The second stage begins within several weeks to months of the skin lesion and is characterized by exacerbation of migratory musculoskeletal pains as well as cardiac and neurologic abnormalities. In 10% of cases, conduction abnormalities, particularly atrioventricular block, result from myocarditis. Neurologic abnormalities, most commonly meningitis and facial nerve palsies, occur in 15% of patients.
- **Stage 3:** The third stage of Lyme disease begins months to years after the initial infection and is manifested by joint, skin, and neurologic abnormalities, which range from tingling paresthesias to slowly progressive encephalomyelitis, transverse myelitis, organic brain syndromes, and dementia. Joint abnormalities develop in over half of infected persons and in-

clude severe arthritis of the large joints, especially the knee. The histopathology of affected joints is virtually indistinguishable from that of rheumatoid arthritis, with villous hypertrophy and a conspicuous mononuclear infiltrate in the subsynovial lining area. Treatment with tetracycline or erythromycin is effective in eliminating early Lyme disease. In later stages, high doses of intravenous penicillin G and other combinations of antibiotic regimens for long periods are necessary.

CHLAMYDIAL INFECTIONS

Chlamydiae are obligate intracellular parasites that are smaller than most other bacteria. They lack the enzymatic capacity to generate adenosine triphosphate (ATP) and must parasitize the metabolic machinery of a host cell to reproduce. The chlamydial life cycle involves two distinct morphologic forms, the **reticulate and elementary bodies**. The former is metabolically active and commandeers host cell metabolism to fuel chlamydial replication. The reticulate body divides repeatedly, forming daughter elementary bodies and destroying the host cell. Necrotic debris elicits inflammatory and immunologic responses that further damage infected tissue. Chlamydial infections are widespread among birds and mammals, and as many as 20% of humans are infected. Three species of chlamydiae (Chlamydia *trachomatis,* Chlamydia *psittaci,* and Chlamydia *pneumoniae*) cause human infection.

Chlamydia Trachomatis Infection

The species *C. trachomatis* contains a variety of strains, which cause three distinct types of disease: (1) genital and neonatal disease; (2) lymphogranuloma venereum; and (3) trachoma.

- Genital disease: C. trachomatis *causes a genital epithelial infection that is now the most common venereal disease in North America.* Chlamydial infection elicits an infiltrate of neutrophils and lymphocytes. Lymphoid aggregates, with or without germinal centers, may appear at the site of infection. In men, *C. trachomatis* infection produces urethritis and sometimes epididymitis or proctitis. In women, it usually begins with cervicitis, which can progress to endometritis, salpingitis, and generalized infection of the pelvic adnexal organs (pelvic inflammatory disease).
- **Neonatal Disease:** Perinatal transmission of *C. trachomatis* by passage through an infected birth canal causes neonatal conjunctivitis in about two thirds of exposed neonates. Infected conjunctival epithelium often contains characteristic vacuolar cytoplasmic inclusions, and the disease is frequently called **inclusion conjunctivitis**. Chlamydial pneumonia manifests in the second or third month with tachypnea and paroxysmal cough, usually without fever.
- **Lymphogranuloma venereum** is a sexually transmitted disease that begins as a genital ulcer, spreads to lymph nodes and may cause local scarring. The disease is uncommon in developed countries, but is endemic in the tropics and subtropics. The organism is introduced through a break in the skin. After an incubation period of 4 to 21 days, an ulcer appears, usually on the penis, vagina, or cervix. The organisms are transported by lymphatics to regional lymph nodes, where a necrotizing lymphadenitis and abscess formation occurs. The abscesses have a granulomatous appearance, containing neutrophils and necrotic debris in the center, surrounded by palisading epithelioid cells, macrophages, and occasional giant cells. Abscesses are rimmed by lymphocytes, plasma cells, and fibrous tissue. The nodal architecture is eventually effaced by fibrosis. The intense inflammatory process can result in severe scarring, which may produce chronic lymphatic obstruction, ischemic necrosis of overlying structures, or strictures and adhesions.

- **Trachoma:** This chronic infection causes progressive scars of the conjunctiva and cornea. Trachoma is worldwide, associated with poverty, and most prevalent in dry or sandy regions of Africa, Asia, and the Middle East. In endemic areas, infection is acquired early in childhood, becomes chronic, and eventually progresses to blindness. The agent reproduces in the conjunctival epithelium, inciting a mixed acute and chronic inflammatory infiltrate. Progressive scarring distorts the eyelids thereby leading to corneal abrasions and secondary bacterial infections. Ultimately, the combination of chronic inflammation, infection, scarring, and abrasion produces blindness.

Psittacosis (Ornithosis)

Psittacosis is a self-limited pneumonia transmitted to humans from birds. The causative agent, *Chlamydia psittaci,* is spread to humans by the excreta, dust, and feathers of infected birds. Treatment and quarantine of imported tropical birds has limited the spread of disease, and fewer than 50 cases of psittacosis are reported annually in the United States.

 PATHOLOGY: *C. psittaci* first infects pulmonary macrophages, which carry the organism to the phagocytic cells of the liver and spleen, where it reproduces. The organism is then distributed by the bloodstream, producing systemic infection, particularly diffuse involvement of the lungs. The pneumonia is predominantly interstitial, with a lymphocytic inflammatory infiltrate and hyperplasia of type II pneumocytes, which may show characteristic chlamydial cytoplasmic inclusions. Dissemination of the infection is characterized by foci of necrosis in the liver and spleen as well as diffuse mononuclear cell infiltrates in the heart, kidneys, and brain.

RICKETTSIAL INFECTIONS

The rickettsiae are small, gram-negative, coccobacillary bacteria that are obligate intracellular pathogens and cannot replicate outside a host. Humans are accidental hosts for most species of *Rickettsia.* The organisms reside in animals and insects and do not require humans for perpetuation. Human rickettsial infection results from insect bites. Many species of *Rickettsia* cause different human diseases often localized to a geographic region (Table 9-4), although rickettsial infections have many features in common. *The human target cell for all rickettsiae is the endothelial cell of capillaries and other small blood vessels.* The organisms reproduce within these cells, killing them in the process and produce a necrotizing vasculitis. Human rickettsial infections are traditionally divided into the "spotted fever group" and the "typhus group."

Rocky Mountain Spotted Fever

Rocky Mountain spotted fever is an acute, potentially fatal, systemic vasculitis, usually manifested by headache, fever, and rash. The causative organism, *Rickettsia rickettsii,* is transmitted to humans by tick bites. About 1,500 cases are reported annually in the United States, mostly from the eastern seaboard (Georgia to New York) westward to Texas, Oklahoma, and Kansas. Although the disease is uncommon in the Rocky Mountain region, it was discovered in Idaho.

 PATHOGENESIS AND PATHOLOGY: *R. rickettsii* in salivary glands of ticks is introduced into the skin while the ticks feed. The organisms spread via lymphatics and small blood vessels to the systemic and pulmonary circulation, where the agent attaches to and is engulfed by endothelial cells. The organisms reproduce and are shed into the vascular and lymphatic systems. Destruction of vascular endothelium causes a systemic vasculitis. Vessel walls are infiltrated, initially with neutrophils and macrophages, and later with lymphocytes and plasma cells. Microscopic infarctions and extravasation of blood into surrounding tissues are common. The rash is the most visible manifestation of the generalized phenomenon of vascular injury, which may eventuate in disseminated intravascular coagulation and shock. Damage to pulmonary capillaries can produce pulmonary edema and acute alveolar injury.

The disease manifests with fever, headache, and myalgias, followed by a rash. Skin lesions begin as a maculopapular eruption but rapidly become petechial, spreading centripetally from the distal extremities to the trunk. If untreated, more than 20% to 50% of infected

TABLE 9–4			
Rickettsial Infections			
Disease	**Organism**	**Distribution**	**Transmission**
	Spotted-Fever Group (genus *Rickettsia*)		
Rocky Mountain spotted fever	*R. rickettsii*	Americas	Ticks
Queensland tick fever	*R. australis*	Australia	Ticks
Boutonneuse fever, Kenya tick fever	*R. conorii*	Mediterranean, Africa, India	Ticks
Siberian tick fever	*R. sibirica*	Siberia, Mongolia	Ticks
Rickettsialpox	*R. akari*	United States, Russia, Central Asia, Korea, Africa	Mites
	Typhus Group		
Louse-borne typhus (epidemic typhus)	*R. prowazekii*	Latin America, Africa, Asia	Lice
Murine typhus (endemic typhus)	*R. typhi*	Worldwide	Fleas
Scrub typhus	*R. tsutsugamushi*	South Pacific, Asia	Mites
Q fever	*Coxiella burnetii*	Worldwide	Inhalation

persons die within 8 to 15 days. Prompt diagnosis and antibiotic treatment (usually with doxycycline) is life saving, and the mortality rate in the United States is less than 5%.

Epidemic (Louse-Borne) Typhus

Epidemic typhus is a severe systemic vasculitis transmitted by the bite of infected lice. The disease is caused by *Rickettsia prowazekii*, an organism that has a human-louse-human life cycle (Fig. 9-15). The bacteria are transmitted from one infected person to another by the bite of an infected body louse. Devastating epidemics of typhus were as-

sociated with conditions of social stress, such as war or famine, which led to louse infestation of human populations. Currently, the disease is limited to mountainous areas of Africa, the Andes in South America, and is very uncommon in the US.

PATHOGENESIS AND PATHOLOGY: A person becomes infected when the contaminated louse feces penetrate an abrasion or scratch or when the person inhales airborne rickettsiae. The disease begins with localized infection of capillary endothelium and progresses to a systemic vasculitis with many similarities to Rocky Mountain spotted fever. Focal necrosis is associated with an infiltrate of mast cells, lympho-

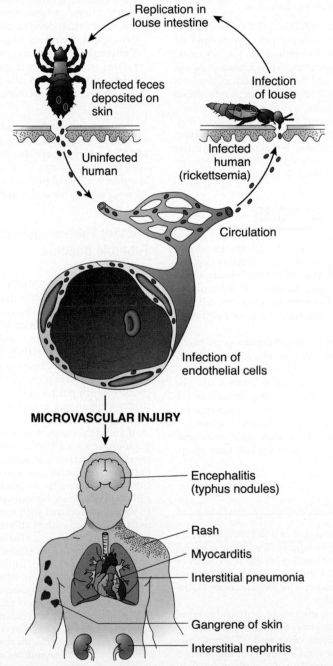

FIGURE 9-15. **Epidemic typhus (louse-borne typhus).** *Rickettsia prowazekii* has a man-louse-man life cycle. The organism multiplies in endothelial cells, which detach, rupture, and release organisms into the circulation (rickettsemia). A louse taking a blood meal becomes infected with rickettsiae, which enter the epithelial cells of its midgut, multiply, and rupture the cells, thereby releasing rickettsiae into the lumen of the louse intestine. Contaminated feces are deposited on the skin or clothing of a second host, penetrate an abrasion, or are inhaled. The rickettsiae then enter endothelial cells, multiply and rupture the cells, thus completing the cycle.

cytes, plasma cells, and macrophages, frequently arranged as **typhus nodules** around arterioles and capillaries.

MYCOPLASMAL INFECTIONS: MYCOPLASMA PNEUMONIA

At less than 0.3 μm in greatest dimension, mycoplasmas are the smallest free-living prokaryotes, and they lack the rigid cell walls of more complex bacteria. M. pneumoniae *produces acute, self-limited lower respiratory tract infections, affecting mostly children and young adults.* The organism is spread by aerosol transmission, mostly in small groups of persons who have frequent close contact. *M. pneumoniae* infection occurs worldwide, and in developed countries, the organism causes 15% to 20% of all pneumonias.

PATHOGENESIS AND PATHOLOGY: *M. pneumoniae* initiates infection by attaching to a glyco-lipid on the surface of the respiratory epithelium. The organism remains outside the cells, where it reproduces and causes progressive dysfunction and eventual death of the host cells. Pneumonia caused by *M. pneumoniae* usually shows patchy consolidation of a single segment of a lower lung lobe. The alveoli show a largely interstitial process, with reactive alveolar lining cells and mononuclear infiltration. Pulmonary changes are often complicated by bacterial superinfection. *Mycoplasma* pneumonia tends to be milder than other bacterial pneumonias and is sometimes called "walking pneumonia."

MYCOBACTERIAL INFECTIONS

Mycobacteria are distinctive organisms, 2 to 10 μm in length, which share the cell wall architecture of gram-positive bacteria but also contain large amounts of lipid. Mycobacteria are structurally gram-positive; however, this property is difficult to demonstrate by routine staining. The waxy lipids of the cell wall make the mycobacteria "**acid fast**" (i.e., they retain carbolfuchsin after rinsing with acid alcohol).

The mycobacteria grow more slowly than other pathogenic bacteria and cause chronic, slowly progressive illnesses. Most mycobacterial pathogens replicate within cells of the monocyte/macrophage lineage and elicit granulomatous inflammation. The outcome of mycobacterial infection is largely determined by the host's capacity to contain the organism through delayed-type hypersensitivity mechanisms and cell-mediated immune responses.

The two main mycobacterial pathogens, *Mycobacterium tuberculosis* and *Mycobacterium leprae,* infect only humans and have no environmental reservoir.

Tuberculosis

Tuberculosis is a chronic, communicable disease in which the lungs are the prime target, although any organ may be infected. The disease is mainly caused by M. tuberculosis hominis (Koch bacillus) but also occasionally by M. tuberculosis bovis. The characteristic lesion is a spherical granuloma with central caseous necrosis. M. tuberculosis is an obligate aerobe, a slender, beaded, nonmotile, acid-fast bacillus.

Tuberculosis is one of the most important human bacterial diseases. The World Health Organization estimates a worldwide annual incidence of 140 tuberculosis cases and 27 deaths per 100,000. By comparison, the US annual incidence is currently 5 tuberculosis cases and 0.2 deaths per 100,000, with more than half of the cases occurring in foreign-born individuals. This represents a greater than 10-fold reduction in incidence in the last 50 years. The HIV-infected, homeless, and malnourished persons in impoverished areas are highly susceptible, as are immigrants from areas where the disease is endemic. In the United States, tu-

berculosis is most common in the elderly, with a case rate of 8 per 100,000 in the population over the age of 65, accounting for about 20% of the patients with the disease. This may reflect reactivation of infections acquired early in life before the decline in the prevalence of the disease.

M. tuberculosis is transmitted from person to person by aerosolized droplets. Coughing, sneezing, and talking all create aerosolized respiratory droplets; usually, droplets evaporate, leaving an organism (droplet nucleus) that is readily carried in the air.

PATHOGENESIS: The course of tuberculosis depends on age and immune competence, as well as the total burden of organisms (Fig. 9-16). Some patients have only an indolent, asymptomatic infection, whereas in others, tuberculosis is a destructive, disseminated disease. Many more persons are infected with *M. tuberculosis* than develop clinical symptoms. Thus, one must distinguish between infection and active tuberculosis. **Tuberculous infection** refers to growth of the organism in a person, whether there is symptomatic disease or not. **Active tuberculosis** denotes the subset of tuberculous infections manifested by destructive and symptomatic disease.

Primary tuberculosis occurs on first exposure to the organism and can pursue either an indolent or aggressive course (Fig. 9-16). **Secondary tuberculosis** develops long after a primary infection, mostly as a result of reactivation of a primary infection. Secondary tuberculosis can also be produced by exposure to exogenous organisms and is always an active disease.

Primary Tuberculosis is a First Exposure to the Tubercle Bacillus

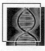

PATHOGENESIS AND PATHOLOGY: Inhaled *M. tuberculosis* is deposited in alveoli. The organisms are phagocytosed by alveolar macrophages but resist killing; cell wall lipids of *M. tuberculosis* apparently block fusion of phagosomes and lysosomes, allowing the bacilli to proliferate within macrophages. Development of activated lymphocytes responsive to *M. tuberculosis* antigen produces a type IV hypersensitivity response to the organism, which results in the emergence of activated macrophages that can ingest and destroy the bacilli. The process requires 3 to 6 weeks to come into play.

If an infected person is immunologically competent, a vigorous granulomatous reaction is produced. Microscopically, the classic lesion of tuberculosis is a caseous granuloma (Fig. 9-17), a lesion that has a soft, semisolid core surrounded by epithelioid macrophages, Langhans giant cells, lymphocytes, and peripheral fibrous tissue. Although not invariably caused by *M. tuberculosis*, caseous necrosis is so strongly associated with tuberculosis, that its discovery in tissue must raise a suspicion of this disease. The lung lesion of primary tuberculosis is known as a **Ghon focus**. It is found in the subpleural area of the upper segments of the lower lobes or in the lower segments of the upper lobes. Initially, it is a small, ill-defined area of inflammatory consolidation, which then drains to hilar lymph nodes. The combination of a peripheral Ghon focus and involved mediastinal or hilar lymph nodes is called the **Ghon complex**. *In more than 90% of normal adults, tuberculous infection is self-limited.* In both lungs and lymph nodes, the Ghon complex heals, undergoing shrinkage, fibrous scarring, and calcification, the latter visible radiographically. Small numbers of organisms may remain viable for years. Later, if immune mechanisms wane or fail, resting bacilli may proliferate and break out, causing serious secondary tuberculosis.

In immunologically immature subjects (a young child or immunosuppressed patient), granulomas are poorly formed or not formed at all, and infection progresses at the primary site in the lung, in the regional lymph nodes, or in multiple sites of dissemi-

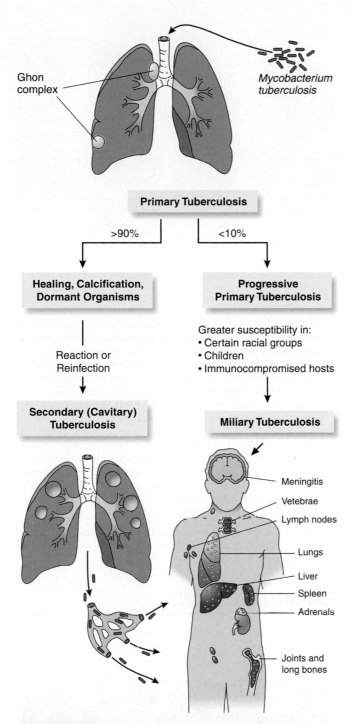

Primary Tuberculosis

>90%   <10%

Healing, Calcification, Dormant Organisms

Progressive Primary Tuberculosis

Greater susceptibility in:
• Certain racial groups
• Children
• Immunocompromised hosts

Reaction or Reinfection

Secondary (Cavitary) Tuberculosis

Miliary Tuberculosis

Meningitis
Vetebrae
Lymph nodes
Lungs
Liver
Spleen
Adrenals
Joints and long bones

FIGURE 9-16. **Stages of tuberculosis. Primary** tuberculosis (in a person lacking previous contact or immune responsiveness). **Progressive primary** tuberculosis develops in less than 10% of infected normal adults but more frequently in children and immunosuppressed patients. **Secondary** (cavitary) tuberculosis results from reactivation of dormant endogenous bacilli or reinfection with exogenous bacilli. **Miliary** tuberculosis is caused by dissemination of tubercle bacilli to produce numerous, minute, yellow-white lesions (resembling millet seeds) in distant organs.

nation. This process produces **progressive primary tuberculosis**, in which the immune response fails to control the tubercle bacilli. The Ghon focus enlarges and may even erode into the bronchial tree. Affected hilar and mediastinal lymph nodes also enlarge. In some instances, the infected lymph nodes erode into an airway to spread organisms throughout the lungs.

FIGURE 9-17. **Primary tuberculosis.** Photomicrograph of a hilar lymph node shows a tuberculous granuloma with central caseation.

Miliary tuberculosis occurs when infection disseminates to produce multiple, small, yellow, nodular lesions in several organs (Fig. 9-18). The term "miliary" refers to the resemblance of these lesions to millet seeds. The lungs, lymph nodes, kidneys, adrenals, bone marrow, spleen, and liver are common sites of miliary lesions. Progressive disease may involve the meninges and cause tuberculous meningitis.

Secondary (Cavitary) Tuberculosis Results from Proliferation of *M. tuberculosis* in Someone Who Has Previously Contained the Infection

The mycobacteria in secondary tuberculosis may be either dormant organisms from old granulomas (which is usually the case) or newly acquired bacilli. Various conditions, including cancer, antineoplastic chemotherapy, immunosuppressive therapy, AIDS, and old age, predispose to the re-emergence of endogenous dormant *M. tuberculosis*. Secondary tuberculosis may develop even decades after primary infection.

 PATHOGENESIS AND PATHOLOGY: Any location may be involved, but the lungs are by far the most common site for secondary tuberculosis. In the lungs, secondary tuberculosis usually begins in the apical–posterior segments of the upper lobes, where organisms are commonly seeded during primary infection. There, the bacilli proliferate and elicit an inflammatory response, causing localized consolidation. *Ensuing T-cell-mediated immune responses to the now-familiar tuberculous antigens leads to tissue necrosis and production of tuberculous cavities* (Fig. 9-19). These cavities contain necrotic material teeming with mycobacteria and are surrounded by a granulomatous response.

The pulmonary lesions of secondary tuberculosis may be complicated by a variety of secondary effects: (1) scarring and calcification; (2) spread to other areas; (3) pleural fibrosis and adhesions; (4) rupture of a caseous lesion, spilling bacilli into the pleural cavity; (5) erosion into a bronchus, which seeds bronchioles, bronchi, and trachea; and (6) implantation of bacilli in the larynx, causing hoarseness and pain on swallowing. Tubercle bacilli may also spread throughout the body through the lymphatics and bloodstream to cause miliary tuberculosis. Tuberculosis is discussed in further detail in Chapter 12.

Leprosy

Leprosy (Hansen disease) is a chronic, slowly progressive, destructive process involving peripheral nerves, skin, and mucous membranes,

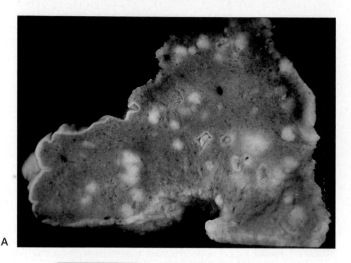

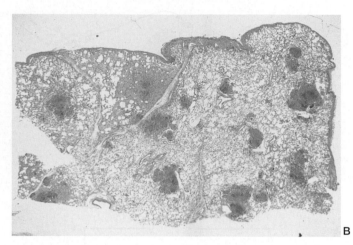

A   B

FIGURE 9-18.   **Miliary tuberculosis. A.** The cut surface of the lung reveals numerous uniform, white nodules. **B.** A low-power photomicrograph discloses many foci of granulomatous inflammation.

caused by Mycobacterium leprae. This agent is a slender, weakly acid-fast rod. Leprosy is transmitted from person to person, usually as a result of years of intimate contact. Although leprosy is now rare in developed countries, about 500,000 persons are reported to be infected worldwide, primarily in tropical areas, including tropical Africa, Brazil, and Southeastern Asia. Vigorous international programs aimed at discovery and therapy have been successful in reducing the incidence of new cases. In the United States, about 100 cases are diagnosed yearly, mostly in immigrants from endemic areas.

PATHOGENESIS AND PATHOLOGY: Most (95%) persons have a natural protective immunity to *M. leprae* and are not infected, despite intimate and prolonged exposure. Susceptible individuals span a broad immunologic spectrum from anergy to hyperergy and may develop symptomatic infection. *At one end of the spectrum, anergic patients have little or no resistance and develop* **lepromatous leprosy**, whereas hyperergic patients with high resistance contract **tuberculoid leprosy**. Most patients, in between these extremes, have **borderline leprosy**.

- **Tuberculoid leprosy** is characterized by a single lesion or very few lesions of the skin, usually on the face, extremities, or trunk. Microscopically, lesions show well-formed, circumscribed, dermal, noncaseating granulomas with epithelioid macrophages, Langhans giant cells, and lymphocytes. Skin lesions form well-demarcated, hypopigmented or erythematous, dry, hairless patches, with raised outer edges that are characterized by decreased sensation. The lesions of tuberculoid leprosy cause minimal disfigurement and are not infectious.

- **Lepromatous leprosy** exhibits multiple, tumor-like lesions of the skin, eyes, testes, nerves, lymph nodes, and spleen. Nodular or diffuse infiltrates of foamy macrophages contain myriad bacilli (Fig. 9-20). Foamy macrophages exhibit numerous organisms, which appear as aggregates of acid-fast material, called "globi." The dermal infiltrates expand slowly to distort and disfigure the face, ears, appendages, and upper airway and to destroy the eyes, eyebrows and eyelashes, nerves, and testes. Involvement of the upper airways leads to chronic nasal discharge and voice change.

Multidrug therapy using a combination of rifampicin, dapsone, and other agents is critical, as monodrug therapy always results in the development of resistance.

FUNGAL INFECTIONS

Of more than 100,000 known fungi, only a few cause human disease. Of these, most are "opportunists," that is, they only infect peo-

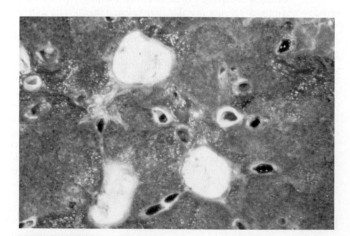

FIGURE 9-19.   **Secondary pulmonary tuberculosis.** A cross-section of lung shows several tuberculous cavities filled with necrotic, caseous material.

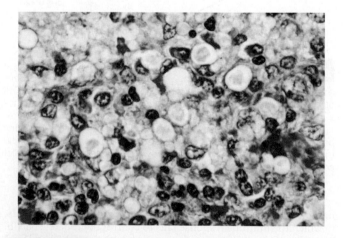

FIGURE 9-20.   **Lepromatous leprosy.** A section of skin shows a tumor-like mass of foamy macrophages. The faint masses within the vacuolated macrophages are enormous numbers of lepra bacilli.

ple with impaired immune mechanisms. *Thus, corticosteroid administration, antineoplastic therapy, and congenital or acquired T-cell deficiencies all predispose to mycotic infections.*

Fungi are larger and more complex than bacteria. They vary from 2 to 100 μm and are eukaryotes meaning that they possess nuclear membranes and cytoplasmic organelles, such as mitochondria and endoplasmic reticulum.

Pneumocystis Jiroveci Pneumonia

Pneumocystis jiroveci (*formerly, carinii*) *causes progressive, often fatal, pneumonia in persons with impaired cell-mediated immunity and is a common opportunistic pathogen in persons with AIDS.* P. jiroveci is distributed worldwide. It is likely that the organisms are omnipresent, because 75% of the population has acquired antibodies to Pneumocystis by the age of 5. In persons with intact cell-mediated immunity, infection is rapidly contained without producing symptoms. However, 80% of AIDS patients developed Pneumocystis pneumonia prior to the use of modern agents (see this chapter).

 PATHOGENESIS: *P. jiroveci* reproduces in association with alveolar type 1 lining cells, and active disease is confined to the lungs. If the process is not checked by the host immune system or antibiotic therapy, the infected alveoli eventually fill with organisms and proteinaceous fluid. Microscopically, the alveoli contain a frothy eosinophilic material, composed of alveolar macrophages and cysts and trophozoites of *P. jiroveci* (Fig. 9-21). The progressive filling of alveoli prevents adequate gas exchange, and the patient slowly suffocates. Therapy is with trimethoprim-sulfamethoxazole, pentamidine, atovaquone or several other regimens.

Candida

The genus *Candida,* comprising over 20 species of yeasts, includes the most common opportunistic pathogens. Many *Candida* species are endogenous human flora, well adapted to life on or in the human body. However, they can cause disease when host defenses are compromised. Although the forms of candidiasis vary in clinical severity, most are localized superficial diseases, limited to a particular mucocutaneous site, such as oral infections (thrush), esophagitis, vulvovaginitis, and others. Superficial infections may be linked to eradication of resident bacterial fauna (such as by antibiotic use)

because such fauna are important in host defense against candida. Candidal infections of deep tissues with concomitant sepsis and dissemination occur only in immunologically compromised persons and are often fatal. *Candida albicans* resides in small numbers in the oropharynx, gastrointestinal tract, and vagina and is the most frequent candidal pathogen, being responsible for more than 95% of infections. Candidal infections of specific organs are discussed in Chapters 13 and 25.

Aspergillosis

Aspergillus species are common environmental fungi that cause opportunistic infections, usually involving the lungs. Of these species, *Aspergillus fumigatus* is by far the most frequent human pathogen. There are three types of pulmonary aspergillosis: (1) allergic bronchopulmonary aspergillosis; (2) colonization of a pre-existing pulmonary cavity (aspergilloma or fungus ball); and (3) invasive aspergillosis.

ALLERGIC BRONCHOPULMONARY ASPERGILLOSIS: The disease is acquired by inhalation of the widely distributed spores thereby exposing the airway and alveoli to fungal antigens. Subsequent contact initiates an allergic response in susceptible persons. Bronchi and bronchioles show infiltrates of lymphocytes, plasma cells, and variable numbers of eosinophils. Airways may be impacted with mucus and fungal hyphae. The condition is virtually restricted to asthmatics, 20% of whom eventually develop this disorder.

ASPERGILLOMA: This condition occurs in persons with pulmonary (commonly old tuberculous) cavities or bronchiectasis. Inhaled spores germinate in the warm humid atmosphere provided by these hollows and fill them with masses of noninvasive hyphae.

INVASIVE ASPERGILLOSIS: Invasion may occur whenever neutrophil number or activity is compromised (such as by high-dose steroid or cytotoxic therapy or acute leukemia). Inhaled spores germinate to produce hyphae, which invade through bronchi into the lung parenchyma, from where the fungi spread widely. *Aspergillus* readily invades blood vessels and produces thrombosis.

Cryptococcosis

Cryptococcosis is a systemic mycosis caused by Cryptococcus neoformans, *which principally affects the meninges and lungs* (Fig. 9-22). The

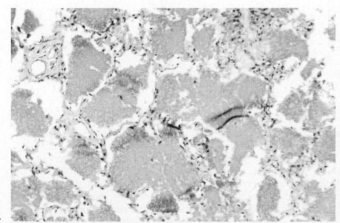
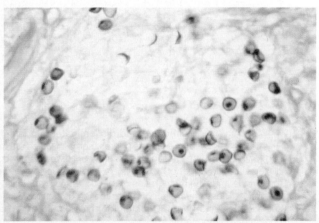

A   B

FIGURE 9-21. *Pneumocystis jiroveci* **pneumonia. A.** The alveoli contain a frothy eosinophilic material that is composed of alveolar macrophages and cysts and trophozoites of *P. carinii*. **B.** A silver stain shows crescent-shaped organisms, which are collapsed and degenerated. Some have a characteristic dark spot in their walls.

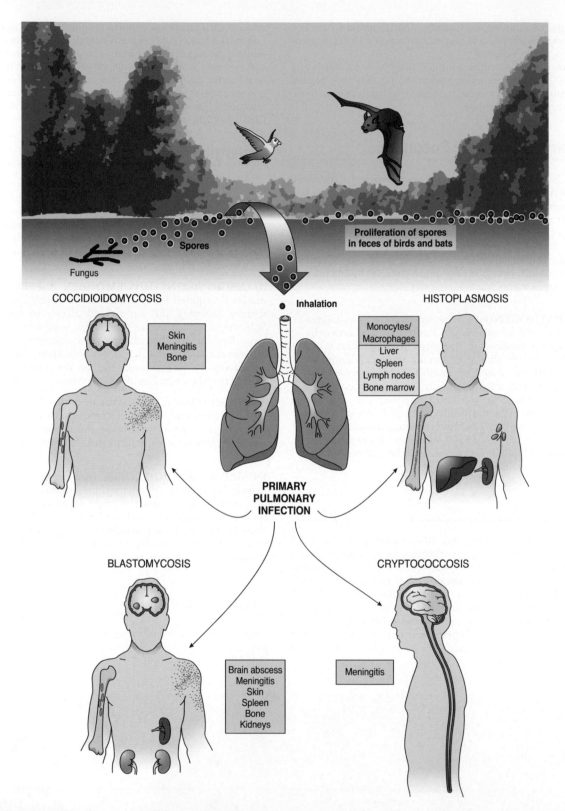

FIGURE 9-22. **Pulmonary and disseminated fungal infection.** Fungi grow in soil, air, and in the feces of birds and bats; they produce spores, some of which are infectious. When inhaled, spores cause primary pulmonary infection. In a few patients, the infection disseminates. **Histoplasmosis.** Primary infection is in the lung. In susceptible patients, the fungus disseminates to target organs, namely, the monocyte/macrophage system (liver, spleen, lymph nodes, and bone marrow) and the tongue, mucous membranes of mouth, and the adrenals. **Cryptococcosis.** Primary infection of the lung disseminates to the meninges. **Blastomycosis.** Primary infection of the lung disseminates widely. The principal targets are the brain, meninges, skin, spleen, bone, and kidney. **Coccidioidomycosis.** Primary infection of the lung may disseminate widely. The skin, meninges, and bone are common targets.

main reservoir for the fungus is pigeon droppings, and when inhaled, the organisms reach the terminal bronchioles.

Cryptococcus *almost exclusively affects persons with impaired cell-mediated immunity.* Although the organism is ubiquitous and exposure is common, cryptococcosis is rare in the absence of predisposing illness. Cryptococcosis occurs in patients with AIDS, lymphomas (particularly Hodgkin disease), leukemias, sarcoidosis, and in those treated with high doses of corticosteroids.

PATHOGENESIS: In immunologically intact persons, neutrophils and alveolar macrophages kill *C. neoformans*, and no clinical disease develops. By contrast, in a patient with defective cell-mediated immunity, the cryptococci survive, reproduce locally, and then disseminate. Although the lung is the entry site, the CNS is the most common site of disease. More than 95% of cryptococcal infections involve the meninges and brain. In meningoencephalitis, the entire brain is swollen and soft, and leptomeninges are thickened and gelatinous from infiltration by the thickly encapsulated organisms. Inflammatory responses are variable and often minimal, with large numbers of cryptococci infiltrating tissue. Because of its thick capsule, *C. neoformans* stains poorly with routine hematoxylin and eosin and appears as bubbles or holes in tissue sections (Fig. 9-23A). Untreated cryptococcal meningitis is invariably fatal. Therapy requires prolonged systemic administration of antifungal agents.

Histoplasmosis

Histoplasmosis is caused by Histoplasma capsulatum. *The disease is usually self-limited but may lead to a systemic granulomatous disease.* Although most cases of histoplasmosis are asymptomatic, progressive disseminated infections occur in persons with impaired cell-mediated immunity. Histoplasmosis is acquired by inhaling infectious spores of *H. capsulatum* (see Fig. 9-22). The reservoir for the fungus is bird and bat droppings and soil. The organism is endemic along the Ohio and Mississippi river valleys of the central and eastern US and also occurs in other areas of the Americas.

PATHOGENESIS AND PATHOLOGY: Histoplasmosis resembles tuberculosis in many ways. Acute self-limited histoplasmosis is characterized by necrotizing granulomas in the lung, mediastinal and hilar lymph nodes, spleen, and liver. Yeast forms of *H. capsulatum* can be demonstrated within macrophages and in the caseous material. Eventually, the cellular components of the granuloma largely disappear, and the caseous material calci-

fies, forming a "fibrocaseous nodule" (Fig. 9-24A). Disseminated histoplasmosis develops in persons who fail to mount an effective immune response to *H. capsulatum* and is characterized by progressive organ infiltration with macrophages carrying *H. capsulatum* (see Fig. 9-24B). Infants, those with AIDS, and patients treated with corticosteroids are at particular risk. Most infections are asymptomatic, but with extensive disease, patients present with fever, headache, and cough. Disseminated disease may persist for years, but in cases of profound immunodeficiency, there is rapid progress of the disease with high fever, cough, pancytopenia, and changes in mental status. Disseminated histoplasmosis is treated with systemic antifungal agents.

Coccidioidomycosis

Coccidioidomycosis is a chronic, necrotizing mycotic infection that clinically and pathologically resembles tuberculosis. The disease, caused by *Coccidioides immitis,* includes a spectrum of infections that begin as focal pneumonitis. Most are mild and asymptomatic and are limited to the lungs and regional lymph nodes. Occasionally, *C. immitis* infections spread outside the lungs to produce life-threatening disease.

C. immitis is present in the soil in restricted climatic regions, particularly areas with sparse rainfall, hot summers, and mild winters, including large portions of California, Arizona, New Mexico, and Texas. Infection is particularly common in the San Joaquin Valley of California. Epidemics have been associated with sandstorms and earthquakes, which produce airborne spores. The disease is not contagious.

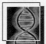

PATHOGENESIS: *Most infections are produced by small inocula of organisms in immunologically competent hosts and are acute and self-limited.* Coccidioidomycosis begins with focal bronchopneumonia where the spores are deposited. Affected alveoli are infiltrated by neutrophils and macrophages (Fig. 9-25). As in tuberculosis and histoplasmosis, the host controls *C. immitis* infection only when inflammatory cells become immunologically activated. Necrotizing granulomas form with the onset of specific hypersensitivity. Subsequent cell-mediated immune responses kill or contain the fungi—a process followed by healing of the granuloma. The course of coccidioidomycosis depends on the size of the infecting dose and the immune status of the host. Extensive pulmonary involvement and fulminant disease may occur in persons from a nonendemic region exposed to large numbers of organisms. **Disseminated coccidioidomycosis** occurs in immunocompromised persons either from a primary infection or reacti-

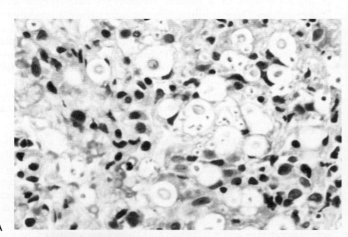

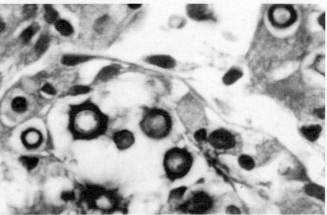

A ... B

FIGURE 9-23. **Cryptococcosis. A.** In a section of the lung stained with hematoxylin and eosin, *C. neoformans* appears as holes or bubbles. **B.** The same section stained with mucicarmine illustrates the capsule of the organism.

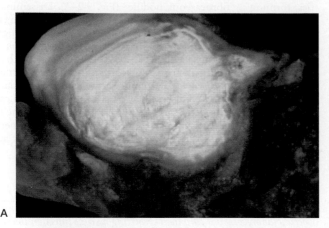
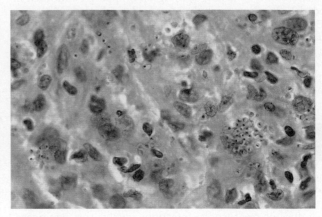

A

B

FIGURE 9-24. **Histoplasmosis. A.** A section of lung shows an encapsulated, subpleural, fibrocaseous nodule. **B.** A section of liver from a patient with disseminated histoplasmosis reveals Kupffer cells containing numerous yeasts of *H. capsulatum* (periodic acid-Schiff [PAS] stain).

vation of old disease. Disseminated disease may involve almost any body site and may manifest as a single extrathoracic site or as widespread disease, including lesions of the skin, bones, meninges, liver, spleen, and genitourinary tract. Certain racial groups, including Filipinos, other Asians, and blacks, are particularly susceptible to dissemination of coccidioidomycosis, probably because of a specific immunologic defect. Even with prolonged amphotericin B therapy, the prognosis is poor in acute disseminated coccidioidomycosis, although the response rate can be quite good with some of the newer azole antifungal agents.

Blastomycosis

Blastomycosis is a chronic granulomatous and suppurative pulmonary disease, which is often followed by dissemination to other body sites, principally the skin and bone. The causative organism, *Blastomyces dermatitidis,* is a dimorphic fungus that grows as a mold in warm moist soil, rich in decaying vegetable matter. In North America, the fungus is endemic along the distributions of the Mississippi and Ohio Rivers, the Great Lakes, and the St. Lawrence River. Disturbance of the soil, either by construction or by leisure activities such as hunting or camping, leads to the formation of aerosols containing fungal spores.

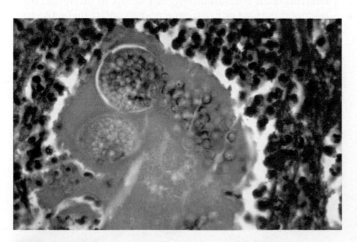

FIGURE 9-25. **Coccidioidomycosis.** A photomicrograph of the lung from a patient with acute coccidioidal pneumonia shows an acute inflammatory infiltrate surrounding spherules and endospores of *Coccidioides immitis.*

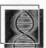**PATHOGENESIS AND PATHOLOGY:** Inhaled spores of *B. dermatitidis* germinate to form yeasts, which reproduce by budding. The host responds to the proliferating organisms with a mixed suppurative and granulomatous inflammatory response, producing a focal bronchopneumonia. Infected areas contain numerous yeasts of *B. dermatitidis,* which are spherical and 8 to 14 μm across, with broad-based buds and multiple nuclei in a central body. With hematoxylin and eosin stains, the yeast are rings with thick, sharply defined cell walls. They may be found in epithelioid cells, macrophages, or giant cells, or they may lie free in microabscesses. Organisms persist until the onset of specific hypersensitivity and cell-mediated immunity, when activated neutrophils and macrophages kill them. Pulmonary disease usually is self-limited and resolves by scarring, but some patients develop progressive miliary lesions or cavities. The skin and bones are the most common sites of extrapulmonary involvement. Symptomatic acute infection presents as a flu-like illness, with fever, arthralgias, and myalgias. Progressive pulmonary disease is characterized by low-grade fever, weight loss, cough, and predominantly upper-lobe infiltrates on the chest radiograph.

Dermatophyte Infections

Dermatophytes are fungi that cause localized superficial infections of keratinized tissues, including skin, hair, and nails. There are about 40 species of dermatophytes in 3 genera: *Trichophyton, Microsporum,* and *Epidermophyton.* Dermatophyte infections are named according to the sites of involvement (e.g., scalp, tinea capitis; feet, tinea pedis, "athlete's foot"; nails, tinea unguium; intertriginous areas of the groin, tinea cruris, "jock itch"). Dermatophyte infections are minor illnesses but are among the most common skin diseases for which persons seek medical help. Dermatophytes are resident in the soil, on animals, and on other humans. The disease is usually acquired by direct contact with persons who have infected hairs or skin scales.

PATHOLOGY: Dermatophytes proliferate within the superficial keratinized tissues. They spread centrifugally from the initial site, producing round, expanding lesions with sharp margins. The appearance once suggested that a worm was responsible for the disease, hence the names **ringworm** and **tinea** (from the Latin *tinea,* "worm"). Infections produce thickening of the squamous epithelium, with increased numbers of keratinized cells. Hyphae and spores are confined to the nonviable portions of skin, hair, and nails.

PROTOZOAL INFECTIONS

Protozoa cause human disease by diverse mechanisms. Some, such as *Entamoeba histolytica,* are extracellular parasites capable of digesting and invading human tissues. Others, such as plasmodia, are obligate intracellular parasites that replicate in, and kill, human cells. Still others, such as trypanosomes, damage human tissue largely by eliciting inflammatory and immunologic responses. Some protozoa (e.g., *Toxoplasma gondii*) can establish latent infections and cause reactivation disease in immunocompromised hosts.

Malaria

Malaria is a mosquito-borne, hemolytic, febrile illness that infects more than 300 million individuals and kills more than 1 million yearly. Four species of *Plasmodium* cause malaria: *Plasmodium falciparum, Plasmodium vivax, Plasmodium ovale, and Plasmodium malariae.* They infect and destroy human erythrocytes, producing chills, fever, anemia, and splenomegaly. *P. falciparum* causes more severe disease than the others and accounts for most malarial deaths. It is estimated that 40% of the world's population concentrated in tropical and subtropical areas, especially Africa, South and Central America, India, and Southeast Asia, are at risk of the disease. Although malaria has been eradicated in developed countries, more than 1,000 cases of malaria are detected yearly in the US, most imported by returning travelers or immigrants. *P. falciparum* and *P. ovale* predominate in Africa where *P. vivax* infection is rare because much of the black population lacks the erythrocyte cell-surface receptors required for infection.

 PATHOGENESIS: The complex life cycle of the *Plasmodium* species responsible for human malaria requires both human and mosquito hosts and is summarized in Figure 9-26. The anopheles mosquito inoculates the sporozoites into a human's bloodstream, where the organisms ultimately invade erythrocytes, inside of which they grow and reproduce. Within 2 to 4 days, the organisms burst from infected erythrocytes, invade naïve red cells, and so initiate another cycle of erythrocytic parasitism. The rupture of infected erythrocytes releases pyrogens and causes the recurrent **paroxysms** of chills and high fever characteristic of malaria. Paroxysms recur for weeks, eventually subsiding as an immunologic response is mounted. Each paroxysm reflects another round of the rupture of infected erythrocytes and release of daughter organisms. Anemia results both from loss of circulating infected erythrocytes and sequestration of cells by fixed mononuclear phagocytes in the enlarging spleen. Liver, spleen, and lymph nodes are darkened by macrophages filled with hemosiderin and malarial pigment, the end-product of parasitic digestion of hemoglobin.

 P. falciparum causes **malignant malaria**, the most aggressive form of the disease. The organism alters flow characteristics and adhesive properties of infected erythrocytes, which adhere to the endothelial cells of small blood vessels. Obstruction of small blood vessels frequently produces severe tissue ischemia of the brain, kidneys, and lungs, which is probably the most important factor in the virulence of *P. falciparum.* Brains of persons who die of cerebral malaria show congestion and thrombosis of small blood vessels in the white matter, which are rimmed with edema and hemorrhage ("ring hemorrhages") (Fig. 9-27). Ischemic brain injury causes symptoms ranging from somnolence, hallucinations, and behavioral changes, to seizures and coma. CNS disease has a mortality of 20% to 50%. Therapy for malaria varies depending on the disease type and degree of the organism's drug resistance. Current therapeutic guidelines may be found in *Guidelines for Treatment of Malaria in the United States* available from the Centers for Disease Control (www.cdc.gov/malaria/diagnosis_ treatment/clinicians2.htm).

Toxoplasmosis

Toxoplasmosis is a worldwide infectious disease caused by a protozoan, Toxoplasma gondii. *Most infections are asymptomatic, but if they occur in a fetus or immunocompromised host, devastating necrotizing disease may result.* Exposure to the organism is common. In the United States, more than 20% of adolescents and adults have serological evidence of having been infected. *T. gondii* has an extremely complex life cycle. The final host is the cat, which becomes infected by ingesting cysts of the organism from an infected mouse, bird, human, or other intermediate host. The organism multiplies within the intestinal epithelial cells of the cat and is shed in the feces. Humans become infected by ingestion of infected meat, from environments contaminated by infected cat feces (such as litter boxes or garden soil), and by maternal-fetal transmission (see Chapter 6).

 PATHOGENESIS: In acute infections, multiplying organisms spread from the gut through the lymphatics to regional lymph nodes and through the blood to the liver, lungs, heart, brain, and other organs. In most infections, little significant tissue destruction occurs before the immune response brings the active phase of the infection under control. Infected persons suffer few clinical effects, the most frequent of which is lymphadenopathy. *T. gondii* establishes latent infection, however, by forming dormant tissue cysts in some infected cells, which survive for decades in the host. If an infected person loses cell-mediated immunity, the organism can emerge from its encysted form and re-establish a destructive infection.

Congenital Toxoplasma Infections Principally Affect the Brain

T. gondii infection in a fetus is far more destructive than is postnatal infection (see Chapter 6).

 PATHOGENESIS: The most severe fetal disease is produced by infection early in pregnancy and often terminates in spontaneous abortion. The developing brain and eyes are readily infected, and the fetus lacks the immunologic capacity to contain the infection. CNS infection causes a necrotizing meningoencephalitis, which in the most severe cases leads to loss of brain parenchyma, cerebral calcifications, and marked hydrocephalus (Fig. 9-28). Ocular infection causes chorioretinitis (i.e., necrosis and inflammation of the choroid and retina).

Toxoplasmosis in Immunocompromised Hosts Produces Encephalitis

Devastating *T. gondii* infections occur in persons with decreased cell-mediated immunity (e.g., patients with AIDS or those receiving immunosuppressive therapy). In most cases, the disease represents reactivation of a latent infection. The brain is the most commonly affected organ, where infection with *T. gondii* produces a multifocal necrotizing encephalitis. Patients with encephalitis present with paresis, seizures, alterations in visual acuity, and changes in mentation. *Toxoplasma* encephalitis in immunocompromised patients is fatal if not treated with effective antiprotozoal agents.

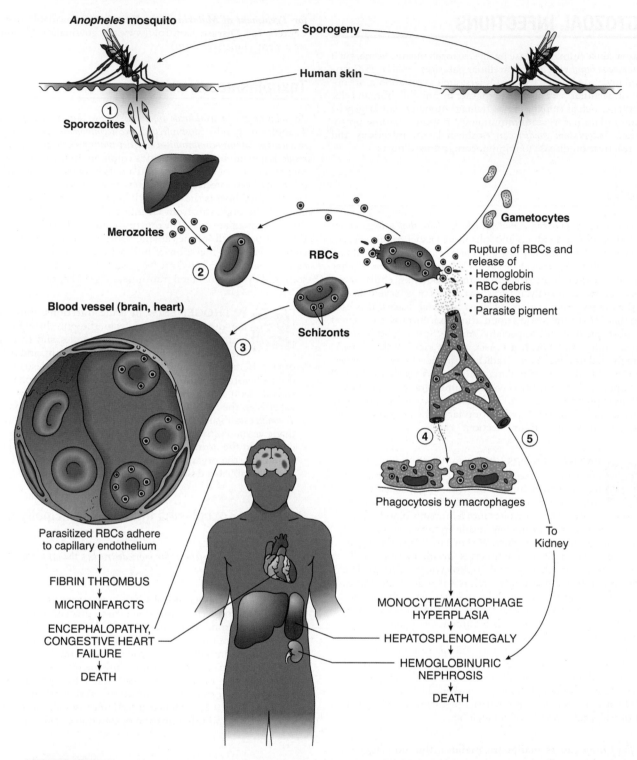

FIGURE 9-26. **Life cycle of malaria.** An *Anopheles* mosquito bites an infected person, taking blood that contains micro- and macrogametocytes (sexual forms). In the mosquito, sexual multiplication (sporogony) produces infective sporozoites in the salivary glands. *(1)* During the mosquito bite, sporozoites are inoculated into the bloodstream of the vertebrate host. Some sporozoites leave the blood and enter the hepatocytes, where they multiply asexually (exoerythrocytic schizogony) and form thousands of uninucleated merozoites. *(2)* Rupture of hepatocytes releases merozoites, which penetrate erythrocytes and become trophozoites, which then divide to form numerous schizonts (intraerythrocytic schizogony). Schizonts divide to form more merozoites, which are released on the rupture of erythrocytes and re-enter other erythrocytes to begin a new cycle. After several cycles, subpopulations of merozoites develop into micro- and macrogametocytes, which are taken up by another mosquito to complete the cycle. *(3)* Parasitized erythrocytes obstruct capillaries of the brain, heart, kidney, and other deep organs. Adherence of parasitized erythrocytes to capillary endothelial cells causes fibrin thrombi, which produce microinfarcts. These result in encephalopathy, congestive heart failure, pulmonary edema, and frequently death. Ruptured erythrocytes release hemoglobin, erythrocyte debris, and malarial pigment. *(4)* Phagocytosis leads to monocyte/macrophage hyperplasia and hepatosplenomegaly. *(5)* Released hemoglobin produces hemoglobinuric nephrosis, which may be fatal. RBCs, red blood cells.

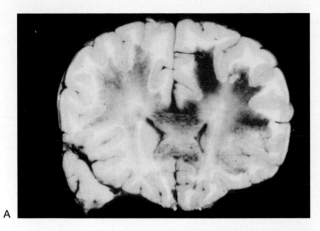

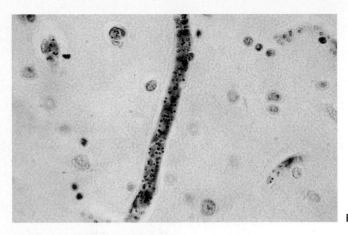

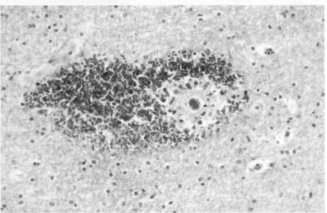

FIGURE 9-27. **Acute falciparum malaria of the brain. A.** There is severe diffuse congestion of the white matter and focal hemorrhages. **B.** A section of **(A)** shows a capillary packed with parasitized erythrocytes. **C.** Another section of **(A)** displays a ring hemorrhage around a thrombosed capillary, which contains parasitized erythrocytes in a fibrin thrombus.

Amebiasis

Amebiasis is infection with Entamoeba histolytica, *which principally involves the colon and occasionally, the liver. E. histolytica is named for its lytic actions on tissue.* Intestinal infection ranges from asymptomatic colonization to severe invasive infections with bloody diarrhea. Humans are the only known reservoir for *E. histolytica,* which reproduces in the colon. Disease is acquired by

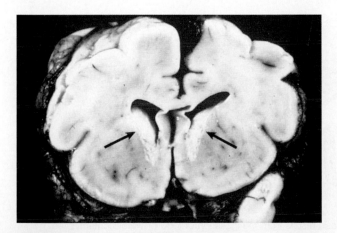

FIGURE 9-28. **Congenital toxoplasmosis.** The brain of a premature infant reveals subependymal necrosis with calcification appearing as bilaterally symmetric areas of whitish discoloration *(arrows).*

ingestion of fecally contaminated material. Amebiasis is most prevalent in developing countries with poor sanitation. In the United States, the disease is uncommon and associated with travelers, immigrants, and male homosexuals (Fig. 9-29).

 PATHOGENESIS AND PATHOLOGY: Colitis begins with attachment of the invasive stage of the organism (trophozoites) to a colonic epithelial cell. The organism kills the target cell by elaborating a lytic protein that breaches the cell membrane. Progressive death of mucosal cells produces small foci of necrosis that progress to ulcers (Fig. 9-30A). Undermining of the ulcer margin and confluence of expanding ulcers lead to irregular sloughing of the mucosa. The ulcer bed is gray and necrotic, with fibrin and cellular debris. The exudate raises the undermined mucosa, producing chronic amebic ulcers, with a shape that has been described as resembling a flask or a bottle neck. Trophozoites are found on the surface of the ulcer, in the exudate, and in the crater (see Fig. 9-30B). They are also frequent in the submucosa, muscularis propria, serosa, and small veins of the submucosa. There is little inflammatory response in early amebic ulcers. However, as the ulcer enlarges, acute and chronic inflammatory cells accumulate. Intestinal amebiasis ranges from completely asymptomatic to a severe dysenteric disease. Nausea, vomiting, malodorous flatus, and intermittent constipation are typical features. Liquid stools (up to 25 a day) contain bloody mucus, but diarrhea is rarely prolonged enough to cause dehydration. Amebic colitis often persists for months or years, and patients may become emaciated and anemic. Transmission of disease is by cystic forms of the organism, which are spread in

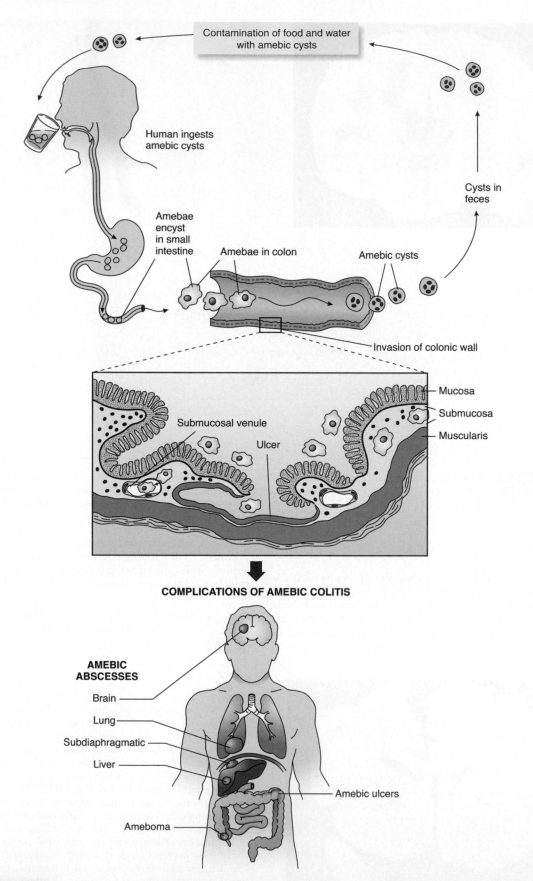

FIGURE 9-29. **Amebic colitis and its complications.** Amebiasis results from the ingestion of food or water contaminated with amebic cysts. In the colon, the amebae penetrate the mucosa and produce flask-shaped ulcers of the mucosa and submucosa. The organisms may invade submucosal venules, thereby disseminating the infection to the liver and other organs. The liver abscess can expand to involve adjacent structures.

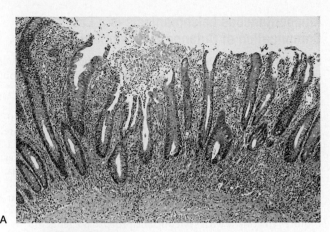
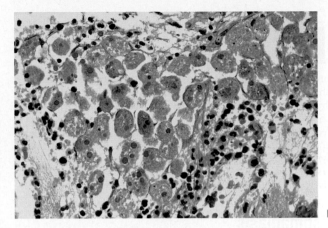

A

B

FIGURE 9-30. **Intestinal amebiasis. A.** The colonic mucosa shows superficial ulceration beneath a cluster of trophozoites of *Entamoeba histolytica*. The lamina propria contains excess acute and chronic inflammatory cells, including eosinophils. **B.** Higher-power view shows numerous trophozoites in the luminal exudate.

stool and persist in the environment. Therapy for symptomatic intestinal amebiasis includes metronidazole or tinidazole, which act against trophozoites, followed by diloxanide, paromomycin, or iodoquinol, which are effective against cysts.

Amebic liver abscess is a major complication of amebiasis that can occur when trophozoites invade the submucosal veins of the colon, enter the portal circulation, and reach the liver. Here the organisms kill hepatocytes, producing a slowly expanding necrotic cavity filled with a dark brown, odorless, semisolid material. Neutrophils are rare within the cavity, and trophozoites are found along the edges adjacent to hepatocytes (Fig. 9-31). An amebic liver abscess may expand and rupture through the capsule, extending into the peritoneum, diaphragm, pleural cavity, lungs, or pericardium.

Cryptosporidiosis

Cryptosporidiosis is a recently recognized enteric infection with protozoa of the genus Cryptosporidium *that cause diarrhea.* The infection varies from a self-limited gastrointestinal infection in immunocompetent individuals to a potentially life-threatening illness in the im-

munocompromised. It is acquired by ingesting *Cryptosporidium* oocysts, which are shed in the feces of infected humans and animals. Many domesticated animals harbor the parasite and are a large reservoir for human infection. Water-borne outbreaks have infected large numbers of persons.

 PATHOGENESIS: *Cryptosporidium* oocysts are extremely stable in the environment, survive passage through the stomach, and release forms that attach to the microvillous surface of the small bowel. In that location, they form a complex structure involving both the host and parasite cell membranes. The organisms reproduce on the luminal surface of the gut, from stomach to rectum, forming progeny that also attach to the epithelium. In the small intestine (the most common site of infection), there may be moderate or severe chronic inflammation in the lamina propria and some villous atrophy directly related to the density of the parasites. In immunologically competent persons, infection is terminated by immune responses. Patients with AIDS and some congenital immunodeficiencies cannot contain the parasite and develop chronic infections, which sometimes spread from the bowel to involve the gallbladder and intrahepatic bile ducts.

Cryptosporidiosis presents as profuse, watery diarrhea, sometimes accompanied by cramping abdominal pain or low-grade fever. Extraordinary volumes of fluid can be lost as diarrhea, and intensive fluid replacement is required. In immunologically competent individuals, diarrhea resolves spontaneously in 1 to 2 weeks. In immunocompromised patients, diarrhea persists indefinitely and may contribute to death. Therapy in such cases relies on attempting to re-establish immunocompetence.

Giardiasis

Giardiasis is an infection of the small intestine caused by the flagellated protozoan Giardia lamblia *and characterized by abdominal cramping and diarrhea.* The organism has a worldwide distribution. Giardiasis is acquired by ingesting infectious cyst forms of the organism, which are shed in the feces of infected humans and animals. Infection spreads directly from person to person and also in contaminated water or food. *Giardia* is often acquired from wilderness water sources, where infected animals, such as beavers and bears, serve as the reservoir of infection.

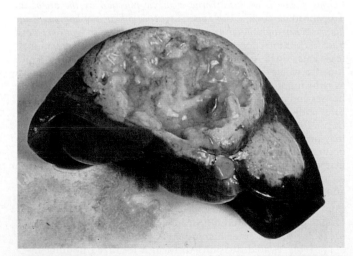

FIGURE 9-31. **Amebic abscesses of the liver.** The cut surface of the liver shows multiple abscesses containing "anchovy paste" material.

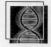 **PATHOGENESIS:** *Giardia* cysts survive gastric acidity and rupture within the duodenum and jejunum to release trophozoites. The latter attach to the small bowel epithelial microvilli and reproduce. Giardiasis produces no grossly visible alterations. Microscopic examination shows *Giardia* trophozoites on the surface of villi and within crypts, with minimal associated mucosal changes. Organisms encyst as the parasites transit toward the colon and are shed in feces. Acute giardiasis occurs with the abrupt onset of abdominal cramping and frequent foul-smelling stools. In some patients, symptoms resolve spontaneously in 1 to 4 weeks, whereas in others, the disease is more chronic. The infection is treated effectively with various antibiotics, including metronidazole.

Leishmaniasis

Leishmaniae are protozoans that are transmitted to humans by Phlebotomuss and flies. The organisms cause a spectrum of clinical syndromes, ranging from indolent, self-resolving cutaneous ulcers to fatal disseminated disease. There are numerous species of *Leishmania*, which differ in their natural habitats and the types of disease that they produce. In many subtropical and tropical areas, leishmanial infection is endemic in animal populations; dogs, ground squirrels, foxes, and jackals are reservoirs and potential sources for transmission to humans. It is mainly a disease found in less-developed countries where humans live in close proximity to animal hosts and the fly vector, although the disease is occasionally found in the Mediterranean area, including Spain, France, Italy, and Malta. Leishmaniasis is becoming associated with HIV coinfection. There are estimated to be 12 million persons infected worldwide, with 2 million new cases per year.

 PATHOGENESIS: Infection begins when the organisms are inoculated into human skin by the bite of the sandfly and are phagocytosed by mononuclear phagocytes. The organisms reproduce within macrophages, which rupture and yield a cluster of infected macrophages at the site of inoculation. From this initial local infection, the disease may take widely divergent courses, depending on the immunologic capabilities of the host and the infecting species of *Leishmania*. Three distinct clinical entities are recognized: (1) localized cutaneous leishmaniasis; (2) mucocutaneous leishmaniasis; and (3) visceral leishmaniasis.

Localized and Diffuse Cutaneous Leishmaniasis is an Ulcerating Disorder

Several *Leishmania* species, predominantly found in Afghanistan, other Middle Eastern countries, Iran, Brazil, and Peru, produce localized cutaneous disease, also known as "oriental sore" or "tropical sore."

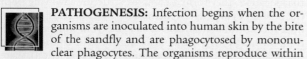 **PATHOGENESIS AND PATHOLOGY: Localized cutaneous leishmaniasis** begins as an itching, solitary papule, which erodes to form a shallow ulcer with a sharp, raised border. This ulcer can grow to 6 to 8 cm in diameter. With progressive development of cell-mediated immunity, macrophages become activated and kill the intracellular parasites. The lesion slowly assumes a more mature granulomatous appearance, with epithelioid macrophages, Langhans giant cells, plasma cells, and lymphocytes. Over the course of months, the cutaneous ulcer heals spontaneously.

Diffuse cutaneous leishmaniasis develops in some patients who lack specific cell-mediated immune responses to leishmaniae. The disease begins as a single nodule, but adjacent satellite nodules slowly form, eventually involving much of the skin. These lesions so closely resemble lepromatous leprosy that some patients have been cared for in leprosaria. The nodule of anergic leishmaniasis is caused by enormous numbers of macrophages replete with leishmaniae.

Mucocutaneous Leishmaniasis is a Late Complication of Cutaneous Leishmaniasis

Mucocutaneous leishmaniasis is caused by infection with *Leishmania braziliensis*. Most cases occur in Central and South America, where rodents and sloths are reservoirs.

 PATHOGENESIS: The early course and pathologic changes of mucocutaneous leishmaniasis are similar to those of localized cutaneous leishmaniasis. Years after a primary lesion has healed, an ulcer develops at a mucocutaneous junction, such as the larynx, nasal septum, anus, or vulva. The mucosal lesion is slowly progressive, highly destructive, and disfiguring, eroding mucosal surfaces and cartilage. Mucocutaneous leishmaniasis requires treatment with systemic antiprotozoal agents.

Visceral Leishmaniasis (Kala Azar) is a Potentially Fatal Infection of the Monocyte/Macrophage System

Kala azar is produced by several subspecies of Leishmania donovani. Reservoirs of the agent and susceptible age groups vary in different parts of the world. Humans are the reservoir in India and dogs in the Mediterranean basin.

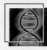 **PATHOGENESIS:** Most persons destroy *L. donovani* by cell-mediated immune responses, but 5% develop visceral leishmaniasis. Young children and malnourished persons are especially susceptible. The liver (Fig. 9-32A), spleen, and lymph nodes become massively enlarged, as macrophages in these organs fill with proliferating organisms. Normal organ architecture is gradually replaced by sheets of parasitized macrophages (see Fig. 9-32B). Eventually, these cells accumulate in other organs, including the heart and kidney. Over the course of months, a patient with visceral leishmaniasis becomes profoundly cachectic and displays massive splenomegaly. The untreated disease is invariably fatal. Treatment entails systemic antiprotozoal therapy.

Chagas Disease (American Trypanosomiasis)

Chagas disease is an insect-borne, zoonotic infection by the protozoan Trypanosoma cruzi, *which causes a systemic infection of humans. Acute manifestations and long-term sequelae occur in the heart and gastrointestinal tract. T. cruzi* infection is endemic in wild and domesticated animals (e.g., rats, dogs, goats, cats, armadillos) in Central and South America, where the parasite is transmitted by triatomine (also known as reduviid or "kissing") bugs. The insects hide in cracks of rickety houses and in vegetal roofing, emerge at night, feed on sleeping victims, and discharge infective forms of *T. cruzi* in their feces. The infective forms penetrate at the site of the bite or other abrasions or may penetrate the mucosa of the eyes or lips. Congenital infection occurs upon passage of the parasite from mother to fetus. It is estimated that approximately 20 million individuals in Latin America are infected with *T. cruzi*, more than half of whom live in Brazil. An annual total of 50,000 deaths are attributable to the disease.

 PATHOGENESIS: Once in the body, the organisms enter macrophages, where they undergo repeated divisions to form a localized nodular inflammatory lesion, a **chagoma**. The organisms also invade other sites, including cardiac myocytes and the brain. Within host cells, organisms differentiate and divide, break out and enter the bloodstream, from where they may be passed to the insect vector. Parasitemia and widespread

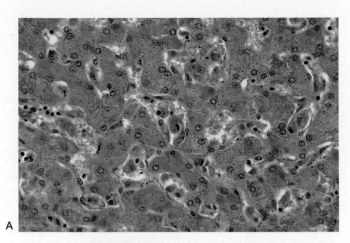
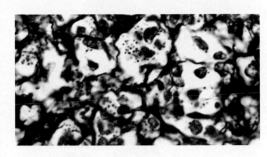

A

B

FIGURE 9-32. **Visceral leishmaniasis. A.** A photomicrograph of an enlarged liver shows prominent Kupffer cells distended by leishmanial amastigotes. **B.** A section of bone marrow subjected to silver impregnation shows macrophages filled with proliferating leishmanial amastigotes.

cellular infection are responsible for the systemic symptoms of acute Chagas disease. The onset of cell-mediated immunity eliminates the acute manifestations, but chronic tissue damage may continue. Progressive destruction of cells at sites of infection—particularly the heart, esophagus, and colon—causes organ dysfunction, manifested decades after the acute infection. Antiprotozoal chemotherapy is effective for acute Chagas disease but not for its chronic sequelae.

- **Acute Chagas disease** generally causes a mild illness. Myocarditis may result from the presence of numerous parasites in the heart where they are evident as pseudocysts within myofibers. There is extensive chronic inflammation and, in fatal cases, the heart is enlarged and dilated, with a pale, focally hemorrhagic myocardium.
- **Chronic Chagas disease** develops in 10% to 40% of acutely infected persons. *T. cruzi* is no longer present in blood or tissue. Infected organs have been damaged, however, by a chronic, progressive inflammatory process. This results in ***chronic myocarditis***, in which the heart displays extensive interstitial fibrosis, hypertrophied myofibers, and focal lymphocytic inflammation. Progressive cardiac fibrosis causes dysrhythmia or congestive heart failure. ***Megaesophagus and megacolon*** result from the destruction of parasympathetic ganglia in the wall of the lower esophagus and the myenteric plexus of the colon. The massive dilation of these areas leads to difficulty in swallowing and severe constipation.
- **Congenital Chagas disease** occurs in some pregnant women with parasitemia. Infection of the placenta and fetus leads to spontaneous abortion. In the infrequent live births, the infants die of encephalitis within a few days or weeks.

African Trypanosomiasis

African trypanosomiasis, popularly termed **sleeping sickness**, *is an infection with* Trypanosoma brucei gambiense *or* Trypanosoma brucei rhodesiense, *which produces a life-threatening meningoencephalitis.* Gambian trypanosomiasis is a chronic infection often lasting more than a year, for which humans appear to be the only significant reservoir. By contrast, East African (Rhodesian) trypanosomiasis is a rapidly progressive infection that kills the patient in 3 to 6 months. Game animals and domestic cattle are natural reservoirs for *T. rhodesiense*. Hence, rural populations engaged in animal husbandry and agriculture are at high risk (Fig. 9-33).

PATHOGENESIS: *T. brucei* multiplies at sites of inoculation by tsetse flies, occasionally producing localized nodular lesions called "primary chancres." Generalized involvement of lymph nodes and spleen is prominent early in the disease. The organisms disseminate to the bone marrow and tissue fluids where they produce systemic disease. Some eventually invade the CNS. Bloodstream invasion is marked by intermittent fever, for up to a week, often accompanied by splenomegaly and local and generalized lymphadenopathy. The evolving illness is marked by remitting irregular fevers, headache, joint pains, lethargy, and muscle wasting. Differences between the forms of sleeping sickness are primarily a matter of time scale, especially with regard to invasion of the brain. This feature develops early (weeks or months) in Rhodesian trypanosomiasis and late (months or years) in the Gambian form. Brain invasion is marked by apathy, daytime somnolence, and sometimes coma.

HELMINTHIC INFECTIONS

Helminths, or worms, are among the most common human pathogens. At any given time, 25% to 50% of the world's population carries at least one helminth species. Although most infections cause little harm, some produce significant disease. Schistosomiasis, for instance, ranks among the leading global causes of morbidity and mortality.

Most helminths that infect humans are well adapted to human parasitism, causing limited or no host tissue damage. Helminths gain entry by ingestion, skin penetration, or insect bites. The parasites cause disease in various ways. A few compete with their human host for certain nutrients. Some grow to block vital structures, producing disease by mass effect. Most, however, cause dysfunction through the destructive inflammatory and immunologic responses that they elicit. For example, morbidity in schistosomiasis, the most destructive helminthic infection, results from the granulomatous response to the schistosome eggs deposited in tissue. Eosinophils contain basic proteins toxic to some helminths and are a major component of inflammatory responses to these organisms.

- **Roundworms (nematodes)** are elongate cylindrical organisms with tubular digestive tracts.
- **Flatworms (trematodes)** are dorsoventrally flattened organisms with digestive tracts that end in blind loops.
- **Tapeworms (cestodes)** are segmented organisms with separate head and body parts; they lack a digestive tract and absorb nutrients through their outer walls.

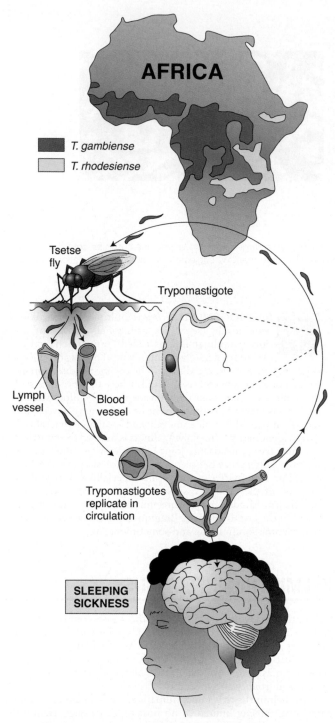

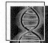

FIGURE 9-33. **African trypanosomiasis (sleeping sickness).** The distribution of Gambian and Rhodesian trypanosomiasis is related to the habitats of the vector tsetse flies (*Glossina* spp.). A tsetse fly bites an infected animal or human and ingests trypomastigotes, which multiply into infective, metacyclic trypomastigotes. During another fly bite, these are injected into lymphatic and blood vessels of a new host. A primary chancre develops at the site of the bite (stage 1a). Trypomastigotes replicate further in the blood and lymph, causing a systemic infection (stage 1b). Another fly ingests hypomastigotes to complete the cycle. In stage 2, invasion of the central nervous system by trypomastigotes leads to meningoencephalomyelitis and associated symptoms, including lethargy and daytime somnolence. Patients with Rhodesian trypanosomiasis may die within a few months. *T. gambiense, Trypanosoma brucei gambiense, T. rhodeseince, Trypanosoma* brucei rhodesiense.

Filarial Nematodes

Lymphatic Filariasis Results in Massive Lymphedema (Elephantiasis)

Lymphatic filariasis (bancroftian and Malayan filariasis) is an inflammatory parasitic infection of lymphatic vessels caused by the roundworms *Wuchereria bancrofti* and *Brugia malayi*. Adult worms inhabit the lymphatics, most frequently in inguinal, epitrochlear and axillary lymph nodes, testis, and epididymis, where they cause acute lymphangitis. In a minority of infected subjects, lymphatic obstruction leads to severe lymphedema, in its most severe form termed elephantiasis (Fig. 9-34). Humans, the only definitive host of these filarial nematodes, acquire infection from the bites of at least 80 species of mosquitoes. *W. bancrofti* infection is widespread in southern Asia, the Pacific, Africa, and portions of South America. *B. malayi* is localized to coastal southern Asia and western Pacific islands. Worldwide, 120 million persons are estimated to be infected, and 40 million have serious disease.

PATHOGENESIS AND PATHOLOGY: Mosquito bites transmit infectious larvae that migrate to lymphatics and lymph nodes. After maturing into adult forms over several months, worms mate and the female releases microfilariae into lymphatics and the bloodstream. Lymphatic vessels harboring adult worms are dilated, and their endothelial lining is thickened. In adjacent tissue, a chronic inflammatory infiltrate including eosinophils surrounds the worms. A granulomatous reaction may develop, and degenerating worms can provoke acute inflammation. The manifestations of filariasis result from the repeated inflammatory responses in the lymphatics that over years result in extensive scarring and obstruction of lymphatics. This blockage causes localized dependent edema, most commonly affecting legs, arms, genitalia, and breasts. Elephantiasis occurs in less than 5% of the infected population.

Onchocerciasis Causes Blindness

Onchocerciasis ("river blindness") is a chronic inflammatory disease of the skin, eyes, and lymphatics caused by the filarial nematode *Onchocerca volvulus*. Onchocerciasis is one of the world's major

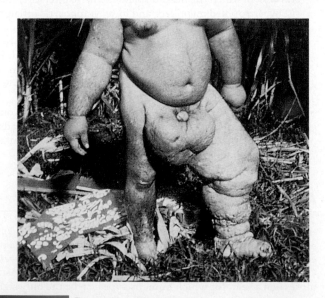

FIGURE 9-34. **Bancroftian filariasis.** Massive lymphedema (elephantiasis) of the scrotum and left lower extremity are present.

causes of blindness, afflicting an estimated 18 million individuals, of whom half a million are blind. Humans are the only definitive host. On biting, water breeding blackflies transmit infectious larvae to humans. Onchocerciasis is thus endemic along rivers and streams (hence, "**river blindness**"). About 90% of cases occur in tropical Africa, the rest in southern Mexico, Central America, and South America.

PATHOGENESIS: Adult worms live as coiled tangled masses in the deep fascia and subcutaneous tissues. They do not cause tissue damage or elicit inflammatory responses, but gravid females release millions of microfilariae, which migrate into the skin, eyes, lymph nodes, and deep organs, producing corresponding onchocercal lesions. Ocular onchocerciasis results from migration of microfilariae into all regions of the eye, from the cornea to the optic nerve head. When microfilariae die, they incite vigorous inflammatory and immune responses, characterized by chronic inflammation, including eosinophils. Inflammatory damage to the cornea, choroid, or retina leads to partial or total loss of vision. Systemic antihelminthic therapy, particularly with ivermectin, is effective in treatment. Aggressive fly eradication programs have also been successful in reducing endemic disease.

Intestinal Nematodes

The adult forms of several nematode species (Table 9-5) reside in the human bowel but rarely cause overt symptomatic disease. Clinical symptoms most often occur in persons who carry unusually large numbers of worms or who are immunocompromised. *It must be emphasized however, that soil-transmitted nematode infestation (in particular ascariasis, trichuriasis, and hookworm) is, on a population basis, a highly significant contributor to malnutrition, growth retardation, and cognitive deficits in children living in developing countries.* Humans are the exclusive or primary host for all of intestinal nematodes, and infection spreads from person to person via eggs or larvae passed in the stool or deposited in the perianal region. Infection is most prevalent in settings where hand-washing and hygienic disposal of feces are lacking. Warm, moist climates are required for survival of the infectious forms of many of the intestinal nematodes outside the body. These worms are, therefore, endemic in tropical and subtropical environments. Bisimidazole drugs, such as mebendazole and albendazole, are highly effective therapeutic agents.

Ascariasis is Usually an Asymptomatic Infestation of the Small Bowel

Ascariasis refers to infection by the large roundworm Ascaris lumbricoides. It is the most common helminth infection of humans, affecting about 10% of the population in developing countries, usually without causing symptoms. However, severe infestation is estimated to result in the death of about 60,000 children annually. Ascariasis is found worldwide, but infection is most common in areas with warm climates and poor sanitation.

PATHOGENESIS: Adult worms live in the small intestine where gravid females discharge eggs that pass in the feces. These eggs hatch when ingested. *Ascaris* larvae emerge in the small intestine, penetrate the bowel wall, and reach the lungs through the venous circulation. From the pulmonary capillaries, they enter alveolar spaces and migrate up the trachea to the glottis, where they are swallowed and again reach the small bowel. There, they mature and live as adult worms within the lumen for 1 to 2 years. Adult worms (15 to 35 cm long) usually cause no pathologic changes. Heavy infections may cause vomiting, malnutrition, and sometimes intestinal obstruction.

Trichuriasis is a Superficially Invasive Infection of the Large Bowel

Trichuriasis is caused by the intestinal nematode Trichuris trichiura *("whipworm").* Whipworm infection is found worldwide, affecting more than 700 million people. Parasitism is most common in warm, moist places with poor sanitation, including the southern US and in some recent immigrant groups. Children are especially susceptible. Adult worms live in the cecum and upper colon where female worms produce eggs that pass in the feces. Eggs embryonate in moist soil and become infective in 3 weeks. Humans are infected by ingesting eggs in contaminated soil, food, or drink.

TABLE 9–5			
Intestinal Nematodes			
Species	Common Name	Site of Adult Worm	Clinical Manifestations
Ascaris lumbricoides	Roundworm	Small bowel	Allergic reactions to lung migration; intestinal obstruction
Ancylostoma duodenale	Hookworm	Small bowel	Allergic reactions to cutaneous inoculation and lung migration; intestinal blood loss
Necator americanus	Hookworm	Small bowel	Allergic reactions to cutaneous inoculation and lung migration; intestinal blood loss
Trichuris trichiura	Whipworm	Large bowel	Abdominal pain and diarrhea; rectal prolapse (rare)
Strongyloides stercoralis	Threadworm	Small bowel	Abdominal pain and diarrhea; dissemination to extraintestinal sites in immunocompromised persons
Enterobius vermicularis	Pinworm	Cecum, appendix	Perianal and perineal itching

PATHOGENESIS: Larvae emerge from ingested eggs in the small bowel and migrate to the cecum and colon, where the adult worms burrow their anterior portions into the superficial mucosa. This invasion causes small erosions, focal active inflammation, and a continuous loss of small quantities of blood. Heavy infestation of worms may produce chronic colitis resembling inflammatory bowel disease, with cramping abdominal pain, bloody diarrhea, weight loss, and anemia.

Hookworms Cause Intestinal Blood Loss and Anemia

Necator americanus *and* Ancylostoma duodenale *(American and Old-World "hookworms," respectively) are intestinal nematodes that infect the human small bowel. They lacerate the bowel mucosa, causing intestinal blood loss, which can produce symptomatic disease in heavy infestations.* Hookworm infections are found in moist, warm, temperate, and tropical areas and cause serious public health problems with about 700 million people infected worldwide. The disease was once common in the southeastern US but has been largely eradicated.

 PATHOGENESIS: On contact with human skin, larvae directly penetrate the epidermis and enter the venous circulation. They travel to the lungs, where they lodge in alveolar capillaries. After rupturing into the alveoli, larvae migrate up the trachea to the glottis and are then swallowed. They molt in the duodenum, attach to the mucosal wall with tooth-like buccal plates, clamp off a section of the villus, and ingest it without producing associated inflammation. With extensive worm infections, blood loss can cause clinical disease. Infection with this parasite is the most important cause of chronic anemia worldwide. Skin penetration is sometimes associated with a pruritic eruption ("ground itch"), and the phase of larval migration through the lungs occasionally causes asthma-like symptoms.

Strongyloidiasis May Become Disseminated in Immunocompromised Hosts

Strongyloidiasis is a small intestinal infection with a nematode, Strongyloides stercoralis *("threadworm"). Although most cases are asymptomatic, the infection can progress to lethal disseminated disease in immunocompromised persons.* Infection is most frequent in areas with warm, moist climates and poor sanitation. However, endemic pockets of strongyloidiasis still exist in the United States. The disease has been common in recent immigrant groups, particularly those from the Sudan.

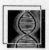 **PATHOGENESIS:** Adult females are buried in the crypts of the duodenum or jejunum but produce no visible alterations. The larvae are passed into the soil from the feces where they become filariform, the infective stage that penetrates human skin. The organism travels in the bloodstream to the lungs and then to the small bowel, in a manner similar to that of hookworms. Unlike other intestinal nematodes, S. stercoralis may reproduce by a mechanism known as **autoinfection**. This occurs when larvae become infective within a host's intestine and re-penetrate either the intestinal wall or the perianal skin, thereby starting a new parasitic cycle within a single host.

Most infected persons are completely asymptomatic, but moderate eosinophilia is common. **Disseminated strongyloidiasis or hyperinfection syndrome** occurs in patients with suppressed immunity, particularly those receiving corticosteroids. In such patients, the rate of internal autoinfection is greatly increased, and extraordinary numbers of filariform larvae penetrate intestinal

walls and disseminate to distant organs. The gut may exhibit ulceration, edema, and severe inflammation with subsequent sepsis. Untreated, disseminated strongyloidiasis is fatal; even with prompt treatment only one-third of infected patients survive.

Tissue Nematodes: Trichinellosis

Trichinellosis (formerly trichinosis) is a myositis produced by the round-worm Trichinella spiralis, *which humans acquire by eating infected wild or domesticated animals (predominantly pork)* (Fig. 9-35). Infection with *T. spiralis* occurs worldwide. Humans acquire trichinellosis by ingesting inadequately cooked meat containing encysted *T. spiralis* larvae. The larvae are found in the skeletal muscles of various carnivorous or omnivorous wild and domesticated animals, including pigs, rats, bears, and walruses. Pork is the most common source of human trichinellosis. Meat inspection programs and restriction of feeding practices have largely eliminated *T. spiralis* from domesticated pigs in many developed countries. Wild game is an increasingly common source in the US, where fewer than 20 cases of trichinellosis are reported annually.

 PATHOGENESIS: In the small bowel, *T. spiralis* larvae emerge from the ingested tissue cysts and burrow into the intestinal mucosa where they develop into adult worms. The adults mate, and the female worm liberates larvae that penetrate the intestinal wall and enter the circulation. The larvae can invade nearly any tissue but can survive only in striated skeletal muscle. The resulting myositis is especially prominent in the diaphragm, extrinsic ocular muscles, tongue, intercostal muscles, gastrocnemius, and deltoids. Sometimes the CNS or heart is also involved in the inflammatory response, producing meningoencephalitis or myocarditis. When a larva infects a myocyte, the cell undergoes basophilic degeneration and swelling. Early myocyte infection elicits an intense inflammatory infiltrate rich in eosinophils and macrophages. The larva grows to 10 times its initial size, folds on itself, and develops a capsule. With encapsulation, the inflammatory infiltrate subsides. Several years later, the larva dies, and the cyst calcifies. Symptomatic trichinellosis is usually self-limited, and patients recover in a few months. If large numbers of cysts are eaten, abdominal pain and diarrhea may result from small-bowel invasion by the worms. Major symptoms usually develop several days later when skeletal muscles are invaded. Patients suffer severe pain and tenderness of affected muscles, fever, and weakness. Eosinophilia may be extreme (more than 50% of all leukocytes).

Trematodes (Flukes)

Schistosomiasis Produces Diseases of the Liver and Bladder

Schistosomiasis (bilharziasis) is the most important helminthic disease of humans, in whom intense inflammatory and immune responses damage the liver, intestine, or urinary bladder. Three species of schistosomes, *Schistosoma mansoni, Schistosoma haematobium, and Schistosoma japonicum, are the causative agents. Schistosomiasis causes greater morbidity and mortality than all other worm infections.* The disease affects about 10% of the world's population and ranks second only to malaria as a cause of disabling disease. The three schistosomal pathogens inhabit distinct geographic regions, dictated by the distribution of their specific host snail species. *S. mansoni* is found in much of tropical Africa, parts of southwest Asia, South America, and the Caribbean islands. *S. haematobium* is endemic in large regions of tropical Africa and parts of the Middle East. *S. japonicum* occurs in parts of China, the Philippines, Southeast Asia, and India.

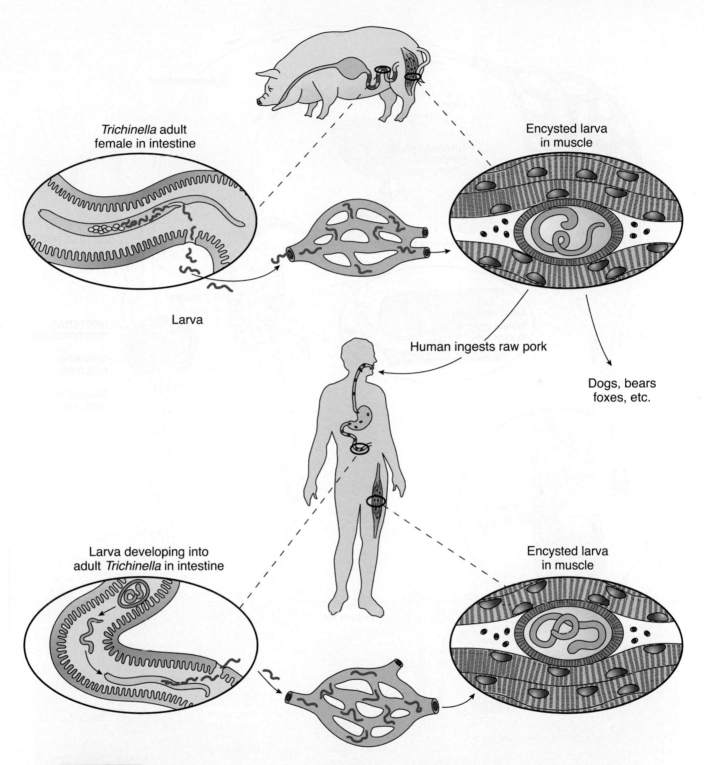

FIGURE 9-35. **Trichinosis.** After being ingested by the pig, cysts of *Trichinella* are digested in the gastrointestinal tract, liberating larvae that mature to adult worms. Female worms release larvae that penetrate the intestinal wall, enter the circulation, and lodge in striated muscle, where they encyst. When humans ingest inadequately cooked pork, the cycle is repeated, resulting in the muscle disease characteristic of trichinosis.

PATHOGENESIS AND PATHOLOGY: The schistosomes have complicated life cycles, alternating between asexual generations in the invertebrate host (snail) and sexual generations in the vertebrate host (Fig. 9-36). A schistosome egg hatches in fresh water, liberating a motile form that penetrates a snail, where it develops into the final larval stage which escapes into the water and penetrates the skin of the human host. The larvae migrate through tissues, penetrate blood vessels, and are transported to the lung and liver. In the intestinal venules of the portal drainage, the organisms mature, forming pairs of male and female worms. The females of *S. mansoni* and *S. japonicum* deposit eggs in intestinal venules, whereas *S. haematobium* lays eggs in those of the urinary bladder. *The basic lesion is a circumscribed granuloma or a cellular infiltrate of eosinophils and neutrophils around an egg as a result of host reaction to egg antigens.* Eosinophils often predominate in early granulomas. In older granulomas, epithelioid macrophages and giant cells are conspicuous,

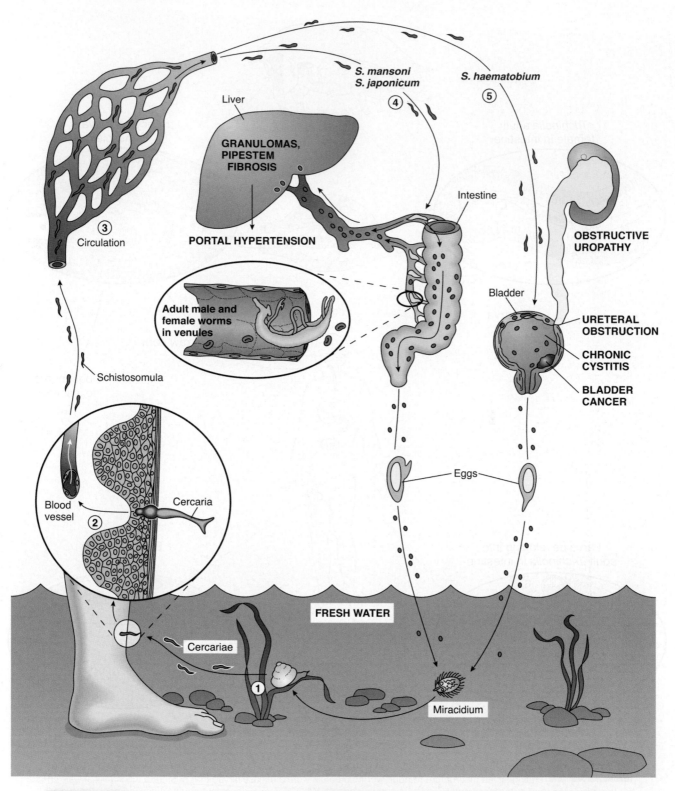

FIGURE 9-36. **Life cycle of *Schistosoma* and clinical features of schistosomiasis.** The schistosome egg hatches in water, liberates a miracidium that penetrates a snail, and develops through two stages to a sporocyst to form the final larval stage, the cercaria. *(1)* The cercaria escapes from the snail into water, "swims," and penetrates the skin of a human host. *(2)* The cercaria loses its forked tail to become a schistosomulum, which migrates through tissues, penetrates a blood vessel, and *(3)* is carried to the lung and later to the liver. In hepatic portal venules, the schistosomula become sexually mature and form pairs, each with a male and a female worm, the female worm lying in the gynecophoral canal of the male worm. The organism causes lesions in the liver, including granulomas, portal ("pipestem") fibrosis, and portal hypertension. *(4)* The female worm deposits immature eggs in small venules of the intestine and rectum (*S. mansoni* and *S. japonicum*) or *(5)* of the urinary bladder (*S. haematobium*). The bladder infestation leads to obstructive uropathy, ureteral obstruction, chronic cystitis, and bladder cancer. Embryos develop during passage of the eggs through tissues, and larvae are mature when eggs pass through the wall of the intestine or urinary bladder. Eggs hatch in water and liberate miracidia to complete the cycle.

and the oldest granulomas are densely fibrotic. Granulomas that form about the eggs also obstruct the microvascular blood supply and produce ischemic damage to adjacent tissue. The result is progressive scarring and dysfunction in the affected organs.

LIVER DISEASE: *S. mansoni* and *S. japonicum* are responsible for liver disease, which begins as periportal granulomatous inflammation (Fig. 9-37) and progresses to dense periportal fibrosis (**pipestem fibrosis**) (Fig. 9-38). In severe cases of hepatic schistosomiasis, this effect results in obstruction of portal blood flow and portal hypertension. *S. mansoni* and *S. japonicum* may also damage the intestine, where the granulomatous response produces inflammatory polyps and foci of mucosal and submucosal fibrosis.

UROGENITAL DISEASE: *S. haematobium* infection features eggs that are most numerous in the bladder, ureter, and seminal vesicles, although they may also reach the lungs, colon, and appendix. Eggs in the bladder and ureters lead to a granulomatous reaction, inflammatory protuberances, and patches of mucosal and mural fibrosis. These can obstruct urine flow, thus producing secondary inflammatory damage to the bladder, ureters, and kidneys. *The bladder disease produced by* S. haematobium *is a major risk factor for squamous cell carcinoma of the bladder.*

Although schistosomes are effectively killed by systemic antihelminthic agents such as praziquantel, the structural changes resulting from extensive fibrosis and scarring are irreversible.

Clonorchiasis Leads to Biliary Obstruction

Clonorchiasis is an infection of the hepatic biliary system by the Chinese liver fluke, Clonorchis sinensis, *which results from the ingestion of undercooked infected freshwater fish.* Although the fluke usually causes only mild symptoms, it is sometimes associated with bile duct stones, cholangitis, and bile duct cancer. Clonorchiasis is endemic in east Asia, from Vietnam to Korea. The disease frequency has recently tripled in China to 15 million cases in association with an increase in fresh water aquaculture.

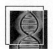
PATHOGENESIS AND PATHOLOGY: When humans eat infected fish, the organisms emerge in the duodenum, enter the common bile duct through the ampulla of Vater, and mature in the distal bile ducts to an adult fluke. The presence of *Clonorchis* in the bile ducts elicits an inflammatory response, which fails to eliminate the worm but causes dilation and fibrosis of the ducts. Microscopically, the epithelial duct lining is initially hyperplastic and then

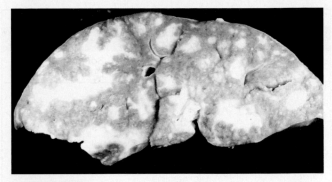

FIGURE 9-38. **Hepatic schistosomiasis.** Chronic infection of the liver with *S. japonicum* has led to the characteristic "pipestem" fibrosis.

becomes metaplastic. The surrounding stroma is fibrotic. Secondary bacterial infection is common and may be associated with suppurative cholangitis. Eggs deposited in the hepatic parenchyma are surrounded by a fibrous and granulomatous reaction. Masses of eggs may become lodged in the bile ducts and cause cholangitis. Sometimes the worms cause calculus formation within the hepatic bile ducts, leading to ductal obstruction. The adult *Clonorchis* persists in the ducts for decades, and long-standing infection is associated with an increased incidence of carcinoma of the bile duct epithelium (cholangiocarcinoma). In heavy *Clonorchis* infections, the liver may be up to three times normal size. Dilated bile ducts are seen through the capsule, and the cut surface is punctuated with thick-walled dilated bile ducts (Fig. 9-39). The pancreatic ducts may also be invaded and become dilated, thickened, lined by metaplastic epithelium, and eventually surrounded by scar tissue. The infestation is treated effectively with systemic antihelminthic agents.

Cestodes: Intestinal Tapeworms

Taenia saginata, Taenia solium, and *Diphyllobothrium latum* are tapeworms that infect humans, growing to their adult forms within the intestine (Table 9-6). The presence of these adult worms rarely damages the human host. Intestinal tapeworm infections are acquired by eating inadequately cooked beef (*T. saginata*), pork (*T. solium*), or fish (*D. latum*) containing larval forms of these organisms. Modern cattle and pig farming practices, plus meat inspection, have largely eliminated beef and pork tapeworms in industrialized countries, but infection remains common in developing

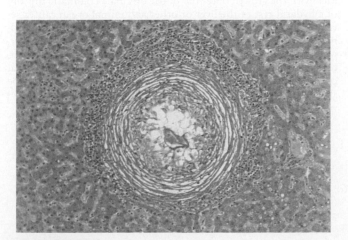

FIGURE 9-37. **Hepatic schistosomiasis.** A hepatic granuloma surrounds a degenerating egg of *S. mansoni*.

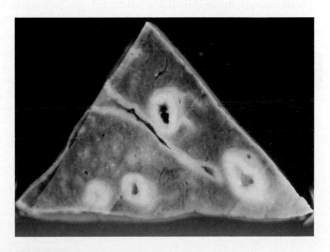

FIGURE 9-39. **Clonorchiasis of the liver.** The bile ducts are greatly thickened and dilated because of the presence of adult flukes (*Clonorchis sinensis*).

TABLE 9-6

Tapeworm Infections

Species	Human Disease	Source of Human Infection
Taenia saginata	Adult tapeworm in intestine	Beef
Taenia solium	Adult tapeworm in intestine; cysticercosis	Pork; human feces
Diphyllobothrium latum	Adult tapeworm in intestine	Fish
Echinococcus granulosus	Hydatid cyst disease	Dog feces

countries. Fish tapeworm infection is prevalent in regions where raw, pickled, or partly cooked freshwater fish are common fare. Tapeworm infections are usually asymptomatic, although it may be distressing when an infected person passes portions of the worm in the stool. The fish tapeworm *(D. latum)* competes for vitamin B$_{12}$, and a small number (<2%) of infected individuals develop pernicious anemia (see Chapter 20).

Accidental ingestion of *T. solium* eggs from human feces or ingestion of larvally infected pork can lead to **Cysticercosis**, systemic infection by the **larvae** of the pork tapeworm. The consequences may be catastrophic. The eggs release oncospheres, which penetrate the wall of the gut, enter the bloodstream, lodge in tissue, encyst, and differentiate to cysticerci. Cysticercosis of the brain (neurocysticercosis) manifests as headaches or seizures, and symptoms vary according to the sites affected. Massive cysticercosis of the brain causes convulsions and death.

Echinococcosis

Echinococcosis (hydatid disease) is a zoonotic infection caused by larval cestodes of the genus *Echinococcus*. The most common offender is *Echinococcus granulosus,* which causes cystic hydatid disease. Rarely, *Echinococcus multilocularis* and *Echinococcus vogeli* infect humans. Infestation with the tapeworm *E. granulosus* is endemic in sheep, goats, and cattle as well as their attendant dogs. Dogs contaminate their habitats (and their human keepers) with infectious eggs. Humans become infected when they inadvertently ingest the tapeworm eggs. The resulting hydatid disease is present worldwide among herding populations, which live in close proximity to dogs and herd animals. In the United States, hydatid cyst disease is seen among immigrants and among the indigenous sheep-herding populations of the Southwest.

 PATHOGENESIS AND PATHOLOGY: Humans are infected by ingesting material contaminated by the cestode eggs. Larvae released from the eggs penetrate the wall of the gut, enter the bloodstream, and disseminate to deep organs, where they grow to form large cysts containing brood capsules and scolices. The slowly growing hydatid cyst is found by chance or becomes

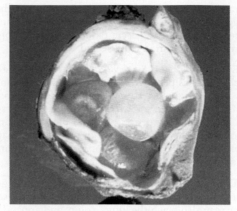

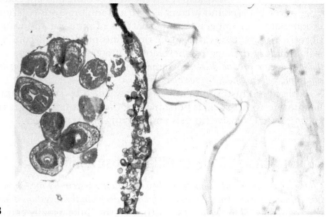

FIGURE 9-40. **Echinococcal cyst. A.** An echinococcal cyst showing daughter cysts was resected from the liver of a patient infected with *E. granulosus*. **B.** A photomicrograph of the cyst wall shows *(from right to left)* a laminated, non-nuclear layer, a nucleated germinal layer with brood capsules attached, and numerous scolices in the cyst cavity.

obvious when its size and position interferes with normal functions. Compression of intrahepatic bile ducts by a hepatic cyst (Fig. 9-40) may lead to obstructive jaundice. Pulmonary cysts are often asymptomatic and discovered incidentally on a chest radiograph.

A major complication of cyst rupture is the seeding of adjacent tissues, which results in the production of many additional cysts, each with the growth potential of the original. Traumatic rupture of a hydatid cyst of the liver or other abdominal organ causes severe diffuse pain, resembling that of peritonitis. Rupture of a pulmonary cyst may lead to pneumothorax and empyema. Moreover, when a hydatid cyst ruptures into a body cavity, release of cyst contents can cause fatal allergic reactions. Treatment of echinococcal cysts frequently requires careful surgical removal. Cysts must be sterilized with formaldehyde before drainage or extirpation to prevent intraoperative anaphylactic shock.

10 Blood Vessels

Avrum I. Gotlieb

At one time, blood vessels were seen as passive conduits serving to distribute blood to organs. However, an appreciation of vascular disease as the most common cause of morbidity and mortality in Western society has led to a dramatically increased understanding of blood vessels as dynamic systems. Most vascular diseases result from dysfunction of endothelial and smooth muscle cells and their interaction with the circulating elements of the blood.

Hemostasis and Thrombosis

Hemostasis is the arrest of hemorrhage and is a response to vascular injury. This process involves vasoconstriction, tissue swelling, coagulation, platelet aggregation, and thrombosis. The hemostatic system comprises (1) a network of activating and inactivating enzymes and (2) cofactors derived from different cells and tissues, some of which are circulating and some locally produced (Table 10-1). Specific disorders of hemostasis are discussed in detail in Chapter 20.

The hemostatic complex can be divided into several functional areas that combine coagulation of blood proteins and aggregation of platelets to form a hemostatic "plug." *Thrombosis* is the formation of a blood clot (thrombus) in the circulation. A thrombus is an

TABLE 10-1

Coagulation Factor Designations

Factor	Standard Name
I	Fibrinogen
II	Prothrombin
III	Tissue factor
IV	Calcium ions
V	Proaccelerin
VII	Proconvertin
VIII	Antihemophilic factor
IX	Plasma thromboplastin
X	Stuart factor
XI	Plasma thromboplastin antecedent
XII	Hageman factor
XIII	Fibrin stabilizing factor
–	Prekallikrein
–	High-molecular-weight kininogen

aggregate of coagulated blood that contains platelets, fibrin, leukocytes, and red blood cells. Its formation involves a balance between those factors that favor clotting and those that inhibit it. *Thrombosis occurs when antithrombotic systems do not balance prothrombotic processes.*

There is a distinct difference between **coagulation** and **thrombosis**. Coagulation can occur *in vitro* by activation of the clotting cascade. By contrast, thrombosis occurs *in situ* and also involves (1) adherence and aggregation of platelets, (2) participation of cellular elements of the monocyte/macrophage system, and (3) active participation of endothelial cells.

Blood Coagulation Occurs When Fibrinogen is Converted to Fibrin

Coagulation of blood entails conversion of soluble plasma fibrinogen to an insoluble fibrillar polymer termed fibrin; this reaction is catalyzed by the proteolytic enzyme thrombin. This event involves a series of finely tuned steps, each mediated by a number of coagulation factors (see Table 10-1), many of which are restricted by specific inhibitors. *The coagulation cascade amplifies an initial signal into the eventual generation of thrombin, the production of which is probably the most important factor in progression and stabilization of a thrombus.* Although historically, the coagulation cascade was divided into "intrinsic" and "extrinsic" pathways, separation of coagulation into two distinct arms does not accurately reflect the underlying mechanisms of clotting.

The current view of coagulation (Fig. 10-1) highlights the importance of **tissue factor** (TF), a membrane-bound glycoprotein not present within undamaged vessels. Hemostasis is initiated when activated factor VII (VIIa) encounters TF at a site of injury. Small amounts of factors X and IX are activated to Xa and IXa. The dynamic association of factor VIIa-TF complexes with TF pathway inhibitor (TFPI) is crucial to the regulation of thrombosis. *The binding of TFPI to Xa and the formation of a TFPI-Xa-TF-VIIa quaternary complex prevents further generation of Xa and IXa by the VIIa-TF complex.* Hence, the pool of TFPI on the surface of endothelial cells regulates the degree but does not prevent the initiation of coagulation. Activation of larger amounts of X to Xa is promoted by factors VIIIa and IXa. Traces of thrombin catalyze the activation of factor XI, which in turn augments conversion of factor IX to IXa. The IXa and VIIIa complex converts more factor X to Xa, which then binds V_a to form the **prothrombinase complex**. This complex then converts prothrombin to thrombin, which is a serine protease. In addition to its role in coagulation and platelet aggregation, thrombin also:

- Participates in fibrinolysis.
- Regulates growth factors and leukocyte adhesion molecules.
- Serves as an anticoagulant by binding to thrombomodulin and subsequently initiating the activation of protein C. Activated protein C down-regulates factors V_a and VIIIa activity.
- Increases endothelial cell permeability.

Platelet Adhesion and Aggregation Occur After Injury to a Blood Vessel

When vascular endothelium is disrupted, platelets respond by creating a platelet plug to minimize bleeding. Platelets are particularly important in sealing damaged blood vessels that are subjected to a high shear rate, such as arteries and arterioles. In certain diseases, platelets respond to activated leukocytes and endothelial cells (see Chapter 2). Disorders of platelet adhesion and aggregation are discussed in Chapter 20.

There are multiple sequential steps in the platelet activation that follow injury to blood vessels and the loss of an intact endothelial cell layer (Fig. 10-2).

1. **Platelet adhesion** to exposed subendothelial matrix proteins, such as collagen and von Willebrand factor (vWF), by specific platelet surface glycoprotein (GP) receptors. GP Ib/IX binds vWF, and integrin receptor α2β1 and GPVI bind collagen.
2. **Shape change**, from discoid to spherical to stellate
3. **Secretion of platelet granule contents**, including adenosine diphosphate, epinephrine, calcium, vWF, and platelet-derived growth factor (PDGF), which promote platelet adhesion and aggregation
4. **Thromboxane A_2 generation by cyclooxygenase 1**
5. **Membrane changes** that expose P-selectin and procoagulant anionic phospholipids, such as phosphatidylserine
6. **Aggregation of platelets** through cross-linking of fibrinogen receptor GP IIb/IIIa

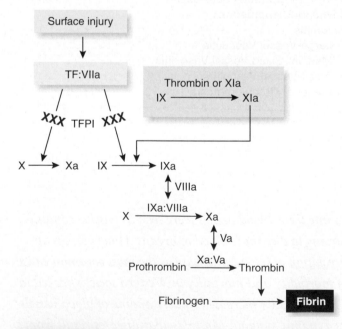

FIGURE 10-1. **Coagulation cascade.** The coagulation cascade is initiated by endothelial injury, which releases tissue factor (TF). The latter combines with activated factor VII (VIIa) to form a complex that activates small amounts of X to Xa and IX to IXa. The complex of IXa with VIIIa further activates X. The complex of Xa with V_a then catalyzes the conversion of prothrombin to thrombin, after which fibrin is formed from fibrinogen. TFPI, tissue factor pathway inhibitor.

Each of these functional steps has specific consequences. Initial adhesion signals promote the activation of platelets. Secreted granule contents and thromboxane A$_2$ provide positive feedback to activate additional platelets via their surface receptors. The stellate shape of activated platelets projects the procoagulant membrane surface and activated GP IIb/IIIa/fibrinogen to the site of interaction with coagulation factors and other platelets. *Thus, the surface of activated platelets is an optimal environment for propagating the assembly of the coagulation factor complex, including the prothrombinase complex. The resulting thrombin has many consequences (see above), particularly further platelet activation.* Finally, P-selectin participates in binding leukocytes and localizing them to participate in healing, together with substances secreted by platelets such as PDGF. *As a result of these concerted steps, activated platelets form a strong primary plug and then an aggregate within a platelet–fibrin meshwork, which stops bleeding and initiates healing.*

Endothelial Factors Regulate Both Anticoagulant and Procoagulant Processes

The major event that triggers most thrombosis is endothelial injury, which imparts a prothrombotic property to the endothelium (see Fig. 10-2). Endothelial cells synthesize vWF and also bind factors IX and X, a process that favors coagulation on the endothelial surface. Finally, inflammatory agents, including cytokines released from monocytes, activate procoagulant activities on the surface of intact endothelium. Thus, thrombi may form when (1) endothelial function is altered, (2) endothelial continuity is lost, or (3) flow in a blood vessel becomes abnormal, such as when turbulent or static.

The endothelium also plays an active role in the control of thrombosis (Table 10-2). A major antithrombotic mechanism of the endothelium is the secretion of **PGI$_2$**, which inhibits platelet aggregation. Endothelial nitric oxide is also a potent inhibitor of platelet aggregation and adhesion to the vessel wall. Endothelial cells metabolize adenosine diphosphate, a strong promoter of thrombogenesis, to metabolites that are antithrombogenic. The luminal surface of the endothelium is coated with heparan sulfate, a molecule that binds a number of clotting factors, including the antiprotease β_2-macroglobulin. Endothelial cells may also lyse some clots as they form through the **plasminogen/plasminogen activator/plasmin system**. Endothelial cells have several other anticoagulant activities. Both protein C and thrombomodulin (see above) are synthesized by endothelial cells. TF and TFPI (see above and Fig. 10-1) are synthesized and secreted by endothelial cells as well as other vascular cells.

Clot Lysis is a Regulatory Mechanism

A thrombus may undergo several fates, including (1) lysis, (2) growth and propagation, (3) embolization, or (4) organization and canalization. The combination of aggregated platelets and clotted blood is made unstable by the activation of the fibrinolytic enzyme plasmin (Fig. 10-3). During clot formation, inactive plasminogen is bound to fibrin and, therefore, is an integral part of the forming platelet mass. Endothelial cells synthesize plasminogen activator, which converts plasminogen to active plasmin. In turn, by digesting fibrin, plasmin lyses clots and disrupts thrombi. Endothelial cells also synthesize plasminogen activator inhibitor-1, and plasmin is inhibited by α_2 antiplasmin. Thus, the regional fibrinolytic balance depends on the ratio of plasminogen activation to inhibition.

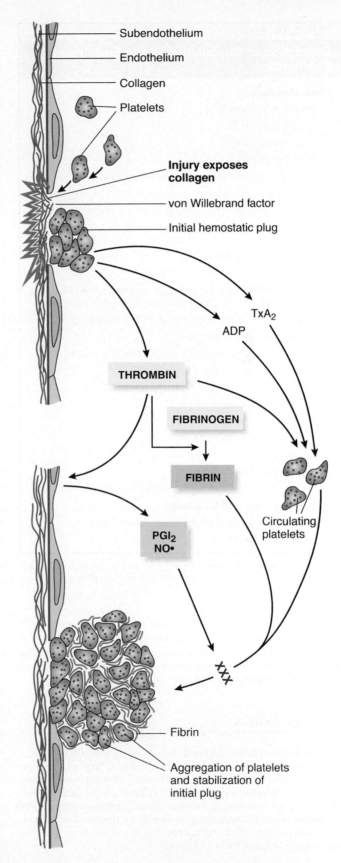

FIGURE 10-2. **The role of platelets in thrombosis.** Following vessel wall injury and alteration in flow, platelets adhere and then aggregate. Adenosine diphosphate (ADP) and thromboxane A$_2$ (TxA$_2$) are released and, along with locally generated thrombin, recruit additional platelets, causing the mass to enlarge. The growing platelet thrombus is stabilized by fibrin. Other elements, including leukocytes and red blood cells, are also incorporated into the thrombus. The release of prostacyclin (PGI$_2$) and nitric oxide (NO) by endothelial cells regulates the process by inhibiting platelet aggregation.

TABLE 10–2

Regulation of Coagulation at the Endothelial Cell Surface

Down-Regulation

1. Thrombin inactivators
   a. Antithrombin III
   b. Thrombomodulin
2. Activated protein C pathway
   a. Synthesis and expression of thrombomodulin
   b. Synthesis and expression of protein S
   c. Thrombomodulin-mediated activation of protein C
   d. Inactivation of factor V_a and factor VIII_a by APC-protein S complex
3. Tissue factor pathway inhibition
4. Fibrinolysis
   a. Synthesis of tissue plasminogen activator, urokinase plasminogen activator, and plasminogen activator inhibitor 1
   b. Conversion of Glu-plasminogen to Lys-plasminogen
   c. APC-mediated potentiation
5. Synthesis of unsaturated fatty acid metabolites
   a. Lipoxygenase metabolites-13-HODE
   b. Cyclooxygenase metabolites PGI_2 and PGE_2

Procoagulant Pathways

1. Synthesis and expression of:
   a. Tissue factor (thromboplastin)
   b. Factor V
   c. Platelet activating factor
2. Binding of clotting factors IX/IX_a, X (prothrombinase complex)
3. Downregulation of APC pathway
4. Increased synthesis of plasminogen activator inhibitor
5. Synthesis of 15-HPETE

APC, activated protein C; 13-HODE, 13-hydroxy-octadeca-dienoic acid; HPETE, hydroperoxy-eicosatetraenoic acid; PGE_2, prostaglandin E2; PGI_2, prostacyclin.

Thrombi may undergo organization and become incorporated into the vessel wall. The process is similar to that seen in wound healing (see Chapter 3) and results in the remodeling of the thrombus to form a fibrous structure with its own new blood vessels. The revascularization process is called **canalization**.

Atherosclerosis

In atherosclerosis, inflammatory cells, smooth muscle cells, lipid, and connective tissue progressively accumulate in the intima of large and medium-sized elastic and muscular arteries. The classical atherosclerotic lesion is best described as a fibroinflammatory lipid plaque (**atheroma**), which develops over several decades. With continued growth, the atheromas result in narrowing (stenosis) of the vascular lumen. The epidemiology of atherosclerosis and subsequent ischemic heart disease are reviewed in Chapter 11.

Our Understanding of the Pathogenesis of Atherosclerosis is Now Based on a Unifying Hypothesis

A hypothetical sequence can be constructed that explains the pathogenesis of atherosclerosis. This unifying hypothesis is di-

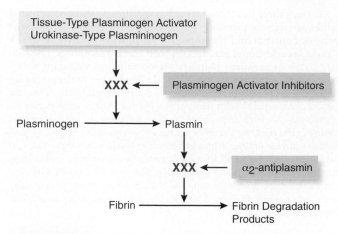

FIGURE 10-3. **Mechanisms of fibrinolysis.** Plasmin formed from plasminogen lyses fibrin. The conversion of plasminogen to plasmin and the activity of plasmin itself are suppressed by specific inhibitors.

vided into three stages: (1) initiation and formation, (2) adaptation, and (3) clinical stage (Figs. 10-4 to 10-7). *The process may begin as early as fetal life, with the formation of intimal cell masses, or perhaps shortly after birth, when fatty streaks begin to evolve. However, the characteristic lesion, which is not initially clinically significant, requires as long as 20 to 30 years to form. Once formed, serious acute complications may occur, or complicated lesions may emerge after several more years of development of the atheromatous lesions.*

Initiation and Formation Stage

1. Intimal lesions initially occur at sites in the circulation where shear stresses are low but fluctuate rapidly, such as at branch points and bifurcations. Endothelial dysfunction or accumulation of subendothelial smooth muscle cells occurs at such locations, particularly in the coronary arteries.
2. Lipid accumulation depends on disruption of the endothelial barrier's integrity through cell loss and dysfunction. Low-density lipoproteins (LDLs) carry lipids into the intima. Macrophages adhere to activated endothelial cells and transmigrate into the intima, bringing lipids with them.
3. Macrophages, in addition to participating in lipid accumulation, release growth factors, thereby stimulating further accumulation of smooth muscle cells. **Oxidized lipoproteins** induce tissue damage and further macrophage accumulation. Monocyte/macrophages synthesize PDGF, fibroblast growth factor, tumor necrosis factor, interleukin-1, interferon-α, and transforming growth factor-β, each of which can stimulate or inhibit growth of smooth muscle or endothelial cells.
4. As a lesion progresses, mural thrombi may form on the damaged intimal surface. This stimulates PDGF release, which accelerates proliferation of smooth muscle and secretion of matrix components.
5. The deeper parts of the thickened intima are poorly nourished and undergo necrosis. This injury initiates angiogenesis within the plaque.
6. The fibroinflammatory lipid plaque contains a central necrotic core and a fibrous cap; the latter separates the core from the blood in the lumen.

Adaptation Stage

7. As the plaque protrudes into the lumen (e.g., in coronary arteries), the wall of the artery remodels to maintain lumen size. When a plaque occupies half the lumen, remodeling can no longer compensate, and the arterial lumen becomes narrowed (stenosis).

Clinical Stage

8. Hemorrhage into a plaque without rupture may increase the size of the lesion as it encroaches upon the lumen. An autoimmune response against oxidized LDL may be important in the progression of atherosclerotic lesions.
9. Complications develop in the now-advanced plaque, including surface ulceration, fissure formation, calcification, and aneurysm formation. Plaque rupture (involving the fibrous cap), ensuing thrombosis, and occlusion may precipitate catastrophic events such as myocardial infarction (MI).

Figure 10-4 shows how these hypothetical mechanisms may operate in the pathogenesis of atherosclerosis.

The Initial Lesion of Atherosclerosis

 PATHOLOGY: Two distinct lesions have been proposed as precursors of atherosclerotic plaques.

FATTY STREAK: Fatty streaks are flat or slightly elevated lesions in the intima that contain macrophages filled with lipid droplets ("foam cells") (see Figs. 10-4 and 10-5) and accumulations of extracellular lipid. Smooth muscle cells also contain fat but in a lesser amount. Significant numbers of fatty streaks may be evident in many parts of the arterial tree of children but appear in a different distribution from the atherosclerotic lesions in adults. Nonetheless, many believe that fatty infiltration is the precursor lesion of atherosclerosis and that other factors control the transition from a fatty streak to a clinically significant atherosclerotic plaque.

INTIMAL CELL MASS: The intimal cell mass is another candidate for the initial lesion of atherosclerosis. Intimal cell masses are white, thickened areas at branch points in the arterial tree. Microscopically, they contain smooth muscle cells and connective tissue but no lipid. The location of these lesions, also known as "cushions," at arterial branch sites correlates well with the locations of later atherosclerotic lesions.

The Characteristic Lesion of Atherosclerosis

The characteristic lesion of atherosclerosis is the fibroinflammatory lipid plaque. **Simple plaques** are focal, elevated, pale yellow, smooth-surfaced lesions, irregular in shape but with well-defined borders. **Fibrofatty plaques** (Fig. 10-6) represent more advanced lesions and tend to be oval, with diameters of 8 to 12 cm. Microscopically, atherosclerotic plaques are initially covered by endothelium and tend to involve the intima and very little of the upper media (see Fig. 10-6). The area between the lumen and the necrotic core—the **fibrous cap**—contains smooth muscle cells, macrophages, lymphocytes, lipid-laden macrophages, smooth muscle cells (foam cells), and connective tissue components. The central core of the atheroma contains necrotic debris. Cholesterol crystals, foam cells, and foreign body giant cells may be present within the fibrous tissue and within the necrotic areas. Numerous inflammatory and immune cells, especially T cells, are also present within a plaque. Neovascularization is an important contributor to plaque growth and its subsequent complication (Fig. 10-7). Newly formed vessels are fragile and may rupture, resulting in acute expansion of the plaque from intraplaque hemorrhage. Foci of hemosiderin-laden macrophages are often present in plaques, indicating a remote intraplaque hemorrhage.

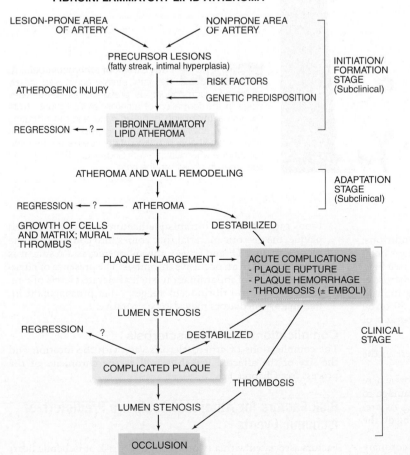

FIGURE 10-4. A unifying hypothesis for the pathogenesis of atherosclerosis.

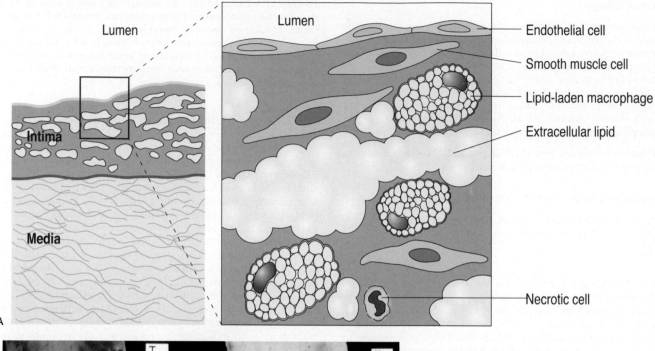

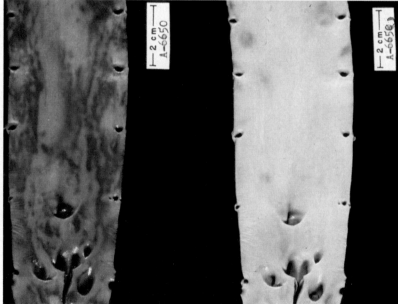

FIGURE 10-5. **Fatty streak of atherosclerosis. A.** The fatty streak, composed largely of foamy macrophages, is presumed to be an early stage in the formation of atherosclerotic lesions. Note the intimal thickening in the *left panel* and the infiltrating cells in the enlargement on the *right*. **B.** The aorta of a young man shows numerous fatty streaks on the luminal surface when stained with Sudan red. The unstained specimen is shown on the *right*.

Complicated Atherosclerotic Plaques

The term **complicated** plaque describes several conditions: erosion, ulceration, or fissuring of the plaque surface; plaque hemorrhage; mural thrombosis; calcification; and aneurysm (see Figs. 10-7 and 10-8). Progression from a simple fibrofatty atherosclerotic plaque to a complicated lesion may occur while some individuals are still in their 20s, but most affected people are 50 or 60 years of age. Cellular interactions involved in the progression of atherosclerotic lesions are summarized in Figure 10-9.

- **Calcification** occurs in areas of necrosis and elsewhere in the plaque.
- **Mural thrombosis** results from turbulent blood flow where the plaque protrudes into the lumen, resulting in damage to and loss of thromboresistance by the endothelial lining. As a result, thrombi often form at sites of erosion and fissuring on the surface of the fibrous cap.
- **Atheroma destabilization**, often resulting in acute coronary syndromes, may occur consequent to mural thrombosis, fi-

brous cap rupture, or intraplaque hemorrhage. In a ruptured plaque, the necrotic material that comes into contact with the blood contains TF and is very thrombogenic; as a result, it is likely to result in an occlusive thrombus. The presence of circulating markers of inflammation (such as elevated levels of c-reactive protein and fibrinogen) suggests that procoagulant inflammatory mediators may also be operative.

Complications of Atherosclerosis

The complications of atherosclerosis vary with the location and the size of the affected vessel as well as the chronicity of the process (see Chapter 11).

Risk Factors for Atherosclerosis are Predictors of Ischemic Events

Factors associated with a twofold or greater risk of ischemic heart disease include the following:

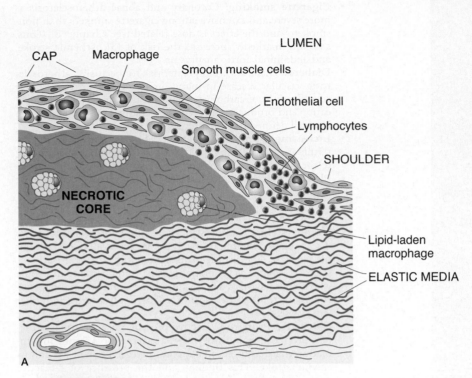
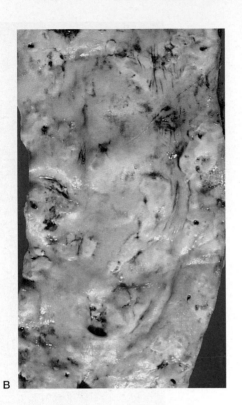

FIGURE 10-6. **Fibrofatty plaque of atherosclerosis.** **A.** In this fully developed fibrous plaque, the core contains lipid-filled macrophages and necrotic smooth muscle cell debris. The "fibrous" cap is composed largely of smooth muscle cells, which produce collagen, small amounts of elastin, and glycosaminoglycans. Also shown are infiltrating macrophages and lymphocytes. Note that the endothelium over the surface of the fibrous cap frequently appears intact. **B.** The aorta shows discrete, raised, tan plaques. Focal plaque ulcerations are also evident.

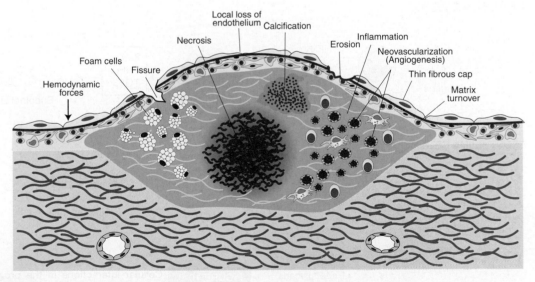

FIGURE 10-7. Factors involved in the pathogenesis of complicated atherosclerotic plaques.

- **Hypertension:** High blood pressure is consistently associated with a greater risk of MI. Although this increased risk was previously associated solely with the diastolic component, recent evidence suggests that the systolic hypertension is equally important. Men with blood pressures of 140/90 mm Hg have almost three times the incidence of MI as those with systolic pressures under 120 mm Hg. Control of hypertension has significantly decreased the incidence of MI and stroke.

- **Blood cholesterol level:** Serum cholesterol levels have been directly correlated with ischemic heart disease. *Serum cholesterol seems to be the most important determinant of the geographic differences in incidence of atherosclerotic coronary artery disease.* In the absence of genetic disorders of lipid metabolism (see below), the amount of cholesterol in the blood is strongly related to the dietary intake of saturated fat. The incidence of MI is reduced by treatment with cholesterol-lowering drugs.

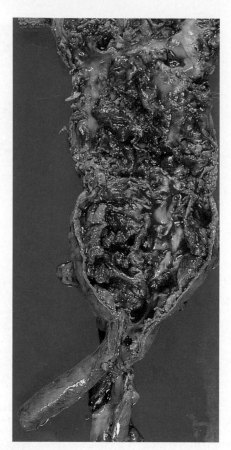

FIGURE 10-8. Complicated lesions of atherosclerosis. The luminal surface of the abdominal aorta and the common iliac arteries shows numerous fibrous plaques and raised, ulcerated lesions containing friable, atheromatous debris. The distal portion of the aorta displays a small aneurysmal dilation.

- **Cigarette smoking:** Coronary and aortic atherosclerosis is more severe and extensive among cigarette smokers than non-smokers, and the effect is dose related (see Chapter 8). Thus, smoking markedly increases the risk of MI, ischemic stroke, and abdominal aortic aneurysms.
- **Diabetes:** Diabetics are at greater risk for occlusive, atherosclerotic vascular disease in many organs. However, the relative contributions of carbohydrate intolerance itself, advanced glycation end-products, and secondary changes in blood lipids are not well defined (see Chapter 22).
- **Increasing age and male gender:** These factors are strong determinants of the risk for MI but both are probably secondary to the accumulated effects of other risk factors.
- **Physical inactivity and stressful life patterns:** Both of these factors have been said to correlate with increased risk of ischemic heart disease, but their precise relationship to the evolution of atherosclerosis is not established.
- **Homocysteine:** Homocystinuria is a rare autosomal recessive disease caused by mutations in the gene encoding cystathionine synthase. The disorder causes premature and severe atherosclerosis. Milder elevations of plasma homocysteine in people who do not have this disease are common and are an independent risk factor for atherosclerosis of coronary arteries and other large vessels.
- **C-Reactive Protein:** C-reactive protein, an acute phase reactant produced by hepatocytes, is a marker for systemic inflammation that has been linked to an increased risk of MI and ischemic stroke. This finding, and the presence of c-reactive protein in atherosclerotic plaques, suggest that systemic inflammation may contribute to atherogenesis.
- **Infection:** Seroepidemiologic studies have suggested that some infectious agents may contribute to atherosclerosis. *Chlamydia pneumoniae* and cytomegalovirus have been the most studied, and there is also interest in *Helicobacter pylori,* herpesvirus, and other organisms.

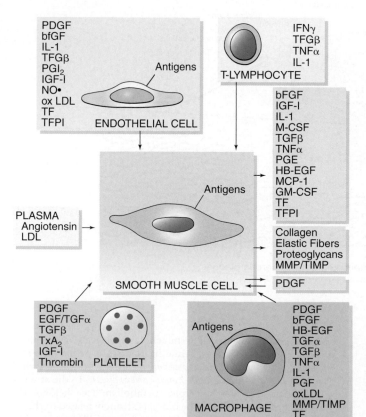

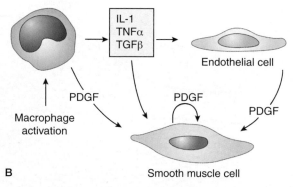

FIGURE 10-9. Cellular interactions in the progression of the atherosclerotic plaque. **A.** Endothelium, platelets, macrophages, T lymphocytes, and smooth muscle cells elaborate a variety of cytokines, growth factors, and other substances. The scheme illustrated here emphasizes their influence on smooth muscle cells. **B.** The cellular interactions that promote the proliferation of smooth cells. bfGF, basic fibroblast growth factor; EGF, endothelial growth factor; HB-EGF, heparin-binding epidermal growth factor-like growth factor; IFN, interferon; IGF-1, insulin-like growth factor; IL, interleukin; MCP-1, monocyte chemotactic protein-1; M-CSF, macrophage colony-stimulating factor; MMP, matrix metalloproteinase; NO, nitric oxide; ox LDL, oxidated low-density lipoprotein; PDGF, platelet-derived growth factor; PGE, prostaglandin; PGI$_2$, prostacyclin; TF, tissue factor; TGF, tumor growth factor; TFPI, tissue factor pathway inhibitor; TNF, tumor necrosis factor; TMIP, inhibitors of MMPs; TxA$_2$, thromboxane A$_2$.

Lipid Metabolism is the Major Factor in Atherosclerosis

The insolubility of cholesterol and other lipids (mainly triglycerides) necessitates a special transport mechanism, a function served by a system of lipoprotein particles (Table 10-3). These particles are categorized according to density:

- Chylomicrons
- Very-low-density lipoproteins (VLDLs)
- Low-density lipoproteins (LDLs)
- High-density lipoproteins (HDLs)

Each of these particles consists of a lipid core with associated proteins (apolipoproteins), as indicated in Table 10-3. The metabolic pathways for lipoproteins containing the B apolipoproteins (apoB) are two major lipoprotein cascades, one from the intestine and the other from the liver (Fig. 10-10).

EXOGENOUS PATHWAY: Fatty acids (linked with glycerol to form triglycerides) and cholesterol from foods that have been absorbed through the intestine are packaged into chylomicrons, which contain apoB-48 secreted by the intestine. These particles serve to transport lipid from the intestine to liver. Following secretion, chylomicrons rapidly acquire apoCII and apoE from HDL. The triglycerides in chylomicrons are hydrolyzed at the surface of capillary endothelial cells by lipoprotein lipase that is activated by ApoCII. This results in the removal of triglycerides, converting chylomicrons to "remnants," and finally to intermediate-density lipoproteins (IDLs). The chylomicron remnants are removed by hepatocytes through an apoE-mediated (remnant) receptor process.

ENDOGENOUS PATHWAY: This network of reactions involves triglyceride-rich lipoproteins, which contain apoB-100 secreted by the liver. Liver VLDL particles acquire apoCII and apoE from HDL shortly after their secretion. The triglycerides on VLDL are hydrolyzed by lipoprotein lipase as above. The lipoproteins containing apoB-100 are initially converted to IDLs and finally to LDLs, in part by hepatic lipoprotein lipase. At this point, most apoCII and apoE dissociates from the particles and reassociates with HDL. Lipoprotein lipase acts both as a triglyceride hydrolase and, more importantly, as a phospholipase. LDL, which contains apoB-100, interacts with high-affinity receptors on hepatocytes and on peripheral cells, including smooth muscle cells, fibroblasts, and adrenal cells (see Fig. 10-10). The interaction of LDL with its receptor initiates receptor-mediated endocytosis, which is followed by catabolism of LDL.

HDL: HDL containing apoAI and apoAII is either secreted by the intestine and liver or created by the transfer of lipid and apolipoprotein constituents released during lipolysis of lipoproteins that contain apoB. Two major functions have been proposed for HDL: (1) a reservoir for apolipoproteins, particularly apoCII and apoE and (2) interaction with cells in the transport system to carry extrahepatic cholesterol, including that in the arterial wall, to the liver for ultimate removal from the body. The latter function has been termed **reverse cholesterol transport**. The cholesterol removed from cells is principally free cholesterol, which rapidly undergoes esterification to cholesteryl esters by the enzyme lecithin:cholesterol acyltransferase. Cholesteryl esters are transferred to the core of the lipoprotein particle or are exchanged to VLDL and LDL. Transfer of cholesteryl esters between lipoprotein particles is mediated by specific transfer proteins, such as cholesterol ester transfer protein. Defects in cholesteryl ester transfer and exchange lead to dyslipoproteinemia, increased intracellular cholesteryl ester concentrations, and premature atherosclerosis.

LDL: LDL cholesterol has numerous effects on endothelial cells, smooth muscle cells, and monocyte/macrophages. For example, it regulates prostacyclin formation in vitro, and each of these cell types in atherosclerotic lesions can oxidize LDL. This change facilitates LDL recognition by the macrophage scavenger receptor and causes massive uptake of cholesterol by macrophages. Autoantibodies to oxidized LDL are present in patients with atherosclerosis in both plasma and plaques and may be important in the pathogenesis of plaques. Oxidized LDL is toxic to vascular wall cells, may disrupt endothelial integrity, and may lead to the accumulation of cell debris within the atheroma. Oxidized LDL is also chemotactic for macrophages, thereby further promoting their accumulation in atheromas. Epidemiologic studies suggest that dietary intake of antioxidants is inversely correlated with the risk of atherosclerosis, implying that oxidized LDL may be an important mediator of vascular disease.

Several Heritable Dyslipoproteinemias are Now Recognized

Familial clustering of ischemic heart diseases is well documented.

FAMILIAL HYPERCHOLESTEROLEMIA: The LDL receptor is a cell-surface glycoprotein that regulates plasma cholesterol by

TABLE 10-3				
The Apolipoproteins				
Apolipoprotein	Approximate Molecular Weight	Major Density Class	Major Sites of Synthesis in Humans	Major Function in Lipoprotein Metabolism
AI	28,000	HDL	Liver, intestine	Activates lecithin: cholesterol acyltransferase
AII	18,000	HDL	Liver, intestine	
AIV	45,000	Chylomicrons	Intestine	
B-100	250,000	VLDL, IDL, LDL	Liver	Binds to LDL receptor
B-48	125,000	Chylomicrons, VLDL IDL	Intestine	
CI	6500	Chylomicrons, VLDL, HDL	Liver	Activates lecithin: cholesterol acyltransferase
CII	10,000	Chylomicrons, VLDL, HDL	Liver	Activates lipoprotein lipase
CIII	10,000	Chylomicrons	Liver	Inhibits lipoprotein uptake by the liver
D	20,000	HDL		Cholesteryl ester exchange protein
E	40,000	Chylomicrons, VLDL, HDL	Liver, macrophage	Binds to E receptor system

HDL, high-density lipoprotein; IDL, intermediate-density lipoprotein; LDL, low-density lipoprotein; VLDL, very low-density lipoprotein.

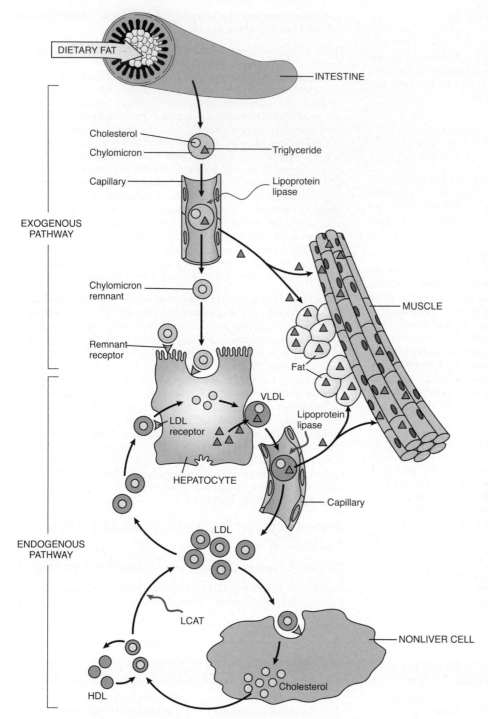

DIETARY FAT

INTESTINE

Cholesterol

Chylomicron

Triglyceride

Capillary

Lipoprotein lipase

EXOGENOUS PATHWAY

Chylomicron remnant

MUSCLE

Remnant receptor

Fat

VLDL

LDL receptor

Lipoprotein lipase

HEPATOCYTE

Capillary

LDL

ENDOGENOUS PATHWAY

LCAT

NONLIVER CELL

HDL

Cholesterol

FIGURE 10-10. **Exogenous and endogenous cholesterol transport pathway.** In the exogenous pathway, cholesterol and fatty acids from food are absorbed through the intestinal mucosa. Fatty acid chains are linked to glycerol to form triglycerides. Triglycerides and cholesterol are packaged into chylomicrons that are returned via the lymph to the blood. The lipids are coupled to proteins by enzymes such as the microsomal transfer protein complex. In the capillaries (mainly of fat tissue and muscle, but also other tissues), the ester bonds holding the fatty acids in triglycerides are split by lipoprotein lipase. Fatty acids are removed, leaving cholesterol-rich lipoprotein remnants. These bind to special remnant receptors and are taken up by liver cells. The cholesterol of the remnant is either secreted into the intestine, largely as bile acids, or packaged as very low-density lipoprotein (VLDL) particles, which are then secreted into the circulation. This is the first step in the endogenous cycle. In fat or muscle tissue, the triglyceride is removed from the VLDL with the aid of lipoprotein lipase. The intermediate-density lipoprotein (IDL) particles (not shown) remain in the circulation. Some IDL is immediately taken up by the liver via the mediation of LDL receptors for ApoB/E. The remaining IDL in the circulation is either taken up by nonliver cells or converted to LDL. Most of the LDL in the circulation binds to hepatocytes or other cells and is removed from the circulation. High-density lipoproteins (HDLs) take up cholesterol from cells. This cholesterol is esterified by the enzyme lecithin:cholesterol acyltransferase (LCAT), after which the esters are transferred to LDL and taken up by cells.

mediating endocytosis and recycling of apoE, the major plasma cholesterol transport protein. Mutations in the LDL receptor gene are discussed in detail in Chapter 6.

APOLIPOPROTEIN E (apoE): Genetic variations in various apoproteins are also known to be accompanied by alterations in LDL levels. Polymorphisms in apoE and variants of apolipoprotein AI and AII have been observed. Approximately 20% of the variability in serum cholesterol has been attributed to apoE polymorphism. In men, the apoE 3/2 phenotype is associated with a 20% lower LDL level than the most common phenotype, apoE 3/3. By contrast, the E4 allele is associated with elevated serum cholesterol. Interestingly, the presence of the E2 allele is increased and that of E4 decreased among male octogenarians.

HDL: An inverse correlation between ischemic heart disease and HDL cholesterol levels has been established. Polymorphisms of apoAI, an HDL-associated apolipoprotein that activates lecithin:cholesterol acyltransferase, are associated with premature atherosclerosis, as are rare cases of hereditary apoAI deficiency.

LIPOPROTEIN (a) (Lp[a]): High circulating levels of Lp(a) are associated with an augmented risk of atherosclerotic disease of the coronary arteries and larger cerebral vessels. Plasma levels of this cholesterol-rich lipoprotein vary greatly (<1 to >140 mg/dL) and appear to be independent of LDL levels. The Lp(a)-specific protein, apo(a), has been detected in atherosclerotic lesions, and high Lp(a) levels correlate with target organ damage in hypertensive patients. Apo(a) is encoded by a gene on chromosome 6 (6q2.7), close to the gene for plasminogen, with which apo(a) is highly homologous. Lp(a) enhances cholesterol delivery to injured blood vessels, suppresses generation of plasmin, and promotes smooth muscle proliferation. Thus, it may be an important link between atherosclerosis and thrombosis.

Hypertensive Vascular Disease

The World Health Organization defines hypertension as systolic pressure above 160 mm Hg and/or diastolic pressure above 90 (see also Chapter 11 for clinical details). Hypertension affects up to 20% of the population in industrial countries and is seen in more than half of cases of MI, stroke, and chronic renal disease. Blacks are particularly plagued by hypertension and are more likely than whites to experience severe complications. Three fourths of patients with dissecting aortic aneurysm, intracerebral hemorrhage, or myocardial wall rupture also have elevated blood pressure. In 95% of patients with hypertension, the cause is not clearly identifiable. Thus, most hypertensive persons are said to have **essential** or **primary** hypertension. Whatever the etiology, treatment of hypertension prolongs life.

 PATHOGENESIS: Blood pressure is the product of cardiac output and systemic vascular resistance to blood flow. Both of these functions are critically influenced by renal function and sodium homeostasis. The most widespread hypothesis holds that primary hypertension results from an imbalance in the interactions between these mechanisms (Fig. 10-11).

A complex endocrine axis centers on the renin–angiotensin system. Renal artery occlusion or dietary salt restriction leads to increased renal secretion of renin. Renin is a protease that cleaves angiotensinogen to a decapeptide, angiotensin I. In turn, angiotensin I is converted to angiotensin II by the endothelial surface protein angiotensin-converting enzyme. Angiotensin II causes vasoconstriction and also affects centers in the brain that control sympathetic outflow and stimulate adrenal aldosterone release. Aldosterone acts on renal tubules to increase sodium reabsorption. The net effect of all these actions is increased total body fluid volume. Thus, the **renin–angiotensin** system elevates blood pressure by three mechanisms:

- Increased sympathetic output
- Increased mineralocorticoid secretion
- Direct vasoconstriction

This axis is antagonized by atrial natriuretic factor (ANF), a hormone secreted by specialized cells in the cardiac atria. ANF binds specific receptors in the kidneys and increases urinary sodium excretion, thereby opposing angiotensin II-induced vasoconstriction. Secretion of ANF may be controlled by atrial distention, a consequence of increased volume, or by as-yet undefined endocrine interactions.

It has proved difficult to identify a central defect in the renin–angiotensin axis in hypertension, because the vasculature responds quickly to hemodynamic changes in the tissues by autoregulation. *Nevertheless, in the case of hypertension, the end result of autoregulation is always increased peripheral resistance.* Many cases of hypertension may also result from a process that begins with alterations in cardiac output, salt metabolism, or ANF release.

 PATHOLOGY: The central lesion in most cases of hypertension is compromised lumina of small muscular arteries and arterioles. These resistance vessels control blood flow through the capillary beds. The lumen may be restricted by active contraction of the vessel wall, increased mass of the vessel wall, or both. Structural changes in hypertension have been shown by morphometric analysis of arterial walls. Structurally thicker vessel walls would be expected to narrow vascular lumina more than would normal thinner walls. The rapid drop in blood pressure produced by smooth muscle relaxants suggests that active constriction is very important.

Acquired Causes of Hypertension

Acquired causes of hypertension are identifiable in a small proportion of cases. These include renal artery stenosis, most forms of chronic renal disease (including diabetes mellitus), primary elevation of aldosterone levels (Conn syndrome), Cushing syndrome, pheochromocytoma, hyperthyroidism, coarctation of the aorta, and renin-secreting tumors. In addition, those with severe atherosclerosis may have high systolic pressures, because a sclerotic aorta cannot properly absorb the kinetic energy of the pulse wave. In such patients, renovascular hypertension is also more common.

Arteriosclerosis

Chronic hypertension leads to reactive changes in smaller arteries and arterioles throughout the body, collectively termed **arteriosclerosis**. In the arterioles, the alterations are known as *arteriolosclerosis*.

BENIGN ARTERIOSCLEROSIS: This condition reflects mild chronic hypertension, and the major change is a variable increased arterial wall thickness (Fig. 10-12A). In the smallest arteries and arterioles, these lesions are referred to as **hyaline arteriosclerosis** and **arteriolosclerosis**. "Hyaline" refers to the glassy, scarred appearance of the blood vessel walls as seen by light microscopy. Arteriolar walls are thickened by the deposition of basement membrane material and the accumulation of plasma proteins (see Fig. 10-12B). The small muscular arteries display new layers of elastin, manifested as a reduplication of the intimal elastic lamina and increased connective tissue. The vascular lesions of benign arteriosclerosis are particularly evident in the kidney, where they result in the loss of renal parenchyma, a condition termed **benign nephrosclerosis** (see Chapter 16).

MALIGNANT (ACCELERATED) HYPERTENSION: In malignant hypertension, elevated blood pressure causes rapidly progressive vascular compromise, with the onset of symptomatic diseases of the brain, heart, or kidney. Although malignant hypertension cannot be defined strictly by the degree of blood pressure elevation, it is ordinarily not associated with blood pressures below 160/110 mm Hg. Modern antihypertensive therapy has made malignant hypertension a rare disorder.

Malignant hypertension produces dramatic microvascular pathologic changes, allowing for diagnosis by ophthalmoscopy. If blood pressure rises rapidly, retinal arterioles show microaneurysms, focal hemorrhages, and scarring of the retina. Ischemic necrosis and edema of the retina are visible with the ophthalmoscope as "cotton wool spots" (see Chapter 29). These retinal changes are typical of those in other resistance vessels when the pressure rises rapidly. In malignant hypertension, small muscular

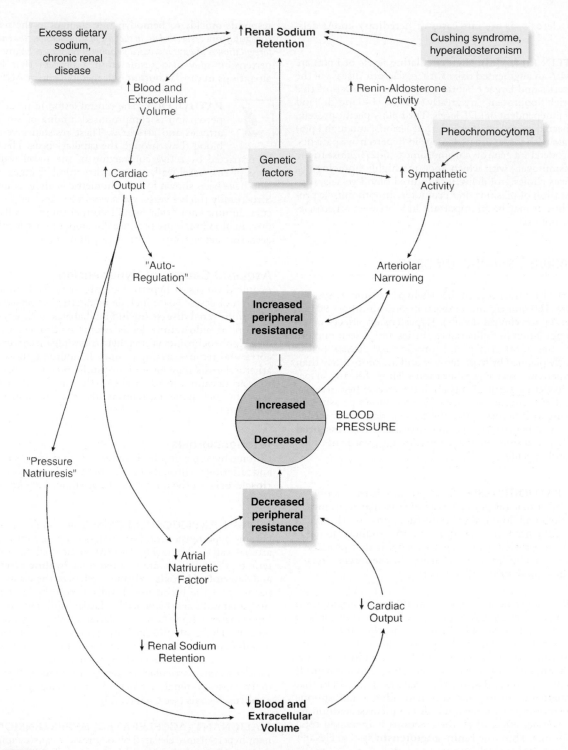

FIGURE 10-11. **Factors contributing to hypertension and the counterregulatory factors that lower blood pressure.** An imbalance in these factors results in the increased peripheral resistance that is responsible for most cases of essential (primary) hypertension. Note the central role of peripheral resistance.

arteries show segmental dilation due to necrosis of smooth muscle cells. Endothelial integrity is lost in these regions, and increased vascular permeability leads to the entry of plasma proteins into the vessel wall, deposition of fibrin, and an appearance termed **fibrinoid necrosis**. The period of acute injury is rapidly followed by smooth muscle proliferation and a striking concentric increase in the number of layers of smooth muscle cells, which yields the so-called onion-skin appearance (Fig. 10-13). Together, these changes are labeled **malignant arteriosclerosis** or **arteriolosclerosis**, depending on the size of the vessels affected. In the kidney, lesions of malignant hypertension are known as **malignant nephrosclerosis**.

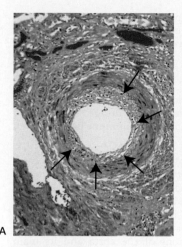
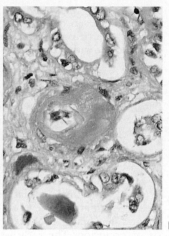

FIGURE 10-12. **Benign arteriosclerosis. A.** A cross-section of a renal intralobular artery shows irregular thickening of the intima (*arrows*). **B.** A renal arteriole exhibits hyalin arteriolosclerosis.

Mönckeberg Medial Sclerosis

Mönckeberg medial sclerosis refers to degenerative calcification of the media of large and medium-sized muscular arteries. The disorder occurs principally in older persons and most often involves arteries of the upper and lower extremities.

 PATHOLOGY: The involved arteries are hard and dilated. Microscopically, the smooth muscle of the media is focally replaced by pale-staining, acellular, hyalinized fibrous tissue, with concentric dystrophic calcification. Osseous metaplasia in calcified areas is occasionally observed. Mönckeberg medial sclerosis is distinct from atherosclerosis and ordinarily does not lead to any clinical disorder.

Raynaud Phenomenon

Raynaud phenomenon refers to intermittent, bilateral attacks of ischemia of the fingers or toes and sometimes the ears or nose. It is characterized by severe pallor of the affected structures and is often accompanied by paresthesias and pain. Symptoms are precipitated by cold or emotional stimuli and relieved by heat. Raynaud phenomenon may occur as an isolated disorder or as a part of a number of systemic diseases of connective tissue (collagen vascular disorders), particularly scleroderma and systemic lupus erythematosus. Whatever the cause, Raynaud phenomenon reflects arterial vasospasm in the skin.

Vasculitis

Vasculitis refers to inflammation and necrosis of blood vessels and may affect arteries, veins, and capillaries (Table 10-4). Arteries or veins may be damaged by immune mechanisms, infectious agents, mechanical trauma, radiation, or toxins. However, in many cases, no specific cause is determined. The classification of vasculitides is most often based on the size of the affected vessel (The Chapel Hill Consensus System):

- **Large-vessel vasculitis:** chronic granulomatous inflammation of the aorta and its larger branches
- **Medium-sized vessel vasculitis:** necrotizing inflammation of mid-sized arteries
- **Small-vessel vasculitis:** necrotizing inflammation of small arteries, arterioles, venules, and capillaries

 PATHOGENESIS: Vasculitic syndromes are thought to involve immune mechanisms including (1) deposition of immune complexes, (2) direct attack on vessels by circulating antibodies, (3) antineutrophil cytoplasmic antibodies (ANCA) and resultant neutrophil degranulation, and (4) various forms of cell-mediated immunity.

Viral antigens may cause vasculitis. For example, chronic infection with hepatitis B virus is associated with some cases of polyarteritis nodosa. In this case, circulating viral antigen–antibody complexes are deposited in the vascular lesions.

ANCA are associated with small-vessel vasculitides (e.g., Wegener granulomatosis and microscopic polyangiitis; see below). ANCA cause endothelial damage by activating neutrophils. P-ANCA, which is directed mainly against myeloperoxidase, and C-ANCA, directed mainly against proteinase 3, can be distinguished by the pattern of immunoreactivity shown by the patient's serum toward neutrophils. Both myeloperoxidase and proteinase 3 are expressed on the surface of neutrophils activated by cytokines, and

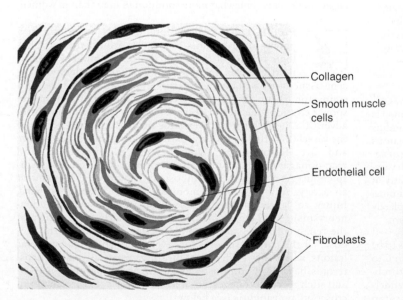

Collagen

Smooth muscle cells

Endothelial cell

Fibroblasts

FIGURE 10-13. **Arteriolosclerosis.** In cases of hypertension, the arterioles exhibit smooth muscle cell proliferation and increased amounts of intercellular collagen and glycosaminoglycans, resulting in an "onion-skin" appearance. The mass of smooth muscle and associated elements tends to fix the size of the lumen and restrict the arteriole's capacity to dilate.

ANCA binding to such molecules leads to subsequent degranulation of neutrophils and vascular damage.

Large-Vessel Vasculitis is Associated with Granulomatous Inflammation

Giant cell arteritis, the most common vasculitis, is difficult to distinguish from **Takayasu arteritis** based solely on tissue pathology. The former is predominantly a disease of older patients, whereas the latter is uncommon after the age of 50 years.

Giant Cell Arteritis (Temporal Arteritis, Granulomatous Arteritis)

Giant cell arteritis is a focal, chronic, granulomatous inflammation often found in the temporal arteries. It may also involve additional cranial arteries, the aorta and its branches, and occasionally other arteries. Aortic aneurysm and dissection occur. The average age at onset is 70 years, and it is rare before age 50.

 PATHOGENESIS: The etiology of giant cell arteritis is obscure. Its association with HLA-DR4 and its occurrence in first-degree relatives support a genetic component in its pathogenesis. The morphologic alterations, including the presence of activated CD4$^+$ T-helper cells and macrophages, and an association of giant cell arteritis with a specific polymorphism of the leukocyte adhesion molecule ICAM-1, suggest an immunologic reaction.

 PATHOLOGY: In giant cell arteritis, the affected vessels are cord-like and show nodular thickening. The lumen is reduced to a slit or may be obliterated by a thrombus (Fig. 10-14A). Microscopically, there is granulomatous inflammation of the adventitia, media and intima, consisting of aggregates of macrophages, lymphocytes, and plasma cells, with varying admixtures of eosinophils and neutrophils. Giant cells vary in number and tend to be distributed at the internal elastic lamina, which is often swollen and fragmented, and may even completely disappear (see Fig. 10-14B). Fibrinoid necrosis is usually absent.

 CLINICAL FEATURES: Giant cell arteritis tends to be benign and self-limited, and symptoms subside in 6 to 12 months. Patients present with headache and throbbing temporal pain accompanied by swelling, tenderness, and redness in the overlying skin. Visual symptoms occur in almost half of patients and may proceed from transient to permanent blindness in one or both eyes, sometimes rapidly. The response to corticosteroid therapy is usually dramatic, and symptoms subside within days.

Takayasu Arteritis

This form of arteritis is seen worldwide and mainly affects women (90%), most of whom are under 30 years of age. The cause of Takayasu arteritis is unknown, but an autoimmune basis has been proposed.

 PATHOLOGY: Takayasu arteritis is classified according to the extent of aortic involvement. The pulmonary artery is also occasionally affected, and involvement of the retinal vasculature is often a prominent feature. On gross examination, the aorta is thickened by intimal focal plaques. The branches of the aorta often display localized stenosis or occlusion. The early lesions of the aorta and its main branches begin in the media and progress to an acute panarteritis, with infiltrates of neutrophils, mononuclear cells, and occasional Langhans giant cells. Late lesions exhibit fibrosis and severe intimal proliferation.

 CLINICAL FEATURES: Patients with early Takayasu arteritis complain of constitutional symptoms, dizziness, visual disturbances, dyspnea, and occasionally syncope. As the disease progresses, cardiac symptoms become more severe, and intermittent claudication of the arms or legs may occur. Asymmetric differences in blood pressure may develop, and the pulse in one extremity may actually disappear, accounting for the synonym "**pulseless disease**." They may lose visual acuity, ranging from field defects to total blindness. Most patients eventually suffer congestive heart failure. Early Takayasu arteritis responds to corticosteroids, but the later lesions require surgical reconstruction.

Medium-Sized Vessel Vasculitis is Characterized by Necrotizing Vasculitis

Polyarteritis nodosa and Kawasaki disease affect medium-sized arteries and are distinguished from a variety of other vasculitides that demonstrate necrotizing lesions in venules, capillaries, and arterioles.

Polyarteritis Nodosa (PAN)

PAN affects medium-sized and smaller muscular arteries and occasionally larger arteries. It is somewhat more common in men than in women.

 PATHOLOGY: The lesions of PAN are found in a patchy distribution. The most prominent morphologic feature of the affected artery is an area of fibrinoid necrosis, in which the medial muscle and adjacent tissues are fused into a structureless eosinophilic mass that stains for fibrin. Initially, a vigorous acute inflammatory response envelops the area of necrosis, usually involving the entire adventitia (periarteritis) and extends through the other coats of the vessel (Fig. 10-15). In early disease, neutrophils predominate and are followed by lymphocytes, plasma cells, and macrophages in varying proportions. Eosinophils are often conspicuous. As a result of thrombosis in the affected segment of an artery, infarcts are commonly found in involved organs. Injury to larger arteries causes small aneurysms (pseudoaneurysms) (<0.5 cm in diameter), particularly in branches of the renal, coronary, and cerebral arteries, hence the term "nodosa." If the patient survives for several months, many vascular lesions will show evidence of healing, especially if corticosteroids have been administered. ANCA is uncommon in PAN, and such reactivity suggests a small-vessel vasculitis, such as microscopic polyangiitis (see below).

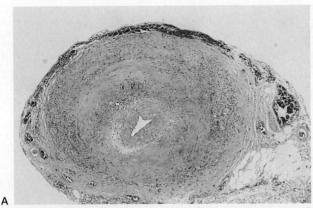

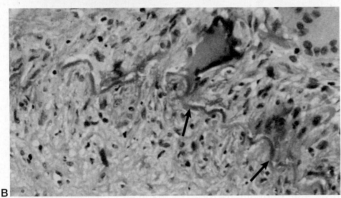

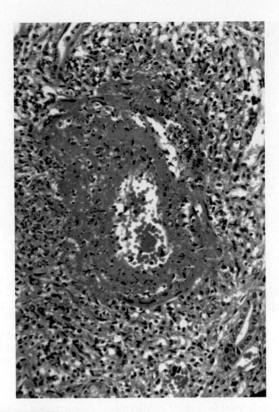

FIGURE 10-15. **Polyarteritis nodosa.** The intense inflammatory cell infiltrate in the arterial wall and surrounding connective tissue is associated with fibrinoid necrosis and disruption of the vessel wall.

FIGURE 10-14. **Temporal arteritis. A.** A photomicrograph of a temporal artery shows chronic inflammation throughout the wall, giant cells, and a lumen severely narrowed by intimal thickening. **B.** A high-power view shows giant cells adjacent to the fragmented internal elastic lamina *(arrows)*.

 CLINICAL FEATURES: Clinical manifestations of PAN are highly variable and depend on the locations of lesions in different organs. Kidneys, heart, skeletal muscle, skin, and mesentery are most frequently involved, but lesions may occur in almost any organ, including the bowel, pancreas, lungs, liver, and brain. Constitutional symptoms such as fever and weight loss are common. Without treatment, PAN is usually fatal, but anti-inflammatory and immunosuppressive therapy in the form of corticosteroids and cyclophosphamide leads to remission or cure in most patients.

Kawasaki Disease (Mucocutaneous Lymph Node Syndrome)

Kawasaki disease is an acute necrotizing vasculitis of infancy and early childhood characterized by high fever, rash, conjunctival and oral lesions, and lymphadenitis. In 70% of patients, the vasculitis affects the coronary arteries and leads to coronary artery aneurysms (Fig. 10-16), which cause death in 1% to 2% of cases.

 PATHOGENESIS: Kawasaki disease is usually self-limited. Although an infectious cause has been sought, none has been conclusively proved. Infection with *parvovirus B19* or with *New Haven coronavirus* has been implicated in some cases, and there is evidence for various bacterial infections, including staphylococcus, streptococcus, and chlamydia. The common theme seems to be the massive activation of the immune system by viral or bacterial superantigens in an antigen-nonspecific manner. Autoantibodies to endothelial and smooth muscle cells have been identified in some patients.

Small-Vessel Vasculitis is Associated with Either Immune Complexes or is "Pauci-Immune"

Small-vessel vasculitides that demonstrate immune complex deposition in the vascular wall such as Henoch-Schönlein purpura and cryoglobulinemic vasculitis, are briefly discussed in Chapter 16. Both of these conditions have skin lesions characterized as **leukocytoclastic vasculitis** (referring to the nuclear debris from disintegrating neutrophils), **cutaneous vasculitis**, *or* **cutaneous necrotizing venulitis** (emphasizing the predominant involvement of the venules). Small-vessel vasculitides that lack evidence of immune complex deposition (pauci-immune vasculitis), such as microscopic polyangiitis, Wegener granulomatosis, and Churg-Strauss syndrome, are often associated with circulating ANCA reactivity.

Microscopic Polyangiitis

Microscopic polyangiitis affects many of the same organs as PAN, but most patients have disease that is not restricted to small arteries and arterioles.

 PATHOLOGY: In addition to arterial involvement, venules and capillaries may be affected. Pulmonary and renal lesions are common and are expressed as necrotizing glomerulonephritis and alveolar capillaritis. Segmental fibrinoid necrosis is initially associated with neutrophilic infiltration, which is followed by monocytes, macrophages, and lymphocytes. The disease is strongly associated with both P-ANCA and C-ANCA activity.

CLINICAL FEATURES: Constitutional symptoms such as fever, weight loss, and myalgia are common. Skin involvement is seen as a rash with "palpable purpura." Pulmonary symptoms may include cough, dyspnea, and hemoptysis. The most feared complication of micro-

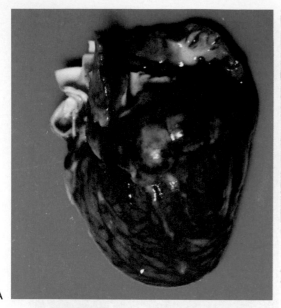
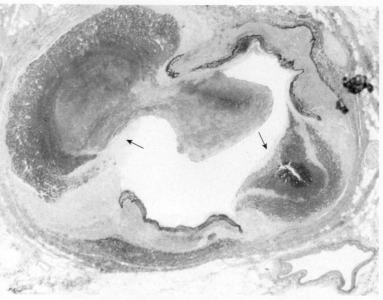

A B

FIGURE 10-16. **Kawasaki disease. A.** The heart of a child who died from Kawasaki disease shows conspicuous coronary artery aneurysms. **B.** A microscopic section of a coronary artery from the same patient shows two large defects (arrows) in the internal elastic lamina, with two small aneurysms filled with thrombus.

scopic polyarteritis is renal involvement, characterized by rapidly progressive glomerulonephritis and renal failure (see Chapter 16).

Churg-Strauss Syndrome (Allergic Granulomatosis and Angiitis)

Churg-Strauss Syndrome occurs in young patients and is characterized by asthma and eosinophilia.

PATHOLOGY: Widespread necrotizing lesions of small and medium-sized arteries, arterioles, and veins are found in the lungs, spleen, kidney, heart, liver, central nervous system, and other organs. These lesions are granulomatous and show intense eosinophilic infiltrates in and around blood vessels. The resulting fibrinoid necrosis, thrombosis, and aneurysm formation may simulate PAN, although Churg-Strauss syndrome seems to be a distinct entity. Glomerulonephritis does occur, but is less severe than in other small-vessel vasculitis. Two thirds of patients have C-ANCA or P-ANCA. Untreated persons with Churg-Strauss syndrome have a poor prognosis, but corticosteroids are now almost always successful in treating the disease.

Wegener Granulomatosis

Wegener granulomatosis is a systemic necrotizing vasculitis of unknown etiology characterized by granulomatous lesions of the nose, sinuses, and lungs and renal glomerular disease. Men are affected more often than women, usually in the fifth and sixth decades of life. The etiology of the disease is unknown. More than 90% of patients with Wegener granulomatosis exhibit ANCA, of whom 75% have C-ANCA. The response to immunosuppressive therapy supports an immunologic basis for the disease.

PATHOLOGY: The lesions of Wegener granulomatosis feature parenchymal necrosis, vasculitis, and a granulomatous inflammation composed of neutrophils, lymphocytes, plasma cells, macrophages, and eosinophils. Vasculitis involving arterioles, venules, and capillaries may be seen anywhere but occurs most frequently in the respiratory tract, kidney, and spleen (Fig. 10-17). Small-vessel vasculitis is characterized principally by chronic inflammation, although acute inflamma-

tion, necrotizing and nonnecrotizing granulomatous inflammation, and fibrinoid necrosis are frequently present. The most prominent pulmonary feature is persistent bilateral pneumonitis with nodular infiltrates that undergo cavitation reminiscent of tuberculous lesions (although the mechanisms are clearly different). Chronic sinusitis and ulcers of the nasopharyngeal mucosa are

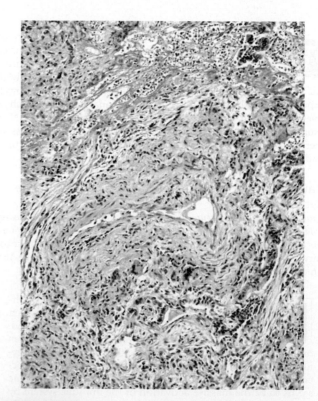

FIGURE 10-17. **Wegener granulomatosis.** A photomicrograph of the lung shows vasculitis of a pulmonary artery. There are chronic inflammatory cells and Langhans giant cells in the wall, together with thickening of the intima.

common. The kidney at first shows focal necrotizing glomeru-lonephritis, which progresses to crescentic glomerulonephritis (see Chapter 17).

 CLINICAL FEATURES: Most patients (>90%) present with symptoms referable to the respiratory tract, particularly pneumonitis and sinusitis. Glomerular disease can progress to renal failure. In untreated Wegener granulomatosis, most individuals (80%) die within a year of onset, with a mean survival of 5 to 6 months. Treatment with cyclophosphamide produces both complete remissions and substantial disease-free intervals in most patients.

Aneurysms

Arterial aneurysms are localized dilations of blood vessels caused by a congenital or acquired weakness of the media. They are not rare, and their incidence tends to rise with age. Aneurysms of the aorta and other arteries are found in as many as 10% of autopsies. The wall of an aneurysm is formed by the stretched remnants of the arterial wall.

Aneurysms are classified by location, configuration, and etiology (Fig. 10-18). The location refers to the type of vessel involved—artery or vein—and the specific vessel affected, such as the aorta or popliteal artery. The gross morphology of aneurysms reveals several different pathologic features.

- **Fusiform aneurysm** is an ovoid swelling parallel to the long axis of the vessel.
- **Saccular aneurysm** is a bubble-like arterial wall outpouching at a site of weakened media.
- **Dissecting aneurysm** is actually a dissecting hematoma, in which hemorrhage into the media separates the layers of the vascular wall.
- **Arteriovenous aneurysm** is a direct communication between an artery and a vein.

Abdominal Aortic Aneurysms are Complications of Atherosclerosis

Abdominal aortic aneurysms are dilations that increase vessel wall diameter by at least 50%. They are the most frequent aneurysms, usually developing after the age of 50 and are associated with severe atherosclerosis of the artery. Aortic aneurysms occur much more often in men than in women, and half of the patients are hypertensive. Occasionally, aneurysms are found in ascending, arch, and descending parts of the thoracic aorta and in iliac and popliteal arteries.

Although abdominal aortic aneurysms occur in the context of atherosclerosis, it is thought that the disease is actually multifactorial, as familial clustering suggests a genetic predisposition. Changes in the extracellular matrix of the aortic wall, inflammation or alterations in cell-mediated immune responses, and hemodynamic factors, especially hypertension, have all been implicated in the pathogenesis of abdominal aortic aneurysms.

 PATHOLOGY: Most abdominal aortic aneurysms are distal to the renal arteries and proximal to the bifurcation (Fig. 10-19). They are usually fusiform, although saccular varieties are occasionally encountered. Symptomatic aneurysms are generally more than 5 to 6 cm in diameter. Aneurysms that extend above the renal arteries may occlude the origin of the superior mesenteric artery and the celiac axis. Most abdominal aortic aneurysms are lined by raised, ulcerated, and calcified (complicated) atherosclerotic lesions. They tend to contain mural thrombi of varying degrees of organization, portions of which may embolize to peripheral arteries. Infrequently, the thrombus itself may enlarge enough to compromise the lumen of the aorta. Microscopically, complicated atherosclerotic lesions show destruction of the normal arterial wall and its replacement by fibrous tissue. Remnants of normal media

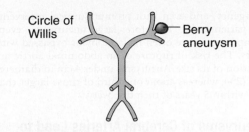
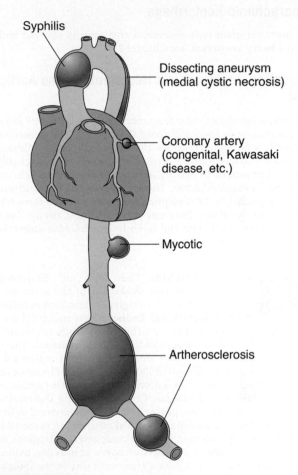

FIGURE 10-18. **The locations of aneurysms.** Syphilitic aneurysms are the common variety in the ascending aorta, which is usually spared by the atherosclerotic process. Atherosclerotic aneurysms can occur in the abdominal aorta or muscular arteries, including the coronary and popliteal arteries and other vessels. Berry aneurysms are seen in the circle of Willis, mainly at branch points; their rupture leads to subarachnoid hemorrhage. Mycotic aneurysms occur almost anywhere that bacteria can deposit on vessel walls.

are seen focally, and atheromatous lesions extend to variable depths. The adventitia is thickened and focally inflamed as a response to severe atherosclerosis.

 CLINICAL FEATURES: Many abdominal aortic aneurysms are asymptomatic and are discovered only by palpation of a mass in the abdomen or on nonrelated radiologic examination. In some cases, the condition is brought to medical attention by the onset of abdominal pain, which reflects aneurysmal expansion. Abrupt occlusion of a peripheral artery by an embolus from the mural thrombus presents as sudden ischemia of a lower limb. The most dreaded complication is rupture and exsanguinating retroperitoneal (or thoracic) hemorrhage, in which case the patient presents with pain, shock, and a pulsatile mass in the abdomen. Such a situation is an acute emergency, and even with prompt surgical intervention, half of the patients die. Therefore, large aneurysms, even if entirely asymptomatic, are often replaced by or bypassed with prosthetic grafts. The risk of rupture of an abdominal aortic aneurysm is a function of its size. Aneurysms under 4 cm in diameter rarely rupture (2%), whereas about one third of those larger than 5 cm rupture within 5 years of their discovery.

Aneurysms of Cerebral Arteries Lead to Subarachnoid Hemorrhage

The most common type of cerebral aneurysm is saccular and is called a **berry aneurysm** (see Chapter 28).

Dissecting Aneurysm is a Hematoma of the Aortic Wall

Hemorrhage into the arterial wall separates the layers of the wall as it dissects a path along the length of the vessel (Fig. 10-20). The dissection is essentially a false lumen within the wall of the artery. Although this lesion is conventionally termed an aneurysm, it is actually a form of hematoma. Dissecting aneurysms most often affect the aorta and its major branches. Their frequency has been estimated to be as high as 1 in 400 autopsies, with men affected three times as frequently as women. They may occur at almost any age but are most common in the sixth and seventh decades. *Most patients have histories of hypertension.*

 PATHOGENESIS: The basis of dissecting aneurysms is usually weakening of the aortic media. The changes were originally described as **cystic medial necrosis (of Erdheim)** because focal loss of elastic and muscle fibers in the media leads to "cystic" spaces filled with a metachromatic myxoid material. These spaces are not true cysts but are rather pools of matrix collected between the cells and tissues of the media. The cause of medial degeneration is not known. Some cases are complications of Marfan syndrome, (see Chapter 6). Aging also results in mild degenerative changes in the aorta, characterized by focal elastin loss and medial fibrosis. Taken together, these data suggest that the common factor in these several situations is a defect that leads to weakness of aortic connective tissue. More than 95% of cases have a transverse tear in the intima and internal media, and it is widely held that spontaneous laceration of the intima allows blood from the lumen to enter and dissect the media.

 PATHOLOGY: Most intimal tears are in the ascending aorta, 1 or 2 cm above the aortic ring. Dissection in the media occurs within seconds and separates the inner two thirds of the aorta from the outer third. It can also involve coronary arteries, great vessels of the neck, and renal, mesenteric, or iliac arteries. Because the outer wall of the false channel of the dissecting aneurysm is thin, hemorrhage into the extravascular space, including the pericardium, mediastinum, pleural space, and retroperitoneum, frequently causes death.

 CLINICAL FEATURES: The typical patient with an aortic dissection presents with the acute onset of severe, "tearing" pain in the anterior chest, which is sometimes misdiagnosed as MI. Loss of one or more arterial pulses is common, and a murmur of aortic regurgitation is often present. Whereas many patients suffer from hypertension, hypotension is an ominous sign, suggesting aortic rupture. Cardiac tamponade or congestive heart failure may occur. Surgical intervention and control of hypertension have reduced overall mortality to less than 20%.

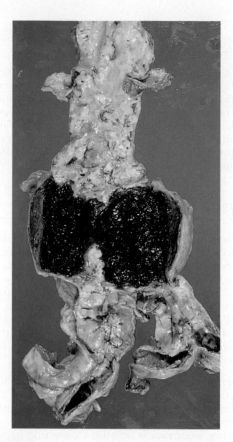

FIGURE 10-19. **Atherosclerotic aneurysm of the abdominal aorta.** The aneurysm has been opened longitudinally to reveal a large mural thrombus in the lumen. The aorta and common iliac arteries display complicated lesions of atherosclerosis.

Syphilitic Aneurysms are due to Inflammation of Aortic Vasa Vasorum

Syphilis was once the most common cause of aortic aneu-rysms, but as this infection has become less common, so has syphilitic vascular disease, including aortitis and aneurysms. Syphilitic aneurysms mainly affect the ascending aorta, where microscopic examination shows endarteritis and periarteritis of the vasa vasorum (see Chapter 9 for additional details).

Veins

Varicose Veins of the Legs Involve the Superficial Saphenous System

A varicose vein is an enlarged and tortuous vein. Superficial varicosities of leg veins are usually in the saphenous system and are very common. They vary from a trivial knot of dilated veins to disabling distention of the whole venous system of the leg. It is estimated that as much as 10% to 20% of the population has some varicosities in the leg veins, but only a fraction of these individuals develop symptoms.

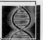 **PATHOGENESIS:** There are a number of risk factors for varicose veins:

- **Age:** Varicose veins increase in frequency with age and may reach 50% in persons over 50.

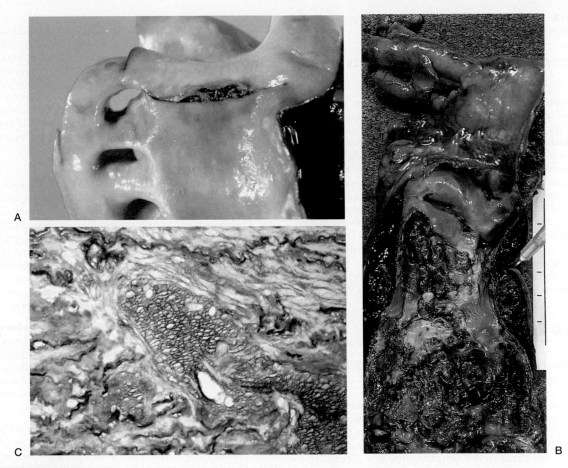

FIGURE 10-20. **Dissecting aneurysm of the aorta. A.** A transverse tear is present in the aortic arch. The orifices of the great vessels are on the *left*. **B.** The thoracic aorta has been open longitudinally and reveals clotted blood dissecting the media of the vessel. The luminal surface shows extensive complicated lesions of atherosclerosis. **C.** A section of the aortic wall stained with aldehyde fuchsin shows pools of metachromatic material characteristic of the degenerative process known as cystic medial necrosis.

- **Gender:** Among 30- to 50-year-olds, women are more often affected by varicose veins than men, particularly those who have experienced pregnancy.
- **Heredity:** There is a strong familial predisposition to varicose veins, possibly due to inherited configurations or structural weakness of the walls or valves of the veins.
- **Posture:** Leg vein pressure is 5 to 10 times higher when a person is erect, rather than recumbent. As a result, the incidence of varicose veins and its complications are greater in people whose occupations require them to stand in one place for long periods.
- **Obesity:** Excessive body weight increases the incidence of varicose veins, possibly because of increased intra-abdominal pressure or poor support provided by the subcutaneous fat to vessel walls.

Other factors that raise venous pressure in the legs can cause varicose veins, including pelvic tumors, congestive heart failure, and thrombotic obstruction of the main venous trunks of the thigh or pelvis.

In the pathogenesis of varicose veins, it is not clear whether incompetence of the valves or dilation of the vessels comes first. Whatever the case, the two reinforce each other. The vein increases in length and diameter, so that tortuousities develop. Once the process begins, the varicosity extends progressively throughout the length of the affected vein.

 PATHOLOGY: Microscopically, varicose veins show variations in wall thickness. Thinning due to dilation is present in some areas, whereas others are thickened by smooth muscle hypertrophy, subintimal fibrosis, and incorporation of mural thrombi into the wall. Patchy calcification is frequently seen. Valvular deformities consist of thickening, shortening, and rolling of the cusps.

 CLINICAL FEATURES: Most varicose veins are without clinical effects and are mainly cosmetic problems. The principal symptoms are aching in the legs, aggravated by standing and relieved by elevation. Severe varicosities may lead to alterations in the skin drained by the affected veins, termed stasis dermatitis. Surgical intervention is mandated if the overlying skin has ulcerated or if the patient has spontaneous bleeding or extensive thrombosis (which may lead to pulmonary embolism).

Varicose Veins also Occur at Other Sites

HEMORRHOIDS: These are dilations of the veins of the rectum and anal canal, which may occur inside or outside the anal sphincter (see Chapter 13).

ESOPHAGEAL VARICES: This complication of portal hypertension is caused mainly by cirrhosis of the liver (see Chapter 14). Hemorrhage from esophageal varices is one of the most common causes of death in cirrhosis.

VARICOCELE: This palpable mass in the scrotum represents varicosities of the pampiniform plexus (see Chapter 17).

Deep Venous Thrombosis Principally Affects Leg Veins

- **Thrombophlebitis** is inflammation and secondary thrombosis of small veins and sometimes larger ones, commonly as part of a local reaction to bacterial infection.
- **Phlebothrombosis** is the term for venous thrombosis that occurs without an initiating infection or inflammation.
- **Deep venous thrombosis** now refers to both phlebothrombosis and thrombophlebitis. Because most cases of venous thrombosis are not associated with inflammation or infection, the condition is most commonly associated with prolonged bed rest, reduced cardiac output, or other prothrombotic states such as protein C or antithrombin III deficiency. It is most frequent in deep leg veins and can be a major threat to life because of pulmonary embolization (witness the well-known phenomenon of sudden death with ambulation after surgery). Deep venous thrombosis is discussed more fully in Chapter 7.

Lymphatic Vessels

Lymphangitis Refers to Infection and Inflammation in Lymphatic Vessels

Transport of infectious material to regional lymph nodes leads to intranodal inflammation termed **lymphadenitis**. The periphery of a focus of inflammation reveals dilated lymphatics filled with fluid exudate, cells, cellular debris, and bacteria. Almost any virulent pathogen can cause acute lymphangitis, but β-hemolytic streptococci (*S. pyogenes*) are common offenders. Draining lymph nodes are regularly enlarged and inflamed. Painful subcutaneous red streaks, often accompanied by tender regional lymph nodes, characterize acute lymphangitis.

Lymphatic Obstruction Causes Lymphedema

Lymphatics may be obstructed by scar tissue, intraluminal tumor cells, pressure from surrounding tumor tissue, or plugging with parasites. As collateral lymphatic routes are abundant, **lymphedema** (distention of tissue by lymph) usually occurs only when major trunks, most commonly in the axilla or groin, are obstructed. For example, when radical mastectomy for breast cancer was routine, axillary lymph node dissection frequently disrupted lymphatic channels and led to lymphedema of the arm. Prolonged lymphatic obstruction causes progressive dilation of lymphatic vessels, termed **lymphangiectasia**, and overgrowth of fibrous tissue. The term **elephantiasis** describes a lymphedematous limb that has become grossly enlarged. An important cause of elephantiasis in the tropics is filariasis, in which a parasitic worm invades the lymphatics (see Chapter 9). *Milroy disease* is *an inherited type of lymphangiectasia that is present at birth.* It usually affects only one limb, but it may be more extensive and involve the eyelids and lips. Affected tissues show hugely dilated lymphatic channels, and the entire area appears honeycombed or spongy.

Benign Tumors of Blood Vessels

Hemangiomas are Common Benign Tumors of Vascular Channels

Hemangiomas usually occur in the skin but may also be found in internal organs.

 PATHOGENESIS: Although hemangiomas are clearly benign, their origin is uncertain; they represent either true neoplasms or hamartomas. The evidence favoring hamartoma (i.e., a malformation) includes (1) the lesion is present at birth, (2) it grows only as the rest of the body grows and remains limited in size, and (3) after growth ceases, it usually remains unchanged indefinitely in the absence of trauma, thrombosis, or hemorrhage. At present, hemangiomas are classified by histologic type and location.

PATHOLOGY:
CAPILLARY HEMANGIOMA: *This lesion is composed of vascular channels with the size and structure of normal capillaries.* Capillary hemangiomas may be located in any tissue. The most common sites are skin, subcutaneous tissues, mucous membranes of lips and the mouth, and internal viscera, including spleen, kidneys, and liver. Capillary hemangiomas vary from a few millimeters to several centimeters in diameter. They are bright red to blue, depending on the degree of oxygenation of the blood. In the skin, capillary hemangiomas are known as **birthmarks** or **ruby spots**. The only disability is cosmetic.

JUVENILE HEMANGIOMA: Also called **strawberry hemangiomas**, these benign lesions are found on the skin of newborns. They grow rapidly in the first months of life, begin to fade at 1 to 3 years of age, and completely regress in most (80%) cases by 5 years of age. Juvenile hemangiomas contain packed masses of capillaries separated by connective tissue stroma. The endothelium-lined channels are usually filled with blood.

CAVERNOUS HEMANGIOMA: *This designation is reserved for lesions consisting of large vascular channels, frequently interspersed with small, capillary-type vessels.* Cavernous hemangiomas occur in the skin, where they are termed **port wine stains**. They also appear on mucosal surfaces and visceral organs, including the spleen, liver, and pancreas. Occasionally, they are encountered in the brain, where they may slowly enlarge and cause neurologic symptoms. A cavernous hemangioma is a red-blue, soft, spongy mass, with a diameter of up to several centimeters. Unlike the capillary hemangioma, a cavernous hemangioma does not regress spontaneously. Although the lesion is demarcated by a sharp border, it is not encapsulated. Large endothelial-lined, blood-containing spaces are separated by sparse connective tissue.

MULTIPLE HEMANGIOMATOUS SYNDROMES: More than one hemangioma may occur in a single tissue. Two or more tissues may be involved, such as skin and nervous system or spleen and liver. **von Hippel-Lindau syndrome** is a rare entity in which cavernous hemangiomas occur in the cerebellum or brainstem and the retina. **Sturge-Weber syndrome** involves a developmental disturbance of blood vessels in the brain and skin.

Glomus Tumor (Glomangioma) is a Painful Arteriolar–Venous Anastomosis

A glomus tumor is a benign neoplasm of the glomus body. Glomus bodies are normal neuromyoarterial receptors that are sensitive to temperature and regulate arteriolar flow. They are widely distributed in the skin, mostly in the distal regions of fingers and toes. This pattern is reflected in the location of glomus tumors at these sites, typically in a subungual location.

 PATHOLOGY: The lesions are small, usually under 1 cm in diameter; many are smaller than a few millimeters. In the skin, they are slightly elevated, rounded, red-blue, and firm (Fig. 10-21). The two main histologic components are branching vascular channels in a connective tissue stroma and aggregates or nests of the specialized glomus cells.

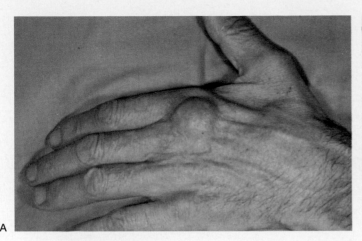
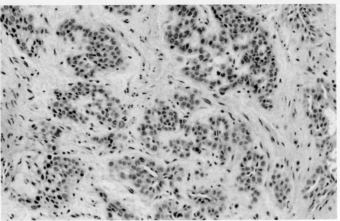

A | B

FIGURE 10-21. **Glomus tumor. A.** The dorsal surface of the hand displays a prominent tumor nodule on the proximal third finger. **B.** A photomicrograph of **(A)** reveals nests of glomus tumor cells embedded in a fibrovascular stroma.

The latter are regular, round-to-cuboidal cells that reveal typical smooth muscle cell features by electron microscopy.

Hemangioendothelioma Has Some Malignant Characteristics

Hemangioendothelioma is a vascular tumor of endothelial cells that is intermediate between benign hemangiomas and frankly malignant angiosarcomas. **The epithelioid or histiocytoid variant** displays endothelial cells with considerable eosinophilic, often vacuolated, cytoplasm. Vascular lumina are evident, and there are few mitoses. These tumors occur in almost all locations. Surgical removal is generally curative, but about one fifth of patients develop metastases. **Spindle cell hemangioendothelioma** occurs principally in males of any age, usually in the dermis and subcutaneous tissue of the distal extremities. It features vascular, endothelial-lined spaces into which papillary projections extend. Although the lesion may recur locally after excision, it rarely metastasizes.

Malignant Tumors of Blood Vessels

Malignant vascular neoplasms are rare and may sometimes arise in pre-existing benign tumors.

Angiosarcoma is a Rare, Highly Malignant Tumor of Endothelial Cells

The lesions occur in either gender and at any age and begin as small, painless, sharply demarcated, red nodules. The most common locations are skin, soft tissue, breast, bone, liver, and spleen. Eventually, most lesions enlarge to become pale gray, fleshy masses without a capsule. Often, these tumors undergo central necrosis, with softening and hemorrhage.

 PATHOLOGY: Angiosarcomas exhibit varying degrees of differentiation, ranging from those composed mainly of distinct vascular elements to undifferentiated tumors with few recognizable blood channels. The latter display frequent mitoses, pleomorphism, giant cells, and tend to be more aggressive. Almost half of patients with angiosarcoma die of the disease.

Angiosarcoma of the liver is of special interest because of its association with environmental carcinogens, particularly arsenic (a component of pesticides) and vinyl chloride (used in the production of plastics). Hepatic angiosarcoma was associated with the administration of thorium dioxide, a radioactive contrast medium (Thorotrast) used by radiologists prior to 1950. The earliest detectable changes are atypism and diffuse hyperplasia of the cells lining the hepatic sinusoids. The tumors are frequently multicentric and may arise in the spleen as well. Hepatic angiosarcomas are highly malignant and show both local invasion and metastatic spread.

Kaposi Sarcoma is a Complication of Acquired Immunodeficiency Syndrome (AIDS)

Kaposi sarcoma is a malignant angioproliferative tumor derived from endothelial cells.

 EPIDEMIOLOGY: Originally described as uncommon, Kaposi sarcoma now appears in epidemic form in association with AIDS and in immunosuppressed patients. Human herpesvirus 8, also termed Kaposi sarcoma-associated herpes virus, is thought to be responsible for this tumor. Only a small faction of individuals infected with Kaposi sarcoma-associated herpes virus develop Kaposi sarcoma.

 PATHOLOGY: Kaposi sarcoma begins as painful purple or brown cutaneous nodules, 1 mm to 1 cm in diameter. They appear most often on the hands or feet but may occur anywhere. The histologic appearance is highly variable. One form resembles a simple hemangioma with tightly packed clusters of capillaries and scattered hemosiderin-laden macrophages. Other forms are highly cellular, and the vascular spaces are less prominent. These lesions may be difficult to distinguish from fibrosarcomas, but the characteristic features of endothelial cells can be demonstrated immunochemically and by electron microscopy. Although Kaposi sarcoma is considered a malignant lesion and may be widely disseminated in the body, it is only exceptionally a cause of death.

11 The Heart

Jeffrey E. Saffitz

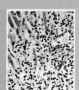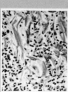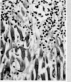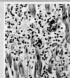

The heart is a fist-sized muscular pump that has a remarkable capacity to work unceasingly for the 80 or more years of a human lifetime. As demand requires, it can increase its output manyfold, in part because the coronary circulation can augment its blood flow to more than 10 times normal. The ventricles also respond to short-term increases in workload by dilating, in accordance with Starling law of the heart. When an increased workload is imposed for a longer period (e.g., in cases of essential hypertension), the left ventricle hypertrophies, an adaptation that increases its work capacity. However, when this compensatory mechanism reaches its limits, the heart no longer provides an adequate supply of blood to peripheral tissues, and the result is congestive heart failure. Damage to the myocardium, caused mostly by ischemic heart disease, also limits the capacity of the left ventricle to pump blood and similarly results in heart failure.

Coronary Arteries Supply Blood to the Heart

The right and left main coronary arteries originate in, or immediately above, the sinuses of Valsalva of the aortic valve. The left main coronary artery bifurcates within 1 cm of its origin into the left anterior descending (LAD) and left circumflex coronary arteries. The left circumflex coronary artery rests in the left atrioventricular groove and supplies the lateral wall of the left ventricle (Fig. 11-1). The LAD coronary artery lies in the anterior interventricular groove and provides blood to the (1) anterior left ventricle, (2) adjacent anterior right ventricle, and (3) anterior half to two thirds of the interventricular septum. In the apical region, the LAD artery supplies the ventricles circumferentially (see Fig. 11-1).

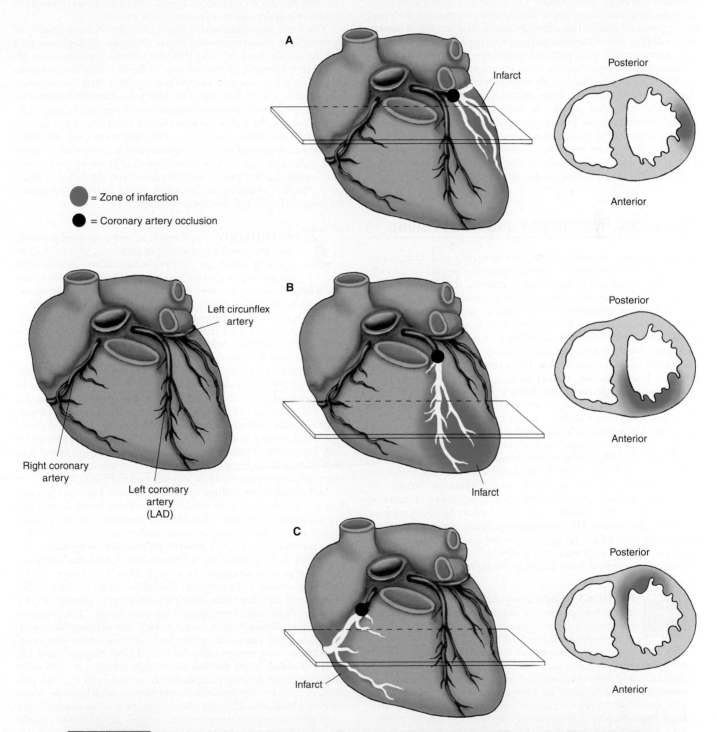

● = Zone of infarction

● = Coronary artery occlusion

FIGURE 11-1. **Position of left ventricular infarcts resulting from occlusion of each of the three main coronary arteries.** **A.** Posterolateral infarct, which follows occlusion of the left circumflex artery and is present in the posterolateral wall. **B.** Anterior infarct, which follows occlusion of the anterior descending branch (left anterior descending, LAD) of the left coronary artery. The infarct is located in the anterior wall and adjacent two thirds of the septum. It involves the entire circumference of the wall near the apex. **C.** A posterior ("inferior" or "diaphragmatic") infarct results from occlusion of the right coronary artery and involves the posterior wall, including the posterior third of the interventricular septum and the posterior papillary muscle in the basal half of the ventricle.

The right coronary artery travels along the right atrioventricular groove and nourishes the bulk of the right ventricle and posteroseptal left ventricle (see Fig. 11-1), including the posterior third to half of the interventricular septum at the base of the heart (also referred to as the "inferior" or "diaphragmatic" wall). From these distributions, one can predict the location of infarcts that result from occlusion of any of the three major epicardial coronary arteries. The epicardial coronary arteries are usually arranged in a so-called right coronary-dominant distribution. The pattern of dominance is determined by the coronary artery that contributes most of the blood to the posterior descending coronary artery. Ten percent of human hearts display a left-dominant pattern with the left circumflex coronary artery supplying the posterior descending coronary artery.

Blood flow in the myocardium occurs inward from epicardium to endocardium. Thus, as a general rule, the endocardium is most vulnerable to ischemia when flow through a major epicardial coronary artery is compromised. The epicardial portion of each coronary artery fills and expands during systole and empties and narrows during diastole. The intramyocardial arteries have the opposite action and are narrowed by the systolic muscular pressure. As a result, blood flow within myocardium, especially in the subendocardial ventricular regions, is decreased or absent during systole.

Myocardial Hypertrophy and Heart Failure

During systole, ventricles contract vigorously and eject about 60% of the blood present in the ventricle at the end of diastole (ejection fraction). When a heart is injured, the clinical consequences are similar, regardless of the cause of cardiac dysfunction. *If the initial impairment is severe, cardiac output is not maintained despite compensatory changes, and the result is acute, life-threatening,* **cardiogenic shock.** When the functional impairment is less, compensatory mechanisms (see below) maintain cardiac output by increasing diastolic ventricular filling pressure and end-diastolic volume. This situation results in the characteristic signs and symptoms of **congestive heart failure.** Because of the heart's capacity to compensate, congestive heart failure is often tolerated for years. The heart's ability to adapt to injury is based on the same mechanisms that allow cardiac output to increase in response to stress. *The fundamental compensatory mechanism is the Frank-Starling mechanism: the cardiac stroke volume is a function of diastolic fiber length and, within certain limits, a normal heart will pump whatever volume is brought to it by the venous circulation.* Stroke volume, a measure of ventricular function, is enhanced by increasing ventricular end-diastolic volume secondary to an increase in atrial filling pressure. *The most prominent feature of heart failure is the abnormally high atrial filling pressure relative to stroke volume.* However, the absolute values of stroke volume and cardiac output are generally well maintained in the failing heart.

 PATHOGENESIS: Myocardial hypertrophy is an adaptive response that augments myocyte contractile strength. It develops as a compensatory response to hemodynamic overload, which occurs in association with chronic hypertension or valvular stenosis (pressure overload), myocardial injury, valvular insufficiency (volume overload), and other stresses that increase heart workload. A distinction must be made between **physiologic hypertrophy** of a heart that develops in highly trained athletes and **pathologic hypertrophy** that occurs in response to injury or overload. Hypertrophic responses feature enlargement of cardiac myocytes and accumulation of sarcomeric proteins without an increase in the number of cardiac myocytes. Hypertrophy initially reflects a compensatory and potentially reversible mechanism, but faced with persistent stress, the myocardium becomes irreversibly enlarged and dilated (Fig. 11-2).

Receptor-mediated myocardial events that are triggered by a stimulus promote the hypertrophic response by autocrine and paracrine mechanisms. Contractile cells respond to mechanical stimuli, such as stretching, by activating receptor-mediated signaling pathways that produce hypertrophy. Among the most important ligands that activate these pathways are (1) angiotensin II, (2) endothelin-1, and (3) various growth factors, including insulin-like growth factor-1 and transforming growth factor-β. Some of these mediators may also act on interstitial fibroblasts in the heart to promote synthesis and deposition of extracellular matrix.

The heart has traditionally been thought of as incapable of growing new myocytes to regenerate or repair damage due to a lack of cardiac stem cells. In this view, cardiac myocytes can respond to injury only by hypertrophy or death. Many controversies remain, but there is now compelling evidence that cardiac stem cells exist in adults. For example, male transplant recipients who have received female hearts exhibit fully differentiated cardiac myocytes bearing the Y chromosome, which must have been derived from the circulation. Moreover, embryonic stem cells and adult bone marrow-derived cells can experimentally repopulate areas of myocardial injury and differentiate into cardiac myocytes. In addition, *resident* cardiac progenitor cells have been identified in interstitial "niches" in the heart. Thus, the failing heart is a candidate for potential stem cell therapy (see Chapter 3).

 PATHOLOGY: Anything that increases cardiac workload for a prolonged period or produces structural damage may eventuate in myocardial failure. *Ischemic heart disease is by far the most common condition responsible for cardiac failure, accounting for more than 80% of deaths from heart disease.* Most of the remaining deaths are caused by nonischemic forms of heart muscle disease (cardiomyopathies) and congenital heart disease (CHD). Other than changes characteristic of specific disease entities (e.g., ischemic heart disease or cardiac amyloidosis), the morphology of the failing heart is nonspecific.

Ventricular hypertrophy is observed in virtually all conditions associated with chronic heart failure. Initially, only the left ventricle may be hypertrophied, as occurs in compensated hypertensive heart disease. But when the left ventricle fails, some right ventricular hypertrophy usually follows because of the increased workload imposed on the right ventricle by the failing left ventricle. *In most cases of clinically apparent heart failure, the ventricles are conspicuously dilated.* The distribution of end-organ involvement depends on whether the heart failure is predominantly left-sided or right-sided.

Left-sided heart failure is more common, because the most frequent causes of cardiac injury (e.g., ischemic heart disease and hypertension) primarily affect the left ventricle. To compensate for left ventricular failure, left atrial and pulmonary venous pressures increase, resulting in **passive pulmonary congestion**. The capillaries in the alveolar septa fill with blood, and small ruptures allow erythrocytes to escape. As a result, alveoli contain many hemosiderin-laden macrophages (so-called heart failure cells). Moreover, if capillary hydrostatic pressure exceeds plasma osmotic pressure, fluid leaks from capillaries into alveoli. The resultant **pulmonary edema** may be massive, with alveoli being "drowned" in a transudate. Interstitial pulmonary fibrosis results when congestion is present over an extended period (see Chapters 7 and 12).

Right-sided heart failure commonly complicates left-sided failure, or it can develop independently secondary to intrinsic pulmonary disease or pulmonary hypertension, which create resistance to blood flow through the lungs. As a consequence, right atrial pressure and systemic venous pressure both increase, resulting in jugular venous distention, lower-extremity edema, and congestion of the liver and spleen. Hepatic congestion in heart failure is discussed in Chapter 14.

Diastolic heart failure is seen in up to one third of elderly patients with obvious heart failure. As the heart ages, the ventricles become progressively stiffer and require greater filling (diastolic) pressures. Some patients exhibit signs and symptoms of

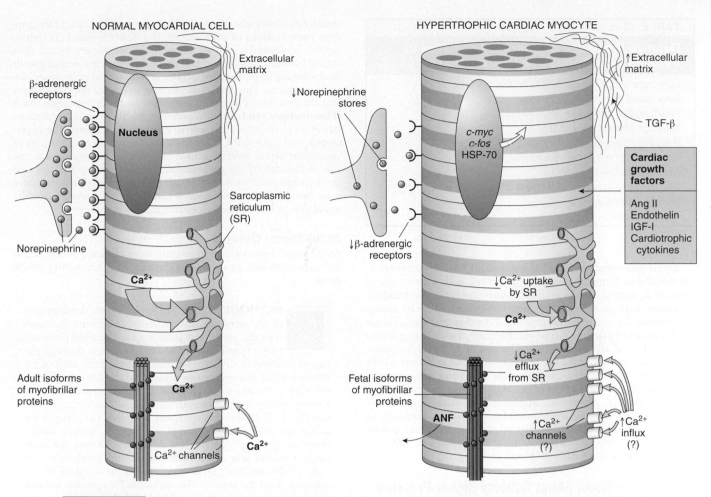

NORMAL MYOCARDIAL CELL

HYPERTROPHIC CARDIAC MYOCYTE

FIGURE 11-2. Biochemical characteristics of myocardial hypertrophy and congestive heart failure. ANF, atrial natriuretic factor; ANG II, angiotensin II; HSP-70, heat shock protein 70; IGF, insulin-like growth factor; TGF, transforming growth factor.

heart failure although their hearts are normal in size, do not show left ventricular hypertrophy, and have normal systolic contractile function. These patients do not easily tolerate increases in blood volume and are susceptible to developing pulmonary edema in response to a fluid challenge. Microscopically, these hearts typically exhibit interstitial fibrosis, which may contribute to the decreased compliance of ventricular myocardium.

 CLINICAL FEATURES: Symptoms of left-sided failure include dyspnea on exertion, orthopnea (dyspnea when lying down), and paroxysmal nocturnal dyspnea. Dyspnea on exertion reflects the increasing pulmonary congestion that accompanies a higher end-diastolic pressure in the left atrium and ventricle. Orthopnea and paroxysmal nocturnal dyspnea result when thoracic blood volume increases, on account of reduced blood volume in the lower extremities during recumbency.

Although much of the clinical presentation of heart failure can be explained by venous congestion (**backward failure**), certain aspects of congestive failure involve inadequate arterial perfusion of vital organs (**forward failure**). Most patients with left-sided heart failure retain sodium and water (edema), owing to decreased renal perfusion, decreased glomerular filtration rate, and activation of the renin–angiotensin–aldosterone system (see Chapters 7 and 10). Inadequate cerebral perfusion can lead to confusion, memory loss, and disorientation. Reduced perfusion of skeletal muscle is associated with fatigue and weakness.

Congenital Heart Disease (CHD)

CHD is a consequence of faulty embryonic development, expressed either as misplaced structures (e.g., transposition of the great vessels) or as an arrest in the progression of a normal structure from an early stage to one that is more mature (e.g., atrial septal defect).

Significant CHD occurs in almost 1% of all live births. This does not include certain common defects that are not functionally important, such as an anatomically patent foramen ovale that is functionally closed by the left atrial flap that covers it. In this circumstance, the foramen ovale remains closed as long as left atrial pressure exceeds that in the right atrium. A bicuspid aortic valve is also common and is usually asymptomatic until adulthood, when it is often associated with calcific aortic stenosis. Estimates of the incidence of particular cardiovascular anomalies vary, depending on many factors. A range derived from several sources is shown in Table 11-1.

 PATHOGENESIS: The causes of CHD are usually not ascertained. Most congenital heart defects reflect both multifactorial genetic and environmental influences. As in other diseases with multifactorial inheritance (see Chapter 6), the risk of recurrence is increased among siblings of an affected child. Moreover, an infant born to a mother with CHD also has an increased risk of cardiac defects.

TABLE 11–1

Relative Incidence of Specific Anomalies in Patients With Congenital Heart Disease

Ventricular septal defects—25% to 30%
Atrial septal defects—10% to 15%
Patent ductus arteriosus—10% to 20%
Tetralogy of Fallot—4% to 9%
Pulmonary stenosis—5% to 7%
Coarctation of the aorta—5% to 7%
Aortic stenosis—4% to 6%
Complete transposition of the great arteries—4% to 10%
Truncus arteriosus—2%
Tricuspid atresia—1%

Single-gene syndromes are rare causes of CHD. Mutations in *Csx/Mkx2-5* in humans have been associated with a spectrum of congenital cardiac malformations. Chromosomal abnormalities associated with an increased incidence of congenital heart anomalies include Down syndrome (trisomy 21), other trisomies, Turner syndrome, and DiGeorge syndrome. Together, these account for no more than 5% of all cases of CHD. The best evidence for intrauterine influence in the occurrence of congenital cardiac defects relates to maternal rubella infection during the first trimester, especially during the first 4 weeks of gestation. Maternal use of certain drugs, including alcohol, phenytoin, amphetamines, lithium, estrogenic steroids and, historically, thalidomide have been associated with an increased risk of CHD, as is maternal diabetes. A contemporary classification divides the cases into the groups shown in Table 11-2 and is based on the pattern of blood shunting.

Early Left-to-Right Shunt Reflects Higher Pressure on the Left Side of the Heart

Ventricular Septal Defect

Ventricular septal defects are the most common congenital heart lesions (see Table 11-1). They occur as isolated defects or in combination with other malformations.

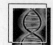 **PATHOGENESIS:** The fetal heart consists of a single chamber until the fifth week of gestation, after which it is divided by the development of interatrial and interventricular septa and by the formation of atrioventricular valves from endocardial cushions. A muscular interventricular septum grows upward from the apex toward the base of the heart (Fig. 11-3). It is joined by the down-growing membranous septum, separating right and left ventricles. *The most common ventricular septal defect is related to failure of the membranous portion of the septum to form in whole or in part.*

 PATHOLOGY: Ventricular septal defects occur as (1) a small hole in the membranous septum, (2) a large defect involving more than the membranous region (perimembranous defects), (3) defects in the muscular portion, which are more common anteriorly but can occur anywhere in the muscular septum, or (4) complete absence of the muscular septum (leaving a single ventricle).

 CLINICAL FEATURES: *A small septal defect may have little functional significance and may actually close spontaneously as the child matures.* Closure is accomplished by either hypertrophy of adjacent muscle or adherence of tricuspid valve leaflets to the margins of the defect. In infants with large septal defects, higher left ventricular pressure initially creates a left-to-right

shunt. Left ventricular dilation and congestive heart failure are common complications of such shunts. If a defect is small enough to permit prolonged survival, augmented pulmonary blood flow caused by shunting of blood into the right ventricle eventually leads to thickening of pulmonary arteries and increased pulmonary vascular resistance. This increased vascular resistance may be so great that the direction of the shunt is reversed and goes from right to left (**Eisenmenger syndrome**). A patient with this condition displays late onset of cyanosis (i.e., tardive cyanosis), right ventricular hypertrophy, and right-sided heart failure. Additional complications of ventricular septal defects include (1) infective endocarditis at the site of the defect, (2) paradoxical emboli (moving right to left through a patent foramen ovale), and (3) prolapse of an aortic valve cusp (with resulting aortic valve insufficiency). Large ventricular septal defects are repaired surgically, usually in infancy.

Atrial Septal Defects

Atrial septal defects range in severity from clinically insignificant and asymptomatic anomalies to chronic, life-threatening conditions.

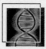 **PATHOGENESIS:** The embryologic development of the atrial septum occurs in a sequence that permits the continued passage of oxygenated placental blood from the right to the left atrium through the patent foramen until birth. Beginning at the fifth week of intrauterine life, the septum primum extends downward from the roof of the atrium to join with the endocardial cushions, thereby closing the incomplete segment, or "ostium primum" (see Fig. 11-3). Before this closure is complete, the midportion of the septum primum develops a defect, or "ostium secundum," so that right-to-left flow continues. During the sixth week, a second septum (septum secundum) develops to the right of the septum primum, passing from the roof of the atrium toward the endocardial cushions. This process leaves a patent foramen at about the midpoint of the septum, known as the **foramen ovale**. The defect persists after birth until it is sealed off by fusion of the septum primum and septum secundum, after which it is termed the **fossa ovalis**.

TABLE 11–2

Classification of Congenital Heart Disease

Initial left-to-right shunt
Ventricular septal defect
Atrial septal defect
Patent ductus arteriosus
Persistent truncus arteriosus
Anomalous pulmonary venous drainage
Hypoplastic left heart syndrome
Right-to-left shunt
Tetralogy of Fallot
Tricuspid atresia
No shunt
Complete transposition of the great vessels
Coarctation of the aorta
Pulmonary stenosis
Aortic stenosis
Coronary artery origin from pulmonary artery
Ebstein malformation
Complete heart block
Endocardial fibroelastosis

PATHOLOGY: The atrial septum may be defective at a number of sites (see Fig. 11-3).

- **Patent foramen ovale:** Tissue derived from the septum primum situated on the left side of the foramen ovale functions as a flap valve that normally fuses with the margins of the foramen ovale, thereby sealing the opening. An incomplete seal of the foramen ovale is found in 25% of healthy adults and is not usually functional. If circumstances increase right atrial pressure, as can occur with recurrent pulmonary thromboemboli, a right-to-left shunt will be produced, and thromboemboli from the right-sided circulation will pass directly into the systemic circulation. These **paradoxical emboli** can produce infarcts in many parts of the arterial circulation, most commonly in the brain, heart, spleen, intestines, kidneys, and lower extremities.
- **Atrial septal defect, ostium secundum type:** This is by far the most common atrial septal defect, accounting for 90% of all cases. It is a true deficiency of the atrial septum and should not be confused with a patent foramen ovale. An ostium secundum defect occurs in the middle portion of the septum and varies from a trivial opening to a large defect of the entire fossa ovalis region. A small defect is usually not functional, but a larger one may allow shunting of sufficient blood from left to right to cause dilation and hypertrophy of the right atrium and ventricle. In this setting, the diameter of the pulmonary artery may exceed that of the aorta.
  - **Lutembacher syndrome,** a variant of the ostium secundum type of atrial septal defect, is the combination of either congenital or rheumatic mitral stenosis and an ostium secundum atrial septal defect.
- **Sinus venosus defect:** This anomaly occurs in the upper portion of the atrial septum, above the fossa ovalis, near the entry of the superior vena cava. It is usually accompanied by drainage of the right pulmonary veins into the right atrium or superior vena cava. This defect represents 5% of atrial septal defects.
- **Atrial septal defect, ostium primum type:** This condition involves the region adjacent to the endocardial cushion and comprises 7% of all atrial septal defects. There are usually clefts in the anterior leaflet of the mitral valve and the septal leaflet of the tricuspid valve, which may be accompanied by an associated defect in the adjacent interventricular septum.
- **Persistent common atrioventricular canal:** This anomaly represents fully developed combined atrial and ventricular septal defects. Although ordinarily uncommon, this defect is frequently encountered in patients with Down syndrome. Incomplete defects are also observed.

 CLINICAL FEATURES: Young children with atrial septal defects are ordinarily asymptomatic, although they may complain of easy fatigability and dyspnea on exertion. Later in life, usually in adulthood, changes in the pulmonary vasculature may reverse the flow of blood through the defect and create a right-to-left shunt. In such cases, cyanosis and clubbing of the fingers ensue. Complications of atrial septal defects include atrial arrhythmias, pulmonary hypertension, right ventricular hypertrophy, heart failure, paradoxical emboli, and bacterial endocarditis. Symptomatic cases are treated surgically or with closure devices, which can be delivered and placed percutaneously.

Patent Ductus Arteriosus (PDA)

The **ductus arteriosus** in the fetus connects the descending aortic arch with the pulmonary artery and conveys most of the pulmonary outflow into the aorta. After birth, the ductus constricts in response to the increased arterial oxygen content and becomes occluded by fibrosis (ligamentum arteriosus).

 PATHOGENESIS: Persistent PDA is one of the most common congenital cardiac defects and is seen frequently in infants whose mothers were infected with the rubella virus early in pregnancy. In full-term infants with PDA, the ductus has an abnormal endothelium and media and only rarely closes spontaneously.

 CLINICAL FEATURES: The luminal diameter of a PDA varies greatly. A small shunt has little effect on the heart, whereas a large shunt leads to considerable diversion of blood from the aorta to the low-pressure pulmonary artery. In severe cases, left ventricular hypertrophy and heart failure ensue because of increased demand for cardiac output. The increased volume and pressure of blood in the pulmonary circulation eventually produce pulmonary hypertension and its cardiac complications. Infective endarteritis is a frequent complication of untreated PDA.

PDA can be corrected surgically or by cardiac catheterization. It can be caused to contract and then close by the instillation of prostaglandin synthesis inhibitors (e.g., indomethacin).

Truncus Arteriosus

Persistent truncus arteriosus refers to a common trunk for the origin of the aorta, pulmonary arteries, and coronary arteries. It results from absent or incomplete partitioning of the truncus arteriosus by the spiral septum. Truncus arteriosus always overrides a ventricular septal defect and receives blood from both ventricles. Several structural variants have been described. The most common (**type 1**) consists of a single trunk that gives rise to a common pulmonary artery and ascending aorta.

 CLINICAL FEATURES: Most infants with truncus arteriosus have torrential pulmonary blood flow, causing heart failure, recurrent respiratory tract infections, and often, early death. Pulmonary vascular disease develops in children with prolonged survival, in which case cyanosis, polycythemia, and clubbing of the fingers appear. Open-heart surgery prior to the development of significant pulmonary vascular changes is an effective treatment.

Tetralogy of Fallot (Dominant Right-to-Left Shunt) is the Most Common Cyanotic CHD

Tetralogy of Fallot represents 10% of all cases of CHD and is the most common cyanotic heart disease in older children and adults.

 PATHOLOGY: The four anatomical changes that define the tetralogy of Fallot are (Fig. 11-4):

- **Pulmonary stenosis**
- **Ventricular septal defect**
- **Dextroposition of the aorta so that it overrides the ventricular septal defect**
- **Right ventricular hypertrophy**

The heart is hypertrophied so as to give it a boot shape. Almost half of patients with tetralogy of Fallot have other cardiac anomalies, including ostium secundum atrial septal defects, PDA, left superior vena cava, and endocardial cushion defects. The aortic arch is on the right side in about 25% of cases of tetralogy of Fallot. Patency of the ductus arteriosus is actually protective, because it provides a source of blood to the otherwise deprived pulmonary vascular bed.

 CLINICAL FEATURES: In the face of severe pulmonary stenosis, right ventricular blood is shunted through the ventricular septal defect into the aorta, resulting in arterial desaturation and cyanosis. Surgical correction is typ-

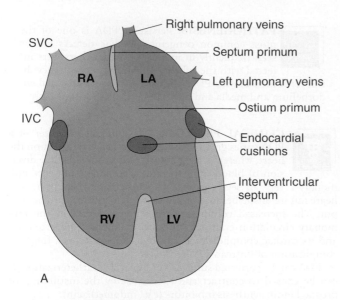

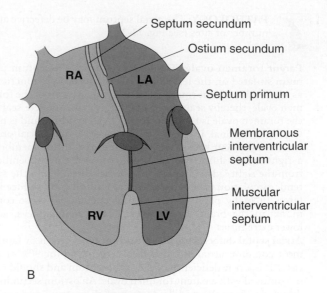

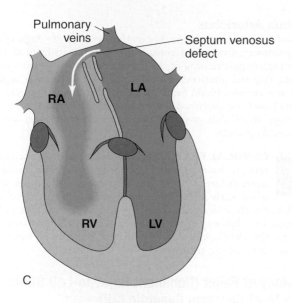

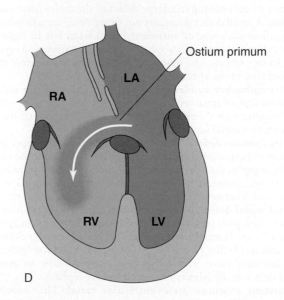

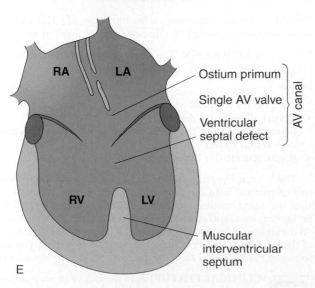

FIGURE 11-3. **Pathogenesis of ventricular and atrial septal defects. A.** The common atrial chamber is being separated into the right and left atria (RA and LA) by the septum primum. Because the septum primum has not yet joined the endocardial cushions, there is an open ostium primum. The ventricular cavity is being divided by a muscular interventricular septum into right and left chambers (right and left ventricles, RV and LV). SVC, superior vena cava; IVC, inferior vena cava. **B.** The septum primum has joined the endocardial cushions but at the same time, has developed an opening in its midportion (the ostium secundum). This opening is partly overlaid by the septum secundum, which has grown down to cover, in part, the foramen ovale. Simultaneously, the membranous septum joins the muscular interventricular septum to the base of the heart, completely separating the ventricles. **C.** The sinus venosus type of atrial septal defect is located in the most cephalad region and is adjacent to the inflow of the right pulmonary veins, which thus tend to open into the RA. **D.** The ostium primum defect occurs just above the atrioventricular (AV) valve ring, sometimes in the presence of an intact valve ring. It may also, in conjunction with a defect of the valve ring and ventricular septum, form an AV canal, as shown in **(E)**. This common opening allows free communication between the atria and the ventricles.

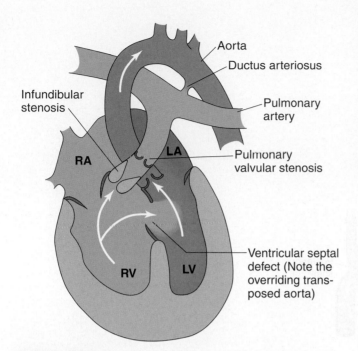

FIGURE 11-4. **Tetralogy of Fallot.** Note the pulmonary stenosis, which is due to infundibular hypertrophy as well as pulmonary valvular stenosis. The ventricular septal defect involves the membranous septum region. Dextroposition of the aorta and right ventricular hypertrophy are shown. Because of the pulmonary obstruction, the shunt is from right to left, and the patient is cyanotic. LA, left atrium; LV, left ventricle; RA, right atrium; RV, right ventricle.

ically performed in the first 2 years of life. In children who are unrepaired, dyspnea on exertion is particularly noticeable, and the affected child often assumes a squatting position to relieve the shortness of breath. Physical development is characteristically retarded. Cerebral thromboses may complicate the disease due to marked polycythemia. Patients are also at risk for bacterial endocarditis and brain abscesses. Without surgical intervention, tetralogy of Fallot has a dismal prognosis. However, total correction is now possible with open-heart surgery, which carries a mortality rate that is less than 10%. After successful surgery, patients are asymptomatic and have an excellent long-term prognosis.

CHDs Without Shunts Involve Various Cardiovascular Sites

Transposition of the Great Arteries (TGA)

In transposition of the great arteries (TGA), the aorta arises from the right ventricle and the pulmonary artery from the left ventricle. In TGA, the aorta is anterior to the pulmonary artery and to its right ("D" or dextrotransposition) all the way from its origin. The condition shows a male predominance and is more common in offspring of mothers with diabetes. TGA is responsible for more than half of deaths in infants with cyanotic heart disease who are younger than 1 year of age.

 PATHOGENESIS: Because the venous blood from the right side of the heart flows to the aorta, and the oxygenated blood from the lungs returns to the pulmonary artery, there are, in effect, two independent and parallel blood circuits for the systemic and pulmonary circulations (Fig. 11-5). Survival is possible only if there is a communication between the circuits. Virtually all infants with TGA have an atrial septal defect. One half of patients exhibit a ventricular septal defect and two thirds have a PDA.

 CLINICAL FEATURES: Before cardiac surgery, the outlook for infants with TGA was hopeless; 90% died in their first year. It is now possible to correct the malformation within the first 2 weeks of life using an arterial-switch operation, with overall survival rate of 90%. Patients in whom corrected TGA is the only malformation are clinically entirely normal. Unfortunately, many cases are complicated by other cardiac anomalies, which require their own specific interventions.

Coarctation of the Aorta

Coarctation of the aorta is a local constriction that almost always occurs immediately below the origin of the left subclavian artery at the site of the ductus arteriosus (Fig. 11-6). Rare coarctations can occur at any point from the aortic arch to the abdominal bifurcation. The condition is two to five times more frequent in males than females and is associated with a bicuspid aortic valve in two thirds of cases. Mitral valve malformations, ventricular septal defects, and subaortic stenosis may also accompany coarctation of the aorta. There is a particular association of coarctation with Turner syndrome, and berry aneurysms in the brain are also more common.

 CLINICAL FEATURES: The clinical hallmark of coarctation of the aorta is a discrepancy in blood pressure between the upper and lower extremities. The pressure gradient produced by the coarctation causes hypertension proximal to the narrowed segment and, occasionally, dilation of that portion of the aorta. Hypertension in the upper part of the body results in left ventricular hypertrophy and may produce dizziness, headaches, and nosebleeds. Hypotension below the coarctation leads to weakness, pallor, and coldness of lower extremities. Radiologic examination of the chest shows **notching of the inner surfaces of the ribs**, produced by increased pressure in markedly dilated intercostal arteries.

Most patients with coarctation of the aorta die by age 40 unless they are treated. Complications include (1) heart failure, (2) rupture of a dissecting aneurysm (secondary to cystic medial necrosis of the aorta), (3) infective endarteritis at the point of narrowing or at the

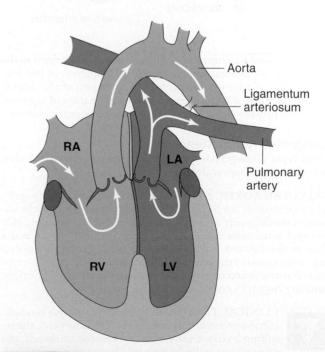

FIGURE 11-5. **Complete transposition of great arteries, regular type.** The aorta is anterior to, and to the right of, the pulmonary artery ("D-transposition") and arises from the right ventricle. In the absence of interatrial or interventricular connections or patent ductus arteriosus, this anomaly is incompatible with life. LA, left atrium; LV, left ventricle; RA, right atrium; RV, right ventricle.

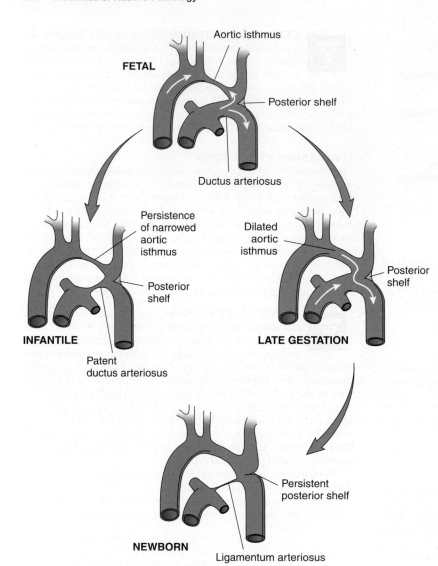

FETAL

Aortic isthmus

Posterior shelf

Ductus arteriosus

INFANTILE

Persistence of narrowed aortic isthmus

Posterior shelf

Patent ductus arteriosus

LATE GESTATION

Dilated aortic isthmus

Posterior shelf

NEWBORN

Persistent posterior shelf

Ligamentum arteriosus

FIGURE 11-6. **Pathogenesis of coarctation of the aorta.** In the fetus, ductal blood is diverted into cephalad and descending streams by the posterior aortic shelf. In late fetal life, the isthmus dilates, and the increased descending blood flow is accommodated by the ductal orifice. After birth, if the shelf does not undergo the normal involution, obliteration of the ductal orifice does not permit free flow around the persistent posterior shelf, thereby creating a juxtaductal obstruction of blood flow to the distal aorta. If the aortic isthmus does not dilate during late fetal life, it remains narrow, resulting in an infantile or preductal coarctation. In this circumstance, the ductus arteriosus usually remains patent.

site of jet stream impingement on the wall immediately distal to the coarctation, (4) cerebral hemorrhage, and (5) stenosis or infective endocarditis of a bicuspid aortic valve. Coarctation of the aorta is successfully treated by surgical excision of the narrowed segment, preferably between 1 and 2 years of age for asymptomatic patients.

Congenital Aortic Stenosis

Three types of congenital aortic stenosis are recognized: valvular, subvalvular, and supravalvular.

VALVULAR AORTIC STENOSIS: The most common congenital aortic stenosis is a bicuspid valve, which arises through the abnormal development of the endocardial cushions. A congenitally bicuspid aortic valve is considerably more frequent (4:1) in males than in females and is associated with other cardiac anomalies (e.g., coarctation of the aorta) in 20% of cases. A bicuspid valve typically features fusion of two of the three semilunar cusps (the right coronary cusp with one of the adjacent two cusps).

CLINICAL FEATURES: Many children with bicuspid aortic stenosis are asymptomatic. Over the years, the resulting bicuspid valve tends to become thickened and calcified, generally leading to symptoms in adulthood. More severe forms of congenital aortic stenosis involving unicommissural or valves without commissures cause symptoms in early life. Exertional dyspnea and angina pectoris may be prominent. Sudden death, principally due to ventricular arrhythmias, is a distinct threat for patients with severe obstruction. Bacterial endo-

carditis sometimes complicates the disease. In symptomatic cases, aortic valvulotomy has had a high degree of success, although valve replacement is occasionally indicated.

SUBVALVULAR AORTIC STENOSIS: This defect accounts for 10% of all cases of congenital aortic stenosis. Stenosis results from a membranous diaphragm or fibrous ring that surrounds the left ventricular outflow tract immediately below the aortic valve. It is twice as common in males as in females. In many persons with subvalvular aortic stenosis, thickening and immobility of the aortic cusps develops, with mild aortic regurgitation. Bacterial endocarditis may occur and also aggravate the regurgitation. Surgical treatment of subvalvular aortic stenosis involves excising the membrane or fibrous ridge.

SUPRAVALVULAR AORTIC STENOSIS: This type of stenosis is much less common than the other two and is often associated with defects in the elastin gene, such as are found in **Williams syndrome**, a congenital disease associated with a deletion of an area of chromosome 7. The syndrome is characterized by idiopathic infantile hypercalcemia, mental retardation, and multiple system disorders.

Ebstein Malformation

Ebstein malformation results from downward displacement of an abnormal tricuspid valve into an underdeveloped right ventricle. One or more tricuspid valve leaflets are plastered to the right ventricular wall for a variable distance below the right atrioventricular annulus.

PATHOLOGY: Septal and posterior tricuspid valve leaflets are usually affected. They are irregularly elongated and adherent to the right ventricular wall, so that the upper part of the right ventricular cavity (inflow region) functions separately from the distal chamber. Thus, the effective tricuspid valve orifice is displaced downward into the ventricle, thereby dividing it into two separate parts: the "atrialized" ventricle (proximal ventricle) and the functional right ventricle (distal ventricle). In two thirds of cases, conspicuous dilation of the functional ventricle hinders its ability to pump blood efficiently through the pulmonary arteries. The degree of insufficiency of the tricuspid valve depends on the severity and configuration of the defect in the leaflets.

 CLINICAL FEATURES: Ebstein malformation leads to heart failure, massive right atrial dilation, arrhythmias with palpitations and tachycardia, and sudden death. Surgical treatment has met with variable success.

Congenital Heart Block

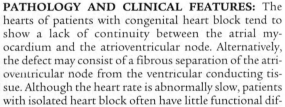 **PATHOGENESIS:** Congenital complete heart block is usually associated with other cardiac anomalies. In such cases, disruption in the continuity of the conduction system is probably caused by the accompanying cardiac abnormality. Congenital heart block in the absence of structural heart disease has been linked to maternal connective tissue disease, especially systemic lupus erythematosus (SLE). If maternal SS-A/Ro or SS-B/La autoantibodies are transplacentally transmitted to the fetus, the incidence of congenital complete heart block approaches 100%.

 PATHOLOGY AND CLINICAL FEATURES: The hearts of patients with congenital heart block tend to show a lack of continuity between the atrial myocardium and the atrioventricular node. Alternatively, the defect may consist of a fibrous separation of the atrioventricular node from the ventricular conducting tissue. Although the heart rate is abnormally slow, patients with isolated heart block often have little functional difficulty. Later in life, cardiac hypertrophy, attacks of Stokes-Adams syncope (dizziness and unexpected fainting), arrhythmias, and heart failure may develop.

Endocardial Fibroelastosis

Endocardial fibroelastosis (EFE) is characterized by thickening of the endocardium of the left ventricle, which may also affect the valves. The disorder is classified as primary or secondary, the latter being far more common.

SECONDARY ENDOCARDIAL FIBROELASTOSIS: This disorder occurs in association with underlying cardiovascular anomalies that lead to left ventricular hypertrophy in the face of an inability to meet the increased myocardial oxygen demands. Thus, secondary EFE is a frequent complication of congenital aortic stenosis (including hypoplastic left ventricle syndrome) and coarctation of the aorta. Presumably, some type of endocardial injury is involved in its pathogenesis.

 PATHOLOGY: On gross examination, the left ventricle endocardium displays irregular, opaque, grey-white patches, which also may be present on the cardiac valves. Microscopically, these plaques are areas of endocardial fibroelastotic thickening, frequently accompanied by degeneration of adjacent subendocardial myocytes. The valves may show collagenous thickening.

PRIMARY ENDOCARDIAL FIBROELASTOSIS: De-fined as fibroelastosis in the absence of any associated lesion, this disorder is now quite rare. It afflicts infants, usually 4 to 10 months of age. Although it has occurred in siblings, no specific mode of inheritance has been established. Recent evidence links primary EFE to mumps infection, which may explain why this condition is now so rarely encountered.

 PATHOLOGY: The left ventricle is usually conspicuously dilated but occasionally contracted and hypertrophic. Diffuse endocardial thickening involves most of the left ventricle as well as the aortic and mitral valve leaflets. The thickened endocardium tends to obscure the trabecular pattern of the underlying myocardium, and papillary muscles and chordae tendineae are thick and short. Mural thrombi may complicate the condition. Infants with primary EFE develop progressive heart failure. The prognosis is dismal, and cardiac transplantation offers the only hope for a cure.

Dextrocardia

Dextrocardia is rightward orientation of the base–apex axis of the heart. It is often associated with a mirror image of the normal left-sided location and configuration. The position of the ventricles is determined by the direction of the embryonic cardiac loop. If the loop protrudes to the right, the future right ventricle develops on the right, and the left ventricle comes to occupy its proper position. If the loop protrudes to the left, the opposite occurs.

 PATHOLOGY: When dextrocardia occurs without abnormal positioning of the visceral organs (situs inversus), the condition is invariably associated with severe cardiovascular anomalies. These include transposition of the great arteries, a variety of atrial and ventricular septal defects, anomalous pulmonary venous drainage, and many others. In dextrocardia that occurs with situs inversus, the heart is functionally normal, although minor anomalies are not uncommon.

Ischemic Heart Disease

Ischemic heart disease is, in most cases, a consequence of coronary artery atherosclerosis. It develops when blood flow is inadequate to meet the oxygen demands of the heart. Ischemic heart disease is responsible for at least 80% of all deaths attributable to heart disease in the United States and other industrialized nations, where it remains the leading cause of death. By contrast, atherosclerotic heart disease is far less frequent in developing countries. The principal effects of ischemic heart disease are angina pectoris, myocardial infarction, chronic congestive heart failure, and sudden death.

ANGINA PECTORIS: *This term refers to the pain resulting from myocardial ischemia. It typically occurs in the substernal portion of the chest and may radiate to the left arm, jaw, and epigastrium. It is the most common symptom of ischemic heart disease.* Coronary atherosclerosis usually becomes symptomatic only when the luminal cross-sectional area of the affected vessel is reduced by more than 75%. A patient with typical angina pectoris exhibits recurrent episodes of chest pain, usually brought on by increased physical activity or emotional excitement. The pain is of limited duration (1 to 15 minutes) and is relieved by reducing physical activity or by treatment with sublingual nitroglycerin (a potent vasodilator).

Although the most common cause of angina pectoris is severe coronary atherosclerosis, decreased coronary blood flow can result from other conditions, including coronary vasospasm, aortic stenosis, or aortic insufficiency. Angina pectoris is not associated with anatomic changes in the myocardium as long as the duration and severity of ischemic episodes are insufficient to cause myocardial cell necrosis.

PRINZMETAL ANGINA (VARIANT ANGINA) *is an atypical form of angina that occurs at rest and is caused by coronary artery spasm.* The responsible mechanisms are not fully understood. Whereas coronary artery spasm may contribute to the pathogenesis of an acute myocardial infarction or to the size of the infarct, it is generally not the principal cause of infarction.

UNSTABLE ANGINA, *a variety of chest pain that has a less predictable relationship to exercise than does stable angina and may occur during rest or sleep, is associated with development of nonocclusive thrombi over atherosclerotic plaques.* In some cases of unstable angina, episodes of chest pain become progressively more frequent and longer in duration over a 3- to 4-day period. Electrocardiographic changes are not characteristic of infarction, and serum levels of cardiac-specific intracellular proteins, such as MB isoform of CK (MB-CK) or cardiac troponin T or I (evidence of myocardial necrosis), remain normal. Unstable angina is also termed **preinfarction angina, accelerated angina,** or **"crescendo" angina**. Without pharmacologic or mechanical intervention to "open up" the coronary narrowing, many patients with unstable angina progress to myocardial infarction.

MYOCARDIAL INFARCT: *A myocardial infarct is a discrete focus of ischemic muscle necrosis in the heart.* This definition excludes patchy foci of necrosis caused by drugs, toxins, or viruses. The development of an infarct is related to the duration of ischemia and the metabolic rate of the ischemic tissue. In experimental coronary artery ligation, foci of necrosis form after 20 minutes of ischemia and become more extensive as the period of ischemia lengthens.

CHRONIC CONGESTIVE HEART FAILURE: Contractile impairment in these patients is due to irreversible loss of myocardium from previous infarcts and hypoperfusion of surviving muscle, which leads to chronic ventricular dysfunction. Many patients will develop progressive pump failure and die of multiorgan failure.

SUDDEN DEATH: In some patients, the first and only clinical manifestation of ischemic heart disease is sudden death occurring within 1 hour of symptom onset due to spontaneous ventricular fibrillation. *Coronary atherosclerosis underlies most of such cases. In many cases, lethal arrhythmia is likely triggered by acute ischemia without overt myocardial infarction.* However, the presence of a healed infarct or ventricular hypertrophy increases the risk that an episode of acute ischemia will initiate a life-threatening ventricular arrhythmia.

 EPIDEMIOLOGY: *The major risk factors that predispose to coronary artery disease are (1) systemic hypertension, (2) cigarette smoking, (3) diabetes mellitus, and (4) elevated blood cholesterol level.* Any one of these factors significantly increases the risk of myocardial infarction, but a combination of multiple factors augments the risk more than sevenfold (see Chapter 8).

In 1950, the age-adjusted death rate from myocardial infarction was 226 per 100,000 cases; 50 years later, it was 150. This shift reflects many factors, including reduced smoking, lower dietary saturated fat, and new drugs that control hypertension, reduce cholesterol, and lyse coronary thrombi. Multiple studies established that elevated serum LDLs increase the risk of myocardial infarction, whereas elevated levels of high-density lipoproteins (HDLs) decrease the risk. The total cholesterol/HDL cholesterol ratio appears to be a better predictor of coronary artery disease than serum cholesterol level alone. Factors other than blood lipid profile have powerful independent effects. A person with a blood pressure of 160/95 mm Hg has twice the risk of ischemic heart disease as one whose blood pressure is 140/75 mm Hg or less. The risk of ischemic heart disease increases in proportion to the number of cigarettes smoked. Increased levels of plasma factors involved in thrombosis or the inhibition of thrombolysis, such as fibrinogen, plasminogen activator inhibitor-1, homocysteine, and decreased fibrinolytic activity, contribute to the risk of myocardial infarction. Levels of selected serum markers of inflammation, such as C-reactive protein, are also predictors of ischemic heart disease.

During the past several years, there has been a remarkable increase in the incidence of type II diabetes in the United States, which mirrors a similar increase in obesity (see Chapter 22). Ischemic heart disease is a consequence of both type 1 and type 2 diabetes, and the risk is two- to threefold greater than in nondiabetic individuals. Conversely, atherosclerotic cardiovascular disease (myocardial infarction, stroke, peripheral vascular disease) accounts for 80% of all deaths in patients with diabetes.

Other risk factors for ischemic heart disease include:

- **Obesity:** In a major, longitudinal study of one population (Framingham Heart Study), obesity was an independent risk factor for cardiovascular disease, with an increased risk for obese persons over those who are lean of 2 to 2.5.
- **Age:** The risk of infarction is greater with increasing age, up to age 80 years.
- **Gender:** Men have an increased risk of ischemic heart disease; 60% of coronary events occur in men. Angina pectoris is considerably more frequent in men than in women; the male: female ratio at ages younger than 50 years is 4:1 and that at age 60 years is 2:1.
- **Family history:** In one study that controlled for other risk factors, relatives of patients with ischemic heart disease had a two- to fourfold increased risk for coronary artery disease. The genetic basis for this familial risk may interact with the other risk factors.
- **Use of oral contraceptives:** Women over 35 years who smoke cigarettes and use oral contraceptives have a modestly increased incidence of myocardial infarction.
- **Sedentary life habits:** Regular exercise reduces the risk of myocardial infarction, perhaps by increasing HDL levels. In one study, the least-fit quartile of persons subjected to exercise testing had six times the risk of myocardial infarction than did those in the fittest quartile.
- **Personality features:** The relationship between coronary artery disease and "type A personality" is controversial, and recent studies have failed to show the strong association previously reported.

Many Conditions Limit the Supply of Blood to the Heart

The heart is an aerobic organ, requiring oxidative phosphorylation to provide energy for contraction. The anaerobic glycolysis used by skeletal muscle under conditions of extreme physical exertion is insufficient to sustain cardiac contraction. Ischemic heart disease is caused by an imbalance between the oxygen demands of the myocardium and the supply of oxygenated blood. Any increase in cardiac workload increases the heart's need for oxygen. Conditions that raise blood pressure or cardiac output, such as exercise or pregnancy, augment oxygen demand by the myocardium, which may lead to angina pectoris or myocardial infarction in the compromised organ. Disorders in this category include valvular disease (mitral or aortic insufficiency, aortic stenosis), infection, and conditions such as hypertension, coarctation of the aorta, and hypertrophic cardiomyopathy (HCM). The increased metabolic rate and tachycardia in patients with hyperthyroidism are also accompanied by increased oxygen demand as well as an increase in the workload of the heart (Table 11-3).

Atherosclerosis and Thrombosis

The pathogenesis of atherosclerosis is detailed in Chapter 10. Here, the features of special importance to ischemic heart disease are briefly discussed. Maximal blood flow to the myocardium is not impaired until about 75% of the cross-sectional area of a coronary artery (~50% of the diameter as assessed during coronary angiography) is compromised by atherosclerosis. However, resting blood flow is not reduced until more than 90% of the lumen is occluded. In patients with long-standing angina pectoris, the extent and distribution of collateral circulation exerts an important influence on the risk of acute myocardial infarction. Although myocardial infarction often occurs during physically demanding activities, such as running or shoveling snow, many infarcts occur at rest or even during sleep. Thus, for most people, conversion of the clinically silent disease of coronary atherosclerosis to the catastrophic event of my-

TABLE 11–3
Causes of Ischemic Heart Disease
Decreased supply of oxygen
Conditions that influence the supply of blood
Atherosclerosis and thrombosis
Thromboemboli
Coronary artery spasm
Collateral blood vessels
Blood pressure, cardiac output, and heart rate
Miscellaneous: arteritis (e.g., periarteritis nodosa), dissecting aneurysm, luetic aortitis, anomalous origin of coronary artery, muscular bridging of coronary artery
Conditions that influence the availability of oxygen in the blood
Anemia
Shift in the hemoglobin-oxygen dissociation curve
Carbon monoxide
Cyanide
Increased oxygen demand (i.e., increased cardiac work)
Hypertension
Valvular stenosis or insufficiency
Hyperthyroidism
Fever
Thiamine deficiency
Catecholamines

ocardial infarction involves a sudden, marked decrease in myocardial blood flow, with or without an increase in myocardial oxygen demand. *It is now well established that coronary artery thrombosis is the event that usually precipitates an acute myocardial infarction. Thrombosis typically results from spontaneous rupture of an atherosclerotic plaque, usually in a region that contains numerous inflammatory cells and a thin fibrous cap. The initiating event may be hemorrhage into or beneath the plaque.*

Myocardial Infarcts May be Mainly Subendocardial or Transmural

PATHOLOGY
Location of Infarcts
There are important differences between these two types of infarction.

A *subendocardial infarct* affects the inner one third to one half of the left ventricle. It may arise within the territory of one of the major epicardial coronary arteries or it may be circumferential, involving subendocardial territories of multiple coronary arteries. Subendocardial infarction generally occurs as a consequence of hypoperfusion of the heart. It may result from atherosclerosis in a specific coronary artery or develop in disorders that limit myocardial blood flow globally, such as aortic stenosis, hemorrhagic shock, or hypoperfusion during cardiopulmonary bypass. Most subendocardial infarcts do not involve occlusive coronary thrombi. In the case of circumferential subendocardial infarction caused by global hypoperfusion of the myocardium, coronary artery stenosis need not be present. Because necrosis is limited to the inner layers of the heart, complications arising in transmural infarcts (e.g., pericarditis and ventricular rupture) are generally not seen in subendocardial infarcts.

A *transmural infarct* involves the full left ventricular wall thickness and usually follows occlusion of a coronary artery. As a result, transmural infarcts typically conform to the distribution of one of the three major coronary arteries (see Fig. 11-1).

- **Right coronary artery:** Occlusion of the proximal portion of this vessel results in an infarct of the posterior basal region of the left ventricle and the posterior third to half of the interventricular septum ("inferior" infarct).
- **LAD coronary artery:** Blockage of this artery produces an infarct of the apical, anterior, and anteroseptal walls of the left ventricle.
- **Left circumflex coronary artery:** Obstruction of this vessel is the least common cause of myocardial infarction and leads to an infarct of the lateral wall of the left ventricle.

Myocardial infarction does not occur instantaneously. Rather, it first develops in the subendocardium and progresses as a wavefront of necrosis from subendocardium to subepicardium over the course of several hours. Transient coronary occlusion may cause only subendocardial necrosis, whereas persistent occlusion eventually leads to transmural necrosis. The goal of acute coronary interventions (pharmacologic or mechanical thrombolysis) is to interrupt this wavefront and limit myocardial necrosis.

Infarcts involve the left ventricle much more commonly and extensively than they do the right ventricle. This difference may be partly explained by the greater workload imposed on the left ventricle by systemic vascular resistance and the greater thickness of the left ventricular wall. Right ventricular hypertrophy (e.g., in pulmonary hypertension) increases the incidence of right ventricular infarction, although infarcts limited to the right ventricle are rare.

Macroscopic Characteristics of Myocardial Infarcts
Total ischemia for up to 20 to 30 minutes results in reversible cyanosis and bulging during systole. On gross examination, an acute myocardial infarct is not identifiable within the first 12 hours.

- **By 24 hours**, the infarct can be recognized on the cut surface of the involved ventricle by its pallor.
- **After 3 to 5 days**, the infarcted area becomes mottled and more sharply outlined, with a central pale, yellowish, necrotic region bordered by a hyperemic zone (Fig. 11-7).
- **Within 2 to 3 weeks**, the infarcted region is depressed and soft, with a refractile, gelatinous appearance.
- **After several months, healed infarcts** are firm and contracted and have the pale-gray appearance of scar tissue (Fig. 11-8).

Microscopic Characteristics of Myocardial Infarcts

THE FIRST 24 HOURS: Electron microscopy is required to discern the earliest morphologic features of ischemic injury. After 30 to 60 minutes of ischemia, when myocyte injury has become irreversible, mitochondria are greatly swollen, with disorganized cristae and amorphous matrix densities. The nucleus shows clump-

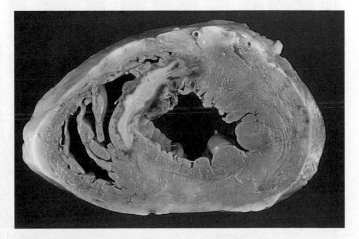

FIGURE 11-7. **Acute myocardial infarct.** A transverse section of the heart of a patient who died a few days after the onset of severe chest pain shows a transmural infarct in the anteroseptal region of the left ventricle (left anterior descending [LAD] coronary artery territory). The necrotic myocardium is soft, yellowish, and sharply demarcated.

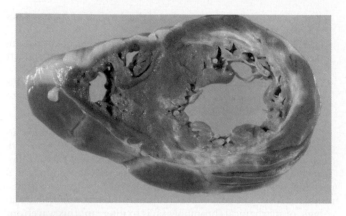

FIGURE 11-8. **Healed myocardial infarct.** A cross-section of the heart from a man who died after a long history of angina pectoris and several myocardial infarctions shows circumferential scarring of the left ventricle.

ing and margination of chromatin, and the sarcolemma is focally disrupted. Loss of sarcolemmal integrity leads to release of intracellular proteins, such as myoglobin, LDH, CK, and troponins I and T. The noncontractile ischemic myocytes are stretched with each systole and by light microscopy become "**wavy fibers**." After 24 hours, myocytes are deeply eosinophilic (Fig. 11-9) and show the characteristic changes of coagulation necrosis (see Chapter 1). However, it takes several days for the myocyte nucleus to disappear totally.

TWO TO 3 DAYS: Polymorphonuclear leukocytes (PMNs) are attracted to necrotic myocytes. The PMNs accumulate at infarct borders where blood flow is maintained and reach maximal concentration after 2 to 3 days (see Figs. 11-9 and 11-10). Interstitial edema and microscopic areas of hemorrhage may also appear. Muscle cells are more clearly necrotic, nuclei disappear, and striations become less prominent. Some of the PMNs that were attracted to the area begin to undergo karyorrhexis.

FIVE TO 7 DAYS: By this time, few, if any, PMNs remain. The periphery of the infarcted region shows phagocytosis of dead muscle by macrophages. Fibroblasts begin to proliferate, and new colla-

gen is deposited. Lymphocytes and pigment-laden macrophages are prominent. The process of replacing necrotic muscle with scar tissue is initiated at about 5 days, beginning at the periphery of the infarct and gradually extending toward the center.

ONE TO 3 WEEKS: Collagen deposition proceeds, the inflammatory infiltrate gradually recedes, and the newly sprouted capillaries are progressively obliterated.

MORE THAN 4 WEEKS: Considerable dense fibrous tissue is present. The debris is progressively removed, and the scar becomes more solid and less cellular as it matures (Fig. 11-11).

In estimating the age of a large infarct, it is more accurate to base the interpretation on the outer border where repair begins, rather than on changes in the central region. In fact, in some large infarcts, rather than being removed, dead myocytes remain indefinitely "mummified."

Reperfusion of Ischemic Myocardium

Blood flow may be restored to regions of evolving infarcts either because of spontaneous thrombolysis or in response to pharmacologic or mechanical means of opening up occluded coronary arteries. When that happens, the infarct's gross and microscopic appearances change. Reperfused infarcts are typically hemorrhagic, the result of blood flow through a damaged microvasculature. One of the most characteristic features of reperfused infarcts is **contraction band necrosis**. Contraction bands are thick, irregular, transverse eosinophilic bands in necrotic myocytes. By electron microscopy, these bands are small groups of hypercontracted and disorganized sarcomeres with thickened Z lines. The bands form as a result of massive infusion of Ca^{2+} into the myocytes as a result of sarcolemmal damage mediated by reactive oxygen species.

CLINICAL FEATURES:
Clinical Diagnosis of Acute Myocardial Infarction May be Complicated by "Silent Disease"

The onset of acute myocardial infarction is often sudden and associated with severe, crushing substernal or precordial pain. These symptoms may be accompanied by sweating, nausea, vomiting, and shortness of breath. In some cases, an acute myocardial infarc-

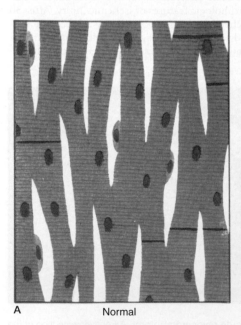

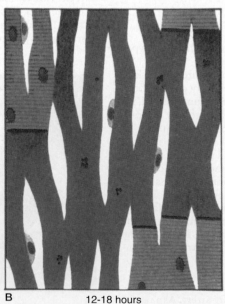

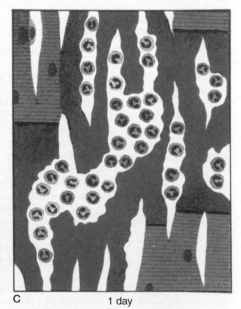

A   Normal   B   12-18 hours   C   1 day

FIGURE 11-9. **Development of a myocardial infarct. A.** Normal myocardium. **B.** After about 12 to 18 hours, the infarcted myocardium shows eosinophilia *(red staining)* in sections of the heart stained with hematoxylin and eosin. **C.** About 24 hours after the onset of infarction, polymorphonuclear neutrophils infiltrate necrotic myocytes at the periphery of the infarct.

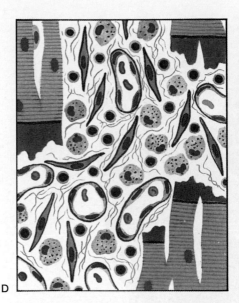
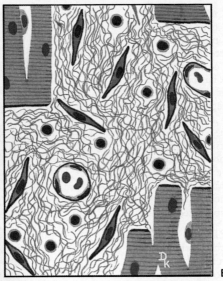

FIGURE 11-9. *Continued.* **Development of a myocardial infarct. D.** After about 3 weeks, peripheral portions of the infarct are composed of granulation tissue with prominent capillaries, fibroblasts, lymphoid cells, and macrophages. The necrotic debris has been largely removed from this area, and a small amount of collagen has been laid down. **E.** After 3 months or more, the infarcted region has been replaced by scar tissue.

tion is preceded by unstable angina of several days' duration. *One fourth to one half of all nonfatal myocardial infarctions occur without any symptoms, and infarcts are identified only later by electrocardiographic changes or at autopsy.* These "clinically silent" infarcts are particularly common among diabetic patients with autonomic dysfunction and also in cardiac transplant patients whose hearts are denervated.

Complications of Myocardial Infarction Influence the Clinical Course

Early mortality in acute myocardial infarction (within 30 days) has dropped from 30% in the 1950s to less than 5% today. Nevertheless,

the clinical course after acute infarction may be dominated by functional or mechanical complications of the infarct.

ARRHYTHMIAS: Virtually all patients who have a myocardial infarct have an abnormal cardiac rhythm at some time during their illness. Arrhythmias still account for half of all deaths caused by ischemic heart disease, although the advent of coronary care units and defibrillators has greatly reduced early mortality.

LEFT VENTRICULAR FAILURE AND CARDIOGENIC SHOCK: The development of left ventricular failure soon after myocardial infarction is an ominous sign that generally indicates massive loss of muscle. Fortunately, cardiogenic shock occurs in less than 5% of cases, owing to the development of techniques that limit the extent of infarction (thrombolytic therapy, angioplasty) or assist damaged myocardium (intra-aortic balloon pump). Cardiogenic shock tends to develop early after infarction, when 40% or more of the left ventricle has been lost; the mortality rate is as high as 90%.

EXTENSION OF THE INFARCT: Clinically recognizable extension of an acute myocardial infarct occurs in the first 1 to 2 weeks in up to 10% of patients. Such a situation is associated with a doubling of mortality.

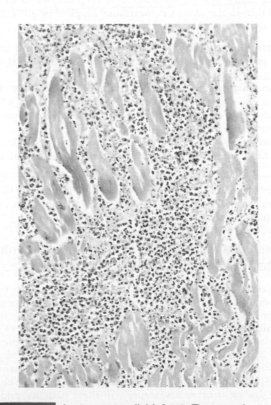

FIGURE 11-10. **Acute myocardial infarct.** The necrotic myocardial fibers, which are eosinophilic and devoid of cross-striations and nuclei, are immersed in a sea of acute inflammatory cells.

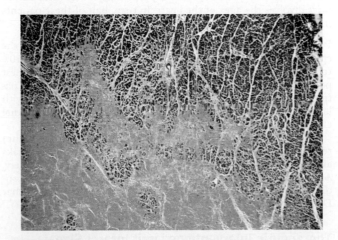

FIGURE 11-11. **Healed myocardial infarct.** A section at the edge of a healed infarct stained for collagen shows dense, acellular regions of collagenous matrix sharply demarcated from the adjacent viable myocardium.

RUPTURE OF THE FREE WALL OF THE MYOCARDIUM:
Myocardial rupture may occur at almost any time during the 3 weeks after acute myocardial infarction but is most common between the first and fourth days, when the infarcted wall is weakest. During this vulnerable period, the infarct is composed of soft, necrotic tissue in which the extracellular matrix has been degraded by proteases released by inflammatory cells but new matrix deposition has not yet occurred. Once scar tissue begins to form, rupture is less likely. Rupture of the free wall is a complication of transmural infarcts. The remaining viable, contractile myocardium adjacent to the infarct produces mechanical forces that can initiate and propagate tearing along the lateral border of the infarct where neutrophils accumulate. Rupture of the left ventricle's free wall most often leads to hemopericardium and death from cardiac tamponade. Myocardial rupture accounts for 10% of deaths after acute myocardial infarction in hospitalized patients.

OTHER FORMS OF MYOCARDIAL RUPTURE: A few patients in whom a myocardial infarct involves the interventricular septum develop **septal perforation**, varying in length from 1 cm or more. The magnitude of the resulting left-to-right shunt and, therefore, the prognosis varies with the size of the rupture. **Rupture of a portion of a papillary muscle** results in mitral regurgitation. In some cases, an entire papillary muscle is transected, in which case, massive mitral valve incompetence may be fatal.

ANEURYSMS: Left ventricular aneurysms complicate 10% to 15% of transmural myocardial infarcts. After acute transmural infarction, the affected ventricular wall tends to bulge outward during systole in one third of patients. Localized thinning and stretching of the ventricular wall in the region of a healing myocardial infarct has been termed "infarct expansion" but is actually an early aneurysm (Fig. 11-12). Such an aneurysm is composed of a thin layer of necrotic myocardium and collagenous tissue, which expands with each contraction of the heart. As the evolving aneurysm becomes more fibrotic, its tensile strength increases. However, the aneurysm continues to dilate with each beat, thereby "stealing" some of the left ventricular output and increasing the workload of the heart. Mural thrombi often develop within aneurysms and are a source of systemic emboli. A distinction should be made between "**true**" aneurysms (as above) and "**false**." **False aneurysms** result from rupture of a portion of the left ventricle that has been walled off by pericardial scar tissue. Thus, the wall of a false aneurysm is composed of pericardium and scar tissue but not left ventricular myocardium.

MURAL THROMBOSIS AND EMBOLISM: Half of all patients who die after myocardial infarction have mural thrombi overlying the infarct at autopsy. This occurs particularly often when the infarct involves the apex of the heart. In turn, half of these patients have some evidence of systemic embolization.

PERICARDITIS: A transmural myocardial infarct involves the epicardium and leads to inflammation of the pericardium in 10% to 20% of patients. Pericarditis is manifested clinically as chest pain and may produce a pericardial friction rub. One fourth of patients with acute myocardial infarction, particularly those with larger infarcts and congestive heart failure, develop a pericardial effusion, with or without pericarditis.

Postmyocardial infarction syndrome (Dressler syndrome) refers to a delayed form of pericarditis that develops 2 to 10 weeks after infarction. A similar disorder may occur after cardiac surgery. Antibodies to heart muscle appear in these patients, and the condition improves with corticosteroid therapy, suggesting that Dressler syndrome may have an immunologic basis.

Therapeutic Interventions Limit Infarct Size

Because the amount of myocardium that undergoes necrosis is an important predictor of morbidity and mortality, any therapy that limits infarct size should be beneficial. **Restoration of arterial**

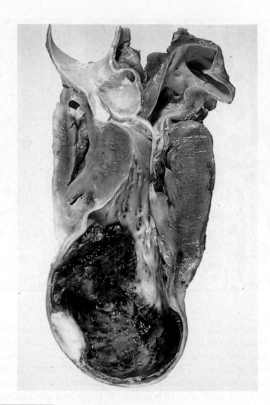

FIGURE 11-12. **Ventricular aneurysm.** The heart of a patient with a history of an anteroapical myocardial infarct who developed a massive ventricular aneurysm. The apex of the heart shows marked thinning and aneurysmal dilation.

blood flow remains the only way to salvage ischemic myocytes permanently, although a number of interventions can delay ischemic injury. Several methods have been developed to restore blood flow to the area of myocardium supplied by an obstructed coronary artery.

- **Thrombolytic enzymes** such as tissue plasminogen activator or streptokinase can be infused intravenously to dissolve the clot causing the obstruction.
- **Percutaneous transluminal coronary angioplasty** is dilation of a narrowed coronary artery by inflation with a balloon catheter. It also allows stent placement in the coronary artery to maintain its patency.
- **Coronary artery bypass grafting** can restore blood flow to the distal segment of a coronary artery with a proximal occlusion.

Procedures that restore blood flow must be performed as quickly as possible, preferably in the first few hours after the onset of symptoms. Beyond 6 hours, it is unlikely that much salvageable ischemic myocardium remains.

Chronic Congestive Heart Failure is Most Commonly Related to Ongoing Coronary Artery Disease

Because the rate of early mortality associated with acute myocardial infarction has fallen to less than 5%, many patients with ischemic heart disease survive longer and eventually develop **chronic congestive heart failure**. In more than 75% of all patients with heart failure, coronary artery disease is the major cause of their condition. Contractile impairment in these patients is due to irreversible loss of myocardium (previous infarcts) and hypoperfusion of surviving muscle. Because coronary artery disease is often so extensive in these patients, and many have already undergone coronary artery bypass surgery, the only treatments available are cardiac transplantation or the use of artificial pumps (ventricular assist devices). In a minority of patients with severe coronary atherosclerosis, myocardial contractility is impaired globally without discrete infarcts. This situation usually reflects a combination of ischemic myocardial dysfunction, diffuse fibrosis, and multiple small healed infarcts. *However, there is a group of patients with left ventricular failure in whom cardiac dysfunction occurs without obvious infarction.* These patients are said to have **ischemic cardiomyopathy**, which is a condition that results from repetitive episodes of ischemic injury, leading to myocyte degeneration.

Hypertensive Heart Disease

Effects of Hypertension on the Heart

Hypertension has been defined by the World Health Organization as a persistent increase of systemic blood pressure above 140 mm Hg systolic or 90 mm Hg diastolic, or both (see Chapter 10). Systemic hypertension is one of the most prevalent and serious causes of coronary artery and myocardial disease in the United States. Chronic hypertension leads to pressure overload and results first in compensatory left ventricular hypertrophy and, eventually, cardiac failure. The term **hypertensive heart disease** is used when the heart is enlarged in the absence of a cause other than hypertension.

 PATHOLOGY: Hypertension causes compensatory left ventricular hypertrophy as a result of the increased cardiac workload. The left ventricular free walls and interventricular septum become thickened uniformly and concentrically (Fig. 11-13), and heart weight increases, exceeding 375 g in men and 350 g in women. Microscopically, hypertrophic myocardial cells have an increased diameter with enlarged, hyperchromatic, and rectangular ("boxcar") nuclei (Fig. 11-14).

 CLINICAL FEATURES: Myocardial hypertrophy clearly adds to the ability of the heart to handle an increased workload. However, there is a limit beyond which additional hypertrophy no longer compensates. This upper limit to useful hypertrophy may reflect increasing diffusion distance between the interstitium and the center of each myofiber; if the distance becomes too great, the oxygen supply to the myofiber will be deficient.

Diastolic dysfunction is the most common functional abnormality caused by hypertension and by itself can lead to congestive heart failure. Some interstitial fibrosis typically develops as part of hypertrophy, which further contributes to left ventricular stiffness. *Hypertension is also associated with increased severity of coronary artery*

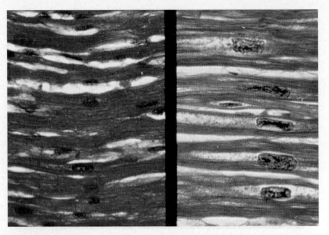

FIGURE 11-14. **Hypertensive heart disease with myocardial hypertrophy.** *(Left)* Normal myocardium. *(Right)* Hypertrophic myocardium shows thicker fibers and enlarged, hyperchromatic, rectangular nuclei.

atherosclerosis. The combination of increased cardiac workload (systolic dysfunction), diastolic dysfunction, and narrowed coronary arteries leads to a greater risk for myocardial ischemia, infarction, and heart failure.

Cause of Death in Patients with Hypertension

Congestive heart failure is the most common cause of death in untreated hypertensive patients. Fatal intracerebral hemorrhage is also common. Death may also result from coronary atherosclerosis and myocardial infarction, dissecting aneurysm of the aorta, or ruptured berry aneurysm of the cerebral circulation. Renal failure may supervene when nephrosclerosis induced by hypertension becomes severe.

Cor Pulmonale

Cor pulmonale is right ventricular hypertrophy and dilation due to pulmonary hypertension. Increased pressure in the pulmonary circulation may reflect a disorder of the lung parenchyma or, more rarely, a primary disease of the vasculature (e.g., primary pulmonary hypertension, recurrent small pulmonary emboli).

Acute cor pulmonale is the sudden occurrence of pulmonary hypertension, most commonly as a result of sudden, massive pulmonary embolization. This condition causes acute right-sided heart failure and is a medical emergency. At autopsy, the only cardiac findings are severe dilation of the right ventricle and sometimes the right atrium.

Chronic cor pulmonale is a common heart disease, accounting for 10% to 30% of all cases of heart failure. This frequency reflects the prevalence of chronic obstructive pulmonary disease, especially chronic bronchitis and emphysema.

 PATHOGENESIS: Chronic cor pulmonale may be caused by any pulmonary disease that interferes with ventilatory mechanics or gas exchange or obstructs the pulmonary vasculature. *The most common causes of chronic cor pulmonale are chronic obstructive pulmonary disease and pulmonary fibrosis.* In addition to the obliteration of blood vessels in the lung, these disorders also lead to pulmonary arteriolar vasoconstriction, which reduces the effective cross-sectional area of the pulmonary vascular bed without destroying the vessels. Hypoxia, acidosis, and hypercapnia directly cause pulmonary vasoconstriction.

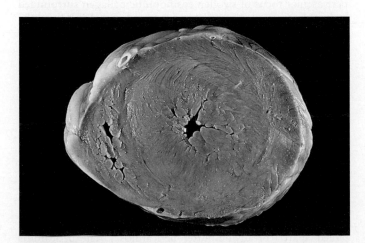

FIGURE 11-13. **Hypertensive heart disease.** A transverse section of the heart shows marked hypertrophy of the left ventricular myocardium without dilation of the chamber. The right ventricle is of normal dimensions.

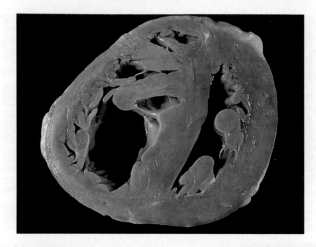

FIGURE 11-15. **Cor pulmonale.** A transverse section of the heart from a patient with primary (idiopathic) pulmonary hypertension shows a markedly hypertrophied right ventricle *(left)*. The right ventricular free wall has a thickness equal to the left ventricular wall. The right ventricle is dilated. The straightened interventricular septum has lost its normal curvature toward the left ventricle as part of the remodeling process in cor pulmonale.

PATHOLOGY: Chronic cor pulmonale is characterized by conspicuous right ventricular hypertrophy (Fig. 11-15) to the extent of exceeding 1.0 cm in thickness (normal range, 0.3 to 0.5 cm). Dilation of the right ventricle and right atrium are often present.

Acquired Valvular and Endocardial Diseases

A variety of inflammatory, infectious, and degenerative diseases damage cardiac valves and impair their function. The valves normally consist of thin flexible membranes, which close tightly to prevent backward blood flow. When they become damaged, leaflets or cusps may be thickened and fused enough to narrow the aperture and obstruct blood flow, a condition labeled **valvular stenosis**. Diseases that destroy valve tissue may also allow retrograde blood flow, termed **valvular regurgitation** or **insufficiency**. In many cases, diseases of the cardiac valves produce both stenosis and insufficiency, but generally one or the other predominates.

Stenosis of a cardiac valve results in hypertrophy of the myocardium proximal (in terms of blood flow) to the obstruction. Once compensatory mechanisms are exhausted, **pressure overload** eventually causes myocardial dilation and failure of the chamber proximal to the valve. Thus, mitral stenosis leads to left atrial hypertrophy and dilation. As the left atrium decompensates and can no longer force the venous return through the stenotic mitral valve, signs of pulmonary congestion develop, followed by right ventricular hypertrophy and even cor pulmonale. Similarly, aortic stenosis causes left ventricular hypertrophy and eventually left heart failure.

Valvular regurgitation or insufficiency also results in hypertrophy and dilation of the chamber proximal to the valve, owing to **volume overload**. In aortic insufficiency, the left ventricle first hypertrophies and then dilates when it can no longer accommodate the regurgitant volume and provide adequate cardiac output. On the other hand, an incompetent mitral valve leads to hypertrophy and dilation of both the left atrium and left ventricle, because both are subjected to volume overload.

Rheumatic Heart Disease Encompasses Acute Myocarditis and Residual Valvular Deformities

Acute Rheumatic Fever

Rheumatic fever (RF) is a multisystem childhood disease that follows a streptococcal infection and is characterized by an inflammatory reaction involving the heart, joints, and central nervous system.

EPIDEMIOLOGY: RF is a complication of an acute streptococcal infection, almost always pharyngitis (i.e., "strep" throat) (see Chapter 9). The offending agent is *Streptococcus pyogenes*, also known as group A β-hemolytic *Streptococcus*. In some epidemics of streptococcal pharyngitis, the incidence of RF has been as high as 3%. RF is principally a disease of childhood, and the median age is 9 to 11 years, although it can occur in adults. *Despite its declining importance in industrialized countries, RF is a leading cause of death of heart disease in persons 5 to 25 years old in less-developed regions.*

PATHOGENESIS: The pathogenesis of RF remains unclear, and with the exception of the link to streptococcal infection, no theory has been proven unequivocally. Most hypotheses relate rheumatic carditis to antibodies against streptococcal antigens that cross-react with heart antigens, an observation that raises the possibility of an autoimmune etiology related to so-called molecular mimicry (Fig. 11-16).

However, it has not been proved that such antibodies are cytotoxic or that they are directly involved in the pathogenesis of the disease. A direct toxic effect of some streptococcal product on the myocardium has not yet been excluded.

PATHOLOGY: Acute rheumatic heart disease is a pancarditis, involving all three layers of the heart (endocardium, myocardium, and pericardium).

MYOCARDITIS: At the most early stage, the heart tends to be dilated and exhibits a nonspecific myocarditis, in which lymphocytes and macrophages predominate, although a few neutrophils and eosinophils may be evident. Fibrinoid degeneration of collagen, in which fibers become swollen, fragmented, and eosinophilic, is characteristic of this early phase. In severe cases, a few patients may die acutely.

The **Aschoff body** is the characteristic granulomatous lesion of rheumatic myocarditis (Fig. 11-17), developing several weeks after symptoms begin. This structure initially consists of a perivascular focus of swollen eosinophilic collagen surrounded by lymphocytes, plasma cells, and macrophages. With time, the Aschoff body assumes a granulomatous appearance, with a central fibrinoid focus associated with a perimeter of lymphocytes, plasma cells, macrophages, and giant cells. Eventually, the Aschoff body is replaced by a nodule of scar tissue. **Anitschkow cells** are unusual cells within the Aschoff body, with nuclei that contain a central band of chromatin (see Fig. 11-17). These cells are macrophages that are normally present in small numbers but accumulate and become prominent in certain types of inflammatory diseases of the heart. Anitschkow cells may become multinucleated, in which case they are termed **Aschoff giant cells**.

PERICARDITIS: Tenacious irregular fibrin deposits are found on both visceral and parietal surfaces of the pericardium during the acute inflammatory phase of RF. These deposits resemble the shaggy surfaces of two slices of buttered bread that have been pulled apart ("bread-and-butter pericarditis"). The pericarditis may be recognized clinically by hearing a friction rub, but it has little functional effect and ordinarily does not lead to constrictive pericarditis.

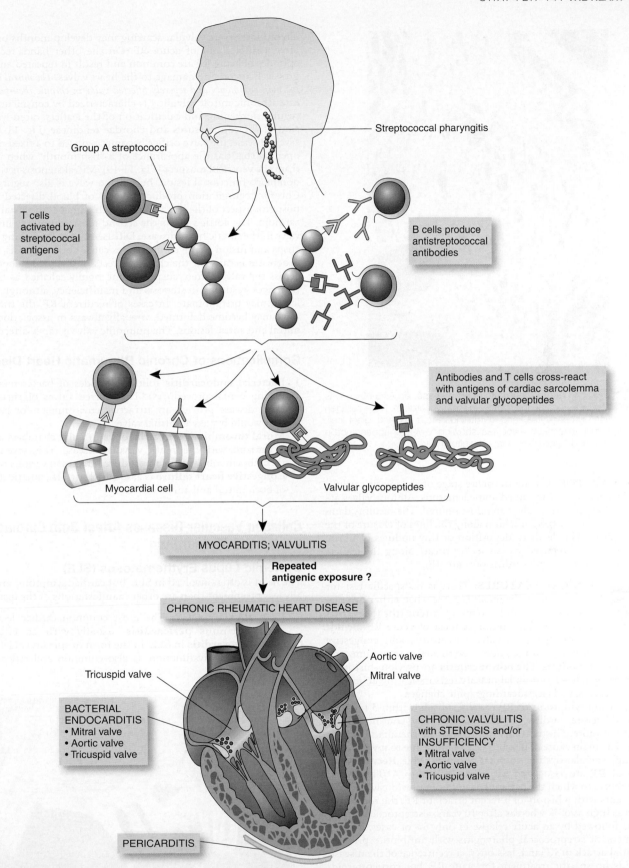

Streptococcal pharyngitis

Group A streptococci

T cells activated by streptococcal antigens

B cells produce antistreptococcal antibodies

Antibodies and T cells cross-react with antigens of cardiac sarcolemma and valvular glycopeptides

Myocardial cell

Valvular glycopeptides

MYOCARDITIS; VALVULITIS

Repeated antigenic exposure ?

CHRONIC RHEUMATIC HEART DISEASE

Aortic valve

Mitral valve

Tricuspid valve

BACTERIAL ENDOCARDITIS
• Mitral valve
• Aortic valve
• Tricuspid valve

CHRONIC VALVULITIS with STENOSIS and/or INSUFFICIENCY
• Mitral valve
• Aortic valve
• Tricuspid valve

PERICARDITIS

FIGURE 11-16. **Biological factors in rheumatic heart disease.** The upper portion illustrates the initiating β-hemolytic streptococcal infection of the throat, which introduces the streptococcal antigens into the body and may also activate cytotoxic T cells. These antigens lead to the production of antibodies against various antigenic components of the streptococcus, which can cross-react with certain cardiac antigens, including those from the myocyte sarcolemma and glycoproteins of the valves. This may be the mechanism of inflammation of the heart in acute rheumatic fever, which involves all cardiac layers (endocarditis, myocarditis, and pericarditis). This inflammation becomes apparent after a latent period of 2 to 3 weeks. Active inflammation of the valves may eventually lead to chronic valvular stenosis or insufficiency. These lesions involve the mitral, aortic, tricuspid, and pulmonary valves, in that order of frequency.

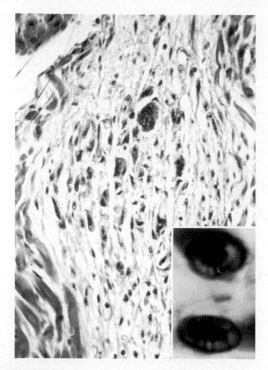

ENDOCARDITIS: During the acute stage of rheumatic carditis, valve leaflets become inflamed and edematous. All four valves are affected, but left-sided valves are most injured. The result is damage and focal loss of endothelium along the lines of closure of the valve leaflets. This leads to deposition of tiny nodules of fibrin, which can be recognized grossly as "verrucae" along the leaflets (so-called verrucous endocarditis of acute RF).

CLINICAL FEATURES: There is no specific test for RF. The clinical diagnosis is made when either two major or one major and two minor criteria (the Jones criteria) are met. The **major criteria** of acute RF include carditis (murmurs, cardiomegaly, pericarditis, and congestive heart failure), polyarthritis, chorea, erythema marginatum, and subcutaneous nodules. **The minor criteria** are previous history of RF, arthralgia, fever, certain laboratory tests indicating an inflammatory process, and electrocardiographic changes.

The acute symptoms of RF usually subside within 3 months, but with severe carditis, clinical activity may continue for 6 months or more. The mortality rate from acute rheumatic carditis is low. The main cause of death is heart failure due to myocarditis, although valvular dysfunction may also play a role. **Recurrent attacks of RF** are associated with types of group A β-hemolytic streptococci to which the patient has not been previously exposed. In patients with a history of a recent attack of RF, the recurrence rate is as high as 65%, whereas after 10 years, a streptococcal infection is followed by an acute relapse in only 5% of cases. Prompt treatment of streptococcal pharyngitis with antibiotics prevents an initial attack of RF and, less often, a recurrence of the disease. There is no specific treatment for acute RF, but corticosteroids and salicylates are helpful in managing the symptoms.

Chronic Rheumatic Heart Disease

PATHOLOGY: The myocardial and pericardial components of rheumatic pancarditis typically resolve without permanent sequelae. By contrast, the acute valvulitis of RF often results in long-term structural and functional alterations. Severe valvular scarring may develop months or years after a single bout of acute RF. On the other hand, recurrent episodes of acute RF are common and result in repeated and progressively increasing damage to the heart valves. *The mitral valve is the most commonly and severely affected valve in chronic rheumatic disease.* Chronic mitral valvulitis is characterized by conspicuous, irregular thickening and calcification of the leaflets, often with fusion of the commissures and chordae tendineae (Fig. 11-18). In severe disease, the valve orifice becomes reduced to a fixed narrow opening that has the appearance of a "fish mouth" when viewed from the ventricular aspect (Fig. 11-19). Mitral stenosis is the predominant functional lesion, but such a valve is also regurgitant. Chronic regurgitation produces a "jet" of blood directed at the posterior aspect of the left atrium, which damages the atrial endocardium. The aortic valve is the second most commonly involved valve in rheumatic heart disease. Diffuse fibrous thickening of the cusps and fusion of the commissures cause aortic stenosis, which progresses because of the chronic effects of turbulent blood flow across the valve. Often, cusps become rigidly calcified as the patient ages, resulting in stenosis and insufficiency, although either lesion may predominate. In cases of recurrent RF, the tricuspid valve may become deformed, virtually always in association with mitral and aortic lesions. The pulmonic valve is rarely affected.

Complications of Chronic Rheumatic Heart Disease

- **Bacterial endocarditis** follows episodes of bacteremia (e.g., during dental procedures). The scarred valves of rheumatic heart disease provide an attractive environment for bacteria that would bypass a normal valve.
- **Mural thrombi** form in atrial or ventricular chambers in 40% of patients with rheumatic valvular disease. They give rise to thromboemboli, which can produce infarcts in various organs.
- **Congestive heart failure** is associated with rheumatic disease of both mitral and aortic valves.

Collagen Vascular Diseases Affect Both Cardiac Valves and Myocardium

Systemic Lupus Erythematosus (SLE)

The heart is often involved in SLE, but cardiac symptoms are usually less prominent than are other manifestations of the disease.

PATHOLOGY: The most common cardiac lesion is **fibrinous pericarditis**, usually with an effusion. **Myocarditis** in SLE, in the form of subclinical left ventricular dysfunction, is also common and reflects the

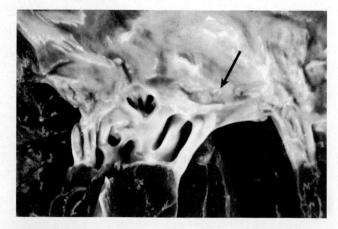

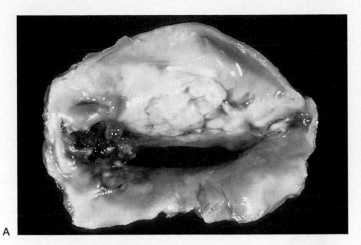

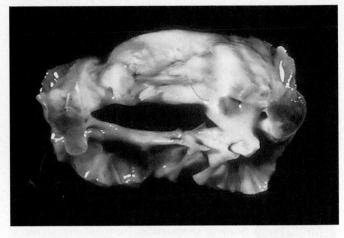

A   B

FIGURE 11-19   **Chronic rheumatic valvulitis.** A view of a surgically excised rheumatic mitral valve from the left atrium **(A)** and left ventricle **(B)** shows rigid, thickened, and fused leaflets with a narrow orifice, creating the characteristic "fish mouth" appearance of rheumatic mitral stenosis. Note that the tips of the papillary muscles (*shown in* **B**) are directly attached to the underside of the valve leaflets, reflecting marked shortening and fusion of the chordae tendineae.

severity of the disease in other organs. Microscopically, fibrinoid necrosis of small vessels and focal degeneration of interstitial tissue are seen.

Endocarditis is the most striking cardiac lesion of SLE. Verrucous vegetations up to 4 mm across occur on endocardial surfaces and are termed **Libman-Sacks endocarditis**. They are most common on the mitral valve. Ordinarily, Libman-Sacks endocarditis heals without scarring and does not produce a functional deficit.

Scleroderma (Progressive Systemic Sclerosis)

Cardiac involvement is second only to renal disease as a cause of death in scleroderma. The myocardium exhibits intimal sclerosis of small arteries, which leads to small infarcts and patchy fibrosis. As a result, congestive heart failure and arrhythmias are common. Cor pulmonale secondary to interstitial fibrosis of the lungs and hypertensive heart disease (caused by renal involvement) are also seen.

Polyarteritis Nodosa

The heart is involved in up to 75% of cases of polyarteritis nodosa. Necrotizing lesions in branches of the coronary arteries result in myocardial infarction, arrhythmias, or heart block. Cardiac hypertrophy and failure secondary to renal vascular hypertension are common.

Bacterial Endocarditis Refers to Infection of the Cardiac Valves

Before the antibiotic era, bacterial endocarditis was untreatable and almost invariably fatal. The infection is classified according to its clinical course as either acute or subacute endocarditis.

Acute bacterial endocarditis is an infection of a normal cardiac valve by highly virulent suppurative organisms, typically *Staphylococcus aureus* and *S. pyogenes*. The affected valve is rapidly destroyed, and prior to modern therapy, the patient died within 6 weeks in acute heart failure or of overwhelming sepsis.

Subacute bacterial endocarditis is a less fulminant disease in which less-virulent organisms (e.g., *Streptococcus viridans* or *Staphylococcus epidermidis*) infect a structurally abnormal valve, which typically had been deformed by rheumatic heart disease. In these cases, patients typically survived for 6 months or more, and infectious complications were uncommon.

Antimicrobial therapy changed the clinical patterns of bacterial endocarditis, and classical presentations described above are now unusual. The disease is currently classified according to the anatomical location and the etiologic agent.

 EPIDEMIOLOGY: *The most common predisposing condition for bacterial endocarditis in children now is CHD.* Under 10% of cases of bacterial endocarditis in children today are attributable to rheumatic heart disease.

The epidemiology of bacterial endocarditis has also changed in adults. *Mitral valve prolapse (MVP) and CHD are today the most frequent bases for bacterial endocarditis in adults, and rheumatic heart disease accounts for few cases.* More than half of adults with bacterial endocarditis have no predisposing cardiac lesion. Other predisposing conditions include:

- **Intravenous drug abuse** related to the injection of pathogenic organisms along with illicit drugs. The most common source of bacteria in intravenous drug abusers is the skin, with *S. aureus* causing more than half of the infections.
- **Prosthetic valves** are sites of infection in 15% of all cases of endocarditis in adults, and 4% of patients with prosthetic valves have this complication. Staphylococci are again responsible for half of these infections, and most of the rest are caused by gram-negative aerobic organisms.
- **Transient bacteremia** from any procedure may lead to infective endocarditis. Examples include dental procedures, urinary catheterization, gastrointestinal endoscopy, and obstetric procedures. Antibiotic prophylaxis is recommended during such maneuvers for patients at increased risk for bacterial endocarditis (e.g., those with a history of RF or a cardiac murmur).
- **The elderly** also have an increasing tendency to develop endocarditis. A number of degenerative changes in heart valves, including calcific aortic stenosis and calcification of the mitral annulus, predispose to endocarditis.

 PATHOGENESIS: Virulent organisms, such as *S. aureus*, can infect apparently normal valves, but the mechanism of such bacterial colonization is poorly understood. The pathogenesis of the infection of a damaged valve by less virulent organisms is initiated by damage to the affected valve's endothelium by turbulent blood flow. The damage leads to focal deposition of platelets and fibrin, creating small sterile vegetations that are hospitable sites for bacterial colonization and growth (Fig. 11-20). Microorganisms that gain access to the circulation can be de-

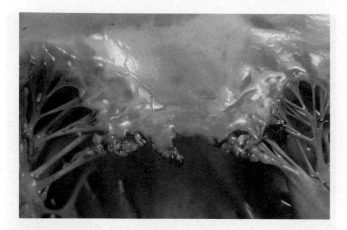

FIGURE 11-20 **Bacterial endocarditis.** The mitral valve shows destructive vegetations, which have eroded through the free margins of the valve leaflets.

posited within the vegetations. In this protected environment, colony counts upon culture may reach 10^{10} organisms per gram of tissue.

 PATHOLOGY: Bacterial endocarditis most commonly involves the mitral valve, the aortic valve, or both. The most common congenital heart lesions that underlie bacterial endocarditis are patent ductus arteriosus, tetralogy of Fallot, ventricular septal defect, and bicuspid aortic valve; the last is an increasingly recognized risk factor, especially in men over 60 years of age. Vegetations are composed of platelets, fibrin, cell debris, and masses of organisms. The underlying valve tissue is edematous and inflamed and may eventually become so damaged that a leaflet perforates, causing regurgitation. Lesions vary in size from a small, superficial deposit to bulky, exuberant vegetations. The infective process may spread locally to involve the valve ring or adjacent mural endocardium and chordae tendineae. **Infected thromboemboli** travel to multiple systemic sites, causing infarcts or abscesses in many organs, including the brain, kidneys, intestine, and spleen.

 CLINICAL FEATURES: Many patients show early symptoms of bacterial endocarditis within a week of the bacteremic episode, and almost all are symptomatic within 2 weeks. Heart murmurs develop almost invariably, often with a changing pattern during the course of the disease. In cases of more than 6 weeks duration, splenomegaly, petechiae, and clubbing of the fingers are frequent. In one third of patients, systemic emboli are recognized at some time during the illness. One third of the victims of bacterial endocarditis manifest some evidence of neurologic dysfunction, owing to the frequency of embolization to the brain.

Antibacterial therapy is effective in limiting the morbidity and mortality of bacterial endocarditis. Most patients defervesce within a week of instituting such therapy. However, the prognosis depends on the offending organism and the stage at which the infection is treated. *One third of cases of S. aureus endocarditis are still fatal. The most common serious complication of bacterial endocarditis is congestive heart failure, usually due to destruction of a valve.* Surgical replacement of a valve destroyed by endocarditis is risky and carries a high surgical mortality.

Nonbacterial Thrombotic Endocarditis (Marantic Endocarditis) is a Complication of Wasting Diseases

Nonbacterial thrombotic endocarditis (NBTE), also known as marantic endocarditis (from the Greek, marantikos, "wasting away"), refers to sterile vegetations on apparently normal cardiac valves, almost always in associa-

tion with cancer or some other wasting disease. NBTE affects mitral and aortic valves with equal frequency. Its gross appearance is similar to that of infective endocarditis, but it does not destroy the affected valve, and on microscopic examination, neither inflammation nor microorganisms can be demonstrated. The cause of NBTE is poorly understood. It is seen commonly in complicating adenocarcinomas (particularly of pancreas and lung) and hematologic malignancies.

Calcific Aortic Stenosis Reflects Chronic Damage to the Valve

Calcific aortic stenosis refers to a narrowing of the aortic valve orifice as a result of calcium deposition in the cusps and valve ring.

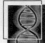 **PATHOGENESIS AND PATHOLOGY:** Calcific aortic stenosis has three main causes.

- **Rheumatic aortic valve disease**, in which it is characterized by diffuse fibrous thickening and scarring of the cusps, commissural fusion, and deposition of calcium, all of which reduce the valve orifice and limit valve mobility. The disorder is now uncommon due to surgical intervention.
- **Degenerative (senile) calcific stenosis** develops in elderly patients as a degenerative process that involves a normal symmetric tricuspid aortic valve. Valve cusps become rigidly calcified, but unlike the case in the rheumatic valve, there is no commissural fusion.
- **Congenital bicuspid aortic stenosis** often develops with age and, as above, shows no commissural fusion (Fig. 11-21).

Calcific aortic stenosis in both congenitally malformed valves as well as normal valves is probably related to the cumulative effect of years of trauma, owing to turbulent blood flow around the valve. In any of the forms of calcific aortic stenosis, calcification produces nodules restricted to the base and lower half of the cusps, rarely involving free margins.

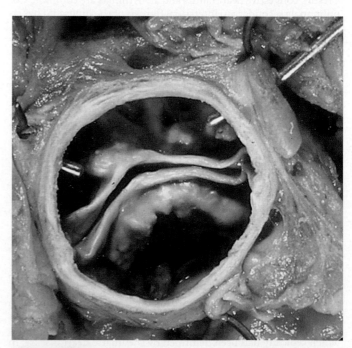

FIGURE 11-21. **Calcific aortic stenosis of a congenitally bicuspid aortic valve.** The two leaflets are heavily calcified, but there is no commissural fusion.

CLINICAL FEATURES: Severe aortic stenosis results in striking concentric left ventricular hypertrophy. Eventually, the heart dilates and fails. The disease is treated with great success (5-year survival rate of 85%) with surgical valve replacement, provided the operation is performed before ventricular dysfunction becomes irreversible. The hypertrophic left ventricle is then restored to its normal size.

Mitral Valve Prolapse (MVP) is the Most Common Indication for Valve Replacement

MVP is a condition in which mitral valve leaflets become enlarged and redundant, and chordae tendineae become thinned and elongated, such that the billowed leaflets prolapse (protrude) into the left atrium during systole (Fig. 11-22A). Also referred to as "floppy mitral valve syndrome," MVP is the most frequent cause of mitral regurgitation that requires surgical valve replacement. As much as 5% of the adult population may show echocardiographic evidence of MVP, although most will not have regurgitation severe enough to warrant surgical intervention.

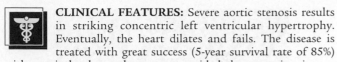 **PATHOGENESIS:** MVP has an important hereditary component and many cases appear to be transmitted as an autosomal dominant trait. Patients with primary MVP exhibit a striking accumulation of myxomatous connective tissue in the center of the valve leaflet (see Fig. 11-22B). Presumably, the extracellular matrix defect allows the leaflets and chordae to enlarge and stretch under the high-pressure conditions they experience during the cardiac cycle.

 PATHOLOGY: On gross examination, mitral valve leaflets are redundant and deformed (see Fig. 11-22A). On cross-section, they have a gelatinous appearance and slippery texture, owing to the accumulation of acid mucopolysaccharides (proteoglycans; Fig. 11-22B). The myxomatous degenerative process also affects the annulus and chordae tendineae, which increases the degree of prolapse and regurgitation. Although the mitral valve is usually the only valve affected, myxomatous degeneration can develop in the other cardiac valves, especially in patients with Marfan syndrome, 90% of whom have some clinical evidence of MVP.

 CLINICAL FEATURES: Most patients with MVP are asymptomatic. Endocarditis, both infective and nonbacterial, is sometimes a serious complication, and cerebral emboli are common. Significant mitral regurgitation develops in 15% of patients after 10 to 15 years of MVP, after which mitral valve replacement is indicated.

Carcinoid Heart Disease Affects Right-Sided Valves

Carcinoid heart disease is an unusual condition that uniquely affects the right side of the heart and produces tricuspid regurgitation and pulmonary stenosis. It arises in patients with carcinoid tumors, usually of the small intestine, that have metastasized to the liver.

 PATHOGENESIS: The pathogenesis of carcinoid heart disease is not fully understood. The valvular and endocardial lesions are thought to be caused by high concentrations of serotonin or other vasoactive amines and peptides produced by the tumor in the liver. Because these moieties are metabolized in the lung, carcinoid heart disease affects the right side of the heart almost exclusively. Use of anorexigenic drugs (such as "fen-phen") and ergot alkaloids, such as methysergide and ergotamine (used to treat migraine headaches), are also associated with cardiac disease strikingly similar to those seen in carcinoid syndrome,

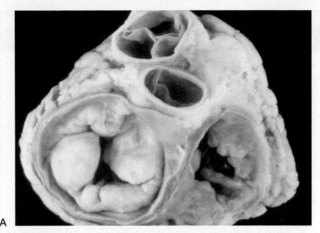

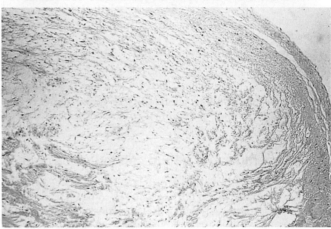

B

FIGURE 11-22. **Mitral valve prolapse. A.** A view of the mitral valve *(left)* from the left atrium shows redundant and deformed leaflets, which billow into the left atrial cavity. **B.** A microscopic section of one of the mitral valve leaflets reveals conspicuous myxomatous connective tissue in the center of the leaflet.

except that lesions develop on the left-sided valves. Because these drugs interfere with serotonin metabolism and signaling, it has been suggested that the pathogenesis of drug-related and carcinoid valvular disease is similar.

 PATHOLOGY: The cardiac lesions are plaque-like deposits of dense, pearly gray, fibrous tissue on the tricuspid and pulmonary valves and on the endocardial surface of the right ventricle. Microscopically, these patches appear "tacked on" to valve leaflets and are not associated with inflammation or apparent damage to underlying valve structures. However, leaflets become deformed, and their surface area is reduced. As a result, the tricuspid leaflets become "stuck down" onto adjacent right ventricular mural endocardium, resulting in tricuspid insufficiency or stenosis. Shrinkage of the pulmonary valve and its annulus leads to pulmonary stenosis.

Myocarditis

Myocarditis is inflammation of the myocardium associated with myocyte necrosis and degeneration. This definition specifically excludes ischemic heart disease. Myocarditis can occur at any age but is most common in children between the ages of 1 and 10. It is one of the few heart diseases that can produce acute heart failure in

TABLE 11–4
Causes of Myocarditis
Idiopathic
Infectious
• Viral: Coxsackievirus, adenovirus, echovirus, influenza virus, human immunodeficiency virus, and many others
• Rickettsial: Typhus, Rocky Mountain spotted fever
• Bacterial: Diphtheria, staphylococcal, streptococcal, meningococcal, Borrelia (Lyme disease), and leptospiral infection
• Fungi and protozoan parasites: Chagas' disease, toxoplasmosis, aspergillosis, cryptococcal, and candidal infection
• Metazoan parasites: *Echinococcus, Trichina*
Noninfectious
• Hypersensitivity and immunologically related diseases: Rheumatic fever, systemic lupus erythematosus, scleroderma, drug reaction (e.g., to penicillin or sulfonamide), and rheumatoid arthritis
• Radiation
• Miscellaneous: Sarcoidosis, uremia

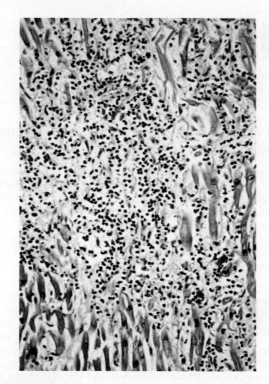

FIGURE 11-23. **Viral myocarditis.** The myocardial fibers are disrupted by a prominent interstitial infiltrate of lymphocytes and macrophages.

previously healthy children, adolescents, or young adults. Severe myocarditis can cause arrhythmias and even sudden cardiac death.

Viral Myocarditis May be Difficult to Demonstrate

Most cases of myocarditis in North America occur without an easily demonstrable cause but are believed to be viral, although the evidence is usually circumstantial. The most common viruses that cause myocarditis are listed in Table 11-4.

 PATHOGENESIS: The pathogenesis of viral myocarditis is thought to involve direct viral cytotoxicity or cell-mediated immune reactions directed against infected myocytes. There is substantial evidence for both mechanisms. The stimulus for the immune attack on myocytes is not established but appears to involve major histocompatibility antigens.

 PATHOLOGY: The hearts of patients with myocarditis who develop clinical heart failure during the active inflammatory phase show biventricular dilation and generalized myocardial hypokinesis. At autopsy, these hearts are flabby and dilated. The histologic changes of viral myocarditis vary with the clinical severity of the disease. Most cases show a patchy or diffuse interstitial, predominantly mononuclear, inflammatory infiltrate composed principally of T lymphocytes and macrophages (Fig. 11-23). Multinucleated giant cells may also be present. The inflammatory cells often surround individual myocytes, and focal myocyte necrosis is seen. During the resolving phase, fibroblast proliferation and interstitial collagen deposition predominate.

 CLINICAL FEATURES: Many persons who develop viral myocarditis may be asymptomatic. When symptoms do occur, they usually begin a few weeks after infection. Most patients recover from acute myocarditis, although a few die of congestive heart failure or arrhythmias. The disease may be unusually severe in infants and pregnant women. Despite resolution of the active inflammatory phase of viral myocarditis, subtle functional impairment may persist for years, and progression to overt cardiomyopathy is well documented. There is no specific treatment for viral myocarditis, and supportive measures usually suffice. In addition to viruses, other microorganisms and parasites that gain access to the bloodstream can infect the heart. Myocarditis may also result from noninfectious etiologies (see Table 11-4).

Metabolic Diseases of the Heart

Hyperthyroidism Causes High-Output Failure

*Hyper*thyroidism causes conspicuous tachycardia and an increased cardiac workload, owing to decreased peripheral resistance and increased cardiac output. It may eventually lead to angina pectoris and high-output failure.

Thiamine Deficiency (Beriberi) Heart Disease is Similar to Hyperthyroidism

In the United States, thiamine deficiency (beriberi) is occasionally seen in alcoholics or neglected individuals who consume an inadequate amount of thiamine (see Chapter 8). Beriberi heart disease results in decreased peripheral vascular resistance and increased cardiac output, a combination similar to that produced by hyperthyroidism. At autopsy, the heart is dilated and shows only nonspecific microscopic changes.

Hypothyroid Heart Disease Diminishes Cardiac Output

Patients with severe *hypo*thyroidism (myxedema) have decreased cardiac output, reduced heart rate, and impaired myocardial contractility—changes that are the reverse of those seen in hyperthyroidism. The hearts of patients with myxedema are flabby and dilated, and the myocardium exhibits myofiber swelling. Basophilic (mucinous) degeneration is common. Interstitial fibrosis may also be present. Despite these changes, myxedema does not produce congestive heart failure in the absence of other cardiac disorders.

Cardiomyopathy

Cardiomyopathy refers to a primary disease of the myocardium and excludes damage caused by extrinsic factors. Dilated cardiomyopathy (DCM) is the most common type of cardiomyopathy and is characterized by biventricular dilation, impaired contractility, and eventually congestive heart failure. DCM can develop in response to a large number of known insults that directly injure cardiac myocytes ("secondary DCM"), or it may be idiopathic (primary).

Idiopathic Dilated Cardiomyopathy is Characterized by Impaired Contractility

 PATHOGENESIS: Numerous etiologies have been implicated in idiopathic DCM, but the pathogenesis is unresolved.

Genetic factors now appear to be more important than previously believed. Among patients with idiopathic DCM, at least one-third have a familial disease. Most familial cases seem to be transmitted as an autosomal dominant trait, but autosomal recessive, X-linked recessive, and mitochondrial inheritance patterns have all been described. Mutations in several known genes including those encoding dystrophin, δ-sarcoglycan, troponin T, β-myosin heavy chain, actin, lamin A/C, and desmin have been identified as causing a dilated cardiomyopathic phenotype. *A current hypothesis holds that defects in force transmission lead to development of a dilated, poorly contracting heart.* Interestingly, mutations in proteins such as actin, troponin T, and β-myosin heavy chain may produce either dilated or hypertrophic cardiomyopathy (HCM) phenotypes, perhaps depending on whether they produce a defect in force generation (HCM) or force transmission (dilated cardiomyopathy).

Viral myocarditis may eventually lead to DCM, but how this would develop has not been clear. Interestingly, a protease expressed by cardiotropic enteroviruses has been shown to cleave dystrophin, thereby providing a potential mechanistic link between viral infection and the development of a dilated cardiomyopathy phenotype.

Immunologic abnormalities involving both cellular and humoral effects have been recognized in both myocarditis and idiopathic DCM. Autoantibodies to cardiac antigens that have been identified include those directed against a variety of mitochondrial antigens, cardiac myosin, and β-adrenergic receptors. However, a pathogenic role for immune mechanisms remains to be proved.

 PATHOLOGY: The pathologic changes in patients with DCM are generally nonspecific and are similar whether the disorder is idiopathic or secondary to a known injurious agent. At autopsy, the heart is invariably enlarged, reflecting conspicuous left and right ventricular hypertrophy. The weight of the heart may be as much as tripled (>900 g). As a rule, all chambers of the heart are dilated, although the ventricles are more severely affected than are the atria (Fig. 11-24). The myocardium is flabby and pale, and small subendocardial scars are occasionally evident. The left ventricular endocardium, especially at the apex (not shown), tends to be thickened. Adherent mural thrombi are often present in this area.

Microscopically, DCM is characterized by atrophic and hypertrophic myocardial fibers. Cardiac myocytes, especially in the subendocardium, often show advanced degenerative changes characterized by myofibrillar loss, an effect that gives cells a vacant, vacuolated appearance. Interstitial and perivascular fibrosis of myocardium is evident, also most prominently in the subendocardial zone.

 CLINICAL FEATURES: The clinical courses of idiopathic and secondary DCM are comparable. The disease begins insidiously with compensatory ventricular hypertrophy and asymptomatic left ventricular dilation. Commonly, exercise intolerance progresses relentlessly to frank congestive heart failure, and 75% of patients die within 5 years of symptom onset. Although supportive treatment is useful, cardiac transplantation or a ventricular assist device eventually becomes the only option.

Secondary Dilated Cardiomyopathy Has Many Causes

Almost 100 distinct myocardial diseases can result in the clinical features of DCM. Thus, secondary DCM is best viewed as a final common pathway for the effects of virtually any toxic, metabolic, or infectious disorder that directly injures cardiac myocytes. In this context, alcohol abuse, hypertension, pregnancy, and viral myocarditis predispose to secondary DCM. Diabetes mellitus and cigarette smoking are also associated with increased incidence of this disorder.

Toxic Cardiomyopathy

Numerous chemicals and drugs cause myocardial injury. Several of the more important substances are discussed here.

ETHANOL: *Alcoholic cardiomyopathy is the single most common identifiable cause of DCM in the United States and Europe.* Ethanol abuse can lead to chronic, progressive cardiac dysfunction, which may be fatal. The typical patient is between 30 and 55 years of age and has been drinking heavily for at least 10 years. Although the short-term action of alcohol on cardiac myocytes is reversible, the cumulative injury eventually becomes irreversible.

CATECHOLAMINES: In high concentrations, catecholamines can cause focal myocyte necrosis. Toxic myocarditis may occur in patients with pheochromocytomas, those who require high doses of inotropic drugs to maintain blood pressure, and in accident victims who sustain massive head trauma.

ANTHRACYCLINES: Doxorubicin (Adriamycin) and other anthracycline drugs are potent chemotherapeutic agents, and their usefulness is limited by cumulative, dose-dependent, cardiac toxicity. The clinical major effect is poor myocyte contractility secondary to chronic, irreversible degeneration of cardiac myocytes. The histopathology of this disorder includes vacuolization and loss of myofibrils. Once severe degeneration occurs, intractable congestive heart failure develops.

COCAINE: Cocaine use is frequently associated with chest pain and palpitations. True DCM is an unusual complication of cocaine abuse, but myocarditis, focal necrosis, and thickening of intramyocardial coronary arteries have been reported. Sudden death

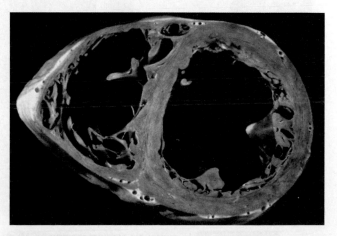

FIGURE 11-24. **Idiopathic dilated cardiomyopathy.** A transverse section of the enlarged heart reveals conspicuous dilation of both ventricles. Although the ventricular wall appears thinned, the increased mass of the heart indicates considerable hypertrophy.

due to spontaneous ventricular tachyarrhythmias is well documented. Mechanisms underlying the arrhythmogenic effects of cocaine include vasoconstriction, sympathomimetic activity, hypersensitivity responses, and direct toxicity.

Cardiomyopathy of Pregnancy

A unique form of DCM develops in the last trimester of pregnancy or the first 6 months after delivery. The disorder is relatively uncommon in the United States, but in some regions of Africa, it is encountered in as many as 1% of pregnant women. The risk of cardiomyopathy of pregnancy is greatest in black, multiparous women, older than 30 years of age. The cause of this form of DCM is unknown. Some patients exhibit inflammatory cells in heart biopsies taken during the symptomatic phase of the illness, consistent with the hypothesis that disordered immunity may underlie the development of DCM in this setting.

In Hypertrophic Cardiomypathy (HCM), Cardiac Hypertrophy is Out of Proportion to the Hemodynamic Load

HCM that develops for no apparent physiologic reason is probably genetically determined in most patients and is identified as an autosomal dominant trait in half of patients. HCM is now known to be far more common than previously appreciated: its prevalence in the United States is about 1 in 500.

PATHOGENESIS: The clinical picture of HCM is caused by more than 100 mutations in at least nine genes encoding proteins of the sarcomere. The mutated genes most commonly involved encode (1) β-myosin heavy chain (35%), (2) myosin-binding protein C (20%), and (3) troponin T (15%). *This proposed mechanism has led to the hypothesis that HCM is related to defects in force generation owing to altered sarcomeric function.*

PATHOLOGY: The heart in HCM is always enlarged, but the degree of hypertrophy varies in different genetic forms. The left ventricular wall is thick, and its cavity is small, sometimes reduced to a slit. Papillary muscles and trabeculae carneae are prominent and encroach on the ventricular lumen. More than half of cases exhibit asymmetric hypertrophy of the interventricular septum, with a ratio of the septum thickness to that of the left ventricular free wall greater than 1.5 (Fig. 11-25A).

*The most notable histologic feature of HCM is **myofiber disarray**,* which is most extensive in the interventricular septum. Instead of the usual parallel arrangement of myocytes into muscle bundles, myofiber disarray is characterized by an oblique and often perpendicular orientation of adjacent hypertrophic myocytes (see Fig. 11-25B).

CLINICAL FEATURES: Most patients with HCM have few if any symptoms, and the diagnosis is commonly made during screening of the family with an affected member. Despite a lack of symptoms, such persons may be at risk for sudden death, particularly during severe exertion. In fact, unsuspected HCM is commonly found at autopsy in young competitive athletes who die suddenly. Clinical recognition of HCM can occur at any age, often in the third, fourth, or fifth decade of life, but the disorder is also encountered in the elderly. Some patients with HCM become incapacitated by cardiac symptoms, of which dyspnea, angina pectoris, and syncope are most common. The clinical course tends to remain stable for many years, although eventually, the disease can progress to congestive heart failure.

Restrictive Cardiomyopathy Impairs Diastolic Function

Restrictive cardiomyopathy describes a group of diseases in which myocardial or endocardial abnormalities limit diastolic filling, while contractile function remains normal. It is the least common category of cardiomyopathy in Western countries, although in some less-devel-

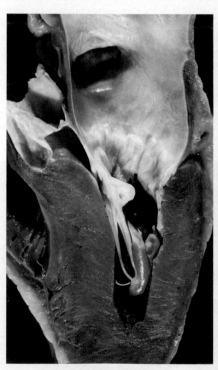
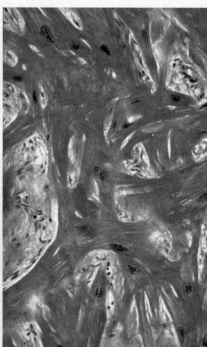
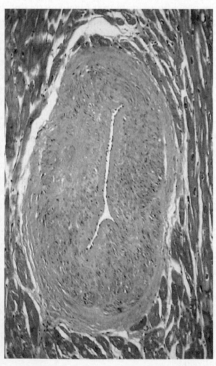

A   B,C

FIGURE 11-25. **Hypertrophic cardiomyopathy (HCM). A.** The heart has been opened to show striking asymmetric left ventricular hypertrophy. The interventricular septum is thicker than the free wall of the left ventricle and impinges on the outflow tract such that it contacts the underside of the anterior mitral valve leaflet. **B.** A section of the myocardium shows the characteristic myofiber disarray and hyperplasia of interstitial cells. **C.** A small intramural coronary artery shows thickened, hypercellular media. This type of remodeling of coronary vessels could contribute to development of angina-like symptoms in some patients with HCM.

oped regions (e.g., parts of equatorial Africa, South America, and Asia), endomyocardial disease related to parasitic infections leads to many cases of restrictive cardiomyopathy.

  PATHOGENESIS AND PATHOLOGY: Restrictive cardiomyopathy is caused by (1) interstitial infiltration of amyloid, metastatic carcinoma, or sarcoid granulomas; (2) endomyocardial disease characterized by marked fibrotic thickening of the endocardium; (3) storage diseases, including hemochromatosis; and (4) markedly increased interstitial fibrous tissue. Many cases of restrictive cardiomyopathy are classified as idiopathic, with interstitial fibrosis as the only histologic abnormality. The disease almost invariably progresses to congestive heart failure, and only 10% of the patients survive for 10 years.

Amyloidosis

The heart is affected in most forms of generalized amyloidosis (see Chapter 23). In fact, restrictive cardiomyopathy is the most common cause of death in AL amyloidosis of plasma cell dyscrasias.

 PATHOLOGY: Amyloid infiltration of the heart results in cardiac enlargement without ventricular dilation, and the gross appearance of the heart may resemble that of HCM. Ventricular walls are typically thickened, firm, and rubbery. Microscopically, amyloid accumulation is most prominent in interstitial, perivascular, and endocardial regions. Endocardial involvement is common in the atria, where nodular endocardial deposits often impart a granular appearance and gritty texture to the endocardial surface. Amyloid deposits can also cause thickening of cardiac valves.

 CLINICAL FEATURES: Cardiac amyloidosis is most often a restrictive cardiomyopathy, with symptoms mainly referable to right-sided heart failure. Infiltration of the conduction system can result in arrhythmias, and sudden cardiac death is not unusual. Cardiomegaly is characteristically prominent. The prognosis is grim; most patients survive less than 1 year once the disease becomes symptomatic.

SENILE CARDIAC AMYLOIDOSIS: *Senile cardiac amyloidosis refers to the deposition of a protein closely related to prealbumin (transthyretin) in the hearts of elderly persons* (see Chapter 23). The disorder may be present to some extent in up to 25% of patients who are 80 years old or older. The functional significance of senile cardiac amyloidosis is often minimal, and it is usually an incidental finding at autopsy.

Endomyocardial Disease

Endomyocardial disease comprises two geographically separate disorders.

ENDOMYOCARDIAL FIBROSIS: This condition is particularly common in equatorial Africa, where it accounts for 10% to 20% of all deaths from heart disease. The malady is also occasionally seen in other tropical and subtropical regions of the world. It is most common in children and young adults but has been reported to occur in persons up to 70 years of age. Endomyocardial fibrosis leads to progressive myocardial failure and has a poor prognosis, although survival for as long as 12 years has been reported.

EOSINOPHILIC ENDOMYOCARDIAL DISEASE (LÖFFLER ENDOCARDITIS): This is a cardiac disorder of temperate regions characterized by hypereosinophilia (as high as 50,000/μL). It is usually encountered in men in the fifth decade and is often accompanied by a rash. Löffler endocarditis typically progresses to congestive heart failure and death, although corticosteroids may improve survival.

 PATHOGENESIS: Endomyocardial fibrosis and Löffler endocarditis were once considered distinct entities, but there is a growing consensus that they represent variants of the same underlying disease. Endomyocardial disease is suspected to result from myocardial injury produced by eosinophils, possibly mediated by cardiotoxic granule components. In the tropics, transient high blood eosinophil counts often result from parasitic infestations; in temperate climates, idiopathic hypereosinophilia is usually persistent.

 PATHOLOGY: At autopsy, a grayish-white layer of thickened endocardium extends from the apex of the left ventricle over the posterior papillary muscle to the posterior leaflet of the mitral valve and for a short distance into the left outflow tract. On cut section of the ventricle, endocardial fibrosis spreads into the inner one-third to one-half of the wall. Mural thrombi in various stages of organization may be present. When the right ventricle is involved, the entire cavity may exhibit endocardial thickening, which may penetrate as far as the epicardium. Microscopically, the fibrotic endocardium contains only a few elastic fibers. Myofibers trapped within the collagenous tissue display nonspecific degenerative changes.

Storage Diseases

The various lysosomal storage diseases are discussed in detail in Chapter 6. Only the cardiac manifestations are reviewed here.

GLYCOGEN STORAGE DISEASES: Of the various forms of glycogen storage disease, types II (Pompe disease), III (Cori disease), and IV (Andersen disease) affect the heart. The most common and severe involvement is with Pompe disease. In infants with this condition, the heart is markedly enlarged (up to seven times normal), and endocardial fibroelastosis is seen in 20% of patients. The myocytes are vacuolated as a result of the large amounts of stored glycogen. The functional changes are those of a restrictive type of cardiomyopathy, and the usual cause of death is cardiac failure.

MUCOPOLYSACCHARIDOSES: Several of the mucopolysaccharidoses involve the heart. Cardiac disease results from lysosomal accumulation of mucopolysaccharides (glycosaminoglycans) in various cells. In general, pseudohypertrophy of the ventricles develops, and contractility gradually diminishes. The coronary arteries may be narrowed by thickening of the intima and media, and in Hurler and Hunter syndromes, myocardial infarction is common.

SPHINGOLIPIDOSES: Fabry disease may result in the accumulation of glycosphingolipids in the heart, with functional and pathologic changes similar to those that complicate the mucopolysaccharidoses.

HEMOCHROMATOSIS: This multiorgan disease is associated with excessive iron deposition in many tissues (see Chapter 14). The degree of iron deposition in the heart varies and only roughly correlates with that in other organs. Cardiac involvement has features of both dilated and restrictive cardiomyopathy, with systolic and diastolic impairment. *Congestive heart failure occurs in as many as one third of patients with hemochromatosis.* At autopsy, the heart is dilated, and ventricular walls are thickened. The brown color seen on gross examination correlates with iron deposition in cardiac myocytes. The severity of myocardial dysfunction seems to be proportional to the quantity of iron deposited.

Cardiac Tumors

Primary cardiac tumors are rare but can result in serious problems when they occur.

Cardiac Myxoma is the Most Common Primary Tumor of the Heart

Cardiac myxoma accounts for about 50% of all primary cardiac tumors. It is usually sporadic, but it is occasionally associated with familial autosomal dominant syndromes.

 PATHOLOGY: Most myxomas (75%) arise in the left atrium, although they can occur in any cardiac chamber or on a valve. The tumor appears as a glistening, gelatinous, polypoid mass, usually 5 to 6 cm in diameter, with a short stalk (Fig. 11-26). It may be sufficiently mobile to obstruct the mitral valve orifice. Microscopically, cardiac myxoma has a loose myxoid stroma containing abundant proteoglycans. Polygonal stellate cells are found within the matrix, occurring singly or in small clusters.

 CLINICAL FEATURES: More than half of patients with left atrial myxoma have clinical evidence of mitral valve dysfunction. Although the tumor does not metastasize in the usual sense, it often embolizes. One third of patients with myxomas of the left atrium or left ventricle die from tumor embolization to the brain. Surgical removal of the tumor is successful in most cases.

Rhabdomyoma is a Childhood Tumor

Rhabdomyoma is the most common primary cardiac tumor in infants and children and forms nodular masses in the myocardium. It may actually be a hamartoma rather than a true neoplasm, although the issue is still debated. Almost all are multiple and involve both ventricles and, in one third of cases, the atria as well. In half of cases, the tumor projects into a cardiac chamber and obstructs the lumen or valve orifices.

 PATHOLOGY: On gross examination, cardiac rhabdomyomas are pale masses, from 1 mm to several centimeters in diameter. Microscopically, tumor cells show small central nuclei and abundant glycogen-rich clear cytoplasm, in which fibrillar processes containing sarcomeres radiate

to the margin of the cell ("spider cell"). Rhabdomyomas often occur in association with tuberous sclerosis (one third to one half of cases). A few cardiac rhabdomyomas have been successfully excised.

Metastatic Tumors to the Heart May Manifest as Restrictive Cardiomyopathy

Metastatic tumors to the heart are seen most frequently in patients with the most prevalent forms of carcinomas—those of the lung, breast, and gastrointestinal tract. Still, only a minority of patients with these tumors will show cardiac metastases. Lymphomas and leukemia may also involve the heart. Of all tumors, the one most likely to metastasize to the heart is malignant melanoma. Metastatic cancer of the myocardium can result in clinical manifestations of restrictive cardiomyopathy, particularly if the cardiac tumors are associated with extensive fibrosis.

Diseases of the Pericardium

Pericardial Effusion Can Cause Cardiac Tamponade

Pericardial effusion is the accumulation of excess fluid within the pericardial cavity, either as a transudate or an exudate. The pericardial sac normally contains no more than 50 mL of lubricating fluid. If the pericardium is slowly distended, it can accommodate up to 2 L of fluid without notable hemodynamic consequences. However, rapid accumulation of as little as 150 to 200 mL of pericardial fluid or blood may significantly increase intrapericardial pressure and restrict diastolic filling, especially of the right ventricle. *Cardiac tamponade is the syndrome produced by the rapid accumulation of pericardial fluid, which restricts the filling of the heart.*

- **Serous pericardial effusion** is often a complication of an increase in extracellular fluid volume, as occurs in congestive heart failure or the nephrotic syndrome. The fluid has a low protein content and few cellular elements.
- **Chylous effusion** (fluid containing chylomicrons) results from a communication of the thoracic duct with the pericardial space secondary to lymphatic obstruction by tumor or infection.
- **Hemopericardium** is bleeding directly into the pericardial cavity. The most common cause is ventricular free wall rupture at a myocardial infarct. Less frequent causes are penetrating cardiac trauma, rupture of a dissecting aneurysm of the aorta, infiltration of a vessel by tumor, or a bleeding diathesis.

The hemodynamic consequences range from a minimally symptomatic condition to abrupt cardiovascular collapse and death. As the pericardial pressure increases, it reaches and then exceeds central venous pressure, thereby limiting return of blood to the heart. Acute cardiac tamponade is almost invariably fatal unless the pressure is relieved by removing pericardial fluid, by either needle pericardiocentesis or surgical procedures.

Acute Pericarditis May Follow Viral Infections

Pericarditis refers to inflammation of the visceral or parietal pericardium.

 PATHOGENESIS: The causes of pericarditis are similar to those for myocarditis (see Table 11-4). In most cases, the cause of acute pericarditis is obscure and (as in myocarditis) is attributed to an undiagnosed viral infection. Bacterial pericarditis is distinctly unusual in the antibiotic era. Metastatic tumors, most commonly breast and lung carcinomas, may involve the pericardium and cause a malignant pericardial effusion. Pericarditis associated with myocardial infarction and rheumatic fever is discussed above.

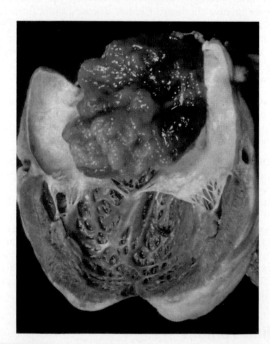

FIGURE 11-26. **Cardiac myxoma.** The left atrium contains a large, polypoid tumor that protrudes into the mitral valve orifice.

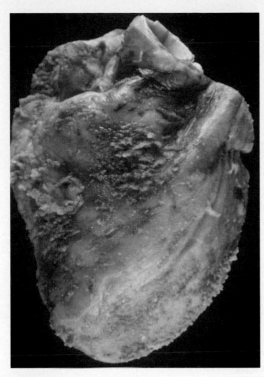

FIGURE 11-27. **Fibrinous pericarditis.** The heart of a patient who died in uremia displays a shaggy, fibrinous exudate covering the visceral pericardium.

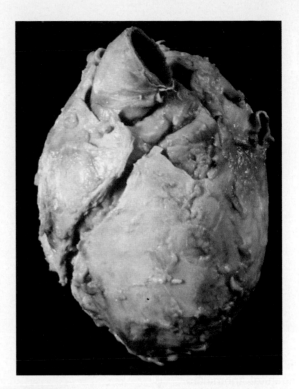

FIGURE 11-28. **Constrictive pericarditis.** The pericardial space has been obliterated, and the heart is encased in a fibrotic, thickened pericardium.

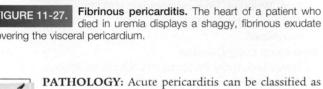 **PATHOLOGY:** Acute pericarditis can be classified as **fibrinous**, **purulent**, or **hemorrhagic**, depending on the gross and microscopic characteristics of the pericardial surfaces and fluid. The most common form is fibrinous pericarditis, in which the normal smooth, glistening appearance of the pericardial surfaces becomes replaced by a dull, granular fibrin-rich exudate (Fig. 11-27). The rough texture of the inflamed pericardial surfaces produces the characteristic friction rub heard by auscultation. The effusion fluid in fibrinous pericarditis is usually rich in protein, and the pericardium contains primarily mononuclear inflammatory cells.

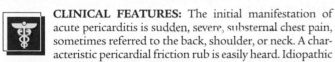 **CLINICAL FEATURES:** The initial manifestation of acute pericarditis is sudden, severe, substernal chest pain, sometimes referred to the back, shoulder, or neck. A characteristic pericardial friction rub is easily heard. Idiopathic or viral pericarditis is a self-limited disorder, although it may infrequently lead to constrictive pericarditis. Corticosteroids are the treatment of choice. The therapy for other specific forms of acute pericarditis varies with the cause.

Constrictive Pericarditis May Mimic Right Heart Failure

Constrictive pericarditis is a chronic fibrosing disease of the pericardium that compresses the heart and restricts inflow.

 PATHOGENESIS AND PATHOLOGY: Constrictive pericarditis results from an exuberant healing response after acute pericardial injury, in which the pericardial space becomes obliterated and visceral, and parietal layers become fused in a dense, rigid mass of fibrous tissue. The scarred pericardium may be so thick (up to 3 cm) that it narrows the orifices of the venae cavae (Fig. 11-28). The fibrous envelope may contain calcium deposits. The condition is infrequent today and, in developed countries, is predominantly idiopathic. Constrictive pericarditis may follow tuberculous infection and is still the major cause in underdeveloped regions.

 CLINICAL FEATURES: Patients with constrictive pericarditis have a small, quiet heart in which venous inflow is restricted, and the rigid pericardium determines the diastolic volume of the heart. These patients have high venous pressure, low cardiac output, small pulse pressure, and fluid retention with ascites and peripheral edema. Total pericardiectomy is the treatment of choice.

12 The Respiratory System

Mary Beth Beasley
William D. Travis
Emanuel Rubin

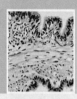

Diseases of the lung are not only important problems for the individual but are major public health concerns. Cancer of the lung, mostly related to smoking, remains the most common cause of cancer-related death in the US, killing more than 160,000 persons per year. Chronic obstructive pulmonary disease, also frequent in smokers, is responsible for at least 120,000 deaths per year in the US. Acute respiratory distress syndrome (ARDS) affects about 150,000 persons a year and even humble respiratory tract infections, mostly benign and self-limited are the most common cause of days lost from work. The growing number of respiratory infections of public concern, including drug-resistant tuberculosis, the potential for the recurrence of SARS, and the threat of pandemic avian influenza, highlight the importance of respiratory disease worldwide.

THE LUNGS

Congenital Anomalies

PULMONARY HYPOPLASIA: This condition reflects incomplete or defective development of the lung. The lung is smaller than normal, owing to the presence of fewer acini or a decrease in their size. Pulmonary hypoplasia, the most common congenital lesion of the lung, is found in 10% of neonatal autopsies. In most cases (90%), it occurs in association with other congenital anomalies, most of which impinge on the thorax. The lesion may be accompanied by hypoplasia of the bronchi and pulmonary vessels if the insult occurs early in gestation, as in congenital diaphragmatic hernia.

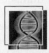 **PATHOGENESIS:** Three major factors have been implicated as causes of pulmonary hypoplasia: (1) **Compression of the lung** is usually caused by a congenital diaphragmatic hernia, typically on the left side, owing to failure of the pleuroperitoneal canal to close; (2) **Oligohydramnios** (inadequate volume of amniotic fluid) is usually due to genitourinary anomalies and is an important cause of pulmonary hypoplasia; (3) **Decreased respiration** has been shown experimentally to produce hypoplastic lungs, which may be caused by a lack of repetitive stretching of the lung.

CONGENITAL CYSTIC ADENOMATOID MALFORMATION: *This common anomaly consists of abnormal bronchiolar structures of varying sizes or distribution.* Most cases are seen in the first 2 years of life. The lesion usually affects one lobe of the lung and consists of multiple cyst-like spaces, which are lined by bronchiolar epithelium and separated by loose fibrous tissue (Fig. 12-1). Some patients with congenital cystic adenomatoid malformation have other congenital anomalies. The most common presenting symptom is respiratory distress and cyanosis. Surgical resection is the treatment of choice.

BRONCHOGENIC CYST: *This lesion is a discrete, extrapulmonary, fluid-filled mass lined by respiratory epithelium and limited by walls that contain muscle and cartilage.* It is most commonly found in the middle mediastinum. In the newborn, a bronchogenic cyst may compress a major airway and cause respiratory distress. Secondary infection of the cyst in older patients may lead to hemorrhage and perforation. Many bronchogenic cysts are asymptomatic and are found on routine chest radiographs.

EXTRALOBAR SEQUESTRATION: *Extralobar sequestration is a mass of lung tissue that is not connected to the bronchial tree and is located outside the visceral pleura.* An abnormal artery, usually arising from the aorta, supplies the sequestered tissue.

 PATHOGENESIS: This lesion is thought to originate from an outpouching of the foregut that later loses its connection to the original foregut. It is three to four times as common in males as in females and is associated with other anomalies in two thirds of patients.

 PATHOLOGY: On gross examination, extralobar sequestration is a pyramidal or round mass covered by pleura, from 1 to 15 cm in greatest dimension. Microscopically, dilated bronchioles, alveolar ducts, and alveoli are noted. Infection or infarction may alter the histologic appearance.

 CLINICAL FEATURES: In the neonatal period, often during the first day of life, the disorder may manifest as dyspnea and cyanosis. In older children, it may come to medical attention because of recurrent bronchopulmonary infections. Surgical excision is curative.

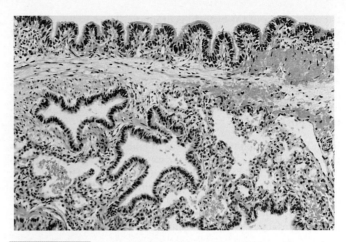

FIGURE 12-1. **Congenital cystic adenomatoid malformation.** Multiple gland-like spaces are lined by bronchiolar epithelium.

INTRALOBAR SEQUESTRATION: *Intralobar sequestration is a mass of lung tissue within the visceral pleura, isolated from the tracheobronchial tree and supplied by a systemic artery.* For many years, it was considered a congenital malformation, but it is now thought to be acquired.

 PATHOLOGY: Intralobar sequestration is found in a lower lobe in almost all cases. Bilateral involvement is distinctly unusual. On gross examination, the sequestered pulmonary tissue shows the result of chronic recurrent pneumonia, with end-stage fibrosis and honeycomb cystic changes. The cysts range up to 5 cm in diameter and lie in a dense fibrous stroma. Microscopically, the cystic spaces are mostly lined by cuboidal or columnar epithelium, and the lumen contains foamy macrophages and eosinophilic material. Interstitial chronic inflammation and hyperplasia of lymphoid follicles is often prominent. Acute and organizing pneumonia may be seen.

 CLINICAL FEATURES: Cough, sputum production, and recurrent pneumonia are noted in almost all patients. Most cases are discovered in adolescents or young adults. Surgical resection is often indicated.

Diseases of the Bronchi and Bronchioles

Most bronchial and bronchiolar diseases deal with acute conditions and their sequelae. Chronic bronchitis will be discussed with chronic obstructive pulmonary disease (COPD).

Airway Infections are Caused by Diverse Organisms

The agents causing pulmonary infections are discussed in detail in Chapter 9. Many infectious agents that involve the intrapulmonary airways tend to affect the more peripheral airways (**bronchiolitis**). The classic examples are adenovirus, respiratory syncytial virus (RSV), and measles. All are more serious in malnourished children and populations not ordinarily exposed to these agents. Severe symptomatic illnesses with these agents are more commonly encountered in infants and children, and recovery is the rule. Symptoms include cough, a feeling of tightness in the chest, and, in extreme cases, shortness of breath and even cyanosis.

INFLUENZA: This is a characteristic example of tracheobronchitis, and in the occasional patient who dies with this infection, the appearance of the bronchi is dramatic. The surface of the airway is fiery red, reflecting acute inflammation and congestion of the mucosa.

ADENOVIRUS: Infection with adenovirus produces the most serious sequelae, including extensive inflammation of bronchioles (Fig. 12-2) and subsequent healing by fibrosis. Bronchioles may become obliterated or occluded by loose fibrous tissue (**obliterative bronchiolitis**).

RSV: RSV infection tends to occur in epidemics in nurseries. It is usually self-limited, but rare fatal cases occur. It can cause nosocomial infection in children and (rarely) in adults. Histologically, one encounters peribronchiolar inflammation and disorganization of the epithelium. Severe overdistention may be found without obvious bronchiolar obstruction, possibly due to displacement of surfactant from the bronchiolar surface.

MEASLES: At one time, a major cause of bronchiolitis, measles is rarely a problem in developed countries since the advent of the measles vaccine. Similar to adenovirus, it may result in bronchiolar obliteration and bronchiectasis.

BORDETELLA PERTUSIS: This bacterium commonly infects the airways and is the cause of whooping cough. With the advent of a pertussis vaccine, the disease has become rare in the United States, but the disease is still a problem in nonvaccinated populations. Clinically, whooping cough is typified by fever and severe prolonged bouts of coughing, followed by a characteristic deep whooping inspiration. Severe bronchial and bronchiolar inflammation has been found in fatal cases. Whooping cough occasionally leads to the development of bronchiectasis.

Bronchocentric Granulomatosis Usually Reflects Allergic Responses to Infection

Bronchocentric granulomatosis refers to nonspecific granulomatous inflammation centered on bronchi or bronchioles. The histologic pattern can be seen in a number of clinical settings and is not a distinct clinical entity. Bronchocentric granulomatosis can be the predominant pulmonary pathologic finding in two groups of patients, namely asthmatics and nonasthmatic patients with tuberculosis or fungi such as *Histoplasma capsulatum*.

Bronchocentric granulomatosis can also be a manifestation of rheumatoid arthritis, ankylosing spondylitis, and Wegener granulomatosis. Patients with bronchocentric granulomatosis of either the allergic or nonallergic type generally respond well to corticosteroid therapy.

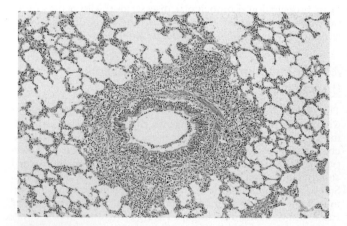

FIGURE 12-2. **Bronchiolitis due to adenovirus.** The wall of this bronchiole shows an intense chronic inflammatory infiltrate with local extension into the surrounding peribronchial tissue.

Constrictive Bronchiolitis May Obliterate the Airway

Constrictive (obliterative) bronchiolitis is an uncommon disorder in which an initial inflammatory bronchiolitis is followed by bronchiolar scarring and fibrosis, resulting in constrictive narrowing and eventually complete obliteration of the airway lumen.

PATHOLOGY: Bronchioles show chronic mural inflammation and varying amounts of submucosal fibrosis. These lesions are often focal and may be difficult to identify. Elastic stains may assist in recognizing the scarred bronchioles. Bronchiolectasis and mucus plugs may be seen in adjacent airways. The surrounding lung is usually normal.

CLINICAL FEATURES: Patients may have dyspnea and wheezing due to severe obstruction of pulmonary function. This pattern of fibrosis is seen in a number of situations, including (1) bone marrow transplantation (graft-versus-host disease), (2) lung transplantation (chronic rejection), (3) collagen vascular diseases (especially rheumatoid arthritis), (4) postinfectious disorders (especially viral infections), (5) after inhalation of toxins (SO_2, ammonia, phosgene), and (6) intake of certain drugs (penicillamine). It may also occur as an idiopathic entity. Most patients have a relentless progressive clinical course. Many are treated with steroids, but no therapy is effective for this disease.

Bronchial Obstruction Leads to Atelectasis

Bronchial obstruction in adults is most often the consequence of the endobronchial extension of primary lung tumors, although mucus plugs from aspirated gastric contents or foreign bodies may be responsible, especially in children. In the case of partial obstruction, the trapped air may lead to overdistention of the distal affected segment; complete obstruction results in atelectasis. Areas distal to the obstruction are also susceptible to pneumonia, pulmonary abscess, and bronchiectasis (see below).

Atelectasis refers to the collapse of expanded lung tissue (Fig. 12-3). If the air supply is obstructed, the loss of gas from the alveoli to the blood causes collapse of the affected region. Atelectasis is an important postoperative complication of abdominal surgery, occurring because of (1) mucus obstruction of a bronchus and (2) diminished respiratory movement resulting from postoperative pain. It is often asymptomatic, but when severe, it results in hypoxemia and a shift of the mediastinum *toward* the affected side. Atelectasis is usually caused by bronchial obstruction but may also result from direct compression of the lung (e.g., hydrothorax or pneumothorax). Such pressure may seriously compromise the function of the affected lung and cause a mediastinal shift *away* from the affected side. In long-standing atelectasis, the collapsed lung becomes fibrotic and bronchi dilate, in part, because of infection distal to the obstruction. Permanent bronchial dilation (bronchiectasis) results.

Bronchiectasis is Irreversible Dilation of Bronchi Caused by Destruction of Bronchial Wall Muscle and Elastic Elements

PATHOGENESIS: Bronchiectasis may be obstructive or nonobstructive.

Obstructive bronchiectasis is localized to a segment of the lung distal to a mechanical obstruction of a central bronchus by a variety of lesions, including tumors, inhaled foreign bodies, mucus plugs (in asthma), and compressive lymphadenopathy. **Nonobstructive bronchiectasis** is usually a complication of respiratory infections or defects in the defense mechanisms that protect the airways from infection. It may be localized or generalized.

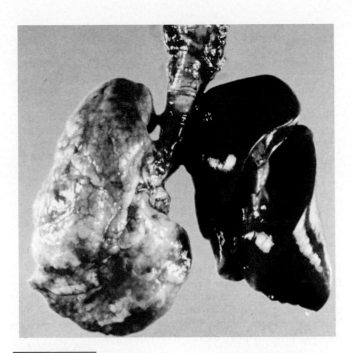

Atelectasis. The right lung of an infant is pale and expanded by air; the left lung is collapsed.

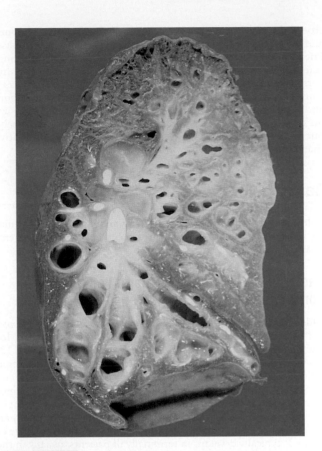

Bronchiectasis. The resected upper lobe shows widely dilated bronchi, with thickening of the bronchial walls and collapse and fibrosis of the pulmonary parenchyma.

Localized nonobstructive bronchiectasis was once common, usually resulting from childhood bronchopulmonary infections. Although reduced in frequency by antibiotics and childhood immunizations, one half to two thirds of all cases still follow a bronchopulmonary infection. At present, adenovirus and RSV infections are frequent causes of bronchiectasis in children.

Generalized bronchiectasis is, for the most part, secondary to inherited impairment in host defense mechanisms or acquired conditions that permit introduction of infectious organisms into the airways. The acquired disorders that predispose to bronchiectasis include (1) neurologic diseases that impair consciousness, swallowing, respiratory excursions and the cough reflex; (2) incompetence of the lower esophageal sphincter, which promotes gastric reflux; (3) nasogastric intubation; and (4) chronic bronchitis. The principal inherited conditions associated with generalized bronchiectasis are cystic fibrosis, the dyskinetic ciliary syndromes, hypogammaglobulinemias, and deficiencies of specific immunoglobulin (Ig)G subclasses.

Kartagener syndrome is one of the immotile cilia (ciliary dyskinesia) syndromes and comprises the triad of dextrocardia (with or without situs inversus), bronchiectasis, and sinusitis. It is caused by absence of inner or outer dynein arms of cilia. In the respiratory tract, ciliary defects lead to repeated upper and lower respiratory tract infections in the lung and, thus, to bronchiectasis.

 PATHOLOGY: Generalized bronchiectasis is usually bilateral and is most common in the lower lobes, the left more commonly involved than the right. Localized bronchiectasis may occur wherever there is obstruction or infection. Bronchi are dilated and have white or yellow thickened walls, and lumina frequently contain thick, mucopurulent secretions (Fig. 12-4). Microscopically, severe inflammation of bronchi and bronchioles results in destruction of all components of the bronchial wall. With the consequent collapse of distal lung parenchyma, the damaged bronchi dilate. The distal bronchi and bronchioles are scarred and often obliterated.

 CLINICAL FEATURES: Patients with bronchiectasis have a chronic productive cough, often with several hundred milliliters of mucopurulent sputum a day. Hemoptysis is common, as bronchial inflammation

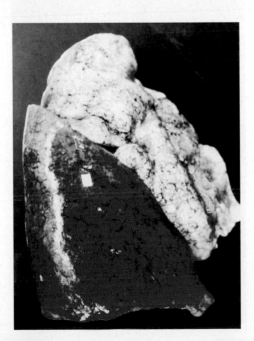

Lobar pneumonia. The entire left lower lobe is consolidated and in the stage of red hepatization. The upper lobe is normally expanded.

erodes through the walls of adjacent bronchial arteries. Dyspnea and wheezing are variable, depending on the extent of the disease. Pneumonia is a common complication, and patients with long-standing cases are at risk of chronic hypoxia and pulmonary hypertension. Acute, reversible dilation of bronchi may occur as a consequence of bacterial or viral bronchopulmonary infection, and it may take months before the bronchi return to normal size. Surgical resection of localized bronchiectasis may be necessary, but in generalized disease, surgical treatment is more palliative than curative.

Bacterial Infections

Pulmonary infections are discussed in detail in Chapter 9. The major pulmonary entities are described below, with particular emphasis on pathologic features.

Bacterial Pneumonia is Inflammation and Consolidation of the Lung Parenchyma

Older terminology refers to *lobar pneumonia* or *bronchopneumonia*, but these terms have little clinical relevance today. In general, **lobar pneumonia** denotes consolidation of an entire lobe (Fig. 12-5), whereas **bronchopneumonia** is characterized by scattered solid foci in the same or several lobes (Fig. 12-6).

Streptococcus pneumoniae was the classic cause of lobar pneumonia, but today, largely due to antibiotic therapy, the involvement of a lobe tends to be incomplete, and more than one lobe is usually affected. By contrast, bronchopneumonia is still a common cause of death. It typically develops in terminally ill patients, usually in the dependent and posterior portions of the lung. Scattered irregular foci of pneumonia are centered on terminal bronchioles and respiratory bronchioles. Bronchiolitis is present, with exudation of polymorphonuclear leukocytes into the adjacent alveoli.

FIGURE 12-6. **Bronchopneumonia.** Scattered foci of consolidation are centered on bronchi and bronchioles.

PATHOGENESIS: Most bacteria that cause pneumonia are normal inhabitants of the oropharynx and nasopharynx and reach the alveoli by aspiration of secretions. Other routes of infection include inhalation from the environment, hematogenous dissemination from an infectious focus elsewhere, and (rarely) spread of bacteria from an adjacent site. A change in oropharyngeal flora from the normal commensals to a virulent organism may proceed to pneumonia in debilitated or immunosuppressed patients in the hospital, in whom nosocomial pneumonia can occur in as many as 25% of cases. A number of conditions predispose to infection by depressing the host's defenses, including cigarette smoking, chronic bronchitis, alcoholism, severe malnutrition, wasting diseases, and poorly controlled diabetes.

Pneumococcal Pneumonia

Despite the impact of antibiotic therapy, pneumonia caused by *Streptococcus pneumoniae* (pneumococcus) remains a significant problem. It is principally a disease of young to middle-aged adults. The disease is rare in infants, less common in the elderly, and considerably more frequent in men than in women.

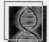

PATHOGENESIS: Pneumococcal pneumonia is mostly a consequence of altered defense barriers in the respiratory tract. Frequently, it follows a viral infection of the upper respiratory tract (e.g., influenza). The bronchial secretions stimulated by a viral infection provide a hospitable environment for proliferation of *S. pneumoniae*, which are normal flora of the nasopharynx. The aspiration of pneumococci is also promoted by factors that impair the epiglottic reflex, including exposure to cold, anesthesia, and alcohol intoxication. Lung injury caused by factors such as congestive heart failure and irritant gases also renders the lung more susceptible to pneumococcal pneumonia.

PATHOLOGY: In the earliest stage of pneumococcal pneumonia, protein-rich edema fluid containing numerous organisms fills the alveoli. Marked capillary congestion leads to massive outpouring of polymorphonuclear leukocytes and intra-alveolar hemorrhage (Fig. 12-7). Because the firm consistency of the affected lung is reminiscent of the liver, this stage has been aptly named "red hepatization" (Fig. 12-8). The next phase, occurring after 2 or more days, depending on the success of treatment, involves lysis of polymorphonuclear leukocytes and appearance of macrophages, which phagocytose the fragmented neutrophils and other inflammatory debris. At this stage, the congestion has diminished, but the lung is still firm ("grey hepatization") (see Fig. 12-8). The alveolar exudate is then removed, and the lung gradually returns to normal.

A number of complications may follow pneumococcal pneumonia:

- **Pleuritis**, often painful, is common, because the pneumonia readily extends to the pleura.
- **Pleural effusion** occurs frequently but usually resolves.
- **Pyothorax** results from an infection of a pleural effusion and may heal with extensive fibrosis.
- **Empyema** (a loculated collection of pus with fibrous walls) results from the persistence of pyothorax.
- **Bacteremia** is present in more than 25% of patients in the early stages of pneumococcal pneumonia and may lead to endocarditis or meningitis. Patients whose spleens have been removed often die of this bacteremia.

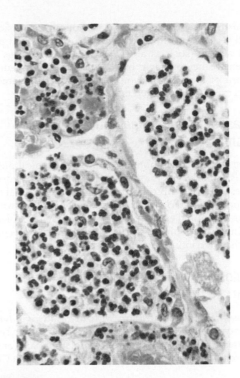

FIGURE 12-7. **Pneumococcal pneumonia.** The alveoli are packed with an exudate composed of polymorphonuclear leukocytes and occasional macrophages.

 CLINICAL FEATURES: The onset of pneumococcal pneumonia is acute, with fever and chills. Chest pain secondary to pleural involvement is common. Hemoptysis is frequent and is characteristically "rusty," because it is derived from altered blood in alveolar spaces. Pneumococcal pneumonia is treated effectively with antibiotics. Although symptoms of pneumonia respond rapidly to antibiotics, the lesion still takes several days to resolve radiologically.

Klebsiella Pneumonia

Other than *S. pneumoniae*, *Klebsiella pneumoniae* is the only organism that causes lobar pneumonia with any frequency. However, it accounts for no more than 1% of all cases of community-acquired pneumonia. The disease is commonly associated with alcoholism and is seen most frequently in middle-aged men, although persons with diabetes and chronic pulmonary disease are also at increased risk.

 PATHOLOGY: *K. pneumoniae* has a thick, gelatinous capsule, which is responsible for the characteristic mucoid appearance of the cut surface of the lung. Another distinctive characteristic of *Klebsiella* pneumonia is that the affected lobe increases in size, so that the fissure "bulges" toward the unaffected region. There is a tendency toward tissue necrosis and abscess formation. A serious complication is **bronchopleural fistula**, (i.e., a communication between the bronchial airway and the pleural space). The onset of *Klebsiella* pneumonia is less dramatic than that of pneumococcal pneumonia, but the disease may be more dangerous. Before the antibiotic era, mortality rates in *Klebsiella* pneumonia ranged from 50% to 80%. Even with prompt antibiotic treatment, the mortality is still considerable.

Staphylococcal Pneumonia

Community-acquired staphylococcal pneumonia is uncommon, accounting for only 1% of the bacterial pneumonias. However, pulmonary infection with *Staphylococcus aureus* is a common superinfection after influenza and other viral respiratory tract infec-

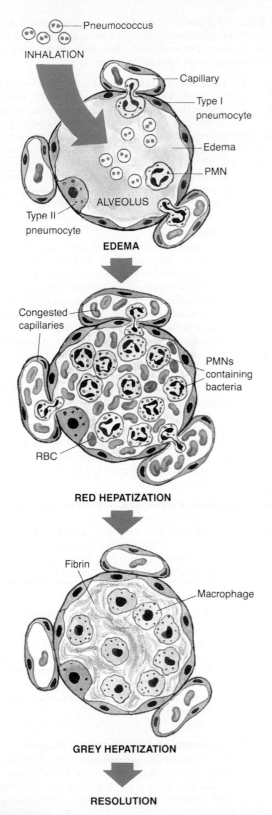

FIGURE 12-8. **Pathogenesis of pneumococcal lobar pneumonia.** Pneumococci, characteristically in pairs (diplococci), multiply rapidly in the alveolar spaces and produce extensive edema. They incite an acute inflammatory response in which polymorphonuclear leukocytes and congestion are prominent (red hepatization). As the inflammatory process progresses, macrophages replace the polymorphonuclear leukocytes and ingest debris (grey hepatization). The process usually resolves, but complications may ensue. PMN, polymorphonuclear neutrophil; RBC, red blood cell.

tions. Repeated episodes of staphylococcal pneumonia are seen in patients with cystic fibrosis. Nosocomial staphylococcal pneumonia typically occurs in weakened, chronically ill patients, who are prone to aspiration and in intubated persons.

PATHOLOGY: Like staphylococcal infection elsewhere, staphylococcal pneumonia is characterized by the production of many small abscesses. In infants and, to a lesser extent, in adults, these may lead to **pneumatoceles** (thin-walled cystic spaces lined primarily by respiratory tissue), which develops when an abscess breaks into an airway. Cavitation and pleural effusions are common complications of staphylococcal pneumonia, but empyema is infrequent. Staphylococcal pneumonia requires aggressive therapy, particularly because *S. aureus* is often antibiotic resistant.

Legionella Pneumonia

In 1976, a mysterious respiratory ailment that carried a high mortality broke out at an American Legion convention in Philadelphia. The responsible organism, *Legionella pneumophila*, was soon identified as a fastidious bacterium, with special requirements for growth in culture. *Legionella* organisms thrive in aquatic environments, and outbreaks of pneumonia have been traced to contaminated water in air-conditioning cooling towers, evaporative condensers, and construction sites. Person-to-person spread does not occur, and there is no animal or human reservoir.

PATHOLOGY: In fatal cases of *Legionella* pneumonia, multiple lobes exhibit a bronchopneumonia, with large confluent areas. Microscopically, alveoli contain fibrin and inflammatory cells, with either neutrophils or macrophages predominating. Necrosis of inflammatory cells (leukocytoclasis) may be extensive. One third of cases have been complicated by empyema. *Legionella* organisms are usually abundant within and outside the phagocytic cells but require special stains for visualization.

CLINICAL FEATURES: The onset of *Legionella* pneumonia tends to be abrupt, with malaise, fever, muscle aches and pains and, curiously, abdominal pain. A productive cough is usual, and chest pain due to pleuritis occasionally occurs. Mortality rates have been high (10% to 20%), especially in immunocompromised patients. Erythromycin is the antibiotic of choice.

Opportunistic Pneumonia Caused by Gram-Negative Bacteria

Pneumonias caused by gram-negative organisms have become more common with the advent of immunosuppressive and cytotoxic therapies, treatment with broad-spectrum antibiotics, and AIDS. The most common bacteria are *Escherichia coli* and *Pseudomonas aeruginosa;* the latter is also a common pathogen in patients with cystic fibrosis.

Anthrax Pneumonia and Pneumonic Plague

Recent world events have refocused attention on infectious agents that may be used as potential weapons of bioterrorism. Chief among these are *Bacillus anthracis* and *Yersinia pestis. B. anthracis*, the causative agent of anthrax, is a gram-positive, spore-forming bacillus. Anthrax occurs in many species of domestic animals, and infection of humans is seen infrequently, most often as a nonfatal cutaneous infection in agricultural workers. Anthrax spores are highly resistant to heat and drying, and when inhaled, they are transported to mediastinal lymph nodes. From there, bacilli emerge and rapidly disseminate. In the lungs, the disease is manifested by hemorrhagic bronchitis and confluent areas of hemorrhagic pneumonia. Anthrax is susceptible to antibiotic therapy.

Yersinia pestis, the causative agent of plague, produces three forms of infection, namely a bubonic form, a pneumonic form, and a rarely encountered septicemic form. In pneumonic plague,

the organisms are inhaled directly without transmission by an arthropod vector, and the disease may be spread from person to person or animal (such as a cat) to person. The lungs typically show extensive hemorrhagic bronchopneumonia, pleuritis, and enlargement of mediastinal lymph nodes. The untreated disease progresses rapidly and is often fatal.

Mycoplasma Pneumoniae Causes Atypical Pneumonia

In contrast to lobar pneumonia, the onset of atypical pneumonia is insidious, leukocytosis is absent or slight, and the course is prolonged. Respiratory symptoms may range from minimal to severe. The infection characteristically causes a bronchiolitis with a neutrophilic intraluminal exudate and an intense lymphoplasmacytic infiltrate in the bronchiolar wall (Fig. 12-9). Erythromycin is effective, and the infection is only rarely fatal.

Tuberculosis is the Classic Granulomatous Infection

Tuberculosis represents infection with *Mycobacterium tuberculosis,* although atypical mycobacterial infections may mimic tuberculosis. The disease is divided into primary and secondary (or reactivation) tuberculosis. The infection is discussed in detail in Chapter 9.

Fungal Infections May be Geographic or Opportunistic

Fungal infections of the lung, including **Histoplasmosis, Coccidioidomycosis, Cryptococcosis, North American blastomycosis,** *Aspergillosis*, and **Pneumocystis,** all cause pulmonary infections, which are discussed in detail in Chapter 9.

Viral Infections of the Lung Produce Diffuse Alveolar Damage or Interstitial Pneumonia

PATHOLOGY: Viral infections initially affect the alveolar epithelium and result in a mononuclear infiltrate in the interstitium of the lung (Fig. 12-10). Necrosis of type I epithelial cells and the formation of hyaline membranes result in an appearance that is indistinguishable from diffuse alveolar damage from other causes (see below). In some instances, alveolar damage may be indolent, and the disease is characterized by hyperplasia of type II pneumocytes and interstitial inflammation. This appearance contrasts with that of most

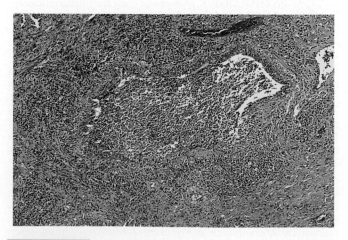

FIGURE 12-9. **Mycoplasma pneumonia.** Chronic bronchiolitis with a neutrophilic luminal exudate.

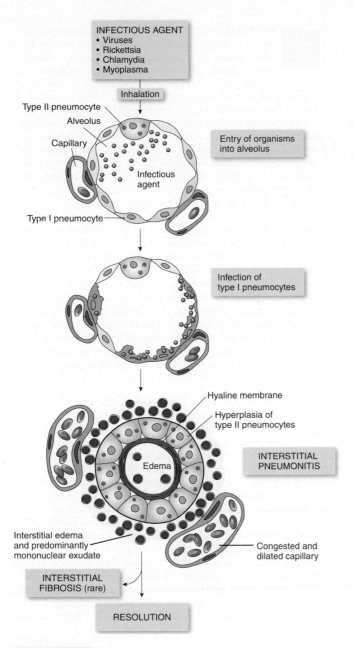

FIGURE 12-10. **Pathogenesis of interstitial pneumonia.** Although interstitial pneumonia is most commonly caused by viruses, other organisms may also cause significant interstitial inflammation. Type I cells are the most sensitive to damage, and loss of their integrity leads to intra-alveolar edema. The proteinaceous exudate and cell debris form hyaline membranes, and type II cells multiply to line the alveoli. Interstitial inflammation is characterized mainly by mononuclear cells. The disease generally resolves completely but occasionally progresses to interstitial fibrosis.

bacterial infections, in which intra-alveolar exudates predominate and the interstitium is only incidentally involved.

Cytomegalovirus produces a characteristic pneumonia that features an intense interstitial lymphocytic infiltrate. The alveoli are lined by type II cells that have regenerated to cover the epithelial defect left by necrosis of type I cells. The infected alveolar cells are very large (cytomegaly) and display a single, dark, basophilic nuclear inclusion with a peripheral halo and multiple indistinct cytoplasmic, basophilic inclusions.

Measles infection, which involves both the airways and the parenchyma, is characterized by very large (100 μm across) multinucleated giant cells that have nuclear inclusions and large

eosinophilic cytoplasmic inclusions. Although interstitial pneumonia is a well-characterized complication of measles, it is rarely fatal, except in immunocompromised, previously unexposed persons.

Varicella infection (both chickenpox and herpes zoster) produces disseminated, focally necrotic lesions in the lung as well as interstitial pneumonia. Pulmonary involvement is usually asymptomatic; however, in immunocompromised persons, it may be fatal. The viral inclusions are nuclear, eosinophilic, refractile and are surrounded by a clear halo. Multinucleation can occur.

Herpes simplex can cause necrotizing tracheobronchitis as well as diffuse alveolar damage. The viral inclusions are identical to those seen in varicella infection.

Adenovirus pneumonia results in a necrotizing bronchiolitis and bronchopneumonia. It can cause two types of nuclear inclusions: eosinophilic nuclear inclusions surrounded by a clear halo and "smudge cells," with indistinct, basophilic, nuclear inclusions that fill the entire nucleus and are surrounded by only a thin rim of chromatin.

Lung Abscess

Lung abscess is a localized accumulation of pus accompanied by the destruction of pulmonary parenchyma, including alveoli, airways, and blood vessels, which is most often caused by aspiration of anaerobic bacteria from the oropharynx. Infections are typically polymicrobial, with fusiform bacteria and *Bacteroides* species often isolated.

PATHOGENESIS: The aspiration that leads to pulmonary abscesses often occurs in the setting of depressed consciousness. Not surprisingly, alcoholism is the single most common predisposing condition. The deposition of enough bacteria to produce a lung abscess requires two conditions. A large number of

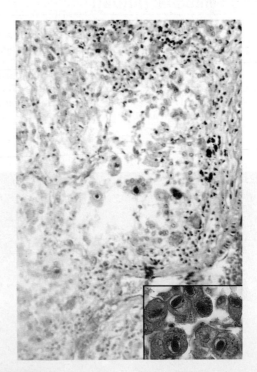

FIGURE 12-11. **Cytomegalovirus pneumonitis.** The infected alveolar cells are enlarged and display the typical dark-blue nuclear inclusions. *(Inset)* A higher-power view shows infected alveolar cells that display a single basophilic nuclear inclusion with a perinuclear halo and multiple, indistinct, basophilic, cytoplasmic inclusions.

anaerobic bacteria must be present in the oral flora, as in persons with poor oral hygiene or periodontal disease. In addition, the cough reflex or tracheobronchial clearance must be impaired, as is the case in alcoholics, those suffering from drug overdose, epileptics, and neurologically impaired persons. Other causes of lung abscess include necrotizing pneumonias, bronchial obstruction, infected pulmonary emboli, penetrating trauma, and extension of infection from tissues adjacent to the lung.

PATHOLOGY: Lung abscesses mostly range from 2 to 6 cm in diameter, and 10% to 20% have multiple cavities. They exhibit abundant polymorphonuclear leukocytes and, depending on the age of the lesion, variable numbers of macrophages. Debris from necrotic tissue may be evident. The abscess is surrounded by hemorrhage, fibrin, and inflammatory cells. As the abscess ages, a fibrous wall forms around the margin. The cavity thus formed contains air, necrotic debris, and inflammatory exudate (Fig. 12-12), creating a fluid level that is easily seen radiographically.

CLINICAL FEATURES: Almost all patients with lung abscess present with cough, fever, and the production of large amounts of foul-smelling sputum. Many patients complain of pleuritic chest pain, and 20% develop hemoptysis. Complications of lung abscess include rupture into the pleural space, with resulting empyema and severe hemoptysis. The abscess may drain into a bronchus, with subsequent dissemination of the infection to other parts of the lung. Despite vigorous antimicrobial therapy, principally directed against anaerobic bacteria, the mortality rate of lung abscess remains 5% to 10%.

Diffuse Alveolar Damage (Acute Respiratory Distress Syndrome [ARDS])

Diffuse alveolar damage (DAD) refers to a pattern of reaction to injury of alveolar epithelial and endothelial cells from a variety of acute insults. The clinical counterpart of DAD is ARDS. In this disorder, a patient with apparently normal lungs sustains pulmonary damage and then develops rapidly progressive respiratory failure. The overall mortality rate of DAD is more than 50%, and in patients older than 60 years, it is as high as 90%.

PATHOGENESIS: DAD is the common pathological endpoint of a large variety of pulmonary insults. These include respiratory tract infections, sepsis, shock, aspiration of gastric contents, inhalation of toxic gases, near-drowning, radiation pneumonitis, and a large assortment of drugs and other chemicals. These diverse conditions share the ability to injure the epithelial and endothelial cells of the alveoli, thereby producing DAD. *Hence, the precise cause of DAD cannot be determined from the morphologic appearance of the lung alone, unless caused by a specific identifiable infectious agent.* Some patients have an idiopathic form of DAD referred to clinically as **acute interstitial pneumonia**. The mechanism of pulmonary injury resulting in DAD is not entirely clear. It is thought that activation of complement (e.g., by endotoxin in the case of gram-negative septicemia) results in the sequestration of neutrophils and their subsequent activation. In turn, the neutrophils release oxygen radicals and hydrolytic enzymes, which damage the capillary endothelium of the lung. However, ARDS has also been reported to occur in severely neutropenic patients. In DAD produced by inhalation of toxic gases or near-drowning, the damage occurs primarily at the alveolar epithelial surface. The alveolar epithelial junctions are usually very tight; damage to the epithelium disrupts these junctions, permitting exudation of fluid and proteins from the interstitium into the alveolar spaces.

PATHOLOGY: As DAD evolves, the initial exudative phase is followed by an organizing phase.

The exudative phase of DAD develops during the first week after the pulmonary insult and features edema, leakage of plasma proteins, accumulation of inflammatory cells, and hyaline membranes (Fig. 12-13). The earliest alveolar injury is characterized by degenerative changes in endothelial cells and type I pneumocytes. This is followed by sloughing of type I cells, leaving alveolar basement membranes denuded. Interstitial and alveolar edema is prominent by the first day but soon recedes. "Hyaline membranes" begin to appear by the second day and are the most conspicuous morphologic feature of the exudative phase after 4 to 5 days. These eosinophilic, glassy "membranes" consist of precipitated plasma proteins as well as cytoplasmic and nuclear debris from sloughed epithelial cells. Interstitial inflammation, consisting of lymphocytes, plasma cells, and macrophages, is apparent early and reaches its maximum in about a week. Toward

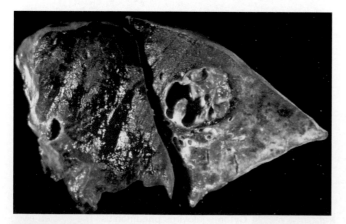

FIGURE 12-12. Pulmonary abscess. A large, cystic abscess contains a purulent exudate and is contained by a fibrous wall. Pneumonia is present in the surrounding pulmonary parenchyma.

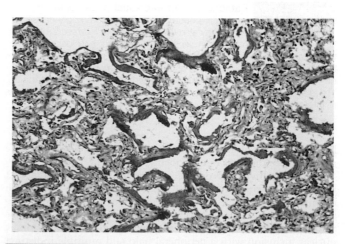

FIGURE 12-13. Diffuse alveolar damage, acute (exudative) phase. The alveolar septa are thickened by edema and a sparse inflammatory infiltrate. The alveoli are lined by eosinophilic hyaline membranes.

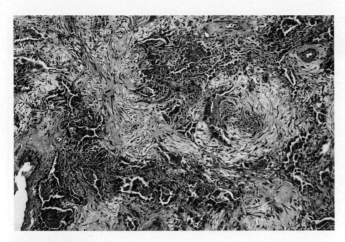

FIGURE 12-14. Diffuse alveolar damage, acute and organizing phase. In addition to hyaline membranes, the alveolar walls are thickened by fibroblasts and loose connective tissue.

the end of the first week and persisting during the subsequent organizing stage, regularly spaced, cuboidal type II pneumocytes become arrayed along the denuded alveolar septa. The alveolar capillaries and pulmonary arterioles may exhibit fibrin thrombi. In fatal cases of DAD, the lungs are heavy, edematous, and virtually airless.

The organizing phase of DAD, beginning about a week after the initial injury, is marked by the proliferation of fibroblasts within alveolar walls (Fig. 12-14). Interstitial inflammation and proliferated type II pneumocytes persist, but hyaline membranes are no longer formed. Alveolar macrophages digest the remnants of hyaline membranes and other cellular debris. Loose fibrosis thickens the alveolar septa. This fibrosis resolves in mild cases. In patients who do not recover, DAD can progress to end-stage fibrosis; remodeling of the lung architecture produces multiple cyst-like spaces throughout the lung (**honeycomb lung**). These spaces are separated from each other by fibrous tissue and lined by type II pneumocytes, bronchiolar epithelium, or squamous cells.

 CLINICAL FEATURES: Patients destined to develop ARDS have a symptom-free interval for a few hours after the initial insult, after which tachypnea and dyspnea mark the onset of the syndrome. As ARDS progresses, dyspnea worsens, and the patient becomes cyanotic. Diffuse, bilateral, interstitial, and alveolar infiltrates are noted radiologically. Arterial hypoxemia at this stage cannot be reversed simply by increasing oxygen tension in the inspired air, and mechanical ventilation becomes necessary. Fatal cases eventuate in alveolar hypoventilation, progressive hypoxemia, and increasing P_{CO_2}. Patients who survive ARDS may recover normal pulmonary function but, in severe cases, are left with scarred lungs, respiratory dysfunction, and in some instances, pulmonary hypertension.

Diffuse Alveolar Damage May Have Specific Causes

Specific noninfectious etiologies of DAD include the following:

- **Oxygen:** It is usually safe to breathe 40% to 50% oxygen for long periods, but normal persons breathing 75% oxygen for as little as 24 hours have shown evidence of early signs of pulmonary toxicity. Such toxicity is thought to be caused by increased production of activated oxygen species in the lung (see Chapter 1).
- **Shock:** ARDS often follows shock from any cause, including gram-negative sepsis, trauma, or blood loss, in which case the pulmonary condition is colloquially referred to as "shock lung." The pathogenesis of DAD associated with shock is poorly understood and is likely multifactorial.

- **Aspiration:** Aspiration of gastric contents introduces acid with a pH less than 3.0 into the alveoli. The severe chemical injury to the alveolar-lining cells leads to DAD. In near drowning, aspiration of water produces pulmonary injury and DAD.
- **Drug-Induced Diffuse Alveolar Damage:** Many drugs cause DAD, especially cytotoxic chemotherapeutic agents such as bleomycin. Bizarre, atypical, hyperchromatic nuclei in type II cells are particularly common in cases of alveolar damage from chemotherapy. Damage progresses despite discontinuation of the offending agent, although it may be modified by administering corticosteroids. Progressive interstitial fibrosis occurs, usually with retention of lung structure. Drugs other than chemotherapeutic agents (e.g. nitrofurantoin, amiodarone, and penicillamine) may also cause DAD.
- **Radiation Pneumonitis:** Radiation pneumonitis occurs in two forms: acute DAD and chronic pulmonary fibrosis. Alveolar injury is believed to be caused by oxygen radicals generated by the radiolysis of water (see Chapter 1). **Acute radiation pneumonitis** occurs in as many as 10% of patients irradiated for cancer of the lung or breast or for mediastinal lymphoma. DAD caused by radiation is mostly dose related, appears 1 to 6 months after radiation therapy, and is usually followed by recovery. **Chronic radiation pneumonitis** is characterized by interstitial fibrosis and may follow acute DAD or may develop insidiously. The disease remains asymptomatic unless a substantial volume of the lung is affected.
- **Paraquat:** The ingestion of the widely used herbicide paraquat is associated with DAD. Pulmonary disease becomes apparent 4 to 7 days after ingestion, as ARDS develops. Patients rarely recover once pulmonary complications have evolved. The intra-alveolar exudate organizes in such a way that the alveolar framework persists, and the airspaces are filled with loose granulation tissue.

Respiratory Distress Syndrome of the Newborn is a Counterpart of ARDS

The counterpart of ARDS in the neonatal period is termed **newborn respiratory distress syndrome (NRDS)**. NRDS, also called **hyaline membrane disease**, is a result of immaturity in the surfactant system at birth, usually as a consequence of severe prematurity. NRDS and bronchopulmonary dysplasia are discussed in detail in Chapter 6.

Diffuse Pulmonary Hemorrhage Syndromes

Diffuse alveolar hemorrhage can occur in diverse clinical settings (Table 12-1). Histologically, the diseases are characterized by acute hemorrhage (intra-alveolar red blood cells) or chronic hemorrhage (hemosiderosis). In virtually all of these disorders, a neutrophilic infiltrate of the alveolar wall (**neutrophilic capillaritis**) is present. This lesion tends to be most prominent in hemorrhagic syndromes associated with Wegener granulomatosis or systemic lupus erythematosus. A linear pattern of fluorescence is seen in antibasement membrane antibody disease, termed Goodpasture syndrome. A granular pattern is present in immune complex–associated diseases, such as systemic lupus erythematosus. Pauci-immune disorders consist of antineutrophil cytoplasm antibody-associated diseases (e.g., Wegener granulomatosis or idiopathic pulmonary hemorrhage syndromes), in which no etiology or immunologic mechanism can be determined (see Table 12-1). For additional details, see Chapters 10 and 16.

TABLE 12-1

Conditions of Pulmonary Hemorrhage

Disease	Immunological Mechanism	Immunofluorescence Pattern
Goodpasture syndrome	Antibasement membrane antibody	Linear
Systemic lupus erythematosus	Immune complexes	Granular
Mixed cryoglobulinemia		
Henoch-Schönlein purpura		
IgA disease		
Wegener granulomatosis	Antineutrophil cytoplasmic antibody	Negative or pauci-immune
Idiopathic glomerulonephritis		
Idiopathic pulmonary hemorrhage	No immunological marker	

Obstructive Pulmonary Diseases

Several different diseases, including chronic bronchitis, emphysema, asthma, and in some classifications, bronchiectasis and cystic fibrosis, are grouped together as obstructive pulmonary diseases because they have in common an obstruction to air flow in the lungs. Chronic obstructive pulmonary disease applies to chronic bronchitis and emphysema, in which forced expiratory volume, measured by spirometry, is decreased. In the lung, narrowed airways produce increased resistance, whereas loss of elastic recoil results in diminished pressure. Airway narrowing occurs in chronic bronchitis or asthma, and emphysema causes loss of recoil.

Chronic Bronchitis is a Chronic Productive Cough for More Than half of the Time Over 2 Years

Chronic bronchitis is primarily a disease of cigarette smokers (see Chapter 8), and 90% of cases occur in persons who smoke. The frequency and severity of acute respiratory tract infections are increased in patients with chronic bronchitis. Conversely, infections have been incriminated in the etiology and progression of the disorder. Although chronic bronchitis is more common among urban dwellers in areas of substantial air pollution and in workers exposed to toxic industrial inhalants, the effects of cigarette smoking far outweigh other contributing factors.

 PATHOLOGY: The main morphologic finding in chronic bronchitis is an increase in size of the bronchial mucus-secreting apparatus (Fig. 12-15). Two types of cells line the mucous glands: pale mucous cells, which are more common, and serous cells, which are more basophilic and contain granules. *Chronic bronchitis is characterized by hyperplasia and hypertrophy of the mucous cells and an increased ratio of mucous to serous cells.* Thus, both the individual acini and the glands enlarge (Fig. 12-16).

Other morphologic changes in chronic bronchitis are variable and include:

- Thickening of the bronchial wall by mucous gland enlargement and edema, which leads to encroachment on the bronchial lumen
- An increase in the number of goblet cells (hyperplasia) in the bronchial epithelium
- Increased smooth muscle, which may indicate bronchial hyperreactivity
- Squamous metaplasia of the bronchial epithelium, reflecting epithelial damage from tobacco smoke, which is probably independent of the other changes seen in chronic bronchitis

 CLINICAL FEATURES: Chronic bronchitis is often accompanied by emphysema (see below); it is often difficult to separate the relative contribution of each disease to the clinical presentation. In general, patients with predomi-

nantly chronic bronchitis have had a productive cough for many years that is initially more severe in the winter months. As the malady becomes more chronic, coughing becomes constant, exertional dyspnea and cyanosis supervene, and cor pulmonale may ensue. The combination of cyanosis and edema secondary to cor pulmonale has led to the label "blue bloater" for such patients. Acute respiratory failure in patients with advanced chronic bronchitis consists of progressive hypoxemia and hypercapnia.

Emphysema Causes Overinflation of the Lungs in Smokers

Emphysema is a chronic lung disease characterized by enlargement of air spaces distal to the terminal bronchioles, with destruction of their walls but

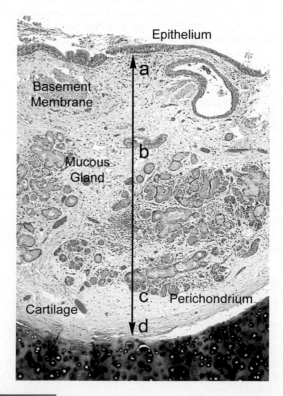

FIGURE 12-15. **Chronic bronchitis.** The bronchial submucosa is greatly expanded by hyperplastic submucosal glands that compose well over 50% of the thickness of the bronchial wall. The Reid index equals the maximum thickness of the bronchial mucous glands internal to the cartilage *(b to c)* divided by the bronchial wall thickness *(a to d)*.

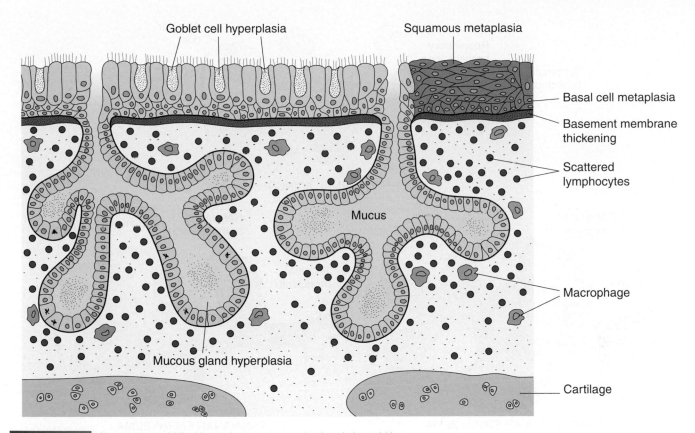

Goblet cell hyperplasia

Squamous metaplasia

Mucus

Basal cell metaplasia

Basement membrane thickening

Scattered lymphocytes

Macrophage

Mucous gland hyperplasia

Cartilage

FIGURE 12-16. **Chronic bronchitis.** Morphological changes in chronic bronchitis.

without fibrosis. Although emphysema is classified in anatomical terms, *the severity of emphysema is more important than the type.*

 PATHOGENESIS: *The major cause of emphysema is cigarette smoking, and moderate-to-severe emphysema is rare in nonsmokers (see Chapter 8).* A balance exists between elastin synthesis and catabolism in the lung. Emphysema results when elastolytic activity increases or when antielastolytic activity is reduced. Increased numbers of neutrophils, which contain serine elastase and other proteases, are found in the bronchoalveolar lavage fluid of smokers. Smoking also interferes with α_1-antitrypsin (α_1-AT) activity by oxidizing methionine residues in α_1-antitrypsin. Hence, unopposed and increased elastolytic activity leads to destruction of elastic tissue in the walls of distal air spaces, thereby impairing elastic recoil.

A_1-AT DEFICIENCY: A hereditary deficiency in α_1-AT, which is coded for by the Pi (protease inhibitor) locus, accounts for only about 1% of all patients with COPD, but most patients with emphysema under age 40 have this deficiency. α_1-AT, circulating glycoprotein produced in the liver, is a major inhibitor of a variety of proteases, including elastase, trypsin, chymotrypsin, thrombin, and bacterial proteases. In fact, this protein accounts for 90% of antiproteinase activity in the blood. In the lung, it inhibits neutrophil elastase, an enzyme that digests elastin and other structural components of the alveolar septa.

The most serious abnormality is associated with the *PiZ* allele, which occurs in approximately 5% of the population. It is more common in persons of Scandinavian origin and is rare in the Jewish population, blacks, and Japanese. *PiZZ* homozygotes have only 15% to 20% of the normal plasma concentration of α_1-AT because the abnormal protein is poorly secreted by the liver. These persons are at risk for both cir-

rhosis of the liver (see Chapter 14) and emphysema. In fact, *PiZZ* homozygotes who do not smoke show a mean age at onset of emphysema between ages 45 and 50 years; those who smoke develop it at about age 35. However, two thirds of nonsmoking *PiZZ* homozygotes show no evidence of emphysema.

PATHOLOGY: Emphysema is morphologically classified according to the location of the lesions within the pulmonary acinus (Fig. 12-17). Only the proximal part of the acinus (respiratory bronchiole) is selectively involved in centrilobular emphysema, whereas the entire acinus is destroyed in panacinar emphysema.

CENTRILOBULAR EMPHYSEMA: This form of emphysema is most frequent and is usually associated with cigarette smoking and with clinical symptoms. Centrilobular emphysema is characterized by the destruction of the cluster of terminal bronchioles near the end of the bronchiolar tree in the central part of the pulmonary lobule (Fig. 12-18A). Dilated respiratory bronchioles form enlarged air spaces, which are separated from each other and from the lobular septa by normal alveolar ducts and alveoli. As centrilobular emphysema progresses, bronchioles proximal to the emphysematous spaces are inflamed and narrowed (see Fig. 12-18B). Centrilobular emphysema is most severe in the upper lobes and the superior segments of the lower lobes.

PANACINAR EMPHYSEMA: In panacinar emphysema, the acinus is uniformly involved, with destruction of the alveolar septa from the center to the periphery of the acinus. The loss of alveolar septa is illustrated in the histologic comparison of lung affected by α_1-AT deficiency with a normal lung at the same magnification (Fig. 12-19). In the final stage, panacinar emphysema leaves behind a lacy network of supporting tissue ("cotton-candy lung").

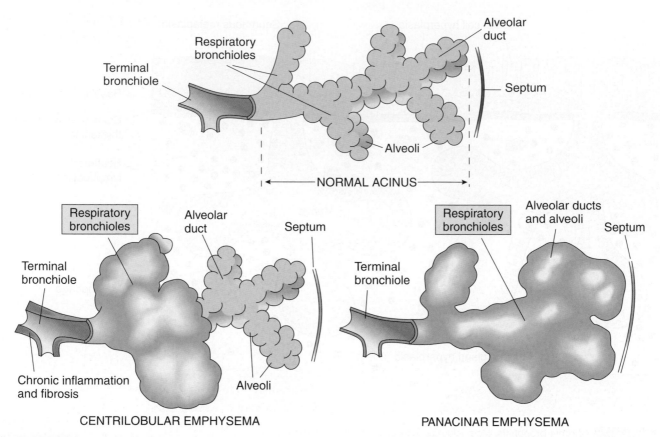

FIGURE 12-17. **Types of emphysema.** The acinus is the unit gas-exchanging structure of the lung distal to the terminal bronchiole. It consists of (in order) respiratory bronchioles, alveolar ducts, alveolar sacs, and alveoli. In centrilobular (proximal acinar) emphysema, the respiratory bronchioles are predominantly involved. In paraseptal (distal acinar) emphysema, the alveolar ducts are particularly affected. In panacinar (panlobular) emphysema, the acinus is uniformly damaged.

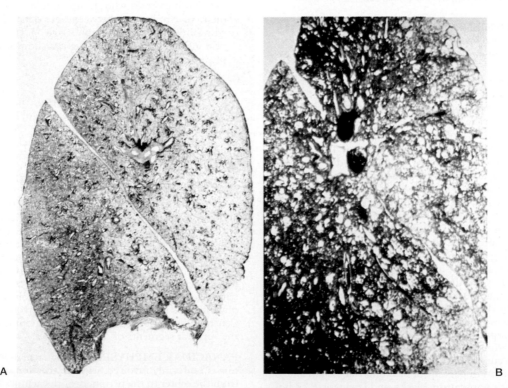

FIGURE 12-18. **Centrilobular emphysema. A.** A whole mount of the left lung of a smoker with mild emphysema shows enlarged air spaces scattered throughout both lobes, which represent destruction of the terminal bronchioles in the central part of the pulmonary lobule. These abnormal spaces are surrounded by intact pulmonary parenchyma. **B.** In a more advanced case of centrilobular emphysema, the destruction of the lung has progressed to produce large, irregular air spaces.

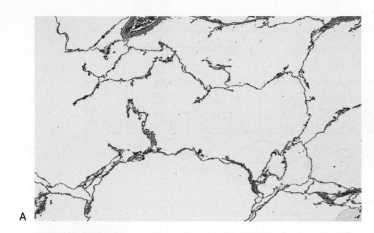
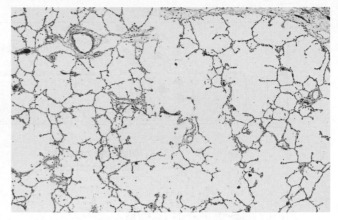

A   B

FIGURE 12-19. **Panacinar emphysema. A.** This lung, from a patient with α_1-antitrypsin deficiency, shows large, irregular air spaces and a markedly reduced number of alveolar walls. **B.** The extensive loss of alveolar walls in **A** is emphasized by comparison with this section of normal lung at the same magnification.

Diffuse panacinar emphysema is typically associated with α_1-AT deficiency, but it is also often found in cigarette smokers in association with centrilobular emphysema. In such cases, the panacinar pattern tends to occur in the lower zones of the lung, whereas centrilobular emphysema is seen in the upper regions.

LOCALIZED EMPHYSEMA: This condition, previously known as "paraseptal emphysema," is characterized by destruction of alveoli and resulting emphysema in only one, or at most, a few locations. The remainder of the lungs is normal. The lesion is usually found at the apex of an upper lobe, although it may occur anywhere in the pulmonary parenchyma, such as in a subpleural location. Although it is of no clinical significance itself, rupture of an area of localized emphysema produces spontaneous pneumothorax (see below). Progression of localized emphysema can result in a large area of destruction, termed a **bulla**, which ranges in size from as small as 2 cm to a large lesion that occupies much of a hemothorax.

CLINICAL FEATURES: Most patients with symptomatic emphysema are seen at age 60 years or older with a prolonged history of exertional dyspnea but with a minimal, nonproductive cough. Tachypnea and a prolonged expiratory phase are typical. The most prominent radiologic abnormality is overinflation of the lung, as evidenced by enlarged lungs, depressed diaphragms, and an increased posteroanterior diameter (barrel chest). Because these patients have a higher respiratory rate and an increased minute volume, they can maintain arterial hemoglobin saturation at near-normal levels and so are called "pink puffers." The clinical course of emphysema is marked by inexorable decline in respiratory function and progressive dyspnea, for which no treatment is adequate.

Asthma is Characterized by Episodic Airflow Obstruction

Patients who suffer from asthma typically have paroxysms of wheezing, dyspnea, and cough. Acute episodes of asthma may alternate with asymptomatic periods or may be superimposed on a background of chronic airway obstruction. Severe acute asthma unresponsive to therapy is termed **status asthmaticus**. Most asthmatic patients, even when apparently well, have some persistent airflow obstruction and morphologic lesions.

In the United States, bronchial asthma affects up to 10% of children and 5% of adults. For unknown reasons, the prevalence of asthma in the United States has doubled since 1980. Although the initial attack of the disease can occur at any age, half of the cases appear in patients younger than 10 years, and the incidence is twice as high in boys as in girls. By age 30, both genders are affected equally.

PATHOGENESIS: Asthma was classically divided into extrinsic (allergic) and intrinsic (idiosyncratic) categories, depending on inciting factors. *The consensus hypothesis attributes bronchial hyperresponsiveness in asthma to an inflammatory reaction produced by diverse stimuli.* After exposure to an inciting factor (e.g., allergens, drugs, cold, exercise), inflammatory mediators released by activated macrophages, mast cells, eosinophils, and basophils induce bronchoconstriction, increased vascular permeability, and mucus secretion, and serve to recruit additional effector cells. Inflammation of the bronchial walls also may injure the epithelium, stimulating nerve endings and initiating neural reflexes that further aggravate and propagate the bronchospasm.

The best-studied situation associated with the induction of asthma is that of inhaled allergens. In a sensitized person, an inhaled allergen interacts with T_H2 cells and IgE antibody bound to the surface of mast cells, which are interspersed among the epithelial cells of the bronchial mucosa (Fig. 12-20). As a result, T_H2 cells and mast cells release mediators of type I (immediate) hypersensitivity, including histamine, bradykinin, leukotrienes, prostaglandins, thromboxane A_2, and platelet-activating factor (PAF), as well as cytokines such as interleukin (IL)-4 and IL-5. The inflammatory mediators cause (1) smooth muscle contraction, (2) mucous secretion, and (3) increased vascular permeability and edema. Each of these effects is a potent, albeit reversible, cause of airway obstruction. IL-5 produces terminal differentiation of eosinophils in the bone marrow. Chemotactic factors, including leukotriene B_4 as well as neutrophil and eosinophil chemotactic factors, attract neutrophils, eosinophils, and platelets to the bronchial wall. In turn, eosinophils release leukotriene B_4 and PAF, thereby aggravating bronchoconstriction and edema. The discharge of eosinophil granules, which contain eosinophil cationic protein and major basic protein, into the bronchial lumen further impairs mucociliary function and damages epithelial cells. Epithelial cell injury is suspected to stimulate nerve endings in the mucosa, initiating an autonomic discharge that contributes to airway narrowing and mucous secretion. Moreover, leukotriene B_4 and PAF recruit more eosinophils and other effector cells, and so continue the vicious circle that prolongs and amplifies the asthmatic attack. Recent evidence suggests that activated T lymphocytes also help propagate the inflammatory response through various cytokine networks.

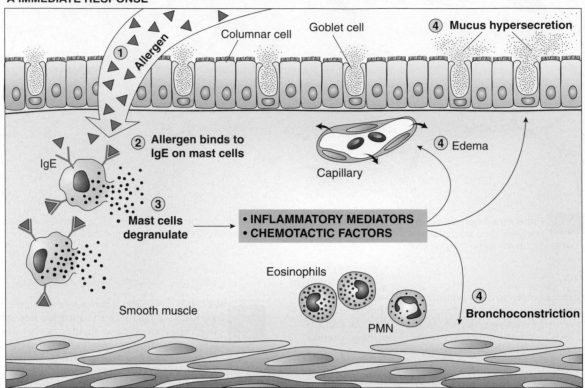

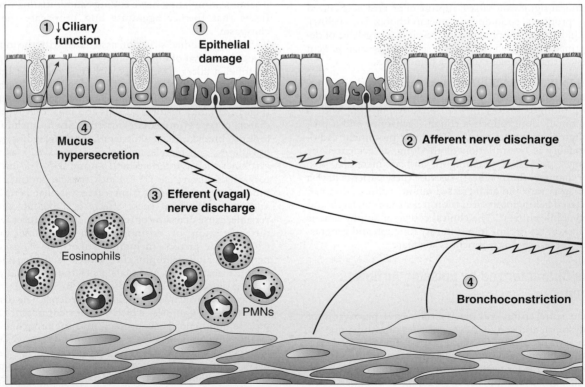

FIGURE 12-20. **Pathogenesis of asthma. A.** Immunologically mediated asthma. Allergens interact with immunoglobulin E (IgE) on mast cells, either on the surface of the epithelium or, when there is abnormal permeability of the epithelium, in the submucosa. Mediators are released and may react locally or by reflexes mediated through the vagus. **B.** The discharge of eosinophilic granules further impairs mucociliary function and damages epithelial cells. Epithelial cell injury stimulates nerve endings in the mucosa, thereby initiating an autonomic discharge that contributes to airway narrowing and mucus secretion. PMNs, polymorphonuclear neutrophils.

ALLERGIC ASTHMA: This is the most common form of asthma and is usually seen in children. One third to one half of all patients with asthma have known or suspected reactions to allergens such as pollens, animal hair, or fur, and house dust contaminated with mites.

INFECTIOUS ASTHMA: A common precipitating factor in childhood asthma is a viral respiratory tract infection. In children under 2 years of age, RSV is the usual agent; in older children, rhinovirus, influenza, and parainfluenza are common inciting organisms.

EXERCISE-INDUCED ASTHMA: Exercise can precipitate bronchospasm in more than half of all asthmatics. In some patients, exercise is the only inciting factor. Exercise-induced asthma is related to the magnitude of heat or water loss from the airway epithelium. The more rapid the ventilation (severity of exercise) and the colder and drier the air breathed, the more likely is an attack of asthma. The condition may be the consequence of mediator release or vascular congestion in the bronchi secondary to rewarming of the airways after the exertion.

OCCUPATIONAL ASTHMA: More than 80 different occupational exposures have been linked to the development of asthma. In some instances, these substances provoke allergic asthma via IgE-related hypersensitivity. Examples are animal handlers, bakers, and workers exposed to wood and vegetable dusts, metal salts, pharmaceutical agents, and industrial chemicals. In other cases, occupational asthma seems to result from direct release of mediators of smooth muscle contraction after contact with an offending agent. Such a mechanism is postulated in byssinosis ("brown lung"), an occupational lung disease in cotton workers.

DRUG-INDUCED ASTHMA: Drug-induced bronchospasm occurs mostly in patients with known asthma. The best-known offender is aspirin, but other nonsteroidal anti-inflammatory agents have also been implicated. It is estimated that up to 10% of adult asthmatics are sensitive to aspirin.

AIR POLLUTION: Massive air pollution, usually in episodes associated with temperature inversions, is associated with bronchospasm in patients with asthma and other pre-existing lung diseases. Sulfur dioxide, oxides of nitrogen, and ozone are the commonly implicated environmental pollutants.

EMOTIONAL FACTORS: Psychological stress can aggravate or precipitate an attack of bronchospasm in as many as half of all asthmatics. It is believed that vagal efferent stimulation is the underlying mechanism.

 PATHOLOGY: Most information on the pathology of asthma has been derived from autopsies on patients who have died in status asthmaticus, and thus only the most severe lesions are described. On gross examination, the lungs are remarkably distended with air, and airways are filled with thick, tenacious, adherent mucus plugs. Microscopically, these plugs (Fig. 12-21A) contain strips of epithelium and many eosinophils. **Charcot-Leyden crystals,** derived from phospholipids of the eosinophil cell membrane, are also seen. In some cases, the mucoid exudate forms a cast of the airways (**Curschmann spirals**), which may be expelled with coughing.

One of the most characteristic features of status asthmaticus is hyperplasia of bronchial smooth muscle. Bronchial submucosal mucous glands are also hyperplastic (see Fig. 12-21A). The submucosa is edematous and contains a mixed inflammatory infiltrate, with variable numbers of eosinophils. The epithelium does not display the normal pseudostratified appearance and may be denuded, with only basal cells remaining (see Fig. 12-21B). The basal cells are hyper-

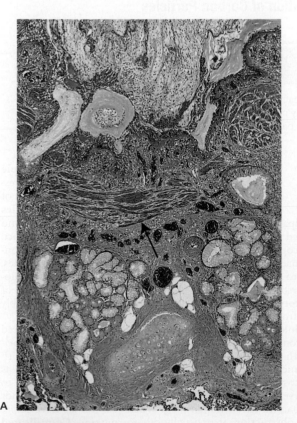

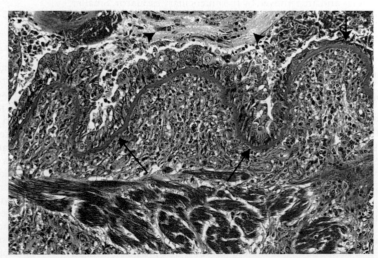

FIGURE 12-21. **Asthma. A.** A section of lung from a patient who died in status asthmaticus reveals a bronchus containing a luminal mucus plug, submucosal gland hyperplasia, and smooth muscle hyperplasia *(arrows)*. **B.** Higher magnification shows hyaline thickening of the subepithelial basement membrane and marked inflammation of the bronchiolar wall with numerous eosinophils. The mucosa exhibits an inflamed and metaplastic epithelium *(arrowheads)*. The epithelium is focally denuded *(short arrows)*.

plastic, and squamous metaplasia is seen. Goblet cell hyperplasia is also apparent. Characteristically, the epithelial basement membrane appears thickened.

 CLINICAL FEATURES: A typical asthma attack begins with a feeling of tightness in the chest and nonproductive cough. Both inspiratory and expiratory wheezes appear, the respiratory rate increases, and the patient becomes dyspneic. Characteristically, the expiratory phase is particularly prolonged. The end of the attack is often heralded by severe coughing and expectoration of thick, mucus-containing Curschmann spirals, eosinophils, and Charcot–Leyden crystals. *Status asthmaticus refers to severe bronchoconstriction that does not respond to the drugs that usually abort the acute attack.* This situation is potentially serious and requires hospitalization. Patients in status asthmaticus have hypoxemia and often hypercapnia, and in particularly severe episodes, they may die.

The cornerstone of asthma treatment includes administration of β-adrenergic agonists, inhaled corticosteroids, cromolyn sodium, methylxanthines, and anticholinergic agents. Systemic corticosteroids are reserved for status asthmaticus or resistant chronic asthma. The inhalation of bronchodilators often provides dramatic relief.

Pneumoconioses

The pneumoconioses are pulmonary diseases caused by dust inhalation. Most inhaled dusts are innocuous and simply accumulate in the lung. However, some lead to crippling pulmonary diseases. The specific types of pneumoconioses are named according to the substance inhaled (e.g., silicosis, asbestosis, talcosis) or, if the offending agent is uncertain, the occupation is simply cited (e.g., "arc welder's lung").

 PATHOGENESIS: *The most important factor in the production of symptomatic pneumoconioses is the capacity of inhaled dusts to stimulate fibrosis* (Fig. 12-22). Thus, small amounts of silica may produce extensive fibrosis, whereas coal and iron are only weakly fibrogenic. In general, lung lesions produced by inorganic dusts reflect the dose and size of the particles that reach the lung. The most dangerous particles are those that reach the peripheral zones (i.e., the smallest bronchioles and the acini). Particles greater than 10 μm in diameter deposit on bronchi and bronchioles and are removed by the mucociliary escalator. Smaller particles reach the acinus, and the smallest ones behave as a gas and are exhaled.

Silicosis is Caused by Inhalation of Silicon Dioxide (Silica)

Silicosis was described historically as a disease of sandblasters. Mining also involves exposure to silica, as do numerous other occupations. The use of air-handling equipment and face masks has substantially reduced the incidence of silicosis.

 PATHOGENESIS: After their inhalation, silica particles are ingested by alveolar macrophages. Silicon hydroxide groups on the surface of the particles form hydrogen bonds with phospholipids and proteins, an interaction that is presumed to damage cellular membranes and thereby kill the macrophages. The dead cells release free silica particles and fibrogenic factors. The released silica is ruben reingested by macrophages, and the process is amplified.

 PATHOLOGY:

SIMPLE NODULAR SILICOSIS: This is the most common form of silicosis and is almost inevitable in any worker with long-term exposure to silica. Ten to 40 years after the initial exposure to silica, the lungs contain silicotic nodules, which are less than 1 cm in diameter (usually 2 to 4 mm). On histologic examination, they have a characteristic whorled appearance, with concentrically arranged collagen that forms the largest part of the nodule (Fig. 12-23). At the periphery, there are aggregates of mononuclear cells, mostly lymphocytes and fibroblasts. Polarized light reveals doubly refractile needle-shaped silicates within the nodule. Hilar nodes may become enlarged and calcified, often at the periphery of the node ("eggshell calcification"). Simple silicosis is not ordinarily associated with significant respiratory dysfunction.

PROGRESSIVE MASSIVE FIBROSIS: Progressive massive fibrosis is defined radiologically as nodular masses of more than 2 cm diameter in a background of simple silicosis. These larger lesions represent the coalescence of smaller nodules. Most of these lesions are 5 to 10 cm across and are usually in the upper zones of the lungs bilaterally (Fig. 12-24). Morphologically, they often exhibit central cavitation. Disability is caused by destruction of lung tissue that has been incorporated into the nodules.

 CLINICAL FEATURES: Simple silicosis is usually a radiologic diagnosis without significant symptoms. Dyspnea on exertion and later at rest suggests progressive massive fibrosis or other complications of silicosis. *It is well recognized that tuberculosis is much more common in patients with silicosis than in the general population.* Silicosis does not predispose to lung cancer.

Coal Workers' Pneumoconiosis (CWP) Reflects Inhalation of Carbon Particles

PATHOGENESIS: Coal dust is composed of amorphous carbon and other constituents including variable amounts of silica. Amorphous carbon by itself is not fibrogenic because of its inability to kill alveolar macrophages and produces only an innocuous anthracosis. By contrast, silica is highly fibrogenic, and inhaled anthracotic particles may thus lead to **anthracosilicosis**.

 PATHOLOGY: CWP is typically divided into **simple CWP** and **complicated CWP** (also known as progressive massive fibrosis). The characteristic lung lesions of simple CWP include nonpalpable **coal-dust macules** and palpable **coal-dust nodules**. Both are typically multiple and scattered throughout the lung as 1- to 4-mm black foci. Microscopically, a coal-dust macule exhibits numerous carbon-laden macrophages that surround distal respiratory bronchioles, extend to fill adjacent alveolar spaces, and infiltrate peribronchiolar interstitial spaces. There is an accompanying mild dilation of respiratory bronchioles (focal dust emphysema), which probably results from atrophy of smooth muscle.

Nodules are round or irregular, may or may not be associated with bronchioles, and consist of dust-laden macrophages associated with a fibrotic stroma. They occur when coal is admixed with fibrogenic dusts, such as silica and are more properly classified as anthracosilicosis. Although simple CWP was once thought to cause severe disability, it is now clear that at worst, it causes minor pulmonary function impairment. When coal miners have severe airflow obstruction, it is usually due to smoking. **Complicated CWP** occurs on a background of simple CWP and is defined as a lesion 2.0 cm or greater in size. Patients with complicated CWP may have significant respiratory impairment.

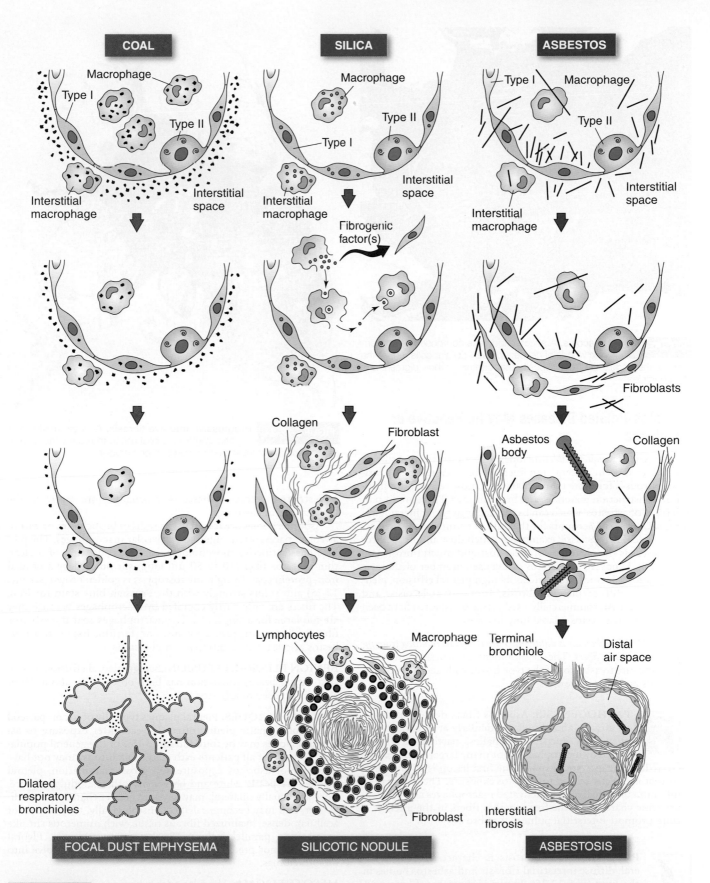

COAL

Macrophage

Type I

Type II

Interstitial macrophage

Interstitial space

SILICA

Macrophage

Type I

Type II

Interstitial macrophage

Interstitial space

Fibrogenic factor(s)

ASBESTOS

Type I

Macrophage

Type II

Interstitial macrophage

Interstitial space

Fibroblasts

Collagen

Fibroblast

Asbestos body

Collagen

Dilated respiratory bronchioles

Lymphocytes

Macrophage

Fibroblast

Terminal bronchiole

Distal air space

Interstitial fibrosis

FOCAL DUST EMPHYSEMA

SILICOTIC NODULE

ASBESTOSIS

FIGURE 12-22. **Pathogenesis of pneumoconioses.** The three most important pneumoconioses are illustrated. In simple coal workers' pneumoconiosis, massive amounts of dust are inhaled and engulfed by macrophages. The macrophages pass into the interstitium of the lung and aggregate around the respiratory bronchioles. Subsequently, the bronchioles dilate. In silicosis, the silica particles are toxic to macrophages, which die and release a fibrogenic factor. In turn, the released silica is again phagocytosed by other macrophages. The result is a dense fibrotic nodule, the silicotic nodule. Asbestosis is characterized by little dust and much interstitial fibrosis. Asbestos bodies are the classic features.

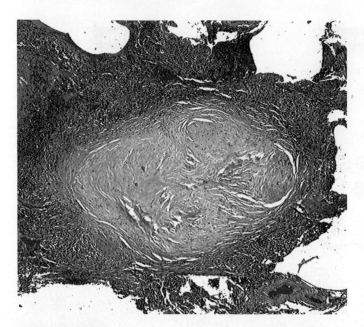

FIGURE 12-23. **Silicosis.** A silicotic nodule is composed of concentric whorls of dense, sparsely cellular collagen. At the edge of the nodule are dust deposits that contain carbon pigment and silica particles.

Asbestos-Related Diseases May be Reactive or Neoplastic

Asbestos (Greek, *unquenchable*) includes a group of fibrous silicate minerals that occur as long, thin fibers. It has been used for a variety of purposes for more than 4,000 years, most recently, for insulation, construction materials, and brake linings. There are six natural types of asbestos, which can be divided into two mineralogical groups. **Chrysotile** accounts for the bulk of commercially used asbestos. If coal is the classic example of much dust and little fibrosis, asbestos is the prototype of little dust and much fibrosis (see Fig. 12-22). Exposure to asbestos can cause a number of thoracic complications, including asbestosis, benign pleural effusion, pleural plaques, diffuse pleural fibrosis, rounded atelectasis, and mesothelioma. All commercially used forms of asbestos have been associated with asbestos-related lung diseases.

ASBESTOSIS: *Asbestosis is diffuse interstitial fibrosis resulting from inhalation of asbestos fibers.* The development of asbestosis requires heavy exposure to asbestos of the type historically seen in asbestos insulators and factory workers.

PATHOGENESIS: Asbestos fibers deposit in distal airways and alveoli, particularly at bifurcations of alveolar ducts. The smallest particles are engulfed by macrophages, but many larger fibers penetrate into the interstitial space. The first lesion is an alveolitis that is directly related to asbestos exposure. The release of inflammatory mediators by activated macrophages and the fibrogenic character of the free asbestos fibers in the interstitium promote interstitial pulmonary fibrosis.

PATHOLOGY: Asbestosis is characterized by bilateral, diffuse interstitial fibrosis and asbestos bodies in the lung (Fig. 12-25). In the early stages, fibrosis occurs in and around alveolar ducts and respiratory bronchioles, as well as in the periphery of the acinus. When asbestos fibers deposit in bronchioles and respiratory bronchioles, they incite a fibrogenic response that leads to mild chronic airflow obstruction. Thus, asbestos may produce obstructive as well

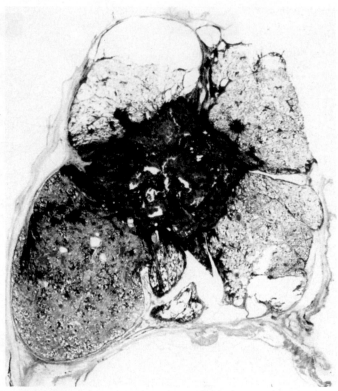

FIGURE 12-24. **Progressive massive fibrosis.** A whole mount of a silicotic lung from a coal miner shows a large area of dense fibrosis containing entrapped carbon particles.

as restrictive defects. Asbestosis is usually more severe in the lower zones of the lung.

Asbestos bodies are found in the walls of bronchioles or within alveolar spaces, often engulfed by alveolar macrophages. The particle has distinctive morphologic features, consisting of a clear, thin asbestos fiber (10 to 50 μm long) surrounded by a beaded iron–protein coat. By light microscopy, it is golden brown (see Fig. 12-25) and stains strongly with the Prussian blue stain for iron. The fibers are only partly engulfed by macrophages because they are too large for a single cell. The macrophages coat the asbestos fiber with protein, proteoglycans, and ferritin. Exposure to asbestos also leads to additional complications.

BENIGN PLEURAL EFFUSION: Benign pleural effusion associated with asbestos inhalation has been observed in about 3% of workers exposed to asbestos.

PLEURAL PLAQUES: Pleural plaques typically occur on parietal and diaphragmatic pleura, often 20 years after exposure to asbestos. Plaques may be found in up to 15% of the general population, and half of all patients with plaques at autopsy may not have a history of asbestos exposure. On gross examination, pleural plaques are pearly white and have a smooth or nodular surface. They are usually bilateral, may measure greater than 10 cm in diameter, and may become calcified. Histologically, they consist of acellular, dense, hyalinized fibrous tissue, with numerous slit-like spaces in a parallel fashion ("basket-weave pattern"). Pleural plaques are not predictors of asbestosis, nor do they evolve into mesotheliomas.

MESOTHELIOMA: The relationship between asbestos exposure and malignant mesothelioma is firmly established. Sometimes, exposure is indirect and slight, for example, wives of asbestos workers who wash their husbands' clothes. More often, mesothelioma is seen in workers heavily exposed to asbestos. This disease is discussed below with diseases of the pleura.

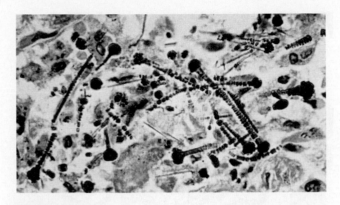

FIGURE 12-25. **Asbestos bodies.** These ferruginous bodies are golden brown and beaded, with a central, colorless, nonbirefringent core fiber. Asbestos bodies are encrusted with protein and iron.

CARCINOMA OF THE LUNG: In asbestos workers who smoke, the incidence of carcinoma of the lung is increased to up to 60 times that of the nonsmoking population or up to three times that of smokers. The link between asbestos is thought to require asbestosis (diffuse interstitial fibrosis).

Berylliosis Displays Noncaseating Granulomas

Berylliosis refers to the pulmonary disease that follows inhalation of beryllium. Today, this metal is used principally in structural materials in aerospace industries, in the manufacture of industrial ceramics, and in nuclear reactors. Exposure to beryllium may also occur in those who mine and extract beryllium ores.

 PATHOLOGY: Berylliosis occurs as an acute chemical pneumonitis or a chronic pneumoconiosis. In the acute form, symptoms begin within hours or days after inhalation of metal particles and manifest pathologically as diffuse alveolar damage. Of all persons with acute beryllium pneumonitis, 10% progress to chronic disease, although chronic berylliosis is often encountered in workers without any history of an acute illness.

Chronic berylliosis differs from other pneumoconioses in that the amount and duration of exposure may be small. The lesion is thus suspected to be a hypersensitivity reaction. Pathologically, the pulmonary lesions are indistinguishable from those of sarcoidosis (see below). Multiple noncaseating granulomas are distributed along the pleura, septa, and bronchovascular bundles. Disease progression can lead to end-stage fibrosis and honeycomb lung. Patients with chronic berylliosis have an insidious onset of dyspnea 15 or more years after the initial exposure. The disease appears to be associated with an increased risk of lung cancer.

Interstitial Lung Disease

A large number of pulmonary disorders are grouped as interstitial, infiltrative, or restrictive diseases because they are characterized by inflammatory infiltrates in the interstitial space and have similar clinical and radiologic presentations. The conditions vary from minimally symptomatic to severely incapacitating and sometimes lethal interstitial fibrosis.

Hypersensitivity Pneumonitis (Extrinsic Allergic Alveolitis) is a Response to Inhaled Antigens

Inhalation of many antigens leads to hypersensitivity pneumonitis (i.e., acute or chronic interstitial inflammation in the lung). Most of the responsible antigens are encountered in occupational settings, and the diseases are often labeled according to a specific

vocation. Thus, **farmer's lung** occurs in farmers exposed to *Micropolyspora faeni* from moldy hay, **bagassosis** results from exposure to *Thermoactinomyces sacchari* in moldy sugar cane, **maple bark–stripper's disease** is seen in persons exposed to the fungus *Cryptostroma corticale* from moldy maple bark, and **bird fancier's lung** affects bird keepers with long-term exposure to proteins from bird feathers, blood, and excrement. Hypersensitivity pneumonitis may also be caused by fungi growing in stagnant water in air conditioners, swimming pools, hot tubs, and central heating units. In many cases, especially in the chronic form of hypersensitivity pneumonitis, the inciting antigen is never identified.

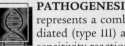 **PATHOGENESIS:** Hypersensitivity pneumonitis represents a combination of immune complex-mediated (type III) and cell-mediated (type IV) hypersensitivity reactions, although the precise contribution of each is still debated. Importantly, most persons with serum precipitins to inhaled antigens do not develop hypersensitivity pneumonitis on exposure, a fact that suggests a genetic component in host susceptibility.

 PATHOLOGY: Acute hypersensitivity pneumonitis is characterized by a neutrophilic infiltrate in alveoli and respiratory bronchioles. Most cases have serum IgG precipitating antibodies against the offending agent. The main microscopic features of chronic hypersensitivity pneumonitis include bronchiolocentric cellular interstitial pneumonia, poorly formed noncaseating granulomas, and organizing pneumonia (Fig. 12-26A,B). The bronchiolocentric interstitial infiltrate varies from subtle to severe and consists of lymphocytes, plasma cells, and macrophages; eosinophils are distinctly uncommon. Poorly formed noncaseating granulomas are present in two thirds of cases (see Fig. 12-26B). Organizing pneumonia is found in two thirds of cases and may form the lesion of bronchiolitis obliterans (see Fig. 12-26A). In the end stage, interstitial inflammation recedes, leaving pulmonary fibrosis, which may resemble usual interstitial pneumonia.

 CLINICAL FEATURES: Hypersensitivity pneumonitis may be first seen as acute, subacute, or chronic pulmonary disease, depending on the frequency and intensity of exposure to the offending antigen. The prototype of hypersensitivity pneumonitis is "farmer's lung." Typically, a farm worker enters a barn where hay has been stored for winter feeding. After a lag period of 4 to 6 hours, the worker rapidly develops dyspnea, cough, and mild fever. Symptoms remit within 24 to 48 hours but return on re-exposure; with time, they become chronic. Patients with the chronic form of hypersensitivity pneumonitis have a more nonspecific presentation, with an indolent onset of dyspnea and cor pulmonale. Removal of the environmental antigen is the only adequate long-term treatment for hypersensitivity pneumonitis. Steroid therapy may be effective in acute forms and for some chronically affected patients.

Sarcoidosis is a Granulomatous Disease of Unknown Etiology

In sarcoidosis, the lung is the organ most frequently involved, but lymph nodes, skin, spleen, liver, and the eye are also common targets.

EPIDEMIOLOGY: Sarcoidosis is a worldwide disease, affecting all races and both genders. The differences in prevalence among racial and ethnic groups are remarkable. In North America, sarcoidosis is much more common in blacks than in whites; the ratio is reported to be as high as 10:1. By contrast, the disease is uncommon in tropical Africa. The incidence of pediatric cases is particularly high among blacks in the southeastern United States.

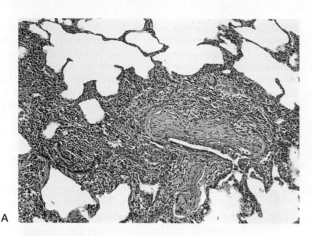
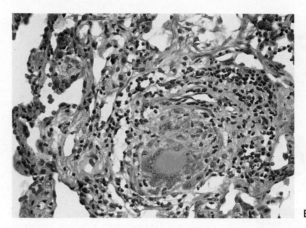

FIGURE 12-26. **Hypersensitivity pneumonitis. A.** A lung biopsy specimen shows a mild peribronchiolar chronic inflammatory interstitial infiltrate, with a focus of intraluminal organizing fibrosis. **B.** Focal poorly formed granulomas were scattered in the lung biopsy specimen.

PATHOGENESIS: Although the exact pathogenesis of sarcoidosis remains obscure, there is a consensus that it represents an exaggerated helper/inducer T-lymphocyte response to exogenous or autologous antigens. These cells accumulate in the affected organs, where they secrete lymphokines and recruit macrophages, which participate in the formation of noncaseating granulomas. The organs that contain sarcoid granulomas have CD4+ to CD8+ T-cell ratios of 10:1, compared with 2:1 in uninvolved tissues. The basis for this abnormal accumulation of helper/inducer T lymphocytes is unclear. Nonspecific polyclonal activation of B cells by T-helper cells leads to hyperglobulinemia, a characteristic feature of active sarcoidosis.

PATHOLOGY: Pulmonary sarcoidosis most commonly affects the lung and hilar lymph nodes, although either involvement may occur separately. Histologically, multiple sarcoid granulomas are scattered in the interstitium of the lung (Fig. 12-27). The distribution is distinctive—along the pleura and interlobular septa and around bronchovascular bundles (see Fig. 12-27A). Fibrosis may be observed at the periphery of the granuloma and may show an onion-skin pattern of lamellar fibrosis around the giant cells. Vasculitis can be demonstrated in two

thirds of open lung biopsy specimens from patients with sarcoidosis. **Asteroid bodies** (star-shaped crystals) and **Schaumann bodies** (small lamellar calcifications) may be seen in the granulomas (see Fig. 12-27B), although they are not specific for sarcoidosis and may be present in most granulomatous process.

CLINICAL FEATURES: Sarcoidosis most often occurs in young adults of both genders. **Acute sarcoidosis** has an abrupt onset, usually followed by spontaneous remission within 2 years and an excellent response to steroids. **Chronic sarcoidosis** has an insidious onset, and patients are more likely to have persistent or progressive disease. The malady may also affect the skin. Black patients tend to have more severe uveitis, skin disease, and lacrimal gland involvement. Cough and dyspnea are the major respiratory complaints. **No laboratory test is specific for the diagnosis of sarcoidosis**. Serum levels of angiotensin-converting enzyme are elevated in two thirds of patients with active sarcoidosis, and 24-hour urine calcium is frequently increased. The laboratory data, together with the clinical and radiologic findings, allow the diagnosis of sarcoidosis to be established with a high probability. The prognosis in pulmonary sarcoidosis is favorable, and most patients do not develop clinically significant sequelae. Resolution occurs in 60% of patients with pulmonary sarcoidosis, but the disease directly accounts for the patient's death in 10% of cases. Corticosteroid therapy is effective for active sarcoidosis.

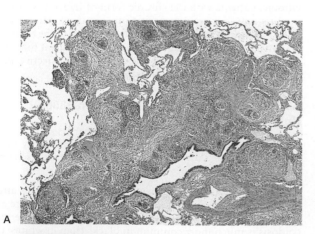

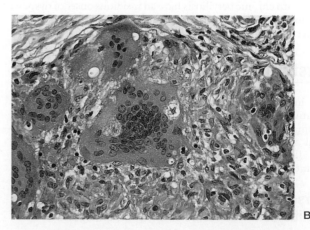

FIGURE 12-27. **Sarcoidosis. A.** Multiple noncaseating granulomas are present along the bronchovascular interstitium. **B.** Noncaseating granulomas consist of tight clusters of epithelioid macrophages and multinucleated giant cells. Several asteroid bodies are present.

Usual Interstitial Pneumonia (UIP) Refers Clinically to Idiopathic Pulmonary Fibrosis

UIP is one of the most common types of interstitial pneumonia, with an annual incidence of 6 to 14.6 cases per 100,000 persons. It has a slight male predominance and a mean age at onset of 50 to 60 years. The clinical terms *idiopathic pulmonary fibrosis* or *cryptogenic fibrosing alveolitis* are often applied.

 PATHOGENESIS: The etiology of UIP is unknown, but viral, genetic, and immunologic factors are thought to play a role. A viral etiology is favored by a history of flu-like illness in some patients. A genetic role is suggested by cases of familial UIP and the association of UIP-like diseases in patients with inherited disorders such as neurofibromatosis and Hermansky-Pudlak syndrome. An immunologic component has been proposed because collagen vascular diseases such as rheumatoid arthritis, systemic lupus erythematosus, and progressive systemic sclerosis may also occur in about 20% of cases. UIP also appears in the context of other autoimmune disorders, and patients frequently exhibit circulating autoantibodies (e.g., antinuclear antibodies and rheumatoid factor). Immune complexes have been demonstrated in the circulation, the inflamed alveolar walls, and bronchoalveolar-lavage specimens, although the antigen has not been identified. It has been postulated that alveolar macrophages become activated upon phagocytosis of immune complexes, after which they release cytokines that recruit neutrophils. These in turn damage alveolar walls, setting in motion a series of events that culminates in interstitial fibrosis.

 PATHOLOGY: *UIP demonstrates a histologic pattern that occurs in a variety of clinical settings, including collagen vascular disease, chronic hypersensitivity pneumonitis, drug toxicity, and asbestosis.* Grossly, fibrosis is often patchy, with areas of dense scarring and honeycomb cystic change (Fig. 12-28A). The histologic hallmark of UIP is patchy chronic inflammation and interstitial fibrosis, with zones of normal lung adjacent to fibrotic regions (see Fig. 12-28B). Areas of loose fibroblastic tissue (fibroblast foci) are found adjacent to dense collagen (see Fig. 12-28C). Dense scarring fibrosis causes remodeling of the lung architecture, resulting in collapse of alveolar walls and formation of cystic spaces (see Fig. 12-28A). Lymphoid aggregates, sometimes containing germinal centers, are occasionally noted, particularly in UIP associated with rheumatoid arthritis. Extensive vascular changes, especially intimal fibrosis and thickening of the media, may be associated with pulmonary hypertension.

 CLINICAL FEATURES: UIP begins insidiously, with the gradual onset of dyspnea on exertion and dry cough, usually over a period of 1 to 3 years. The classic auscultatory finding is late inspiratory crackles and fine ("Velcro") rales at the lung bases. Tachypnea at rest, cyanosis, and cor pulmonale eventually ensue. The prognosis is bleak, with a mean survival of 4 to 6 years. Patients are treated with corticosteroids and sometimes cyclophosphamide, but lung transplantation generally offers the only hope of a cure. A rapidly progressive variant of UIP is termed **acute interstitial pneumonia** and is often fatal.

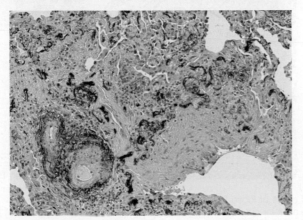

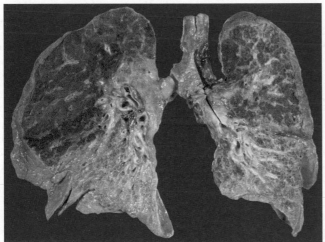

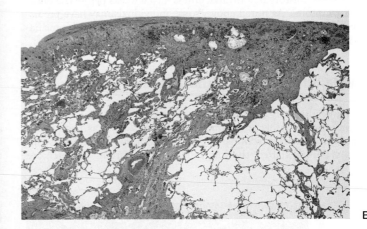

FIGURE 12-28. **Usual interstitial pneumonitis. A.** A gross specimen of the lung shows patchy dense scarring with extensive areas of honeycomb cystic change, predominantly affecting the lower lobes. This patient also had polymyositis. **B.** A microscopic view shows patchy subpleural fibrosis with microscopic honeycomb fibrosis. The areas of dense fibrosis display remodeling, with loss of the normal lung architecture. **C.** Movat stain highlights the fibroblastic focus in green, which contrasts with the adjacent area of yellow staining of dense collagen and black staining of collapsed elastic fibers.

Organizing Pneumonia Features Polypoid Plugs of Tissue that Fill the Bronchiolar Lumen and Surrounding Alveolar Spaces

Organizing pneumonia pattern was previously referred to as "bronchiolitis obliterans–organizing pneumonia". It is not specific for any particular etiologic agent, and the cause cannot be determined from the morphologic appearance. The disorder is observed in many settings, including respiratory tract infections (particularly viral bronchiolitis), inhalation of toxic materials, administration of a number of drugs, and several inflammatory processes (e.g., collagen vascular diseases). Importantly, a substantial number of cases remain idiopathic and are referred to as **cryptogenic organizing pneumonia** (or idiopathic bronchiolitis obliterans–organizing pneumonia).

 PATHOLOGY: Histologically, the organizing pneumonia pattern features patchy areas of loose organizing fibrosis and chronic inflammatory cells in the distal airways adjacent to normal lung. Plugs of organizing fibroblastic tissue occlude bronchioles (bronchiolitis obliterans), alveolar ducts, and surrounding alveoli (organizing pneumonia; Fig. 12-29). The pattern is predominantly one of patchy alveolar organizing pneumonia, and bronchiolitis obliterans may not be seen in all cases. The architecture of the lung is preserved, with none of the remodeling or honeycomb changes seen in UIP. An obstructive or endogenous lipid pneumonia demonstrating foamy lipid-laden macrophages may develop if there is significant bronchiolitis obliterans due to the occlusion of the distal airways. The alveolar septa are only slightly thickened with chronic inflammatory cells, and hyperplasia of type II pneumocytes is mild.

 CLINICAL FEATURES: Organizing pneumonia pattern generally presents in the 5th decade. Onset is acute, with fever, cough, and dyspnea. Many patients have a history of a flu-like illness 4 to 6 weeks before the onset of symptoms. As noted above, some individuals may have predisposing conditions. Corticosteroid therapy is effective, and some patients recover within weeks to months even without therapy.

Vasculitis and Granulomatosis

Many pulmonary conditions result in vasculitis, most of which are secondary to other inflammatory processes, such as necrotizing granulomatous infections. Only a few primary idiopathic vasculitis syndromes affect the lung, the most important of which are Wegener granulomatosis, Churg-Strauss granulomatosis, and necrotizing sarcoid granulomatosis. The vasculitides are discussed in detail in Chapter 10.

Pulmonary Hypertension

In fetal life, the pulmonary arterial walls are thick, and pulmonary arterial pressure is correspondingly high. Blood is oxygenated through the placenta, not the lungs. Thus, the high fetal pulmonary arterial pressure serves to shunt the output of the right ventricle through the ductus arteriosus into the systemic circulation, effectively bypassing the lungs. After birth, the lungs are responsible for oxygenating venous blood, and the ductus arteriosus closes. The lungs must thus adapt to accept the entire cardiac output, a situation that demands the high-volume and low-pressure system of the mature lung. Accordingly, by 3 days after birth, pulmonary arteries dilate, their walls become thin, and pulmonary arterial pressure declines.

Increases in either pulmonary blood flow or vascular resistance may lead to higher pulmonary arterial pressure. Whatever the cause, characteristic morphologic abnormalities result from increased pulmonary artery pressure (Fig. 12-30). Grades 1, 2, and 3 are generally reversible; grades 4 and above are usually not.

- **Grade 1: Medial hypertrophy** of muscular pulmonary arteries and appearance of smooth muscle in pulmonary arterioles
- **Grade 2: Intimal proliferation** with increasing medial hypertrophy
- **Grade 3: Intimal fibrosis of muscular pulmonary arteries** and arterioles, which may be occlusive (Fig. 12-31A).
- **Grade 4: Formation of plexiform lesions together with dilation and thinning of pulmonary arteries.** These nodular lesions are composed of irregular interlacing blood channels and impose a further obstruction in the pulmonary circulation (see Fig. 12-31B).
- **Grade 5: Plexiform lesions in combination with dilation or angiomatoid lesions. Rupture of dilated thin-walled vessels,** with parenchymal hemorrhage and hemosiderosis, is also present.
- **Grade 6: Fibrinoid necrosis** of arteries and arterioles

Even mild atherosclerosis of the pulmonary artery is uncommon when pulmonary arterial pressure is normal. However, with all grades of pulmonary hypertension, atherosclerosis is seen in the largest pulmonary arteries. Increased pressure in the lesser circulation leads to hypertrophy of the right ventricle (**cor pulmonale**).

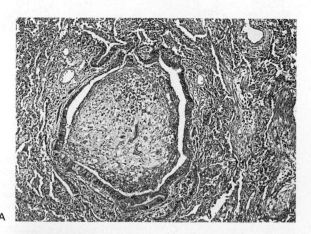
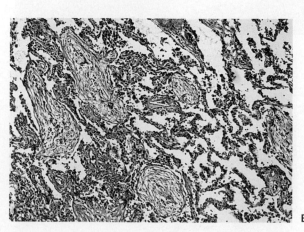

FIGURE 12-29. **Organizing pneumonia pattern. A.** Polypoid plugs of loose fibrous tissue are present in a bronchiole and the adjacent alveolar ducts and alveoli. **B.** The alveolar spaces contain similar plugs of loose organizing connective tissue.

SMALL PULMONARY ARTERIES

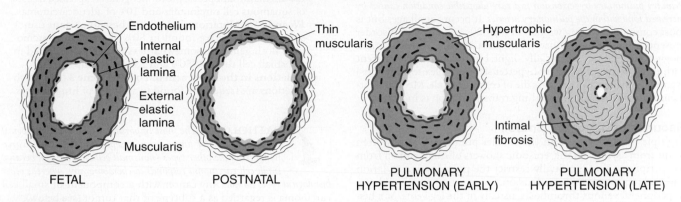

FIGURE 12-30. **Histopathology of pulmonary hypertension.** In late gestation, the pulmonary arteries have thick walls. After birth, the vessels dilate, and the walls become thin. Mild pulmonary hypertension is characterized by thickening of the media. As pulmonary hypertension becomes more severe, there is extensive intimal fibrosis and muscle thickening.

Pulmonary Hypertension May be Considered Precapillary or Postcapillary in Origin

The primary source of increased flow or resistance, whether proximal or distal to the pulmonary capillary bed, may be used to understand the pathophysiology of pulmonary hypertension. Precapillary hypertension includes left-to-right cardiac shunts as well as primary pulmonary hypertension, thromboembolic pulmonary hypertension, and hypertension secondary to fibrotic lung disease and hypoxia. Postcapillary hypertension includes pulmonary veno-occlusive disease, as well as hypertension secondary to left-sided cardiac disorders, such as mitral stenosis and aortic coarctation. (See Chapter 11 for discussion of the role of cardiac disease in pulmonary hypertension.)

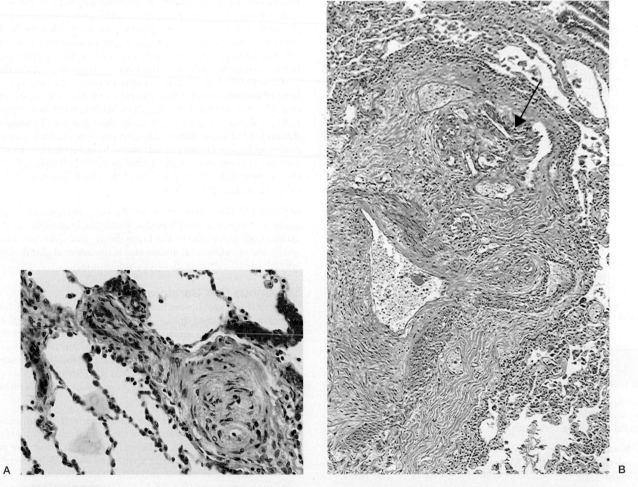

FIGURE 12-31. **Pulmonary arterial hypertension. A.** A small pulmonary artery is virtually occluded by concentric intimal fibrosis and thickening of the media. **B.** A plexiform lesion *(arrow)* is characterized by a glomeruloid proliferation of thin-walled vessels adjacent to a parent artery, which shows marked hypertensive changes of intimal fibrosis and medial thickening.

Primary Pulmonary Hypertension

Primary pulmonary hypertension is a rare idiopathic condition caused by increased tone within the pulmonary arteries. It occurs at all ages but is most common in young women in their 20s and 30s. The disorder presents as an insidious onset of dyspnea. Physical signs and radiologic abnormalities are initially slight, but become more apparent with time. Severe pulmonary hypertension (i.e., plexiform lesions) eventually ensues, and patients die of cor pulmonale. Medical treatment is ineffective, and heart–lung transplantation is indicated.

Recurrent Pulmonary Emboli

Multiple thromboemboli in the smaller pulmonary vessels often result from asymptomatic, episodic showers of small emboli from the periphery. They gradually restrict the pulmonary circulation and lead to pulmonary hypertension. Some patients have evidence of peripheral venous thrombosis, usually in the leg veins, or a history of circumstances predisposing to venous thrombosis. If the condition is diagnosed during life, placement of a filter in the inferior vena cava usually prevents further embolization.

Hypoxemia Can Result in Constriction of Small Pulmonary Arteries and Pulmonary Hypertension

Predisposing conditions that are likely to produce hypoxemia-associated pulmonary hypertension include chronic airflow obstruction (chronic bronchitis), infiltrative lung disease, and living at a high altitude. Severe kyphoscoliosis or extreme obesity **(Pickwickian syndrome)** may mechanically interfere with ventilation and result in pulmonary hypertension.

Cardiac Disease May Result in Pulmonary Hypertension

Left ventricular failure increases pulmonary venous pressure and, to some extent, pulmonary arterial pressure. By contrast, mitral stenosis produces severe venous pulmonary hypertension and significant pulmonary artery hypertension. In such cases, the lungs exhibit lesions of both pulmonary hypertension and chronic passive congestion (see Chapter 7).

Carcinoma of the Lung

EPIDEMIOLOGY: Regarded as a rare tumor as late as 1945, carcinoma of the lung is today the most common cause of cancer death worldwide. In the United States, it is the most common cause of cancer death in both men and women. Approximately 85% of lung cancers occur in cigarette smokers (see Chapter 8). The peak age for lung cancer is between 60 and 70 years, and most patients are between 50 and 80 years old. The former male predominance is decreasing, because of increased smoking among women.

PATHOGENESIS: Individual carcinomas of the lung have multiple genetic alterations that are likely be to the result of a stepwise progression from a normal cell toward a malignant tumor. Carcinogenic products in tobacco are clearly involved in this process. Some of the more common genetic alterations associated with lung carcinoma are as follows:

- **K-*ras* oncogene:** Mutations in this oncogene are found in adenocarcinomas (25%), large cell tumors (20%), and less commonly in squamous cell carcinoma (5%). The mutations correlate with smoking and a poor prognosis.
- *Myc* **oncogene:** Overexpression of this gene occurs in 10% to 40% of small cell carcinomas but is rare in other types.

- *Bcl-2*: This antiapoptotic protooncogene is expressed in 25% of squamous cell carcinomas and 10% of adenocarcinomas.
- *Rb* and *p53*: Mutations in both of these important tumor suppressor genes are found in 80% of small cell carcinomas. Both genes are somewhat less frequently mutated in nonsmall cell tumors (50% and 25%, respectively).
- **Deletions in the short arm of chromosome 3 (3p):** Such deletions are frequently found in all types of lung cancers.

PATHOLOGY: *The most important issue in the histological subclassification of lung cancer is separating small cell carcinoma from the other types (nonsmall cell carcinoma), because small cell carcinoma responds to chemotherapy, whereas other histological types do not.* Any cancer with a component of small cell carcinoma is regarded as a subtype of that tumor (see below).

CLINICAL FEATURES: The overall 5-year survival rate for all patients with lung cancer has remained at 15% for the past 2 decades. The 5-year survival rate at all stages is 42% for bronchioloalveolar carcinoma, 17% for adenocarcinoma, 15% for squamous cell carcinoma, 11% for large cell carcinoma, and 5% for small cell carcinoma. Tumor stage remains the single most important predictor of prognosis.

Some Clinical Features are Common to All Subtypes

LOCAL EFFECTS: Most central endobronchial tumors produce symptoms related to bronchial obstruction, such as cough, dyspnea, hemoptysis, chest pain, obstructive pneumonia, and pleural effusion. Tumors arising peripherally are more likely to be discovered either on routine chest radiographs or after they have become advanced and invaded the chest wall, with resulting chest pain, superior vena cava syndrome, and nerve-entrapment syndromes.

Growth of a lung cancer (usually squamous) in the apex of the lung **(Pancoast tumor)** may extend to involve the eighth cervical and first and second thoracic nerves, leading to shoulder pain that radiates down the arm in an ulnar distribution **(Pancoast syndrome)**. A Pancoast tumor may also paralyze cervical sympathetic nerves and cause **Horner syndrome**, characterized on the affected side by (1) depression of the eyeball (enophthalmos), (2) ptosis of the upper eyelid, (3) constriction of the pupil (miosis), and (4) absence of sweating (anhidrosis).

METASTASES: Carcinomas of the lung metastasize most frequently to regional lymph nodes, particularly the hilar and mediastinal nodes, but also to the brain, bone, and liver. The most frequent site of extranodal metastases is the adrenal gland, although adrenal insufficiency is distinctly uncommon.

Squamous Cell Carcinoma

Squamous cell carcinoma accounts for 30% of all invasive lung cancers in the United States. After injury to the bronchial epithelium, such as occurs with cigarette smoking, regeneration from the pluripotent basal layer commonly occurs in the form of squamous metaplasia. The metaplastic mucosa follows the same sequence of dysplasia, carcinoma in situ, and invasive tumor as that observed in sites that are normally lined by squamous epithelium, such as the cervix or skin.

PATHOLOGY: Most squamous cell carcinomas arise in the central portion of the lung from the major or segmental bronchi, although 10% originate in the periphery. They tend to be firm, grey-white, 3- to 5-cm ulcerated lesions, which extend through the bronchial wall into the adjacent parenchyma (Fig. 12-32A). The appearance of the cut surface is variable, depending on the degree of necrosis and hemorrhage. Central cavitation is frequent. On occasion, a central squamous carcinoma occurs as an endobronchial tumor.

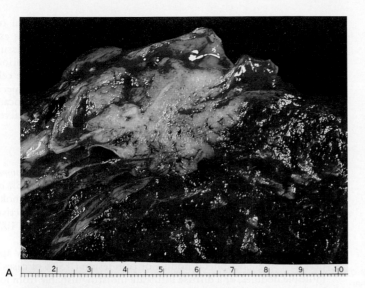

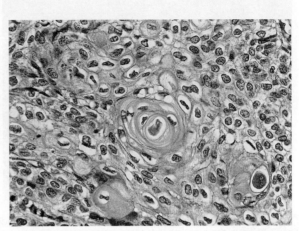

FIGURE 12-32. **Squamous cell carcinoma of the lung. A.** The tumor grows within the lumen of a bronchus and invades the adjacent intrapulmonary lymph node. **B.** A photomicrograph shows well-differentiated squamous cell carcinoma with a keratin pearl composed of cells with brightly eosinophilic cytoplasm.

The microscopic appearance of squamous cell carcinoma is highly variable. Well-differentiated squamous cell carcinomas display keratin "pearls," which are eosinophilic aggregates of keratin surrounded by concentric ("onion skin") layers of squamous cells (see Fig. 12-32B). Individual cell keratinization also occurs, in which a cell's cytoplasm assumes a glassy, intensely eosinophilic appearance. Intercellular bridges are identified in some well-differentiated squamous cancers as slender gaps between adjacent cells, which are traversed by fine strands of cytoplasm. By contrast, some squamous tumors are so poorly differentiated that they show no foci of keratinization and are difficult to distinguish from large cell, small cell, or spindle cell carcinomas. Tumor cells may be readily found in the sputum, in which case the diagnosis is made by exfoliative cytology.

Adenocarcinoma

Adenocarcinoma of the lung comprises one third of all invasive lung cancers in the United States. It tends to arise in the periphery

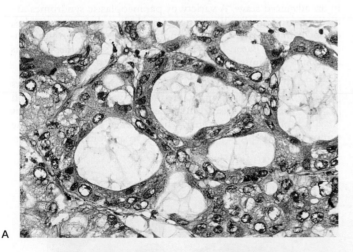

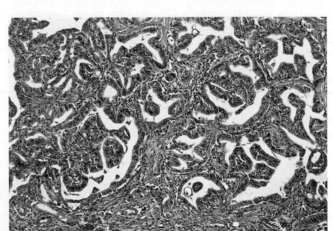

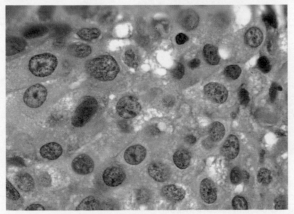

FIGURE 12-33. **Adenocarcinoma of the lung. A.** The malignant epithelial cells of an acinar adenocarcinoma form glands. **B.** A papillary adenocarcinoma consists of malignant epithelial cells growing along thin fibrovascular cores. **C.** A tumor grows in the pattern of solid adenocarcinoma with mucin formation. Several intracytoplasmic mucin droplets stain positively with the mucicarmine stain.

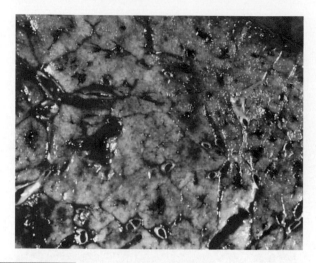

FIGURE 12-34. **Bronchioloalveolar carcinoma.** The cut surface of the lung is solid, glistening, and mucoid, an appearance that reflects a diffusely infiltrating tumor.

and is often associated with pleural fibrosis and subpleural scars, which can result in pleural puckering. In nonsmokers who develop lung cancer, the proportion of adenocarcinomas is greater.

PATHOLOGY: At initial presentation, adenocarcinomas of the lung most often appear as irregular masses 2 to 5 cm in diameter, although they may be so large as to replace an entire lobe. On cut section, the tumor is grayish-white and often glistening, depending on the amount of mucus production. Central adenocarcinomas may have predominantly endobronchial growth and invade bronchial cartilage.

There are four major subtypes of adenocarcinoma, as defined by the World Health Organization (Fig. 12-33; see Figs. 12-34 and 12-35): (1) acinar, (2) papillary, (3) solid with mucus formation, and (4) bronchioloalveolar. However, it is common to encounter a mixture of these histologic subtypes. Bronchioloalveolar carcinoma is distinctive and is discussed below.

Pulmonary adenocarcinoma may reflect the architecture and cell population of any part of the respiratory mucosa, from the large bronchi to the smallest bronchioles. The neoplastic cells may resemble ciliated or nonciliated columnar epithelial cells, goblet cells, cells of bronchial glands, or Clara cells. The most common histologic type of adenocarcinoma features the acinar pattern, which is distinguished by regular glands lined by cuboidal or columnar cells (see Fig. 12-33A). Papillary adenocarcinomas exhibit a single cell layer on a core of fibrovascular connective tissue (see Fig. 12-33B). Solid adenocarcinomas with mucus formation are poorly differentiated tumors, distinguishable from large cell carcinomas by demonstrating mucin with mucicarmine or periodic acid–Schiff (see Fig. 12-33C). Patients with stage I adenocarcinomas (localized to the lung) who undergo complete surgical removal have a 5-year survival rate of 50% to 80%.

Bronchioloalveolar Carcinoma

Bronchioloalveolar carcinoma is a distinctive subtype of adenocarcinoma that grows along pre-existing alveolar walls and accounts for 1% to 5% of all invasive lung tumors. It has not been definitively linked to smoking. Copious mucin in the sputum (bronchorrhea) is a distinctive sign of bronchioloalveolar carcinoma but is seen in fewer than 10% of patients.

On gross examination, bronchioloalveolar carcinoma may appear as a single peripheral nodule or coin lesion (>50% of cases), multiple nodules, or a diffuse infiltrate indistinguishable from lobar pneumonia (Fig. 12-34). Two thirds of tumors are nonmucinous, consisting of Clara cells and type II pneumocytes, in which cuboidal cells grow along the alveolar walls (Fig. 12-35); the remaining one-third are mucinous tumors featuring columnar goblet cells filled with mucus (see Fig. 12-35B). Patients with stage I bronchioloalveolar carcinomas have a good prognosis; but those who have multiple nodules or diffuse lung involvement are more likely to have a poor outcome.

Small Cell Carcinoma

Small cell carcinoma (previously "oat cell" carcinoma) is a highly malignant epithelial tumor of the lung that exhibits neuroendocrine features. It accounts for 20% of all lung cancers and is strongly associated with cigarette smoking. The male-to-female ratio is 2:1. The tumor grows and metastasizes rapidly, and 70% of patients are first seen in an advanced stage. A variety of paraneoplastic syndromes are distinctive for small cell carcinoma, including diabetes insipidus, ectopic adrenocorticotropic hormone (ACTH, corticotropin) syndrome, and the Eaton-Lambert (myasthenic) syndrome, which is associated with muscle weakness in the lower extremities.

PATHOLOGY: Small cell carcinoma usually appears as a perihilar mass, frequently with extensive lymph node metastases. On cut section, it is soft and white but often shows extensive hemorrhage and necrosis. The tumor typically spreads along bronchi in a submucosal and cir-

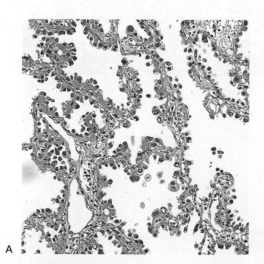
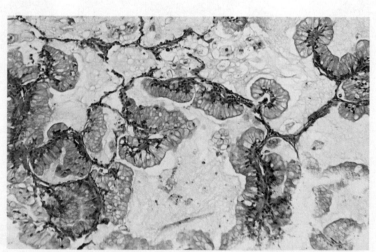

FIGURE 12-35. **Bronchioloalveolar carcinoma. A.** Nonmucinous bronchioloalveolar carcinomas consist of atypical cuboidal to low columnar cells proliferating along the existing alveolar walls. **B.** Mucinous bronchioloalveolar carcinoma consists of tall columnar cells filled with apical cytoplasmic mucin that grow along the existing alveolar walls.

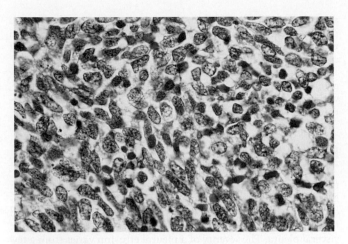

FIGURE 12-36. **Small cell carcinoma of the lung.** This tumor consists of small oval to spindle-shaped cells with scant cytoplasm, finely granular nuclear chromatin, and conspicuous mitoses.

cumferential fashion. Histologically, small cell carcinoma consists of sheets of small, round, oval or spindle-shaped cells with scant cytoplasm. Their nuclei are distinctive, featuring finely granular nuclear chromatin and absent or inconspicuous nucleoli (Fig. 12-36). A high mitotic rate is characteristic, with an average of 60 to 70 mitoses per 10 high-power fields. Necrosis is frequent and extensive. Unlike other lung cancers, small cell carcinomas show marked sensitivity to chemotherapy. From an oncologist's standpoint, all other lung cancers are grouped together as "nonsmall cell carcinoma."

Large Cell Carcinoma

Large cell carcinoma is a diagnosis of exclusion in a poorly differentiated tumor that does not show features of squamous or glandular differentiation and has been shown not to be a small cell carcinoma (Fig. 12-37). This tumor type accounts for 10% of all invasive lung tumors. The cells are large and exhibit ample cytoplasm. The nuclei frequently show prominent nucleoli and vesicular chromatin. Some large cell carcinomas exhibit pleomorphic giant cells or spindle cells.

Carcinoid Tumors

Carcinoid tumors of the lung comprise two subtypes of neuroendocrine neoplasms and are thought to arise from the resident neuroendocrine cells nor-

mally found in the bronchial epithelium. These neoplasms account for 2% of all primary lung cancers, show no gender predilection, and are not related to cigarette smoking. Although neuropeptides are readily demonstrated in the tumor cells, most are endocrinologically silent.

 PATHOLOGY: Carcinoid tumors are characterized histologically by an organoid growth pattern and uniform cytologic features, including eosinophilic, finely granular cytoplasm and nuclei with finely granular chromatin (Fig. 12-38).

 CLINICAL FEATURES: Carcinoid tumors grow so slowly that half of patients are asymptomatic at presentation. Such tumors are often discovered as a mass in a chest radiograph. Patients with typical carcinoids have an excellent prognosis, with a 90% 5-year survival rate after surgery.

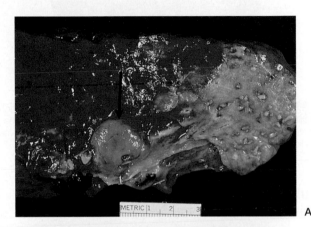

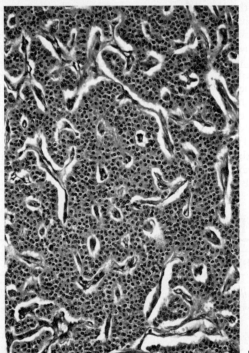

FIGURE 12-38. **Carcinoid tumor of the lung. A.** A central carcinoid tumor *(arrow)* is circumscribed and protrudes into the lumen of the main bronchus. The compression of the bronchus by the tumor caused the postobstructive pneumonia seen in the distal lung parenchyma *(right).* **B.** A microscopic view shows ribbons of tumor cells embedded in a vascular stroma.

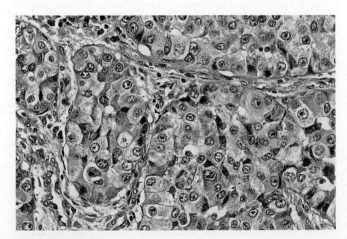

FIGURE 12-37. **Large cell carcinoma of the lung.** This poorly differentiated tumor is growing in sheets. The tumor cells are large and contain ample cytoplasm and prominent nucleoli.

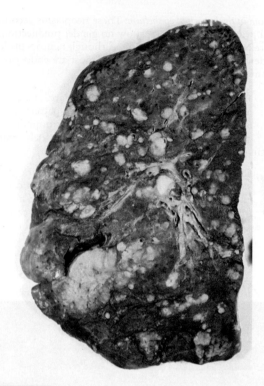

FIGURE 12-39. **Metastatic carcinoma of the lung.** A section through the lung shows numerous nodules of metastatic carcinoma corresponding to "cannon ball" metastases seen radiologically.

Pulmonary Metastases are More Common than Primary Lung Tumors

In one third of all fatal cancers, pulmonary metastases are evident at autopsy. Metastatic tumors in the lung are typically multiple and circumscribed. When large nodules are seen in the lungs radiologically, they are called "cannon ball" metastases (Fig. 12-39). The histologic appearance of most metastases resembles that of the primary tumor. Uncommonly, metastatic tumors may mimic bronchioloalveolar carcinoma, in which cases the usual primary site is the pancreas or stomach. In **lymphangitic carcinoma**, a metastatic tumor spreads widely through pulmonary lymphatic channels to form a sheath of tumor around the bronchovascular tree and veins. Clinically, patients suffer from cough and shortness of breath and display a diffuse reticulonodular pattern on the chest radiograph. The common primary sites are the breast, stomach, pancreas, and colon.

THE PLEURA

Pneumothorax

Pneumothorax is defined as the presence of air in the pleural cavity. It may occur with traumatic perforation of the pleura or may be "spontaneous." Traumatic causes include penetrating wounds of the chest wall (e.g., a stab wound or a rib fracture). Traumatic pneumothorax is most commonly iatrogenic and is seen after aspiration of fluid from the pleura (thoracentesis), pleural or lung biopsies, transbronchial biopsies, and positive pressure-assisted ventilation.

Spontaneous pneumothorax is typically encountered in young adults. For example, while exercising vigorously, a tall young man develops acute chest pain and shortness of breath. A chest radiograph shows collapse of the lung on the side of the pain

and a large collection of air in the pleural space. The condition is usually due to rupture of a subpleural emphysematous bleb. In most cases, spontaneous pneumothorax subsides by itself, but some patients require withdrawal of the air.

Tension pneumothorax refers to unilateral pneumothorax extensive enough to shift the mediastinum to the opposite side, with compression of the opposite lung. The condition may be life-threatening and must be relieved by immediate drainage.

Pleural Effusion

Pleural effusion is the accumulation of excess fluid in the pleural cavity. Normally, only a small amount of fluid in the pleural cavity lubricates the space between the lungs and chest wall. Fluid secreted into the pleural space from the parietal pleura is absorbed by the visceral pleura. The severity of a pleural effusion varies from a few milliliters of fluid to a massive accumulation that shifts the mediastinum and the trachea to the opposite side.

HYDROTHORAX: *This term refers to an effusion that resembles water and would be regarded as edema elsewhere.* It may be due to increased hydrostatic pressure within the capillaries, as occurs in patients with heart failure or in any condition that produces systemic or pulmonary edema.

PYOTHORAX: *A turbid effusion containing many polymorphonuclear leukocytes (pyothorax) results from infections of the pleura.* This may occasionally be caused by an external penetrating wound that introduces pyogenic organisms into the pleural space. More commonly, it is a complication of bacterial pneumonia that extends to the pleural surface, the classic example of which is pneumococcal pneumonia.

EMPYEMA: *This disorder is a variant of pyothorax in which thick pus accumulates within the pleural cavity, often with loculation and fibrosis.*

HEMOTHORAX: *This term refers to blood in the pleural cavity as a result of trauma or rupture of a vessel (e.g., dissecting aneurysm of the aorta).*

CHYLOTHORAX: *Chylothorax is the accumulation of milky, lipid-rich fluid (chyle) in the pleural cavity as a result of lymphatic obstruction.* It has an ominous portent, because lymphatic obstruction suggests disease of the lymph nodes in the posterior mediastinum.

Tumors of the Pleura: Malignant Mesothelioma

Malignant mesothelioma is a neoplasm of mesothelial cells that is most common in the pleura but also occurs in the peritoneum, pericardium, and the tunica vaginalis of the testis.

 EPIDEMIOLOGY: Approximately 2,000 persons develop these tumors yearly in the United States. *In the United States, Great Britain and South Africa, the large majority of patients report exposure to asbestos.* The latency period between asbestos exposure and the appearance of malignant mesothelioma is about 20 years, with a range of 12 to 60 years.

 PATHOLOGY: Grossly, pleural mesotheliomas often encase and compress the lung, extending into fissures and interlobar septa, a distribution often referred to as a "pleural rind" (Fig. 12-40A). Invasion of the pulmonary parenchyma is generally limited to the periphery adjacent to the tumor, and lymph nodes tend to be spared. Microscopically, classic mesotheliomas show a biphasic appearance, with epithelial and sarcomatous patterns (see Fig. 12-40B). Glands and tubules that resemble adenocarcinoma are admixed with sheets of spindle cells that are similar to a fibrosarcoma.

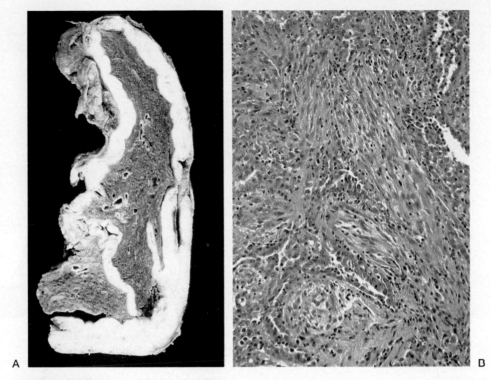

A   B

FIGURE 12-40. **Pleural malignant mesothelioma. A.** The lung is encased by a dense pleural tumor that extends along the interlobar fissures but does not involve the underlying lung parenchyma. **B.** This mesothelioma is composed of a biphasic pattern of epithelial and sarcomatous elements.

Useful criteria for diagnosing mesothelioma include the absence of mucin, presence of hyaluronic acid (positive Alcian blue staining), and demonstration of long, slender microvilli by electron microscopy.

 CLINICAL FEATURES: The average age of patients with mesothelioma is 60 years. Patients are first seen with a pleural effusion or a pleural mass, chest pain, and nonspecific symptoms, such as weight loss and malaise. Pleural mesotheliomas tend to spread locally within the chest cavity, invading and compressing major structures. Metastases can occur to the lung parenchyma and mediastinal lymph nodes, as well as to extrathoracic sites such as the liver, bones, peritoneum, and adrenals. Treatment is largely ineffective, and prognosis is poor. Few patients survive longer than 18 months after diagnosis.

13 The Gastrointestinal Tract

Frank A. Mitros
Emanuel Rubin

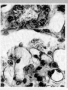
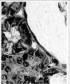
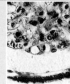

The Esophagus

Congenital Disorders

Tracheoesophageal Fistula

*Tracheoesophageal fistula is the most common esophageal anomaly (Fig. 13-1). It is frequently combined with some form of **esophageal atresia**. In some cases, it is associated with a complex of anomalies identified by the acronym **Vater syndrome** (vertebral defects, anal atresia, tracheoesophageal fistula, and renal dysplasia). Esophageal atresia and fistulas are often associated with congenital heart disease.*

PATHOLOGY: In 90% of tracheoesophageal fistulas, the upper portion of the esophagus ends in a blind pouch, and the superior end of the lower segment communicates with the trachea. *In this type of atresia, the upper blind sac soon fills with mucus, which the infant then aspirates.* Surgical correction is feasible, albeit difficult. Among the remaining 10% of fistulas, the most common is a communication between the proximal esophagus and the trachea; the lower esophageal pouch communicates with the stomach. *Infants with this condition develop aspira-*

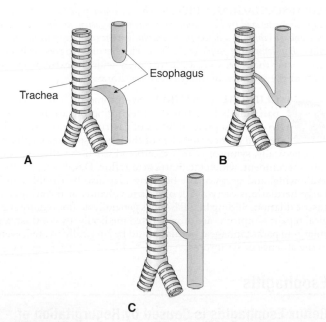

FIGURE 13-1. Congenital tracheoesophageal fistulas. **A.** The most common type is a communication between the trachea and the lower portion of the esophagus. The upper segment of the esophagus ends in a blind sac. **B.** In a few cases, the proximal esophagus communicates with the trachea. **C.** The least common anomaly, the H type, is a fistula between a continuous esophagus and the trachea.

tion immediately after birth. In another variant, termed an *H-type fistula,* a communication exists between an intact esophagus and an intact trachea. In some cases (see Fig. 13-1C), the lesion becomes symptomatic only in adulthood, when repeated pulmonary infections call attention to it.

Rings and Webs Cause Dysphagia

ESOPHAGEAL WEBS: Occasionally, a thin mucosal membrane projects into the esophageal lumen. Webs are usually single but may be multiple and can occur anywhere in the esophagus. They are often successfully treated by dilation with large rubber bougies; occasionally, they can be excised with biopsy forceps during endoscopy.

PLUMMER-VINSON (PATERSON-KELLY) SYNDROME: *This disorder is characterized by (1) a cervical esophageal web, (2) mucosal lesions of the mouth and pharynx, and (3) iron-deficiency anemia.* Dysphagia, often associated with aspiration of swallowed food, is the most common clinical manifestation. Ninety percent of cases occur in women. *Carcinoma of the oropharynx and upper esophagus is a recognized complication.*

SCHATZKI RING: *This lower esophageal narrowing is usually seen at the gastroesophageal junction.* The upper surface of the mucosal ring has stratified squamous epithelium; the lower, columnar epithelium. Although it has been noted in up to 14% of barium meal examinations, Schatzki ring is usually asymptomatic. Patients with narrow Schatzki rings, however, may complain of intermittent dysphagia.

Esophageal Diverticula Often Reflect Motor Dysfunction

A **true esophageal diverticulum** is an outpouching of the wall that contains all layers of the esophagus. If a sac has no muscular layer, it is a **false** diverticulum. Esophageal diverticula occur in the hypopharyngeal area above the upper esophageal sphincter, in the middle esophagus, and immediately proximal to the lower esophageal sphincter.

ZENKER DIVERTICULUM: *Zenker diverticulum is an uncommon lesion that appears high in the esophagus and affects men more than women.* Disordered function of cricopharyngeal musculature is generally thought to be involved in the pathogenesis of this false diverticulum. Most affected persons who come to medical attention are older than 60 years, suggesting that this diverticulum is acquired. The typical symptom is regurgitation of food eaten some time previously (occasionally days), in the absence of dysphagia. Recurrent aspiration pneumonia may be a serious complication. When symptoms are severe, surgical intervention is the rule.

TRACTION DIVERTICULA: *Traction diverticula are outpouchings that occur principally in the midportion of the esophagus.* They were so named because of their now-uncommon finding of attachment to adjacent tuberculous mediastinal lymph nodes. It is now believed that these pouches most often reflect a disturbance in the motor function of the esophagus. A diverticulum in the midesophagus ordinarily has a wide stoma, and the pouch is usually higher than its orifice. Thus, it does not retain food or secretions and remains asymptomatic, with only rare complications.

EPIPHRENIC DIVERTICULA: *These diverticula are located immediately above the diaphragm.* Motor disturbances of the esophagus (e.g., achalasia, diffuse esophageal spasm) are found in two thirds of patients with this true diverticulum. Reflux esophagitis may play a role in the pathogenesis of this condition. Unlike other diverticula, epiphrenic diverticula are encountered in young persons. Nocturnal regurgitation of large amounts of fluid stored in the diverticulum during the day is typical. When symptoms are severe, surgical intervention is directed toward correcting the motor abnormality (e.g., myotomy).

Motor Disorders

The automatic coordination of muscular movement during swallowing is a motor function that results in free passage of food through the esophagus. The hallmark of motor disorders is difficulty in swallowing, termed **dysphagia**. Dysphagia is often an awareness that a bolus of food is not moving downward and in itself is not painful. Pain on swallowing is **odynophagia**. Motor disorders can be caused by either esophageal or systemic defects in striated muscle function, neurological diseases affecting afferent nerves, or peripheral neuropathies occurring in association with diabetes or alcoholism.

Achalasia Features Impaired Function of the Lower Esophageal Sphincter

*Achalasia, at one time termed **cardiospasm**,* is characterized by failure of the lower esophageal sphincter to relax in response to swallowing and the absence of peristalsis in the body of the esophagus. As a result of these defects in both the outflow tract and the pumping mechanisms of the esophagus, food is retained within the esophagus, and the organ hypertrophies and dilates conspicuously (Fig. 13-2). Achalasia is associated with the loss or absence of

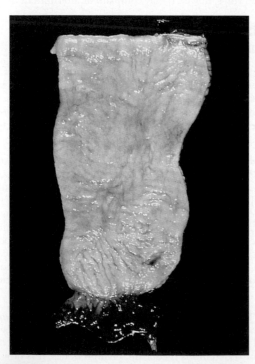

FIGURE 13-2. **Esophagus and upper stomach of a patient with advanced achalasia.** The esophagus is markedly dilated above the esophagogastric junction, where the lower esophageal sphincter is located. The esophageal mucosa is redundant and has hyperplastic squamous epithelium.

ganglion cells in the esophageal myenteric plexus. In Latin America, achalasia is a common complication of **Chagas disease**, in which the ganglion cells are destroyed by the protozoa *Trypanosoma cruzi*. Dysphagia, occasionally odynophagia, and regurgitation of material retained in the esophagus are common symptoms of achalasia. Squamous carcinoma of the esophagus is also a complication.

Scleroderma Causes Fibrosis of the Esophageal Wall

Scleroderma (progressive systemic sclerosis) leads to fibrosis in many organs and produces a severe abnormality of esophageal muscle function (see Chapter 4). The disease mainly affects the lower esophageal sphincter, which may become so impaired that the lower esophagus and upper stomach are no longer distinct functional entities and are visualized as a common cavity. In addition, there may be a lack of peristalsis in the entire esophagus.

Microscopically, fibrosis of esophageal smooth muscle (especially the inner layer of the muscularis propria) and nonspecific inflammatory changes are seen. Intimal fibrosis of small arteries and arterioles is common and may play a role in the pathogenesis of the fibrosis. Clinically, patients have dysphagia and heartburn caused by peptic esophagitis, due to reflux of acid from the stomach (see below).

Hiatal Hernia

Hiatal hernia is a herniation of the stomach through an enlarged esophageal hiatus in the diaphragm. Two basic types of hiatal hernia are observed (Fig. 13-3).

SLIDING HERNIA: *An enlargement of the diaphragmatic hiatus and laxity of the circumferential connective tissue allows a cap of gastric mucosa to move upward to a position above the diaphragm.* This condition is common. Sliding hiatal hernia is asymptomatic in most patients; only 5% of patients diagnosed radiologically complain of symptoms referable to gastroesophageal reflux.

PARAESOPHAGEAL HERNIA: *This uncommon form of hiatal hernia is characterized by herniation of a portion of gastric fundus alongside the esophagus through a defect in the diaphragmatic connective tissue membrane that defines the esophageal hiatus.* The hernia progressively enlarges, and the hiatus grows increasingly wide. In extreme cases, most of the stomach herniates into the thorax.

 CLINICAL FEATURES: Symptoms of hiatal hernia, particularly heartburn and regurgitation, are attributed to gastroesophageal reflux of gastric contents, primarily related to incompetence of the lower esophageal sphincter. Classically, symptoms are exacerbated when the affected person is recumbent, which facilitates acid reflux. Dysphagia, painful swallowing, and occasionally bleeding may also be troublesome. Large herniations carry a risk of gastric volvulus or intrathoracic gastric dilation. Sliding hiatal hernias generally do not require surgical repair; symptoms are often treated medically. By contrast, an enlarging paraesophageal hernia should be surgically treated, even in the absence of symptoms.

Esophagitis

Reflux Esophagitis is Caused by Regurgitation of Gastric Contents

Reflux esophagitis, by far the most common type of esophagitis, is often found in conjunction with a sliding hiatal hernia, although it may occur through an incompetent lower esophageal sphincter without any demonstrable anatomical lesion.

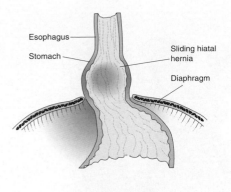

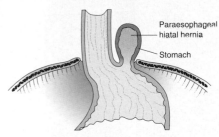

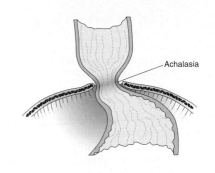

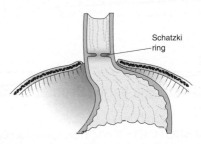

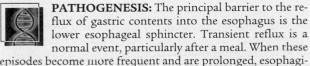

FIGURE 13-3. Disorders of the esophageal outlet.

PATHOGENESIS: The principal barrier to the reflux of gastric contents into the esophagus is the lower esophageal sphincter. Transient reflux is a normal event, particularly after a meal. When these episodes become more frequent and are prolonged, esophagitis results. Agents that decrease the pressure of the lower esophageal sphincter (e.g., alcohol, chocolate, fatty foods, cigarette smoking) are also associated with reflux. Certain central nervous system depressants (e.g., morphine, diazepam), pregnancy, estrogen therapy, and the presence of a nasogastric tube may lead to reflux esophagitis. Although acid is damaging to the esophageal mucosa, the combination of acid and pepsin may be particularly injurious. Moreover, gastric fluid often contains refluxed bile from the duodenum, which is harmful to the esophageal mucosa. Alcohol, hot beverages, and spicy foods may also damage the mucosa directly.

PATHOLOGY: The first grossly evident change caused by gastroesophageal reflux is hyperemia. Areas affected by reflux are susceptible to superficial mucosal erosions and ulcers, which often appear as vertical linear streaks. Microscopically, mild injury to the squamous epithelium is manifested by cell swelling (hydropic change). The basal region of the epithelium is thickened, and the papillae of the lamina propria are elongated and extend toward the surface because of reactive proliferation. Capillary vessels within the papillae are often dilated. An increase in lymphocytes is seen in the squamous epithelium, and eosinophils and neutrophils may be present. Esophageal stricture may eventuate in those patients in whom the ulcer persists and damages the esophageal wall deep to the lamina propria. In this circumstance, reactive fibrosis can narrow the esophageal lumen.

Barrett Esophagus is Replacement of Esophageal Squamous Epithelium by Columnar Epithelium

Barrett esophagus is a result of chronic gastroesophageal reflux. This disorder occurs in the lower third of the esophagus but may extend higher. There is a slight male predominance and a more than twofold increased risk for Barrett esophagus among smokers. Patients with Barrett esophagus are placed in a regular surveillance program to detect early microscopic evidence of dysplastic mucosa.

PATHOLOGY: Metaplastic Barrett epithelium may partially involve the circumference of short segments or may line the entire lower esophagus (Fig. 13-4A). Microscopically, the sine qua non of Barrett esophagus is the presence of a distinctive type of epithelium, referred to as "specialized epithelium." It consists of an admixture of intestine-like epithelium characterized by well-formed goblet cells interspersed with gastric foveolar cells (see Fig. 13-4B). Complete intestinal metaplasia, with Paneth cells and absorptive cells, occurs occasionally. Inflammatory changes are often superimposed on the epithelial alterations. *Barrett esophagus may transform into adenocarcinoma, the risk correlating with the length of the involved esophagus and the degree of dysplasia* (see below).

Infective Esophagitis is Associated with Immunosuppression

CANDIDA ESOPHAGITIS: This fungal infection has become commonplace because of an increasing number of immunocompromised persons. Esophageal candidiasis also occurs in patients with diabetes, those receiving antibiotic therapy, and uncommonly in persons with no known predisposing factors. Dysphagia and severe pain on swallowing are usual.

PATHOLOGY: In mild cases of candidiasis, a few small, elevated white plaques surrounded by a hyperemic zone are present on the mucosa of the middle or lower third of the esophagus. In severe cases, confluent pseudomembranes lie on a hyperemic and edematous mucosa. Microscopically, *Candida* sometimes involves only the superficial layers of the squamous epithelium. The candidal pseudomembrane contains fungal mycelia, necrotic debris, and fibrin. Involvement of deeper layers of the esophageal wall can lead to disseminated candidiasis or fibrosis, sometimes severe enough to create a stricture.

HERPETIC ESOPHAGITIS: Esophageal infection with herpesvirus type I is most frequently associated with lymphomas and leukemias and is often manifested by odynophagia. However, on occasion, it may occur in otherwise healthy individuals.

PATHOLOGY: The well-developed lesions of herpetic esophagitis grossly resemble those of candidiasis. Microscopically, lesions are superficial, and epithelial cells exhibit typical nuclear herpetic inclusions and occasional multinucleation. Necrosis of infected cells leads to ulcera-

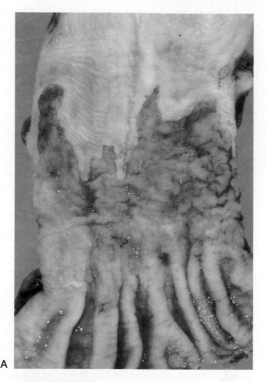

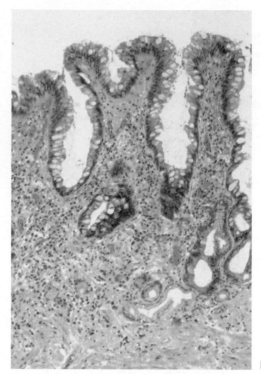

FIGURE 13-4. **Barrett esophagus. A.** The presence of the tan tongues of epithelium interdigitating with the more proximal squamous epithelium is typical of Barrett esophagus. **B.** The specialized epithelium has a villiform architecture and is lined by cells that are foveolar gastric type cells and intestinal goblet type cells.

tion, and candidal and bacterial superinfection results in the formation of pseudomembranes.

Esophageal Varices

Esophageal varices are dilated veins immediately beneath the mucosa (Fig. 13-5) *that are prone to rupture and hemorrhage* (also see Chapter 14). They arise in the lower third of the esophagus, virtually always in patients with cirrhosis and portal hypertension. The lower esophageal veins are linked to the portal system through gastroesophageal anastomoses. If portal system pressure exceeds a critical level, these anastomoses become prominent in the upper stomach and lower esophagus. When varices are greater than 5 mm in diameter, they are prone to rupture, leading to life-threatening hemorrhage. Reflux injury or infective esophagitis can contribute to variceal bleeding.

Neoplasms

Esophageal Carcinoma Varies Geographically and Histologically

EPIDEMIOLOGY: Worldwide, most esophageal cancers are squamous cell carcinomas, but adenocarcinoma is now more common in the United States (see below). Geographic variations in the incidence of esophageal carcinoma are striking. There is an esophageal cancer belt extending across Asia from the Caspian Sea region of northern Iran and through Central Asia and Mongolia to northern China. In parts of China, the mortality rate from esophageal cancer in men may be 70 times that in the United States. Esophageal cancer is uncommon in the United States and accounts for only about 2% of cancer deaths. American blacks, however, have a much higher incidence than whites.

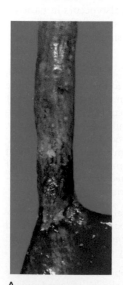

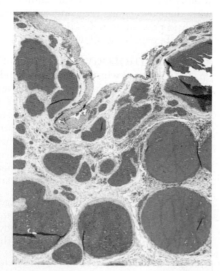

FIGURE 13-5. **Esophageal varices. A.** Numerous prominent blue venous channels are seen beneath the mucosa of the everted esophagus, particularly above the gastroesophageal junction. **B.** Section of the esophagus reveals numerous dilated submucosal veins.

PATHOGENESIS: Geographic variations in esophageal cancer, even in relatively homogeneous populations, suggest that environmental factors contribute strongly to its development. However, no single factor has been incriminated.

• **Cigarette smoking** increases risk of esophageal cancer 5- to 10-fold. The number of cigarettes smoked correlates with the frequency of esophageal dysplasia.

- **Excessive consumption of alcohol** is a major risk factor in the United States, even when cigarette smoking is taken into account.
- **Nitrosamines** and aniline dyes produce esophageal cancer in animals, but direct evidence for their contribution to human esophageal cancer is lacking.
- **Diets low in fresh fruits, vegetables, animal protein, and trace metals** are described in areas with endemic esophageal cancer. However, the close proximity of endemic and nonendemic areas renders a causative role for these dietary factors unlikely.
- **Plummer-Vinson syndrome, celiac sprue, and achalasia** for unknown reasons are associated with an increased incidence of esophageal cancer.
- **Chronic esophagitis** has been related to esophageal cancer in areas in which this tumor is endemic.
- **Chemical injury with esophageal stricture** is a risk factor. Of persons who have an esophageal stricture after ingestion of lye, 5% develop cancer 20 to 40 years later.
- **Webs, rings, and diverticula** are sometimes associated with esophageal cancer.

 PATHOLOGY: About half of cases of esophageal cancer involve the lower third of the esophagus; the middle and upper thirds account for the remainder. Grossly, the tumors are of three types: (1) ulcerating (Fig. 13-6A), (2) polyploid, which project into the lumen (Fig. 13-6B), and (3) infiltrating, in which the principal plane of growth is in the wall. The bulky polyploid tumors tend to obstruct early, whereas those that are ulcerated tend to be smaller and are more likely to bleed.

Infiltrating tumors gradually narrow the lumen by circumferential compression. Local extension of tumor into mediastinal structures is commonly a major problem.

Microscopically, neoplastic squamous cells range from well differentiated, with epithelial "pearls," to poorly differentiated tumors that lack evidence of squamous differentiation. Occasional tumors have a predominant spindle cell population of tumors cells (metaplastic carcinoma). The rich lymphatic drainage of the esophagus provides a route for most metastases. Metastases to liver and lung are common, but almost any organ may be involved.

CLINICAL FEATURES: The most common presenting complaint is dysphagia, but by this time, most tumors are unresectable. Patients with esophageal cancer are almost invariably cachectic, due to anorexia, difficulty in swallowing, and the remote effects of a malignant tumor. Surgery and radiation therapy are useful for palliation, but the prognosis remains dismal. Many patients are inoperable, and of those who undergo surgery, only 20% survive for 5 years.

Adenocarcinoma of the Esophagus

As its incidence has recently increased, adenocarcinoma of the esophagus is now more common (60%) in the United States than is squamous carcinoma. *Virtually all adenocarcinomas arise in the background of Barrett esophagus*, although a rare case may originate in submucosal mucous glands. Endoscopic surveillance for adenocarcinoma is now commonly done in patients with Barrett esophagus, particularly in those with dysplasia. The symptoms and clinical course of esophageal adenocarcinoma are similar to those of squamous cell carcinoma.

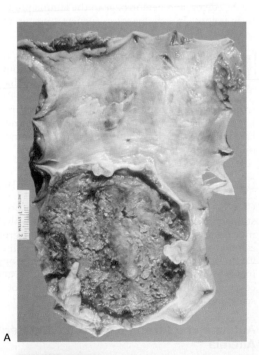

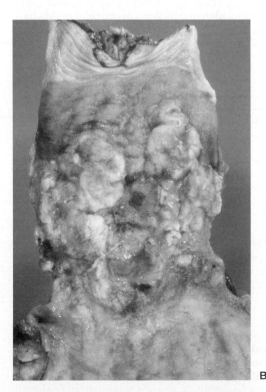

FIGURE 13-6. **Esophageal carcinoma. A.** Squamous cell carcinoma. There is a large ulcerated mass present in the squamous mucosa with normal squamous mucosa intervening between the carcinoma and the stomach. **B.** Adenocarcinoma. There is a large exophytic ulcerated mass lesion just proximal to the gastroesophageal junction. The well-differentiated adenocarcinoma was separated from the most proximal squamous epithelium by a tan area representing Barrett esophagus.

THE STOMACH

Congenital Disorders: Congenital Pyloric Stenosis

Congenital pyloric stenosis is concentric enlargement of the pyloric sphincter and narrowing of the pyloric canal that obstructs the gastric outlet. This disorder is the most common indication for abdominal surgery in the initial 6 months of life. It is four times more common in boys than in girls and affects first-born children more than subsequent ones. Pyloric stenosis occurs in 1 in 250 white infants but is rare in blacks and Asians.

 PATHOGENESIS: Congenital pyloric stenosis may have a genetic basis; there is a familial tendency, and the condition is more common in identical than in fraternal twins. It also occurs with Turner syndrome, trisomy 18, and esophageal atresia. Embryopathies associated with rubella infection and maternal intake of thalidomide have also been associated with congenital pyloric stenosis.

 PATHOLOGY: Gross examination of the stomach shows concentric pyloric enlargement and narrowing of the pyloric canal. The only consistent microscopic abnormality is extreme hypertrophy of the circular muscle coat. After pyloromyotomy, the lesion disappears, although occasionally a small mass remains.

 CLINICAL FEATURES: Projectile vomiting is the main symptom and is usually seen within the first month of life. Consequent loss of hydrochloric acid leads to hypochloremic alkalosis in one third of infants. A palpable pyloric lesion and visible peristalsis are common. Surgical incision of hypertrophied pyloric muscle is curative.

Gastritis

Acute Hemorrhagic Gastritis is Associated with Drugs and Stress

Acute hemorrhagic erosive gastritis is characterized by mucosal necrosis. Erosion of the mucosa may extend into the deeper tissues to form an ulcer. The necrosis is accompanied by an acute inflammatory response and hemorrhage, which may be severe enough to result in exsanguination.

 PATHOGENESIS: Acute hemorrhagic gastritis is most commonly associated with the intake of aspirin, other NSAIDs, excess alcohol, or ischemic injury. These agents injure the gastric mucosa directly and exert their effects topically. Oral administration of corticosteroids may also be complicated by acute hemorrhagic gastritis. **Any serious illness that is accompanied by profound physiologic alterations that require substantial medical or surgical intervention renders the gastric mucosa more vulnerable to acute hemorrhagic gastritis because of mucosal ischemia.** The factor common to all forms of acute hemorrhagic gastritis is thought to be the breakdown of the mucosal barrier, which permits acid-induced injury.

Stress ulcers and erosions occur in severely burned persons (**Curling ulcer**) and commonly result in bleeding. Ulceration may be deep enough to cause perforation of the stomach. Patients occasionally exhibit both gastric and duodenal ulcers.

Central nervous system trauma, accidental or surgical (**Cushing ulcer**), may also cause stress ulcers. These ulcers, which may also occur in the esophagus or duodenum, are characteristically deep and carry a substantial risk of perforation.

Severe trauma, especially if accompanied by **shock, prolonged sepsis, and incapacitation** from many debilitating chronic diseases, also predisposes to development of acute hemorrhagic gastritis.

Hypersecretion of gastric acid has been incriminated in the pathogenesis of acute hemorrhagic gastritis, but its role is not clear. Nevertheless, gastric acid plays a permissive role, because inhibition of gastric acid secretion (e.g., with histamine-receptor antagonists) protects against the development of stress ulcers.

Microcirculatory changes in the stomach induced by shock or sepsis suggest that ischemic injury may contribute to the development of acute hemorrhagic gastritis. Failure of defense mechanisms of the gastric mucosa are also likely to play a role. For example, prostaglandin deficiency caused by nonsteroidal anti-inflammatory drugs (NSAIDs) that inhibit prostaglandin synthesis, has been postulated to decrease mucosal resistance to gastric contents. Both steroids and NSAIDs may lead directly to decreased mucus production. Decreasing the intraluminal pH of the gastric mucosa is protective in hemorrhagic shock, supporting the role of acid in the pathogenesis of certain erosions.

 PATHOLOGY: Acute hemorrhagic gastritis is characterized grossly by widespread petechial hemorrhages in any portion of the stomach or regions of confluent mucosal or submucosal bleeding. Lesions vary from 1 to 25 mm across and appear occasionally as sharply punched-out ulcers. Microscopically, patchy mucosal necrosis, which can extend to the submucosa, is visualized adjacent to normal mucosa. Fibrinous exudate, edema, and hemorrhage in the lamina propria are present in early lesions. In extreme cases, penetrating ulcers may reach the serosa.

 CLINICAL FEATURES: Symptoms of acute hemorrhagic gastritis range from vague abdominal discomfort to massive, life-threatening hemorrhage and clinical manifestations of gastric perforation. Patients with gastritis induced by aspirin and other NSAIDs may be seen with hypochromic, microcytic anemia caused by undetected chronic bleeding. Treatment with antacids and histamine-receptor antagonists has proved useful.

Chronic Gastritis is Autoimmune or Environmental

Chronic gastritis refers to chronic inflammatory diseases of the stomach, which range from mild superficial involvement of gastric mucosa to severe atrophy. This heterogeneous group of disorders exhibits distinct anatomical distributions within the stomach, varying etiologies, and characteristic complications. The predominant symptom is dyspepsia. The diseases are also commonly discovered in asymptomatic persons undergoing routine endoscopic screening.

Autoimmune Atrophic Gastritis and Pernicious Anemia

Autoimmune atrophic gastritis is a chronic, diffuse inflammatory disease of the stomach that is restricted to the body and fundus. This disorder typically exhibits:

- Diffuse atrophic gastritis in the body and fundus of the stomach, with lack of, or minimal involvement of, the antrum
- Antibodies to parietal cells and intrinsic factor

- Significant reduction in or absence of gastric secretion, including acid
- Increased serum gastrin, owing to G-cell hyperplasia of the antral mucosa
- Enterochromaffin-like cell hyperplasia in the atrophic oxyntic mucosa, secondary to gastrin stimulation

Pernicious anemia *is a megaloblastic anemia caused by malabsorption of vitamin B$_{12}$, owing to a deficiency of intrinsic factor. In most cases, pernicious anemia is a complication of autoimmune gastritis.* The latter disorder is also associated with extragastric autoimmune diseases such as chronic thyroiditis, Graves' disease, Addison disease, vitiligo, diabetes mellitus type I, and myasthenia gravis (see also Chapter 20).

 PATHOGENESIS: Autoimmune gastritis is so named because of the presence of autoantibodies and the association with other diseases that have a similar pathogenesis. Circulating antibodies to parietal cells, some of which are cytotoxic in the presence of complement, occur in 90% of patients with pernicious anemia. Importantly, about 20% of individuals over 60 years have parietal cell antibodies, although few have pernicious anemia. The majority of patients also have intrinsic factor autoantibodies that interfere with vitamin B$_{12}$ absorption. In addition, anti-thyroid antibodies are common.

Multifocal Atrophic Gastritis (Environmental Metaplastic Atrophic Gastritis)

Multifocal atrophic gastritis is a disease of uncertain etiology that typically involves the antrum and adjacent areas of the body. This form of chronic gastritis has these features:

- It is considerably more common than the autoimmune variety of atrophic gastritis and is four times as frequent among whites as in other races.
- It is not linked to autoimmune phenomena.
- Like autoimmune gastritis, it is often associated with reduced acid secretion (hypochlorhydria).
- Complete absence of gastric secretion (achlorhydria) and pernicious anemia are uncommon.

 EPIDEMIOLOGY AND PATHOGENESIS: *The age and geographic distribution of environmental metaplastic atrophic gastritis parallel those of gastric carcinoma; this type of gastritis seems to be a precursor of this cancer.* The disease exhibits a striking localization to certain populations and is particularly common in Asia, Scandinavia, and parts of Europe and Latin America. It also increases in incidence with age in all populations in which it is prevalent. Offspring of emigrants from areas of high risk for stomach cancer to those of low risk lose their predisposition to this tumor, suggesting the importance of environmental factors such as diet and *Helicobacter pylori* (see below).

 PATHOLOGY: The pathologic features of autoimmune and multifocal atrophic gastritis are similar, except for the localization of the autoimmune type to the fundus and body and the multifocal variety mainly to the antrum.

ATROPHIC GASTRITIS: This condition is characterized by prominent chronic inflammation in the lamina propria. Occasionally, lymphoid cells are arranged as follicles, an appearance that has led to an erroneous diagnosis of lymphoma, especially in patients with *H. pylori* infection (see below). Involvement of gastric glands leads to degenerative changes in their epithelial cells and ultimately to a conspicuous reduction in the number of glands (thus the name **atrophic gastritis**). Eventually, inflammation may abate, leaving only a thin atrophic mucosa, in which case the term **gastric atrophy** is applied.

INTESTINAL METAPLASIA: *This lesion is a common and important histopathologic feature of both autoimmune and multifocal types of atrophic gastritis.* In response to injury of the gastric mucosa, the normal epithelium is replaced by one composed of cells of the intestinal type. Numerous mucin-containing goblet cells and enterocytes line crypt-like glands. Paneth cells, which are not normal inhabitants of the gastric mucosa, are present. Intestinal-type villi may occasionally form. The metaplastic cells also contain enzymes characteristic of the intestine but not of the stomach (e.g., alkaline phosphatase, aminopeptidase).

Atrophic Gastritis and Stomach Cancer

Persons with autoimmune or multifocal atrophic gastritis have an elevated risk of carcinoma of the stomach. Patients with pernicious anemia, who invariably have atrophic gastritis, have a threefold greater risk for gastric adenocarcinoma and a 13-fold higher risk of carcinoid (neuroendocrine) tumors. Cancer arises in the antrum several times more frequently than in the body of the stomach, suggesting that antral gastritis is related to gastric carcinogenesis.

Intestinal metaplasia of the stomach has been identified as a preneoplastic lesion for several reasons: (1) gastric cancer arises in areas of metaplastic epithelium, (2) half of all stomach cancers are of the intestinal cell type, and (3) many gastric cancers show aminopeptidase activity similar to that seen in areas of intestinal metaplasia.

Helicobacter pylori Gastritis

H. pylori *gastritis is a chronic inflammatory disease of the antrum and body of the stomach caused by* H. pylori *and occasionally by* Helicobacter heilmannii. It is the most common type of chronic gastritis in the United States. *H. pylori* infection is also strongly associated with peptic ulcer disease of the stomach and duodenum (see below).

 PATHOGENESIS: *Helicobacter* species are small, curved, gram-negative rods (Proteobacteria) with polar flagella and a corkscrew-like motion. The prevalence of infection with this organism increases with age: by age 60 years, half the population has serologic evidence of infection. Twin studies have shown genetic influences in susceptibility to infection with *H. pylori*. Intrafamilial clustering of *H. pylori* infection suggests that these bacteria may spread from person to person. Two thirds of those who have been infected with *H. pylori* show histologic evidence of chronic gastritis.

H. pylori is considered to be the pathogen responsible for chronic antral gastritis rather than a commensal organism that colonizes injured gastric mucosa because (1) gastritis develops in healthy persons after ingesting the organism, (2) *H. pylori* attaches to the epithelium in areas of chronic gastritis and is absent from uninvolved areas of the gastric mucosa, (3) eradicating the infection with bismuth or antibiotics cures the gastritis, (4) antibodies against *H. pylori* are routinely found in persons with chronic gastritis, and (5) the increasing prevalence of *H. pylori* infection with age parallels that of chronic gastritis. Chronic infection with *H. pylori* also predisposes to the development of mucosa-associated lymphoid tissue (MALT) lymphoma of the stomach and is associated with adenocarcinoma of the stomach (see below).

 PATHOLOGY: The curved rods of *H. pylori* are found in the surface mucus of epithelial cells and in gastric foveolae (Fig. 13-7). Active gastritis features polymorphonuclear leukocytes in glands and their lumina as

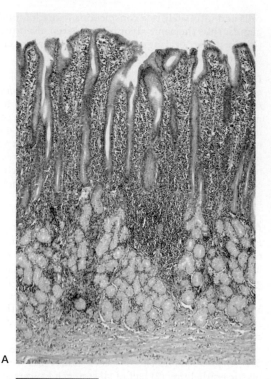
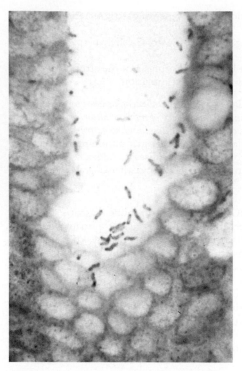

A   B

FIGURE 13-7. **Helicobacter pylori-associated gastritis. A.** The antrum shows an intense lymphocytic and plasma cell infiltrate, which tends to be heaviest in the superficial portions of the lamina propria. **B.** The microorganisms appear on silver staining as small, curved rods on the surface of the gastric mucosa.

well as increased numbers of plasma cells and lymphocytes in the lamina propria (see Fig. 13-7A). Lymphoid hyperplasia with germinal centers is frequent and is the setting for the development of MALT lymphoma.

Peptic Ulcer Disease

Peptic ulcer disease refers to focal destruction of gastric mucosa and the small intestine, principally the proximal duodenum, caused by the action of gastric secretions. About 10% of the population of Western industrialized countries may develop such ulcers at some time during their lives. However, both the incidence and prevalence of duodenal ulcers have declined substantially during the past 30 years.

Gastric and Duodenal Ulcer Disease Have Unique Features

For practical purposes, peptic ulcer disease affects the distal stomach and proximal duodenum. Many clinical and epidemiologic features distinguish gastric from duodenal ulcers; *the common factor that unites them is the gastric secretion of hydrochloric acid.*

 EPIDEMIOLOGY: The peak age for peptic ulcer disease has progressively increased in the past 50 years, and for duodenal ulcer disease, it is now between 30 and 60 years of age, although the disorder may occur in persons of any age and even in infants. Gastric ulcers afflict the middle-aged and elderly more than the young. For duodenal ulcers, there is a male predominance. By contrast, the incidence of gastric ulcers is similar in men and women.

 PATHOGENESIS: Numerous etiologic factors have been implicated in the pathogenesis of peptic ulcers, but no single agent seems to be responsible.

Environmental Factors

DIET: Little evidence supports the contention that any food or beverage, including coffee and alcohol, contributes to the development or persistence of peptic ulcers. However, cirrhosis from any cause is associated with an increased incidence of peptic ulcers.

DRUGS: Aspirin, other NSAIDs, and analgesics are important contributing factors for peptic ulcers.

CIGARETTE SMOKING: Smoking is a definite risk factor, particularly for gastric ulcers.

Genetic Factors

First-degree relatives of people with duodenal or gastric ulcers have a threefold increased risk of developing an ulcer, but only at the same site. Identical twins show a 50% concordance, indicating that environmental factors are also involved.

BLOOD GROUP ANTIGENS: The risk of duodenal (but not gastric) ulcer is 30% higher in persons with type O blood than in those with other types. People who do not secrete blood-group antigens in saliva or gastric juice (nonsecretors) carry a 50% increased risk for duodenal ulcers.

PEPSINOGEN I: A person with a high circulating level of pepsinogen I has five times the normal risk of developing a duodenal ulcer. Serum levels of this proenzyme correlate with the capacity for gastric acid secretion and are considered a measure of parietal cell mass. Elevated levels of pepsinogen I occur in half of children of ulcer patients with hyperpepsinogenemia and has been attributed to autosomal dominant inheritance.

Physiologic Factors in Duodenal Ulcers

Hydrochloric acid secretion is necessary for the formation and persistence of peptic ulcers in the stomach and duodenum. The maximal capacity for gastric acid production is reflected in total parietal cell mass. Patients with duodenal ulcers may have up to double normal parietal cell mass and maximal acid secretion. However, there is a large overlap with normal values, and only one third of these patients secrete excess acid. Acid secretion in people with duodenal ulcers may also be more sensitive than normal to gastric secretagogues such as gastrin, possibly as the result of increased vagal tone or increased affinity of parietal cells for gastrin.

Accelerated gastric emptying has been noted in patients with duodenal ulcers. This condition might lead to excessive acidification of the duodenum. However, as with other factors, there is an overlap with normal rates. Normally, duodenal bulb acidification inhibits further gastric emptying. In most patients with duodenal ulcers, this inhibitory mechanism is absent; duodenal acidification leads to continued, rather than delayed, gastric emptying.

The pH of the duodenal bulb reflects the balance between delivery of gastric juice and its neutralization by biliary, pancreatic, and duodenal secretions. In ulcer patients, duodenal pH after a meal decreases to a lower level and remains depressed for a longer time than in normal persons. Such duodenal hyperacidity reflects the gastric factors discussed above.

Impaired mucosal defenses have been invoked as contributing to peptic ulceration. These mucosal factors, including prostaglandin function, may or may not be similar to those protecting the gastric mucosa.

Physiologic Factors In Gastric Ulcers

Gastric ulcers almost invariably arise in the setting of epithelial injury by H. pylori *or chemical gastritis.* The mechanisms by which chronic gastritis predisposes to gastric ulceration are obscure. *Most patients with gastric ulcers secrete less acid than do those with duodenal ulcers and even less than normal persons.* The concurrence of gastric ulcers and gastric hyposecretion implies: (1) the gastric mucosa may in some way be particularly sensitive to low concentrations of acid; (2) something other than acid may damage the mucosa, such as NSAIDs; or (3) the gastric mucosa may be exposed to potentially injurious agents for unusually long periods.

The Role of *Helicobacter pylori*

H. pylori *is isolated from the gastric antrum of virtually all patients with duodenal ulcers.* The converse is not true; that is, only a small minority of persons infected with this bacterium have duodenal ulcer disease. Thus, *H. pylori* infection may be a necessary, but not sufficient, condition for the development of peptic ulcers in the duodenum.

Just how *H. pylori* infection predisposes to duodenal ulcers is not completely known, but several mechanisms have been proposed. Cytokines produced by inflammatory cells that respond to *H. pylori* infection stimulate gastrin release and suppress somatostatin secretion. The release of histamine metabolites from the organism itself may stimulate basal gastric acid secretion. There is some evidence that *H. pylori* infection might indirectly cause an increased acid load in the duodenum, thereby contributing to duodenal ulceration. Acidification of the duodenal bulb leads to islands of metaplastic gastric mucosa in the duodenum in many patients with a peptic ulcer. It has been postulated that infection of the metaplastic epithelium by *H. pylori* renders the mucosa more susceptible to peptic injury (Fig. 13-8).

Infection with H. pylori *is probably also important in the pathogenesis of gastric ulcers,* because this organism is responsible for most cases of the chronic gastritis that underlies this disease. About 75% of patients with gastric ulcers harbor *H. pylori.* The remaining 25% of cases may represent an association with other types of chronic gastritis. The various gastric and duodenal factors that have been implicated as possible mechanisms in the pathogenesis of duodenal ulcers are summarized in Figure 13-9.

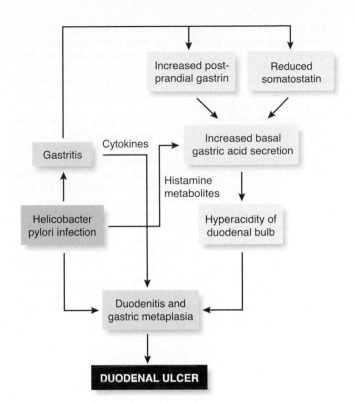

FIGURE 13-8. Possible mechanisms in the pathogenesis of duodenal ulcer disease associated with *Helicobacter pylori* infection.

Several Diseases are Associated with Peptic Ulcers

CIRRHOSIS: The incidence of duodenal ulcers in patients with cirrhosis is 10 times greater than that in normal individuals.

CHRONIC RENAL FAILURE: End-stage renal disease with hemodialysis increases the risk of peptic ulceration. Patients subjected to renal transplantation also show a substantially increased incidence of peptic ulceration and its complications, such as bleeding and perforation.

HEREDITARY ENDOCRINE SYNDROMES: There is an increased incidence of peptic ulcers in persons with **multiple endocrine neoplasia, type I** (see Chapter 21). Zollinger-Ellison syndrome, a cause of severe peptic ulceration, is characterized by gastric hypersecretion caused by a gastrin-producing islet cell adenoma of the pancreas.

α_1**-ANTITRYPSIN DEFICIENCY:** Almost one third of patients with this disease have peptic ulcers, the incidence of which is even higher if patients also have lung disease. Moreover, peptic ulcer is increased in people heterozygous for mutant α_1-antitrypsin.

CHRONIC PULMONARY DISEASE: Long-standing pulmonary dysfunction significantly increases the risk of ulcers, and it is estimated that fully one fourth of those with such disorders have peptic ulcer disease. Conversely, chronic lung disease is increased two- to threefold in persons who have peptic ulcers.

Gastric and Duodenal Ulcers are Similar Microscopically

PATHOLOGY: Most peptic ulcers arise in the lesser gastric curvature, in the antral and prepyloric regions, and in the first part of the duodenum.

Gastric ulcers (Fig. 13-10) are usually single and smaller than 2 cm in diameter. Ulcers on the lesser curvature are commonly associated with chronic gastritis, whereas those on the greater curvature are often related to NSAIDs. The edges of the ulcers tend to be sharply punched out, with overhanging margins. Deeply penetrating ulcers produce a serosal exudate that may cause adherence of the stomach to surrounding structures. Scarring of ulcers in the prepyloric region may be severe enough to produce pyloric stenosis. *Grossly, chronic peptic ulcers may closely resemble ulcerated gastric carcinomas.*

Duodenal ulcers (Fig. 13-11) are ordinarily on the anterior or posterior wall of the first part of the duodenum, close to the pylorus. The lesions are usually solitary, but it is not uncommon to find paired ulcers on both walls, so-called kissing ulcers.

Microscopically, gastric and duodenal ulcers are similar (Fig. 13-12). From the lumen outward, the following are noted: (1) a superficial zone of fibrinopurulent exudate; (2) necrotic tissue; (3) granulation tissue; and (4) fibrotic tissue at the base of the ulcer, which exhibits variable degrees of chronic inflammation. Ulceration may penetrate the muscle layers, causing them to be interrupted by scar tissue after healing. Blood vessels on the margins of the ulcer are often thrombosed. The mucosa at the margins tends to be hyperplastic; as the ulcer heals, the mucosa grows over the ulcerated area as a single layer of epithelium. Duodenal ulcers are usually accompanied by peptic duodenitis, with Brunner gland hyperplasia and gastric mucin cell metaplasia.

 CLINICAL FEATURES: The symptoms of gastric and duodenal ulcers are sufficiently similar that the two conditions are generally not distinguishable by history or physical examination. The classic case of duodenal ulcer is characterized by epigastric pain 1 to 3 hours after a meal or pain that awakens the patient at night. Both alkali and food relieve the symptoms. Dyspeptic symptoms commonly associated with gallbladder disease, including fatty food intolerance, distention, and belching, occur in half of patients with peptic ulcers. The major complications of peptic ulcer disease are hemorrhage, perforation with peritonitis, and obstruction.

HEMORRHAGE: The most common complication of peptic ulcers is bleeding, which occurs in up to 20% of patients. Bleeding is often occult and, in the absence of other symptoms, may manifest as iron-deficiency anemia or occult blood in stools. *Massive life-threatening bleeding is a well-known complication of active peptic ulcers.*

PERFORATION: Perforation is a serious complication of peptic ulcers, which occurs in 5% of patients. In one third of the cases, there are no antecedent symptoms of a peptic ulcer. Perforations occur more often with duodenal than with gastric ulcers, mostly on the anterior wall of the duodenum. *Perforation carries a high mor-*

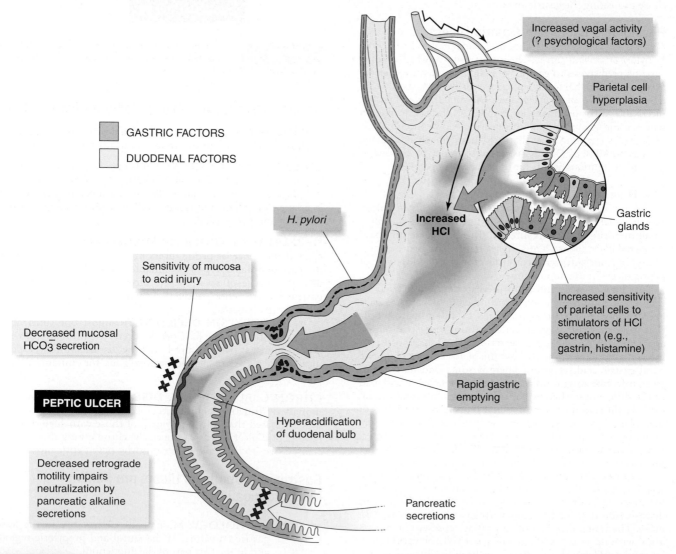

FIGURE 13-9. Gastric and duodenal factors in the pathogenesis of duodenal peptic ulcers. *H. pylori, Helicobacter pylori;* HCl, hydrochloric acid; HCO₃⁻, bicarbonate.

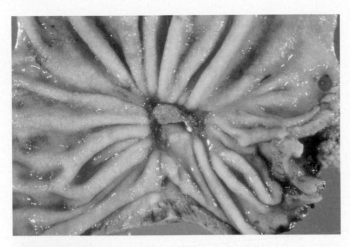

FIGURE 13-10. Gastric ulcer. There is a characteristic sharp demarcation from the surrounding mucosa, with radiating gastric folds. The base of the ulcer is gray because of fibrin deposition.

tality rate. The risk of death for perforated gastric ulcers is 10% to 40%, which is two to three times more than for duodenal ulcers (~10%). Perforations are occasionally complicated by hemorrhage. Although shock, abdominal distention, and pain are common symptoms, perforations are occasionally diagnosed for the first time at autopsy, particularly in institutionalized, elderly patients.

MALIGNANT TRANSFORMATION OF BENIGN GASTRIC ULCERS: *Malignant transformation of a duodenal ulcer is very uncommon.* However, although cancers originating in benign peptic ulcers probably account for less than 1% of all malignant tumors in the stomach, such tumors have been well documented.

TREATMENT: In the past, peptic ulcers were treated by subtotal gastrectomy. However, the disease is now cured by using antibiotics to eliminate *H. pylori* and by blocking gastric acid secretion with histamine receptor blockers and proton pump inhibitors.

Benign Neoplasms

Stromal Tumors in the Stomach Tend to be Nonaggressive

Nearly all gastrointestinal stromal tumors (GISTs) are derived from the pacemaker cells of Cajal embedded in the muscular tis-

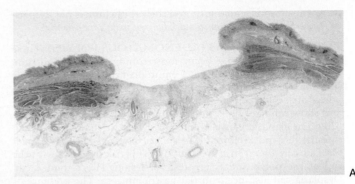

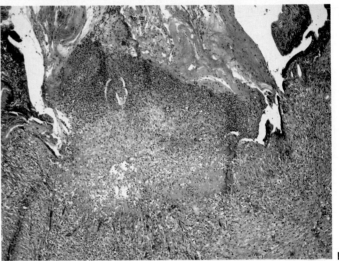

FIGURE 13-12. Gastric ulcer. **A.** There is full-thickness replacement of the gastric muscularis with connective tissue. **B.** Photomicrograph of a peptic ulcer with superficial exudate over necrosis, granulation tissue, and fibrosis.

sue of the GI tract. GISTs include the vast majority of mesenchymal-derived stromal tumors of the entire GI tract. The pacemaker cells and the tumor cells express the *c-kit* oncogene (CD117), which encodes a tyrosine kinase that promotes cell proliferation. Many of gastric GISTs, independently of size, tend to behave in a nonaggressive fashion, as opposed to small and large bowel tumors, which more commonly behave in a malignant manner.

Gastric GISTs are usually submucosal and covered by intact mucosa or, when they project externally, by peritoneum. The cut surface is whorled. Microscopically, the tumors are variably cellular and are composed of spindle-shaped cells with cytoplasmic vacuoles embedded in a collagenous stroma. The cells are disposed in whorls and interlacing bundles. With few exceptions, GISTs are considered tumors of low malignant potential. Treatment of GISTs consists mainly of surgical resection and administering an inhibitor of the specific tyrosine kinase.

Epithelial Polyps May Represent Either Hyperplasia or a Neoplastic Process

HYPERPLASTIC POLYPS: These lesions are by far the most common of the gastric polyps. They may be single or multiple and are seen as pedunculated or sessile lesions of variable sizes. Hyperplastic polyps are common in the hydrochloric acid– secreting mucosa of the body and fundus of patients with autoimmune metaplastic atrophic gastritis, but they also occur in the antrum of patients with *H. pylori* gastritis. Microscopically, the polyps consist of elongated, branched crypts lined by foveolar epithelium, beneath which pyloric or gastric glands are present. They appear to

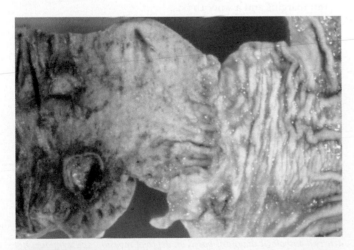

FIGURE 13-11. Duodenal ulcer. There are two sharply demarcated duodenal ulcers surrounded by inflamed duodenal mucosa. The gastroduodenal junction is in the midportion of the photograph.

represent a response to injury, and their epithelium is not dysplastic. *Hyperplastic polyps of the stomach have no malignant potential.*

TUBULAR ADENOMAS (ADENOMATOUS POLYPS): These are true neoplasms that occur most commonly in the antrum. They range from smaller than 1 cm in diameter to a considerable size; the average dimension is about 4 cm. Most adenomatous polyps are sessile and are usually solitary. Microscopically, adenomas show tubular or a combination of tubular and villous structures. The glands are usually lined by dysplastic epithelium, which is sometimes intestinalized. *Adenomatous polyps manifest a malignant potential, variably reported at 5% to 75%.* This risk increases with the size of the polyp and is greatest for lesions larger than 2 cm. Dysplasia can also occur in flat gastric mucosa. The presence of multiple tubular adenomas in the stomach of patients with familial adenomatous polyposis greatly increases the risk of developing adenocarcinoma.

FUNDIC GLAND POLYPS: Fundic gland polyps are characterized by dilated acid-producing glands lined by parietal and chief cells and by mucous cell metaplasia. They are mostly seen in patients treated with proton pump inhibitors. These polyps are not considered preneoplastic, and patients have no increased risk of gastric carcinoma.

Malignant Tumors

Carcinoma of the Stomach is Associated with Many Environmental Factors

 EPIDEMIOLOGY: About 50 years ago, gastric carcinoma was the most common cause of cancer deaths, but in a surprising reversal, in men in the United States, it now accounts for only about 3% of such deaths. The incidence of stomach cancer remains exceedingly high in such countries as Japan and Chile, where rates are seven to eight times that in the United States. Emigrants from high-risk to low-risk areas show a decline in the incidence of cancer of the stomach (see Chapter 5), which strongly implicates environmental factors in the carcinogenic process.

 PATHOGENESIS: Although correlations have been demonstrated with a number of factors, the causes of gastric cancer remain elusive.

DIETARY FACTORS: Gastric cancer is more common among persons who eat large amounts of starch, smoked fish and meat, and pickled vegetables. Benzpyrene, a potent carcinogen, has been detected in smoked foods.

NITROSAMINES: Nitrosamines are potent carcinogens in animals, and secondary amines are converted to nitrosamines in the presence of nitrates or nitrites. High concentrations of nitrate have been found in the soil and water in certain areas that feature a high incidence of gastric cancer, and processed meats and vegetables contain considerable amounts of nitrates and nitrites. The decrease in gastric cancer in the United States parallels the increased use of refrigeration, which inhibits conversion of nitrates to nitrites and also obviates the need for such food preservatives. Consumption of whole milk and fresh vegetables rich in vitamin C is inversely related to the occurrence of stomach cancer. Vitamin C inhibits the nitrosation of secondary amines in vivo.

GENETIC FACTORS: Heredity is not thought to play an important role in most cases of gastric carcinoma, but the disease occurs with higher frequency in persons who suffer hereditary nonpolyposis colorectal cancer (HNPCC) syndrome (see below). Blood type A is found in 38% of the general population, whereas half of patients with gastric cancer display this blood type.

AGE AND GENDER: Gastric cancer is uncommon in persons younger than 30 years of age and shows a sharp peak in incidence in individuals over 50. In countries with a high incidence of this tumor, the male-to-female ratio is about 2:1, but the United States demonstrates only a slight male predominance.

HELICOBACTER PYLORI: Serologic studies have shown a high prevalence of gastric infection with H. pylori *many years before the appearance of stomach cancer.* Because gastric adenocarcinoma develops in only a small proportion of persons infected with *H. pylori,* and because some stomach cancers are found in uninfected persons, *H. pylori* alone is neither sufficient nor necessary for gastric carcinogenesis.

Atrophic gastritis, pernicious anemia, subtotal gastrectomy, and gastric adenomatous polyps are discussed above as factors associated with a high risk of stomach cancer.

 PATHOLOGY: Gastric adenocarcinoma accounts for more than 95% of malignant gastric tumors. It occurs in two major but overlapping types: diffuse and intestinal. *Most intestinal type gastric cancers originate from areas of intestinal metaplasia.* By contrast, less-differentiated and anaplastic tumors of the diffuse type are more likely to derive from the necks of gastric glands without intestinal metaplasia. Cancers are most common in the distal stomach, the lesser curvature of the antrum, and the prepyloric region. Adenocarcinoma may occur anywhere, but is rare in the fundus.

ADVANCED GASTRIC CANCER: By the time most gastric cancers in the Western world are detected, they have penetrated beyond the submucosa into the muscularis propria and may extend through the serosa. The macroscopic appearance of these advanced cancers is of great importance in distinguishing carcinomas from benign lesions and assessing the degree of spread.

Advanced gastric cancers are divided into three major macroscopic types (Figure 13-13).

- **Polypoid (fungating) adenocarcinoma** accounts for one third of advanced cancers. The tumor is a solid mass, often several centimeters in diameter, that projects into the stomach lumen. The surface may be partly ulcerated, and deeper tissues may or may not be infiltrated.
- **Ulcerating adenocarcinomas** comprise another third of all gastric cancers. They have shallow ulcers of variable size. Surrounding tissues are firm, raised, and nodular. Characteristically, the lateral margins of the ulcer are irregular and the base is ragged. This appearance stands in contrast to that of the usual benign peptic ulcer, which exhibits punched-out margins and a smooth base.
- **Diffuse or infiltrating adenocarcinoma** accounts for one tenth of all stomach cancers. No true tumor mass is seen; instead, the wall of the stomach is thickened and firm. If the entire stomach is involved, it is called **linitis plastica**. In the diffuse type of gastric carcinoma, invading tumor cells induce extensive fibrosis in the submucosa and muscularis. Thus, the wall is stiff and may be more than 2 cm thick.

Microscopically, the histologic pattern of advanced gastric cancer varies from a well-differentiated adenocarcinoma with gland formation (intestinal type) to a poorly differentiated carcinoma without glands. Tumor cells may contain cytoplasmic mucin that displaces the nucleus to the periphery of the cell, resulting in the so-called signet ring cell (Fig. 13-14).

EARLY GASTRIC CANCER: Early gastric cancer is defined as a tumor limited to the mucosa or submucosa. *Early gastric cancer is strictly a pathologic diagnosis based on depth of invasion; the term does not refer to the duration of the disease, its size, presence of symptoms, absence of metastases, or curability.* Early gastric cancer may sometimes demonstrate a more benign course and greater curability because it has an inherently lower biological potential for invasion.

EARLY GASTRIC CANCER

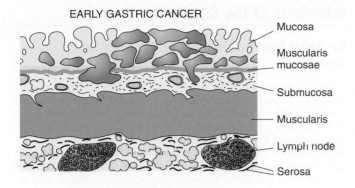

- Mucosa
- Muscularis mucosae
- Submucosa
- Muscularis
- Lymph node
- Serosa

POLYPOID CARCINOMA

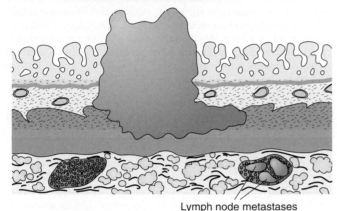

Lymph node metastases

ULCERATING CARCINOMA

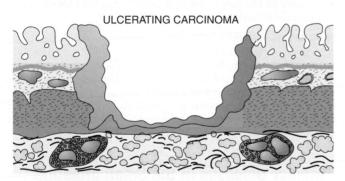

INFILTRATING CARCINOMA (LINITIS PLASTICA)

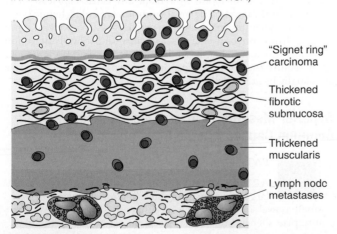

- "Signet ring" carcinoma
- Thickened fibrotic submucosa
- Thickened muscularis
- Lymph node metastases

FIGURE 13-13. The major types of gastric cancer.

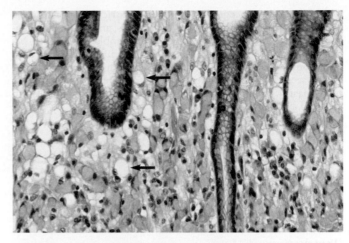

A

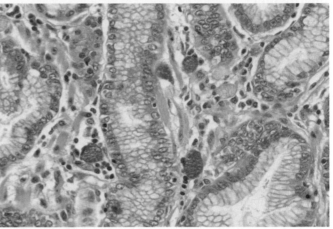

B

FIGURE 13-14. **Infiltrating gastric carcinoma. A.** Numerous signet ring cells (*arrows*) infiltrate the lamina propria between intact crypts. **B.** Mucin stains highlight the presence of mucin within the neoplastic cells.

Gastric cancer metastasizes mainly via lymphatics to regional lymph nodes of the lesser and greater curvature, porta hepatis, and subpyloric region. Distant lymphatic metastases also occur; the most common is an enlarged supraclavicular node, called a **Virchow node**. Hemato-genous spread may seed any organ, including the liver, lung, or brain. Direct extension to nearby organs is often seen. The tumor can also spread to the ovaries, where it commonly elicits a desmoplastic response, which is termed a **Krukenberg tumor**.

 CLINICAL FEATURES: In the United States and Europe, most patients with gastric cancer have metastases when they are first seen for examination. The most frequent initial symptom is weight loss, usually with anorexia and nausea. Most patients complain of epigastric or back pain, a symptom that mimics benign gastric ulcer and is often relieved by antacids or H_2-receptor antagonists. However, as the disease advances, symptomatic amelioration with medical therapy disappears. Gastric outlet obstruction may occur with large tumors of the antrum or prepyloric region. Massive bleeding is uncommon, but chronic bleeding often leads to anemia and finding occult blood in the stools. Tumors involving the esophagogastric junction cause dysphagia and may mimic achalasia and esophageal adenocarcinoma.

Gastric Lymphoma is the Most Common Extranodal Lymphoma

Primary lymphoma of the stomach accounts for about 5% of all gastric malignancies and 20% of all extranodal lymphomas.

Clinically and radiologically, it mimics gastric adenocarcinoma. The age at diagnosis is usually 40 to 65 years, and there is no gender predominance. The tumors grossly resemble carcinomas, because they may be polypoid, ulcerating, or diffuse. Most gastric lymphomas are low-grade B-cell neoplasms of the MALToma type and arise in the setting of chronic *H. pylori* gastritis with lymphoid hyperplasia. Some of the tumors actually regress after eradication of the *H. pylori* infection.

THE SMALL INTESTINE

Congenital Disorders

Atresia and Stenosis Cause Neonatal Intestinal Obstruction

ATRESIA: Atresia is defined as a complete occlusion of the intestinal lumen, which may manifest as (1) a thin intraluminal diaphragm, (2) blind proximal and distal sacs joined by a cord, or (3) disconnected blind ends.

STENOSIS: This is an incomplete stricture, which narrows but does not occlude, the lumen. Stenosis may also be caused by an incomplete diaphragm. It is usually symptomatic in infancy, but cases presenting in middle-aged adults have been recorded. Intestinal atresia or stenosis is diagnosed on the basis of persistent vomiting of bile-containing fluid within the first day of life. Meconium is not passed. The obstructed fetal intestine is dilated and filled with fluid, which can be detected radiologically. Surgical correction is usually successful, but there are often other complicating anomalies.

Meckel Diverticulum Causes Bleeding, Obstruction, and Perforation

Meckel diverticulum, caused by persistence of the vitelline duct, is an outpouching of the gut on the antimesenteric border of the ileum, 60 to 100 cm from the ileocecal valve in adults. It is the most common and the most clinically significant congenital anomaly of the small intestine. Two thirds of patients are younger than 2 years of age.

 PATHOLOGY: In adults, Meckel diverticulum is about 5 cm long, slightly narrower than the ileum. A fibrous cord may hang freely from the apex of the diverticulum or may be attached to the umbilicus. The anomaly is a true diverticulum, possessing all the coats of normal intestine; the mucosa is similar to that of the adjoining ileum. Most Meckel diverticula are asymptomatic and discovered only as incidental findings at laparotomy for other causes or at autopsy. Of the minority that becomes symptomatic, about half contain ectopic gastric, duodenal, pancreatic, biliary, or colonic tissue.

 CLINICAL FEATURES: The potential complications of Meckel diverticulum include hemorrhage, perforation, obstruction and diverticulitis, the last presenting with symptoms indistinguishable from appendicitis.

Meconium Ileus is an Early Complication of Cystic Fibrosis

Neonatal intestinal obstruction in cystic fibrosis is caused by the accumulation of tenacious meconium in the small intestine. The abnormal consistency of the meconium reflects a deficiency in pancreatic enzymes and the high viscosity of intestinal mucus. In half of affected infants, meconium ileus is complicated by (1) volvulus, (2) perforation with meconium peritonitis, or (3) intestinal atresia.

Infections of the Small Intestine

Bacterial Diarrhea is a Major Cause of Death Worldwide

Infectious diarrhea is particularly lethal in infants living in underdeveloped countries. The small bowel normally has few bacteria (usually $<10^4$/mL), which are mostly aerobic (such as lactobacilli) and ordinarily do not colonize the small intestine. Infectious diarrhea is caused by bacterial colonization, for example, with toxigenic strains of *Escherichia coli* and *Vibrio cholerae*. *The most significant factor in infectious diarrhea is increased intestinal secretion, stimulated by bacterial toxins and enteric hormones.* Decreased absorption and increased peristaltic activity contribute less to the diarrhea.

The agents of infectious diarrhea are conveniently classified into toxigenic organisms such as *V. cholerae* and toxigenic strains of *E. coli*, which produce diarrhea by elaborating toxins and invasive bacteria, of which *Shigella, Salmonella,* and certain strains of *E. coli, Yersinia,* and *Campylobacter* are the most widely recognized. Individual agents responsible for infectious diarrhea are discussed in Chapter 9.

Rotavirus and Norwalk Virus are the Most Common Causes of Viral Gastroenteritis in the United States

ROTAVIRUS: Rotavirus infection is a common cause of infantile diarrhea. It accounts for about half of acute diarrhea in hospitalized children younger than 2 years of age. Rotavirus has been demonstrated in duodenal biopsy specimens and is associated with injury to the surface epithelium and impaired intestinal absorption for periods of up to 2 months.

NORWALK VIRUSES: These agents account for one third of the epidemics of viral gastroenteritis in the United States. The virus targets the upper small intestine, where it causes patchy mucosal lesions and malabsorption. Vomiting and diarrhea are usual, and the symptoms resolve within 2 days.

Other viruses implicated as etiological agents of infective diarrhea include echovirus, coxsackievirus, cytomegalovirus, adenovirus, and coronavirus.

Vascular Diseases of the Small Intestine

Decreased intestinal blood flow from any cause can lead to **ischemic bowel disease**. The most common type of ischemic bowel disease is acute intestinal ischemia, which is associated with injury ranging from mucosal necrosis to transmural bowel infarction. Chronic intestinal ischemic syndromes are less common and generally require the severe compromise of two or more major arteries, usually by atherosclerosis.

Superior Mesenteric Artery Occlusion is the Most Common Cause of Acute Intestinal Ischemia

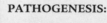 **PATHOGENESIS:**

ARTERIAL OCCLUSION: Sudden occlusion of a large artery by thrombosis or embolization leads to small bowel infarction before collateral circulation comes into play. Depending on the size of the artery, infarction may be segmental or may lead to gangrene of virtually the entire small bowel (Fig. 13-15). Occlusive intestinal infarction is most often caused by embolic or thrombotic occlusion of the superior mesenteric artery or its larger branches. Less com-

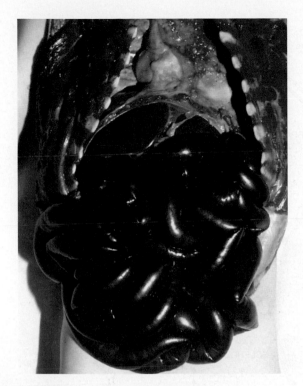

FIGURE 13-15. **Infarct of the small bowel.** This infant died after an episode of intense abdominal pain and shock. Autopsy demonstrated volvulus of the small bowel that had occluded the superior mesenteric artery. The entire small bowel is dilated, gangrenous, and hemorrhagic.

monly, ischemic necrosis of the bowel results from vasculitis, which often involves small arteries. In addition to intrinsic vascular lesions, volvulus, intussusception, and incarceration of the intestine in a hernial sac may all lead to arterial as well as venous occlusion.

NONOCCLUSIVE INTESTINAL ISCHEMIA: Nonocclusive intestinal infarction may be extensive and is seen in hypoxic patients with reduced cardiac output secondary to shock from a variety of causes, including hemorrhage, sepsis, and acute myocardial infarction. Shock leads to redistribution of blood flow to the brain and other vital organs. The drastically lowered perfusion pressure in the arterioles causes their collapse, thereby aggravating the ischemia.

THROMBOSIS OF MESENTERIC VEINS: Causes of mesenteric vein thrombosis include hypercoagulable states, stasis, and inflammation (pylephlebitis). Almost all thromboses affect the superior mesenteric vein; only 5% involve the inferior mesenteric vein.

 PATHOLOGY: Infarcted bowel is edematous and diffusely purple. The demarcation between infarcted bowel and normal tissue is usually sharp, although venous occlusion may feature a more diffuse appearance. Extensive hemorrhage is seen in the mucosa and submucosa and is especially prominent in venous occlusion (e.g., mesenteric vein thrombosis). The mucosal surface shows irregular white sloughs, the wall becomes thin and distended, and bubbles of gas (pneumatosis) may be present in the bowel wall and mesenteric veins. The serosal surface is cloudy and covered by an inflammatory exudate. Dysfunction of smooth muscle interferes with peristalsis and leads to **adynamic ileus**, in which the bowel proximal to the lesion is dilated and filled with fluid. Intestinal organisms may pass

through the damaged wall and cause **peritonitis** or **septicemia**. If the patient survives the episode of hypoperfusion, the bowel may be completely repaired, or it may heal with granulation tissue and fibrosis, with eventual **stricture formation**.

 CLINICAL FEATURES: Mesenteric artery occlusion is heralded the by abrupt onset of abdominal pain. Bloody diarrhea, hematemesis, and shock are common. In untreated cases, perforation is frequent. *As infarction progresses, systemic manifestations become more severe (multiple organ dysfunction syndrome).* In extensive infarction, as a result of occlusion in the proximal portion of the superior mesenteric artery, almost the entire small bowel must be resected, which is a situation incompatible with ultimate survival.

Chronic Intestinal Ischemia Leads to Recurrent Abdominal Pain

Atherosclerotic narrowing of major splanchnic arteries produces chronic intestinal ischemia and is associated with intermittent abdominal pain, termed **intestinal (abdominal) angina**. Characteristically, the pain begins within a half hour of eating and lasts for a few hours.

 PATHOLOGY: Chronic small-bowel ischemia may promote fibrosis and stricture formation, and the latter may produce intestinal obstruction or, occasionally, malabsorption due to stasis and bacterial overgrowth.

Malabsorption

Malabsorption is a general term that describes a number of clinical conditions in which important nutrients are inadequately absorbed by the GI tract. Although some nutrient absorption occurs in the stomach and colon, only absorption from the small intestine, mainly in the proximal portion, is clinically important. Normal intestinal absorption is characterized by a luminal phase and an intestinal phase (Fig. 13-16). The **luminal phase**, consisting of those processes that occur within the lumen of the small intestine, alters the physicochemical state of the various nutrients so that they can be taken up by the small-bowel absorptive cells. In the luminal phase of intestinal absorption, **pancreatic enzymes** and **bile acids** must be secreted into the duodenal lumen in adequate amounts and in a normal physicochemical condition (e.g., a regulated flow of gastric contents into the duodenum at an appropriately high pH). The **intestinal phase** includes those processes that occur in the cells and transport channels of the intestinal wall.

Luminal-Phase Malabsorption Often Reflects Insufficient Bile Acids or Pancreatic Enzymes

- **Interruption of the normal continuity of the distal stomach and duodenum** occurs after gastroduodenal surgery (gastrectomy, antrectomy, pyloroplasty).
- **Pancreatic dysfunction** can occur as a result of chronic pancreatitis, pancreatic carcinoma, or cystic fibrosis.
- **Deficient or ineffective bile salts** may result from three possible causes:
  1. **Impaired excretion of bile** resulting from liver disease.
  2. **Bacterial overgrowth** from a disturbance in gut motility. This is seen in such conditions as blind-loop syndrome, multiple diverticula of the small bowel, and muscular or neurogenic defects of the intestinal wall (e.g., amyloidosis, scleroderma, diabetic enteropathy). When GI motility is defective, bile salts are deconjugated by the excess bacterial flora, after which they cannot form micelles, which are essential for normal absorption of monoglycerides and free fatty acids.

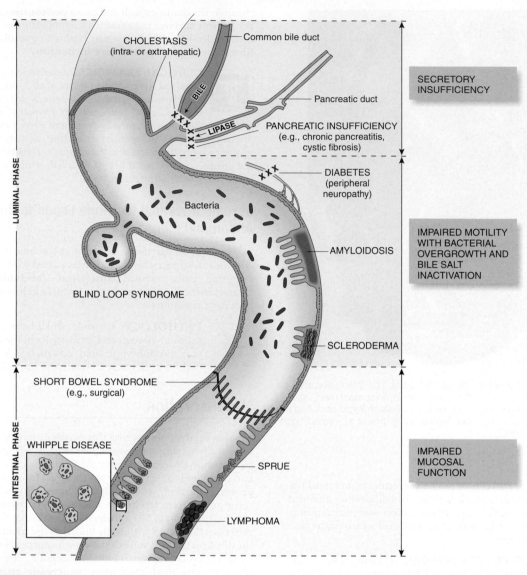

FIGURE 13-16. Causes of malabsorption.

3. **Deficient bile salts** due to the absence or bypass of the distal ileum caused by surgical excision, surgical anastomoses, fistulas, or ileal disease (e.g., Crohn disease, lymphoma).

Intestinal-Phase Malabsorption Frequently Reflects Specific Enzyme Defects or Impaired Transport

Although abnormalities in any one of the four components of the intestinal phase may cause malabsorption, some diseases affect more than one of these components. Figure 13-16 summarizes the major causes of malabsorption.

PATHOGENESIS:

MICROVILLI: The intestinal disaccharidases and oligopeptidases are integrally bound to the microvillous membranes. Disaccharidases are essential for sugar absorption, because only monosaccharides can be absorbed by intestinal epithelial cells. Abnormal function of the microvilli may be primary (as in primary disaccharidase deficiencies) or secondary, when there is damage to the villi, as in celiac disease (sprue). The various enzyme deficiencies (e.g., of lactase) are characterized by intolerance for the corresponding disaccharides.

ABSORPTIVE AREA: The considerable length of the small bowel and the amplification of its surface wall by the intestinal folds provide a large absorptive surface. Severe diminution in this area may result in malabsorption. The surface area may be diminished by (1) small-bowel resection (short-bowel syndrome), (2) gastrocolic fistula (bypassing the small intestine), or (3) mucosal damage secondary to a number of small intestinal diseases (celiac disease, tropical sprue, and Whipple disease).

METABOLIC FUNCTION OF THE ABSORPTIVE CELLS: For their subsequent transport to the circulation, nutrients within the absorptive cells depend on their metabolism within these cells. Monoglycerides and free fatty acids are reassembled into triglycerides and coated with proteins (apoproteins) to form chylomicrons and lipoprotein particles. Specific metabolic dysfunction is seen in abetalipoproteinemia, a disorder in which the absorptive cells cannot synthesize the apoprotein required for the assembly of lipoproteins and chylomicrons. Nonspecific damage to small intestinal epithelial cells occurs in celiac disease, tropical sprue, Whipple disease, and hyperacidity due to gastrinoma.

TRANSPORT: Nutrients are transported from the intestinal epithelium through the intestinal wall by way of blood capillaries and lymphatic vessels. Impaired transport of nutrients through these conduits is probably an important factor in the malabsorption associated with Whipple disease, intestinal lymphoma, and congenital lymphangiectasia.

 CLINICAL FEATURES: Malabsorption may be either specific or generalized.

- *Specific or isolated malabsorption refers to an identifiable molecular defect that causes malabsorption of a single nutrient.* Examples of this group are the disaccharidase deficiencies (notably lactase deficiency) and deficiency of gastric intrinsic factor, which causes malabsorption of vitamin B_{12} and consequently pernicious anemia.
- *Generalized malabsorption describes a condition in which absorption of several or all major nutrient classes is impaired.* It leads to generalized malnutrition.

Lactase Deficiency Causes Intolerance to Milk Products

The intestinal brush border contains disaccharidases that are important for the absorption of carbohydrates. As a prominent constituent of milk and many other dairy products, lactose is one of the most common disaccharides in the diet. Typically, the symptoms of lactase deficiency begin in adolescence, and patients complain of abdominal distention, flatulence, and diarrhea after the ingestion of dairy products. Eliminating milk and its products from the diet relieves these symptoms. Diseases that injure the intestinal mucosa (e.g., celiac disease) may also lead to acquired lactase deficiency.

Celiac Disease Reflects an Immune Response to Gluten in Cereals

Celiac disease (celiac sprue, gluten-sensitive enteropathy) is characterized by (1) generalized malabsorption, (2) small intestinal mucosal lesions, and (3) a prompt clinical and histopathologic response to the withdrawal of gluten-containing foods from the diet.

 EPIDEMIOLOGY: Celiac disease is worldwide and affects all ethnic groups. There is a slight female predominance, 1.3:1. Most cases are diagnosed during childhood.

 PATHOGENESIS: Genetic predisposition and gluten exposure are crucial factors in the development of celiac disease.

ROLE OF CEREAL PROTEINS: The ingestion of gluten-containing cereals such as wheat, barley, or rye flour by persons with quiescent celiac sprue is followed by the clinical and histopathologic features of active disease. Gliadin, the alcohol soluble fraction of gluten, has the same effect.

GENETIC FACTORS: Concordance for celiac disease in first-degree relatives ranges between 8% and 18% and reaches 70% in monozygotic twins. About 90% of patients with celiac disease carry HLA-B8, and a comparable frequency has been reported for HLA DR8 and DQ2.

IMMUNOLOGIC FACTORS: The intestinal lesion in celiac disease is characterized by damage to the epithelial cells and a marked increase in the number of T lymphocytes within the epithelium and of plasma cells in the lamina propria. Gliadin challenge of persons with treated celiac sprue stimulates local immunoglobulin synthesis. Serum antigliadin antibodies are present in almost all patients, but their role in pathogenesis is unknown.

A region of amino acid sequence homology has been found between α-gliadin and a protein of an adenovirus (serotype 12) that infects the human GI tract. Most (90%) untreated patients with celiac disease have serologic evidence of prior infection with this virus. Exposure of a genetically susceptible person to gluten-containing cereals might then stimulate an immune reaction to the protein at the intestinal epithelial cell surface.

ASSOCIATION WITH DERMATITIS HERPETIFORMIS: Celiac disease is occasionally associated with dermatitis herpetiformis, a vesicular skin disease that typically affects extensor surfaces and exposed parts of the body. Almost all patients with dermatitis herpetiformis have a small-bowel mucosal lesion similar to that of celiac disease, although only 10% have overt malabsorption. Treatment with a strict gluten-free diet leads to improvement in both GI symptoms and skin lesions.

Malabsorption in celiac disease probably results from multiple factors, including reduced intestinal mucosa surface area (due to blunting of villi and microvilli) and impaired intracellular metabolism within damaged epithelial cells.

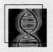 **PATHOLOGY:** The hallmark of fully developed celiac disease is a flat mucosa, with (1) blunting or total disappearance of villi, (2) damaged mucosal surface epithelial cells with numerous intraepithelial lymphocytes (T cells), and (3) increased plasma cells in the lamina propria but not in deeper layers (Fig. 13-17). The most severe histologic abnormalities in untreated celiac disease usually occur in the duodenum and proximal jejunum. There is a progressive decrease in disease manifestations distally, and in some cases, the ileal mucosa appears virtually normal. The clinical severity of the disease is related to the length of the affected intestine.

 CLINICAL FEATURES: *Fully developed celiac disease is characterized by generalized malabsorption.* The signs and symptoms of generalized malabsorption are often initially manifested in older children and adults. Growth retardation is more frequently encountered in young children.. Late complications in some cases include ulcerative jejunitis, small-bowel T-cell lymphoma, and other malignancies of the GI tract. Treatment with a strict gluten-free diet is usually followed by a complete and prolonged clinical and histopathologic remission.

Whipple Disease is a Rare Infection of the Small Bowel

Malabsorption is the most prominent feature of Whipple disease. White men in their 30s and 40s are most affected. The disease is systemic, and other clinical findings include fever, increased skin pigmentation, anemia, lymphadenopathy, arthritis, pericarditis, pleurisy, endocarditis, and central nervous system involvement.

PATHOGENESIS: Whipple disease typically shows infiltration of the small-bowel mucosa by macrophages packed with small, rod-shaped bacilli. The causative organism is one of the actinomycetes, *Tropheryma whippelii.* The results of several studies suggest that host susceptibility factors, possibly defective T-lymphocyte function, may be important in predisposing to the disease. Macrophages from patients with Whipple disease exhibit a decreased ability to degrade intracellular microorganisms. Dramatic clinical remissions occur with antibiotic therapy.

PATHOLOGY: The bowel wall is thickened and edematous, and mesenteric lymph nodes are usually enlarged. *Villi are flat and thickened, and the lamina propria is extensively infiltrated with large foamy macrophages (Fig. 13-18A) with cytoplasm that is filled with large glycoprotein granules that stain strongly with periodic acid–Schiff.* These granules correspond to lysosomes engorged with bacilli in various stages of degeneration (see Fig. 13-18B). The

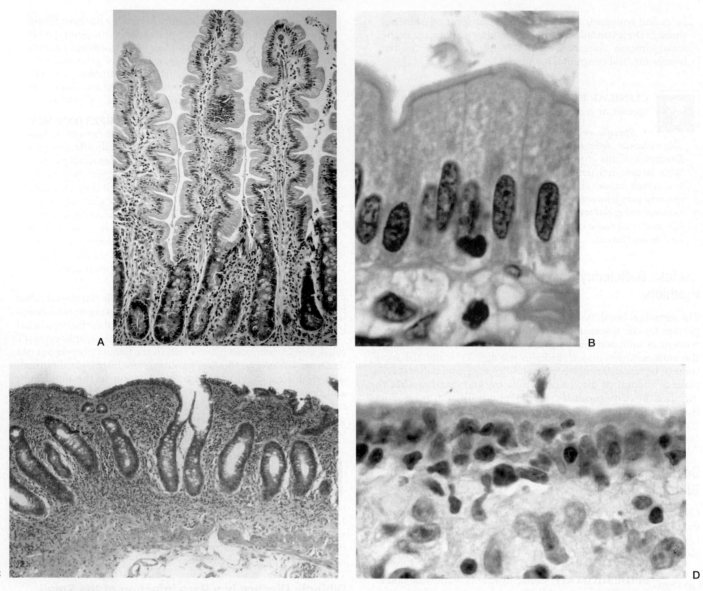

FIGURE 13-17. **Celiac disease. A.** Normal proximal small intestine shows tall slender villi with crypts present at the base. **B.** Normal surface epithelium shows an occasional intraepithelial lymphocyte as well as an intact brush border. **C.** A mucosal biopsy from a patient with advanced celiac disease shows complete loss of the villi with infiltration of the lamina propria by lymphocytes and plasma cells. The crypts are increased in height. **D.** At higher power, the surface epithelium is severely damaged with large numbers of intraepithelial lymphocytes and loss of the brush border.

other normal cellular components of the lamina propria (i.e., plasma cells and lymphocytes) are depleted. The lymphatic vessels in the mucosa and submucosa are dilated, and large lipid droplets are frequently present within lymphatics and in extracellular spaces, a finding that suggests lymphatic obstruction. In contrast to the striking distortion of the villous architecture, epithelial cells show only patchy abnormalities, including attenuation of microvilli and accumulation of lipid droplets within the cytoplasm. Mesenteric lymph nodes draining affected segments of small bowel reveal similar microscopic changes. A characteristic infiltration by macrophages containing bacilli may also be found in most other organs. Whipple disease is treated successfully with appropriate antibiotics.

Mechanical Obstruction

Mechanical obstruction to the passage of intestinal contents can be caused by (1) a luminal mass, (2) an intrinsic lesion of the bowel wall, or (3) extrinsic compression.

INTUSSUSCEPTION: *In this form of intraluminal small-bowel obstruction, a segment of bowel (intussusceptum) protrudes distally into a surrounding outer portion (intussuscipiens).* Intussusception usually occurs in infants or young children, in whom it often occurs without a known cause. In adults, the leading point of an intussusception is usually a lesion in the bowel wall, such as Meckel diverticulum, or a tumor. Once the leading point is entrapped in the intussuscipiens, peristalsis drives the intussusceptum forward. In addition to acute intestinal obstruction, intussusception compresses the blood supply to the intussusceptum, which may become infarcted. If the obstruction is not relieved spontaneously, surgical treatment is required.

VOLVULUS: *This is a cause of an acute abdomen and is an example of intestinal obstruction in which a segment of gut twists on its mesentery, kinking the bowel and usually interrupting its blood supply.* Volvulus often indicates an underlying congenital abnormality.

ADHESIONS: Fibrous scars caused by previous surgery or peritonitis cause obstruction by kinking or angulating the bowel or directly compressing the lumen.

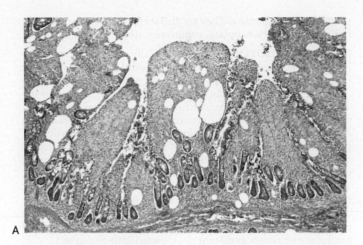

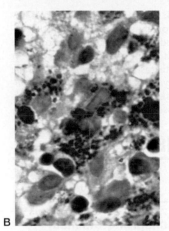 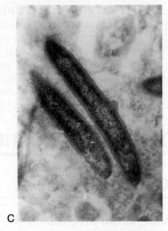

FIGURE 13-18. **Whipple disease. A.** A photomicrograph of a section of jejunal mucosa shows distortion of the villi. The lamina propria is packed with large, pale-staining macrophages. Dilated mucosal lymphatics are prominent. **B.** A periodic acid-Schiff (PAS) reaction shows numerous macrophages filled with cytoplasmic granular material. **C.** An electron micrograph shows small bacilli in a macrophage.

HERNIAS: Loops of small bowel may be incarcerated in an inguinal or femoral hernia, in which case, the lumen may become obstructed and the vascular supply compromised.

Neoplasms

Less than 5% of all GI tumors arise in the small intestine.

Benign Tumors Include Adenomas and Peutz-Jeghers Polyps

Adenomas

Small-bowel adenomas resemble those of the colon. Depending on the predominant component, adenomatous polyps of the small intestine may be tubular, villous, or tubulovillous (see later under Polyps of the Colon and Rectum). Villous adenoma is rare in the small intestine, usually occurring in the duodenum, especially the periampullary region. Adenomas, especially the villous type, may undergo malignant transformation. Benign adenomas are frequently asymptomatic, but bleeding and intussusception are occasional complications.

Peutz-Jeghers Syndrome

Peutz-Jeghers syndrome is an autosomal dominant hereditary disorder characterized by intestinal hamartomatous polyps and mucocutaneous

melanin pigmentation, which is particularly evident on the face, buccal mucosa, hands, feet, and perianal, and genital areas. Except for the buccal pigmentation, the freckle-like macular lesions usually fade at puberty. The polyps occur mostly in the proximal small intestine but are sometimes seen in the stomach and the colon. Patients have symptoms of obstruction or intussusception; in as many as one fourth of cases, however, the diagnosis is often suggested by pigmentation in an otherwise asymptomatic person. Peutz-Jeghers syndrome is associated with inactivating mutations of a gene *(LKB1)* on chromosome 19p that encodes a protein kinase. Carriers of the defective gene are also at increased risk for cancers of the breast, pancreas, testis, and ovary.

 PATHOLOGY: Peutz-Jeghers polyps are hamartomas, with branching networks of smooth muscle fibers continuous with the muscularis mucosae that supports the glandular epithelium of the polyp. Peutz-Jeghers polyps are generally considered benign, but 3% of patients develop adenocarcinoma, although not necessarily in the hamartomatous polyps.

Malignant Tumors of the Small Bowel are Uncommon

Adenocarcinoma

 EPIDEMIOLOGY: Although small intestinal adenocarcinomas are a minute proportion of all GI tumors, they account for half of all malignant small-bowel tumors. Most are located in the duodenum and jejunum. The majority occur in middle-aged persons, and there is a moderate male predominance. *Crohn disease of the small bowel is a risk factor for adenocarcinoma in that location.* Familial adenomatous polyposis, Hereditary nonpolyposis colon cancer syndrome (Lynch syndrome), and celiac disease are additional risk factors.

 PATHOLOGY AND CLINICAL FEATURES: Adenocarcinoma of the small intestine may be polypoid, ulcerative, or simply annular and stenosing. In addition to causing intestinal obstruction directly, a polypoid tumor may be the lead point of an intussusception. Adenocarcinomas originate from crypt epithelium, rather than the villi and, therefore, resemble colorectal cancers. The symptoms of small-bowel adenocarcinoma commonly relate to progressive intestinal obstruction. Occult bleeding is common and often leads to iron-deficiency anemia. If adenocarcinoma of the duodenum involves the papilla of Vater, it is termed **ampullary carcinoma**. This tumor causes obstructive jaundice or pancreatitis. By the time the patient becomes symptomatic, most adenocarcinomas have metastasized to local lymph nodes, and the overall 5-year survival rate is less than 20%.

Primary Intestinal Lymphoma

Primary lymphoma originates in nodules of lymphoid tissue normally present in the mucosa and superficial submucosa (MALT). Lymphoma is the second most common malignant tumor of the small intestine in industrialized countries, where it accounts for about 15% of small-bowel cancers. Another type of primary lymphoma comprises more than two thirds of all cancers of the small intestine in less-developed countries. The latter variety of intestinal lymphoma was originally described in Mediterranean populations, but it is now clear that it is distributed throughout the poorer parts of the world. These two types of lymphoma have distinct epidemiologic, clinical, and pathologic features and are respectively termed **Western type** and **Mediterranean lymphoma**.

The cause of primary lymphoma of the small bowel is unknown, but an association with celiac disease is well documented, occurring in as many as one tenth of patients with primary lymphoma. The persistent activation of lymphocytes in the bowel is thought to predispose to subsequent development of T-cell lymphoma. However, although a gluten-free diet usually improves the inflammatory component of the enteropathy, T-cell lymphoma can still occur. The risk of intestinal lymphoma is also increased in conditions that favor the development of nodal lymphoma, particularly immunodeficiency following treatment with immunosuppressive drugs.

MEDITERRANEAN LYMPHOMA: Mediterranean lymphoma typically occurs in poor countries in young men of low socioeconomic status; it is therefore thought to have an environmental cause. This neoplasm is associated with α-heavy chain disease, a proliferative disorder of intestinal B lymphocytes, which secrete the heavy chain of IgA without light chains. Mediterranean lymphoma and α-chain disease are considered to be the same disorder, termed **immunoproliferative small intestinal disease**.

Mediterranean intestinal lymphoma predominantly involves the duodenum and proximal jejunum. A long segment of small intestine, or even the entire small bowel, is characteristically affected. Typically, a diffuse infiltrate of plasmacytoid lymphocytes or plasma cells is seen in the mucosa and submucosa. Lymphomatous infiltration of the mucosa leads to mucosal atrophy and severe malabsorption.

WESTERN-TYPE INTESTINAL LYMPHOMA: This disorder usually affects adults older than 40 years of age and children younger than 10. It is most common in the ileum, where it is seen as (1) a fungating mass that projects into the lumen, (2) an elevated ulcerated lesion, (3) a diffuse segmental thickening of the bowel wall, or (4) plaque-like mucosal nodules. Intestinal obstruction, intussusception, and perforation are important complications. Occult bleeding is common, and massive acute hemorrhage may also occur. Microscopically, all varieties of malignant lymphoma are encountered. When extraintestinal spread is present, the 5-year survival rate is less than 10%.

Chronic abdominal pain, diarrhea, and clubbing of fingers are the most frequent clinical signs of intestinal lymphoma. Diarrhea and weight loss reflect the underlying malabsorption. Patients with Mediterranean lymphoma tend to survive longer than those with the Western type of lymphoma.

Carcinoid Tumor (Neuroendocrine Tumors)

The term carcinoid tumor has been largely replaced by the term **neuroendocrine tumors** (NETs). These tumors are all considered malignant but usually with low metastatic potential. *NETs account for about 20% of all small intestinal malignancies.* Important considerations include the site of origin size, depth of invasion, hormonal responsiveness, and presence or absence of function. The appendix is the most common GI site of origin, followed by the rectum. Tumors at these sites are usually small and rarely aggressive. The next most common site is the ileum, where they are often multi-

ple, and more aggressive. They are also seen in association with the multiple endocrine neoplasia syndromes, usually type I.

 PATHOLOGY: Macroscopically, small carcinoid tumors present as submucosal nodules covered by intact mucosa. Large carcinoids may grow in a polypoid, intramural, or annular pattern (Fig. 13-19A) and often undergo secondary ulceration. As they enlarge, carcinoid tumors invade the muscular coat and penetrate the serosa, often causing a conspicuous desmoplastic reaction. This fibrosis is responsible for peritoneal adhesions and kinking of the bowel, which may lead to intestinal obstruction. Microscopically, these neoplasms appear as nests, cords, and rosettes of uniform, small, round cells, (see Fig. 13-19B). Occasional gland-like structures are also seen. Nuclei are remarkably regular, and mitoses are rare. Abundant eosinophilic cytoplasm contains cytoplasmic granules. NETs metastasize first to regional lymph nodes. Subsequently, hematogenous spread produces metastases at distant sites, particularly the liver.

 CLINICAL FEATURES: Carcinoid syndrome is an uncommon clinical condition caused by the release of a variety of active tumor products. Most NETs are to some extent functional, but this syndrome mainly occurs in patients with extensive hepatic metastases. *Classic symptoms include diarrhea (often the most distressing symptom), episodic flushing, bronchospasm, cyanosis, telangiectasia, and skin lesions.* Half of patients also have right-sided cardiac valvular disease.

THE LARGE INTESTINE

Congenital Disorders

Congenital Megacolon (Hirschsprung Disease) Reflects a Segmental Absence of Ganglion Cells

Hirschsprung disease is a disorder in which dilation of the colon results from the congenital absence of ganglion cells, in most cases, in the wall of the rectum (Fig. 13-20). In one fourth of cases, ganglion cells are deficient in more proximal portions of the colon. The incidence of the disorder is estimated to be 1 in 5,000 live births, and 80% of patients are male.

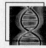 **PATHOGENESIS:** The pathogenesis of Hirschsprung disease can be traced to an interruption of the developmental sequence that leads to innervation of the colon. Given that the aganglionic rec-

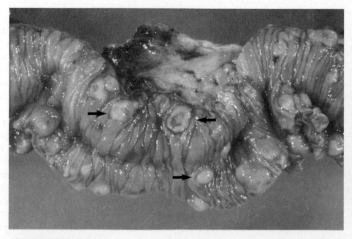
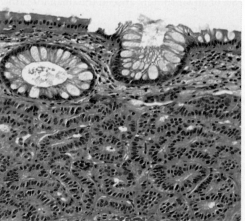

FIGURE 13-19. **Neuroendocrine tumor of small intestine. A.** A resected segment of distal ileum shows multiple neuroendocrine tumors (*arrows*). **B.** A photomicrograph of the lesion in *A* demonstrates cords of uniform small, round cells.

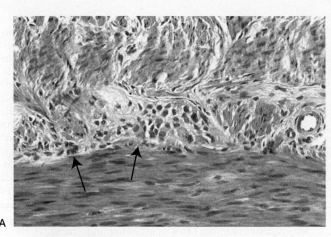
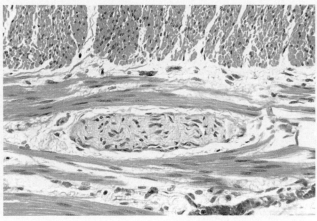

A   B

FIGURE 13-20. **Hirschsprung disease. A.** A photomicrograph of ganglion cells in the wall of the rectum. **B.** A rectal biopsy specimen from a patient with Hirschsprung disease shows a nonmyelinated nerve in the mesenteric plexus and an absence of ganglion cells.

tum (and occasionally the adjacent colon) is permanently contracted because of the absence of relaxation stimuli, the fecal contents do not readily enter this stenotic area, and the proximal bowel becomes dilated.

Most cases of Hirschsprung disease are sporadic, but 10% of cases are familial. Half of the familial cases and 15% of sporadic cases reflect inactivating mutations of the RET receptor tyrosine kinase gene on chromosome 10q (see multiple endocrine neoplasia 2 syndrome, Chapter 21). Some cases involve mutations in the endothelin-B receptor or in genes that encode ligands of the RET receptor and endothelin-B receptor. The incidence of congenital megacolon is elevated 10-fold in infants with **Down syndrome**.

 PATHOLOGY: The large intestine in Hirschsprung disease has a constricted and spastic segment that represents the aganglionic zone. Proximal to this region, the bowel is very dilated. The definitive diagnosis of Hirschsprung disease is made on the basis of absence of ganglion cells in a rectal biopsy specimen (see Fig. 13-20B).

 CLINICAL FEATURES: Hirschsprung disease is the most common cause of congenital intestinal obstruction. The clinical signs are delayed passage of meconium by a newborn and vomiting in the first few days of life. In children who have short rectal segments lacking ganglion cells and who have only partial obstruction, constipation, abdominal distention, and recurrent fecal impactions are characteristic. The most serious complication of congenital megacolon is an enterocolitis, in which necrosis and ulceration affect the dilated proximal segment of the colon and may extend into the small intestine. The treatment for Hirschsprung disease is surgical removal of the aganglionic segment.

Anorectal Malformations are Common Developmental Defects

These malformations vary from minor narrowing to serious and complex defects and result from arrested development of the caudal region of the gut in the first 6 months of fetal life. Malformations include anorectal agenesis or stenosis and imperforate anus. Fistulas between the malformation and the bladder, urethra, vagina, or skin may occur in all types of anorectal anomalies.

Infections of the Large Intestine

The principal infections of the colon, including tuberculosis and amebiasis, are discussed in Chapter 9 or above in the context of

small intestine infectious diarrhea. Most of the remaining infectious diseases are transmitted sexually and involve the anorectal region, often in male homosexuals, including gonorrhea, syphilis, lymphogranuloma venereum, anorectal herpes, and venereal warts (condylomata acuminata). Immunosuppressed people have a high incidence of colonic infections (e.g., amebiasis and shigellosis). Bone marrow transplant recipients often contract cytomegalovirus and herpes infection of the GI tract.

Pseudomembranous Colitis Usually Follows Antibiotic Treatment

Pseudomembranous colitis is a generic term for an inflammatory disease of the colon that is characterized by exudative plaques on the mucosa.

 PATHOGENESIS: *Clostridium difficile,* which is also implicated in neonatal necrotizing enterocolitis, is the offending organism in pseudomembranous colitis associated with antibiotic therapy. The organism is not invasive but produces toxins that damage the colonic mucosa. The mechanism by which *C. difficile* becomes pathogenic is not entirely clear, although alteration of fecal flora by antibiotics contributes. Only 2% to 3% of healthy adults harbor the organism, whereas 10% to 20% of those who were recently treated with antibiotics are infected. The microbe can be isolated from the stools of 95% of patients with antibiotic-associated pseudomembranous colitis.

 PATHOLOGY: Macroscopically, the colon, particularly the rectosigmoid region, shows raised yellowish plaques up to 2 cm in diameter, which adhere to the underlying mucosa (Fig. 13-21). The intervening mucosa appears congested and edematous but is not ulcerated. In severe cases, plaques coalesce into extensive pseudomembranes. Necrosis of the superficial epithelium is believed to be the initial pathologic event. Subsequently, the crypts become disrupted and expanded by mucin and neutrophils. The pseudomembrane consists of the debris of necrotic epithelial cells, mucus, fibrin, and neutrophils.

 CLINICAL FEATURES: Antibiotic-associated infections with *C. difficile* are virtually always accompanied by diarrhea, but in most cases, the disorder does not progress to colitis. In patients with pseudomembranous colitis, fever, leukocytosis, and abdominal cramps are superimposed on the diarrhea. Before the use of antibiotics, many patients with this form of colitis died within hours or days from ileus and irreversible shock. Today, pseudomembranous colitis, although

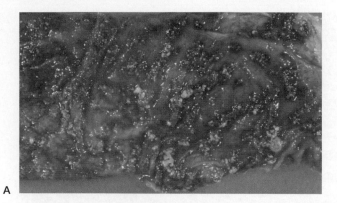

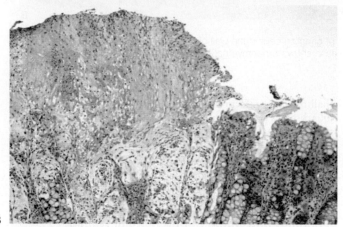

FIGURE 13-21. **Pseudomembranous colitis. A.** The colon shows variable involvement ranging from erythema to yellow-green areas of pseudomembrane. **B.** Microscopically, the pseudomembrane consists of fibrin, mucin, and inflammatory cells (largely neutrophils).

still serious, is usually controlled with appropriate antibiotics and supportive fluid and electrolyte therapy.

Neonatal Necrotizing Enterocolitis Complicates Prematurity

Necrotizing enterocolitis is one of the most common acquired surgical emergencies in newborns. It is particularly common in premature infants after oral feeding and is likely related to an ischemic event involving the intestinal mucosa, which is followed by bacterial colonization, usually with *C. difficile*. The lesions vary from those of typical pseudomembranous enterocolitis to gangrene and perforation of the bowel.

Diverticular Disease

Diverticular disease refers to two entities: a condition termed **diverticulosis** and an inflammatory complication called **diverticulitis**.

Diverticulosis Reflects Environmental and Structural Factors

Diverticulosis is an acquired herniation (diverticulum) of the mucosa and submucosa through the muscular layers of the colon.

 EPIDEMIOLOGY: Diverticulosis shows a striking geographic variation and is common in Western societies and infrequent in Asia, Africa, and developing countries. Diverticulosis increases in frequency with age. In Western countries, about 10% of persons are affected.

 PATHOGENESIS: The striking variation in the prevalence of diverticulosis implies that environmental factors are primarily responsible for the disease. Western populations consume a diet in which refined carbohydrates and meat have replaced crude cereal grains. It is widely assumed that the lack of indigestible fibers in some way predisposes to the formation of diverticula in susceptible persons. In this respect, the larger fecal mass in those who ingest a high-fiber diet diminishes spontaneous motility and intraluminal pressure in the colon; the latter is hypothesized as important in the process of herniation. In addition to pressure, defects in the wall of the colon are required for the formation of a diverticulum. The circular muscle of the colon is interrupted by connective tissue clefts at the sites of penetration by the nutrient vessels. With increasing age, this connective tissue loses its resilience and, therefore, its resistance to the effects of increased intraluminal pressure.

 PATHOLOGY: The abnormal structures in diverticulosis are, in a strict sense, pseudodiverticula, in which only the mucosa and submucosa are herniated through the muscle layers. True diverticula involve all layers of the intestinal wall. The sigmoid colon is affected in 95% of cases, but diverticulosis can affect any segment of the colon, including the cecum. Diverticula vary in number from a few to hundreds. Most appear in parallel rows between the mesenteric and lateral taeniae. They measure up to 1 cm in depth and are connected to the intestinal lumen by necks of varying length and caliber. The muscular wall of the affected colon is consistently thickened.

Microscopically, a diverticulum characteristically is seen as a flask-like structure that extends from the lumen through the muscle layers (Fig. 13-22). Its wall is continuous with the surface mucosa and thus has an epithelium *and* a submucosa. The base of the diverticulum is formed by serosal connective tissue.

 CLINICAL FEATURES: *Diverticulosis is generally asymptomatic, and 80% of affected persons remain symptom free.* Many patients complain of episodic colicky abdominal pain. Both constipation and diarrhea, sometimes alternating, may occur, and flatulence is common. Sudden, painless, and severe bleeding from colonic diverticula is a cause of serious lower GI hemorrhage in the elderly, occurring in as many as 5% of persons with diverticulosis. Chronic blood loss may lead to anemia.

Diverticulitis Refers to Inflammation at the Base of a Diverticulum

Diverticulitis presumably results from irritation caused by retained fecal material. In 10% to 20% of patients with diverticulosis, diverticulitis supervenes at some point.

 PATHOLOGY: Diverticulitis produces inflammation of the wall of the diverticulum, an event that may lead to perforation and release of fecal bacteria into the peridiverticular tissues. The resulting abscess is usually contained by the appendices epiploicae and the pericolonic tissue. Infrequently, free perforation leads to generalized peritonitis. Fibrosis in response to repeated episodes of diverticulitis may constrict the bowel lumen, causing obstruction. Fistulas may form between the colon and adjacent organs, including the bladder, vagina, small intestine, and skin of the abdomen. Additional complications include pylephlebitis and liver abscesses.

 CLINICAL FEATURES: The most common symptoms of diverticulitis, usually following microscopic or gross perforation of the diverticulum, are persistent lower abdominal pain and fever. Changes in bowel habits, ranging from diarrhea to constipation, are frequent, and dysuria indicates bladder irritation. Most patients have tenderness

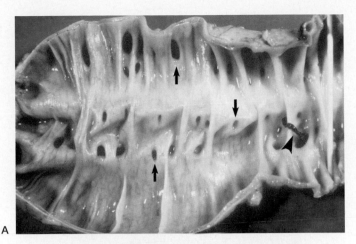

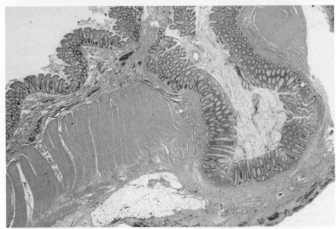

FIGURE 13-22. **Diverticulosis of the colon. A.** The colon was inflated with formalin. The mouths of numerous diverticula are seen between the taenia (*arrows*). There is a blood clot seen protruding from the mouth of one of the diverticula (*arrowhead*). This was the source of massive GI bleeding. **B.** Sections show mucosa including mucularis mucosae, which has herniated through a defect in the bowel wall producing a diverticulum.

in the left lower quadrant, where a mass may be palpated. Leukocytosis is the rule. Antibiotic treatment and supportive measures usually alleviate acute diverticulitis, but about 20% of patients eventually require surgical intervention.

Inflammatory Bowel Disease

Inflammatory bowel disease is a term that describes two diseases: **Crohn disease** and **ulcerative colitis**. Although these two disorders have different clinical courses as well as natural histories and are usually clearly distinguishable, they have certain common features.

Crohn Disease Features Chronic, Segmental, Transmural Inflammation of the Intestine

Crohn disease occurs principally in the distal small intestine but may involve any part of the digestive tract and even extraintestinal tissues. The colon, particularly the right colon, may be affected.

 EPIDEMIOLOGY: Crohn disease occurs worldwide, with an annual incidence of 0.5 to 5 per 100,000. Reports from various countries indicate that the incidence has increased dramatically over the past 30 years.

The disease usually appears in adolescents or young adults and is most common among persons of European origin, with a considerably higher frequency in the Jewish population. There is a slight female predominance (1.6:1).

 PATHOGENESIS: Concordance rates in twin pairs and siblings strongly implicate a genetic predisposition to Crohn disease. A family history of inflammatory bowel disease is more common for Crohn disease than for ulcerative colitis. A putative susceptibility locus for Crohn disease has been assigned to the centromeric region of chromosome 16 where it is associated with the *NOD2/CARD15* locus, which codes for an intracellular receptor for bacterial products involved in innate immunity. The possibility that Crohn disease reflects immunologically mediated damage to the intestine is suggested by (1) the chronic and recurrent nature of the inflammation and (2) its association with systemic manifestations that are suggestive of autoimmune disease. Most recent immunologic studies focus on the possible role of cell-mediated cytotoxicity.

The fecal stream appears to be of prime importance in the pathogenesis of Crohn disease, as evidenced by (1) the beneficial effects of surgical bypass, (2) the pattern of preanastomotic recurrence in patients with side-to-end anastomotic sites, and (3) the frequency of early inflammatory lesions (aphthoid erosions) in the epithelium in association with mucosal lymphoid tissue.

 PATHOLOGY: Two major characteristics of Crohn disease differentiate it from other GI inflammatory diseases. First, the inflammation usually involves all layers of the bowel wall and is, therefore, referred to as **transmural inflammatory disease**. Second, the involvement of the intestine is discontinuous; that is, segments of inflamed tissue are separated by apparently normal intestine.

It is convenient to classify Crohn disease into four broad macroscopic patterns. The disease involves (1) mainly the ileum and cecum in about 50% of cases, (2) only the small intestine in 15%, (3) only the colon in 20%, and (4) mainly the anorectal region in 15%. In women with anorectal Crohn disease, the inflammation may spread to involve the external genitalia.

The macroscopic and microscopic features of Crohn disease are variable. Grossly, the bowel and adjacent mesentery are thickened as well as edematous, and mesenteric fat often wraps around the bowel ("creeping fat"). Mesenteric lymph nodes are frequently enlarged, firm, and matted together. The intestinal lumen is narrowed by a combination of edema and fibrosis. Nodular swelling, fibrosis, and mucosal ulceration lead to a "cobblestone" appearance (Fig. 13-23A). In early cases, ulcers have either an aphthous or a serpiginous appearance; later, they become deeper and appear as linear clefts or fissures (see Fig. 13-23B).

The cut surface of the bowel wall shows the transmural nature of the disease, with thickening, edema, and fibrosis of all layers. Involved loops of bowel are often adherent, and fistulas between such segments are frequent. These fistulas may also penetrate from the bowel into other organs, including the bladder, uterus, vagina, and skin. Lesions in the distal rectum and anus may create perianal fistulas, a well-known presenting feature.

Microscopically, Crohn disease appears as a chronic inflammatory process. During early phases of the disease, the inflammation may be confined to the mucosa and submucosa. Small, superficial mucosal ulcerations (aphthous ulcers) are seen. Later, long, deep, fissure-like ulcers are seen, and vascular hyalinization and fibrosis become apparent.

The microscopic hallmark of Crohn disease is transmural, nodular, lymphoid aggregates (Fig. 13-24). *Discrete, noncaseating granulomas, mostly in the submucosa, may be present. Although the pres-*

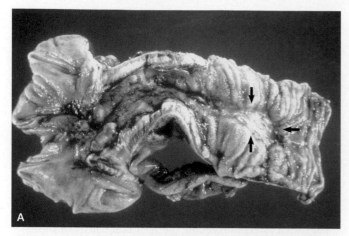

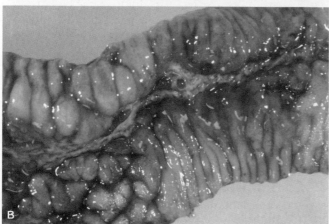

FIGURE 13-23. **Crohn disease. A.** The terminal ileum shows striking thickening of the wall of the distal portion with distortion of the ileocecal valve. A longitudinal ulcer is present (*arrows*). **B.** Another longitudinal ulcer is seen in this segment of ileum. The large rounded areas of edematous damaged mucosa give a "cobblestone" appearance to the involved mucosa. A portion of the mucosa to the lower right is uninvolved.

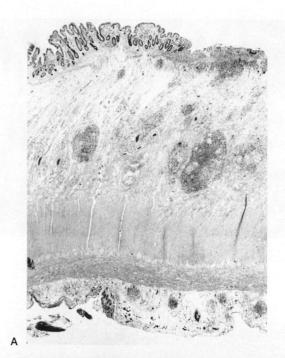

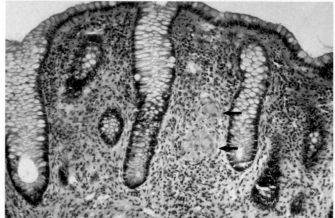

FIGURE 13-24. **Crohn disease. A.** The colon involved with Crohn disease shows an area of mucosal ulceration, an expanded submucosa with lymphoid aggregates, and numerous lymphoid aggregates in the subserosal tissues immediately adjacent to the muscularis externa. **B.** This mucosal biopsy in Crohn disease shows a small epithelioid granuloma (*arrows*) between two intact crypts.

ence of granulomas is strong evidence in favor of Crohn disease, less than half of the cases show these lesions. The pathologic features of Crohn disease are summarized in Figure 13-25.

 CLINICAL FEATURES: The clinical manifestations and natural history of Crohn disease are highly variable and relate to the anatomical sites involved by the disease. The most frequent symptoms are **abdominal pain** and **diarrhea**, which are seen in more than 75% of patients, and recurrent **fever**, evident in 50%. When the small intestine is diffusely involved, **malabsorption** and malnutrition may be major features. Crohn disease of the colon leads to **diarrhea** and sometimes **colonic bleeding**. In a few patients, the major site of involvement is the anorectal region, and recurrent anorectal fistulas may be the presenting sign.

Intestinal obstruction and **fistulas** are the most common intestinal complications of Crohn disease. Occasionally, free perforation of the bowel occurs. **Small bowel cancer** is at least threefold more common in patients with Crohn disease, and the disease also predisposes to **colorectal cancer**.

No cure for Crohn disease is available. Several medications suppress the inflammatory reaction, including corticosteroids, sulfasalazine, metronidazole, 6-mercaptopurine, cyclosporine, and anti-TNF antibodies. Surgical resection of obstructed areas or of

severely involved portions of intestine and drainage of abscesses caused by fistulas are often required.

Ulcerative Colitis is a Chronic Superficial Inflammation of the Colon and Rectum

Ulcerative colitis is characterized by chronic diarrhea and rectal bleeding, with a pattern of exacerbations and remissions and with the possibility of serious local and systemic complications.

 EPIDEMIOLOGY: In Europe and North America, the incidence of ulcerative colitis is 4 to 7 per 100,000 population, and its prevalence is 40 to 80 per 100,000. It usually begins in early adult life, with a peak incidence in the third decade. However, it also occurs in childhood and old age. In the United States, whites are affected more commonly than blacks.

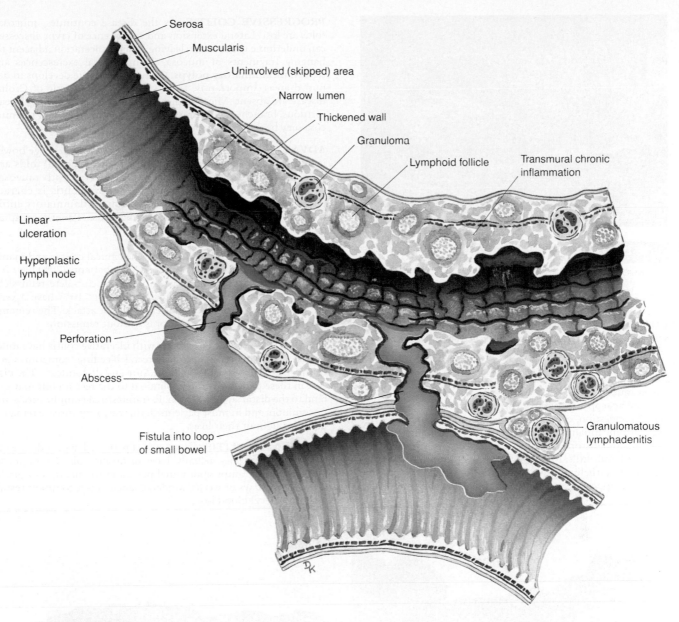

Serosa
Muscularis
Uninvolved (skipped) area
Narrow lumen
Thickened wall
Granuloma
Lymphoid follicle
Transmural chronic inflammation
Linear ulceration
Hyperplastic lymph node
Perforation
Abscess
Fistula into loop of small bowel
Granulomatous lymphadenitis

FIGURE 13-25. **Crohn disease.** A schematic representation of the major features of Crohn disease in the small intestine.

 PATHOGENESIS: *The cause of ulcerative colitis is unknown.* In some families as many as six patients with this disease have been described, and concordance has been reported in monozygotic twins. However, available family studies do not suggest any distinct mode of genetic transmission.

The possibility that an abnormal immune response may be involved has been studied extensively. There is abundant lymphoid tissue throughout the colon, and ulcerative colitis may occur with autoimmune-like conditions, such as uveitis, erythema nodosum, and vasculitis. Increased circulating antibodies against antigens in colonic epithelial cells and against cross-reacting antigens in enterobacteria may occur. Antineutrophil cytoplasmic antibodies are found in 80% of patients with ulcerative colitis. However, these abnormalities are neither unique for ulcerative colitis, nor are they a prerequisite for the development of the disease.

 PATHOLOGY: Three major pathologic features characterize ulcerative colitis and help to differentiate it from other inflammatory conditions:

- **Ulcerative colitis is a diffuse disease.** It usually extends from the most distal part of the rectum for a variable distance proximally (Fig. 13-26). Sparing of the rectum or involvement of the right side of the colon alone is rare and suggests the possibility of another disorder, such as Crohn disease.
- **Inflammation in ulcerative colitis is generally limited to the colon and rectum.** It rarely involves the small intestine, stomach, or esophagus.
- **Ulcerative colitis is essentially a mucosal disease.** *Deeper layers are uncommonly involved,* mainly in fulminant cases and usually in association with toxic megacolon.

The following morphologic sequence may develop rapidly or over a course of years.

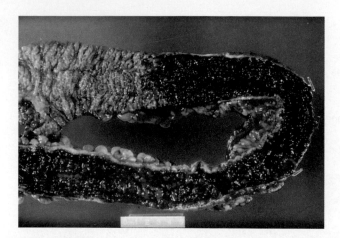

FIGURE 13-26. **Ulcerative colitis.** Prominent erythema and ulceration of the colon begin in the ascending colon and are most severe in the rectosigmoid area.

EARLY COLITIS: Early in the evolution of the disease, the mucosal surface is raw, red, and granular. It is frequently covered with a yellowish exudate and bleeds easily. Later small, superficial erosions or ulcers may appear. These occasionally coalesce to form irregular, shallow, ulcerated areas that appear to surround islands of intact mucosa.

The microscopic features of early ulcerative colitis include (1) mucosal congestion, edema, and microscopic hemorrhages; (2) a diffuse chronic inflammatory infiltrate in the lamina propria; and (3) damage and distortion of the colorectal crypts, which are often surrounded and infiltrated by neutrophils. Suppurative necrosis of the crypt epithelium gives rise to the characteristic **crypt abscess**, which appears as a dilated crypt filled with neutrophils (Fig. 13-27).

PROGRESSIVE COLITIS: As the disease continues, mucosal folds are lost. Lateral extension and coalescence of crypt abscesses can undermine the mucosa, leaving areas of ulceration adjacent to hanging fragments of mucosa. Such mucosal excrescences are termed **inflammatory polyps**. Granulation tissue develops in denuded areas. Importantly, the strictures characteristic of Crohn disease are absent. Microscopically, colorectal crypts may appear tortuous, branched, and shortened in the late stages, and the mucosa may be diffusely atrophic.

ADVANCED COLITIS: In long-standing cases, the large bowel is often shortened, especially in the left side. Mucosal folds are indistinct and are replaced by a granular or smooth mucosal pattern. Microscopically, advanced ulcerative colitis is characterized by mucosal atrophy and a chronic inflammatory infiltrate in the mucosa and superficial submucosa. Paneth metaplasia is common.

 CLINICAL FEATURES: The clinical course and manifestations are very variable. Most patients (70%) have intermittent attacks, with partial or complete remission between attacks. A small number (<10%) have a very long remission (several years) after their first attack. The remaining 20% have continuous symptoms without remission.

MILD COLITIS: Half of patients with ulcerative colitis have mild disease. Their major symptom is rectal bleeding, sometimes accompanied by tenesmus (rectal pressure and discomfort). The disease in these patients is usually limited to the rectum but may extend to the distal sigmoid colon. Extraintestinal complications are uncommon, and in most patients in this category, disease remains mild throughout their lives.

MODERATE COLITIS: About 40% of patients have moderate ulcerative colitis. They usually have recurrent episodes of loose bloody stools, crampy abdominal pain, and frequently low-grade fever, lasting days or weeks. Moderate anemia is a common result of chronic fecal blood loss.

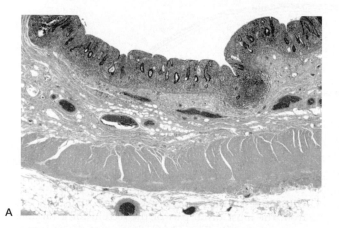

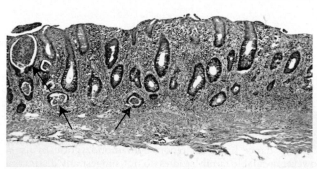

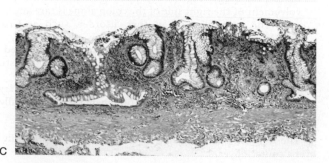

FIGURE 13-27. **Ulcerative colitis. A.** A full-thickness section of colon resected for ulcerative colitis shows inflammation affecting the mucosa with sparing of the submucosa and muscularis propria. **B.** Sections of a mucosal biopsy from a patient with active ulcerative colitis show expansion of the lamina propria and several crypt abscesses (*arrows*). **C.** Chronic ulcerative colitis shows significant crypt distortion and atrophy.

SEVERE COLITIS: About 10% of patients have severe or fulminant ulcerative colitis, often during a flare of activity. They may have more than 6 and sometimes more than 20 bloody bowel movements daily, often with fever and other systemic manifestations. Blood and fluid loss rapidly leads to anemia, dehydration, and electrolyte depletion. Massive hemorrhage may be life-threatening. A particularly dangerous complication is **toxic megacolon**, which is characterized by extreme dilation of the colon and an associated high risk for perforation. Fulminant ulcerative colitis is a medical emergency requiring immediate, intensive medical therapy, and, in some cases, prompt colectomy. About 15% of patients with fulminant ulcerative colitis die of the disease.

The distinction between ulcerative colitis and Crohn colitis is based on different anatomical localization and histopathology (Table 13-1). The medical treatment of ulcerative colitis depends on the sites involved and the severity of the inflammation. The 5-aminosalicylate–based compounds are the mainstays of treatment for patients with mild-to-moderate ulcerative colitis. Corticosteroids and immunosuppressive and immunoregulatory agents (azathioprine or mercaptopurine) are used in patients who have severe and refractory disease.

Extraintestinal Manifestations

Arthritis is seen in 25% of patients with ulcerative colitis. Eye inflammation (mostly **uveitis**) and skin lesions develop in about 10%. The most common cutaneous lesions are **erythema nodosum** and **pyoderma gangrenosum**; the latter is a serious, noninfective disorder characterized by deep, purulent, necrotic ulcers in the skin. Liver disease occurs in about 4% of patients, most commonly **primary sclerosing cholangitis**. Thromboembolic phenomena, usually deep vein thromboses of the lower extremities, occur in 6% of ulcerative colitis patients.

Ulcerative Colitis and Colorectal Cancer

People with long-standing ulcerative colitis have a higher risk of colorectal cancer than the general population. Colorectal **epithelial dysplasia** is a neoplastic epithelial proliferation and precursor to colorectal carcinoma in patients with long-term ulcerative colitis. High-grade epithelial dysplasia reflects a significant risk for the development of colorectal cancer, and when identified in a biopsy, it is a strong indication for colectomy.

TABLE 13-1

Comparison of the Pathologic Features in the Colon of Crohn Disease and Ulcerative Colitis

Lesion	Crohn Disease	Ulcerative Colitis
Macroscopic		
Thickened bowel wall	Typical	Uncommon
Luminal narrowing	Typical	Uncommon
"Skip" lesions	Common	Absent
Right colon predominance	Typical	Absent
Fissures and fistulas	Common	Absent
Circumscribed ulcers	Common	Absent
Confluent linear ulcers	Common	Absent
Pseudopolyps	Absent	Common
Microscopic		
Transmural inflammation	Typical	Uncommon
Submucosal fibrosis	Typical	Absent
Fissures	Typical	Rare
Granulomas	Common	Absent
Crypt abscesses	Uncommon	Typical

Vascular Diseases

The Colon is Subject to the Same Types of Ischemic Injury as the Small Intestine

Unlike the small bowel, extensive infarction of the colon is uncommon, and chronic segmental disease is the rule. Most cases of ischemic colitis are caused by atherosclerosis of major intestinal arteries, and the disease usually occurs in individuals older than 50 years of age. The most vulnerable areas are those between adjacent arterial distributions such as the splenic flexure, the so-called **watershed areas**.

PATHOLOGY: Most patients do not require immediate surgical intervention, as acute signs often stabilize. On endoscopy, multiple ulcers, hemorrhagic nodular lesions, or pseudomembranes are seen. Biopsy reveals ischemic necrosis of the bowel: mucosal ulceration, crypt abscesses, edema, and hemorrhage. Such patients may recover completely or may develop a colonic stricture.

CLINICAL FEATURES: Ischemic disease of the rectosigmoid area typically manifests as abdominal pain, rectal bleeding, and a change in bowel habits. On clinical grounds alone, ischemic colitis often cannot be distinguished from some forms of infective colitis, ulcerative colitis, and Crohn colitis.

Angiodysplasia (Vascular Ectasia) May Cause Intestinal Bleeding

Angiodysplasia (vascular ectasia) refers to localized arteriovenous malformations, mainly in the cecum and ascending colon, which produce lower intestinal bleeding. The mean age at presentation is 60 years. Younger persons preferentially exhibit lesions at other sites, including the rectum, stomach, and small bowel. The diagnosis is difficult and often requires selective mesenteric arteriography or colonoscopy. Surgical removal of the affected segment is curative.

PATHOLOGY: The resected specimen displays small, often multiple vascular lesions, usually smaller than 0.5 cm in diameter. Microscopically, the submucosal veins and capillaries are tortuous, thin walled, and dilated. The attenuated walls of these vessels are presumably responsible for their propensity to bleed.

Hemorrhoids are Associated with Rectal Bleeding

Hemorrhoids are dilated venous channels of the hemorrhoidal plexuses. They result from downward displacement of the anal cushions. Internal hemorrhoids arise from the superior hemorrhoidal plexus above the pectinate line, whereas external hemorrhoids originate from the inferior hemorrhoidal plexus below that line. *Hemorrhoids are common in Western countries, to some degree afflicting at least half of the population over 50 years old.* They are common in pregnancy, presumably because of the increased abdominal pressure.

PATHOLOGY: Microscopic examination of hemorrhoidectomy specimens discloses dilated vascular spaces with excess smooth muscle in their walls. Hemorrhage and thrombosis of varying severity are common.

CLINICAL FEATURES: The salient clinical feature of hemorrhoids is bleeding. Chronic blood loss may lead to **iron-deficiency anemia. Rectal prolapse** often develops. Prolapsed hemorrhoids may become irreducible and lead to painful strangulated hemorrhoids. **Thrombosis** of external hemorrhoids is exquisitely painful and requires evacuation of the intravascular clot.

Polyps of the Colon and Rectum

A GI polyp is defined as a mass that protrudes into the lumen of the gut. Polyps are subdivided according to their attachment to the bowel wall (e.g., sessile or pedunculated, with a discrete stalk), their histopathologic appearance (e.g., hyperplastic or adenomatous), and their neoplastic potential (i.e., benign or malignant). *By themselves, polyps are only infrequently symptomatic and their clinical importance lies in their potential for malignant transformation.*

Adenomatous Polyps are Premalignant Lesions

Adenomatous polyps (tubular adenomas) are neoplasms that arise from the mucosal epithelium. They are composed of neoplastic epithelial cells that have migrated to the surface and have accumulated beyond the needs for replacement of the cells that are sloughed into the lumen.

 EPIDEMIOLOGY: The prevalence of adenomatous polyps of the colon is highest in industrialized countries. As in diverticular disease, the diet is the only consistent environmental difference between high-risk and low-risk populations that has been identified. In the United States, it appears that at least one adenomatous polyp is present in half of the adult population, a figure that increases to more than two-thirds among individuals older than 65 years of age. There is a modest male predominance (1.4:1), and blacks have a higher proportion of right-sided adenomas and cancers.

 PATHOLOGY: *Almost half of all adenomatous polyps of the colon in the United States are located in the rectosigmoid region and can, therefore, be detected by digital examination or by sigmoidoscopy.* The remaining half are evenly distributed throughout the rest of the colon. The macroscopic appearance of an adenoma varies from a barely visible nodule or small, pedunculated adenoma to a large, sessile (flat) adenoma. Adenomas are classified by architecture into tubular, villous, and tubulovillous types.

TUBULAR ADENOMAS: These constitute two thirds of benign large bowel adenomas. Tubular adenomas are typically smooth-surfaced lesions, usually less than 2 cm in diameter, which often have a stalk (Fig. 13-28). Some tubular adenomas, particularly the smaller ones, are sessile. Microscopically, tubular adenoma has closely packed epithelial tubules, which may be uniform or irregular and excessively branched (see Fig. 13-28C). The tubules are embedded in a fibrovascular stroma similar to that in the normal lamina propria. Although most tubular adenomas show little epithelial dysplasia, one-fifth (particularly larger tumors) may have dysplastic features, which vary from mild nuclear pleomorphism to invasive carcinoma (Fig. 13-29). In high-grade dysplasia, glands become crowded and highly irregular in size and shape. Papillary or cribriform (sieve-like or perforated) growth patterns are common. *As long as the dysplastic focus is confined to the mucosa, the lesion is cured by resection of the polyp.* The risk of invasive carcinoma correlates with the size of the tubular adenoma. Only 1% of tubular adenomas smaller than 1 cm display invasive cancer at the time of resection; among those between 1 and 2 cm, 10% harbor malignancy; and among those larger than 2 cm, 35% are cancerous.

VILLOUS ADENOMAS: These polyps constitute one tenth of colonic adenomas and are found predominantly in the rectosigmoid region. They are typically large, broad-based, elevated lesions with a shaggy, cauliflower-like surface (Fig. 13-30A), although they can be small and pedunculated. Most are larger than

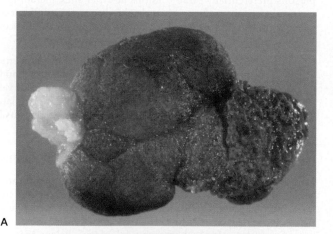

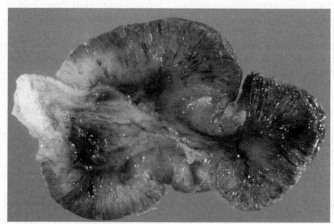

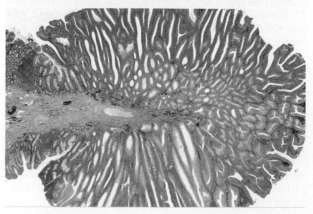

FIGURE 13-28. **Tubular adenoma of the colon. A.** The adenoma shows a characteristic stalk and bosselated surface. **B.** The bisected adenoma shows the stalk covered by the adenomatous epithelium. The ashen white color is cautery at the polypectomy resection margin from the polypectomy. **C.** Microscopically, the adenoma shows a repetitive pattern that is largely tubular. The stalk, which is in continuity with the submucosa of the colon, is not involved and is lined by normal colonic epithelium.

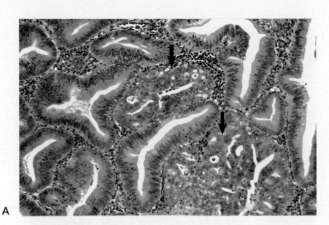

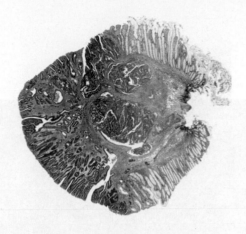

A   B

FIGURE 13-29. **Adenocarcinoma arising in a pedunculated adenomatous polyp. A.** Both low-grade dysplasia and high-grade dysplasia are present. The latter is characterized by a cribriform pattern and increased nuclear pleomorphism (*arrows*). **B.** Trichrome stain showing tumor invading the stalk (blue). Because there was a margin of resection of greater than 1 mm, polypectomy was sufficient therapy.

2 cm in diameter. Microscopically, villous adenomas are composed of thin, tall, finger-like processes that superficially resemble the villi of the small intestine. They are lined externally by neoplastic epithelial cells and are supported by a core of fibrovascular connective tissue corresponding to the normal lamina propria (see Fig. 13-30B).

The histopathology of dysplasia in villous adenomas is comparable to that in tubular adenomas. *However, villous adenomas contain foci of carcinoma more often than do tubular adenomas. In polyps smaller than 1 cm across, the risk is 10 times higher than that for comparably sized tubular adenomas.* Of greater importance is the fact that 50% of villous adenomas larger than 2 cm harbor invasive carcinoma. *Given that most villous adenomas measure more than 2 cm in greatest dimension, more than one third of all resected villous adenomas contain invasive cancer.*

TUBULOVILLOUS ADENOMAS: Many adenomatous polyps have both tubular and villous features. Polyps with more than 25% and less than 75% villous architecture are termed tubulovillous. These adenomas tend to be intermediate in distribution and size between the tubular and villous forms, and one-fourth to one-third are larger than 2 cm across. Tubulovillous polyps are also intermediate between tubular and villous adenomas in the risk of invasive carcinoma.

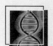 **PATHOGENESIS:** The pathogenesis of adenomas of the colon and rectum involves neoplastic alteration of crypt epithelial homeostasis, which includes (1) diminished apoptosis, (2) persistent cell replication, and (3) failure to mature and differentiate as the epithelial cells migrate toward the surface of the crypts (Fig. 13-31). Normally, DNA synthesis ceases when cells reach the upper third of the crypts, after which they mature, migrate to the surface, and become senescent. They then undergo apoptosis or are sloughed into the lumen. Adenomas represent focal disruption of this orderly sequence. Mitotic figures are initially visualized not only along the entire length of the crypt but also on the mucosal surface. As the lesion evolves, cell proliferation exceeds the rate of apoptosis and sloughing, and cells begin to accumulate in the upper crypts and on the surface. Eventually, the accumulated cells on the mucosal surface form tubules or villous structures, in concert with stromal elements. **Prophylactic polypectomies** have significantly reduced the risk of subsequent cancer development.

Hyperplastic Polyps are Frequent in the Rectum

Hyperplastic polyps are small, sessile mucosal excrescences that display exaggerated crypt architecture. They are the most common polypoid lesions of the colon and are particularly frequent in the rectum. Hyperplastic polyps are present in 40% of rectal specimens in persons younger than 40 years of age and in 75% of older persons. They are more common than usual in colons with adenomatous polyps and in populations with higher rates of colorectal cancer.

 PATHOGENESIS: Hyperplastic polyps are believed to arise due to a defect in proliferation and maturation of normal mucosal epithelium. In a hyperplastic polyp, proliferation occurs at the base of the crypt, and upward migration of the cells is slowed. Thus, epithelial cells differentiate and acquire absorptive characteristics lower in the crypts. Moreover, cells persist at the surface longer do than normal cells.

 PATHOLOGY: Hyperplastic polyps are small, sessile, raised mucosal nodules, up to 0.5 cm in diameter but occasionally larger. They are almost always multiple. Histologically, the crypts of hyperplastic polyps are elongated and may show cystic dilation. The epithelium contains goblet cells and absorptive cells, with no dysplasia. The surface cells are elongated and exhibit a tufted appearance, which accounts for the serrated contour of the glands near the surface.

Familial Adenomatous Polyposis (FAP) is an Autosomal Dominant Trait that Invariably Leads to Cancer

Also termed **adenomatous polyposis coli** (APC), FAP accounts for less than 1% of colorectal cancers. It is caused by a mutation of the *APC* gene on the long arm of chromosome 5 (5q21-22) (see below). Most cases are familial, but 30% to 50% reflect new mutations. FAP is characterized by hundreds to thousands of adenomas carpeting the colorectal mucosa, sometimes throughout its length, but particularly in the rectosigmoid area. The adenomas are mostly of the tubular variety, although tubulovillous and villous adenomas are also present. Microscopic adenomas, sometimes involving a single

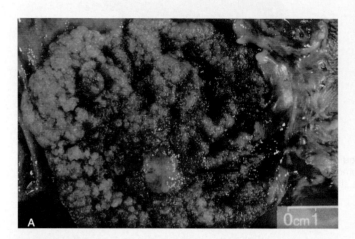

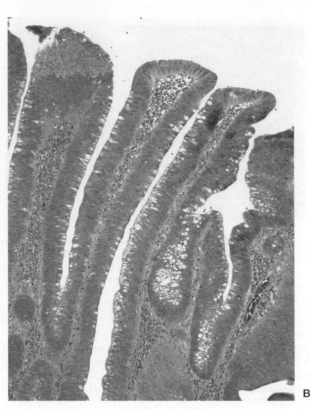

FIGURE 13-30. **Villous adenoma of the colon. A.** The colon contains a large, broad-based, elevated lesion that has a cauliflower-like surface. A firm area near the center of the lesion proved on histologic examination to be an adenocarcinoma. **B.** Microscopic examination shows finger-like processes with fibrovascular cores lined by hyperchromatic nuclei.

crypt, are numerous. A few polyps are usually present by age 10, but the mean age for occurrence of symptoms is 36 years, by which time cancer is often already present. *Carcinoma of the colon and rectum is inevitable, and the mean age of onset is 40 years.* Total colectomy before the onset of cancer is curative, but some patients also have tubular adenomas in the small intestine and stomach that have the same malignant potential as those in the colon. Genetic testing for FAP is available, but mutations are found in only 75% of familial cases. **Gardner syndrome** is a phenotypic variant of FAP defined by extracolonic lesions, including osteomas and congenital hypertrophy of the retinal pigmented epithelium.

Non-Neoplastic Polyps are Acquired Lesions

Non-neoplastic polyps are entirely different entities and are grouped together solely because of their gross appearance as raised lesions of the colonic mucosa.

Juvenile Polyps (Retention Polyps)

Juvenile polyps are hamartomatous proliferations of the colonic mucosa. They are most common in children younger than 10 years of age, although one-third occur in adults.

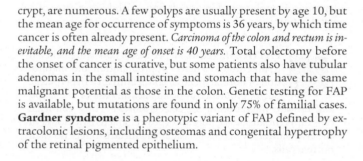

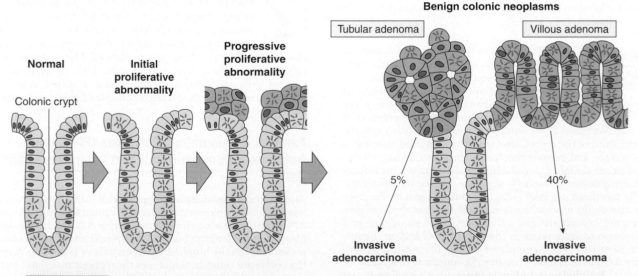

Benign colonic neoplasms

Tubular adenoma

Villous adenoma

Normal

Initial proliferative abnormality

Progressive proliferative abnormality

Colonic crypt

5%

40%

Invasive adenocarcinoma

Invasive adenocarcinoma

FIGURE 13-31. **The histogenesis of adenomatous polyps of the colon.** The initial proliferative abnormality of the colonic mucosa, the extension of the mitotic zone in the crypts, leads to the accumulation of mucosal cells. The formation of adenomas may reflect epithelial–mesenchymal interactions.

PATHOLOGY: Juvenile polyps are single or (rarely) multiple. They mostly occur in the rectum, but may be seen anywhere in the small or large bowel. Grossly, most are pedunculated lesions up to 2 cm in diameter. They have smooth, rounded surfaces, unlike the fissured surfaces of adenomatous polyps. Microscopically, dilated and cystic epithelial tubules filled with mucus (hence the name "retention polyp") are embedded in a fibrovascular lamina propria (Fig. 13-32). Surface epithelial erosion is common, and reactive epithelial proliferation is evident, but the epithelium usually lacks dysplasia. Patients with five or more juvenile polyps, or juvenile polyps present outside the colon along with a family history of juvenile polyps, have a high likelihood of the syndrome of **familial juvenile polyposis**. These patients have an increased risk for GI carcinoma, not necessarily arising from the polyps or even the segment of the GI tract in which they are located.

Inflammatory Polyps

Inflammatory polyps are not neoplasms but are elevated nodules of inflamed, regenerating epithelium. They are commonly found in association with ulcerative colitis and Crohn disease, but they are also encountered in cases of amebic colitis and bacterial dysentery. Microscopically, inflammatory polyps are composed of a variable component of distorted and inflamed mucosal glands, often intermixed with granulation tissue. As healing proceeds, epithelial regeneration characterized by large, basophilic epithelial cells restores mucosal architecture. Although these lesions are not precancerous, they occur in chronic inflammatory diseases that are associated with a high incidence of cancer (e.g., ulcerative colitis) and must thus be distinguished from adenomatous polyps.

Malignant Tumors

Adenocarcinoma of the Colon and Rectum is an Example of Multistep Carcinogenesis

In Western societies, colorectal cancer is the most common cause of cancer deaths that are not directly attributable to tobacco use. Approximately 5% of Americans develop this cancer during their lifetime. Although the widely used term **colorectal** implies a common biology, the differences between cancers of the colon and rectum seem to be more fundamental than simple location. For instance, whereas colon cancer is much more common in the United States than in Japan, the incidence of rectal cancer in the two populations is nearly the same. Moreover, colon cancer shows a slight female preponderance, whereas rectal cancer is somewhat more common in men.

Molecular Genetics of Colorectal Cancer

In 85% of cases of colorectal carcinoma, it has been estimated that at least 8 to 10 mutational events must accumulate before an invasive cancer with metastatic potential develops. This process is initiated in histologically normal mucosa, proceeds through an adenomatous precursor stage, and ends as invasive adenocarcinoma.

The most important mutational events are illustrated in Figure 13-33 and involve:

- **APC gene:** As noted above, germline mutations in APC (adenomatous polyposis coli), a putative tumor-suppressor gene, lead to familial adenomatous polyposis. In most sporadic colorectal cancers, the same gene is mutated. Some tumors with normal APC have mutations in the β-catenin gene (its product binds to the APC protein). APC mutations are seen in normal colonic mucosa preceding development of sporadic adenomas. These data suggest an important role for APC in the early development of most colorectal neoplasms.

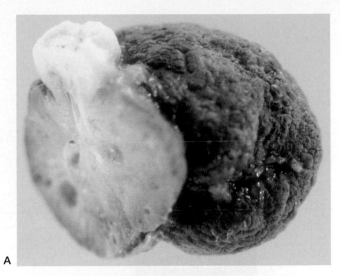

A

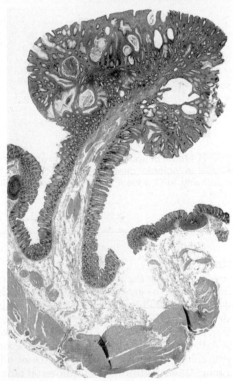

B

FIGURE 13-32. **Juvenile polyp. A.** The resected specimen shows a rounded surface that is dark because of hemorrhage and ulceration. The cut surface is cystic. **B.** Microscopically, the polyp displays cystically dilated glands.

- ***Ras* oncogene:** Activating mutations of the *ras* protooncogene occur early in tubular adenomas of the colon.
- ***DCC* gene:** A putative tumor-suppressor gene, *DCC* ("deleted in colon cancer") is located on chromosome 18 and is often missing in colorectal cancers.
- ***p53* tumor-suppressor gene:** In the most common type of adenocarcinoma of the colon, mutation of *p53* participates in the transition from adenoma to carcinoma and is a late event in the carcinogenic pathway.
- **Mismatch repair associated genes:** In 15% of colorectal cancers, DNA repair is impaired, leading to deficient correction of spontaneous replication errors, particularly in simple repetitive sequences (microsatellites).

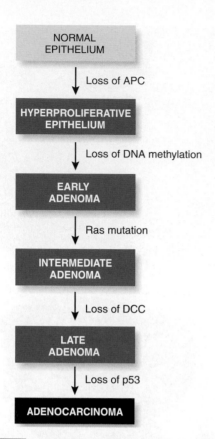

NORMAL
EPITHELIUM

↓ Loss of APC

HYPERPROLIFERATIVE
EPITHELIUM

↓ Loss of DNA methylation

EARLY
ADENOMA

↓ Ras mutation

INTERMEDIATE
ADENOMA

↓ Loss of DCC

LATE
ADENOMA

↓ Loss of p53

ADENOCARCINOMA

FIGURE 13-33. Model of some of the genetic alterations involved in colonic carcinogenesis following the tumor suppressor pathway. APC, adenomatous polyposis coli; DCC, "deleted in colon cancer."

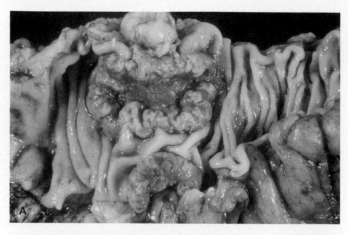

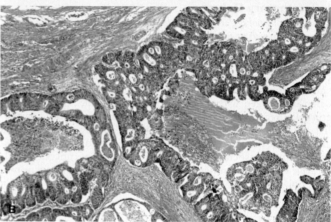

FIGURE 13-34. Adenocarcinoma of the colon. **A.** A resected colon shows an ulcerated mass with enlarged, firm, rolled borders. **B.** Microscopically, this colon adenocarcinoma consists of moderately differentiated glands with a prominent cribriform pattern and frequent central necrosis.

Risk Factors

Increasing age is probably the single most important risk factor for colorectal cancer in the general population. Risk is low before age 40 and increases steadily to age 50, after which it doubles with each decade. Chronic inflammatory bowel disease, prior colorectal cancer, diet, and genetic factors are all risk factors (as discussed above). Persons with two or more first- or second-degree relatives with colorectal cancer constitute 20% of all patients with this tumor. About 5% to 10% of all colorectal cancers are inherited as autosomal dominant traits.

 PATHOLOGY: Grossly colorectal cancers resemble adenocarcinomas elsewhere in the gut. *They tend to be polypoid and ulcerating or infiltrative and may be annular and constrictive* (Fig. 13-34A). Polypoid cancers are more common in the right colon, particularly in the cecum, where the large caliber of the colon allows unimpeded intraluminal growth. Annular constricting tumors are more common in the distal colon. Ulceration of tumors, regardless of growth pattern, is common. *The vast majority of colorectal cancers are adenocarcinomas* (see Fig. 13-34B), which are microscopically similar to their counterparts in other parts of the digestive tract. Approximately 10% to 15% secrete large quantities of mucin; these are called **mucinous** adenocarcinomas.

Colorectal cancer spreads by direct extension or vascular/lymphatic invasion. The connective tissues of the serosa offer little resistance to tumor spread, and cancer cells are often found in the fat and serosa at some distance from the primary tumor. The peritoneum is occasionally involved, in which case, there may be multiple deposits throughout the abdomen. *Colorectal cancer invades lymphatic channels and initially involves the lymph nodes immediately underlying the tumor.* Venous invasion leads to blood-borne metastases, which involve the liver in most patients with metastatic disease. The prognosis of colorectal cancer is more closely related to the degree of tumor extension through the large bowel wall than to its size or histopathological characteristics.

Current staging of colorectal carcinomas uses the TNM classification (tumor, lymph nodes, metastasis). In this system, a T1 tumor invades the submucosa; a T2 tumor infiltrates into, but not through, the muscularis propria; a T3 tumor invades into the subserosal tissue; and T4 tumors penetrate the serosa or involve adjacent organs. N refers to the presence or absence of nodal metastases, and M indicates the presence or absence of extranodal metastases.

 CLINICAL FEATURES: Initially, colorectal cancer is clinically silent. As the tumor grows, the most common sign is **occult blood in the feces** when the tumor is in the proximal portions of the colon. Both occult blood and **bright red blood** in the feces may occur if a lesion is in the distal colorectum. Cancers on the left side of the colon, where the caliber of the lumen is small and the fecal contents are more solid, often constrict the lumen, producing **obstructive symptoms**. These are manifested as changes in bowel habits and abdominal pain. Occasionally, colorectal cancer **perforates** early and induces peritonitis. By contrast, on the right side of the colon, particularly in the cecum, the lumen is large and fecal contents are liquid. As a result, tumors can grow to a large size without causing symptoms of obstruction. In this situation, chronic asymptomatic bleeding may cause **iron-deficiency anemia**, which is often the first indication of colorectal cancer. Periodic fiberoptic colonoscopy and testing for occult blood in the feces improves the prognosis of colorectal cancer, because these methods can often detect the disease at an early stage.

The only curative treatment for colorectal cancer is surgery. Small polyps are easily removed endoscopically; large lesions require segmental resection. Tumors close to the anal verge often necessitate abdominal–perineal resection and colostomy, although newer surgical techniques may allow sphincter preservation. In rectal cancers, the use of adjuvant chemotherapy and radiotherapy before surgery improves the prognosis.

Hereditary Nonpolyposis Colon Cancer (HNPCC)

HNPCC, or Warthin-Lynch syndrome, is an autosomal dominant inherited disease that accounts for 3% to 5% of all colorectal cancers. It is characterized by (1) the onset of colorectal cancer at a young age, (2) few adenomas (hence "nonpolyposis"), (3) a high frequency of carcinomas proximal to the splenic flexure (70%), (4) multiple synchronous or metachronous colorectal cancers, and (5) extracolonic cancers, including endometrial and ovarian cancers, adenocarcinomas of the stomach, small intestine, and hepatobiliary tract, and transitional cell carcinomas of the renal pelvis and ureter.

 PATHOGENESIS AND PATHOLOGY: HNPCC is caused by a germline mutation followed by a second somatic mutation in DNA mismatch repair genes, most commonly *hMSH2* (human MutS homolog 2) on chromosome 2p and *hMLH1* (human MutL homolog 1) on chromosome 3p. These mutations lead to widespread genomic instability, particularly in simple repetitive sequences (microsatellites), which are particularly prone to replication errors. Histologically, HNPCC-related colorectal cancers are characterized by a high frequency of mucinous, signet ring cell and solid (medullary) carcinomas.

Cancers of the Anal Canal are Epidermoid Carcinomas

Carcinomas of the anal canal, which constitute 2% of cancers of the large bowel, may arise at or above the dentate line. These tumors occur in both genders but are more common in women and in blacks.

 PATHOLOGY: Anal cancers have various histologic patterns, such as squamous, basaloid (cloacogenic), or mucoepidermoid. However, the different tumor types exhibit similar clinical behavior and so are all classed as **epidermoid carcinomas**. Carcinoma of the anus penetrates directly into surrounding tissues, including internal and external sphincters, perianal soft tissues, prostate, and vagina.

CLINICAL FEATURES: Infection with human papilloma virus and chronic inflammatory disease of the anus (e.g., venereal disease), fissures, and trauma predispose to anal cancer. Factors associated with genital carcinoma, poor hygiene, indiscriminate sexual practices, and genital warts also contribute to the development of anal cancer.

The usual symptoms of anal cancers include bleeding, pain, and an anal or rectal mass. Often, a tumor is not clinically recognized as a malignant lesion and may be discovered only in a hemorrhoidectomy specimen. Combined chemotherapy and radiation therapy is the customary treatment, although abdominal–perineal

resection is sometimes carried out. More than half of the patients survive for at least 5 years.

THE APPENDIX

Appendicits

Acute appendicitis is an inflammatory disease of the wall of the vermiform appendix that leads to transmural inflammation and perforation with peritonitis. This condition is by far the most common disease of the appendix and is the most frequent cause of an abdominal emergency. Although the incidence peaks in the second and third decades, acute appendicitis may occur in individuals of any age.

 PATHOGENESIS: *Acute appendicitis relates to obstruction of its orifice, with secondary distention of the lumen and bacterial invasion of the wall.* Mechanical obstruction by fecaliths or solid fecal material in the cecum is found only in one third of cases, and the factor that precipitates the disease in the other two thirds of the patients is unknown. As secretions distend an obstructed appendix, intraluminal pressure increases and eventually exceeds the venous pressure. This causes venous stasis, ischemia, and invasion by intestinal bacteria.

 PATHOLOGY: The appendix is congested, tense, and covered by a fibrinous exudate. Its lumen often contains purulent material. A fecalith may be evident (Fig. 13-35). Microscopically, early cases show mucosal microabscesses and a purulent exudate in the lumen. As infection progresses, the entire wall becomes infiltrated with neutrophils, which eventually reach the serosa. Perforation of the wall releases the luminal contents into the peritoneal cavity. *The complications of appendicitis are principally related to perforation,* which occurs in one third of children and young adults. Almost all children under 2 years have a perforated appendix at the time of operation, as do three fourths of patients over 60.

 CLINICAL FEATURES: Acute appendicitis is typically manifested as epigastric or periumbilical cramping pain, but the pain may be diffuse or initially restricted to the right lower quadrant. Shortly thereafter, nausea and vomiting occur, and the patient develops a low-grade fever and moderate leukocytosis. The pain shifts to the right lower quadrant, where point tenderness is the rule. Treatment is surgical

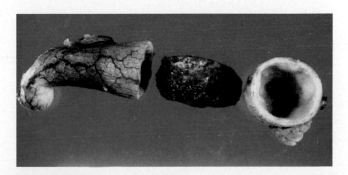

FIGURE 13-35. **Acute appendicitis.** The lumen of this acutely inflamed appendix is dilated and contains a large fecalith.

in the vast majority of cases. As perforation carries a much higher risk of death than does laparoscopic surgery, early surgical intervention is warranted, even if the diagnosis of acute appendicitis is not entirely secure.

Mucocele

Mucocele refers to a dilated mucus-filled appendix. The pathogenesis may be neoplastic or non-neoplastic. In the non-neoplastic variety, chronic obstruction leads to retention of mucus in the appendiceal lumen. Most mucoceles are associated with neoplastic epithelium. In the presence of a **mucinous cystadenoma** or a **mucinous cystadenocarcinoma**, the dilated appendix is lined by a villous adenomatous mucosa. Cystadenocarcinoma exhibits infiltrating neoplastic glands into the wall of the appendix. When a mucocele results from mucus secretion by a cystadenoma or cystadenocarcinoma of the appendix, perforation may lead to seeding of the peritoneum by mucus-secreting tumor cells, a condition known as **pseudomyxoma peritonei**.

Neoplasms of the Appendix: Carcinoid Tumors

Carcinoid tumors of the appendix are common, and are unlikely to metastasize except in the rare case when they are larger than 1.5 cm in size.

14 The Liver and Biliary System

Raphael Rubin
Emanuel Rubin

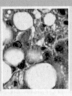

The liver lobule is a polyhedral structure (Fig. 14-1), classically depicted as a hexagon. **Portal triads** *(or portal tracts) are found peripherally at the angles of the polygon and are so named because they contain intrahepatic branches of the (1)* **bile ducts**, *(2)* **hepatic artery**, *and (3)* **portal vein**. *However, from a functional point of view, the lobule should be thought of as an acinus with its center in the portal tract (see Fig. 14-1). Such a concept takes into account the functional gradients that exist within the lobule.*

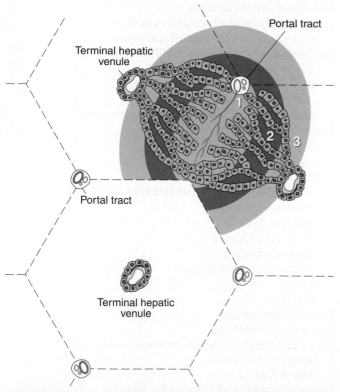

FIGURE 14-1. **Morphologic and functional concepts of the liver lobule.** In the classic, morphologic liver lobule, the periphery of the hexagonal lobule is anchored in the portal tracts, and the terminal hepatic venule is in the center. The functional liver lobule is an acinus derived from the gradients of oxygen and nutrients in the sinusoidal blood. In this scheme, the portal tract, with the richest content of oxygen and nutrients, is in the center (zone 1). The region most distant from the portal tract (zone 3) is poor in oxygen and nutrients and surrounds the terminal hepatic venule.

THE LIVER

The functions served by the liver can be broadly categorized as metabolic, synthetic, storage, catabolic, and excretory.

METABOLIC FUNCTIONS: The liver is the central organ of **glucose homeostasis, maintaining blood glucose levels** by glycogenolysis and gluconeogenesis.

SYNTHETIC FUNCTIONS: Most serum proteins, including albumin and blood coagulation factors, are synthesized in the liver. In addition, complement, other acute phase reactants, and binding proteins for iron, copper, and vitamin A are liver products.

STORAGE FUNCTIONS: The liver is an important storage site for glycogen, triglycerides, iron, copper, and lipid-soluble vitamins.

CATABOLIC FUNCTIONS: Endogenous substances, including hormones and serum proteins, are catabolized by the liver to maintain a balance between their production and their elimination. The liver is also the principal site for the **detoxification of foreign compounds** (xenobiotics).

EXCRETORY FUNCTIONS: The principal excretory product of the liver is **bile**, an aqueous mixture of conjugated bilirubin, bile acids, phospholipids, cholesterol, and electrolytes. Bile not only provides a repository for the products of heme catabolism but is also vital for fat absorption in the small intestine.

Bilirubin Metabolism and the Mechanics of Jaundice

Bilirubin is the End Product of Heme Catabolism

Bilirubin has no known physiologic function, although a role as an antioxidant has been suggested. *Up to 85% of bilirubin is derived from senescent erythrocytes, which are removed from the circulation by mononuclear phagocytes of the spleen, bone marrow, and liver.* The remaining bilirubin arises from the degradation of heme produced from other sources, the most important of which is the premature breakdown of hemoglobin in developing erythroid cells in the bone marrow. Circulating bilirubin is bound to albumin for transport to the liver.

The transfer of bilirubin from the blood to the bile involves four steps:

1. **Uptake:** The albumin–bilirubin complex is dissociated, and bilirubin is transported across the sinusoidal hepatocyte plasma membrane. This transport likely involves specific recognition of bilirubin by a plasma membrane receptor.
2. **Binding:** Within the hepatocyte, bilirubin is bound to a group of cytosolic proteins known collectively as **glutathione-S-transferases** (also termed ligandins).
3. **Conjugation:** For its excretion, bilirubin is complexed with glucuronic acid by the uridine diphosphate glucuronyl trans-

ferase (UGT) system The reaction forms bilirubin diglucuronide and a small amount (<10%) of the monoglucuronide.

4. **Excretion:** Conjugated bilirubin diffuses through the cytosol to the bile canaliculus, where it is excreted into the bile by an energy-dependent carrier-mediated process.

Hyperbilirubinemia refers to an increased concentration of bilirubin in the blood (>1.0 mg/dL) and may be associated with:

- **Jaundice** or **icterus** describes yellow skin and sclerae (Fig. 14-2), with color that becomes apparent when the circulating bilirubin concentration exceeds 2.0 to 2.5 mg/dL.
- **Cholestasis** is the presence of plugs of inspissated bile in dilated bile canaliculi and visible bile pigment in hepatocytes.
- **Cholestatic jaundice** is characterized by histologic cholestasis and hyperbilirubinemia.

As shown in Figure 14-3, many conditions are associated with hyperbilirubinemia.

Overproduction of bilirubin, interference with hepatic uptake or intracellular metabolism of bilirubin, and impairment of bile excretion are all causes of jaundice.

Overproduction of Bilirubin Can Lead to Unconjugated Hyperbilirubinemia

*An increased production of bilirubin results from increased destruction of erythrocytes (i.e., hemolytic anemia) or ineffective erythropoiesis (**dyserythropoiesis**).* In unusual circumstances, the breakdown of erythrocytes in a large hematoma (e.g., after trauma) may also provide excess bilirubin.

The hyperbilirubinemia of uncomplicated hemolytic disease principally involves unconjugated bilirubin, whereas in parenchymal liver disease, both conjugated and unconjugated bilirubin participate. Although the unconjugated hyperbilirubinemia of hemolytic disease is of little clinical significance in the adult, hemolytic disease of the newborn may be catastrophic and result in concentrations of unconjugated bilirubin high enough to cause kernicterus characterized by damage to the infantile central nervous system (see Chapter 6). Kernicterus has generally been associated with bilirubin concentrations greater than 20 mg/dL, but subtle psychomotor retardation may follow considerably lower bilirubin concentrations.

Decreased Hepatic Uptake of Bilirubin is a Common Cause of Jaundice

Hyperbilirubinemia can result from impaired hepatic uptake of unconjugated bilirubin. Such a situation occurs in generalized liver cell injury, exemplified by viral hepatitis. Certain drugs (e.g.,

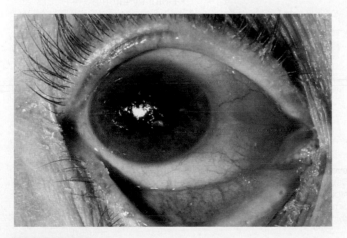

FIGURE 14-2. **Jaundice.** A patient in hepatic failure displays a yellow sclera.

rifampin and probenecid) interfere with the net uptake of bilirubin by the liver cell and may produce a mild unconjugated hyperbilirubinemia.

Decreased Bilirubin Conjugation Occurs in a Number of Hereditary Syndromes

Three syndromes demonstrating hyperbilirubinemia are associated with either a total lack or decreased levels of hepatic UGT activity. The clinical differentiation is based on total serum bilirubin levels, which range from 1 to 6 mg/dL in Gilbert syndrome (which is essentially asymptomatic) to 20 to 45 mg/dL in Crigler-Najjar syndrome type I (which is lethal in infancy without intervention).

Crigler-Najjar Syndrome

Crigler-Najjar syndrome type I is a rare, recessively inherited malady characterized by chronic, severe, unconjugated hyperbilirubinemia, owing to the complete absence of hepatic UGT activity (see above). A variety of mutations in the *UGT* gene lead to the synthesis of a completely inactive enzyme. The bile in this condition is colorless and contains no conjugated bilirubin and no more than trace amounts of unconjugated bilirubin. *The morphologic appearance of the liver is normal.* Infants with Crigler-Najjar syndrome type I invariably develop bilirubin encephalopathy and usually die in the first year of life if not treated by liver transplantation. *Crigler-Najjar syndrome type II is similar to but less severe than type I and manifests only a partial decrease in the activity of UGT.*

Gilbert Syndrome

*Gilbert syndrome is an inherited, mild, chronic unconjugated hyperbilirubinemia (<6 mg/dL) that is caused by **impaired clearance of bilirubin** in the absence of any detectable functional or structural liver disease.* The disease is most often inherited as an autosomal recessive and is related to reduced expression of the UGT gene (often but not exclusively related to mutations in the promoter region). *Gilbert syndrome is exceptionally common, occurring in 3% to 7% of the population.* It is seen more often in men than in women and is usually recognized after puberty. Gilbert syndrome is harmless and, for the most part, without symptoms other than cosmetic.

Decreased Transport of Conjugated Bilirubin Often Involves Mutations in the Multidrug Resistance Protein (MRP) Family

MRPs are molecules that mediate organic ion transport across membranes, including conjugated bilirubin, bile acids, and phospholipids. Mutations in these proteins, as well as an array of other canalicular transporters, impair hepatocellular secretion of bilirubin glucuronides and other organic anions into the canalicular lumen. The diseases vary in severity from innocuous to lethal, owing to the heterogeneity of the mutations.

Dubin-Johnson Syndrome

Dubin-Johnson syndrome is a benign autosomal recessive disease characterized by chronic conjugated hyperbilirubinemia and conspicuous deposition of melanin-like pigment in the liver. The disease is linked to mutations that result in the complete absence of MRP2 protein (also referred to as the canalicular multispecific organic anion transporter, cMOAT) in hepatocytes. The syndrome is rare, but certain groups, such as the Iranian Jewish population, have a considerably higher incidence.

 PATHOLOGY: The microscopic appearance of the liver is entirely normal in Dubin-Johnson syndrome, except for the accumulation of coarse, iron-free, **dark-brown granules** in hepatocytes and Kupffer cells, primarily in the centrilobular zone. By electron microscopy, the pigment is seen in enlarged lysosomes. The accumulation of this intracellular pigment is reflected in a grossly pigmented, or "black," liver.

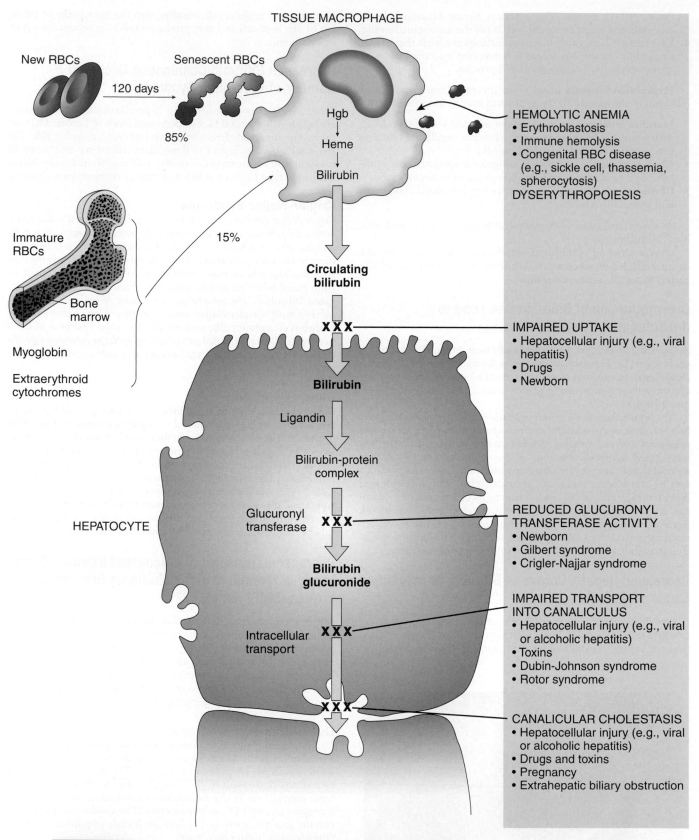

FIGURE 14-3. **Mechanisms of hyperbilirubinemia at the level of the hepatocyte.** Bilirubin is derived principally from the senescence of circulating red blood cells (RBCs), with a smaller contribution from the degradation of erythropoietic elements in the bone marrow, myoglobin, and extra erythroid cytochromes. Hyperbilirubinemia and jaundice result from overproduction of bilirubin (hemolytic anemia), dyserythropoiesis, impaired bilirubin uptake, or defects in its hepatic metabolism. The locations of specific blocks in the metabolic pathway of bilirubin in the hepatocyte are illustrated. Hgb, hemoglobin.

CLINICAL FEATURES: Except for mild intermittent jaundice, most patients with Dubin-Johnson syndrome do not complain of any symptoms, although vague nonspecific complaints are common. Half of those affected have dark urine. The serum bilirubin value varies from 2 to 5 mg/dL, although it may be much higher transiently.

Neonatal (Physiologic) Jaundice Occurs in Most Newborns

Infants who exhibit hyperbilirubinemia in the absence of any specific disorder are said to suffer from physiologic jaundice.

 PATHOGENESIS: The liver of the newborn assumes the responsibility for bilirubin clearance before its conjugating and excretory capacities are fully developed. Moreover, the demands on the liver in the newborn are actually increased because of augmented destruction of circulating erythrocytes during this period. *As a consequence, 70% of normal newborns exhibit transient unconjugated hyperbilirubinemia.* This physiologic jaundice is more pronounced in premature infants, both because the hepatic clearance of bilirubin is less developed and because the turnover of erythrocytes is more pronounced than in the term infant. The hepatic bilirubin-conjugating capacity reaches adult levels about 2 weeks after birth; the ligandin level takes somewhat longer to reach adult values. As a result of this hepatic maturation, serum bilirubin levels rapidly decline to adult values. Absorption of light by unconjugated bilirubin generates water-soluble bilirubin isomers. Thus, phototherapy of the skin is now routinely used in cases of neonatal jaundice.

Impaired Canalicular Bile Flow Accompanied by Visible Biliary Pigment (Cholestasis) Reflects Either Extrahepatic or Intrahepatic Biliary Obstruction

Functionally, cholestasis represents decreased bile flow through the canaliculus and reduced secretion of water, bilirubin, and bile acids by the hepatocyte. Cholestasis may be produced by intrinsic liver disease, in which case the term **intrahepatic cholestasis** is used (see Fig. 14-4) or by obstruction of the large bile ducts, a condition known as **extrahepatic cholestasis**.

The inability to excrete bile acids into the canaliculus results in elevated serum and hepatocellular bile acid concentrations. Much of the hepatic injury and progression to cirrhosis associated with cholestasis is due to the accumulation of bile acids within hepatocytes. Bile acids induce injury by their detergent action and by direct activation of apoptotic pathways. Elevated serum bile acid concentrations are the likely cause of severe itching (pruritus).

The extrahepatic biliary system may be obstructed by a number of lesions. These include gallstones passing through the cystic duct to lodge in the common bile duct, cancer of the bile duct or surrounding tissues (pancreas or ampulla of Vater), external compression by enlarged neoplastic lymph nodes in the porta hepatis (as in Hodgkin disease), benign strictures (postoperative scarring or primary sclerosing cholangitis), and congenital biliary atresia.

 PATHOGENESIS: The biochemical basis of cholestasis is not entirely clear. In the case of extrahepatic biliary obstruction, the effects clearly begin with increased pressure in the bile ducts. However, in the early stages, the biochemical and morphologic events at the canalicular level are similar to those that occur with intrahepatic cholestasis, including *a centrilobular predilection for the appearance of canalicular bile plugs* (Fig. 14-4). The invariable presence of bile constituents in the blood of persons with cholestasis implies regurgitation of conjugated bilirubin from the hepatocyte into the bloodstream.

 PATHOLOGY: *The morphologic hallmark of cholestasis is the presence of brownish bile pigment within dilated canaliculi and in hepatocytes* (see Fig. 14-4). The canaliculus is enlarged. In the hepatocyte, bile stasis is reflected in the presence of large, bile-laden lysosomes. When cholestasis persists, secondary morphologic abnormalities develop. Scattered necrotic hepatocytes probably reflect a toxic effect of excess intracellular bile. Within the sinusoids, the macrophages and Kupffer cells contain bile pigment and cellular debris. *Whereas early cholestasis is restricted almost exclusively to the central zone, chronic cholestasis is also marked by the appearance of bile plugs in the periphery of the lobule.*

In extrahepatic biliary obstruction, the liver is swollen and bile stained. Initially, centrilobular cholestasis is accompanied by edema of the portal tracts. As obstruction proceeds, mononuclear inflammatory cells infiltrate the portal tracts. Tortuous and distended bile ductules, characterized by a high cuboidal epithelium, proliferate. Damaged hepatocytes containing large amounts of bile manifest (1) hydropic swelling, (2) diffuse impregnation with bile pigment, and (3) a reticulated appearance. This triad is termed **feathery degeneration**. Dilated bile ducts may rupture, promoting the formation of **bile lakes** (Fig. 14-5), which appear as focal, golden-yellow deposits that are surrounded by degenerating hepatocytes. Within bile ducts and proliferated ductules, biliary concretions may be conspicuous.

With time, the portal tracts become enlarged and fibrotic. Typically, the periductal fibrosis is concentric, giving rise to the term "onion-skin fibrosis." In untreated extrahepatic biliary obstruction, septa eventually extend between the portal tracts of contiguous lobules to form **micronodular cirrhosis** (discussed below).

 CLINICAL FEATURES: Cholestasis usually presents with jaundice, regardless of its underlying cause. **Pruritus** (itching) is common and can be severe and intractable. Cholesterol accumulates in the skin in the form of **xanthomas**. **Malabsorption** may develop in cases of protracted cholestasis (see Chapter 13).

Cirrhosis

Cirrhosis, the end stage of chronic liver disease, is defined as the destruction of the normal liver architecture by fibrous septa that encompass regenerative nodules of hepatocytes. This morphologic pattern invariably results from persistent liver cell necrosis. Advanced cases of cirrhosis all tend to have a similar appearance, and often the cause can no longer be ascertained by morphologic examination alone. During earlier stages,

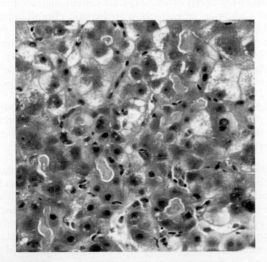

FIGURE 14-4. **Bile stasis.** A photomicrograph of the liver shows prominent bile plugs in dilated bile canaliculi.

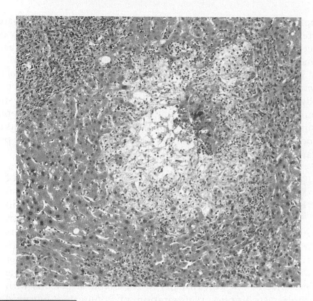

FIGURE 14-5. **Bile infarct (bile lake).** A photomicrograph of the liver in a patient with extrahepatic biliary obstruction shows an area of necrosis and the accumulation of extravasated bile.

on the other hand, the characteristic features of the inciting pathogenic insult may be evident. For example, fat and Mallory bodies are typical of alcoholic liver injury, whereas chronic inflammation and periportal necrosis define chronic hepatitis.

A spectrum of nodular patterns has been defined in cirrhosis. At one end is **micronodular cirrhosis** usually found early in the course of a disease. At the other end of the spectrum, ordinarily late in the progression of the disease, is **macronodular cirrhosis**. Between these two extremes are many cases that show features of both types.

MICRONODULAR CIRRHOSIS: Micronodular cirrhosis exhibits nodules scarcely larger than a lobule, measuring less than 3 mm in diameter. The micronodules show no landmarks of lobular architecture in the form of portal tracts or central venules. The connective tissue septa separating the nodules are usually thin, but irregular focal collapse of parenchyma may lead to the presence of wider septa. In active stages of the cirrhotic process, numerous mononuclear inflammatory cells and proliferated bile ductules inhabit the septa. *The prototype of micronodular cirrhosis is alcoholic cirrhosis, but this pattern may also be observed in cirrhosis from many other causes.*

MACRONODULAR CIRRHOSIS: Macronodular cirrhosis is classically associated with chronic hepatitis. It also occasionally results from submassive confluent hepatic necrosis (see below), in which case the liver may be grossly misshapen. The liver demonstrates grossly visible, coarse, irregular nodules, which are mirrored histologically by large nodules of varying size and shape that are encircled by bands of connective tissue (Fig. 14-6). The connective tissue septa in macronodular cirrhosis are characteristically broad and contain elements of pre-existing portal tracts, mononuclear inflammatory cells, and proliferated bile ductules. *Micronodular cirrhosis can be converted into a macronodular pattern by continued regeneration and expansion of existing nodules.* This is particularly true of alcoholics who are persuaded to abstain from drinking.

 PATHOGENESIS: The diseases associated with cirrhosis are listed in Table 14-1. They have little in common except that they are all accompanied by persistent liver cell necrosis. Most cases of cirrhosis are attributable to alcoholism or chronic viral hepatitis. Despite advances in diagnostic modalities, approximately 15% of cases are of unknown origin and are classified as **cryptogenic cirrhosis**.

Hepatic Failure

Hepatic failure is the clinical syndrome that occurs when the mass of liver cells or their function is inadequate to sustain the vital activities of the liver. Liver failure may develop acutely, most commonly as a result of viral hepatitis or toxic liver injury. By contrast, chronic liver diseases, such as chronic viral hepatitis or cirrhosis, may lead to an insidious onset of hepatic failure. The consequences of acute and chronic hepatic failure are depicted in Figure 14-8, which deals with the complications of cirrhosis, the most common cause of hepatic failure. Although advances in supportive care have improved survival in acute hepatic failure, the mortality rate for this condition remains above 50%.

Inadequate Clearance of Bilirubin by the Liver Causes Jaundice

Hepatic failure is always associated with jaundice as a result of inadequate clearance of bilirubin by the diseased liver. Hyperbilirubinemia associated with hepatic failure is for the most part conjugated, although the level of unconjugated bilirubin also tends to increase. On occasion, increased erythrocyte turnover may add to unconjugated hyperbilirubinemia, thereby aggravating the jaundice.

Hepatic Encephalopathy Refers to Neurologic Signs and Symptoms of Liver Failure

Hepatic encephalopathy progresses from sleep disturbance and irritability (stage I) to coma (stage IV) in patients who suffer chronic unrelenting liver failure or the diversion of the portal circulation. Progression may occur over a period of many months or may evolve rapidly in days or weeks in cases of fulminant hepatic failure.

PATHOGENESIS: The pathogenesis of hepatic encephalopathy remains elusive. It is probable that the condition is caused in part by injurious compounds absorbed from the intestine that have escaped hepatic detoxification either because of hepatocyte dysfunction or the existence of structural or functional vascular shunts. The latter mechanism is particularly evident after the surgical construction of a portal–systemic anastomosis for the relief of portal hypertension (see below), in which the resultant neurological abnormality is termed **portasystemic encephalopathy**.

Substances proposed to account for hepatic encephalopathy include:

AMMONIA: Levels of ammonia are usually increased in the blood and brain of patients with hepatic encephalopathy. The brain detoxifies ammonia by using it to synthesize glutamate and glutamine. Excess levels of these molecules may alter neurotransmission and brain osmolality. However, the correlation between the increased concentration of blood ammonia and the severity of hepatic encephalopathy is inexact.

GABA: Neural inhibition, mediated by the γ-aminobutyric acid (GABA)–benzodiazepine receptor complex, is accentuated in hepatic encephalopathy by increased levels of benzodiazepine-like molecules.

OTHER SUBSTANCES: These include **mercaptans** that result from the breakdown of sulfur-containing amino acids in the colon. The characteristic breath odor of patients with hepatic failure, termed **fetor hepaticus**, reflects the presence of mercaptans in saliva. Increased blood levels of aromatic amino acids, may lead to decreased synthesis of normal neurotransmitters (such as norepinephrine) and augmented production of **false neurotransmitters** (e.g., octopamine), which may also play a role in encephalopathy.

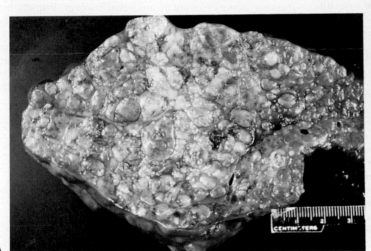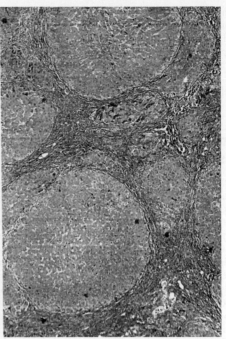

A B

FIGURE 14-6. **Macronodular cirrhosis. A.** The liver is misshapen, and the cut surface reveals irregular nodules and connective tissue septa of varying width. **B.** A photomicrograph shows nodules of varying size and irregular fibrous septa.

PATHOLOGY: In patients who have died with chronic liver disease and hepatic coma, the most striking changes are found in the astrocytes. These brain cells are increased in number and size and show swelling, nuclear enlargement, and nuclear inclusions characteristic of **Alzheimer type II astrocytes.** The deep layers of the cerebral cortex and subcortical white matter, the basal ganglia, and the cerebellum exhibit laminar necrosis and a spongiform appearance.

In patients with acute hepatic failure, **cerebral edema** is the major cause of death, occurring in more than half of the cases, often in conjunction with uncal and cerebellar herniation. This edema is not simply a terminal event but is rather a specific lesion associated with hepatic coma, although the precise mechanism is obscure.

Defects of Coagulation Often Cause Bleeding

Reduced hepatic synthesis of coagulation factors and thrombocytopenia are the principal causes for the impaired hemostasis in liver failure. Decreased production of most clotting factors (fibrinogen; prothrombin; factors V, VII, IX, and X) reflects the generalized impairment of protein synthesis by the liver.

Thrombocytopenia ($<80,000/\mu L$) occurs commonly in hepatic failure and is accompanied by qualitative abnormalities in platelet function. Thrombocytopenia may result from (1) hypersplenism, (2) bone marrow depression, or (3) the consumption of circulating platelets by intravascular coagulation.

Disseminated intravascular coagulation occurs frequently in liver failure. Intravascular coagulation may be stimulated by necrosis of liver cells, activation of factor XII (Hageman factor) by endotoxin, or inadequate hepatic clearance of activated clotting factors from the circulation.

Hypoalbuminemia Complicates Hepatic Failure

A decreased level of circulating albumin is secondary to impaired hepatic synthesis of albumin and is an important factor in the pathogenesis of edema, which often complicates chronic liver disease.

Hepatorenal Syndrome Refers to Renal Failure Secondary to Hepatic Failure

Hepatorenal syndrome is characterized by the features of renal hypoperfusion, namely, oliguria, azotemia, and increased plasma creatinine levels. The syndrome usually occurs in the setting of cirrhosis and indicates a poor prognosis. Curiously, the kidneys clearly maintain the ability to function normally. Kidneys from patients who have died of the hepatorenal syndrome function well when trans-

---

TABLE 14–1

Major Causes of Cirrhosis

Alcoholic liver disease

Nonalcoholic fatty liver disease

Chronic hepatitis

Chronic viral hepatitis

Autoimmune hepatitis

Drugs

Biliary disease

Extrahepatic biliary obstruction

Primary biliary cirrhosis

Sclerosing cholangitis

Metabolic disease

Hemochromatosis

Wilson disease

α_1-Antitrypsin deficiency

Tyrosinemia

Glycogen storage disease

Hereditary fructose intolerance

Hereditary storage diseases

Galactosemia

Cryptogenic

planted into recipients with chronic renal failure. Conversely, in patients with the hepatorenal syndrome, liver transplantation can restore renal function. Vasoactive substances produced by the failing liver or inadequately cleared by it seem to contribute to the renal hemodynamic changes. In any event, the hepatorenal syndrome is caused by *inadequate perfusion of the kidneys* when local vasodilation can no longer counteract the effects of vasoconstriction.

Endocrine Complications are Associated with Cirrhosis

It is important to distinguish between the direct effects of alcohol abuse, a common cause of liver disease, and changes that are better attributed to hepatic dysfunction. Chronic liver failure in men leads to feminization, characterized by **gynecomastia**, a female body habitus, and a female distribution of pubic hair (female escutcheon). In addition, vascular manifestations of **hyperestrogenism** are common and include **spider angiomas** in the territory drained by the superior vena cava (upper trunk and face) and **palmar erythema** (Fig. 14-7). **Feminization** is attributed to reduced hepatic catabolism of estrogens and weak androgens. The weak androgens (androstenedione and dehydroepiandrosterone) are converted to estrogenic compounds in peripheral tissues, thereby adding to the burden of circulating estrogens.

Portal Hypertension

Portal hypertension is defined as a sustained increase in portal venous pressure and results from obstruction to blood flow somewhere in the portal circuit. The major complications of increased portal pressure and the opening of collateral channels are bleeding from gastroesophageal varices, ascites, and splenomegaly.

For the sake of convenience, obstruction to the flow of portal blood can be pictured as (1) **prehepatic**, occurring before the blood enters the liver; (2) **intrahepatic**, occurring during transit through the portal tracts and lobules; and (3) **posthepatic**, occurring after the exit of the blood from the lobules (Fig. 14-8).

Intrahepatic Portal Hypertension is Usually Caused by Cirrhosis

Regenerative nodules in the cirrhotic liver impinge on the hepatic veins, thereby obstructing blood flow distal to the lobules. The small portal veins and venules are trapped, narrowed, and often obliterated by scarring of the portal tracts. Moreover, blood flow through the hepatic artery is increased, and small arteriovenous communications become functional. In this way, portal hypertension due to obstruction of blood flow distal to the sinusoid is augmented by increased arterial blood flow. In addition, increased splanchnic arterial blood flow, the cause of which is unclear, is an important factor in the maintenance of portal hypertension. Intrahepatic vasoconstriction in cirrhosis may further exacerbate portal hypertension. Central vein sclerosis and sinusoidal fibrosis also contribute to the development of portal hypertension in alcoholic liver disease. In fact, portal hypertension can result from **alcoholic central sclerosis** alone, even in cases that do not progress to cirrhosis.

Worldwide, **hepatic schistosomiasis** is a major cause of intrahepatic portal hypertension (see Chapter 9 for details).

Idiopathic portal hypertension refers to occasional cases of intrahepatic portal hypertension with spleno-megaly that occur in the absence of any demonstrable intrahepatic or extrahepatic disease. In some countries (e.g., England, Japan), idiopathic portal hypertension accounts for 15% to 35% of all cases that require surgery to decompress the portal circulation.

Prehepatic Portal Hypertension is Often Caused by Portal Vein Thrombosis

Portal vein thrombosis occurs most commonly in the setting of cirrhosis. Other causes of portal vein thrombosis include tumors, infections, hypercoagulability states, pancreatitis, and surgical trauma. Some cases are of unknown etiology. Primary hepatocellular carcinoma characteristically invades branches of the portal vein and occasionally occludes the main portal vein. Portal hypertension may also occur in patients with splenomegaly from a variety of causes, including polycythemia vera, myeloid metaplasia, and chronic myelogenous leukemia. In cirrhosis, the accompanying splenomegaly that augments blood flow in the splenic vein may further aggravate portal hypertension.

Posthepatic Portal Hypertension Refers to Obstruction to Blood Flow Beyond the Liver Lobules: Budd-Chiari Syndrome

Budd-Chiari syndrome is a congestive disease of the liver caused by occlusion of the hepatic veins and their tributaries.

 PATHOGENESIS: The principal cause of the Budd-Chiari syndrome is thrombosis of the hepatic veins, in association with such diverse conditions as polycythemia vera (10% to 40% of cases) and other myeloproliferative disorders, hypercoagulable states associated with malignant tumors, the use of oral contraceptives, pregnancy, bacterial infections, paroxysmal nocturnal hemoglobinuria, metastatic and primary tumors in the liver, and surgical trauma. In 20% of cases, no specific cause is evident. Thrombosis is most common in the large hepatic veins close to their exit from the liver and in the intrahepatic portion of the inferior vena cava.

Hepatic veno-occlusive disease is a variant of the Budd-Chiari syndrome and is caused by occlusion of the central venules and small branches of the hepatic veins. Most commonly, this disorder is traced to the ingestion of toxic pyrrolizidine alkaloids present in plants of the *Crotalaria* and *Senecio* genera, which are sometimes used in the formulation of herbal teas (comfrey is the most common in Europe and North America). It is also seen in patients treated with certain antineoplastic chemotherapeutic agents and after hepatic irradiation. Veno-occlusive disease is also reported in association with bone marrow transplantation, possibly as a manifestation of graft-versus-host disease.

 PATHOLOGY: In the acute stage of **hepatic vein thrombosis**, the liver is swollen and tense, and the cut surface exhibits a mottled appearance and oozes blood. In the chronic stage, the cut surface is paler, and the liver is firm, because of an increase in connective tissue. Microscopically, the hepatic veins display thrombi in varying stages of evolution, from recent clots to well-organized thrombi that have been canalized.

In the acute stage of both the Budd-Chiari syndrome and veno-occlusive disease, the sinusoids of the central zone are dilated and packed with erythrocytes. The liver cell plates are compressed, and there is necrosis of centrilobular hepatocytes. In long-standing venous congestion, fibrosis of the central zone radiating into the more peripheral portions of the lobules is conspicuous. The sinusoids are dilated, and the central-to-midzonal hepatocytes show pressure atrophy. Eventually, connective tissue septa link adjacent central zones to form nodules with a single portal tract in the center, a process known as *reverse lobulation.* The fibrosis is usually not severe enough to justify a label of cirrhosis.

 CLINICAL FEATURES: *Complete thrombosis of the hepatic veins presents as an acute illness characterized by abdominal pain, enlargement of the liver, ascites, and mild jaundice.* Acute hepatic failure and death often occur rapidly. The more

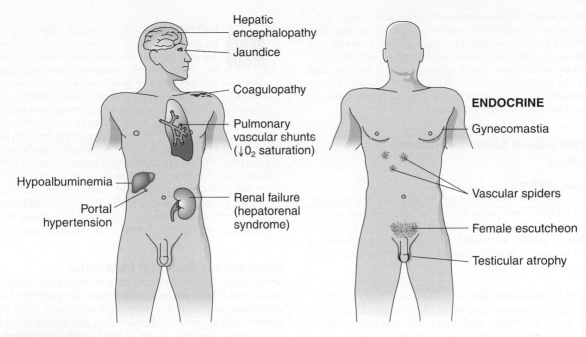

Hepatic
encephalopathy

Jaundice

Coagulopathy

Pulmonary
vascular shunts
($\downarrow O_2$ saturation)

Hypoalbuminemia

Portal
hypertension

Renal failure
(hepatorenal
syndrome)

ENDOCRINE

Gynecomastia

Vascular spiders

Female escutcheon

Testicular atrophy

FIGURE 14-7. **Complications of** cirrhosis and hepatic failure.

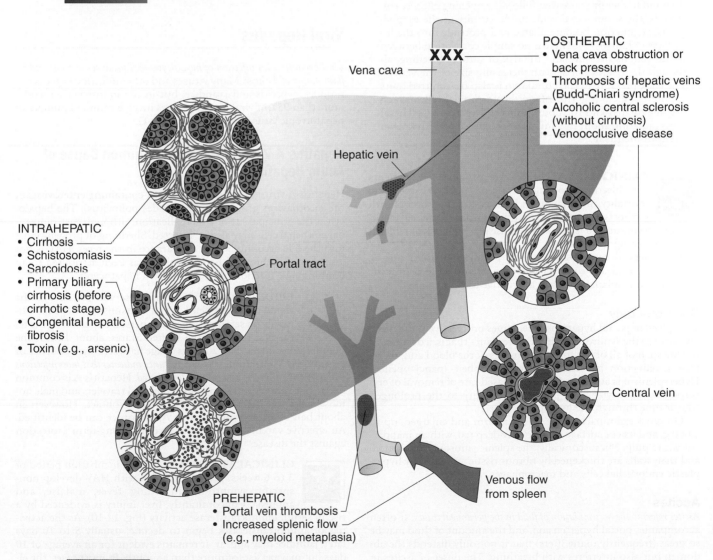

POSTHEPATIC
• Vena cava obstruction or
  back pressure
• Thrombosis of hepatic veins
  (Budd-Chiari syndrome)
• Alcoholic central sclerosis
  (without cirrhosis)
• Venoocclusive disease

Vena cava

XXX

Hepatic vein

INTRAHEPATIC
• Cirrhosis
• Schistosomiasis
• Sarcoidosis
• Primary biliary
  cirrhosis (before
  cirrhotic stage)
• Congenital hepatic
  fibrosis
• Toxin (e.g., arsenic)

Portal tract

Central vein

Venous flow
from spleen

PREHEPATIC
• Portal vein thrombosis
• Increased splenic flow
  (e.g., myeloid metaplasia)

FIGURE 14-8. Causes of portal hypertension.

usual course, in which the obstruction of the hepatic venous circulation is incomplete, is marked by similar symptoms but may pursue a protracted course over periods ranging from a month to a few years. More than 90% of patients with Budd-Chiari syndrome develop ascites, usually severe, and splenomegaly is seen in more than 30%. Most patients eventually die in hepatic failure or from the complications of portal hypertension. Liver transplantation has been successful in curing the disease.

Portal Hypertension Leads to Systemic Complications

Esophageal Varices

Esophageal varices arise from the opening of portal–systemic collaterals as an adaptation to decompress the portal venous system. One of the most common causes of death in patients with cirrhosis and other disorders associated with portal hypertension is exsanguinating upper gastrointestinal tract hemorrhage from **bleeding esophageal varices**.

PATHOGENESIS: The collaterals of most clinical significance are located in the submucosa of the lower esophagus and upper stomach and are the result of communications between the portal vein and the gastric coronary vein. Because of the increased blood flow and higher pressure that follow the opening of these collaterals, the submucosal veins in the vicinity of the esophagogastric junction become dilated and protrude into the lumen (see Chapter 13). There is no simple correlation between portal venous pressure and the risk of variceal bleeding, although the risk does rise with increasing size of the varices. The back-pressure in the portal vein is also transmitted to its tributaries, including the inferior hemorrhoidal veins, which become dilated and tortuous (**anorectal varices**). Collateral veins radiating about the umbilicus produce a pattern known as **caput medusae**.

CLINICAL FEATURES: The prognosis in patients with bleeding esophageal varices is poor, and the acute mortality rate may be as high as 40%. In patients with cirrhosis who survive an initial episode of variceal bleeding, long-term survival is unlikely because of a high risk of rebleeding or worsening liver failure.

Permanent decompression of the portal circulation can be achieved by surgically constructed portasystemic shunts. In some cases, liver transplantation is an alternative to shunt surgery.

Splenomegaly

The spleen in portal hypertension enlarges progressively and often gives rise to the syndrome of **hypersplenism**—that is, a decrease in the life span of all of the formed elements of the blood and, therefore, a reduction in their circulating numbers (pancytopenia). Hypersplenism is attributed to an increased rate of removal of erythrocytes, leukocytes, and platelets secondary to the prolonged transit time through the hyperplastic spleen.

On gross examination, the spleen is firm and enlarged, up to 1,000 g, and its cut surface is uniformly deep red, with an inapparent white pulp. Microscopically, the splenic sinusoids are dilated, and their walls are thickened by fibrous tissue and lined by hyperplastic endothelial cells and macrophages.

Ascites

Ascites refers to the accumulation of fluid in the peritoneal cavity. It often accompanies portal hypertension, and the amount of fluid may be so great (frequently many liters) that it not only distends the abdomen but also interferes with breathing. The onset of ascites in cirrhosis is associated with a poor prognosis.

PATHOGENESIS: Although clearly important in the pathogenesis of cirrhosis, the mechanisms of renal sodium and water retention remain controversial. Hypovolemia resulting from transudation of water and sodium into the peritoneal space, intrinsic defects in volume regulation not secondary to decreased intravascular volume, and peripheral arterial vasodilation have all been suggested to play a role (Fig. 14-9). Other factors contribute to the formation of ascites in cirrhosis. Portal hypertension increases the hydrostatic pressure in the mesenteric capillaries. At the same time, the low serum albumin characteristic of cirrhosis is associated with decreased plasma oncotic pressure. The resulting imbalance in Starling forces leads to transudation of fluid into the peritoneal cavity. Finally, the rate of formation of hepatic lymph exceeds the capacity of the lymphatics to remove it, and the liver "weeps" lymph into the abdomen.

Spontaneous Bacterial Peritonitis

Spontaneous bacterial peritonitis is an important complication in patients with both cirrhosis and ascites. The infection is extremely dangerous and carries a very high mortality rate, even when treated with antibiotics. Presumably, the ascitic fluid is seeded with bacteria from the blood or lymph or by the passage of bacteria through the bowel wall.

Viral Hepatitis

Viral hepatitis is an infection of hepatocytes that produces necrosis and inflammation of the liver. Many viruses and other infectious agents can produce hepatitis and jaundice, but in the industrialized world, more than 95% of viral hepatitis cases involve a limited number of hepatotropic viruses, named from A to G.

Hepatitis A Virus is the Most Common Cause of Acute Hepatitis

Hepatitis A virus (HAV) is a small RNA-containing enterovirus of the picornavirus group (which includes poliovirus). The hepatocyte is the principal site of viral replication, although gastrointestinal epithelial cells may also be infected. Shedding of progeny virus into the bile accounts for its appearance in the feces. HAV is not directly cytopathic, and hepatic injury has been attributed to an immunologic reaction to virally infected hepatocytes.

EPIDEMIOLOGY: The only reservoir for HAV is the acutely infected person, and transmission depends primarily on serial passage from person to person by the fecal–oral route. In the United States, about 10% of the population younger than 20 years of age have serologic evidence of previous HAV infection. *This circumstance indicates that most infections with HAV are anicteric and remain undetected.* Hepatitis A is common in day care centers and among international travelers and male homosexuals, the latter reflecting oral–anal contact. However, in about half of all cases of hepatitis A, no source can be identified. An effective vaccine for hepatitis A confers long-term protection against the disease.

CLINICAL FEATURES: After an incubation period of 3 to 6 weeks, persons infected with HAV develop nonspecific symptoms, including fever, malaise, and anorexia. Concomitantly, liver injury is evidenced by a rise in serum aminotransferase activity (Fig. 14-10). As the activities of aminotransferases begin to decline, usually 5 to 10 days later, jaundice may appear. It remains evident for an average of 10 days but may persist for more than a month. In most cases, the elevated levels of aminotransferases return to normal by the time

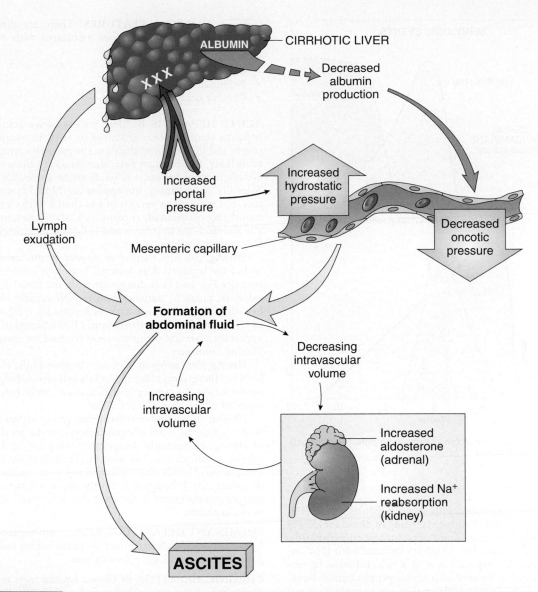

Pathogenesis of ascites. In addition to the other factors depicted, the traditional concept holds that renal retention of sodium is a response to a decreased "effective" blood volume. An alternative view (overflow hypothesis) considers the increased renal reabsorption of sodium to be a primary effect of cirrhosis that precedes the formation of ascites. Peripheral vasodilation should also considered. Na$^+$, sodium.

jaundice has disappeared. *Hepatitis A never pursues a chronic course. There is no carrier state, and infection provides lifelong immunity.* Fatal fulminant hepatitis occurs only rarely.

Hepatitis B Virus is a Major Cause of Acute and Chronic Liver Disease

Hepatitis B virus (HBV) is a hepatotropic DNA hepadnavirus. The DNA of HBV is predominantly double-stranded and consists of one long circular strand containing the entire genome and a shorter complementary strand that varies from 50% to 85% of the length of the longer strand. The HBV genome contains four genes:

- **Core (C) gene:** The core of the virus contains the **core antigen (HBcAg)** and the **e antigen (HBeAg),** both products of the C gene.
- **Surface gene:** The core of HBV is enclosed in a coat that expresses an antigen termed **hepatitis B surface antigen (HBsAg).** The surface coat is synthesized by infected hepato-

cytes independently from the viral core and is secreted into the blood in vast amounts. **HBsAg particles are immunogenic but not infectious. The intact and infectious virus** is also synthesized in the hepatocyte (Dane particle).

- **Polymerase gene:** The *P* gene encodes the DNA polymerase.
- **X gene:** The small X protein activates viral transcription and probably plays a role in the pathogenesis of hepatocellular carcinoma associated with chronic HBV infection.

 EPIDEMIOLOGY: It is estimated that there are about 200 million chronic carriers of HBV in the world, constituting an enormous reservoir of infection. Carrier rates vary from as low as 0.3% (United States and Western Europe) to 20% in Southeast Asia, sub-Saharan Africa, and Oceania, where the high rate is sustained by vertical transmission of the virus from a carrier mother to her newborn.

In the United States, it is estimated that there are 1.3 million chronic HBV carriers, and 50,000 persons are newly infected with HBV annually. Of these new cases, only one-fourth are clinically

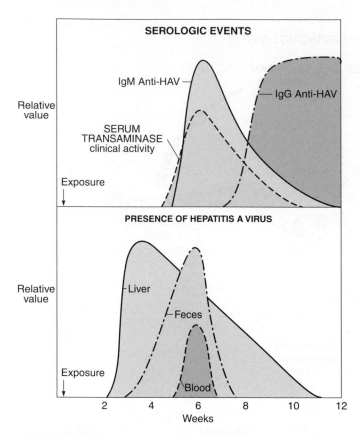

FIGURE 14-10. Typical serologic events associated with hepatitis A (HAV).

CLINICAL FEATURES: There are three well-recognized clinical courses associated with HBV infection (Fig. 14-11):

* Acute hepatitis
* Fulminant hepatitis
* Chronic hepatitis

ACUTE HEPATITIS B: Most patients have acute, self-limited hepatitis similar to that produced by HAV, in which complete recovery and lifelong immunity are the rule. The symptoms of hepatitis B are, for the most part, also similar to those of hepatitis A, although acute hepatitis B tends to be somewhat more severe. Typically, symptoms do not appear until 2 to 3 months after exposure, but incubation periods of less than 6 weeks and as long as 6 months are occasionally encountered. Many cases, including virtually all infections in infants and children, are anicteric and, therefore, not clinically apparent.

HBsAg, the first marker to appear in the serum of patients with acute hepatitis B, is detected 1 week to 2 months after exposure (see Fig. 14-11). It disappears from the blood during the convalescent phase in patients who recover rapidly from the acute hepatitis. Simultaneously with, or shortly after, the disappearance of HBsAg, antibody to HBsAg (anti-HBs) is found in the blood. Its appearance heralds complete recovery, and its presence provides lifelong immunity.

HBcAg (core antigen) does not circulate in the blood, but antibody to HBcAg (anti-HBc) appears shortly after HBsAg. Anti-HBcAg does not clear the virus or protect against reinfection, although it is a marker of previous HBV infection.

HBeAg, the second circulating antigen to appear in hepatitis B, is seen before the onset of clinical disease and after the appearance of HBsAg. It generally disappears within about 2 weeks while HBsAg is still present. *The presence of HBeAg in the serum correlates with a period of intense viral replication and, hence, maximal infectivity of the patient.* Anti-HBe appears shortly after the disappearance of the antigen and is detectable for up to 2 or more years after resolution of the hepatitis.

FULMINANT HEPATITIS B: Rarely, acute hepatitis B pursues a fulminant course, characterized by massive liver cell necrosis, hepatic failure, and a high mortality rate.

CHRONIC HEPATITIS B: *Chronic hepatitis refers to the presence of necrosis and inflammation in the liver for more than 6 months.* In 5% to 10% of patients with hepatitis B, HBs antigenemia does not resolve, in which case the infection persists, and the disease progresses to chronic hepatitis B. For unknown reasons, 90% of patients with chronic hepatitis B are male.

Patients with chronic hepatitis B do not have detectable anti-HBs in the blood, although some manifest circulating HBsAg–anti-HBs complexes. These immune complexes cause a variety of **extrahepatic** ailments, including a serum sickness-like syndrome (fever, rash, urticaria, acute arthritis), polyarteritis, glomerulonephritis, and cryoglobulinemia. In fact, one third to one half of patients with polyarteritis nodosa are carriers of HBV. Some chronic carriers who were initially negative for anti-HBs eventually develop measurable antibody (often after many years), clear the virus, and are restored to full health. Others (no more than 3% of all patients with hepatitis B) never develop anti-HBs and suffer from relentless and progressive chronic hepatitis that leads to cirrhosis. Hepatitis associated with persistent HBsAg antigenemia is often accompanied by the continued presence of HBeAg. As is discussed in detail under the heading of Hepatocellular Carcinoma, chronic hepatitis B is associated with a significant risk of liver cancer. *The possible outcomes of infection with HBV are summarized in Figure 14-12.*

recognized because of jaundice. Fulminant hepatitis B results in 250 to 300 deaths per year. Routine screening of blood for HBsAg has essentially eliminated the hazard of posttransfusion hepatitis.

Whereas no more than 10% of adults infected with HBV become carriers, neonatal hepatitis B is, as a rule, followed by persistent infection in the absence of immunoprophylaxis at birth. In the United States, chronic HBV carriers are particularly common among male homosexuals and drug addicts. Humans are the only significant reservoir of HBV. Unlike hepatitis A, hepatitis B is neither transmitted by the fecal–oral route nor does it contaminate food and water supplies. *Although HBsAg is found in most secretions, infectious virus has been demonstrated only in blood, saliva, and semen.* Hepatitis B is transmitted by shared blood (often by drug abusers) and frequently by hetero- or homosexual contact.

Synthetic vaccines for hepatitis B, composed of recombinant HBsAg or its immunogenic epitopes, are highly effective, confer lifelong immunity, and have greatly reduced the prevalence of the disease. It is now routine in the United States to administer the vaccine to infants. Prompt neonatal immunization of infants born to infected mothers is highly effective in preventing vertical transmission.

PATHOGENESIS: HBV is not directly cytopathic, as reflected in the fact that asymptomatic chronic carriers of the virus maintain a large burden of infectious virus in the liver for years without functional or biochemical evidence of liver cell injury. Cytotoxic (CD8+) T lymphocytes directed against multiple HBV epitopes are the major mediators of the destruction of hepatocytes and consequent clinical liver disease. Although the intact viral genome is not integrated into the host DNA, genomic fragments are progressively integrated, after which they produce a variety of viral antigens. Thus, despite declining infectivity of the blood, chronic hepatitis tends to persist.

Hepatitis D Virus (HDV) is a Defective RNA Virus

Infection with HDV must occur either simultaneously with HBV infection (coinfection) or after HBV infection (superinfection). HDV and HBsAg are cleared together, and the clinical

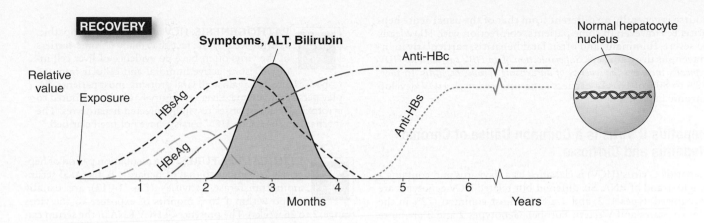

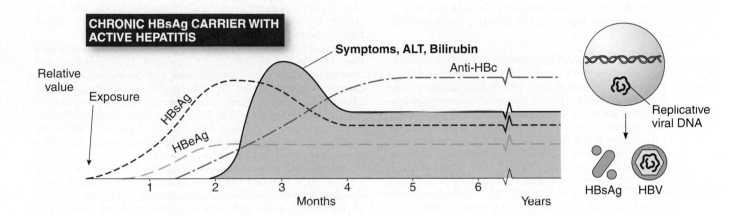

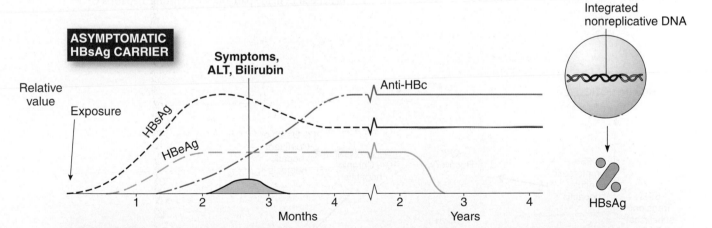

FIGURE 14-11. **Typical serologic events in three distinct outcomes of hepatitis B.** *(Top panel)* In most cases, the appearance of antibody to HBsAg (anti-HBs) ensures complete recovery. Viral DNA disappears from the nucleus of the hepatocyte. *(Middle panel)* In about 10% of cases of hepatitis B, HBs antigenemia is sustained for longer than 6 months, due to the absence of anti-HBs. Patients in whom viral replication remains active, as evidenced by sustained high levels of HBeAg in the blood, develop active hepatitis. In such cases, the viral genome persists in the nucleus but is not integrated into host DNA. *(Lower panel)* Patients in whom active viral replication ceases or is attenuated, as reflected in the disappearance of HBeAg from the blood, become asymptomatic carriers. In these individuals, fragments of the hepatitis B virus (HBV) genome are integrated into the host DNA, but episomal DNA is absent.

course is generally no different from that of the usual acute hepatitis B. However, in some patients, coinfection with HDV leads to severe, fulminant, and often fatal hepatitis, particularly in intravenous drug abusers. *Superinfection of an HBV carrier with HDV typically increases the severity of an existing chronic hepatitis.* In fact, 70% to 80% of HBsAg carriers superinfected with HDV develop chronic hepatitis.

Hepatitis C Virus is a Common Cause of Chronic Hepatitis and Cirrhosis

Hepatitis C virus (HCV) is classified as a flavivirus and contains a single strand of RNA. Six different but related HCV genotypes are recognized; types 1, 2, and 3 are the most common (72% in the United States and Western Europe). Genotypes 2 and 3 are more responsive to antiviral therapy than is type 1. In an individual patient, many mutant HCV strains arise, which likely accounts for several features of infection, including (1) the inability of anti-HCV IgG antibodies to clear the infection, (2) persistent and relapsing infection (chronic hepatitis), and (3) lack of progress in developing a vaccine.

 EPIDEMIOLOGY: The prevalence of HCV is variable, ranging from 1.6% in the United States to 22% in Egypt. It is estimated that 200 million people are infected worldwide. HCV is the most common indication for liver transplantation, accounting for up to half of all patients on the waiting list. HCV infection is transmitted by contact with infected blood and is particularly associated with intravenous drug abuse and high-risk sexual behavior (particularly among male homosexuals). The risk from blood transfusions has been almost completely eliminated, owing to screening of the blood supply for anti-HCV antibodies. Vertical transmission of HCV from an infected mother to her newborn baby is infrequent (about 5%), although it is more common in the case of women infected with HIV. About 40% of cases occur in the absence of known risk factors.

 PATHOGENESIS: HCV is not directly cytopathic, as evidenced by the fact that many chronic carriers of the virus often have no evidence of liver cell injury. Despite active humoral and cellular immune responses directed against all viral proteins, most patients display persistent viremia. Liver cell injury has been attributed to cytotoxic T-cell responses to virally infected hepatocytes. The mechanisms by which HCV persists have not been clarified.

 CLINICAL FEATURES: The incubation period of hepatitis C is similar to that of hepatitis B. Elevated serum aminotransferase activities (Fig. 14-13) are usually found within 1 to 3 months of exposure to the virus (range, 2 to 26 weeks). The presence of HCV RNA in the serum can be detected by the polymerase chain reaction within 2 weeks of infection. Anti-HCV antibodies usually appear 7 to 8 weeks after HCV infection and persist during the chronic infection phase. The clinical course of **acute** hepatitis C is surprisingly mild and is only very rarely complicated by fulminant hepatitis. In fact, only 10% of patients become jaundiced in the acute phase.

The major consequences of infection with HCV relate to chronic disease (Fig. 14-14). The probability of persistent HCV infection and chronic hepatitis is at least 80% and may be higher. Moreover, chronic hepatitis ensues in 50% to 70% of infected persons. Clinical morbidity in most patients remains mild for at least 10 years and in many cases, for 20 or more years. Importantly, approximately 20% of patients with chronic hepatitis C eventually develop cirrhosis. *In patients with well-established cirrhosis, up to 5% a year develop primary hepatocellular carcinoma.*

Extrahepatic manifestations of hepatitis C are well recognized. Chronic HCV infection has been associated with essential mixed cryoglobulinemia, membranoproliferative glomerulonephritis, porphyria cutanea tarda, and sicca syndrome. A higher incidence of lymphoma has also been described in patients with chronic hepatitis C. Treatment with α-interferon and antiviral agents has been beneficial in many patients with chronic hepatitis C.

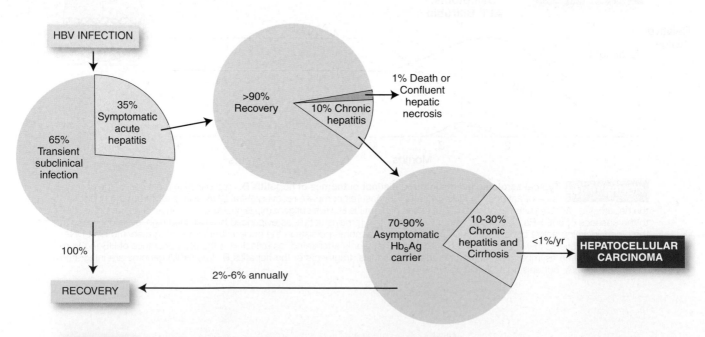

FIGURE 14-12. Possible outcomes of infection with the hepatitis B virus (HBV).

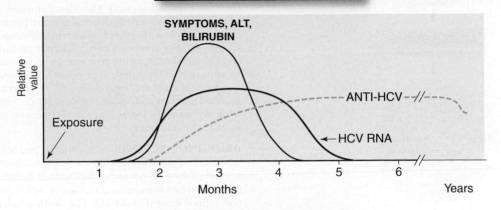

ACUTE RESOLVING HEPATITIS C

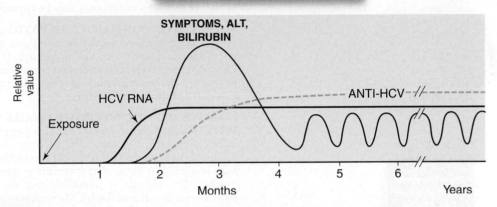

CHRONIC HEPATITIS C

FIGURE 14-13. **Clinical course of hepatitis C.** Typical serologic events in two distinct outcomes. *(Top panel)* About 20% of the patients with acute hepatitis C have a self-limited infection that resolves in a few months. Anti-HCV appears at the end of the clinical course and persists. *(Bottom panel)* The remaining patients with hepatitis C develop chronic illness, with exacerbations and remissions of clinical symptoms. The development of anti-HCV does not affect the clinical outcome. Chronic hepatitis often eventuates in cirrhosis. ALT, alanine aminotransferase.

Hepatitis E Virus is a Major Cause of Epidemics of Hepatitis in Underdeveloped Countries

Hepatitis E virus (HEV) is an enteric RNA virus transmitted by the fecal–oral route. It accounts for more than half of cases of acute viral hepatitis in young to middle-aged persons in poor regions of the world. The disease is similar to hepatitis A and is icteric, self-limited, and acute. Jaundice, hepatomegaly, fever, and arthralgias are common and usually resolve within 6 weeks. Mortality rates range from 1% to 12% but may reach 20% to 40% in pregnant women.

Pathology of Viral Hepatitis

Acute Hepatitis is Morphologically Similar in all Forms of Viral Hepatitis

 PATHOLOGY: The hallmark of acute viral hepatitis is liver cell death (Fig. 14-15). Within the hepatic lobule, scattered necrosis of single cells or of small clusters of hepatocytes is seen. A few apoptotic liver cells appear as small, deeply eosinophilic bodies (**Council-man or acidophilic bodies**), sometimes containing pyknotic nuclear material, which have been extruded from the liver cell plates into the sinusoids.

Although acidophilic bodies are characteristic of viral hepatitis, they are also encountered in other liver diseases. In acute viral hepatitis, many liver cells appear normal, but others show varying degrees of hydropic swelling and differences in size, shape, and staining qualities. Concomitantly, regenerative liver cells that display a larger nucleus and expanded basophilic cytoplasm are also seen. The resulting irregularity of the liver cell plates is termed **lobular disarray**.

Chronic Inflammatory Cells in Acute Hepatitis

Chronic inflammatory cells, principally lymphoid, infiltrate the lobule diffusely, surround individual necrotic liver cells, and accumulate in areas of focal necrosis. In addition, macrophages may be prominent, and eosinophils and polymorphonuclear leukocytes are not uncommon. Character-istically, lymphoid cells infiltrate between the wall of the central vein and the liver cell plates, an appearance termed **central phlebitis**. Swelling and proliferation of the endothelial cells of the central vein (**endophlebitis**) often develop. The Kupffer cells are enlarged, project into the lumen of the sinusoid, and contain lipofuscin pigment and phagocytosed debris. Cholestasis is common, and when severe, is termed **cholestatic hepatitis**.

Confluent Hepatic Necrosis

*The term **confluent hepatic necrosis** refers to particularly severe variants of acute viral hepatitis, which are characterized by the

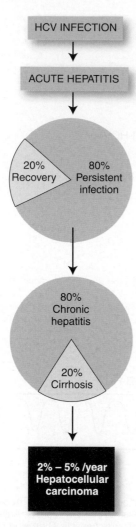

HCV INFECTION

↓

ACUTE HEPATITIS

↓

20% Recovery | 80% Persistent infection

↓

80% Chronic hepatitis

20% Cirrhosis

↓

2% – 5% /year Hepatocellular carcinoma

FIGURE 14-14. Possible outcomes of infection with the hepatitis C virus (HCV).

death of numerous hepatocytes in a geographical distribution and, in extreme cases, by the demise of almost all the liver cells (massive hepatic necrosis). The most common cause is acute hepatitis B, and only rarely does confluent hepatic necrosis result from infection with other hepatotropic viruses. Importantly, the lesions are not confined to viral hepatitis but may also be encountered after exposure to a variety of hepatotoxic agents and in autoimmune hepatitis (see below). *In contrast to the most common forms of acute viral hepatitis, in which the necrosis of hepatocytes appears to be random and patchy, confluent hepatic necrosis typically affects whole regions of the lobule.* Specific variants of confluent necrosis include the following:

BRIDGING NECROSIS: At the milder end of the spectrum of lesions that constitute confluent hepatic necrosis are bands of necrosis (bridging necrosis) that stretch between adjacent portal tracts, between adjacent central veins, and between portal tracts and central veins (Fig. 14-16). The death of adjacent plates of hepatocytes results in the collapse of the collagenous stroma to form bands of connective tissue, best visualized with a reticulin stain. When such bands encircle an area of liver cells, a nodular pattern, similar to that seen in cirrhosis, may be apparent.

SUBMASSIVE CONFLUENT HEPATIC NECROSIS: This form of acute hepatitis defines an even more severe injury involving necrosis of entire lobules or groups of adjacent lobules. Clinically, these patients manifest severe hepatitis, which may rapidly proceed to hepatic failure, in which case the disease is classed clinically as **fulminant hepatitis**.

MASSIVE HEPATIC NECROSIS (ACUTE YELLOW ATROPHY): Although uncommon, massive hepatic necrosis is the most feared variant of acute viral hepatitis, because it is a form of fulminant hepatitis that is almost invariably fatal. Grossly, the liver is shrunken to as small as 500 g (one third of normal weight). The capsule is wrinkled, and the mottled, red-tan parenchyma is soft and flabby. Microscopic examination reveals that virtually all the hepatocytes are dead, and the hepatic lobule is represented only by the collagenous framework, which in many areas has collapsed. Macrophages, erythrocytes, and necrotic debris fill the sinusoids. For unknown reasons, massive hepatic necrosis does not elicit a vigorous inflammatory response in either the parenchyma or the portal tracts. Liver transplantation is a mainstay of therapy for severe forms of confluent hepatic necrosis.

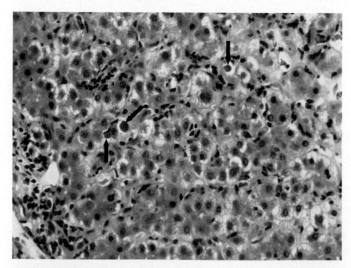

FIGURE 14-15. **Acute viral hepatitis.** A photomicrograph shows disarray of liver cell plates, swollen (ballooned) hepatocytes, and an infiltrate of lymphocytes and scattered mononuclear inflammatory cells. The remnants of necrotic hepatocytes have been extruded into the sinusoids, where they appear as acidophilic, or Councilman, bodies *(arrows)*.

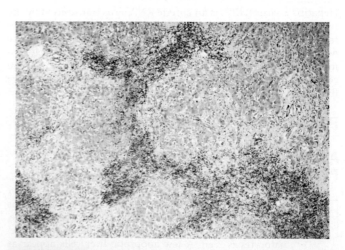

FIGURE 14-16. **Confluent hepatic necrosis.** Hemorrhagic zones of necrosis bridge adjacent portal tracts (bridging necrosis).

Chronic Hepatitis is a Complication of Hepatitis B and C, and of a Number of Metabolic and Immune Disorders

The morphologic spectrum of chronic hepatitis ranges from mild portal inflammation, with little or no evidence of liver cell necrosis, to a widespread inflammatory, necrotizing, and fibrosing condition that often eventuates in cirrhosis (Fig. 14-17).

PIECEMEAL NECROSIS: This lesion is essentially periportal and refers to focal destruction of the limiting plate of hepatocytes. A periportal chronic inflammatory infiltrate creates an irregular border between the portal tracts and the lobular parenchyma (see Fig. 14-17).

PORTAL TRACT LESIONS: Chronic hepatitis is characterized by variable infiltration of the portal tracts by lymphocytes, plasma cells, and macrophages (see Fig. 14-17). The expanded portal tracts often display mild-to-severe proliferation of bile ductules, which represents a nonspecific response to chronic liver injury. In the case of chronic hepatitis C, lymphoid aggregates or follicles with reactive centers are often present.

INTRALOBULAR LESIONS: Focal necrosis and inflammation within the parenchyma are typical of chronic hepatitis. Scattered acidophilic bodies are common, and enlarged Kupffer cells are seen within the sinusoids. The liver in chronic hepatitis B often exhibits scattered hepatocytes with a large granular cytoplasm containing abundant HBsAg (**ground-glass hepatocytes**).

PERIPORTAL FIBROSIS: The progressive erosion of the periportal hepatocytes by piecemeal necrosis leads to the deposition of collagen, which gives the portal tract a star-like appearance. With time, the fibrosis may extend to adjacent portal tracts or into the lobule itself toward the central vein, ultimately developing into cirrhosis.

Autoimmune Hepatitis

Autoimmune hepatitis is a severe type of chronic hepatitis of unknown cause that is associated with circulating autoantibodies and high levels of serum immunoglobulins. Although the disorder occurs predominantly

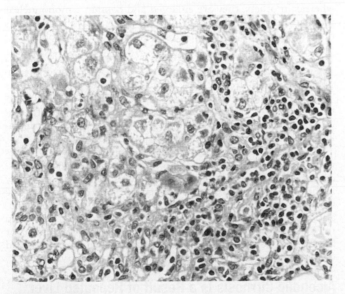

FIGURE 14-17. Severe chronic hepatitis. A photomicrograph discloses a mononuclear inflammatory infiltrate in an expanded portal tract. The inflammation penetrates the limiting plate and surrounds groups of hepatocytes at the border of the portal tract.

among young women, up to one third of patients are men, and the disease may appear at any age. In the United States, autoimmune hepatitis affects up to 200,000 individuals and accounts for 6% of liver transplants.

 PATHOGENESIS: Two distinct types of autoimmune hepatitis have been identified.

- **Type I** autoimmune hepatitis is the most common form of the disease (80% of cases) and features antinuclear and antismooth muscle antibodies. Approximately 70% of cases occur in women younger than 40 years of age, among whom one-third have other autoimmune diseases, including thyroiditis, rheumatoid arthritis, and ulcerative colitis. Importantly, one quarter of patients with type I autoimmune hepatitis present with cirrhosis, indicating that the disease usually has a prolonged asymptomatic course. Susceptibility to the disease is associated with the HLA-DRB1 gene.
- **Type II** autoimmune hepatitis occurs principally in children aged 2 to 14 years and is recognized by the presence of antibody to liver and kidney microsomes (anti-LKM). However, the target autoantigen is a P450-type drug-metabolizing enzyme (CYP 2D6). These patients often suffer from other autoimmune diseases, especially type I diabetes and thyroiditis. The genetic background for this type of autoimmune hepatitis is less well defined than is that for type I.

 PATHOLOGY: In general, the histologic appearance of autoimmune hepatitis resembles that of chronic viral hepatitis, although lobular inflammation and necrosis tends to be more pronounced. An inflammatory infiltrate rich in plasma cells is an important diagnostic feature. Pronounced hyperglobulinemia is characteristic of the disease.

Alcoholic Liver Disease

EPIDEMIOLOGY: *The prevalence of cirrhosis is highest in those countries with the highest per capita consumption of alcohol.* Although only a minority of chronic alcoholics develop cirrhosis, a dose–response relationship between the lifetime dose of alcohol (duration of exposure and the daily amount of alcohol consumed) and the appearance of cirrhosis has been established.

It is estimated that about 5% of the adult male population in the United States abuses alcohol (15% report binge drinking), and this figure is considerably higher in many other countries. *About 15% of alcoholics can be expected to develop cirrhosis, and many of these persons die in hepatic failure or from the extrahepatic complications of cirrhosis.* In fact, in many urban areas of the United States with high alcoholism rates, cirrhosis of the liver is the third or fourth leading cause of death in men younger than 45 years of age.

The amount of alcohol required to produce chronic liver disease varies widely, depending on body size, age, gender, and ethnicity, but the lower range seems to be about 80 g/day (8 ounces [240 mL] of 86 proof [43%] whiskey, two bottles of wine, or six 12-ounce bottles of beer). In general, more than 10 years of alcoholism is required to produce cirrhosis, although a few cirrhotic patients give shorter histories of heavy alcohol use.

Alcoholic liver disease spans three major morphologic and clinical entities: **fatty liver, acute alcoholic hepatitis,** and **cirrhosis**. Although these lesions usually occur sequentially, they may coexist in any combination and seem to be independent entities.

Fatty Liver is Found in Virtually all Chronic Alcoholics

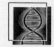 **PATHOGENESIS:** Virtually all chronic alcoholics accumulate fat in hepatocytes (**steatosis**). The pathogenesis of fatty liver is not precisely understood, and the relative contributions of different pathways may vary, depending on the amount of alcohol consumed, dietary lipid content, body stores of fat, hormonal status, and other variables. Nevertheless, the accumulation of fat clearly depends on the intake of ethanol, as it is fully and rapidly reversible on discontinuation of alcohol ingestion.

Most of the fat deposited in the liver after chronic alcohol consumption is derived from the diet. Ethanol increases lipolysis and thus the delivery of free fatty acids to the liver. Within the hepatocyte, ethanol (1) increases fatty acid synthesis, (2) decreases mitochondrial oxidation of fatty acids, (3) increases the production of triglycerides, and (4) impairs the release of lipoproteins. Collectively, these metabolic consequences produce a fatty liver.

 PATHOLOGY: In the alcoholic, the liver becomes yellow and enlarged, sometimes massively, to as much as three times the normal weight. Microscopically, the extent of visible fat accumulation varies from minute droplets scattered in the cytoplasm of a few hepatocytes to distention of the entire cytoplasm of most cells by coalesced droplets (Fig. 14-18).

Increased microsomal function in the liver of the alcoholic augments the metabolism of hepatic toxins, thereby exaggerating the danger produced by agents such as acetaminophen. In contrast to chronic alcohol consumption, which promotes microsomal functions, the presence of ethanol after acute alcohol ingestion inhibits the activity of mixed-function oxidases and acutely reduces the clearance rate of drugs from the body.

 CLINICAL FEATURES: Patients with uncomplicated alcoholic fatty liver have surprisingly few symptoms of liver disease. Despite the striking morphologic change in the liver, alcoholic fatty liver is a fully reversible lesion

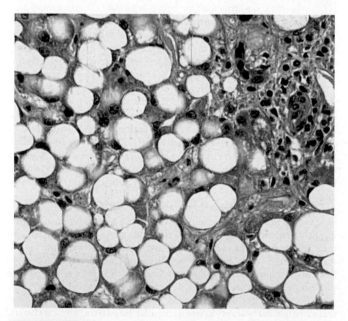

FIGURE 14-18. **Alcoholic fatty liver.** A photomicrograph shows the cytoplasm of almost all hepatocytes distended by fat that displaces the nucleus to the periphery.

and does not by itself progress to more severe disease, notably cirrhosis. A fatty liver, although characteristic of alcoholism, is not restricted to that condition but is also noted in nonalcoholic fatty liver disease (see below), in kwashiorkor, morbid obesity, and following prolonged administration of corticosteroids.

Alcoholic Hepatitis is Associated with Intrahepatic Collagen Deposition

Alcoholic hepatitis is an acute necrotizing lesion characterized by (1) necrosis of hepatocytes, predominantly in the central zone, (2) cytoplasmic hyaline inclusions within hepatocytes, (3) a neutrophilic inflammatory response, and (4) perivenular fibrosis (Fig. 14-19). The pathogenesis of alcoholic hepatitis is mysterious. Alcoholics may have mild fatty liver for many years and, without any change in drinking habits, suddenly develop acute alcoholic hepatitis.

 PATHOLOGY: The hepatic architecture is basically intact, with a normal relation of portal tracts to central venules. The hepatocytes show variable hydropic swelling, which gives them a heterogeneous appearance. Isolated necrotic liver cells or clusters of them exhibit pyknotic nuclei and karyorrhexis. Scattered hepatocytes contain **Mallory bodies** (**alcoholic hyalin**) (see Fig. 14-19). These cytoplasmic inclusions, which are more common in visibly damaged, swollen hepatocytes, are visualized as irregular skeins of eosinophilic material or as solid eosinophilic masses, often in a perinuclear location. Ultrastructurally, they are composed of aggregates of intermediate (cytokeratin) filaments. The damaged, ballooned hepatocytes, particularly those containing Mallory bodies, are surrounded by neutrophils, although a more diffuse, intralobular inflammatory infiltrate is also present. Cholestasis, varying from mild to severe, is present in as many as one third of cases. Alcoholic hepatitis is usually superimposed on an existing fatty liver, although there is no evidence that fat accumulation predisposes or contributes to the development of alcoholic hepatitis.

Collagen deposition is a constant feature of alcoholic hepatitis, especially around the central vein (terminal hepatic venule). In severe cases, the venule and perivenular sinusoids are obliterated and surrounded by dense fibrous tissue, in which case the lesion has been termed **central hyaline sclerosis**.

The appearance of the portal tracts in alcoholic hepatitis is highly variable. In some instances, they are virtually normal, whereas in others, they are enlarged and contain a mononuclear infiltrate and proliferated bile ductules. The altered portal tracts often display spurs of fibrous tissue that penetrate the lobules.

 CLINICAL FEATURES: Alcoholic hepatitis features malaise and anorexia, fever, right upper-quadrant abdominal pain, and jaundice. A mild leukocytosis is common. The serum aminotransferase activities, particularly that of aspartate aminotransferase, are moderately elevated, but not to the levels often noted in viral hepatitis. Serum alkaline phosphatase activity is usually increased.

The prognosis in patients with alcoholic hepatitis correlates with the severity of the liver cell injury. In some patients, the disease rapidly progresses to hepatic failure and death. The mortality in the acute stage of alcoholic hepatitis is about 10%. Among those who abstain from alcohol after recovery from acute alcoholic hepatitis, most recover. However, of those who continue to drink, up to 70% may ultimately develop cirrhosis. No specific treatment for acute alcoholic hepatitis is available, although corticosteroids and dietary supplementation may improve short-term survival.

Alcoholic Cirrhosis is a Result of Repeated Liver Injury, Fibrosis, and Regeneration

In about 15% of alcoholics, hepatocellular necrosis, fibrosis, and regeneration eventually lead to the formation of fibrous septa surrounding hepatocellular nodules, the two features that define cir-

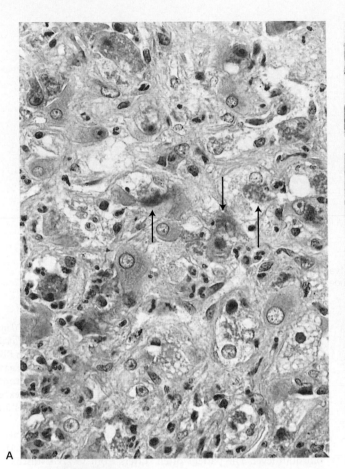

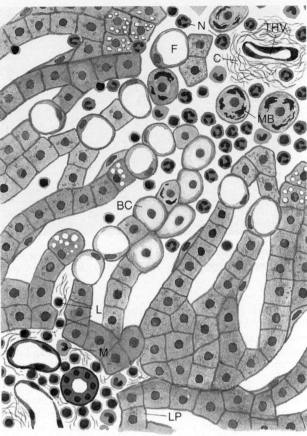

A   B

FIGURE 14-19.   **Alcoholic hepatitis. A.** A photomicrograph shows necrosis and degeneration of hepatocytes, Mallory bodies (eosinophilic inclusions) in the cytoplasm of injured hepatocytes, and infiltration by neutrophils. **B.** Schematic representation of the major pathologic features of alcoholic hepatitis. The lesions are predominantly centrilobular and include necrosis and loss of hepatocytes, ballooned cells *(BC),* and Mallory bodies *(MB)* in the cytoplasm of damaged hepatocytes. The inflammatory infiltrate consists predominantly of neutrophils *(N),* although a few lymphocytes *(L)* and macrophages *(M)* are also present. The central vein, or terminal hepatic venule *(THV),* is encased in connective tissue *(C)* (central sclerosis). Fat-laden hepatocytes *(F)* are evident in the lobule. The portal tract displays moderate chronic inflammation, and the limiting plate *(LP)* is focally breached.

rhosis (Fig. 14-20). The other lesions of alcoholic liver disease—namely, fatty liver and acute or persistent alcoholic hepatitis—are often seen in conjunction with cirrhosis. The prognosis in cases of established alcoholic cirrhosis is considerably better in those who abstain from alcohol abuse. Nevertheless, many patients progress to end-stage liver disease, and alcoholic liver disease is a common indication for liver transplantation.

Primary Biliary Cirrhosis

Primary biliary cirrhosis (PBC) is a chronic progressive cholestatic liver disease characterized by destruction of the intrahepatic bile ducts (nonsuppurative destructive cholangitis). The loss of bile ducts leads to impaired bile secretion, cholestasis, and hepatic damage. PBC occurs principally in middle-aged women (10:1 female predominance). The use of the term *cirrhosis* in this context is somewhat misleading, in that cirrhosis is actually a late complication of the disease. PBC accounts for up to 2% of deaths from cirrhosis.

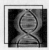 **PATHOGENESIS:** *PBC is associated with many immunologic abnormalities and is, therefore, believed to be an autoimmune disease.* Most (85%) patients with primary biliary cirrhosis have at least one other dis-

ease usually classed as autoimmune, and almost half (40%) have two or more such ailments. Among these disorders are chronic thyroiditis, rheumatoid arthritis, scleroderma, Sjögren syndrome, and systemic lupus erythematosus. *More than 95% of patients have circulating antimitochondrial antibodies, a finding commonly used in the diagnosis of PBC.* Other circulating autoantibodies commonly detected are antinuclear, antithyroid, antiplatelet, anti-acetylcholine receptor, and antiribonucleoprotein antibodies. The complement system is also chronically activated. The cells surrounding and infiltrating the sites of bile duct damage are predominantly suppressor/cytotoxic (CD8+) lymphocytes, suggesting that they mediate the destruction of the ductal epithelium.

 PATHOLOGY: The pathological stages in the evolution of PBC are characterized by ductal lesions, scarring, and cirrhosis.

STAGE I: THE DUCT LESION. Early PBC features a unique lesion, namely a **chronic destructive cholangitis,** that affects the intrahepatic small and medium-sized bile ducts (Fig. 14-21). The injury to the bile ducts is segmental and, therefore, appears focal in histologic sections. The bile ducts are surrounded principally by lymphocytes, but plasma cells and macrophages are also seen. Characteristi-cally, the bile duct epithelium is irregular and hy-

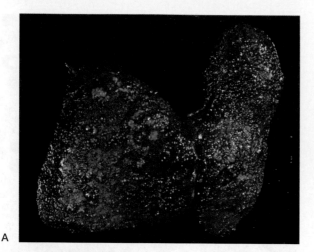

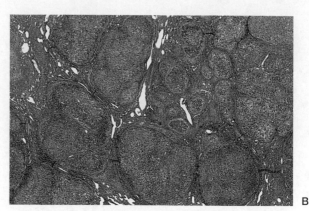

A

B

FIGURE 14-20. **Alcoholic cirrhosis. A.** The surface of the liver displays innumerable small, regular nodules. **B.** A photomicrograph shows small regular nodules surrounded by uniform fibrous septa.

perplastic, with stratification of epithelial cells and occasional papillary ingrowths. In some portal tracts, lymphoid follicles, occasionally containing germinal centers, are conspicuous. Discrete epithelioid granulomas often occur in the portal tracts and may impinge on the bile ducts. The lobular parenchyma tends to be normal.

STAGE II: SCARRING. The small bile ducts virtually disappear, and scarring of medium-sized bile ducts is common. Proliferation of bile ductules within the portal tracts is usual and may be florid. Collagenous septa extend from the portal tracts into the lobular parenchyma and begin to encircle some lobules. Cholestasis, when present, may be severe and is located at the periphery of the portal tracts.

STAGE III: CIRRHOSIS. The end-stage of PBC is cirrhosis, characterized by a dark green, bile-stained liver that exhibits fine nodularity. Microscopically, small bile ducts are scarce, and medium-sized ducts are conspicuously fewer in number. There is little inflammation within either the fibrous septa or the parenchymal nodules.

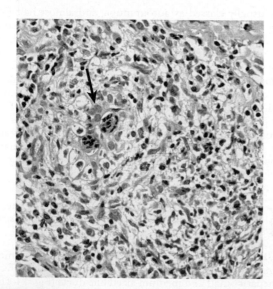

FIGURE 14-21. **Primary biliary cirrhosis (PBC), stage 1.** A photomicrograph shows a portal tract expanded by an inflammatory infiltrate consisting of lymphocytes, plasma cells, and macrophages. A bile duct *(arrow)* is damaged by the inflammation.

CLINICAL FEATURES: *Women, usually between 30 and 65 years of age, constitute about 90% to 95% of those afflicted with PBC.* A substantial proportion of patients with PBC have no symptoms during the early stages of the disease. Fatigue and pruritus are the most common initial symptoms. Some patients remain asymptomatic and appear to have an excellent prognosis; others ultimately develop advanced cirrhosis and its complications.

In a typical case of PBC, high serum alkaline phosphatase activity is accompanied by a normal or only slightly elevated serum bilirubin level. The patient often suffers from severe pruritus. As the disease advances, most patients have a progressive increase in the serum bilirubin level. Serum aminotransferase activities are only moderately elevated. The serum cholesterol level increases strikingly, and an abnormal lipoprotein (lipoprotein-X) appears, which is found in many forms of chronic cholestasis. Cholesterol-laden macrophages accumulate in the subcutaneous tissues, where they appear as localized **xanthomas**. The impairment in the excretion of bile into the intestine often leads to severe **steatorrhea**, owing to fat malabsorption. Because of associated malabsorption of vitamin D and calcium, **osteomalacia** and **osteoporosis** are important complications of PBC. About one third of patients develop gallstones. Patients who eventually develop cirrhosis die in hepatic failure or from the complications of portal hypertension. PBC generally pursues an indolent course, which may be as long as 20 to 30 years. Liver transplantation is highly effective in end-stage PBC.

Primary Sclerosing Cholangitis

Primary sclerosing cholangitis (PSC) is a chronic cholestatic liver disease of unknown cause, in which an inflammatory and fibrosing process narrows and eventually obstructs the intrahepatic and extrahepatic bile ducts. Although the cause of PSC is unknown, two thirds of patients also have ulcerative colitis. Up to 70% of patients are men, with a mean age of 40 years and a prevalence of 14 cases per 100,000 population. Progressive biliary obstruction typically leads to persistent obstructive jaundice and eventually to secondary biliary cirrhosis.

Genetic and immunologic factors contribute to the pathogenesis of PSC. The disease occasionally occurs in families and shows an association with certain HLA haplotypes, including HLA B8 and DR3. Hypergammaglobu-linemia is common, as are circulating antineutrophil cytoplasmic antibodies (perinuclear or P-ANCAs) (see Chapter 16), immune complexes in the serum, and activation of the complement system by the classic pathway. The portal tracts exhibit an increased number of T cells.

PATHOLOGY: The liver disease associated with PSC can be divided into three histologic stages:

- **Stage I:** The initial lesion is periductal inflammation and fibrosis in the portal tracts.
- **Stage II:** Many bile ducts become obliterated, and fibrous septa extend into the parenchyma.
- **Stage III:** Secondary biliary cirrhosis eventually develops.

CLINICAL FEATURES: PSC has a poor prognosis; the mean survival after the appearance of symptoms is 6 years. *Cholangiocarcinoma has been reported to develop in up to 20% of patients with PSC.* Liver transplantation is curative, but recurrence of PSC is not uncommon.

Iron-Overload Syndromes

A number of conditions are characterized by the excessive accumulation of iron in the body (siderosis). Iron overload is divided into two major categories based on the etiology of the increased body iron. **Hereditary hemochromatosis** is caused by a common genetic alteration in the control of the intestinal absorption of iron. **Secondary iron overload** is a condition that (1) complicates certain hematologic disorders; (2) is associated with parenteral iron overload, in which the iron is obtained from multiple blood transfusions or the parenteral administration of iron itself; or (3) is caused by an enormous dietary intake of iron.

Hereditary Hemochromatosis (HH) is a Common Disorder of Iron Metabolism

Type I HH (classic HH) is characterized by excessive iron absorption and the toxic accumulation of iron in parenchymal cells, particularly of the liver, heart, and pancreas. In this disease, 20 to 40 g of iron (i.e., up to 10 times the normal content) accumulates in the body. The excess iron in HH is located exclusively within the storage compartment, and thus iron stores are increased up to 50 times normal. *The clinical hallmarks of advanced HH are cirrhosis, diabetes, skin pigmentation, and cardiac failure.* The disease most often manifests in patients age 40 to 60, and men are afflicted 10 times as often as women. This striking male predilection may be attributed to the increased loss of iron in women during the reproductive years. However, given sufficient time to absorb additional iron, postmenopausal women also seem to be at risk for the development of hemochromatosis. Because maximum daily iron absorption is about 4 mg, hemochromatosis clearly takes years to develop.

PATHOGENESIS: Type I HH (classic HH) is inherited as an **autosomal recessive** disorder, in which increased intestinal absorption of iron occurs even in the presence of excess body stores. The gene involved in type I HH, known as *HFE,* is located on the short arm of chromosome 6 and encodes a transmembrane protein that is similar to MHC class-1 molecules. In populations of European descent, the heterozygous frequency is about 10%, and 1 of 200 to 400 persons is homozygous. However, not all homozygotes develop clinical disease, a finding that represents the effect of multiple mutant alleles at the HFE locus, modifier genes, and host variables (such as sex), all of which are important in controlling the expression of the disease. HFE binds to the transferrin receptor 1(Tfr1), the major receptor for the plasma iron-transporting protein transferrin. In doing so, HFE *facilitates* the uptake of iron-saturated transferrin from the blood by precursors to intestinal enterocytes and macrophages. Mutant HFE *prevents* the uptake of iron-saturated transferrin, thereby signal-

ing the iron-starved enterocyte progeny in the villus to increase gut iron uptake and release the iron into the blood. Hence, paradoxically, the cells that normally store excess iron as ferritin (gut enterocytes and macrophages) are relatively iron deficient in HH.

As noted in Chapter 1, iron is an essential factor in cellular injury mediated by activated oxygen species. The presence of excess iron in cells probably renders them more susceptible to oxidative injury. Genetic variation in antioxidant defense may also control expression of the disease.

PATHOLOGY: HH is characterized pathologically by the accumulation of very large amounts of iron in the parenchymal cells of a variety of organs and tissues.

LIVER: The liver is always affected in HH, containing more than 0.5 g iron per 100 g wet weight in the late stages. The liver is enlarged and reddish brown and exhibits micronodular cirrhosis, which progresses with time to a macronodular pattern. The hepatocytes and bile duct epithelium are filled with iron granules. The excess cellular iron is stored predominantly in lysosomes in the ferric form. Late in the disease, many Kupffer cells contain large deposits of iron derived from the phagocytosis of necrotic hepatocytes. Within the fibrous septa, iron is conspicuous in proliferated bile ductules and macrophages.

SKIN: The skin in patients with HH is typically pigmented, but only half of patients exhibit increased iron deposition in the skin. Most patients display increased melanin in the basal melanocytes.

PANCREAS: Diabetes is a common complication of HH and results from the deposition of iron in the pancreas. Grossly, the organ appears rust-colored and fibrotic. Both exocrine and endocrine cells contain excess iron, and there is degeneration of acinar cells and a reduction in the number of islets of Langerhans. The combination of pigmented skin and glucose intolerance in patients with HH is referred to as **bronze diabetes**.

HEART: Congestive heart failure is a common cause of death in patients with HH. The myocardial fibers contain iron pigment, which is more extensive in the ventricles than in the atria. Necrosis of cardiac myocytes and accompanying interstitial fibrosis are common.

ENDOCRINE SYSTEM: Numerous endocrine glands are involved in HH, including the pituitary, adrenal, thyroid, and parathyroid glands. However, tissue damage is not a usual feature in these organs, except for the pituitary, in which the release of gonadotropins is impaired. As a result, testicular atrophy is seen in one fourth of male patients, even without testicular iron deposition. The disturbance in the pituitary–gonadal axis is characterized by loss of libido and amenorrhea in women and impotence and sparse body hair in men.

JOINTS: Arthropathy, most severe in the fingers and hands, occurs in about half of patients with HH. When arthritis affects the larger joints, such as the knee, it may be severe enough to be disabling.

CLINICAL FEATURES: Symptomatic organ involvement generally starts in midlife. The liver disease in HH generally pursues an indolent and prolonged course, but among untreated patients, one-fourth eventually die in hepatic coma or from gastrointestinal hemorrhage. *Hepatocellular carcinoma is a significant late complication of HH-induced cirrhosis.* In fact, among patients with cirrhosis, the 10-year cumulative probability of developing liver cancer is as high as 30%. By contrast, noncirrhotic patients with HH treated by phlebotomy are not at increased risk of hepatocellular carcinoma.

The treatment of HH, based on the removal of iron from the body by repeated phlebotomy, is impressive. In homozygotes who have neither cirrhosis nor diabetes, iron depletion results in a life expectancy identical to that of the general population. By contrast, the 10-year survival rate of untreated patients with HH is a mere 6%.

Secondary Iron Overload Syndromes Occur in Persons Who Do Not Carry the Gene for HH

PATHOGENESIS: Within certain limits, the amount of iron absorbed bears a relationship to the amount of iron ingested. For example, a low iron content in the diet renders the development of hemochromatosis unlikely. Many patients with secondary iron overload (up to 40%) have a long history of alcohol abuse, and it is thought that alcohol may enhance both the accumulation of iron and its associated cell injury.

Massive iron overload occurs in patients with certain hemolytic anemias, such as sickle cell anemia, thalassemia major, and other anemias associated with ineffective erythropoiesis. Increased iron absorption occurs despite the saturation of transferrin; the release of iron by intravascular hemolysis adds a further burden of iron. Patients with thalassemia often develop secondary iron overload whether or not they have received blood transfusions. Multiple blood transfusions alone are generally insufficient to produce secondary iron overload. In these patients, iron is concentrated principally in mononuclear phagocytes, and cirrhosis is rare.

PATHOLOGY: Cirrhosis with secondary iron overload shows varying degrees of iron accumulation, but iron deposition in the liver is generally less extensive than that in HH and is often restricted to the periphery of the nodules. Transfusional and other types of siderosis are characterized by the uniform, initial deposition of iron in Kupffer cells, with eventual spillover into the hepatocytes.

Heritable Disorders Associated with Cirrhosis

Wilson Disease (Hepatolenticular Degeneration) is a Rare Disorder of Copper Metabolism

Wilson disease (WD) is an autosomal recessive malady in which excess copper is deposited in the liver and brain. The carrier rate is 1 in 100, and the incidence of clinical disease is 1 in 30,000 live births. The mutated gene has a worldwide distribution.

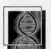

PATHOGENESIS: The intake of copper in the diet usually exceeds requirements, and the liver clears excess copper via excretion into the bile. In addition to biliary secretion, copper is normally bound to ceruloplasmin in the hepatocyte, and the complex is secreted into the blood. The gene for WD, namely *ATP7B*, codes for an ATP-dependent transmembrane cation channel that transports copper within the hepatocytes before it is excreted. *Mutations in the WD gene render copper transport ineffective, and both biliary excretion of copper and its incorporation into ceruloplasmin are deficient.*

WD is most often characterized by a striking reduction in the serum levels of ceruloplasmin. However, this deficiency is thought to be secondary to hepatic copper overload. Excess copper leads to the death of hepatocytes, release of copper into the blood, and subsequent deposits of copper in extrahepatic tissues. The mechanism by which excess copper injures cells remains elusive. Like iron, copper can catalyze the formation of potent oxidizing species from superoxide anions and hydrogen peroxide produced by normal oxygen metabolism. In this regard, copper can replace iron in the Fenton reaction, in which ferrous iron and hydrogen peroxide generate hydroxyl radicals (see Chapter 1).

PATHOLOGY: *Liver disease in WD progresses from mild to severe chronic hepatitis. Cirrhosis may develop rapidly, even in childhood.* The periportal hepatocytes often contain Mallory hyaline, and cholestasis is not infrequent. An initial micronodular cirrhosis eventually assumes a macronodular pattern.

In the brain, the corpus striatum and occasionally the subthalamic nuclei may display a reddish-brown discoloration. The central white matter of the cerebral or cerebellar hemispheres may manifest spongy softening or cavitation, in which case the overlying cortex is atrophic. Astrocytes proliferate in the putamen, and the number of neurons is decreased.

CLINICAL FEATURES: Half of patients with WD display some symptoms by adolescence, and the remainder usually become ill in their early adult years. The presenting symptoms are referable to chronic liver disease in about half of patients; one third initially present with neurologic complaints, and about one tenth are seen because of psychiatric manifestations.

LIVER: The liver disease begins insidiously with nonspecific symptoms and may progress to chronic hepatitis and cirrhosis, with resultant jaundice, portal hypertension, and hepatic failure. Unlike hemochromatosis, WD is not associated with an increased risk of primary hepatocellular carcinoma.

BRAIN: The neurologic disease begins with mild incoordination and tremors. In untreated patients, dysarthria and dysphagia appear, and in late stages, disabling dystonia and spasticity occur.

EYE: Ophthalmic manifestations invariably accompany the neurologic disease. **Kayser-Fleischer ring** is a golden-brown, bilateral discoloration of the cornea that encircles the periphery of the iris and obscures its muscular pattern. It represents a deposition of copper in Descemet membrane.

KIDNEY: Renal glomerular and tubular dysfunction, manifested by proteinuria, lowered glomerular filtration, aminoaciduria, and phosphaturia, are common in WD. These abnormalities are secondary to copper deposition in the renal tubules.

Treatment of WD with copper chelating agents not only prevents the accumulation of tissue copper but also extracts copper that has already been deposited. Both CNS dysfunction and the symptoms of liver disease are often reversed by treatment. For presymptomatic patients, maintenance treatment is with zinc, which may be effective in blocking the intestinal absorption of copper. Liver transplantation is curative for WD.

Cystic Fibrosis May Cause Biliary Obstruction

Biliary obstruction results from the accumulation of tenacious mucous plugs in the intrahepatic biliary tree and may present in the first few weeks of life. *In children who survive to adolescence, clinically symptomatic liver disease develops in about 15%, and secondary biliary cirrhosis is found in 10% of patients who survive beyond the age of 25 years.* See Chapter 6 for additional details.

α_1-Antitrypsin (α_1-AT) Deficiency Leads to Cirrhosis

α_1-AT deficiency is inherited as an autosomal recessive trait and was initially described as a cause of emphysema (see Chapter 12). Thereafter, cases of liver disease, with or without pulmonary involvement, were described. In infants and children, α_1-AT deficiency is the most common genetic cause of liver disease and the most frequent genetic disease for which liver transplantation is indicated. Although the disorder is found in 1 of 2,000 live births, only 10% to 15% of those affected develop liver injury.

PATHOGENESIS: α_1-AT is synthesized in the liver, and both the pulmonary and hepatic disorders result from a defect in the secretion of a mutant variant by the liver. The α_1-AT gene locus is termed *Pi*. The substitution of a lysine for a glutamate in the PiZ variant (95% of all cases) causes the retention of mutant protein within the lumen of the endoplasmic reticulum, where it folds abnormally as an insoluble aggregate, thereby damaging the cell.

PATHOLOGY: *The characteristic feature in the liver of patients with α_1-AT deficiency is the presence of faintly eosinophilic, periodic acid–Schiff-positive cytoplasmic droplets* (Fig. 14-22). α_1-AT deficiency is a cause of hepatitis in the newborn (see below). *Micronodular cirrhosis develops by the age of 2 to 3 years in these children and may ultimately become macronodular.*

CLINICAL FEATURES: The clinical expression of liver disease in α_1-AT deficiency is highly variable, ranging from a rapidly fatal neonatal hepatitis to an absence of any hepatic dysfunction. *Ten percent of infants with the ZZ genotype develop neonatal cholestatic jaundice (conjugated hyperbilirubinemia).* Most infants recover within 6 months, but 10% to 20% develop permanent liver disease. Children with cirrhosis usually die before the age of 10 years from hepatic failure or other complications of α_1-AT deficiency. *The cirrhosis of α_1-AT deficiency is complicated by a high incidence of hepatocellular carcinoma.*

Inborn Errors of Carbohydrate Metabolism Affect the Liver

Glycogen Storage Diseases

The biochemical basis of the glycogen storage diseases is discussed in Chapter 6. *Only glycogenosis type IV (brancher deficiency, Andersen disease) is usually complicated by cirrhosis.* Infants present with severe hepatomegaly and usually die of cirrhosis by the age of 4 years. A slowly developing cirrhosis may occur in glycogenosis type III (debrancher deficiency, Cori disease) but is not inevitable. Glycogenosis type I (glucose-6-phosphatase deficiency, von Gierke disease) is associated with striking hepatomegaly, and type II (acid-glucosidase deficiency, Pompe disease) features mild hepatomegaly. Neither type I nor type II is complicated by cirrhosis.

Galactosemia

Galactosemia, inherited as an autosomal recessive trait, is caused by a deficiency of galactose-1-phosphate uridyl transferase, the enzyme that catalyzes the second step in the conversion of galactose to glucose. As a result of this metabolic defect, galactose and its metabolites accumulate in the liver and other organs. Infants with this disorder who are fed milk rapidly develop **hepatosplenomegaly**, **jaundice**, and **hypoglycemia**. Cataracts and mental retardation are common.

Microscopically, within 2 weeks of birth, the liver shows extensive and uniform fat accumulation and striking proliferation of bile ductules in and around the portal tracts. Cholestasis is often present in canaliculi and bile ductules. Many hepatocytes are arranged around a central space, and bile plugs fill many of these pseudoacini. *At about 6 weeks of age, fibrosis begins to extend from the portal tracts into the lobule and within 6 months progresses to cirrhosis.* A galactose-free diet ameliorates the disease and reverses many of the morphologic alterations.

Hereditary Fructose Intolerance

Hereditary fructose intolerance is an autosomal recessive disease caused by a deficiency of fructose-1-phosphate aldolase. When fructose is fed early in infancy, hepatomegaly, jaundice, and ascites develop. Infants who suffer from liver disease show many of the changes of neonatal hepatitis. Fat accumulation may be marked, in which case the appearance resembles that of galactosemia. Progressive fibrosis culminates in cirrhosis.

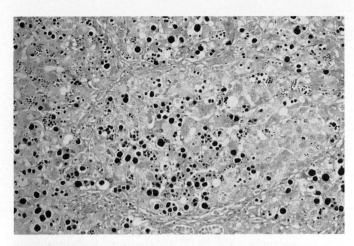

FIGURE 14-22. α_1-**Antitrypsin deficiency.** A photomicrograph of a section of liver stained by the periodic acid-Schiff (PAS) reaction with diastase digestion to remove glycogen reveals numerous cytoplasmic globules in the hepatocytes.

Tyrosinemia

Tyrosinemia is an autosomal recessive trait that interferes with the catabolism of tyrosine to fumarate and acetoacetate. The biochemical defect is a deficiency of fumarylacetoacetate hydrolase (FAH) in the liver caused by mutations in the *FAH* gene. Damage to the liver and kidney is caused by the accumulation of succinyl acetone and succinyl acetoacetate, both of which are potent electrophiles that can react with the sulfhydryl groups of glutathione and proteins.

Acute tyrosinemia, which begins within a few weeks or months of birth, is characterized by hepatosplenomegaly and is associated with liver failure and death, usually before the age of 12 months. The appearance of the liver is remarkably similar to that in galactosemia, including progression to cirrhosis.

Chronic tyrosinemia begins in the first year of life and is characterized by growth retardation, renal disease, and hepatic failure. Death usually supervenes before the age of 10 years. *The incidence of hepatocellular carcinoma associated with chronic tyrosinemia is extraordinarily high.* Tyrosinemia is treated by liver transplantation.

Toxic Liver Injury

Acute, chemically induced hepatic injury spans the entire spectrum of liver disease, from transient cholestasis to fulminant hepatitis to cirrhosis. Chronic toxic injury to the liver is equally diverse; at one extreme is a mild chronic hepatitis and at the other, active cirrhosis. Although hepatic injury caused by drugs accounts for less than 5% of all cases of jaundice, it constitutes up to 25% of cases of fulminant hepatic failure.

Some hepatotoxic chemicals **predictably** produce liver cell necrosis. The defining characteristics of the liver injury produced by **predictable hepatotoxins** are as follows:

- The agent, in sufficiently high doses, always produces liver cell necrosis.
- The extent of hepatic injury is dose dependent.
- These compounds produce the same lesions in different animal species.
- The liver necrosis is characteristically zonal—often, but not exclusively, centrilobular.
- The period between administration of the toxin and the development of liver cell necrosis is brief.

Chapter 1 includes a discussion of the possible mechanisms by which these toxins produce liver necrosis. Briefly, toxic liver necrosis is, in most cases, a consequence of the metabolism of the compound by the mixed-function oxidase system of the liver, yielding activated oxygen species and reactive metabolites.

By contrast, most reactions to therapeutic drugs are **unpredictable** and seem to represent idiosyncratic events or manifestations of unusual sensitivity to a dose-related side effect. Genetic variations in systems of biotransformation or immunologic reaction to drugs, their metabolites, or drug-modified liver cells may play a role in such unexpected reactions.

Zonal Hepatocellular Necrosis is Caused by the Metabolites of Drugs and Chemicals

The centrilobular localization of necrosis presumably reflects the greater activity of drug-metabolizing enzymes in the central zones. Examples of agents that produce such injury are carbon tetrachloride, acetaminophen (Fig. 14-23), and the toxins of the mushroom *Amanita phalloides*. In the affected zones, hepatocytes show coagulative necrosis, hydropic swelling, and variable amounts of fat. Inflammation tends to be sparse. If the dose of the hepatotoxin is sufficiently large, necrosis may extend to involve the entire lobule, leaving only a thin rim of viable hepatocytes surrounding the portal tracts. Patients either die in acute hepatic failure or recover without sequelae.

Fatty Liver is a Response to a Variety of Hepatotoxins

The accumulation of triglycerides within the hepatocytes (i.e., hepatic steatosis or fatty liver) generally occurs in a predictable fashion. Although substantial overlap may exist, two morphologic patterns occur.

Macrovesicular Steatosis

In macrovesicular steatosis, light microscopy shows the cytoplasm of the liver cell to be occupied by fat, seen as a large clear area that distends the cell and displaces the nucleus to the periphery. In addition to its association with chronic ethanol ingestion, macrovesicular fat results from exposure to such direct hepatotoxins as carbon tetrachloride and the poisonous constituents of certain mushrooms. Cortico-steroids and some antimetabolites, such as methotrexate, may also cause macrovesicular steatosis. The presence of fat per se is not injurious to the hepatocyte, but its accumulation reflects the underlying liver cell damage.

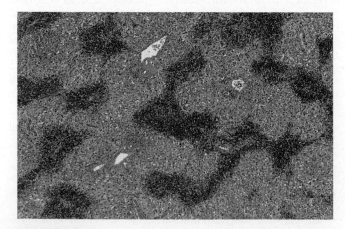

FIGURE 14-23. **Toxic centrilobular necrosis.** The autopsy specimen in a case of acetaminophen overdose discloses prominent hemorrhagic necrosis of the centrilobular zones of all liver lobules.

Microvesicular Steatosis

In contrast to macrovesicular steatosis, which by itself tends to be clinically inconsequential, microvesicular fatty liver is commonly associated with severe, and sometimes fatal, liver disease. Small fat vacuoles are dispersed throughout the cytoplasm of hepatocytes, and the nucleus retains its central position. Again, it is not the presence of fat but the underlying metabolic defects that produce the liver dysfunction.

REYE SYNDROME: *This rare acute disease of children is characterized by microvesicular steatosis, hepatic failure, and encephalopathy.* Cerebral edema and fat accumulation are reported in the brain. The symptoms usually begin after a febrile illness, commonly influenza or varicella infection, and are said to correlate with the administration of aspirin, although the pathogenesis of the syndrome remains unknown. Reye syndrome is now distinctly uncommon, possibly as a result of decreasing use of aspirin in children.

Acute Intrahepatic Cholestasis is a Frequent Manifestation of Drug-Induced Liver Disease

Histologically, the lesions range from bland centrilobular cholestasis with virtually no hepatocellular necrosis or inflammation to panlobular cholestasis with scattered foci of hepatocellular necrosis. Drugs incriminated in this type of liver injury include anabolic steroids and tranquilizing agents. Except for mild jaundice, pruritus, and an elevated serum alkaline phosphatase level, the patients feel well.

Lesions Resembling Viral Hepatitis are Unpredictable

All the features of acute viral hepatitis occasionally occur after administration of a variety of drugs. Historically, the most widely appreciated examples are the inhalation anesthetic halothane, the antituberculosis agent isoniazid, and the antihypertensive drug methyldopa. Although the incidence of these viral hepatitis-like reactions is low, they are far more dangerous than viral hepatitis itself, causing more severe disease and a much higher mortality rate. The entire range of acute liver injury, from mild anicteric hepatitis to rapidly fatal massive hepatic necrosis, is encountered.

Chronic Hepatitis Can Follow the Persistent Intake of Hepatotoxic Drugs

Like chronic hepatitis caused by persistent viral infection, drug-induced chronic hepatitis may progress to cirrhosis, albeit rarely. On discontinuation of drug administration, the lesion usually resolves, although this may require many months. In patients who have progressed to cirrhosis, the scarring remains, but the inflammatory and necrotizing activity is halted. Among the drugs incriminated in the production of chronic hepatitis are the antituberculosis drug isoniazid and certain sulfonamides.

Vascular Lesions May Complicate Hormone Therapy

Occlusion of the hepatic veins **(Budd-Chiari syndrome)** has been reported to follow the use of oral contraceptive agents, presumably reflecting the general hypercoagulable state associated with the use of these steroids. *Peliosis hepatis is a peculiar hepatic lesion, characterized by cystic, blood-filled cavities that are not lined by endothelial cells.* Anabolic sex steroids, contraceptive steroids, and the antiestrogen compound tamoxifen sometimes produce this lesion.

Neoplastic Lesions are Rare Reactions to Drugs

Hepatic adenomas are uncommon benign tumors that arise after the use of oral contraceptives and (uncommonly) of anabolic steroids. **Hemangiosarcomas** of the liver have been associated with chronic exposure to inorganic arsenic, usually in the form of insecticides, the inhalation of vinyl chloride in an industrial setting and the use of Thorotrast, a radioactive agent formerly used in liver imaging.

Vascular Disorders

Congestive Heart Failure is the Major Cause of Liver Congestion

In the face of persistent congestive heart failure, the pressure in the peripheral venous circulation increases, thereby impeding venous outflow from liver and producing **chronic passive congestion** of that organ. The chronically congested liver is often reduced in size. The cut surface exhibits an accentuated lobular pattern, with a mottled appearance of alternating light and dark areas (Fig. 14-24), termed **nutmeg liver**. In severe cases, the centrilobular terminal venules and adjacent sinusoids are markedly dilated and filled with erythrocytes, and the liver cell plates in this zone are thinned by pressure atrophy. In such cases, chronic passive congestion progresses to varying degrees of hepatic fibrosis. Delicate fibrous strands envelop terminal venules, and septa radiate from the centrilobular zones. Fibrous septa may link adjacent central veins, thereby producing a "reverse lobulation." Chronic passive congestion of the liver is of more pathologic than clinical interest, because the condition has little effect on hepatic function.

Shock Results in Decreased Perfusion of the Liver

Shock from any cause often leads to ischemic necrosis of the centrilobular hepatocytes (zone 3, see Fig. 14-1). Microscopically, coagulative necrosis of centrilobular hepatocytes is accompanied by frank hemorrhage.

Infarction of the Liver is Uncommon Because of Its Dual Blood Supply and the Anastomotic Structure of the Hepatic Sinusoids

Acute occlusion of the hepatic artery or its branches is unusual but can occur as a result of embolism, polyarteritis nodosa, or accidental ligation during surgery. Under such circumstances, irregular pale areas, often surrounded by a hyperemic zone, reflect the underlying ischemic necrosis.

Bacterial Infections

Bacterial infections are uncommon causes of liver disease in industrialized countries, and are for the most part, complications of infections elsewhere in the body. The characteristic reactions in the liver are granulomas, abscesses, and diffuse inflammation. Infections associated with granulomatous inflammation elsewhere (e.g., tuberculosis, tularemia, and brucellosis) also cause granulomatous hepatitis.

Pyogenic liver abscesses are produced by staphylococci, streptococci, and gram-negative enterobacteria (particularly the anaerobic *Bacteroides* species). Organisms reach the liver in arterial or portal blood or through the biliary tract. In cases of septicemia, the liver is seeded with organisms from distant sites through the arterial blood.

Pylephlebitic abscesses result from intra-abdominal suppuration, as in peritonitis or diverticulitis, with the organisms being

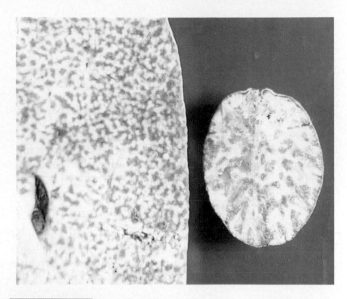

FIGURE 14-24. **Chronic passive congestion of the liver.** The surface of this fixed liver exhibits an accentuated lobular pattern, an appearance resembling that of a nutmeg *(right)*.

transmitted to the liver in portal blood. At one time, pylephlebitis was the most common cause of hepatic abscesses, but the control of abdominal sepsis with antibiotics has rendered this route of infection uncommon.

Cholangitic abscesses in the liver are today the most common form of hepatic abscess in Western countries. Biliary obstruction from any cause is often complicated by bacterial infection of the biliary tree, termed **ascending cholangitis**. The retrograde biliary dissemination of organisms (usually *E. coli*) then leads to the formation of cholangitic abscesses.

 CLINICAL FEATURES: A patient with a hepatic abscess typically presents with high fever, rapid weight loss, right upper-quadrant abdominal pain, and hepatomegaly. Jaundice occurs in one-fourth of cases, but the serum alkaline phosphatase level is almost always elevated. Solitary abscesses are treated with surgical drainage and antibiotics, but multiple abscesses present a difficult therapeutic problem. The mortality rate from hepatic abscess, even in treated cases, remains high, ranging from 40% to 80%.

Parasitic Infestations

Parasitic infestations of the liver are a serious public health problem worldwide, although they are uncommon in industrialized countries. These diseases are discussed in Chapter 9.

Cholestatic Syndromes of Infancy

Diseases characterized by prolonged cholestasis and jaundice in infants represent either diseases primarily affecting the hepatocytes or obstruction of the biliary system.

Neonatal Hepatitis is an Entity of Multiple Causes

Neonatal hepatitis features prolonged cholestasis, morphologic evidence of liver cell injury, and inflammation.

PATHOGENESIS: In about half of all cases of neonatal hepatitis, the cause is discernible (Table 14-2), and about 30% of cases are assigned to α_1-antitrypsin deficiency alone. Most of the other cases with known causes can be attributed to viral hepatitis B and infectious agents such as those of the TORCH group (*toxoplasmosis, "other," rubella, cytomegalovirus, and herpes simplex*). A few cases represent hepatic injury associated with metabolic defects, for instance, galactosemia or fructose intolerance. Occasional cases of neonatal hepatitis are seen in association with Down syndrome and other chromosomal disorders. The remaining half of all cases of neonatal hepatitis are of unexplained etiology.

PATHOLOGY: The characteristic hepatic lesion of neonatal hepatitis is giant cell transformation of hepatocytes, hence the former term **giant cell hepatitis** (Fig. 14-25). The giant cells contain as many as 40 nu-

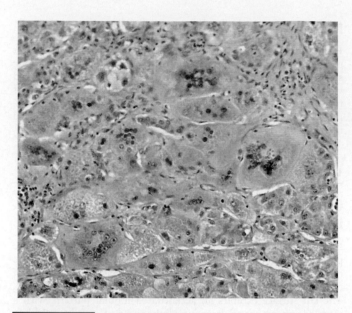

FIGURE 14-25. **Neonatal hepatitis.** A photomicrograph shows multinucleated giant hepatocytes, liver cell injury, and a mild chronic inflammatory infiltrate.

clei and may appear detached from other cells in the liver plate. The pale, distended cytoplasm contains large amounts of glycogen and iron. The number of giant cells decreases with time, and they are rare in children older than 1 year of age. Bile pigment is often prominent within canaliculi and hepatocytes. Ballooned hepatocytes, acinar transformation of hepatocytes, and acidophilic bodies are also typical of neonatal hepatitis. Extramedullary hematopoiesis is often conspicuous. Chronic inflammatory infiltrates are seen in the portal tracts as well as in the lobular parenchyma. Pericellular fibrosis around degenerating hepatocytes, singly or in groups, is common, and fibrous tissue septa extend from the portal tracts.

Biliary Atresia Refers to the Lack of a Lumen in the Biliary Tree

Both extrahepatic and intrahepatic biliary atresias are often associated with the morphologic features of neonatal hepatitis, supporting the concept that all result from a common inflammatory process ("infantile obstructive cholangiopathy").

Extrahepatic Biliary Atresia

Extrahepatic biliary atresia (EXBA) is a cholestatic disease characterized by obliteration of the lumen of all or part of the biliary tree external to the liver, not associated with calculi, neoplasm, or rupture. Although uncommon, EXBA accounts for almost half of all cases of persistent cholestasis in the neonatal period and is the most frequent indication for liver transplantation in children. EXBA is thought to represent the end result of heterogeneous conditions, including congenital anomalies and viral infections during gestational and perinatal development.

PATHOLOGY: EXBA may involve all the extrahepatic bile ducts or may be restricted to segments of the proximal or distal biliary tree. The gallbladder is often atretic. Histologically, cholestasis and periportal bile ductular proliferation in the liver are evident. A minority of cases display multinucleated giant hepatocytes, identical to those seen in neonatal hepatitis. Although the intrahepatic bile ducts may initially appear normal, they are gradually obliterated with the persistence of cholestasis. Eventually, secondary biliary cirrhosis supervenes.

TABLE 14–2

Causes of Neonatal Hepatitis

Idiopathic

Idiopathic neonatal hepatitis

Prolonged intrahepatic cholestasis

    Arteriohepatic dysplasia (Alagille syndrome)

    Paucity of intrahepatic bile ducts not associated with specific syndromes

    Zellweger syndrome (cerebrohepatorenal syndrome)

    Byler disease

Mechanical obstruction of the intrahepatic bile ducts

Congenital hepatic fibrosis

Caroli disease (cystic dilation of intrahepatic ducts)

Metabolic disorders

Defects of carbohydrate metabolism

    Galactosemia

    Hereditary fructose intolerance

    Glycogenosis type IV

Defects in lipid metabolism

    Gaucher disease

    Niemann-Pick disease

    Wolman disease

Tyrosinemia (defect of amino acid metabolism)

α_1-Antitrypsin deficiency

Cystic fibrosis

Parenteral nutrition

Hepatitis

Hepatitis B

TORCH agents (**t**oxoplasmosis, "**o**ther," **r**ubella, **c**ytomegalovirus, and **h**erpes simplex)

Varicella

Syphilis

ECHO viruses

Neonatal sepsis

Chromosomal abnormalities

Down syndrome

Trisomy 18

Extrahepatic biliary obstruction

ECHO, Enteric cytopathic human orphan.

Intrahepatic Biliary Atresia

Intrahepatic biliary atresia refers to a paucity of bile ducts within the liver. The disorder occurs in association with known causes of neonatal hepatitis (see above), as part of **Alagille syndrome** (an uncommon autosomal dominant developmental disease), or as an idiopathic lesion.

 PATHOLOGY: The major histologic feature of intrahepatic biliary atresia is a scarcity of bile ducts in the liver. Cholestasis, giant cell transformation, and bile ductular proliferation are usual. However, cirrhosis is uncommon.

 CLINICAL FEATURES: The majority of patients who have uncomplicated neonatal hepatitis recover without sequelae. By contrast, intrahepatic biliary atresia associated with neonatal hepatitis carries a grave prognosis, given that many of these children progress to biliary cirrhosis. Although surgical correction has been successful in some anatomically favorable cases, most cases of both extrahepatic and intrahepatic biliary atresia are cured only by liver transplantation.

Benign Tumors and Tumor-Like Lesions

Hepatic Adenomas are Benign Tumors of Hepatocytes that Occur Principally in Women

Hepatic adenomas were exceedingly rare before the availability of oral contraceptives, but since their introduction, many such neoplasms have been reported. The incidence has been reduced by the use of newer combinations of estrogen and progesterone.

 PATHOLOGY: Hepatic adenomas usually occur as solitary, sharply demarcated masses, up to 40 cm in diameter and 3 kg in weight (Fig. 14-26). In one fourth of cases, multiple smaller adenomas are present. On gross examination, the tumor is encapsulated and paler than the surrounding parenchyma. Microscopically, the neoplastic hepatocytes resemble their normal counterparts, except that they are not arranged in a lobular architecture (see Fig. 14-26). Portal tracts and central venules are absent. The cells making up the adenoma may be very large and eosinophilic or filled with glycogen, which makes the cytoplasm appear clear. The tumor is circumscribed by a fibrous capsule of variable thickness, and the adjacent hepatocytes appear compressed. Large, thick-walled arteries are often seen in the vicinity of the capsule, and arteries and veins traverse the tumor.

 CLINICAL FEATURES: *In about one third of patients with hepatic adenomas (particularly in pregnant women who have used oral contraceptives), the tumors bleed into the peritoneal cavity and require treatment as a surgical emergency.* Even large adenomas have been reported to disappear after discontinuation of oral contraceptive use. A few adenomas are encountered in men, and they have occasionally been reported in association with the use of anabolic steroids.

Focal Nodular Hyperplasia is a Localized Lesion that Resembles Cirrhosis

The lesion of focal nodular hyperplasia varies from 5 to 15 cm in diameter and weighs as much as 700 g. On occasion, it protrudes from the surface of the liver, and it may even be pedunculated. Focal nodular hyperplasia occurs in both genders and at all ages, but most often in young women. It is not a neoplasm and is not associated with the use of oral contraceptives. The cut surface exhibits a characteristic central scar from which fibrous septa radiate. The division of the mass by multiple fibrous septa accounts for the older term "focal cirrhosis." Microscopically, hepatocytic nodules are circumscribed by fibrous septa, which contain numerous tortuous bile ducts and mononuclear inflammatory cells. Within the nodules, lobular architecture is absent. The lesion exhibits large arteries and veins in the septa, but hemorrhage is uncommon.

Hepatic Hemangiomas are the Most Common Tumors of the Liver

Benign hemangiomas in the liver occur at all ages and in both genders and are found in up to 7% of autopsy specimens. They are ordinarily small and asymptomatic, although larger tumors have

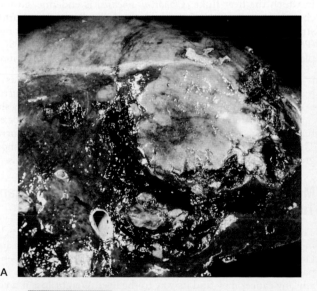

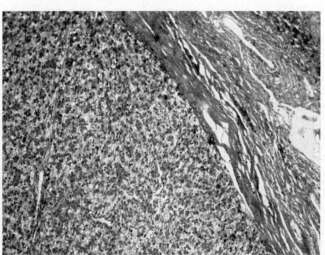

A B

FIGURE 14-26. **Hepatic adenoma. A.** A surgically resected portion of liver shows a tan, lobulated mass beneath the liver capsule. Hemorrhage into the tumor has broken through the capsule and also into the surrounding liver parenchyma. The patient was a woman who had taken birth control pills for a number of years and presented with sudden intraperitoneal hemorrhage. **B.** A fibrous capsule separates normal liver and the adenoma *(left)*. The adenomatous hepatocytes are arranged without discernible lobular architecture and show a clear cytoplasm filled with glycogen.

been reported to cause abdominal symptoms and even hemorrhage into the peritoneal cavity. Grossly, the tumor is usually solitary and less than 5 cm in diameter, but multiple hemangiomas and giant forms have been described. Microscopically, hepatic hemangiomas similar to cavernous hemangiomas are found elsewhere.

Malignant Tumors of the Liver

Hepatocellular Carcinoma (HCC) is a Malignant Tumor that Derives from Hepatocytes or Their Precursors

 EPIDEMIOLOGY AND PATHOGENESIS: HCC is probably the most common malignant tumor of humans. It occurs in all parts of the world, but its incidence shows a striking geographical variability. In Western industrialized countries, the tumor remains uncommon, but its incidence continues to rise owing to the increasing prevalence of HCV infection. Risk factors include the following:

HEPATITIS B: There is a strong association between HBV infection and HCC. Individuals with persistent HBV infection are estimated to have as much as a 200-fold increased risk of developing HCC. One fourth of those with chronic hepatitis B acquired at or near birth ultimately develop HCC. The risk of HCC in men who are positive for HBsAg and HBeAg is about four times as great as in those who are positive only for HBsAg. Most (>80%) cases of HCC associated with HBV infection occur in patients with cirrhosis.

The repeated cycles of liver cell regeneration in chronic hepatitis initiate the emergence of a neoplastic clone (see Chapter 5), although a significant proportion of HBV-associated HCCs develop in patients without cirrhosis. *The genome of HBV is integrated into the host DNA of both the nonneoplastic liver cells and the tumor cells.* The X gene of HBV encodes a viral protein (HBxAg) that inactivates tumor suppressor proteins and transactivates certain oncogenes. Additionally, HBV integration by itself may have oncogenic effects. The worldwide use of a vaccine for HBV should significantly decrease the prevalence of HCC in the future.

HEPATITIS C: Although hepatitis C has a lower global prevalence than does hepatitis B, the former is associated with most cases of HCC in Europe and North America. Hepatitis C has overtaken hepatitis B as a cause of HCC in Japan. In the United States, HCV infection is present in about 50% of cases of HCC. As in hepatitis B, most patients infected with HCV who develop HCC have underlying cirrhosis. The cumulative rate for HCC in persons with HCV-induced cirrhosis is as high as 70% after 15 years. The RNA-dependent RNA polymerase of HCV complexes the hepatocyte Rb gene product, thereby increasing cellular proliferation and potentially contributing to oncogenesis (see Chapter 5).

OTHER CAUSES OF HCC: These include **hemochromatosis**, α_1-AT deficiency, and aflatoxin B_1 (a fungal contaminant of many foods, particularly in less-developed countries). **Alcoholic cirrhosis** may present a small risk, but studies that control for hepatitis B and C are needed.

 PATHOLOGY: HCCs appear grossly as soft, hemorrhagic tan masses in the liver (Fig. 14-27). Occasionally, a green color is present, indicating bile staining. In some cases, a large solitary tumor occupies a portion of the liver; in other instances, many smaller tumors are found. The tumor has a tendency to grow into portal veins and may extend into the vena cava and even the right atrium through the hepatic veins.

Metastases occur widely, although the most common sites are the lungs and portal lymph nodes.

The histologic spectrum of HCC is variable, ranging from a well-differentiated tumor difficult to distinguish from normal liver to an anaplastic or undifferentiated appearance. A number of histologic patterns are recognized, but no prognostic significance can be attributed to any of them. Most HCCs exhibit a "**trabecular pattern**," that is, the tumor cells are arranged in trabeculae or plates that resemble the normal liver. The plates are separated by endothelium-lined sinusoids. A second histologic variant is termed the "**pseudoglandular (adenoid, acinar) pattern**" (see Fig. 14-27B). In this variety, malignant hepatocytes are arranged around a lumen and thus resemble glands. The lumina may contain bile. The acini formed by the tumor cells are not true glands, and the lesion should not be confused with adenocarcinoma.

Fibrolamellar HCC is an uncommon variant that has a distinctive histologic appearance and arises in an apparently normal liver, principally in adolescents and young adults. The tumor is composed of large, eosinophilic, neoplastic hepatocytes arranged in clusters and surrounded by delicate collagen fibers. The prognosis is considered more favorable than in most cases of HCC, although recent data have called this into question.

 CLINICAL FEATURES: HCC usually presents as a painful and enlarging mass in the liver. The prognosis is dismal, and patients die of malignant cachexia, rupture of the tumor with catastrophic bleeding into the peritoneal cavity, or complications of cirrhosis. HCC may be associated with a variety of paraneoplastic manifestations (e.g., polycythemia, hypoglycemia, hypercalcemia) as a result of ectopic hormone production by the tumor. α-Fetoprotein levels are often elevated in HCC (and may also be encountered in other neoplastic and nonneoplastic liver diseases and in some extrahepatic disorders).

Cholangiocarcinoma (Bile Duct Cancer) Arises from Biliary Epithelium

Cholangiocarcinoma originates anywhere in the biliary tree, from the large intrahepatic bile ducts at the porta hepatis to the smallest bile ductules at the periphery of the hepatic lobule. The tumor occurs predominantly in older persons of both genders, with an average age at presentation of 60 years. This cancer is particularly frequent in the parts of Asia in which the liver fluke *(Clonorchis sinensis)* is endemic, although cholangiocarcinoma is encountered in all parts of the world. A strong association exists between primary sclerosing cholangitis (PSC) and cholangiocarcinoma. One quarter of livers with PSC explanted at the time of transplantation have cholangiocarcinoma.

 PATHOLOGY: Peripheral cholangiocarcinomas are composed of small cuboidal cells arranged in a ductular or glandular configuration. Characteris-tically, they show substantial fibrosis, and on liver biopsy, they may be confused with metastatic scirrhous carcinoma of the breast or pancreas. They metastasize to a wide range of extrahepatic sites and show a greater predilection for the portal lymph nodes than do HCCs.

Metastatic Cancer is the Most Common Malignant Tumor of the Liver

The liver is involved in one third of all metastatic cancers, including half of those of the gastrointestinal tract, breast, and lung. Other tumors that characteristically metastasize to the liver are pancreatic carcinoma and malignant melanoma, although virtually any cancer may find its way to the liver. Weight loss is a common early finding in cases of metastatic cancer in the liver. Portal hypertension, with splenomegaly, ascites, and gastrointestinal bleeding may occur. If the patient lives long enough, hepatic failure often ensues. The first indication of a metastatic tumor is frequently an unexplained increase in the serum alkaline phosphatase level. Most patients die within a year of the diagnosis of

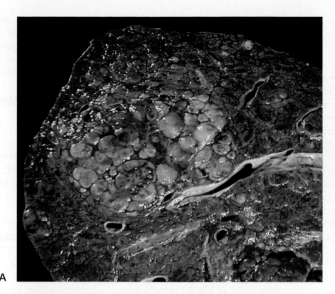
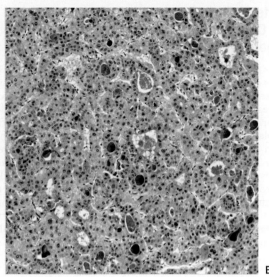

A
B

FIGURE 14-27. **Hepatocellular carcinoma. A.** Cross-section of a cirrhotic liver shows a poorly circumscribed, nodular area of yellow, partially hemorrhagic hepatocellular carcinoma. **B.** A photomicrograph of the tumor shows a trabecular pattern of malignant hepatocytes. Many cells are arranged in an acinar pattern and surround concretions of inspissated bile.

liver metastases. However, surgical resection of a solitary metastasis to the liver has often resulted in cures.

THE GALLBLADDER AND EXTRAHEPATIC BILE DUCTS

Anatomy

The wall of the gallbladder is composed of a mucous membrane, a muscularis, and an adventitia and is covered by a reflection of the visceral peritoneum. The mucosa is thrown into folds and consists of a columnar epithelium and a lamina propria of loose connective tissue. Dipping into the wall of the gallbladder are mucosal diverticula (**Rokitansky-Aschoff sinuses**).

Cholelithiasis

Cholelithiasis is defined as the presence of stones within the lumen of the gallbladder or in the extrahepatic biliary tree. Three fourths of gallstones in industrialized countries consist primarily of cholesterol, and the remainder are composed of calcium bilirubinate and other calcium salts (pigment gallstones). However, pigment stones predominate in the tropics and Asia.

Cholesterol Stones are the Most Common Gallstones

Cholesterol stones are round or faceted, yellow to tan, and single or multiple. They vary from 1 to 4 cm in the greatest dimension (Fig. 14-28). Well over 50% of the stone is composed of cholesterol; the rest consists of calcium salts and mucin.

 EPIDEMIOLOGY: Approximately 20% of American men and 35% of women older than the age of 75 years have gallstones at autopsy. *However, during their reproductive period, women are three times more likely to develop cholesterol gallstones than are men, and the incidence is higher in users of oral contraceptives and in women who have had several pregnancies.*

 PATHOGENESIS: The pathogenesis of cholesterol gallstones is a multifactorial process that involves physicochemical qualities of bile and local factors within the gallbladder itself (Fig. 14-29). The bile of persons afflicted with cholesterol gallstones has more cholesterol and less bile salts as it leaves the liver than does that of normal individuals, and the supersaturated cholesterol precipitates as solid crystals and forms stones (lithogenic bile). In obese persons, cholesterol secretion by the liver is augmented, further adding to the supersaturation of the bile with cholesterol.

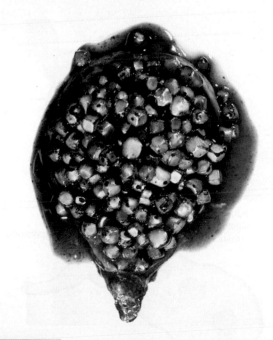

FIGURE 14-28. **Cholesterol gallstones.** The gallbladder has been opened to reveal numerous yellow cholesterol gallstones.

Cholesterol Stone Formation Features Increased Biliary Cholesterol, Decreased Bile Salts, or Inhibition of Bile Discharge

The higher prevalence of gallstones in premenopausal women has been attributed to the fact that estrogens stimulate the formation of lithogenic bile by the liver. Estrogens increase the hepatic secretion of cholesterol and decrease the secretion of bile acids. Progesterone, the predominant hormone of pregnancy, inhibits the discharge of bile from the gallbladder. These mechanisms are also invoked to explain the increased incidence of gallstones in users of oral contraceptives.

Other major risk factors for the development of cholesterol gallstones can be divided into those that relate to increased biliary cholesterol secretion, those that contribute to decreased secretion of bile salts and lecithin, and those that reflect a combination of the two.

Risk factors associated with **increased biliary cholesterol secretion** include the following:

- Increasing age
- Obesity
- Membership in certain ethnic groups
- Familial predisposition
- Diet high in calories and cholesterol
- Certain metabolic abnormalities associated with high blood cholesterol levels (e.g., diabetes, some genetic hyperlipoproteinemias, and primary biliary cirrhosis).

Decreased secretion of bile salts and lecithin occurs in nonobese whites who develop gallstones. Gastrointestinal absorptive disorders that interfere with the enterohepatic circulation of bile acids (e.g., pancreatic insufficiency secondary to cystic fibrosis and Crohn disease) also decrease the secretion of bile acids and favor gallstone formation.

Pigment Stones are Classed as Black or Brown Stones

Black Pigment Stones

Black pigment stones are irregular and measure less than 1 cm across. On cross-section, the surface appears glassy (Fig. 14-30). Black stones contain calcium bilirubinate, bilirubin polymers, calcium salts, and mucin.

 PATHOGENESIS: The incidence of black stones is increased in older and undernourished persons, but no correlations with gender, ethnicity, or obesity have been made. Chronic hemolysis, such as occurs with sickle cell anemia and thalassemia, predisposes to the development of black pigment stones. Cirrhosis, either because it leads to increased hemolysis or because of damage to liver cells, is also associated with a high incidence of black stones. However, in most instances, no predisposing cause for the formation of black pigment stones and the concomitant increased concentration of unconjugated bilirubin in the bile is evident.

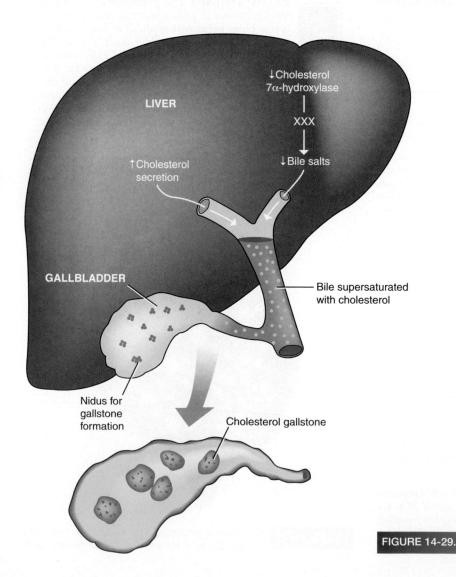

FIGURE 14-29. Pathogenesis of cholesterol gallstones.

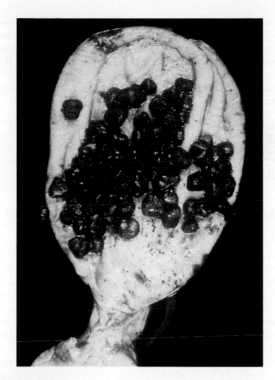

FIGURE 14-30. Pigment gallstones. The gallbladder has been opened to reveal numerous small, dark stones composed of calcium bilirubinate.

Brown Pigment Stones

Brown pigment stones are spongy and laminated and contain principally calcium bilirubinate mixed with cholesterol and calcium soaps of fatty acids. In contrast to the other types of gallstones, brown pigment stones are found more frequently in the intrahepatic and extrahepatic bile ducts than in the gallbladder.

 PATHOGENESIS: Brown stones are almost always associated with bacterial cholangitis, in which *E. coli* is the predominant organism. Rare or uncommon in Western countries, brown stones are not infrequent in Asia, where they are almost entirely restricted to persons infested with *Ascaris lumbricoides* or *Clonorchis sinensis*, helminths that may invade the biliary tract.

The pathogenesis of brown pigment stones also relates to an increased concentration of unconjugated bilirubin in the bile. Conjugated bilirubin is hydrolyzed to unconjugated bilirubin by the action of bacterial β-glucuronidase or other hydrolytic enzymes.

Clinical Features of Gallstones Often Relate to Duct Obstruction

Gallstones may remain "silent" in the gallbladder for many years, and few patients ever die of cholelithiasis itself. The 15-year cumulative probability that asymptomatic stones will lead to biliary pain or other complications is less than 20%. Treatment of gallstones is today most commonly accomplished by laparoscopic cholecystectomy.

Most of the complications of cholelithiasis relate to the obstruction of the cystic duct or common bile duct by gallstones. Passage of a stone into the cystic duct often, but not invariably, causes severe biliary colic and may lead to acute cholecystitis. Repeated episodes of acute cholecystitis then produce chronic cholecystitis. The latter condition

can also result from the presence of stones alone. Gallstones may pass into the common duct (**choledocholithiasis**), where they may lead to obstructive jaundice, cholangitis, and pancreatitis. In fact, in populations in whom alcoholism is not a factor, gallstones are the most common cause of acute pancreatitis. In obstruction of the cystic duct, with or without acute cholecystitis, the bile in the gallbladder is reabsorbed, to be replaced by a clear mucinous fluid secreted by the gallbladder epithelium. The term **hydrops of the gallbladder (mucocele)** is applied to the distended and palpable gallbladder, which may become secondarily infected.

Acute Cholecystitis

Acute cholecystitis is a diffuse inflammation of the gallbladder, usually secondary to obstruction of the gallbladder outlet.

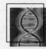 **PATHOGENESIS:** *Approximately 90% of cases of acute cholecystitis are associated with the presence of gallstones.* The remaining cases (**acalculous cholecystitis**) occur in conjunction with sepsis, severe trauma, infection of the gallbladder with *Salmonella typhosa*, and polyarteritis nodosa. Bacterial infection is usually secondary to biliary obstruction, rather than a primary event.

 PATHOLOGY: The external surface of the gallbladder in acute cholecystitis is congested and layered with a fibrinous exudate. The wall is remarkably thickened by edema, and opening the viscus reveals a fiery red or purple mucosa. Gallstones are usually found within the lumen, and a stone is often seen obstructing the cystic duct. On rare occasions, when obstruction of the cystic duct is complete and bacteria have invaded the gallbladder, the cavity may be distended by cloudy, purulent fluid, a condition termed **empyema of the gallbladder**. Microscopically, edema and hemorrhage in the wall are striking, with accompanying acute and chronic inflammation. Secondary bacterial infection may lead to suppuration in the gallbladder wall. The mucosa shows focal ulcerations or, in severe cases, widespread necrosis, in which case the term **gangrenous cholecystitis** is applied.

 CLINICAL FEATURES: The initial symptom of acute cholecystitis is abdominal pain in the right upper quadrant, and most patients have already experienced episodes of biliary colic. Mild jaundice, caused by stones in, or edema of, the common bile duct, is evident in 20% of patients. In most cases, the acute illness subsides within a week, but persistent pain, fever, leukocytosis, and shaking chills indicate progression of acute cholecystitis and the need for cholecystectomy. As the inflammatory process resolves, the gallbladder wall becomes fibrotic and the mucosa heals. However, the function of the gallbladder usually remains impaired.

Chronic Cholecystitis

Chronic cholecystitis, the most common disease of the gallbladder, is a persistent inflammation of the gallbladder wall that is almost invariably associated with gallstones. Chronic cholecystitis may also result from repeated attacks of acute cholecystitis. In the latter case, the pathogenesis probably relates to chronic irritation and chemical injury to the gallbladder epithelium.

 PATHOLOGY: Grossly, the wall of the chronically inflamed gallbladder is thickened and firm, and the serosal surface may show fibrous adhesions to surrounding structures as a result of previous episodes of acute cholecystitis. Gallstones are usually found within the lumen, and the bile often contains gravel or sludge (i.e., fine precipitates of calculous material). The bile is infected with coliform organisms in about half of cases. The mucosa may be focally ulcerated and atrophic or may appear intact. Microscopically, the wall is fibrotic and often penetrated by sinuses of Rokitansky-Aschoff. Chronic inflammation of variable degree may be seen in all layers. In long-standing chronic cholecystitis, the wall of the gallbladder may become calcified (**porcelain gallbladder**).

 CLINICAL FEATURES: Many patients with chronic cholecystitis complain of nonspecific abdominal symptoms, although it is not at all clear that these are necessarily related to the gallbladder disease. On the other hand, pain in the right hypochondrium is typical and often episodic. Cholecystectomy is the definitive treatment.

Tumors

Adenocarcinoma is the Most Common Tumor of the Gallbladder

Adenocarcinoma of the gallbladder is not rare and is incidentally found in 2% of patients who undergo gallbladder surgery. *Because this cancer is usually associated with cholelithiasis and chronic cholecystitis, it is considerably more common in women than in men.* In addition, populations that have a high incidence of cholelithiasis, such as Native Americans, have a higher risk of carcinoma of the gallbladder. The calcified gallbladder (porcelain gallbladder, see above) is particularly prone to the development of gallbladder cancer.

 PATHOLOGY: Gallbladder carcinoma may occur anywhere in the gallbladder but most frequently appears in the fundus. The tumor is characteristically an infiltra-

tive, well-differentiated adenocarcinoma. It is usually desmoplastic, and thus the wall of the gallbladder becomes thickened and leathery. Anaplastic, giant cell, and spindle cell forms of gallbladder carcinoma are reported. The rich lymphatic plexus of the gallbladder provides the most common route of metastasis, although vascular dissemination and direct spread into the liver and contiguous structures occur.

 CLINICAL FEATURES: The symptoms produced by carcinoma of the gallbladder are similar to those encountered with gallstone disease. However, by the time the tumor becomes symptomatic, it is almost invariably incurable; the 5-year survival rate is less than 3%.

Carcinoma of the Bile Duct and the Ampulla of Vater Present as Obstructive Jaundice

Cancer of the extrahepatic bile ducts (extrahepatic cholangiocarcinoma, see above) is almost always adenocarcinoma. It may occur anywhere along the length of the bile duct, including the location where the right and left hepatic ducts join to form the common hepatic duct. The tumor is less common than gallbladder cancer, and the female predominance of gallbladder cancer is not evident. Gallstones are frequently found in those affected, and there is an association with inflammatory disease of the colon. In Asia, bile duct carcinoma is associated with biliary infestation by the fluke *Clonorchis sinensis*. The prognosis is poor, but because symptoms arise early in the course of the disease, the outcome is somewhat better than that of gallbladder carcinoma. *Adenocarcinoma of the ampulla of Vater may also obstruct the bile duct.* The initial symptom is again, obstructive jaundice, although a few patients present with pancreatitis. In contrast to bile duct carcinoma, surgical treatment of cancer of the ampulla of Vater carries a 35% 5-year survival rate.

15 The Pancreas

Gregory Y. Lauwers
Mari Mino-Kenudson
Raphael Rubin

The pancreas comprises two functionally and anatomically distinct "organs," namely the exocrine and the endocrine pancreas. The exocrine pancreas secretes approximately 20 different digestive enzymes, mostly in the form of inactive proenzymes, whereas the endocrine pancreas releases a variety of important hormones that participate in glucose homeostasis and other metabolic activities, some of which are directly or indirectly involved in the control of body weight. Clinically important diseases of the exocrine pancreas are acute and chronic pancreatitis as well as cancer. Dysfunction of beta cells in the islets of Langerhans results in diabetes mellitus (see Chapter 22). The islets are also the site of origin for a variety of functional neoplasms discussed in this chapter.

Pancreatitis

Pancreatitis is an inflammatory condition of the exocrine pancreas that results from injury to acinar cells. At one end of the disease spectrum is a mild, self-limited disorder with acute inflammation and stromal edema, and little or no acinar cell necrosis. At the other extreme is a severe, sometimes fatal, acute hemorrhagic pancreatitis with massive necrosis. Repeated episodes of acute pancreatitis may lead to chronic pancreatitis, which is characterized by recurrent attacks of severe abdominal pain and progressive fibrosis, ultimately leading to pancreatic insufficiency. However, no acute episodes are recognized clinically in about half of the cases of chronic pancreatitis.

Acute Pancreatitis Varies in Clinical Severity

Interstitial or **edematous pancreatitis** is a mild and presumably reversible form of acute pancreatitis. An infiltrate of polymorphonuclear leukocytes and edema of the connective tissue between lobules of acinar cells constitute the initial lesion. There is no necrosis or hemorrhage, and the condition is usually well managed medically.

    Acute hemorrhagic pancreatitis usually occurs in middle age, with a peak incidence at 60 years. Alcoholism (more commonly in men) or chronic biliary disease (more often in women) accounts for more than 80% of cases. Acute pancreatitis erupts abruptly, usually after a heavy meal or excessive alcohol intake and is associated with high morbidity and mortality rates.

PATHOGENESIS: Acinar cell injury and duct obstruction are the major causes of acute pancreatitis. These processes lead to inappropriate extracellular leakage of activated digestive enzymes and consequent autodigestion of pancreatic and extrapancreatic tissues. A number of factors have been implicated in acute pancreatitis, the incidence of which has increased tenfold in the past few decades.

ACTIVATED PANCREATIC ENZYMES: Acinar cells are shielded from the potentially destructive action of their digestive enzymes (proteases, nucleases, amylase, lipase, and phospholipase A). Trypsin activation is central to the pathogenesis of acute pancreatitis. By itself, trypsin does not produce cell necrosis, but it activates other pancreatic proenzymes, including prophospholipase A_2 and proelastase. Phospholipase A_2 attacks membrane phospholipids to cause necrosis, and elastase digests blood vessel walls, causing hemorrhage. Liberation of pancreatic lipase into the interstitium contributes to fat necrosis (see Chapter 1). *Inappropriate activation of pancreatic proenzymes occurs in all forms of pancreatitis.* Four potent protease inhibitors have been identified in human plasma: α_1-antitrypsin, α_2-macroglobulin, C_1 esterase inhibitor, and pancreatic secretory trypsin inhibitor, which serve to constitute a defense against proteolytic enzyme activation. Nevertheless, the protection they render is clearly incomplete in some circumstances.

SECRETION AGAINST OBSTRUCTION: Most enzymes secreted by acinar cells are discharged into the ductal system and enter the duodenum. Any condition that narrows the lumina of pancreatic ducts or impairs the easy outflow of exocrine secretions can raise intraductal pressure and exacerbate back-diffusion across the ducts. This phenomenon is suspected to cause inappropriate activation of digestive proenzymes. Anatomic anomalies and neoplasms (ampullary and pancreatic neoplasms) can also lead to acute pancreatitis by a similar mechanism.

GALLSTONES: Pancreatic duct obstruction may result from gallstones. Approximately 45% of all patients with acute pancreatitis also have cholelithiasis. *About 5% of patients with gallstones develop acute pancreatitis, and the risk of developing this disease in patients with gallstones is 25 times higher than in the general population.* However, fewer than 5% of patients with acute pancreatitis have impacted stones at the ampulla of Vater, and the reason for the association between pancreatitis and cholelithiasis remains obscure. Neither ligation of the pancreatic duct nor its occlusion by tumor causes acute pancreatitis.

ETHANOL CONSUMPTION: *Chronic alcohol abuse accounts for one third of cases of acute pancreatitis, although only 5% of chronic alcoholics develop this complication.* Ethanol is well recognized as a chemical toxin, but a significant injurious effect on pancreatic acinar or duct cells has yet to be demonstrated. Ethanol consumption may adversely affect the pancreas by causing spasm or acute edema of the sphincter of Oddi, especially after an alcoholic binge. It also stimulates secretion from the small intestine, which triggers the exocrine pancreas to release pancreatic juice. When these effects occur together (enhanced secretion into an obstructed duct), the results may be disastrous.

OTHER CAUSES OF PANCREATITIS: Other rare causes of acute pancreatitis include viruses (such as mumps, coxsackievirus, and cytomegalovirus), therapeutic drugs (e.g. azathioprine), blunt trauma, hyperlipidemia, and hypercalcemia. However, **idiopathic pancreatitis** is still the third most common form of the disease, accounting for 10% to 20% of all cases. Factors involved in the pathogenesis of acute hemorrhagic pancreatitis are shown in Figure 15-1.

 PATHOLOGY: In acute hemorrhagic pancreatitis, the pancreas is initially edematous and hyperemic. Within a day, pale, gray foci appear, rapidly becoming friable and hemorrhagic (Fig. 15-2A). *In severe cases, these foci enlarge and become so numerous that most of the pancreas is converted into a large retroperitoneal hematoma, in which pancreatic tissue is barely recognizable.* Yellow-white areas of fat necrosis appear around the pancreas, including the adjacent mesentery (see Fig. 15-2B). These nodules of necrotic fat have a pasty consistency, which becomes firmer and chalk-like as more calcium and magnesium soaps are produced.

The most prominent microscopic findings in acute pancreatitis are (1) acinar cell necrosis, (2) intense acute inflammation, and (3) foci of necrotic fat cells (Fig. 15-3). Necrosis is usually patchy, rarely involving the entire gland. Irregular fibrosis of the pancreas and occasionally, calcification are residuals of healed acute pancreatitis.

As many as half of patients who survive acute pancreatitis are at risk for development of **pancreatic pseudocysts**. These are delimited by connective tissue and contain degraded blood, debris of necrotic pancreatic tissue, and fluid rich in pancreatic enzymes. Pseudocysts may enlarge to compress and even obstruct the duodenum. They may become secondarily infected and form an abscess. Rupture of a pseudocyst is a rare complication that leads to a chemical or septic peritonitis.

 CLINICAL FEATURES: Patients with acute pancreatitis present with severe epigastric pain that is referred to the upper back and is accompanied by nausea and vomiting. Catastrophic peripheral vascular collapse and shock may ensue within hours. If shock is sustained and profound, adult respiratory distress syndrome and acute renal failure may occur within the first week. Early in the disease, pancreatic digestive enzymes are released from injured acinar cells into the blood and the abdominal cavity. *Elevated serum amylase and lipase within 24 to 72 hours is diagnostic for acute pancreatitis.* The necrotic pancreas becomes infected with gram-negative bacteria from the intestinal tract in half of cases of acute pancreatitis, which greatly increases mortality.

Chronic Pancreatitis Results in the Progressive Destruction of the Pancreas

Chronic pancreatitis is the progressive destruction of pancreatic parenchyma, with irregular fibrosis and chronic inflammation. Clinically, the disease manifests as recurrent or persisting abdominal pain or simply as evidence of pancreatic exocrine or endocrine insufficiency.

 PATHOGENESIS: Most factors that cause acute pancreatitis also lead to chronic pancreatitis. The fact that chronic pancreatitis is often characterized by intermittent "acute" attacks and followed by periods of quiescence suggests that it may evolve from repeated bouts of acute pancreatitis. However, about half of patients present without a history of acute episodes, and the pathogenesis of these cases of chronic pancreatitis may relate to persistent but insidious necrosis and scarring, similar to the progression of cirrhosis of the liver.

Long-standing **alcoholism** is the major cause of chronic pancreatitis and is responsible for two thirds of adult cases. In almost half of alcoholics who had no symptoms of chronic pancreatitis during life, autopsy reveals evidence of this disease. The mechanism by which it causes chronic pancreatitis is still debated. Alcohol is a pancreatic secretagogue, so early chronic pancreatitis features hypersecretion of enzyme proteins by acinar cells, without concomitantly increased fluid. As a result, protein plugs precipitate in the small branches of the pancreatic ducts. The plugs are the earliest morphologic abnormality in alcoholic chronic pancreatitis. These deposits initially include degenerating cells within a reticular framework. Intraductal stones then form when calcium carbonate is precipitated in the plugs.

Obstruction of the pancreatic duct by mechanical blockage or congenital defects, by cancer, or by inspissated mucus in cystic fibrosis leads to chronic pancreatitis. However, obstruction by gallstones does not seem to lead to chronic pancreatitis, and cholecystectomy does not alter the course of the disease.

Chronic injury to acinar cells, such as in hemochromatosis, is associated with pancreatic fibrosis and atrophy.

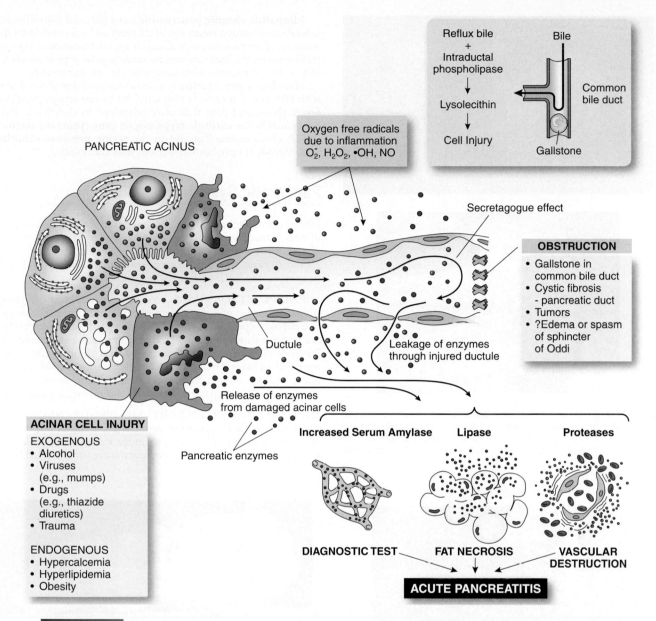

FIGURE 15-1. **The pathogenesis of acute pancreatitis.** Injury to the ductules or the acinar cells leads to the release of pancreatic enzymes. Lipase and proteases destroy tissue, thereby causing acute pancreatitis. The release of amylase is the basis of a test for acute pancreatitis. H_2O_2, hydrogen peroxide; NO•, nitric acid; O_2^-, superoxide ion; •OH, hydroxyl radical.

PATHOLOGY: By the time chronic pancreatitis is clinically evident, it is usually well advanced. Chronic calcifying pancreatitis is the most common type of the disease and is associated with chronic alcoholism in more than 90% of cases. The parenchyma is firm, and the cut surface lacks the usual lobular appearance (Fig. 15-4A). The main pancreatic duct and its tributaries are commonly dilated, owing to obstruction by thick proteinaceous plugs, intraductal stones, or strictures. Pseudocysts or abscess formation are common. Microscopically, large regions of the pancreas show irregular areas of fibrosis, and exocrine and endocrine elements are reduced in number and size (see Fig. 15-4B). Fibrotic areas contain activated fibroblasts, adjacent to which are infiltrates of lymphocytes, plasma cells, and macrophages, particularly around surviving pancreatic lobules. Ductal epithelium may be atrophic or hyperplastic and may show squamous metaplasia.

CLINICAL FEATURES: Half of patients with chronic pancreatitis suffer from repeated episodes of acute pancreatitis. One third of cases are characterized by the gradual onset of continuous or intermittent pain, without any acute attacks. In a few patients, chronic pancreatitis is initially painless but presents with diabetes or malabsorption. Conspicuous weight loss is common, and unrelenting epigastric pain, radiating to the back, may cripple the patient. The mortality rate is 3% to 4% per year and approaches 50% within 20 to 25 years. One fifth of patients die of complications associated with intercurrent attacks of acute pancreatitis. The other deaths are from other causes, particularly alcohol-related disorders.

Cystic Fibrosis and Other Genetic Diseases May Manifest as Chronic Pancreatitis

Cystic fibrosis (CF) (see Chapter 6) is briefly reviewed here because it may present as chronic pancreatitis. In a pancreas of a patient with CF, intraductal secretions are abnormally viscid, accounting for the older name, **mucoviscidosis**. Plugs of inspissated mucus obstruct cystically distended pancreatic ducts, leading to chronic pancreatitis and exocrine pancreatic insufficiency. In its late stages, the entire parenchyma is replaced by adipose tissue.

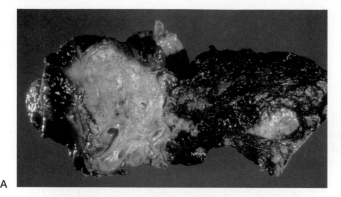

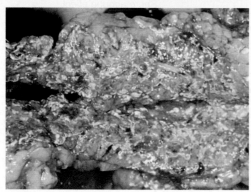

FIGURE 15-2. **Acute hemorrhagic pancreatitis. A.** Large areas of the pancreas are intensely hemorrhagic. **B.** The cut surface of the pancreas in a less severe case of acute pancreatitis and at a somewhat later stage than in **(A)** shows numerous yellow-white foci of fat necrosis.

Idiopathic chronic pancreatitis has a bimodal distribution: a juvenile form with a mean age of 25 years and a second form that occurs in older patients, with a peak at age 60. Mutations in the cystic fibrosis transmembrane conductance regulator gene are seen in 10% to 30% of patients with idiopathic chronic pancreatitis.

Hereditary pancreatitis is a rare autosomal dominant disease with 80% penetrance. It is characterized by recurring episodes of severe abdominal pain that often manifests in childhood. Point mutations in the **cationic trypsinogen gene** (**protease serine 1**, *PRSS1*; chromosome 7q) and in the **serine protease inhibitor gene** (*SPINK 1*) have been associated with the disease.

Pancreatic Cystic Neoplasms

Liberal use of abdominal imaging has led to increased recognition of cystic pancreatic neoplasms. The tumors are large and multiloculated, occurring most frequently in women between the ages of 50 and 70 years. The neoplasms are divided into serous and mucinous types, the latter having malignant potential.

SEROUS CYSTADENOMA: Serous cystic neoplasm is a benign tumor composed of cystic structures uniformly lined by glycogen-rich cuboidal epithelium. It usually occurs in the pancreatic body or tail. Patients with von Hippel-Lindau syndrome are at increased risk for its development. Most patients present with nonspecific symptoms related to local mass effects, but about one-third are asymptomatic. There is often a large, stellate central scar, sometimes with microcalcifications, giving a "sunburst" pattern on imaging studies.

INTRADUCTAL PAPILLARY MUCINOUS NEOPLASM: These tumors are composed of papillary proliferations of neoplastic mucin-secreting cells that arise in the main pancreatic duct or its major branches. The distended duct(s) are usually filled by vis-

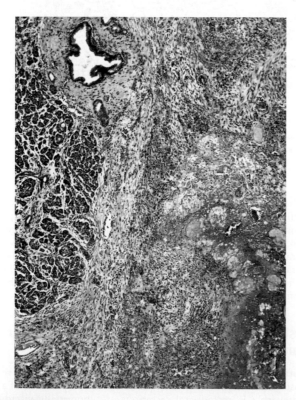

FIGURE 15-3. **Acute hemorrhagic pancreatitis.** A photomicrograph of the pancreas shows areas of acinar cell necrosis, hemorrhage, and fat necrosis (*lower right*). An intact lobule is seen on the left.

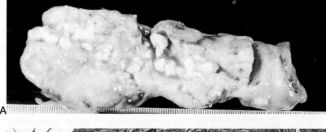

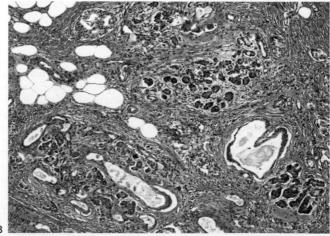

FIGURE 15-4. **Chronic calcifying pancreatitis. A.** The pancreas is shrunken and fibrotic, and the dilated duct contains numerous stones. **B.** Atrophic lobules of acinar cells are surrounded by dense fibrous tissue infiltrated by lymphocytes. The pancreatic ducts are dilated and contain inspissated proteinaceous material.

cous, yellow mucus. Intraductal papillary mucinous neoplasm tumors exhibit varying degrees of epithelial atypia and are classified accordingly: benign (adenoma), borderline, and malignant (either invasive or noninvasive). A focus of invasive adenocarcinoma is found in up to one third of cases.

PANCREATIC MUCINOUS CYSTIC NEOPLASM (MCN): MCN is a uni- or multilocular tumor composed of tall or cuboidal mucin-secreting epithelium, supported by a cellular ovarian-type stroma. Tumors do not communicate with the pancreatic duct system. MCNs have a predilection for the body and tail of the pancreas. The prognosis of MCN (noninvasive) is excellent if it is completely removed.

Pancreatic Cancer

In the United States, pancreatic carcinoma is the fourth most common cause of cancer death in men and the fifth in women. The prognosis is dismal and the 5-year survival is only 5%. The incidence of pancreatic cancer has tripled in the United States over the past 50 years. Ductal adenocarcinoma accounts for 90% of all pancreatic cancers.

 EPIDEMIOLOGY: Pancreatic cancer is seen worldwide. It shows a significant male predominance (up to 3:1) in younger age groups but almost equal gender distribution in old age. In the United States, it is more common in Native Americans and blacks, in whom the incidence is approximately 50% higher than in whites. Pancreatic carcinoma is a disease that occurs later in life, with the greatest incidence in persons older than 60 years of age, although its appearance as early as the third decade is not rare.

 PATHOGENESIS: The factors involved in the development of pancreatic cancer are obscure. Epidemiologic studies have implicated both host and environmental factors as being of possible etiologic significance in cancer of the pancreas.

SMOKING: About 25% of pancreatic cancers are attributable to cigarette smoking, and there is a two- to threefold increased risk of pancreatic cancer in cigarette smokers. Smokers often show hyperplastic pancreatic ducts at autopsy.

CHEMICAL CARCINOGENS: Polycyclic hydrocarbons and a number of nitrosamines are pancreatic carcinogens in rodents. However, epidemiologic studies linking environmental toxins and human pancreatic carcinoma are inconclusive.

BODY MASS INDEX AND DIETARY FACTORS: A diet high in meat and especially fat, may increase the risk of pancreatic cancer. However, confounding factors such as methods of cooking (i.e., frying, boiling, barbecuing) may play a role. A positive association between body mass index and pancreatic cancer has been reported.

DIABETES MELLITUS: Diabetics are at increased risk for carcinoma of the pancreas. Up to 80% of patients with pancreatic cancer have evidence of diabetes mellitus at the time of cancer diagnosis. Patients with diabetes mellitus for 5 or more years have double the risk for pancreatic cancer. Prospective studies of people with abnormal glucose tolerance document a subsequent increased incidence of pancreatic cancer.

CHRONIC PANCREATITIS: Chronic pancreatitis is a risk factor for pancreatic adenocarcinoma, although it accounts for few cases. As chronic pancreatitis may occasionally be mild and clinically silent, its role in the development of pancreatic cancer may be underestimated.

MOLECULAR GENETICS: Pancreatic duct cancers exhibit a number of genetic alterations, and a tumor progression model based on specific gene mutations has been proposed. The concept is supported by the finding of preneoplastic duct epithelial lesions, termed **pancreatic intraductal neoplasia**. An early event is mutational activation of K-*ras* (G→A transition in the second position of codon 12), which is observed in up to 95% of pancreatic carcinomas. Mutational inactivation or deletion of tumor suppressor genes appears later in the sequence of tumor progression, including *p53* (50%), *p16 (MST1)* (85%), and *DPC-4* (deleted in pancreatic cancer, locus 4) (55%). Interestingly, deletions in chromosome 18 are present in 90% of pancreatic cancers. Although *DPC-4* is located on chromosome 18, only half of all pancreatic cancers show loss or inactivation of this gene, suggesting that another nearby tumor suppressor gene contributes to tumor progression. Several familial cancer syndromes have a strong risk for the development of pancreatic carcinoma (Table 15-1; also see Chapter 5).

 PATHOLOGY: Carcinoma arises anywhere in the pancreas; the most frequent focus is in the head (60%), followed by the body (10%), and tail (5%). The pancreas is diffusely involved in the remaining 25%. Carcinomas of the head of the pancreas may cause biliary obstruction and jaundice by compressing the ampulla of Vater and common bile duct. They thus tend to be smaller at diagnosis than those of the body and tail and show more limited spread to regional lymph nodes and distant sites.

On gross examination, pancreatic carcinoma is a firm, gray, poorly demarcated, multinodular mass (Fig. 15-5), often embedded in a dense connective tissue stroma. Tumors of the head of the pancreas may invade the common duct and duodenal wall. They may also obstruct the duct of Wirsung and cause atrophy of the body and tail. Microscopically, more than 75% of pancreatic cancers are well-differentiated **ductal adenocarcinomas** that secrete mucin and are associated with collagen deposition.

Pancreatic cancer metastasizes most commonly to regional lymph nodes and liver. Other frequent metastatic locations include the peritoneum, lungs, adrenals, and bones. Direct extension into neighboring organs (e.g., the stomach and duodenum) occasionally occurs. Perineural infiltration by tumor is charac-

TABLE 15–1			
Familial Cancer Syndromes and Relative Risk for Pancreatic Cancer			
Syndrome	Chromosome	Gene Mutation	Relative Risk of Pancreatic Cancer
Peutz-Jegher syndrome	19p13	*STK11/LKB1*	132-fold
Hereditary pancreatitis	7q35	*PRSS1*	50- to 80-fold
FAMM	9p21	*P16 (CDKN2A)*	9- to 38-fold
HBOC	13q12-13	*BRCA2*	3.5- to 10-fold
HNPCC	3p21, 2p22	*hMLH1, hMSH2*	Unknown

FAMM, familial atypical multiple mole melanoma syndrome; HBOCC, hereditary breast-ovarian cancer syndrome; HNPCC, hereditary nonpolyposis cancer syndrome.

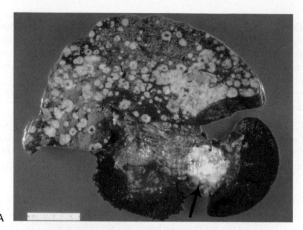

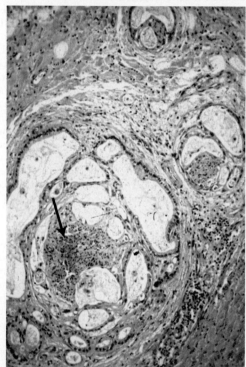

FIGURE 15-5. Carcinoma of the pancreas. **A.** An autopsy specimen shows a large tumor in the tail of the pancreas (*arrow*) and extensive metastases in the liver. **B.** A section of the tumor reveals malignant glands embedded in a dense fibrous stroma. A nerve (*arrow*) shows perineural invasion.

teristic of pancreatic cancer and accounts for the early and persistent pain of this disease.

 CLINICAL FEATURES: Patients with pancreatic cancer present with anorexia, conspicuous weight loss, and a gnawing pain in the epigastrium, which often radiates to the back. *Jaundice is seen in about half of all patients with cancer localized to the head of the pancreas* but in less than 10% of tumors of the body or tail. **Courvoisier sign** is an acute, painless gallbladder dilation accompanied by jaundice, as a result of common bile duct obstruction by tumor. In about one third of patients, it may be the first sign of pancreatic cancer. **Migratory thrombophlebitis** (deep venous thrombosis or Trousseau syndrome) develops in 10% of patients with pancreatic cancer, especially when the tumor involves the body and tail of the pancreas and may also be the first sign of the underlying malignancy. Early diagnosis of pancreatic cancer is unusual because the tumor is not ordinarily symptomatic until it is well advanced. Most have already metastasized at the time of diag-

nosis, and curative surgery is uncommon. Progressive deterioration almost invariably ensues, with intractable pain, cachexia, and death. Half of these patients die within 6 months of diagnosis, and the overall 5-year survival rate is less than 5%.

Acinar Cell Carcinoma

Acinar cell carcinomas are usually large and tend to metastasize to regional lymph nodes and liver and more distantly to the lungs and other body sites. The tumors are uncommon and are usually detected in the seventh decade of life. Some patients develop a curious syndrome of fat necrosis in subcutaneous tissues and bone marrow, polyarthralgia, and occasional constipation. The clinical course is less rapidly fatal than ductal adenocarcinoma.

The Endocrine Pancreas

The Islets of Langerhans Form the Endocrine Pancreas

These islets are scattered throughout the pancreas and consist of richly vascularized globular masses of large epithelioid cells. Six distinct cell types are correlated with specific hormones.

Pancreatic Endocrine Tumors (PETs) Comprise About 10% of Pancreatic Neoplasms

Most of these tumors are nonfunctional and are discovered as incidental findings at autopsy. The tumors are usually composed of monotonous sheets of small round cells with uniform nuclei and infrequent mitoses. *PETs often invade and metastasize, but it is difficult to distinguish between benign and malignant PETs on the basis of histology alone.* Hormone secretion by PETs results in distinctive clinical syndromes (see Fig. 5-8). Functional islet cell tumors may occur alone or as part of the multiple endocrine neoplasia syndrome type I (MEN I) (see Chapter 21). The molecular pathogenesis of sporadic PETs is not well established. The most common chromosomal anomaly is allelic loss of 11q, which includes the *MEN-1* locus.

Insulinomas (Beta Cell Tumors) are the Most Common Islet Cell Neoplasms

Insulinomas (beta cell tumors) comprise 75% of islet cell neoplasms and may release enough insulin to induce severe hypoglycemia. Neoplastic beta cells, unlike their normal counterparts, are not regulated by blood glucose level and continue to secrete insulin autonomously, even when blood glucose is very low.

 PATHOLOGY: *Most insulinomas are benign lesions in the body or tail of the pancreas* (Fig. 15-6). They are generally less than 3 cm in diameter and occasionally as small as 1 mm. Most (90%) are solitary and can be surgically excised. Only a minority (5% to 15%) show malignant behavior. Histologically, insulinoma cells resemble normal beta cells but are dispersed in trabecular or solid patterns (Fig. 15-7). The tumor often elicits a desmoplastic reaction, and amyloid (derived from a peptide hormone secreted with insulin and termed **amylin**) may be found in the stroma. A reliable distinction between benign and malignant insulinomas is difficult on histologic grounds and in most cases awaits the appearance or absence of metastases.

 CLINICAL FEATURES: Low blood sugar produces a syndrome of sweating, nervousness, and hunger, which may progress to confusion, lethargy, and coma. Symptoms can be relieved by eating, so patients with in-

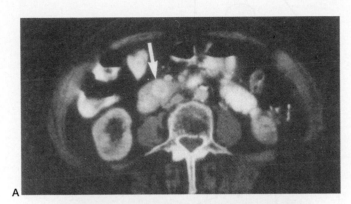

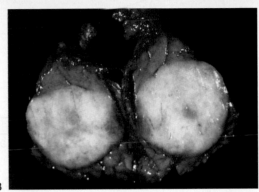

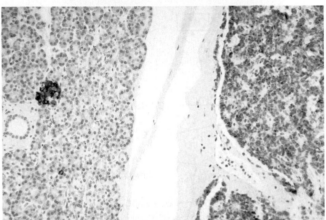

FIGURE 15-6. **Insulinoma. A.** A computed tomography scan of the abdomen shows a solitary insulinoma *(arrow)*. **B.** An insulinoma is embedded in tan, lobular pancreatic tissue.

sulinomas are often overweight. The diagnosis is frequently delayed by abnormal behavior that causes some patients to seek psychiatric care. Most cases are characterized by only a mild hypoglycemia. The diagnosis is established by demonstrating high levels of insulin in the blood and the tumor cells (see Fig. 15-7B).

Pancreatic Gastrinomas (Zollinger-Ellison Syndrome) Induce Gastric Acid Secretion

Pancreatic gastrinoma is an islet cell tumor consisting of so-called G cells, which produce gastrin, a potent hormonal stimulus for gastric acid secretion. The location of this tumor in the pancreas is curious, because gastrin-containing cells do not normally occur in the islets. The pancreatic tumor is believed to arise from multipotent, primitive endocrine cells that have undergone inappropriate differentiation to form G cells in the islets. Pancreatic gastrinoma causes **Zollinger-Ellison syndrome**, a disorder characterized by (1) intractable gastric hypersecretion, (2) severe peptic ulceration of the duodenum and jejunum, and (3) high blood gastrin levels.

Among islet cell tumors, pancreatic gastrinomas are second in frequency only to insulinomas, accounting for one fourth of islet cell tumors. They are most common between the ages of 30 and 50, with a slight male predominance. *Most gastrinomas are malignant (70% to 90%).* The tumor may be solitary or multiple, the latter usually in the context of MEN I. Histologically, gastrinomas are remarkably similar to intestinal carcinoid tumors. Metastases to regional lymph nodes and the liver are often functional.

Glucagonomas (Alpha Cell Tumors) are Rare Islet Cell Tumors Associated with Mild Diabetes and a Characteristic Rash

Alpha cell tumors (glucagonomas) are associated with a syndrome of (1) mild diabetes; (2) a necrotizing, migratory, erythematous rash; (3) anemia;

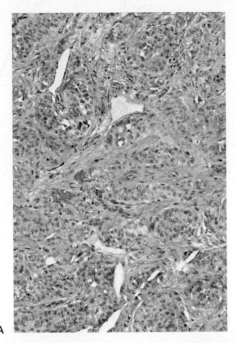

FIGURE 15-7. **A functional insulinoma. A.** Nests of tumor cells are surrounded by numerous capillaries. **B.** Immunochemical localization (brown staining) of insulin in an insulinoma *(right)* and in an islet in the adjacent normal pancreas.

(4) venous thromboses; and (5) severe infections. They are rare (1% of functional islet cell tumors) and occur between the ages of 40 and 70 years, with a slight female predominance. Two thirds of symptomatic glucagonomas are malignant.

Functional glucagonomas are usually large and invade surrounding structures. Microscopically, they show trabecular and solid patterns similar to insulinomas. By immunochemistry, tumor cells contain glucagon. In patients with alpha cell tumors, plasma glucagon levels are elevated up to 30 times above normal. In addition to hyperglycemia, fasting plasma amino acid levels are decreased to as low as 20% of normal.

Somatostatinomas (Delta Cell Tumors) are Associated with Low Blood Insulin and Glucagon

Somatostatinomas are rare and produce a syndrome consisting of mild diabetes, gallstones, steatorrhea, and hypochlorhydria. These effects result from the inhibitory actions of somatostatin on other cells of the pancreatic islets and on neuroendocrine cells of the gastrointestinal tract. Consequently, levels of insulin and glucagon in blood are

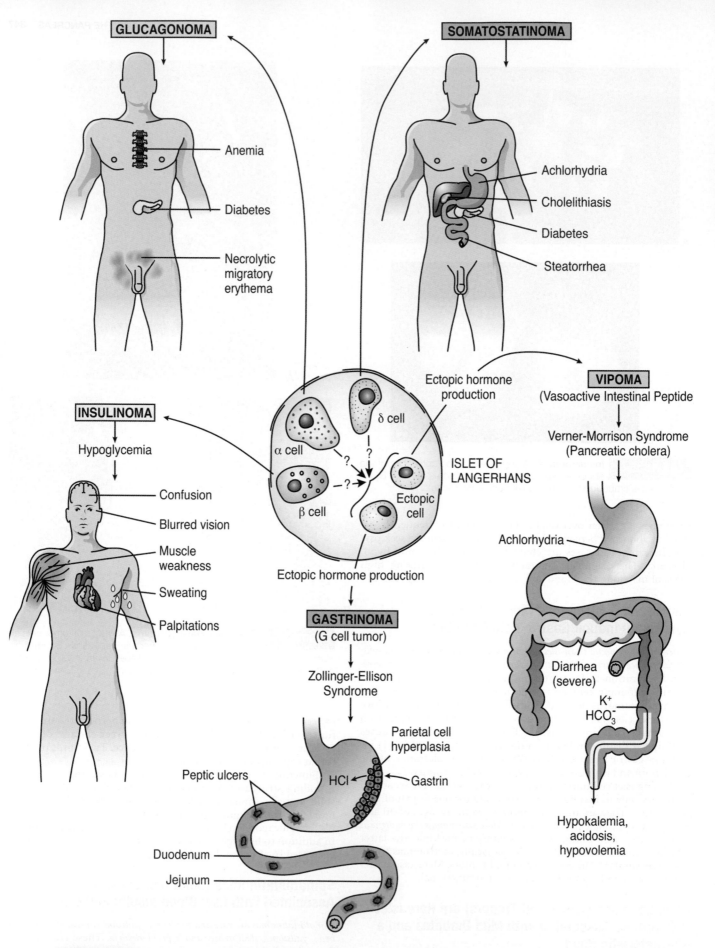

FIGURE 15-8. Syndromes associated with islet cell tumors of the pancreas. HCl, hydrochloric acid; HCO₃⁻, bicarbonate; K⁺, potassium ion.

low. In addition to producing somatostatin, some delta cell tumors also secrete calcitonin or adrenocorticotropic hormone. The tumors are usually solitary. Most are malignant, with metastases already present at the time of diagnosis.

VIPomas (D₁ Tumors) Causes Verner-Morrison Syndrome

Verner-Morrison syndrome is caused by elevated levels of vasoactive intestinal peptide (VIP) and is characterized by explosive and profuse watery diarrhea, accompanied by hypokalemia and hypochlorhydria. The disorder has also been referred to as **pancreatic cholera**. VIPomas are rare tumors (less than 5% of all islet tumors), are usually large and solitary, and in most cases, are malignant. In some patients, MEN I causes Verner-Morrison syndrome.

The syndromes and complications of the major types of islet cell tumors are summarized in Figure 15-8.

MEN I (Multiple Endocrine Neoplasia I) is an Infrequent Familial Disorder

MEN I is characterized by multiple adenomas of the pituitary, parathyroids, and endocrine pancreas. It is frequently associated with the Zollinger-Ellison syndrome, in which case gastrin-secreting islet cell tumors are present. PETs occur in more than 60% of patients with MEN-1. The MEN syndromes are described in detail in Chapter 21.

16 The Kidney

J. Charles Jennette

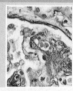

The kidney serves as the principal regulator of the fluid and electrolyte content of the body. The task is accomplished by the complex filtering mechanism of the glomerulus and the selective tubular reabsorption of solutes from the filtrate. The kidney also has endocrine function secreting renin, which regulates sodium me- *tabolism and blood pressure as well as erythropoietin, a hormone that stimulates red cell production in the bone marrow. **The nephron** is the architectural unit of the kidney and includes the glomerulus and its tubule, the latter terminating at the common collecting system (see Fig. 16-1).*

The kidney consists of the glomerular, vascular tubular, and interstitial anatomic compartments (Fig. 16-1). Many renal diseases are best understood in relation to the compartments affected and the associated functional impairment.

Congenital Anomalies

Renal Agenesis is the Complete Absence of Renal Tissue

Most infants born with bilateral renal agenesis are stillborn and have Potter sequence (see Chapter 6). Bilateral agenesis is often associated with other congenital anomalies, especially elsewhere in the urinary tract or lower extremities. Unilateral renal agenesis is not a serious matter if there are no associated anomalies, because the contralateral kidney undergoes sufficient hypertrophy to maintain normal renal function.

Ectopic Kidney is an Abnormal Location of the Organ

The misplaced kidney is usually in the pelvis. Most commonly, this condition results from failure of the fetal kidney to migrate from the pelvis to the flank. Renal ectopia may involve only one kidney, or it may be bilateral.

Horseshoe Kidney is a Single, Large, Midline Organ

Horseshoe kidney results when an infant is born with fused kidneys, usually at the lower poles. This anomaly usually has no clinical consequences but can increase the risk for obstruction and

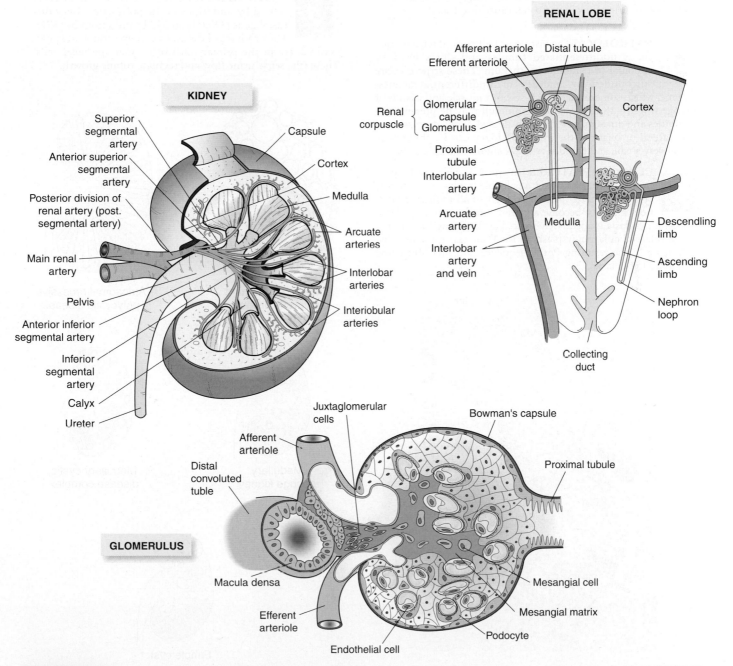

FIGURE 16-1.   The gross and microscopic anatomy of the kidney.

pyelonephritis (see below) because the ureters must cross over the junction between the two kidneys that are fused at their lower pole.

Renal Dysplasia is a Developmental Disorder

Renal dysplasia is characterized by undifferentiated tubular structures surrounded by primitive mesenchyme, sometimes with heterotopic tissue such as cartilage. Cysts often form from the abnormal tubules.

 PATHOGENESIS: Renal dysplasia results from an abnormality in metanephric differentiation that reflects multiple genetic and somatic causes. Some familial forms of dysplasia probably result from abnormal differentiation signals that affect the inductive interactions between the ureteric bud and the metanephric blastema. Many forms of dysplasia are accompanied by other urinary tract abnormalities, especially those that cause obstruction of urine flow. This association suggests that an obstruction to urine flow in utero can cause dysplasia.

 PATHOLOGY: The histologic hallmark of renal dysplasia is undifferentiated tubules and ducts lined by cuboidal or columnar epithelium. These structures are surrounded by mantles of undifferentiated mesenchyme, which sometimes contain smooth muscle and islands of cartilage (Fig. 16-2). Rudimentary glomeruli may be present, and the tubules and ducts may be cystically dilated. Renal dysplasia can be unilateral or bilateral, the involved kidney can be abnormally large or very small, and the kidney may contain multiple cysts.

 CLINICAL FEATURES: In most patients with cystic forms of renal dysplasia, a palpable flank mass is discovered shortly after birth, although small multicystic kidneys may not become apparent until many years later. Unilateral dysplasia is adequately treated by removing the affected kidney. Bilateral aplastic dysplasia in the fetus can cause oligohydramnios and the resulting Potter sequence and life-threatening pulmonary hypoplasia.

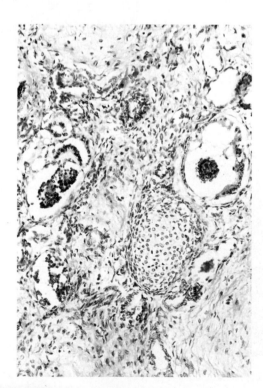

FIGURE 16-2. **Renal dysplasia.** Immature glomeruli, tubules, and cartilage are surrounded by loose, undifferentiated mesenchymal tissue.

Congenital Polycystic Kidney Diseases

Congenital polycystic kidney diseases are a heterogeneous group of genetic disorders that are characterized by distortion of the renal parenchyma by numerous cysts. The diseases vary in age of onset, severity, mode of inheritance, and structure of cysts (Fig. 16-2).

Autosomal Dominant Polycystic Kidney Disease (ADPKD) Features Enlarged Multicystic Kidneys

Autosomal Dominant Polycystic Kidney Disease *(ADPKD) is the most common of a group of congenital diseases that are characterized by numerous cysts within the renal parenchyma (Fig. 16-3). It affects 1:400 to 1:1000 individuals in the United States. Half of all patients with this disease eventually develop end-stage renal failure.*

 PATHOGENESIS: About 85% of ADPKD is caused by mutations in the polycystic kidney disease 1 gene *(PKD1)* and 15% by mutations in *PKD2*. The products of these genes, polycystin-1 and polycystin-2, are in the primary cilia of tubular epithelial cells. These cilia sense urine flow and regulate tubule growth.

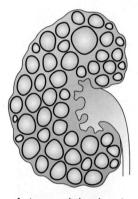
Autosomal dominant
polycystic disease

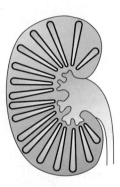
Autosomal recessive
polycystic disease

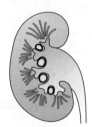
Medullary
sponge kidney

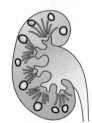
Medullary cystic
disease complex

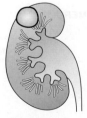
Simple cyst

FIGURE 16-3. **Cystic diseases of the kidney.**

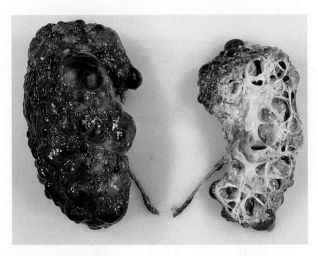

FIGURE 16-4. **Adult polycystic disease.** The kidneys are enlarged, and the parenchyma is almost entirely replaced by cysts of varying size.

Cysts arise in segments of renal tubules and develop from a few cells that proliferate abnormally. The wall of the tubule becomes covered by an undifferentiated epithelium composed of cells with a high nucleus-to-cytoplasm ratio and only few microvilli. Eventually, most of the cysts become disconnected from the tubules. Cyst fluid initially accumulates from glomerular filtrate, followed by fluid derived from transepithelial secretion. Cysts originate in less than 2% of nephrons; therefore, factors other than crowding of normal tissue by the expanding cysts likely contribute to the loss of functioning renal tissue.

 PATHOLOGY: The kidneys in ADPKD are markedly enlarged bilaterally, each weighing as much as 4,500 g (Fig. 16-4). The external contours of the kidneys are distorted by numerous cysts as large as 5 cm in diameter, which are filled with a straw-colored fluid. Microscopically, the cysts are lined by a cuboidal and columnar epithelium. They arise from virtually any point along the nephron, and areas of normal renal parenchyma are found between the cysts.

One third of patients with ADPKD also have **hepatic cysts**, with a lining that resembles bile duct epithelium. One fifth have an associated **cerebral aneurysm**, and intracranial hemorrhage is the cause of death in 15% of patients with ADPKD.

CLINICAL FEATURES: Most patients with ADPKD do not develop clinical manifestations until the fourth decade of life, although a small minority become symptomatic during childhood. Symptoms include a sense of heaviness in the loins, bilateral flank and abdominal masses, and passage of blood clots in the urine. Azotemia (elevated blood urea nitrogen) is common and in half of patients progresses to uremia (clinical renal failure) over a period of several years.

Autosomal Recessive Polycystic Kidney Disease (ARPKD) Occurs in Infants

Autosomal Recessive Polycystic Kidney Disease (ARPKD) is characterized by cystic transformation of collecting ducts. It is rare compared with ADPKD, occurring in about 1 in 10,000 to 50,000 live births. Seventy-five percent of these infants die in the perinatal period, often because of pulmonary hypoplasia caused by oligohydramnios (Potter sequence). ARPKD is caused by mutations in the *PKHD1* gene. The gene product, **fibrocystin**, is found in the kidney, liver, and pancreas, and appears to be involved in the regulation of cell

proliferation and adhesion. Mutations of *PKHD1* also result in pancreatic cysts, hepatic biliary dysgenesis, and fibrosis.

 PATHOLOGY: In contrast to ADPKD, the external kidney surface in the infantile disorder is smooth. The disease is invariably bilateral. The cysts are fusiform dilations of cortical and medullary collecting ducts and have a striking radial arrangement perpendicular to the renal capsule. Interstitial fibrosis and tubular atrophy are common, particularly in children whose disease presents at an older age. The liver usually is affected by **congenital hepatic fibrosis**.

Nephronophthisis–Medullary Cystic Disease Complex Manifests as Tubulointerstitial Injury and Medullary Cysts

Nephronophthisis–medullary cystic disease complex comprises a group of autosomal recessive and autosomal dominant diseases that affect a number of distinct genetic loci and have different ages of onset.

 PATHOLOGY: The kidneys are small and when sectioned often display multiple, variably sized cysts (up to 1 cm) at the corticomedullary junction (see Fig. 16-3). The cysts arise from the distal portions of the nephron. Atrophic tubules with markedly thickened and laminated basement membranes and loss of tubules out of proportion to the glomerular loss are early histologic features of the disease. Eventually, corticomedullary cysts may develop, and the remainder of the parenchyma becomes increasingly atrophic. Secondary glomerular sclerosis, interstitial fibrosis, and nonspecific inflammatory infiltrates dominate the late histologic picture.

 CLINICAL FEATURES: Medullary cystic disease complex accounts for 10% to 25% of renal failure in childhood. Patients present initially with deteriorating tubular function. Progressive azotemia and renal failure follow, usually within 5 years of symptom onset.

Acquired Cystic Kidney Disease

Simple renal cysts are usually incidental findings at autopsy and are rarely clinically symptomatic unless they are very large. These fluid-filled cysts may be solitary or multiple and are usually located in the outer cortex, where they expand the capsule. Simple cysts less commonly occur in the medulla. Microscopically, they are lined by a flat epithelium.

Long-term dialysis is often associated with the formation of multiple cortical and medullary cysts. The cysts are initially lined by a flat to cuboidal epithelium but hyperplastic and neoplastic proliferation may develop.

Glomerular Diseases

The glomerulus is a specialized network of capillaries forming a convoluted glomerular tuft covered by epithelial cells and supported by modified smooth muscle cells called **mesangial cells** (see Figs. 16-1, 16-5, 16-6, and Fig. 16-7). The glomerular capillaries are lined by fenestrated endothelial cells lying on a basement membrane. The outer surface of this basement membrane is covered by specialized epithelial cells called **podocytes** or **visceral epithelial cells**. Podocytes line the glomerular side of **Bowman space**, whereas the **parietal epithelial cells** line **Bowman capsule** on the opposite side.

An extensive variety of renal disorders is caused by injury to the glomerulus. The glomerulus may be the only major site of disease (**primary glomerular disease**; e.g., immunoglobulin [Ig]A nephropathy) or may be a component of a disease that affects multiple organs (**secondary glomerular disease**; e.g., lupus glomeru-

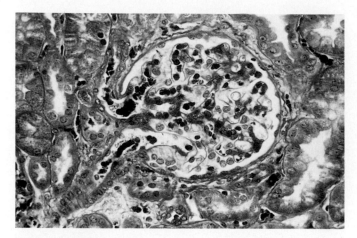

FIGURE 16-5. Normal glomerulus, light microscopy. The Masson trichrome stain shows a glomerular tuft with delicate blue capillary wall basement membranes, small amounts of blue matrix surrounding mesangial cells, and the hilum on the left. The afferent arteriole enters below and the efferent arteriole exits above.

lonephritis). *Renal biopsy evaluation is often the only means of definitive diagnosis for glomerular diseases, although clinical and laboratory data may provide presumptive evidence for a specific illness.*

Nephrotic Syndrome Features Severe Proteinuria

Nephrotic syndrome is characterized by severe proteinuria (>3.5 g of protein/24 hours), hypoalbuminemia, edema, hyperlipidemia, and lipiduria. **Proteinuria**, the major pathogenetic abnormality, results from increased glomerular capillary permeability, allowing protein to be lost from the plasma into the urine (Fig. 16-8).

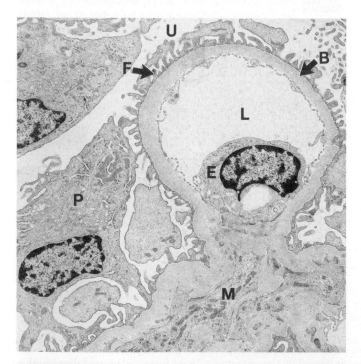

FIGURE 16-6. Normal glomerulus. In this electron micrograph of a single capillary loop and adjacent mesangium, the capillary wall portion of the lumen *(L)* is lined by a thin layer of fenestrated endothelial cytoplasm that extends out from the endothelial cell body *(E)*. The endothelial cell body is in direct contact with the mesangium, which includes the mesangial cell *(M)* and adjacent matrix. The outer aspect of the basement membrane *(B)* is covered by foot processes *(F)* from the podocyte *(P)* that line the urinary space *(U)*. Compare this figure with Figure 16-7.

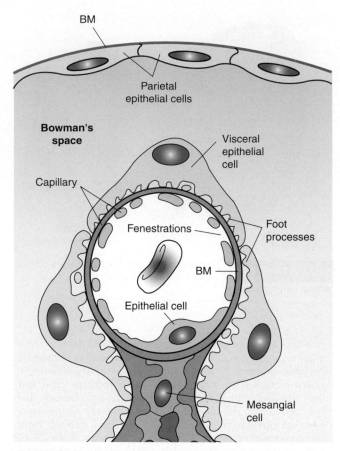

FIGURE 16-7. Normal glomerulus. The relationship of the different glomerular cell types to the basement membrane and mesangial matrix is illustrated using a single glomerular loop. The entire outer aspect of the glomerular basement membrane (BM) (peripheral loop and stalk) is covered by the visceral epithelial cell (podocyte) foot processes. The outer portions of the fenestrated endothelial cell are in contact with the inner surface of the basement membrane, whereas the central part is in contact with the mesangial cell and adjacent mesangial matrix. Compare this figure with Figure 16-6.

There are important differences in the rates of specific glomerular diseases that produce nephrotic syndrome in adults versus those in children. For example, minimal-change glomerulopathy is responsible for most (70%) cases of nephrotic syndrome in children but only 15% in adults. Table 16-1 lists the major causes and frequency of the nephrotic syndrome in adults and children. Table 16-2 details selected pathologic features of some of these diseases (discussed below).

Nephritic Syndrome is an Inflammatory Disease

Nephritic syndrome is characterized by hematuria (either microscopic or visible grossly), variable degrees of proteinuria, and decreased glomerular filtration rate. It results in elevated blood urea nitrogen and serum creatinine, oliguria, salt and water retention, edema, and hypertension. The proteinuria and hematuria associated with the nephritic syndrome are caused by inflammatory changes in glomeruli, such as infiltration by leukocytes, hyperplasia of glomerular cells, damage to capillaries, and, in severe lesions, necrosis. The inflammatory damage may also impair glomerular flow and filtration, resulting in renal insufficiency, fluid retention, and hypertension. Nephritis may be characterized as:

- **Acute glomerulonephritis**, which develops rapidly and is irreversible
- **Rapidly progressive glomerulonephritis**, which may resolve with aggressive treatment

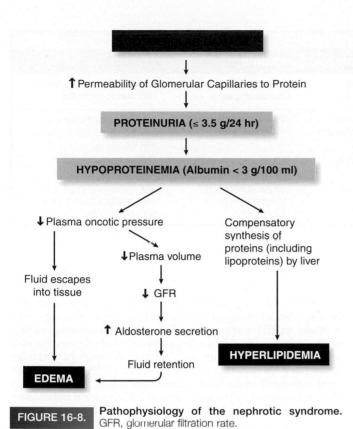

↑Permeability of Glomerular Capillaries to Protein

↓

PROTEINURIA (≤ 3.5 g/24 hr)

↓

HYPOPROTEINEMIA (Albumin < 3 g/100 ml)

↓Plasma oncotic pressure

Compensatory synthesis of proteins (including lipoproteins) by liver

↓Plasma volume

Fluid escapes into tissue

↓ GFR

↑ Aldosterone secretion

HYPERLIPIDEMIA

Fluid retention

EDEMA

FIGURE 16-8. Pathophysiology of the nephrotic syndrome. GFR, glomerular filtration rate.

- **Chronic glomerulonephritis**, which may persist for years and proceeds slowly to renal failure

With the possible exception of minimal-change glomerulopathy (which almost always causes the nephrotic syndrome), all glomerular diseases occasionally produce mixed nephritic and nephrotic manifestations that confound clinical diagnosis.

Glomerular Inflammation is Most Frequently Mediated by Immune Mechanisms

PATHOGENESIS: Both antibody-mediated and cell-mediated types of immunity play roles in the production of glomerular inflammation. However, three mechanisms of antibody-induced inflammation have been incriminated as the major pathogenetic processes in most forms of glomerulonephritis (Fig. 16-9):

TABLE 16-1

Frequency of Causes for the Nephrotic Syndrome Induced by Primary Glomerular Diseases in Children and Adults

Cause	Children (%)	Adults (%)
Minimal-change glomerulopathy	75	15
Membranous glomerulopathy	5	30
Focal segmental glomerulosclerosis	10	30
Type I membranoproliferative glomerulonephritis	5	5
Other glomerular diseases*	5	20

*Includes many forms of mesangioproliferative and proliferative glomerulonephritis, such as immunoglobulin (Ig)A nephropathy, which often also cause nephritic features.

- **In situ immune complex formation** involves binding of circulating antibodies to intrinsic antigens or foreign antigens within glomeruli, resulting in inflammatory injury (see Chapter 4).
- **Deposition of circulating immune complexes** in glomeruli leads to inflammation similar to that produced by immune complex formation in situ.
- **Antineutrophil cytoplasmic autoantibodies (ANCAs)** cause a severe glomerulonephritis that exhibits little or no glomerular deposition of immunoglobulins. These patients have a high frequency of circulating autoantibodies specific for antigens in the cytoplasm of neutrophils, which can mediate glomerular inflammation by activating neutrophils.

PATHOLOGY: Many specific glomerular diseases have distinctive pathologic features, as well as different natural histories and appropriate treatments. *Accurate pathologic diagnosis of glomerular diseases requires evaluation of renal tissue by light, immunofluorescence, and electron microscopy, accompanied by integration of the findings with clinical information.* Table 16-3 lists pathologic features that are useful for diagnosing glomerular diseases.

In general, the pathologic features of acute inflammation, such as endocapillary and extracapillary hypercellularity, leukocyte infiltration, and necrosis, are more common in disorders that have predominantly nephritic features than in those with nephrotic attributes. **Glomerular crescent formation** (extracapillary epithelial cell proliferation) is not specific for a *particular* cause of glomerular inflammation. Crescent formation serves as a marker for severe rapidly progressing injury that has resulted in extensive rupture of capillary walls, allowing inflammatory mediators to enter Bowman space and resulting in macrophage infiltration and epithelial proliferation.

Minimal-Change Glomerulopathy Causes Nephrotic Syndrome

Minimal-change glomerulopathy is a disorder that is clinically associated with the nephrotic syndrome. Pathologically, the disease is characterized by effacement of podocyte foot processes.

PATHOGENESIS: The pathogenesis of minimal-change glomerulopathy is unknown. Involvement of the immune system has been postulated because the disease frequently enters remission when treated with corticosteroids and because it may occur in association with an allergic disease or a lymphoid neoplasm such as Hodgkin disease. The heavy proteinuria of minimal-change glomerulopathy is accompanied by a loss of polyanionic sites on the glomerular basement membrane (GBM), which allows anionic proteins, particularly albumin, to pass more easily through the GBM.

PATHOLOGY: *The light microscopic appearance of glomeruli in minimal-change glomerulopathy is essentially normal.* Electron microscopy of glomeruli reveals total **effacement of visceral, epithelial cell foot processes**, an effect caused by their retraction into the parent epithelial cell bodies (compare Fig. 16-6 with Fig. 16-10). Such retraction (presumably resulting from cell swelling) is not specific for minimal-change glomerulopathy and occurs in association with virtually all cases of proteinuria in the nephrotic range. Loss of protein in the urine leads to hypoalbuminemia, and a compensatory increase in lipoprotein secretion by the liver results in hyperlipidemia. The loss of lipoproteins through the glomeruli causes lipid accumulation in the proximal tubular cells, which is reflected histologically as glassy (hyaline) droplets in tubular epithelial cytoplasm, a finding associated with any disease causing

TABLE 16-2

Pathologic Features of Important Causes of the Nephrotic Syndrome

	Minimal Change Glomerulopathy	Focal Segmental Glomerulosclerosis	Membranous Glomerulopathy	Membranoproliferative Glomerulonephritis
Light microscopy	No lesion	Focal and segmental glomerular consolidation	Diffuse global capillary wall thickening	Capillary wall thickening and endocapillary hypercellularity
Immuno-fluorescence microscopy	No immune deposits	No immune deposits	Diffuse capillary wall immunoglobulin	Diffuse capillary wall complement
Electron microscopy	No immune deposits	No immune deposits	Diffuse subepithelial dense deposits	Subendothelial (type I) or intramembranous (type II) dense deposits

the nephrotic syndrome. Immunofluorescence microscopy for immunoglobulins and complement are most often negative, but there is occasional weak mesangial staining for IgM and the complement component C3.

 CLINICAL FEATURES: Minimal-change glomerulopathy causes 90% of nephrotic syndrome cases in young children, 50% in older children, and 15% in adults. Proteinuria is generally more selective (albumin > globulins) than in the nephrotic syndrome caused by other diseases, but there is too much overlap for this selectivity to be used as a diagnostic criterion. More than 90% of children and fewer adults with minimal-change glomerulopathy have a complete remission of proteinuria within 8 weeks of the initiation of corticosteroid therapy. After withdrawal of corticosteroids, most patients suffer intermittent relapses for up to 10 years. In the absence of complications, the long-term outlook for patients with minimal-change glomerulopathy is no different from that of the general population.

Focal Segmental Glomerulosclerosis (FSGS) is a Feature of Multiple Disease Processes

Focal segmental glomerulosclerosis (FSGS) is characterized by glomerular consolidation that affects some (focal), but not all, glomeruli and initially involves only part of an affected glomerular tuft (segmental). The consolidated segments often contain increased collagenous matrix (sclerosis). There are several primary and secondary forms of FSGS.

 PATHOGENESIS: The term **FSGS** is applied to a heterogeneous group of glomerular diseases with different causes, pathologies, responses to treatment, and outcomes. FSGS occurs as an idiopathic (primary) process or secondary to a number of conditions. It is likely that multiple factors leading to podocyte damage may be common to all types of FSGS. FSGS has been associated with the following conditions likely to injure or stress podocytes:

- **Genetic abnormalities of podocyte proteins** such as podocin, α-actinin-4, and transient receptor potential cation channel 6
- **Reductions in renal mass**, which may be congenital (unilateral agenesis) or acquired (reflux nephropathy, see below)
- **Functional overwork** associated with obesity or hypoxia (as in sickle cell disease or congenital cyanotic heart diseases)

Viruses, the drug pamidronate, and serum factors have also been implicated as causes of FSGS. Infection with HIV, especially in blacks, and intravenous drug abuse are associated with a variant of FSGS characterized by a collapsing pattern of sclerosis, possibly associated with viral injury to podocytes. A serum permeability factor has been detected in some patients with FSGS, which suggests a systemic cause for the glomerular injury. This concept is further supported by the recurrence of FSGS in renal transplants, especially in patients who have the permeability factor.

 PATHOLOGY: By light microscopy, varying numbers of glomeruli show segmental obliteration of capillary loops by increased matrix or by the accumulation of cells, or both (Fig. 16-11). Insudation of plasma proteins and lipid into the lesions causes a glassy appearance, called **hyalinosis**. Adhesions to Bowman capsule occur adjacent to the sclerotic lesions. Uninvolved glomeruli may appear entirely normal, although mild mesangial hypercellularity is occasionally present.

By electron microscopy, FSGS exhibits diffuse effacement of epithelial cell foot processes, with occasional focal detachment or loss of podocytes from the GBM. Increased matrix material, folding and thickening of the basement membranes, and capillary collapse are present in sclerotic segments.

Immunofluorescence microscopy demonstrates nonimmune trapping of IgM and C3 in the segmental areas of sclerosis and hyalinosis. IgG, C4, and C1q are less frequently found in sclerotic segments. Nonsclerotic segments have no staining or only trace mesangial staining, usually for IgM and C3.

 CLINICAL FEATURES: FSGS is the cause of 30% of nephrotic syndrome in adults and 10% in children. It is more common in American blacks (where it is the leading cause of nephrotic syndrome) than in whites. For unknown reasons, its frequency has been increasing over the past few decades. The most common clinical presentation is an insidious onset of asymptomatic proteinuria, which frequently progresses to the nephrotic syndrome. Many patients are hypertensive, and microscopic hematuria is frequent.

Most individuals with FSGS show persistent proteinuria and a progressive decline in renal function. Many progress to end-stage renal disease after 5 to 20 years. Some, but not all, patients appear to improve with corticosteroid therapy. Although renal transplantation is the preferred treatment for end-stage renal disease, FSGS recurs in half of transplanted kidneys. The collapsing variant has a particularly poor prognosis, and half of all patients reach end-stage disease within 2 years. Patients with FSGS secondary to obesity or reduced renal mass usually have a more indolent course that benefits from treatment with angiotensin-converting enzyme inhibitors.

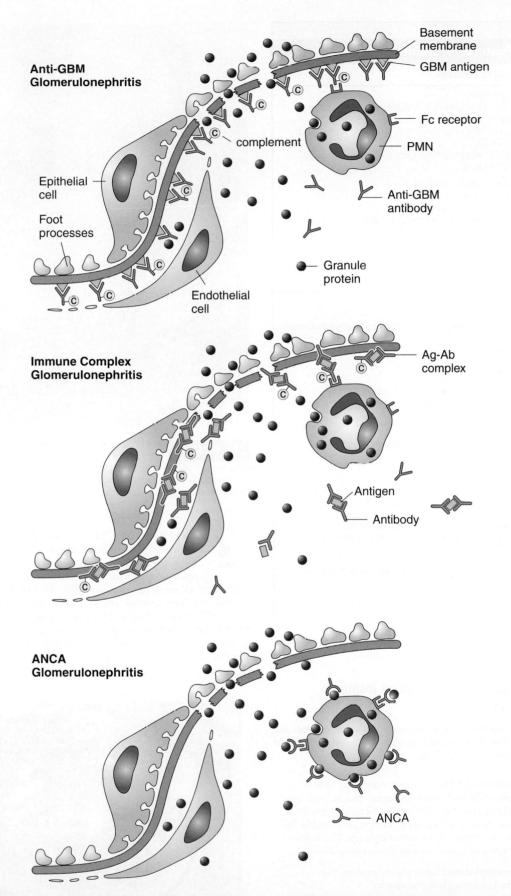

Anti-GBM Glomerulonephritis

Basement membrane
GBM antigen
Fc receptor
PMN
Anti-GBM antibody
complement
Epithelial cell
Foot processes
Endothelial cell
Granule protein

Immune Complex Glomerulonephritis

Ag-Ab complex
Antigen
Antibody

ANCA Glomerulonephritis

ANCA

FIGURE 16-9. **Antibody-mediated glomerulonephritis. Top:** Antiglomerular basement membrane (GBM) antibodies cause glomerulonephritis by binding in situ to basement membrane antigens. This activates complement and recruits inflammatory cells. *Middle:* Immune complexes that deposit from the circulation also activate complement and recruit inflammatory cells. **Bottom:** Antineutrophil cytoplasmic antibodies (ANCA) cause inflammation by activating leukocytes by direct binding of the antibodies to the leukocytes and by Fc receptor engagement of ANCA bound to antigen. PMN, polymorphonecular neutrophil; Ag-Ab complex, antigen-antibody complex.

TABLE 16-3

Diagnostic Features of Glomerular Diseases

I. Light Microscopic Features

A. Increased cellularity
   Infiltration by leukocytes (e.g., neutrophils, monocytes, macrophages)
   Proliferation of "endocapillary" cells (i.e., endothelial and mesangial cells)
   Proliferation of "extracapillary" cells (i.e., epithelial cells) (crescent formation)

B. Increased extracellular material
   Localization of immune complexes
   Thickening or replication of (GBM)
   Increases in collagenous matrix (sclerosis)
   Insudation of plasma proteins (hyalinosis)
   Fibrinoid necrosis
   Deposition of amyloid

II. Immunofluorescence Features

A. Linear staining of GBM
   Anti-GBM antibodies
   Multiple plasma proteins (e.g., in diabetic glomerulosclerosis)
   Monoclonal light chains

B. Granular immune complex staining
   Mesangium (e.g., IgA nephropathy)
   Capillary wall (e.g., membranous glomerulopathy)
   Mesangium and capillary wall (e.g., lupus glomerulonephritis)

C. Irregular (fluffy) staining
   Monoclonal light chains (AL amyloidosis)
   AA protein (AA amyloidosis)

III. Electron Microscopic Features

A. Electron-dense immune complex deposits
   Mesangial (e.g., IgA nephropathy)
   Subendothelial (e.g., lupus glomerulonephritis)
   Subepithelial (e.g., membranous glomerulopathy)

B. GBM thickening (e.g., diabetic glomerulosclerosis)

C. GBM replication (e.g., membranoproliferative glomerulonephritis)

D. Collagenous matrix expansion (e.g., focal segmental glomerulosclerosis)

E. Fibrillary deposits (e.g., amyloidosis)

IgA, immunoglobulin A; GBM, glomerular basement membrane.

Membranous Glomerulopathy is an Immune Complex Disease

Membranous glomerulopathy is a frequent cause of the nephrotic syndrome in adults. It is caused by the accumulation of immune complexes in the subepithelial zone of glomerular capillaries.

 PATHOGENESIS: Immune complexes localize in the **subepithelial zone** (between the visceral epithelial cell and the GBM), most likely as a result of immune complex formation in situ or possibly by the deposition of circulating immune complexes. The following are general causes of membranous glomerulopathy:

- Idiopathic (primary) membranous glomerulopathy
- Secondary membranous glomerulopathy
  - Autoimmune disease (systemic lupus erythematosus [SLE])
  - Infectious disease (hepatitis B)
  - Therapeutic agents (penicillamine)
  - Neoplasms (lung cancer)

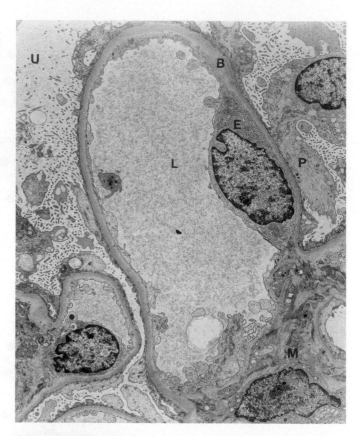

FIGURE 16-10. **Minimal-change glomerulopathy.** In this electron micrograph, the podocyte (*P*) displays extensive effacement of foot processes and numerous microvilli projecting into the urinary space (*U*). B, basement membrane; E, endothelial cell; L, lumen; M, mesangial cell.

 PATHOLOGY: The glomeruli are normocellular. Depending on the duration of the disease, capillary walls are normal or thickened (Fig. 16-12). By electron microscopy, immune complexes appear in capillary walls as electron-dense deposits (Fig. 16-13). As the disease progresses, capillary lumina are narrowed, and glomerular sclerosis eventually ensues. Advanced lesions of membranous glomerulopathy cannot be distinguished from those in other forms of chronic glomerular disease. Atrophy of tubules and interstitial fibrosis parallel the degree of glomerular sclerosis.

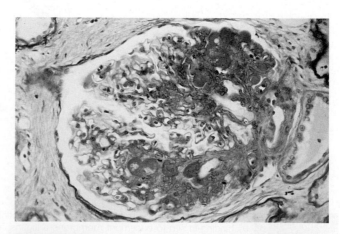

FIGURE 16-11. **Focal segmental glomerulosclerosis.** Periodic acid-Schiff (PAS) staining shows perihilar areas of segmental sclerosis and adjacent adhesions to Bowman's capsule.

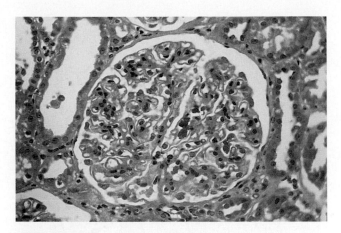

FIGURE 16-12. **Membranous glomerulopathy.** The glomerulus is slightly enlarged and shows diffuse thickening of the capillary walls. There is no hypercellularity.

Immunofluorescence microscopy reveals diffuse granular staining of capillary walls for IgG and C3 (Fig. 16-14). There is intense staining for terminal complement components, including the membrane attack complex, which participate in the induction of glomerular injury.

CLINICAL FEATURES: Membranous glomerulopathy is the most frequent primary glomerular cause of the nephrotic syndrome in white and Asian adults in the United States. (The most common secondary glomerular cause is diabetic glomerulosclerosis.) The course of membranous glomerulopathy is highly variable. Approximately 25% of patients have spontaneous remission within 20 years, 50% have persistent proteinuria and stable or only partial loss of renal function, and 25% develop renal failure. Patients with progressive renal failure are treated with corticosteroids or immunosuppres-

sive drugs, or both. The prognosis is better in children because of a higher rate of permanent spontaneous remission.

Diabetic Glomerulosclerosis Results in Proteinuria and Progressive Renal Failure

PATHOGENESIS: Glomerulosclerosis is a part of diabetic vasculopathy that involves small vessels throughout the body (see Chapter 22). Diabetes is complicated by a generalized increase in synthesis of basement membrane material by the microvasculature. Less than half of patients with diabetes develop glomerulosclerosis, suggesting that additional factors are contributory in some, but not all, diabetic patients.

PATHOLOGY: The earliest lesions of diabetic glomerulosclerosis are glomerular enlargement, GBM thickening, and mesangial matrix expansion. Mild mesangial hypercellularity may also be present. With progressive disease, GBM thickening, and especially expansion of the mesangial matrix, result in changes that can be seen by light microscopy. Overt diabetic glomerulosclerosis is characterized by diffuse global thickening of GBMs and diffuse mesangial matrix expansion, accompanied by sclerotic lesions termed **Kimmelstiel-Wilson nodules** (Fig. 16-15). Tubular basement membranes are thickened. Sclerosing and insudative changes also occur in afferent and efferent arterioles, causing hyaline arteriolosclerosis. Generalized arteriosclerosis is usually present in the kidney. Vascular narrowing and reduced blood flow to the medulla predisposes to papillary necrosis and pyelonephritis.

Electron microscopy shows up to 5- to 10-fold widening of the basement membrane lamina densa. Mesangial matrix is increased, particularly in nodular lesions. The insudative lesions appear as electron-dense masses that contain lipid debris. Immunofluorescence microscopy demonstrates diffuse nonimmune linear trapping of IgG, albumin, fibrinogen, and other plasma proteins in the GBM.

CLINICAL FEATURES: Diabetic glomerulosclerosis is the leading cause of end-stage renal disease in the United States, accounting for one-third of all patients with chronic renal failure. It occurs in type 1 and type 2 diabetes mellitus. The earliest manifestation is microalbuminuria (slightly increased proteinuria). Overt proteinuria occurs between 10 and 15 years after the onset of diabetes and often becomes severe

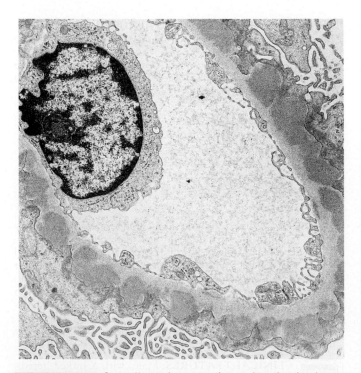

FIGURE 16-13. **Stage II membranous glomerulopathy.** An electron micrograph shows deposits of electron-dense material, with intervening delicate projections of basement membrane material.

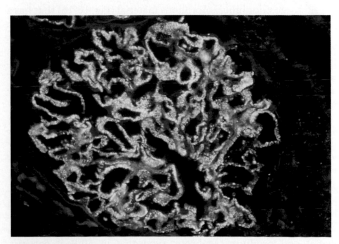

FIGURE 16-14. **Membranous glomerulopathy.** Immunofluorescence microscopy shows granular deposits of IgG outlining the glomerular capillary loops.

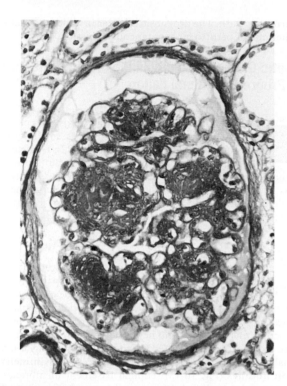

FIGURE 16-15. Diabetic glomerulosclerosis. Periodic acid-Schiff (PAS) staining reveals a prominent increase in the mesangial matrix, forming several nodular lesions. Dilation of glomerular capillaries is evident, and some capillary basement membranes are thickened.

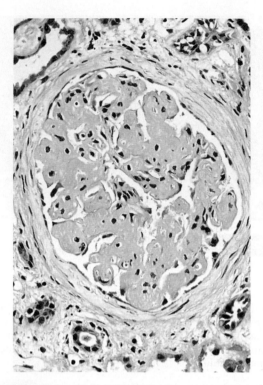

FIGURE 16-16. Amyloid nephropathy. Amorphous acellular material expands the mesangial areas and obstructs the glomerular capillaries. The deposits of amyloid may take on a nodular appearance, somewhat resembling those of diabetic glomerulosclerosis (see Fig. 16-26). However, amyloid deposits are not periodic acid-Schiff–positive and are identifiable by Congo red staining.

enough to cause the nephrotic syndrome. In time, diabetic glomerulosclerosis progresses to renal failure. Strict control of blood glucose reduces the incidence of diabetic glomerulosclerosis and retards progression once it develops. Control of hypertension and restriction of dietary protein also slow progression of the disease.

Amyloidosis Leads to Nephrotic Syndrome and Renal Failure

Renal disease is a frequent complication of primary (AL) and secondary (AA) amyloidosis (see Chapter 23 for details of the pathogenesis of amyloid formation).

PATHOLOGY: Histologically, amyloid is an eosinophilic, amorphous material (Fig. 16-16) that has a characteristic apple-green color in sections stained with Congo red and examined by polarized light microscopy. Acidophilic deposits initially are most apparent in the mesangium but later extend into capillary walls and may destroy capillary lumina (see Fig. 16-16). Glomerular structure is completely obliterated in advanced amyloidosis, and glomeruli appear as large eosinophilic spheres.

Amyloid is composed of nonbranching fibrils, approximately 10 nm in diameter. These fibrils are most prominent in the mesangium but often extend into capillary walls, especially in advanced cases. The epithelial foot processes overlying the GBM are effaced.

CLINICAL FEATURES: Renal involvement is prominent in most cases of systemic AL and AA amyloidosis. Proteinuria is often the initial manifestation. It is nonselective (i.e., both albumin and globulins appear in the urine) and produces nephrotic syndrome in 60% of patients. Eventually, severe infiltration of the glomeruli and blood vessels by amyloid results in renal failure. AL amyloidosis is treated with

chemotherapy analogous to that used for multiple myeloma. AA amyloidosis, especially when caused by familial Mediterranean fever, is ameliorated by colchicine therapy.

Hereditary Nephritis (Alport Syndrome) Reflects Abnormal Type IV Collagen in GBMs

Hereditary nephritis is a proliferative and sclerosing glomerular disease, often accompanied by defects of the ears or the eye, which is caused by mutations in type IV collagen. Alport syndrome is accompanied by a hearing deficit.

PATHOGENESIS: A variety of genetic mutations cause molecular defects in the GBM that produce the renal lesions of hereditary nephritis. The most common defect accounting for 85% of hereditary nephritis is X-linked and is caused by a mutation in the gene for the α5 chain of type IV collagen (*COL4A5* gene).

PATHOLOGY: Early glomerular lesions of hereditary nephritis show mild mesangial hypercellularity and matrix expansion. Renal disease progression is associated with increasing focal and eventually diffuse glomerular sclerosis. Advanced glomerular lesions are accompanied by tubular atrophy, interstitial fibrosis, and the presence of foam cells in the tubules and interstitium. The most diagnostic morphologic lesion is seen only by electron microscopy as an irregularly thickened GBM, with splitting of the lamina densa into interlacing lamellae that surround electron-lucent areas.

CLINICAL FEATURES: Males with X-linked hereditary nephritis develop microscopic hematuria early in childhood, usually followed by proteinuria, and progressive renal failure during the second to fourth decades of life. Females with X-linked (heterozygous) disease generally have a milder form. The slower progression of symptoms varies substantially among patients, possibly related to the degree of random inactivation of the mutated X chromosome. Sensorineural, high-frequency hearing loss affects half of males with X-linked disease.

Thin Glomerular Basement Membrane Nephropathy is a Benign Cause of Hematuria

Thin basement membrane nephropathy, also termed benign familial hematuria, is a common hereditary GBM disorder that typically manifests as asymptomatic microscopic hematuria, and occasionally with intermittent gross hematuria. This disease and IgA nephropathy are the two major diagnostic considerations in patients with asymptomatic glomerular hematuria. Patients with thin basement membrane nephropathy usually do not develop renal failure or substantial proteinuria. By light microscopy, glomeruli are unremarkable. Electron microscopy reveals a reduced thickness of the GBM (150 to 300 nm, compared with the normal 350 to 450 nm). The most common mode of inheritance is autosomal dominant. Heterozygous mutations in the *COL4A3* and *COL4A4* genes lead to thin basement membrane disease, and homozygous mutations lead to a recessive variant of Alport syndrome.

Acute Postinfectious Glomerulonephritis is an Immune Complex Disease of Childhood

Acute postinfectious glomerulonephritis usually occurs after infection with group A (β-hemolytic) streptococci and is caused by deposition of immune complexes in glomeruli.

 PATHOGENESIS: *Acute postinfectious glomerulonephritis is most often caused by certain nephritogenic strains of* group A (β-hemolytic) streptococci. Occasional examples are caused by staphylococcal infection (e.g., acute staphylococcal endocarditis, staphylococcal abscess), and rare cases result from viral (e.g., hepatitis B) or parasitic (e.g., malaria) infections. The exact mechanism by which infection causes the characteristic inflammatory changes in the glomeruli is not completely understood. It is likely that postinfectious glomerulonephritis is caused by glomerular localization of immune complexes composed of antibody plus bacterial, viral, or parasitic antigens. Poststreptococcal glomerulonephritis has a latent period of 9 to 14 days between the time of exposure to the infectious agent and the occurrence of glomerulonephritis. Immune complexes could localize in glomeruli by deposition from the circulation or formation in situ as bacterial antigens trapped in the glomeruli bind circulating antibodies. The specific nephritogenic streptococcal antigens have not been conclusively identified. Immune complexes within glomeruli initiate inflammation by activating complement, as well as other humoral and cellular inflammatory mediators.

 PATHOLOGY: The acute phase of postinfectious glomerulonephritis is characterized by diffuse glomerular enlargement and hypercellularity, which defines acute diffuse proliferative glomerulonephritis. Hypercellularity reflects proliferation of both endothelial and mesangial cells (Fig. 16-17) as well as infiltration by neutrophils and monocytes. Crescents are uncommon. Interstitial edema and mild infiltration of mononuclear leukocytes occur in parallel with the glomerular changes.

The acute phase begins 1 or 2 weeks after the onset of the nephritogenic infection and resolves in more than 90% of patients

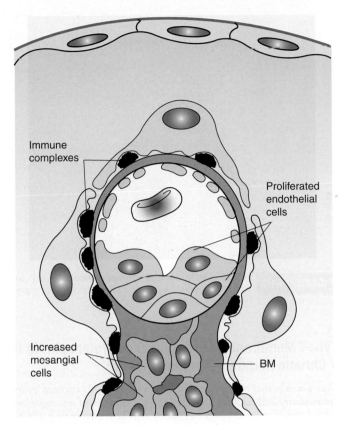

FIGURE 16-17. **Postinfectious glomerulonephritis.** Accumulation of numerous subepithelial immune complexes as hump-like structures is a characteristic feature. Less prominent subendothelial immune complexes are associated with endothelial cell proliferation and are related to increased capillary permeability and narrowing of the lumen. Frequently, proliferation of mesangial cells and a thickened mesangial matrix (BM) result in widening of the stalk and conspicuous trapping of immune complexes.

after several weeks. All histologic changes resolve completely in most patients after several months.

The most distinctive ultrastructural features of acute postinfectious glomerulonephritis are **subepithelial dense deposits** that are shaped like "**humps**" (see Fig. 16-17). These deposits are invariably accompanied by mesangial and subendothelial deposits, which may be more difficult to find but are probably more important in pathogenesis because of their proximity to the inflammatory mediator systems in the blood. In the first few weeks of disease, immunofluorescence microscopy typically reveals granular deposits corresponding to IgG and C3 along the basement membrane, in locations corresponding to the humps. Later in the disease, C3 is present without IgG, possibly because immune complexes containing IgG no longer accumulate in the glomeruli after the infection clears (Fig. 16-18).

 CLINICAL FEATURES: Acute poststreptococcal glomerulonephritis is less common than it was in the past but remains one of the most common childhood renal diseases. The nephritic syndrome begins abruptly with oliguria, hematuria, facial edema, and hypertension. Serum C3 levels are lower during the acute syndrome but return to normal within 1 to 2 weeks. Overt nephritis resolves after several weeks, although hematuria and especially proteinuria may persist for several months. A few patients have abnormal urinary sediment for years after the acute episode, and rare patients (particularly adults) develop progressive renal failure.

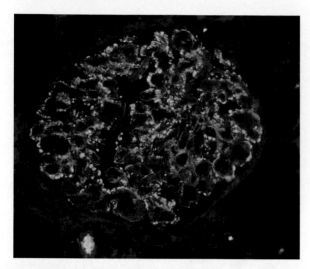

FIGURE 16-18. **Acute postinfectious glomerulonephritis.** An immunofluorescence micrograph demonstrates granular staining for C3 in capillary walls and the mesangium.

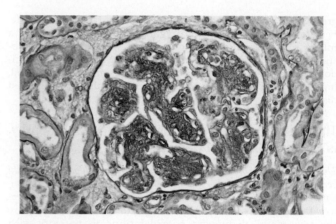

FIGURE 16-19. **Type I membranoproliferative glomerulonephritis.** The glomerular lobulation is accentuated. Increased cells and matrix in the mesangium and thickening of capillary walls are noted.

Type I Membranoproliferative Glomerulonephritis is a Chronic Immune-Complex Disease

Type I membranoproliferative glomerulonephritis is characterized by hypercellularity and capillary wall thickening. Deposition of mesangial and subendothelial immune complexes causes mesangial proliferation and extension into the subendothelial zone.

PATHOGENESIS: Type I membranoproliferative glomerulonephritis, also called **mesangiocapillary glomerulonephritis**, is caused by localization of immune complexes to the mesangium and the subendothelial zone of capillary walls. In most patients, the origin of nephritogenic antigen is unknown, but some have associated conditions that are the apparent source of the antigen. Elimination of disorders such as bacterial endocarditis or osteomyelitis leads to the resolution of glomerulonephritis, which supports a causal relationship between the two. Agents that are responsible for type I membranoproliferative glomerulonephritis cause persistent indolent infections that are associated with chronic antigenemia. This condition leads to chronic localization of immune complexes in glomeruli and resultant hypercellularity and matrix remodeling.

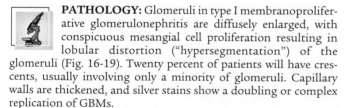

PATHOLOGY: Glomeruli in type I membranoproliferative glomerulonephritis are diffusely enlarged, with conspicuous mesangial cell proliferation resulting in lobular distortion ("hypersegmentation") of the glomeruli (Fig. 16-19). Twenty percent of patients will have crescents, usually involving only a minority of glomeruli. Capillary walls are thickened, and silver stains show a doubling or complex replication of GBMs.

Electron microscopy shows that the capillary wall thickening and replication of GBMs are a consequence of the marked mesangial expansion, with extension of mesangial cytoplasm into the subendothelial zone and deposition of new basement membrane material between the mesangial cytoplasm and endothelial cell (Figs. 16-20 and 16-21). Subendothelial and mesangial electron-dense deposits, corresponding to immune complexes, are the likely stimuli for the mesangial response. Variable numbers of subepithelial dense deposits may also be seen. Immunofluorescence microscopy shows granular deposition of immunoglobulins and complement in glomerular capillary loops and mesangium.

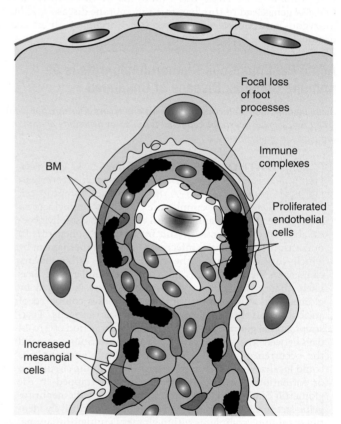

FIGURE 16-20. **Membranoproliferative glomerulonephritis, type I.** In this disease, the glomeruli are enlarged. Hypercellular tufts and narrowing or obstruction of the capillary lumen are seen. Large subendothelial deposits of immune complexes extend along the inner border of the basement membrane. The mesangial cells proliferate and migrate peripherally into the capillary. Basement membrane (BM) material accumulates in a linear fashion parallel to the BM in a subendothelial position. The interposition of mesangial cells and basement membrane between the endothelial cells and the original BM creates a double-contour effect. The accumulation of mesangial cells and stroma in the tufts narrows the capillary lumen. The proliferation of mesangial cells and the accumulation of BM material also widen the mesangium. The entire process leads progressively to lobulation of the glomerulus. Note the proliferation of endothelial cells and focal effacement of foot processes.

Labels in Figure 16-20: Focal loss of foot processes; Immune complexes; Proliferated endothelial cells; BM; Increased mesangial cells

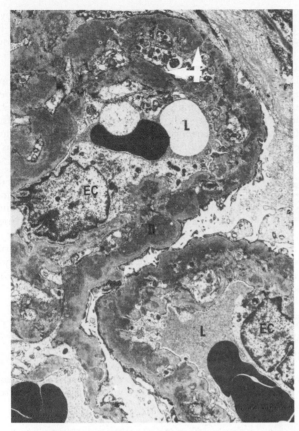

FIGURE 16-21. Type I membranoproliferative glomerulonephritis. An electron micrograph demonstrates a double-contour basement membrane *(arrow)* with mesangial interposition and prominent subendothelial deposits. B, basement membrane; EN, endothelial cell; L, capillary lumen.

 CLINICAL FEATURES: Type I membranoproliferative glomerulonephritis is most frequent in older children and young adults. It may manifest as either nephrotic or nephritic syndrome or a combination of both. Type I disease accounts for 5% of nephrotic syndrome in children and adults in the United States. It is much more common in developing countries that have a high prevalence of chronic infections. Type I membranoproliferative glomerulonephritis is usually a persistent but slowly progressive disease. Half of patients reach end-stage renal disease after 10 years.

Type II Membranoproliferative Glomerulonephritis (Dense Deposit Disease) Features Complement Deposition

Type II membranoproliferative glomerulonephritis is characterized by a pathognomonic electron-dense transformation of GBMs and extensive complement deposition.

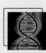 **PATHOGENESIS:** The extensive localization of complement in the GBMs and mesangial matrix, in the absence of significant immunoglobulin deposition, suggests that complement activation via the alternate pathway is a major mediator of the structural and functional abnormalities associated with the disease. A deficiency of, and mutations in, regulatory factors of the alternative complement pathway (e.g., factor H), and the presence in most patients of a serum IgG autoantibody termed **C3**

nephritic factor (which results in the prolongation of C3 cleaving activity), implicate dysregulation of the alternative complement pathway in disease pathogenesis.

 PATHOLOGY: The histologic appearance of type II membranoproliferative glomerulonephritis may be similar to that of type I, with capillary wall thickening and some degree of hypercellularity. The distinctive ribbon-like zone of increased density in the center of a thickened GBM and in the mesangial matrix justifies the alternative name **dense deposit disease**. Immunofluorescence microscopy shows linear staining of capillary walls for C3, with little or no staining for immunoglobulins.

 CLINICAL FEATURES: Type II membranoproliferative glomerulonephritis is rare. It resembles type I disease in clinical presentation and course, except that hypocomplementemia is more common, and the prognosis is slightly worse. No effective treatment has been identified.

Lupus Glomerulonephritis is Associated with Many Autoantibodies

Systemic lupus erythematosus (SLE) is an autoimmune disease characterized by a generalized dysregulation and hyperactivity of B cells, with production of autoantibodies to a variety of nuclear and nonnuclear antigens, including DNA, RNA, nucleoproteins, and phospholipids (see Chapter 4). Nephritis is one of the most common complications of SLE, with a wide range of patterns of immune complex deposition seen in the glomerulus. Mesangial deposition of immune complexes causes less inflammation than subendothelial deposits, which are more exposed to the circulation. Subepithelial localization causes proteinuria but not overt glomerular inflammation.

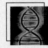 **PATHOGENESIS:** Immune complexes may localize in glomeruli by deposition from the circulation or formation in situ (involving antigens such as DNA bound to GBM or mesangium by charge interaction). Glomerular immune complexes activate complement and initiate inflammatory injury. Immune complexes deposited in other renal compartments may be involved in the tubulointerstitial inflammation seen in patients with lupus nephritis.

 PATHOLOGY: The pathologic and clinical manifestations of lupus nephritis are highly variable because of variable patterns of immune complex accumulation in different patients and in the same patient over time.

- **Class I (minimal mesangial lupus nephritis):** Immune complexes are confined to the mesangium and cause no changes by light microscopy.
- **Class II (mesangial proliferative lupus nephritis):** Immune complexes are confined to the mesangium and produce varying degrees of mesangial hypercellularity and matrix expansion (Fig. 16-22).
- **Class III (focal proliferative lupus nephritis):** Immune complex accumulation in the subendothelial zone and the mesangium stimulates inflammation, with proliferation of mesangial and endothelial cells and the influx of neutrophils and monocytes.
- **Class IV (diffuse proliferative lupus nephritis):** This type is similar to class III but involves more than 50% of glomeruli.
- **Class V (membranous lupus nephritis):** Immune complexes are mostly in the subepithelial zone, but concurrent class III or IV injury may also occur.
- **Class VI (advanced sclerosing lupus nephritis):** This category is the most severe chronic disease.

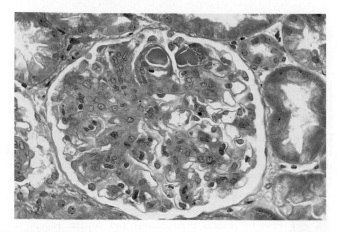

FIGURE 16-22. **Proliferative lupus glomerulonephritis.** Segmental endocapillary hypercellularity and thickening of capillary walls are present.

Electron microscopy demonstrates the varied locations of immune-complex dense deposits in mesangial, subendothelial, and subepithelial locations. About 80% of specimens have **tubuloreticular inclusions** in endothelial cells. Lupus nephritis and HIV-associated nephropathy are the only renal diseases with a high frequency of these structures.

By immunofluorescence, the subepithelial complexes are granular, and the subendothelial deposits appear granular or band-like. The immune complexes often stain most intensely for IgG, but IgA and IgM are also almost always present, as are C3, C1q, and other complement components. Granular staining along tubular basement membranes and interstitial vessels is present in more than 50% of patients.

 CLINICAL FEATURES: Seventy percent of all patients with SLE develop renal disease, which is the major cause for morbidity and mortality in many patients. SLE and associated renal disease is most common in black women. The clinical manifestations and prognosis of renal dysfunction are varied and depend on the pathologic nature of the underlying renal disease. Class III and class IV lupus nephritis have the poorest prognosis and are treated most aggressively, usually with high doses of corticosteroids and other immunosuppressive drugs. Currently, less than 25% of patients with class IV disease reach end-stage renal failure within 5 years.

IgA Nephropathy (Berger Disease) is Caused by Immune Complexes of IgA

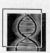 **PATHOGENESIS:** Although the deposition of IgA-dominant immune complexes is the cause of IgA nephropathy, the constituent antigens and mechanism of accumulation are not known. Patients with IgA nephropathy often have elevated blood levels of IgA, and circulating IgA-containing immune complexes have been detected. *Exacerbations of IgA nephropathy are often initiated by respiratory or gastrointestinal infections.* There is evidence for MHC–linked susceptibility to IgA nephropathy, possibly mediated via dysregulation of IgA immune responses. Abnormal glycosylation of the hinge region of IgA appears to be an important predisposing factor in many patients with IgA nephropathy.

IgA-containing immune complexes within the mesangium most likely activate the alternative complement pathway. This concept is supported by the demonstration of C3 and properdin, but not C1q and C4, in the IgA deposits.

 PATHOLOGY: Immunofluorescence microscopy is essential for the diagnosis of IgA nephropathy. The diagnostic finding is mesangial staining for IgA more intense than, or equivalent to, staining for IgG or IgM. This is almost always accompanied by staining for C3.

Depending on the severity and duration of glomerular inflammation, IgA nephropathy manifests a continuum of histologic appearances, ranging from (1) no discernible light microscopic changes, to (2) focal or diffuse mesangial hypercellularity, to (3) focal or diffuse proliferative glomerulonephritis, to (4) chronic sclerosing glomerulonephritis. This spectrum of pathologic changes is analogous to that seen with lupus nephritis but tends to be less severe.

 CLINICAL FEATURES: IgA nephropathy (Berger disease) is the most common form of glomerulonephritis in the world. It accounts for 10% of cases in the United States, has a high frequency in Native Americans, and is rare in blacks. It is most common in young men, with a peak age of 15 to 30 years at diagnosis. The clinical presentations are varied, which reflects the varied pathologic severity. The disease rarely resolves completely, but has a slowly progressive course with 20% of patients reaching end-stage renal failure after 10 years.

Anti-Glomerular Basement Membrane Glomerulonephritis is Often Associated with Pulmonary Hemorrhage

Anti-GBM antibody glomerulonephritis is an uncommon but aggressive form of glomerulonephritis that occurs as a renal-limited disease or is combined with pulmonary hemorrhage (Goodpasture syndrome).

 PATHOGENESIS: Anti-GBM glomerulonephritis is mediated by an autoimmune response against a component of the GBM within the globular non-collagenous domain of the α3 type of collagen IV. Because the target antigen is also expressed on pulmonary alveolar capillary basement membranes, half of patients also have pulmonary hemorrhages and hemoptysis, sometimes severe enough to be life-threatening. If both lungs and kidneys are involved, the eponym **Goodpasture syndrome** is used. Anti-GBM antibodies, anti-GBM T cells, or both, may mediate the injury. Genetic susceptibility to anti-GBM disease is associated with *HLA-DR2* genes. Disease onset often follows viral upper-respiratory tract infections. Pulmonary involvement appears to require prior exposure to other injurious agents, such as cigarette smoke.

 PATHOLOGY: *The pathologic hallmark of anti-GBM glomerulonephritis is diffuse linear staining of GBMs for IgG, which indicates autoantibodies bound to the basement membrane* (Fig. 16-23). *More than 90% of patients with anti-GBM glomerulonephritis have glomerular crescents* (**crescentic glomerulonephritis**) (Figs. 16-24 and 16-25).

 CLINICAL FEATURES: Anti-GBM glomerulonephritis typically presents with rapidly progressive renal failure and nephritic signs and symptoms. It accounts for 10% to 20% of rapidly progressive (crescentic) glomerulonephritis. Treatment consists of high-dose immunosuppressive therapy and plasma exchange. If end-stage renal failure develops, renal transplantation is frequently successful, with little risk of loss of the allograft to recurrent glomerulonephritis.

ANCA Glomerulonephritis Features Neutrophil-Induced Injury

ANCA (antineutrophil cytoplasmic antibodies) glomerulonephritis is an aggressive, neutrophil-mediated disease that is characterized by glomerular necrosis and crescents.

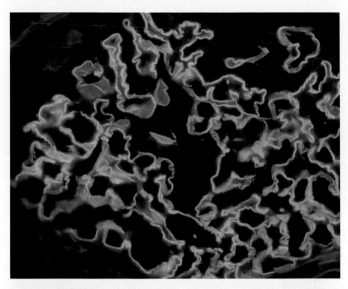

FIGURE 16-23. **Antiglomerular basement membrane (GBM) glomerulonephritis.** Linear immunofluorescence for immunoglobulin G is seen along the GBM. Compare this linear pattern of staining with the granular pattern of immunofluorescence typical for most types of immune complex deposition within capillary walls (see Fig. 16-18).

 PATHOLOGY: More than 90% of patients with ANCA glomerulonephritis have focal glomerular necrosis (Fig. 16-26) and crescent formation. In many patients, more than 50% of glomeruli exhibit crescents. Nonnecrotic segments may appear normal or have slight neutrophil infiltration or mild endocapillary hypercellularity. Immunofluorescence microscopy demonstrates an absence or paucity of staining for immunoglobulins and complement.

 CLINICAL FEATURES: The most common clinical presentation for ANCA glomerulonephritis is rapidly progressive renal failure, with nephritic signs and symptoms. The disease accounts for 75% of rapidly progressive (crescentic) glomerulonephritis in patients over 60 years of age, 45% in middle-aged adults, and 30% in young adults and children. *Three quarters of patients with ANCA glomerulonephritis have systemic small-vessel vasculitis (see below), which has many manifestations, including pulmonary hemorrhage,* a much more frequent cause of **pulmonary–renal vasculitic syndrome** than is Goodpasture syndrome. Without treatment, more than 80% of patients with ANCA glomerulonephritis develop end-stage renal disease within 5 years. Immunosuppressive therapy decreases the development of end-stage disease at 5 years to less than 25%.

Vascular Diseases

Renal Vasculitis May Affect Vessels of All Sizes

The kidney is involved in many types of systemic vasculitis (Table 16-4). *In a sense, glomerulonephritis is a local form of vasculitis that affects*

PATHOGENESIS: ANCA glomerulonephritis was once called *idiopathic crescentic glomerulonephritis* because immunofluorescence microscopy did not demonstrate evidence of glomerular deposition of anti-GBM antibodies or immune complexes. The discovery that 90% of patients with this pattern of glomerular injury have circulating ANCAs led to the demonstration that these autoantibodies cause the disease. *ANCAs are specific for proteins in the cytoplasm of neutrophils and monocytes, usually MPO-ANCA or PR3-ANCA.*

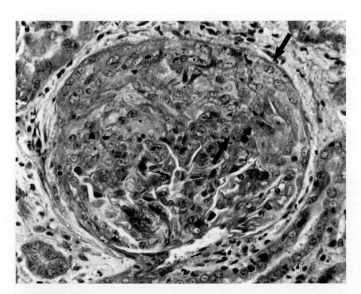

FIGURE 16-24. **Crescentic antiglomerular basement membrane glomerulonephritis.** Bowman's space is filled by a cellular crescent *(between arrows)*. The injured glomerular tuft is at the bottom (Masson trichrome stain).

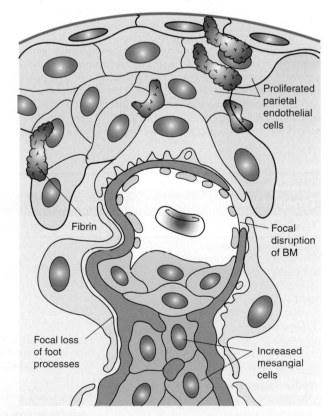

Proliferated parietal endothelial cells

Fibrin

Focal disruption of BM

Focal loss of foot processes

Increased mesangial cells

FIGURE 16-25. **Crescentic (rapidly progressive) glomerulonephritis.** A variety of different pathogenic mechanisms cause crescent formation by disrupting glomerular capillary walls. This allows plasma constituents into Bowman's space, including coagulation factors and inflammatory mediators. Fibrin forms, and there is proliferation of parietal epithelial cells and influx of macrophages, resulting in crescent formation.

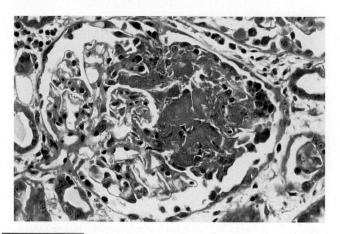

FIGURE 16-26. Antineutrophil cytoplasmic autoantibody glomerulonephritis. Segmental fibrinoid necrosis is illustrated. In time, this lesion stimulates crescent formation.

glomerular capillaries. The glomeruli may be the only site of vascular inflammation, or the renal disease may be a component of a systemic vasculitis.

Small-Vessel Vasculitis

Small-vessel vasculitis affects small arteries, arterioles, capillaries, and venules. Glomerulonephritis, purpura, arthralgias, myalgias, peripheral neuropathy, and pulmonary hemorrhage are common components of the small-vessel vasculitides. Additional details of extrarenal disease may be found in Chapter 10.

Henoch-Schönlein purpura is the most common type of childhood vasculitis. It is caused by vascular localization of immune complexes containing mostly IgA. The glomerular lesion is identical with that to IgA nephropathy.

Cryoglobulinemic vasculitis causes proliferative glomerulonephritis, usually type I membranoproliferative glomerulonephritis. By light microscopy, aggregates of cryoglobulins ("hyaline thrombi") are often seen within capillary lumina.

ANCA vasculitis involves vessels outside the kidneys in 75% of patients with ANCA glomerulonephritis (see Chapter 10). In addition to causing necrotizing and crescentic glomerulonephritis, the

ANCA vasculitides often display necrotizing inflammation in other renal vessels, such as arteries, arterioles, and medullary peritubular capillaries.

Medium-Sized and Large-Vessel Vasculitis

Medium-sized vessel vasculitides such as **polyarteritis nodosa** (in adults) and **Kawasaki disease** (primarily in children) affect arteries, but not arterioles, capillaries, or venules. Large-vessel vasculitides, such as **giant cell arteritis** and **Takayasu arteritis,** affect the aorta and its major branches and may cause renovascular hypertension by involving the main renal arteries or their aortic origin (see Chapter 10).

Hypertensive Nephrosclerosis (Benign Nephrosclerosis) Leads to Obliteration of Glomeruli

 PATHOGENESIS: Sustained systolic pressures over 140 mm Hg and diastolic pressures over 90 mm are generally considered to represent hypertension (see Chapter 10). Mild-to-moderate hypertension causes typical hypertensive nephrosclerosis in approximately 15% of patients and thus is not truly benign.

 PATHOLOGY: The kidneys are smaller than normal (atrophic) and are usually affected bilaterally. The cortical surfaces have a fine granularity (Fig. 16-27), but coarser scars are occasionally present. On cut section, the cortex is thinned. Microscopically, many glomeruli appear normal; others show varying degrees of ischemic change. Initially, glomerular capillaries demonstrate thickening, wrinkling, and collapse of GBMs. Cells of the glomerular tuft are progressively lost, and collagen and matrix material are deposited within Bowman space. Eventually, the glomerular tuft is obliterated by a dense, eosinophilic globular mass within a scar. Tubular atrophy, a consequence of glomerular loss, is associated with interstitial fibrosis and infiltration by chronic inflammatory cells. Sclerotic glomeruli and surrounding atrophic tubules are often clustered in focal subcapsular zones, with adjacent areas of preserved glomeruli and tubules (Fig. 16-28), the basis for the granular surfaces of nephrosclerotic kidneys.

TABLE 16–4		
Types of Vasculitis that Involve the Kidneys		
Type of Vasculitis	**Major Target Vessels in Kidney**	**Major Renal Manifestations**
Small-vessel vasculitis		
Immune-complex vasculitis		
Henoch-Schönlein purpura	Glomeruli	Nephritis
Cryoglobulinemic vasculitis	Glomeruli	Nephritis
Anti-GBM vasculitis		
Goodpasture syndrome	Glomeruli	Nephritis
ANCA-vasculitis		
Wegener granulomatosis	Glomeruli, arterioles, interlobular arteries	Nephritis
Microscopic polyangiitis	Glomeruli, arterioles, interlobular arteries	Nephritis
Churg-Strauss syndrome	Glomeruli, arterioles, interlobular arteries	Nephritis
Medium-sized vessel vasculitis		
Polyarteritis nodosa	Interlobar and arcuate arteries	Infarcts and hemorrhage
Kawasaki disease	Interlobar and arcuate arteries	Infarcts and hemorrhage
Large-vessel vasculitis		
Giant cell arteritis	Main renal artery	Renovascular hypertension
Takayasu arteritis	Main renal artery	Renovascular hypertension

ANCA, antineutrophil cytoplasmic autoantibody; GBM, glomerular basement membrane.

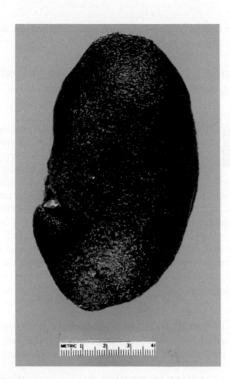

FIGURE 16-27. **Hypertensive nephrosclerosis.** The kidney is reduced in size, and the cortical surface exhibits fine granularity.

The pattern of change in the renal blood vessels depends on the size of the vessel. Arteries down to the size of the arcuate arteries have fibrotic thickening of the intima, with replication of the elastica-like lamina and partial replacement of the muscularis with fibrous tissue. Interlobular arteries and arterioles may develop medial hyperplasia.

Arterioles exhibit concentric hyaline thickening of the wall, often with the loss of smooth muscle cells or their displacement to the periphery. This arteriolar change is termed **hyaline arteriolosclerosis**.

 CLINICAL FEATURES: Although hypertensive nephrosclerosis does not usually lead to significant renal function abnormalities, a few of the many persons with "benign" hypertension develop progressive renal failure, which may terminate in end-stage renal disease. Benign nephrosclerosis is most prevalent and aggressive among blacks. *In fact, among blacks in the United States, hypertension without any evidence of a malignant phase is the leading cause of end-stage renal disease.*

Malignant Hypertensive Nephropathy is a Potentially Fatal Renal Disease

PATHOGENESIS: No specific blood pressure defines malignant hypertension, but diastolic pressures over 130 mm Hg, retinal vascular changes, papilledema, and renal functional impairment are usual criteria. About half of patients have prior histories of benign hypertension, and many others have a background of chronic renal injury caused by many different diseases. Occasionally, malignant hypertension arises *de novo* in apparently healthy persons, particularly young black men. The pathogenesis of the vascular injury is unclear, but it may result from endothelial damage as the blood slams into the narrowed small vessels. At sites of vascular injury, plasma constituents leak into injured walls of arterioles (resulting in fibrinoid necrosis), into intima of arteries (causing edematous intimal thickening), and into the subendothelial zone of glomerular capillaries (leading to glomerular consolidation). At these sites of vascular injury, thrombosis can result in focal renal cortical necrosis (infarcts).

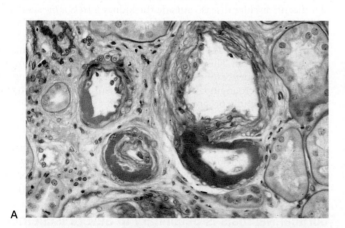

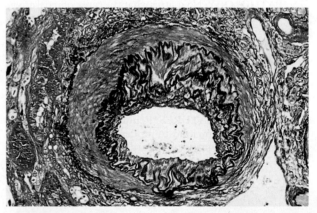

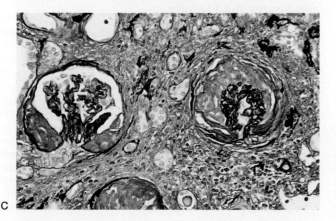

FIGURE 16-28. **Hypertensive nephrosclerosis. A.** Three arterioles with hyaline sclerosis (periodic acid-Schiff stain). **B.** Arcuate artery with fibrotic intimal thickening causing narrowing of the lumen (silver stain). **C.** One glomerulus with global sclerosis and one with segmental sclerosis. Note also the tubular atrophy, interstitial fibrosis, and chronic inflammation (silver stain).

PATHOLOGY: The size of the kidneys in malignant hypertensive nephropathy varies from small to enlarged, depending on the duration of pre-existing benign hypertension. The cut surface is mottled red and yellow and occasionally exhibits small cortical infarcts. Microscopically, malignant hypertensive nephropathy is often superimposed on a background of hypertensive nephrosclerosis, with edematous (myxoid, mucoid) intimal expansion in arteries and fibrinoid necrosis of arterioles. Variable glomerular changes range from capillary congestion to consolidation to necrosis (Fig. 16-29). Severe cases show thrombosis and focal ischemic cortical necrosis (infarction). These pathologic changes are identical to those observed in other forms of thrombotic microangiopathy (see below).

 CLINICAL FEATURES: Malignant hypertension occurs more often in men than in women, typically around the age of 40 years. Patients suffer from headaches, dizziness, and visual disturbances and may develop overt encephalopathy. Hematuria and proteinuria are frequent. Progressive deterioration of renal function develops if the malignant hypertension persists. Aggressive antihypertensive therapy often controls the disease.

Renovascular Hypertension Follows Narrowing of a Renal Artery

 PATHOGENESIS: In patients with renal artery stenosis, hypertension reflects increased production of renin, angiotensin II, and aldosterone. Most (95%) cases are caused by atherosclerosis, which explains why this disorder is twice as common in men as in women and is seen primarily in older age groups. **Fibromuscular dysplasia**, characterized by fibrous and muscular stenosis of the renal artery and vasculitis, are less common causes overall but are the most frequent ones in children.

 PATHOLOGY: No matter what the cause of renal artery stenosis is, the kidney parenchymal changes are the same. The size of the involved kidney is reduced. Glomeruli appear normal but are closer to each other than expected, because the intervening tubules show marked ischemic atrophy without extensive interstitial fibrosis. Many glomeruli lose their attachment to the proximal tubule. The juxtaglomerular apparatus is prominent and reveals hyperplasia and increased granularity.

CLINICAL FEATURES: Renovascular hypertension is characterized by mild-to-moderate blood pressure elevations. A bruit may be heard over the renal artery. In more than half of patients, surgical revascularization, angioplasty, or nephrectomy cures hypertension.

Thrombotic Microangiopathy Refers to Systemic Diseases with Similar Renal Lesions

 PATHOGENESIS: Thrombotic microangiopathy has a variety of causes, all leading to endothelial damage that initiates a final common pathway of vascular changes, which result in narrowing of vessel lumina and ischemia. The injured endothelial surfaces promote thrombosis, which worsens ischemia and may cause focal ischemic necrosis. The passage of blood through the injured vessels leads to a nonimmune (Coombs negative) hemolytic anemia, characterized by misshapen and disrupted erythrocytes (schistocytes) and thrombocytopenia. This hematologic syndrome is termed **microangiopathic hemolytic anemia** (see Chapter 20). The kidneys are ubiquitous targets of thrombotic microangiopathies, but other organs may also be injured.

 PATHOLOGY: The renal pathologic changes are comparable to those in malignant hypertensive nephropathy, which is a form of thrombotic microangiopathy.

 CLINICAL FEATURES: Various clinical presentations and causes allow recognition of different categories of thrombotic microangiopathy. The various clinical disorders share (1) microangiopathic hemolytic anemia, (2) thrombocytopenia, (3) hypertension, and (4) renal failure, although these features are expressed to different degrees.

Hemolytic–Uremic Syndrome

Hemolytic–uremic syndrome (HUS) features microangiopathic hemolytic anemia and acute renal failure, with little or no evidence for significant vascular disease outside the kidneys. *HUS is the most common cause of acute renal failure in children.* Major causes for HUS are Shiga toxin-producing strains of *E coli*, which are ingested in contaminated food such as poorly cooked hamburger or contaminated vegetable products. The toxin injures endothelial cells, setting in motion the sequence of events described above and resulting in thrombotic microangiopathy. Patients present with hemorrhagic diarrhea and rapidly progressive renal failure.

Thrombotic Thrombocytopenic Purpura (TTP)

TTP displays systemic microvascular thrombosis and is characterized clinically by thrombocytopenia, purpura, fever, and changes in mental status. Unlike HUS, renal involvement is often absent or less important than other organ disease (see Chapter 20 for details).

Cortical Necrosis is Secondary to Severe Ischemia and Spares the Medulla

Cortical necrosis affects part or all of the renal cortex. The term **infarct** is used when there is one area (or a few areas) of necrosis caused by occlusion of arteries, whereas **cortical necrosis** implies more widespread ischemic necrosis.

 PATHOGENESIS: Vasa recta that supply arterial blood to the medulla arise from juxtamedullary efferent arterioles, proximal to vessels supplying the outer cortex. Thus, occlusion of outer cortical vessels, for example by vasospasm, thrombi, or thrombotic microangiopathy, leads to cortical necrosis and sparing of the medulla. Historically, the most common cause for renal cortical necrosis was premature separation of the placenta (abruptio placentae) in the third trimester of pregnancy. However, re-

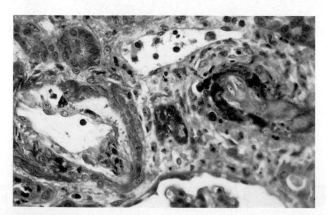

FIGURE 16-29. **Malignant hypertensive nephropathy.** Red fibrinoid necrosis in the wall of the arteriole on the right and clear edematous expansion in the intima of the interlobular artery on the left from a patient with malignant hypertension (Masson trichrome stain).

nal cortical necrosis can complicate any clinical condition associated with hypovolemic or endotoxic shock. Because all forms of shock are associated with acute tubular necrosis (ATN), it is not surprising that there is an overlap between that condition and cortical necrosis, both clinically and pathologically.

 PATHOLOGY: The extent of cortical necrosis varies from patchy to confluent (Fig. 16-30). In the most severely involved areas, all parenchymal elements exhibit coagulative necrosis. The proximal convoluted tubules are invariably necrotic, as are most of the distal tubules. In the adjacent viable portions of the cortex, the glomeruli and distal convoluted tubules are usually unaffected, but many of the proximal convoluted tubules have features of ischemic injury, such as epithelial flattening or necrosis.

With extensive necrosis, the cortex has a marked pallor. The cortex is diffusely necrotic, except for thin rims of viable tissue immediately beneath the capsule and at the corticomedullary junction, which are supplied by capsular and medullary collateral blood vessels, respectively. Patients who survive cortical necrosis may develop striking dystrophic calcification of the necrotic areas.

 CLINICAL FEATURES: Severe cortical necrosis manifests as acute renal failure, which initially may be indistinguishable from that produced by acute tubular necrosis. Recovery is determined by the extent of the disease, but there is a significant incidence of hypertension among survivors.

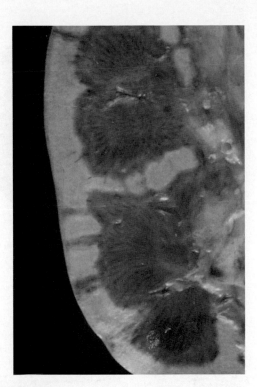

FIGURE 16-30. **Renal cortical necrosis.** The cortex of the kidney is pale yellow and soft due to diffuse cortical necrosis.

Diseases of Tubules and Interstitium

Acute Tubular Necrosis (ATN) Causes Acute Renal Failure

ATN is a severe, but potentially reversible, renal failure due to impairment of tubular epithelial function caused by ischemia or toxic injury. Because necrosis often is not a prominent feature of ATN, this process is also called acute renal injury.

 PATHOGENESIS: Ischemic ATN results from reduced renal perfusion, usually associated with hypotension. Tubular epithelial cells, with their high rate of energy-consuming metabolic activity and numerous organelles, are particularly sensitive to hypoxia and anoxia. Tubular epithelial cells may be simplified (flattened) but not necrotic in some patients with typical clinical ATN.

Nephrotoxic ATN is caused by chemically induced injury to epithelial cells. Tubular epithelial cells are preferred targets because they absorb and concentrate toxins. The high rate of energy consumption by epithelial cells also makes them susceptible to injury by toxins that perturb oxidative or other metabolic pathways. Hemoglobin and myoglobin can be considered endogenous toxins that can induce ATN (**pigment nephropathy**) when they are present in the urine in high concentrations.

The pathophysiology of ATN appears to involve some or all of the perturbations outlined in Figure 16-31, various combinations of which result in a reduced glomerular filtration rate and tubular epithelial dysfunction.

 PATHOLOGY: Ischemic ATN is characterized by swollen kidneys that have a pale cortex and a congested medulla. No pathologic changes are seen in glomeruli or blood vessels. Tubular injury is focal and

is most pronounced in the proximal tubules and the thick limbs of the loop of Henle in the outer medulla. The proximal tubules display focal flattening of the epithelium, with dilation of the lumina and loss of the brush border (epithelial simplification). This results in part from sloughing of the apical cytoplasm, which appears in the distal tubular lumina and urine as brown granular casts. A characteristic feature of **ischemic** ATN is the absence of widespread necrosis of tubular epithelial cells, individual necrotic cells being found within some proximal or distal tubules. These single necrotic cells as well as a few viable cells are shed into the tubular lumen, with resulting focal denudation of tubular basement membrane (Fig. 16-32). Interstitial edema is common. The vasa recta of the outer medulla are congested and frequently contain nucleated cells, which are predominantly mononuclear leukocytes.

Toxic ATN shows more extensive necrosis of tubular epithelium than is usually caused by ischemic ATN (compare Figs. 16-32 and 16-33). In most cases, however, necrosis is limited to certain tubular segments that are most sensitive to the particular toxin. The most common site of injury is the proximal tubule. ATN due to hemoglobin or myoglobin also has many red-brown tubular casts that are colored by heme pigments.

During the recovery phase of ATN, the tubular epithelium regenerates, with mitoses, increased size of cells and nuclei, and cell crowding. Survivors eventually display complete restoration of normal renal architecture.

 CLINICAL FEATURES: *ATN is the leading cause of acute renal failure*. It manifests as a rapidly rising serum creatinine level, usually associated with decreased urine output (oliguria). Urinalysis demonstrates degenerating epithelial cells and **"dirty brown" granular casts** (acute renal failure casts) with cellular debris rich in cytochrome pigments.

The duration of renal failure in patients with ATN depends on many factors, especially the nature and reversibility of the cause. If the cause is immediately removed after the initiation of the injury, renal function often recovers within 1 to 2 weeks, although it may be delayed for months.

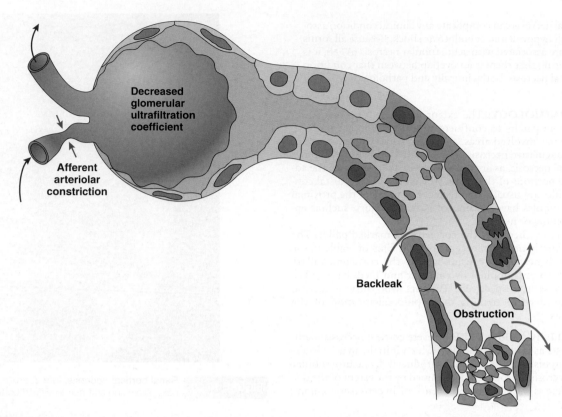

FIGURE 16-31. **Pathogenesis of acute tubular necrosis.** Sloughing and necrosis of epithelial cells result in cast formation. The presence of casts leads to obstruction and increased intraluminal pressure, which reduces glomerular filtration. Afferent arteriolar vasoconstriction, caused in part by tubuloglomerular feedback, results in decreased glomerular capillary filtration pressure. Tubular injury and increased intraluminal pressure cause fluid back leakage from the lumen into the interstitium.

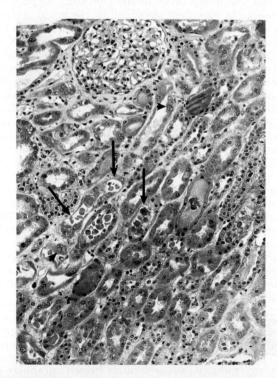

FIGURE 16-32. **Ischemic acute tubular necrosis.** Necrosis of individual tubular epithelial cells is evident both from focal denudation of the tubular basement membrane *(arrows)* and from the individual necrotic epithelial cells present in some tubular lumina. Some enlarged, regenerative-appearing epithelial cells are also present *(arrowheads)*. Note the lack of significant interstitial inflammation.

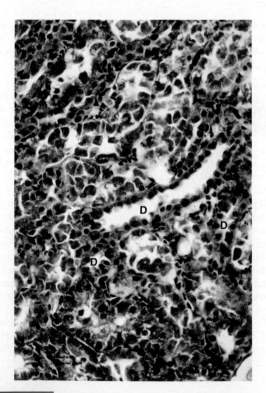

FIGURE 16-33. **Toxic acute tubular necrosis due to mercury poisoning.** There is widespread necrosis of proximal tubular epithelial cells, with sparing of distal and collecting tubules (D). Interstitial inflammation is minimal.

Pyelonephritis Refers to Bacterial Infection of the Kidney

Acute Pyelonephritis

PATHOGENESIS: Gram-negative bacteria from the feces, most commonly *E. coli,* cause 80% of acute pyelonephritis. Infection reaches the kidney by ascending through the urinary tract, a process that depends on several factors:

- Bacterial urinary infection
- Reflux of infected urine up the ureters into the renal pelvis and calyces
- Bacterial entry through the papillae into the renal parenchyma

Bladder infection precedes acute pyelonephritis. It is more common in females because of a short urethra, lack of antibacterial prostatic secretions, and facilitation of bacterial migration by sexual intercourse.

Under some circumstances, the residual urine volume (normally 2 to 3 mL) is increased (e.g., in prostatic obstruction or in an atonic bladder). As a result, the bladder contents are not sufficiently diluted with sterile urine from the kidneys to prevent bacterial accumulation. Diabetic glycosuria also predisposes to infection by providing a rich medium for bacterial growth.

Bacteria in bladder urine usually do not gain access to the kidneys. The ureter commonly inserts into the bladder wall at a steep angle (Fig. 16-34) and in its most distal portion courses parallel to the bladder wall between the mucosa and muscularis. The intravesicular pressure produced by micturition occludes the distal ureteral lumen, preventing urinary reflux. In many individuals who are particularly susceptible to pyelonephritis, an abnormally short passage of the ureter within the bladder wall is associated with an angle of insertion that is more perpendicular to the mucosal surface of the bladder. Thus, on micturition, rather than occluding the lumen, intravesicular pressure forces urine into the patent ureter. This reflux is powerful enough to force the urine into the renal pelvis and calyces.

The simple papillae of the central calyces are convex and do not readily admit reflux urine (see Fig. 16-34). By contrast, the concave

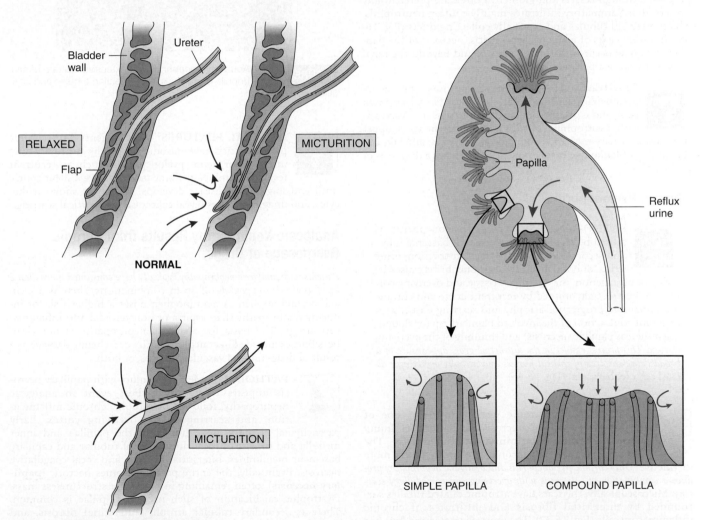

FIGURE 16-34. **Anatomical features of the bladder and kidney in pyelonephritis caused by ureterovesical reflux.** In the normal bladder, the distal portion of the intravesical ureter courses between the mucosa and the muscularis, forming a mucosal flap. On micturition, the elevated intravesicular pressure compresses the flap against the bladder wall, thereby occluding the lumen. Persons with a congenitally short intravesical ureter have no mucosal flap, because the angle of entry of the ureter into the bladder approaches a right angle. Thus, micturition forces urine into the ureter. In the renal pelvis, simple papillae of the central calyces are convex and do not readily allow reflux of urine. By contrast, the peripheral compound papillae are concave and permit entry of refluxed urine.

shapes of peripheral compound papillae allow easier access to the collecting system. However, if the pressure is prolonged, as in obstructive uropathy, even simple papillae are eventually vulnerable to the retrograde entry of urine. From the collecting tubules, bacteria gain access to the interstitial tissue and other tubules of the kidney.

In addition to ascending through urine, bacteria and other pathogens can gain access to the renal parenchyma through the circulation. For example, gram-positive organisms, such as staphylococci, can disseminate from an infected valve in bacterial endocarditis and establish a focus of infection in the kidney. The kidney is commonly involved in miliary tuberculosis. Fungi, such as *Aspergillus,* can seed the kidney in an immunocompromised host. Hematogenous infections of the kidney preferentially affect the cortex.

 PATHOLOGY: The kidneys of acute pyelonephritis have small white abscesses on the subcapsular surface and on cut surfaces. Pelvic and calyceal urothelium may be hyperemic and covered by purulent exudate. *Acute pyelonephritis is often focal, and much of the kidney may appear normal.* Most infections involve only a few papillary systems. Microscopically, the parenchyma, particularly the cortex, typically shows extensive focal destruction by the inflammatory process, although vessels and glomeruli often are preferentially preserved. Inflammatory infiltrates mainly contain neutrophils, which often fill tubules and especially collecting ducts (Fig. 16-35). In severe cases of acute pyelonephritis, necrosis of the papillary tips may occur or infection may extend beyond the renal capsule to cause a perinephric abscess.

 CLINICAL FEATURES: Symptoms of acute pyelonephritis include fever, chills, sweats, malaise, flank pain, and costovertebral angle tenderness. Leukocytosis with neutrophilia is common. Differentiating upper from lower urinary tract infection is often clinically difficult, but the finding of **leukocyte casts** in the urine supports a diagnosis of pyelonephritis.

Chronic Pyelonephritis

 PATHOGENESIS: Chronic pyelonephritis is caused by recurrent and persistent bacterial infection secondary to urinary tract obstruction, urine reflux, or both. In chronic pyelonephritis caused by reflux or obstruction, the medullary tissue and overlying cortex are preferentially injured by recurrent acute and chronic inflammation. Progressive atrophy and scarring ensue, with resultant contraction of the involved papillary tip (or sloughing if there is papillary necrosis) and thinning of the overlying cortex. *This process results in the distinctive gross appearance of a broad depressed area of cortical fibrosis and atrophy overlying a dilated calyx* (**caliectasis**) (Fig. 16-36).

 PATHOLOGY: Chronic pyelonephritis is one of many causes of the microscopic pattern of injury termed **chronic tubulointerstitial nephritis**. The gross appearance of chronic pyelonephritis is more distinctive. *Only chronic pyelonephritis and analgesic nephropathy produce a combination of caliectasis with overlying corticomedullary scarring.* Microscopically, the scars have atrophic dilated tubules surrounded by interstitial fibrosis and infiltrates of chronic inflammatory cells (Fig. 16-37). The most characteristic (but not specific) tubular change is severe epithelial atrophy, with diffuse, eosinophilic, hyaline casts. Such tubules, which are "pinched-off" spherical segments, resemble colloid-containing thyroid follicles, a pattern called "thyroidization." Glomeruli may be completely uninvolved, may show periglomerular fibrosis, or may be sclerotic.

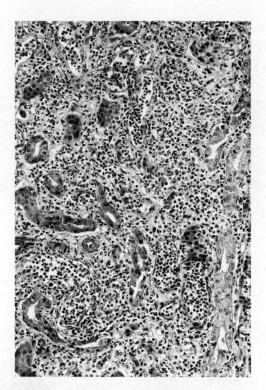

FIGURE 16-35. **Acute pyelonephritis.** An extensive infiltrate of neutrophils is present in the collecting tubules and interstitial tissue.

 CLINICAL FEATURES: Most patients with chronic pyelonephritis have episodic symptoms of urinary tract infection or acute pyelonephritis, such as recurrent fever and flank pain. Some patients have a silent course until end-stage renal disease develops. Urinalysis shows leukocytes, and imaging studies reveal caliectasis and cortical scarring.

Analgesic Nephropathy Results from Chronic Overdosage of Drugs

Patients with analgesic nephropathy typically have consumed more than 2 kg of analgesic compounds, often in combinations, such as aspirin and acetaminophen. Acetaminophen poses a higher risk for inducing nephropathy than aspirin or nonsteroidal anti-inflammatory drugs. The basis for analgesic nephropathy is not clear. Possibilities include direct nephrotoxicity or ischemic damage as a result of drug-induced vascular changes, or both.

 PATHOLOGY: Medullary injury with papillary necrosis appears to be the earliest event in analgesic nephropathy, followed by atrophy, chronic inflammation, and scarring of the overlying cortex. Early parenchymal changes are confined to the papillae and inner medulla and consist of focal thickening of tubular and capillary basement membranes, interstitial fibrosis, and focal coagulative necrosis. Eventually, the entire papilla becomes necrotic (**papillary necrosis**), often remaining in place as a structureless mass. Dystrophic calcification of such necrotic papillae is common. There is secondary tubular atrophy, interstitial fibrosis, and chronic inflammation in the overlying cortex.

 CLINICAL FEATURES: Signs and symptoms occur only in the late stages of analgesic nephropathy and include an inability to concentrate the urine, distal tubular acidosis, hematuria, hypertension, and anemia. Sloughing of necrotic papillary tips into the renal pelvis

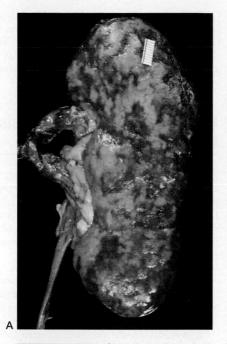 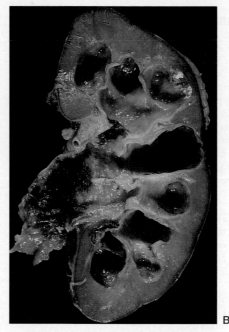

FIGURE 16-36. **Chronic pyelonephritis. A.** The cortical surface contains many irregular, depressed scars (reddish areas). **B.** There is marked dilation of calyces (caliectasis) caused by inflammatory destruction of papillae, with atrophy and scarring of the overlying cortex.

may result in colic as they pass through the ureters. Progressive renal failure often develops and may lead to end-stage renal disease.

Drug-Induced (Hypersensitivity) Acute Tubulointerstitial Nephritis is a Cell-Mediated Immune Response

 PATHOGENESIS: Acute, drug-induced, tubulointerstitial nephritis is characterized histologically by infiltrates of activated T lymphocytes and eosinophils, a pattern that indicates a type IV cell-mediated immune reaction. Drugs most commonly implicated include nonsteroidal anti-inflammatory drugs, diuretics and certain antibiotics, especially β-lactam antibiotics, such as synthetic penicillins and cephalosporins.

 PATHOLOGY: Microscopically, there is patchy infiltration of the cortex and (to a much lesser extent) medulla by lymphocytes and a small number of eosinophils (5% to 10% of the total leukocytes in the tissue). Neutrophils are rare, and their presence should raise suspicion of pyelonephritis or hematogenous bacterial infection. Foci of granulomatous inflammation may be present, especially in the later phase of the disease. Proximal and distal tubules are focally invaded by white blood cells ("tubulitis"). Glomeruli and vessels are not inflamed.

CLINICAL FEATURES: Acute tubulointerstitial nephritis usually manifests as acute renal failure, typically about 2 weeks after drug administration is started. The urine contains erythrocytes, leukocytes (including eosinophils), and sometimes leukocyte casts.

Tubular defects are common, including sodium wasting, glucosuria, aminoaciduria, and renal tubular acidosis. Systemic allergic symptoms such as fever and rash may also be present. Most patients recover fully within several weeks or months if the drug is discontinued.

Light-Chain Cast Nephropathy May Complicate Multiple Myeloma

Light-chain cast nephropathy is renal injury caused by monoclonal immunoglobulin light chains in the urine, which produce tubular epithelial injury and numerous tubular casts.

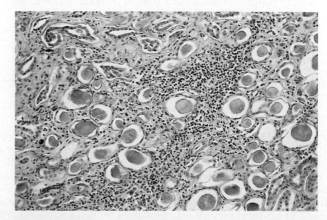

FIGURE 16-37. **A light micrograph** shows tubular dilation and atrophy, with many tubules containing eosinophilic hyaline casts resembling the colloid of thyroid follicles (so-called thyroidization). The interstitium is scarred and contains a chronic inflammatory cell infiltrate.

PATHOGENESIS: Light-chain cast nephropathy is the most common form of renal disease associated with multiple myeloma and is caused by glomerular filtering of circulating light chains. At the acidic pH typical of urine, the light chains bind to Tamm-Horsfall glycoproteins, which are secreted by distal tubular epithelial cells and form casts. Renal dysfunction results from the toxic effects of free light chains on tubular epithelial cells and obstruction from the casts. The molecular structure of light chains determines whether they will induce disease by causing light-chain cast nephropathy, AL amyloidosis, or light-chain deposition disease. Occasional patients show several of these renal diseases.

 PATHOLOGY: The characteristic tubular lesion exhibits numerous dense, hyaline casts in the distal tubules and collecting ducts. These casts are brightly eosinophilic and glassy (hyaline) and often have fractures and angular borders. They may even have a crystalline appearance. Casts may elicit foreign body reactions, with macrophages and multinucleated giant cells. Interstitial chronic inflammatory infiltrates, as well as interstitial edema, typically accompany the tubular lesions.

CLINICAL FEATURES: Light-chain cast nephropathy may manifest as either acute or chronic renal failure. Proteinuria is usually present, although not necessarily in the nephrotic range and most often consists predominantly of immunoglobulin light chains. If a patient has nephrotic-range proteinuria with multiple myeloma, AL amyloidosis or light-chain deposition disease is more likely to occur than light-chain cast nephropathy.

Urate Nephropathy Displays Urate Crystals in the Tubules and Interstitium

Any condition with elevated blood levels of uric acid may cause urate nephropathy. The classic chronic disease in this category is primary gout (see Chapter 26).

 PATHOGENESIS: Chronic urate nephropathy caused by gout is characterized by tubular and interstitial deposition of crystalline monosodium urate. **Acute urate nephropathy** can be caused by increased cell turnover. For example, chemotherapy for malignant neoplasms results in a sudden increase in blood uric acid because of the massive necrosis of cancer cells (**tumor lysis syndrome**). Acute renal failure reflects the obstruction of the collecting ducts by precipitated crystals of uric acid, a result of increased concentrations of uric acid in the acidic pH of the urine. Conditions that interfere with excretion of uric acid can also result in hyperuricemia (e.g., chronic intake of certain diuretics).

 PATHOLOGY: In acute urate nephropathy, the precipitated uric acid in the collecting ducts is seen grossly as yellow streaks in the papillae. Histologically, the tubular deposits appear amorphous, but in frozen sections, birefringent crystals are apparent. The tubules proximal to the obstruction are dilated. Penetration of collecting ducts by uric acid crystals may provoke a foreign-body giant cell reaction.

The basic disease process of chronic urate nephropathy is similar to that of the acute form, but the prolonged course results in more substantial deposition of urate crystals in the interstitium, interstitial fibrosis, and cortical atrophy.

 CLINICAL FEATURES: Acute urate nephropathy manifests as acute renal failure, whereas chronic urate nephropathy causes chronic renal tubular defects. Although histologic renal lesions are found in most persons with chronic gout, fewer than half show significant compromise of renal function.

Renal Stones (Nephrolithiasis and Urolithiasis)

*Nephrolithiasis and urolithiasis are stones within the collecting system of the kidney (**nephrolithiasis**) or elsewhere in the collecting system of the urinary tract (**urolithiasis**).* Renal pelvis and calyces are common sites for calculi to form and accumulate. For unknown reasons, renal stones are more common in men than in women. They vary in size from gravel (<1 mm in diameter) to large stones that dilate the entire renal pelvis.

- **Calcium stones:** Most (75%) kidney stones contain calcium complexed with oxalate or phosphate or a mixture of these anions.
- **Infection stones:** About 15% of stones are caused by infection. Such stones are the most likely to be associated with clinical symptoms. In the presence of urea-splitting bacteria, usually *Proteus* or *Providencia* species, the resulting alkaline urine favors precipitation of magnesium ammonium phosphate (**struvite**) and calcium phosphate (**apatite**). These stones vary from hard to soft and friable. Infection stones occasionally fill the pelvis and calyces to form a cast of these spaces, referred to as a **staghorn calculus** (Fig. 16-38).
- **Uric acid stones:** These stones occur in 25% of patients with hyperuricemia and gout, but most patients with uric acid stones do not have either condition (**idiopathic urate lithiasis**).
- **Cystine stones:** Only 1% of stones overall are of this type, but they represent a significant proportion of childhood calculi and occur exclusively with hereditary cystinuria.

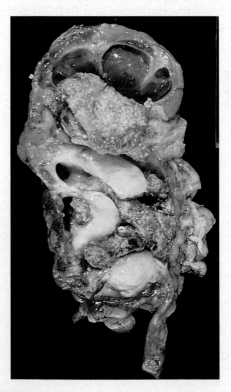

FIGURE 16-38. **Staghorn calculi.** The kidney shows hydronephrosis and stones that are casts of the dilated calyces.

Kidney stones may be well tolerated, but in some cases, they lead to severe hydronephrosis and pyelonephritis. Moreover, they can erode the mucosa and cause hematuria. Passage of a stone into the ureter causes excruciating flank pain, termed **renal colic**.

Obstructive Uropathy and Hydronephrosis

Obstructive uropathy is caused by structural or functional abnormalities in the urinary tract that impede urine flow, which may cause renal dysfunction (obstructive nephropathy) and dilation of the collecting system (hydronephrosis). The causes of urinary tract obstruction are discussed in detail in Chapter 17.

 PATHOLOGY: The most prominent microscopic finding in early hydronephrosis is dilation of the collecting ducts, followed by dilation of proximal and distal convoluted tubules. Eventually, the proximal tubules become widely dilated, and loss of tubules is common. Glomeruli are usually spared. Grossly, progressive dilation of the renal pelvis and calyces occurs, and atrophy of the renal parenchyma ensues (Fig. 16-39). In the presence of hydronephrosis, the kidney is more susceptible to pyelonephritis, which causes additional injury.

 CLINICAL FEATURES: Bilateral acute urinary tract obstruction results in acute renal failure (**postrenal acute renal failure**). Unilateral obstruction is frequently asymptomatic. Left untreated, an obstructed kidney undergoes atrophy. In the case of bilateral obstruction, chronic renal failure ensues.

Renal Transplantation

Renal transplantation is the treatment of choice for most patients with end-stage renal disease. The major obstacle is immunologic rejection, but recurrence of the disease that destroyed the native kidneys and nephrotoxicity from immunosuppressive drugs also injure the renal allograft. For additional details see Chapter 4. The same disease that led to renal failure in native kidneys can recur in a renal transplant.

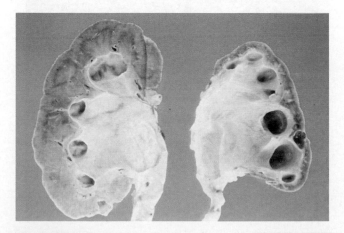

FIGURE 16-39. **Hydronephrosis.** Bilateral urinary tract obstruction has led to conspicuous dilation of the ureters, pelves, and calyces. The kidney on the right shows severe parenchymal atrophy.

Malignant Tumors of the Kidney

Wilms Tumor (Nephroblastoma) is Composed of Embryonal Elements

Wilms tumor is a malignant neoplasm of embryonal nephrogenic elements composed of mixtures of blastemal, stromal, and epithelial tissue. It is the most frequent abdominal solid tumor in children, with a prevalence of 1 in 10,000.

 PATHOGENESIS: In most (90%) cases, Wilms tumor is sporadic and unilateral. About 10% of sporadic cases of Wilms tumor are associated with defects of **WT1**, the Wilms tumor gene located on chromosome 11 (11p13). WT1 is a tumor-suppressor gene that regulates transcription of several other genes, including IGF-2 and PDGF. WT1 protein also forms a complex with the p53 protein. Presumably the presence of a germline mutation and loss of heterozygosity at the WT1 locus are associated with tumor formation in a manner similar to the pathogenesis of hereditary retinoblastoma (see Chapter 5). Two uncommon congenital syndromes associated with Wilms tumor and other developmental defects—WAGR (**W**ilms **A**niridia, **G**enitourinary anomalies, and mental **R**etardation) and Denys-Drash syndrome are also associated respectively with either a deletion of one allele of WT1 or specific mutations within the gene having a dominant negative effect.

Less than 10% of sporadic Wilms tumors exhibit abnormalities at the WT1 locus suggesting that other genes play a role in their genesis. A second gene, WT2, close to, but distinct from the WT1 locus, is implicated in some sporadic tumors. Another uncommon congenital disease, Beckwith-Wiedemann Syndrome, also features Wilms tumor and other abnormalities and is also associated with defects at the WT2 locus. The genetics of defects at the locus are complex and are likely to involve genomic imprinting. Some cases of Beckwith-Wiedemann Syndrome have demonstrated paternal uniparental isodisomy (see Chapter 6).

 PATHOLOGY: Wilms tumor tends to be large when detected, with a bulging, pale tan, cut surface enclosed within a thin rim of renal cortex and capsule (Fig. 16-40). Histologically, the tumor is composed of elements that resemble normal fetal tissue (Fig. 16-41), including (1) metanephric blastema, (2) immature stroma (mesenchymal tissue), and (3) immature epithelial elements.

Although most Wilms tumors contain all three elements in varying proportions, occasionally they contain only two elements or even only one. The component corresponding to blastema is composed of small ovoid cells with scanty cytoplasm, growing in nests and trabeculae. The epithelial component appears as small tubular structures. In some cases, tissues resembling immature glomeruli are found. The stroma between the other elements is composed of spindle cells, which are mostly undifferentiated but occasionally display smooth muscle or fibroblast differentiation.

 CLINICAL FEATURES: Wilms tumor usually presents between 1 and 3 years of age, and 98% of cases occur before 10 years of age. Most often, the diagnosis is made after recognition of an abdominal mass. Additional manifestations include abdominal pain, intestinal obstruction, hypertension, hematuria, and symptoms of traumatic tumor rupture.

A number of histologic and clinical parameters have been used with varying success to predict the behavior of Wilms tumors. Patients younger than 2 years of age tend to have a better

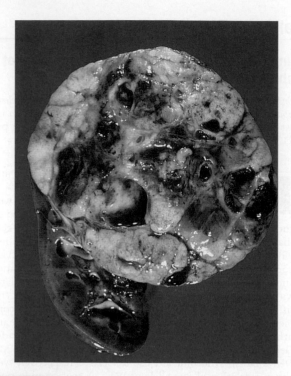

FIGURE 16-40. **Wilms tumor.** A cross-section of a pale tan neoplasm attached to a residual portion of the kidney.

prognosis. Chemotherapy and radiation therapy, combined with surgical resection, have dramatically improved the outlook of patients with this tumor, and a long-term survival rate of 90% is reported.

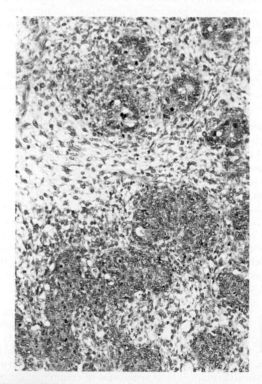

FIGURE 16-41. **Wilms tumor (nephroblastoma).** This photomicrograph of the tumor shows highly cellular areas composed of undifferentiated blastema, loose stroma containing undifferentiated mesenchymal cells, and immature tubules.

Renal Cell Carcinoma (RCC) is the Most Common Primary Cancer of the Kidney

Renal cell carcinoma (RCC) is a malignant neoplasm of renal tubular or ductal epithelial cells. It accounts for 80% of all renal cancers and more than 30,000 cases per year in the United States.

PATHOGENESIS: Most cases of RCC are sporadic, and virtually all such cases are associated with loss of heterozygosity of the tumor suppressor gene VHL, which is located on chromosome 3p. Mutations in VHL are found in more than half of such sporadic RCC tumors. Two uncommon forms of hereditary RCC, **autosomal dominant RCC** and **von Hippel-Lindau disease** (VHL, an autosomal dominant cancer syndrome), are associated with chromosomal translocations involving 3p. The latter disease has mutations in the above-mentioned VHL gene itself. A third uncommon form of hereditary RCC, **hereditary papillary RCC**, shows no association with the *VHL* gene.

Tobacco smoking or chewing is associated with an increased risk of RCC, and one third of these tumors are linked to tobacco use. Both inherited and acquired cystic diseases of the kidney may be complicated by development of RCC, especially papillary RCC. The cancer has also been tied to analgesic nephropathy.

PATHOLOGY: There are pathologic variants of RCC that reflect differences in histogenesis and predict different outcomes.

Clear cell RCC is the most common type and arises from proximal tubular epithelial cells. It is typically yellow-orange and often shows conspicuous focal hemorrhage and necrosis (Fig. 16-42). The tumors are solid or focally cystic. The clear cytoplasm of the neoplastic cells (Fig. 16-43) reflects the removal of abundant cytoplasmic lipids and glycogen during tissue processing. The cells are often arranged in round or elongated collections demarcated by a network of delicate vessels, and little cellular or nuclear pleomorphism is present.

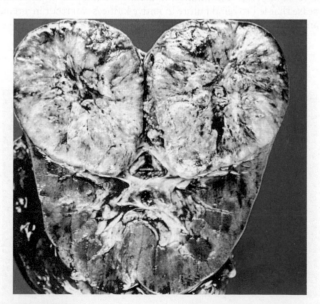

FIGURE 16-42. **Clear cell renal cell carcinoma.** The kidney contains a large irregular neoplasm with a variegated cut surface. Yellow areas correspond to lipid-containing cells.

CLINICAL FEATURES: The incidence of RCC peaks in the sixth decade and is twice as frequent in men as in women. *The classic clinical triad of hematuria, flank pain, and a palpable abdominal mass occurs in less than 10% of patients. Hematuria is the single most common presenting sign.* Often, a patient with RCC initially presents with symptoms due to a metastasis. RCC is a potential source of ectopic hormone production and is frequently associated with fever and paraneoplastic symptoms.

The prognosis for RCC is influenced by many factors, including tumor size, extent of invasion and metastasis, histologic type, and nuclear grade. The 1-year overall survival rate after nephrectomy for clear cell RCC is 50%. Tumor stage is the most important prognostic factor. The 5-year survival rate is 90% if the RCC has not extended beyond the renal capsule, but survival drops to 30% if there are distant metastases. The tumor spreads most frequently to the lungs and bones.

Transitional Cell Carcinoma

Between 5% and 10% of primary neoplasms of the kidney are transitional cell carcinomas of the renal pelvis or calyces (see Chapter 17).

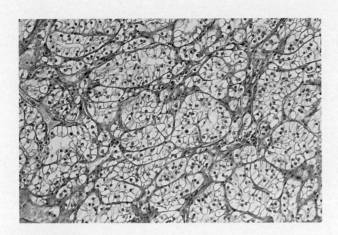

FIGURE 16-43. Clear cell renal cell carcinoma. Photomicrograph showing islands of neoplastic cells with abundant clear cytoplasm.

17 The Lower Urinary Tract and Male Reproductive System

Ivan Damjanov

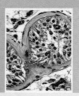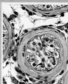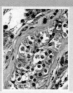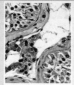

The ureters, urinary bladder, and the urethra—also known as the lower urinary tract—form the outflow part of the urinary system. In males, the lower urinary tract is closely related to the reproductive system.

RENAL PELVIS AND URETER

Congenital Disorders

Developmental anomalies of the renal pelvis and ureters are found in 2% to 3% of all persons. They do not usually cause clinical problems but on occasion may predispose to obstruction and urinary tract infections. The most important developmental anomalies include agenesis (associated with kidney agenesis, see Chapter 16), ectopia, duplications, obstructions, and dilations.

ECTOPIC URETERS: Ureteric buds may develop at the wrong anatomical site during embryogenesis. The lower orifices of ectopic ureters can be found in many anomalous places, such as the midportion of the urinary bladder, seminal vesicles, urethra, or vas deferens.

DUPLICATIONS: Single or multiple ureteric buds may be duplicated on the side of the fetal urinary bladder. There are usually two parallel ureters, each with its own renal pelvis and separate vesical orifice. **Bifid ureters** (subdivided by a septum) and many variations of this anomaly can be encountered but most are not clinically significant.

OBSTRUCTION OF THE UTEROPELVIC JUNCTION: The most common form of hydronephrosis in infants is congenital uteropelvic junction obstruction related to abnormal layering of smooth muscle cells or fibrosis replacing the smooth muscle cells at the ureteropelvic junction. Urinary obstruction in these children is usually unilateral. This form of hydronephrosis is often associated with other urinary tract anomalies and, in some cases, with agenesis of the contralateral kidney.

DILATIONS OF THE RENAL PELVIS OR URETERS: Dilation of the entire ureter, **congenital megaureter**, may be unilateral or bilateral. The ureters are tortuous and lack peristalsis. The resulting stagnation of urine (**hydroureter**) is typically associated with progressive hydronephrosis, ultimately leading to renal failure.

Ureteritis and Ureteral Obstruction

Ureteritis is an inflammation of the ureters. It is a complication of descending infections of kidneys or ascending infections if there is vesicoureteric reflux (VUR). Ureteritis is often associated with ureteral obstruction, which may be either intrinsic or extrinsic (Fig. 17-1).

Ureteral obstruction may also result from diseases that involve the urinary bladder, prostate, and urethra, for example, bladder cancer in the vicinity of the ureteral orifice or bladder neck, neurogenic bladder, and prostatic hyperplasia. Proximal causes of ureteral obstruction tend to be unilateral, whereas more distal causes, such as prostatic hyperplasia, lead to bilateral hydronephrosis, with the possibility of renal failure in untreated cases.

Tumors of the Renal Pelvis and Ureter

Tumors of the renal pelvis and ureter resemble those of urinary bladder except that they are much less common. Histologically, most (>90%) are **transitional cell carcinomas**. The etiologic factors associated with epithelial tumors of the renal pelvis and ureter are similar to those observed in bladder cancer (see below).

Patients most frequently present in their sixth and seventh decades with hematuria (80%) and flank pain (25%). Transitional cell carcinoma of the ureter or renal pelvis requires radical nephroureterectomy. The prognosis is related to the tumor stage at the time of diagnosis.

URINARY BLADDER

Congenital Disorders

EXSTROPHY OF THE BLADDER: *This developmental abnormality is characterized by absence of the anterior bladder wall and part of the anterior abdominal wall.* The estimated frequency is 1 per 50,000 births. In some male infants, it is associated with **epispadias** (i.e., incomplete formation of the penile urethra).

Exstrophy of the bladder results in exposure of the posterior bladder wall to the exterior and transforms the bladder into a cup-like organ that cannot hold urine. The posterior wall of the bladder exposed to mechanical injury undergoes squamous or glandular metaplasia and is prone to frequent infection. Although exstrophy can be surgically repaired, the metaplastic mucosa has an increased risk of malignant transformation. In fact, the incidence of bladder cancer is increased even in persons who have lived for 50 to 60 years after surgical repair of exstrophy.

CONGENITAL INCOMPETENCE OF THE VESICOURE-TERAL VALVE: This anomaly results from an abnormal junction between the ureters and the urinary bladder and results in vesicourinary reflux (VUR) (see also Chapter 16). **VUR** is more common in young girls than in boys and is often familial. In 75% of cases, VUR is asymptomatic, but it may lead to reflux pyelonephritis. Congenital VUR is distinguished from the acquired form that occurs during pregnancy or in conditions associated with bladder hypertrophy.

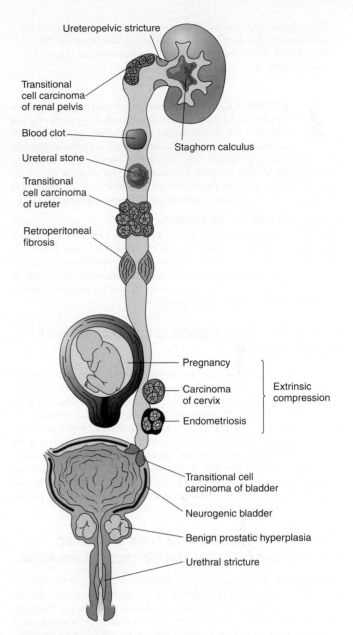

Ureteropelvic stricture

Transitional cell carcinoma of renal pelvis

Blood clot

Staghorn calculus

Ureteral stone

Transitional cell carcinoma of ureter

Retroperitoneal fibrosis

Pregnancy

Carcinoma of cervix — Extrinsic compression

Endometriosis

Transitional cell carcinoma of bladder

Neurogenic bladder

Benign prostatic hyperplasia

Urethral stricture

FIGURE 17-1. Most common causes of ureteral obstruction.

Cystitis

Cystitis is inflammation of the bladder, which may be acute or chronic. It is the most common urinary tract infection and is often seen as a nosocomial infection in hospitalized patients.

 PATHOGENESIS: In most cases, cystitis is secondary to infection of the lower urinary tract. Factors related to bladder infection include the age and gender of the patient, presence of bladder calculi, bladder outlet obstruction, diabetes mellitus, immunodeficiency, prior instrumentation or catheterization, radiation therapy, and chemotherapy. The risk of cystitis is increased in females because of a short urethra, especially during pregnancy. Bladder outlet obstruction secondary to prostatic hyperplasia predisposes men to cystitis.

Coliform bacteria are the most common cause of cystitis, mostly *E. coli, Proteus vulgaris, Pseudomonas aeruginosa,* and

Enterobacter spp. Virtually unknown in the Western world, schistosomiasis as a cause of cystitis is common in North Africa and the Middle East, where *S. haematobium* is endemic (see Chapter 9).

PATHOLOGY: Stromal edema, hemorrhage, and a neutrophilic infiltrate of variable intensity are typical of acute cystitis. Lack of resolution of the inflammatory reaction is associated with the hallmarks of chronic inflammation, including a predominance of lymphocytes (Fig. 17-2) and fibrosis of the lamina propria. Occasionally, the mucosa of the inflamed bladder contains numerous lymphocytic follicles (**follicular cystitis**) or dense infiltrates of eosinophils (**eosinophilic cystitis**).

CLINICAL FEATURES: Virtually all patients with acute or chronic cystitis complain of excessive urinary frequency, painful urination (**dysuria**), and lower abdominal or pelvic discomfort. Examination of urine usually reveals inflammatory cells and the causative agent can be identified by urine culture. Most cases of cystitis respond well to treatment with antimicrobial agents.

Chronic Interstitial Cystitis is a Special Form of Chronic Cystitis

Chronic intersitial cystitis is a disorder of unknown cause, which typically affects middle-aged women, features transmural inflammation of the bladder wall, and is occasionally associated with mucosal ulceration (*Hunner ulcer*). Chronic inflammation, including increased numbers of mast cells, and fibrosis are commonly observed in the mucosa and muscularis. A Hunner ulcer displays an intense acute inflammatory reaction. The most common symptoms of chronic interstitial cystitis are long-standing suprapubic pain, frequency, and urgency, with or without hematuria. Urine cultures are usually negative. The disease is typically persistent and refractory to all forms of therapy.

Malakoplakia is an Unusual Form of Bladder Inflammation Featuring Macrophage Accumulation

Malakoplakia is an uncommon inflammatory disorder of unknown etiology, which is identified by the accumulation of characteristic macrophages. The disorder, originally described in the bladder, has since been seen in numerous other sites, both within and outside the urinary tract. Malakoplakia is found in all age groups, and the peak frequency is in the fifth to seventh decades. There is a marked female preponderance, regardless of the site. Malakoplakia is often associated with urinary tract infection by *E. coli*, although a direct causal relationship is dubious. A clinical background of immunosuppression, chronic infections, or cancer is common.

PATHOLOGY: Malakoplakia is characterized by soft, yellow plaques on the mucosal surface of the bladder (Fig. 17-3). Histologically, the most striking feature is a chronic inflammatory cell infiltrate composed predominantly of large macrophages with abundant, eosinophilic cytoplasm, which contains periodic acid–Schiff positive granules (von Hansemann cells). Some of these macrophages exhibit laminated calcium-salt containing bodies termed **Michaelis-Gutmann bodies**. Ultrastructurally, these granules are engorged lysosomes that contain fragments of bacteria, suggesting that malakoplakia may reflect an acquired defect in lysosomal degradation. The clinical symptomatology of malakoplakia is indistinguishable from that of other forms of chronic cystitis, and treatment is ineffective.

Benign Proliferative and Metaplastic Urothelial Lesions

Benign proliferative and metaplastic lesions of urothelium occur mostly in the urinary bladder but may be found in the entire urinary tract. These nonneoplastic lesions are characterized by hyperplasia or by combined hyperplasia and metaplasia (Fig. 17-4). They are found mostly in association with chronic inflammation caused by urinary tract infections, calculi, neurogenic bladder, and (rarely) bladder exstrophy. They are also occasionally observed in the absence of any pre-existing inflammatory condition.

- **Brunn buds and nests** are bulbous invaginations or nests of the surface urothelium into (or in) the lamina propria. They are found in more than 85% of bladders and are considered normal variants of the urothelium.
- **Cystic lesions of the urinary bladder** (**cystitis cystica**) appear as fluid-filled, grouped, cystic Brunn nests lined by normal transitional epithelium. Similar cysts can be seen in the urethra or the ureter (**urethritis cystica, ureteritis cystica**). Cystitis cystica is common, found histologically in 60% of otherwise normal bladders.
- **Cystitis glandularis** is a mucosal lesion characterized by glandular structures lined by mucin-secreting, columnar epithelial cells, frequently in proximity to Brunn nests and cystitis cystica.
- **Squamous metaplasia** is a reaction to chronic injury and inflammation, particularly when it is associated with calculi. It is now apparent that squamous metaplasia of the urinary tract,

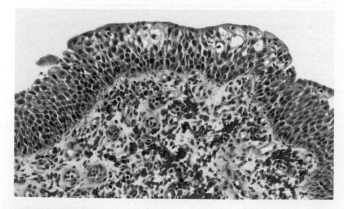

FIGURE 17-2. **Chronic cystitis.** A nonspecific inflammatory infiltrate composed of lymphocytes and plasma cells is present in the edematous lamina propria.

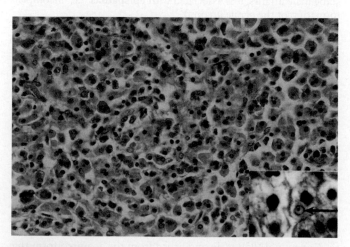

FIGURE 17-3. **Malakoplakia.** Inflammatory cells are composed principally of macrophages, with fewer lymphocytes. *(inset)* A Michaelis-Gutmann body *(arrow)* is seen at high magnification.

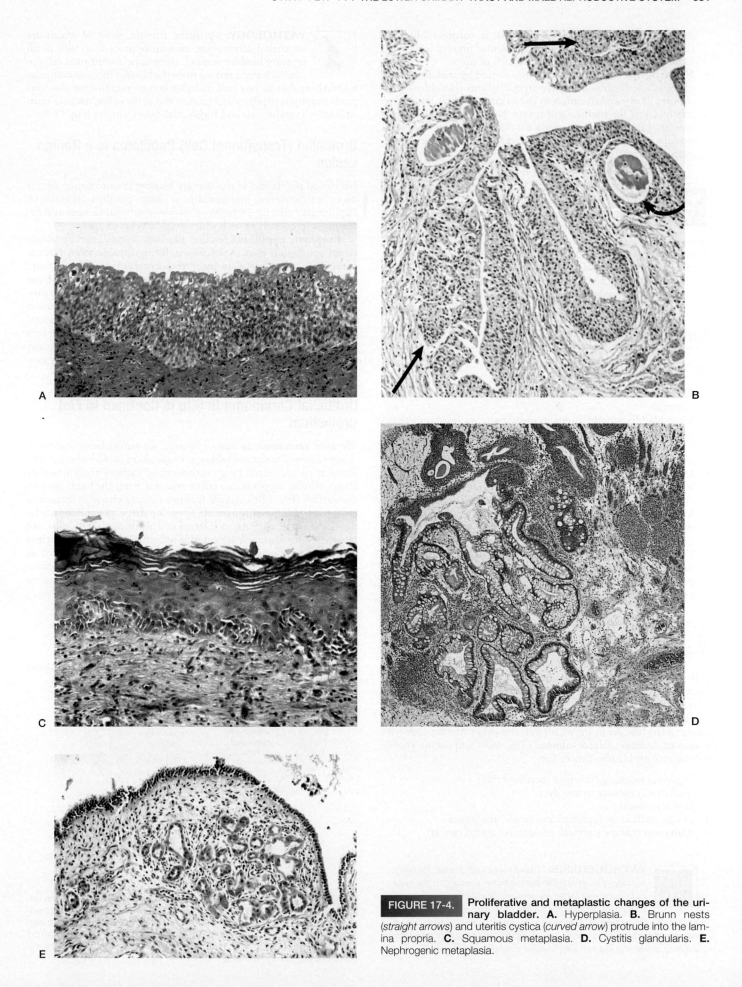

FIGURE 17-4. **Proliferative and metaplastic changes of the urinary bladder. A.** Hyperplasia. **B.** Brunn nests (*straight arrows*) and uteritis cystica (*curved arrow*) protrude into the lamina propria. **C.** Squamous metaplasia. **D.** Cystitis glandularis. **E.** Nephrogenic metaplasia.

presumably associated with infections, is considerably more common than previously appreciated and is present in as many as 50% of normal adult women and 10% of men.

- **Nephrogenic metaplasia** is a lesion caused by transformation of transitional epithelium into an epithelium resembling renal tubules. It is most common in the urinary bladder but is seen less often in the urethra and ureter. Numerous small tubules clustered in the lamina propria produce a papillary exophytic nodule. These may obstruct the ureters, in which case they require surgical treatment.

CLINICAL FEATURES: Proliferative and metaplastic urothelial lesions are of limited clinical significance. However, patients with these changes are at greater risk for urothelial bladder carcinoma and, in the case of cystitis glandularis, of adenocarcinoma as well. Yet there is no evidence to suggest that these lesions themselves are preneoplastic. Rather, the persistence of the injury that leads to the proliferative and metaplastic urothelial lesions is more likely the important factor in the pathogenesis of bladder cancer.

Tumors of the Urinary Bladder

The most important facts about bladder cancer are as follows:

- The urinary bladder is the most common site of urinary tract tumors.
- Most bladder tumors occur in older patients (median age, 65 years) and are rare in individuals under the age of 50 years.
- Tumors are more than three times as common in men as in women.
- Most tumors are microscopically classified as urothelial (transitional cell) neoplasms. Squamous cell carcinomas, adenocarcinomas, neuroendocrine carcinomas, and sarcomas are rare.
- Most tumors are malignant, but their aggressiveness and prognosis vary, depending on the clinical stage and microscopic grade and type of each tumor.
- Tumors are often multifocal and can occur in any part of the urinary tract lined by transitional epithelium, from the renal pelvis to the posterior urethra.
- Surgical treatment is often followed by tumor recurrence.

EPIDEMIOLOGY: Approximately 60,000 new cases of bladder cancer are diagnosed every year in the United States, accounting for 1% to 3% of all cancer-related deaths. Bladder cancer shows significant geographic and gender differences throughout the world. The highest frequencies are among urban white males in the United States and western Europe, whereas a low prevalence occurs in Japan and among American blacks. A high incidence of squamous cell carcinoma of the bladder in Egypt, Sudan, and other African countries is due to endemic schistosomiasis. The most important known risk factors for bladder cancer are:

- Cigarette smoking (fourfold increased risk)
- Industrial exposure to azo dyes
- Schistosomiasis
- Drugs, such as cyclophosphamide and analgesics
- Radiation therapy (cervical, prostate, or rectal cancer)

PATHOGENESIS: *Today, cigarette smoke (possibly because of its polycyclic hydrocarbon content) is the most important risk factor for urinary bladder carcinoma and is likely to account for nearly 50% and 30% of mortality rates from this cancer in American men and women, respectively. A variety of industrial chemicals and dyestuffs, most notably aromatic amines, are also associated with bladder cancer (see Chapter 5).*

PATHOLOGY: Epithelial tumors, most of which are urothelial carcinomas, constitute more than 98% of all primary bladder tumors. Neoplastic transitional cell epithelial lesions arising from the bladder mucosa comprise a spectrum that at one end includes benign papillomas and low-grade exophytic papillary carcinomas and at the other, invasive transitional cell carcinomas and highly malignant tumors (Fig. 17-5).

Urothelial (Transitional Cell) Papilloma is a Benign Lesion

Urothelial papilloma of the urinary bladder is uncommon and is often encountered incidentally or after painless hematuria. Papillomas make up 2% to 3% of bladder epithelial tumors and occur most frequently in men older than 50 years of age.

Exophytic papilloma features papillary fronds lined by transitional epithelium that is virtually indistinguishable from normal urothelium. Tumors that meet this criterion are uncommon. **Inverted papillomas** are covered by normal urothelium, from which cords of transitional epithelium descend into the lamina propria. Recurrences in treated exophytic papillomas are common (70%), and invasive carcinoma develops in 7% of patients. Transitional cell papillomas are not malignant, but they arise in a mucosa that is abnormal. Evolving tumors may be seen on repeated examinations for years. In most cases, "recurrences" represent new tumors that develop elsewhere in the urinary bladder.

Urothelial Carcinoma In Situ is Confined to Flat Urothelium

The term **carcinoma in situ** *is reserved for full-thickness, malignant changes confined to flat urothelium in nonpapillary bladder mucosa.* The lesion is characterized by a urothelium of variable thickness that shows cellular atypia of the entire mucosa, from the basal layer to the surface (Fig. 17-6). Atypia features nuclear changes, including enlargement, hyperchromatism, irregular shape, prominent nucleoli, and coarse chromatin. Occasional multinucleated cells are present. A disorganized appearance reflecting variation in nuclear polarity is a constant feature. In one third of cases, carcinoma in situ of the bladder is associated with subsequent invasive carcinoma. In turn, most invasive transitional cell carcinomas arise

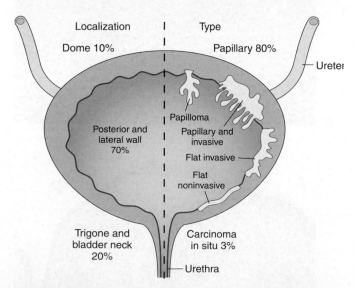

FIGURE 17-5. **Urothelial neoplasms.** Most tumors occur in the urinary bladder and are classified histologically as transitional cell carcinomas (TCCs). Ureters and the posterior urethra are also lined by transitional epithelium and can give rise to TCCs. TCCs can be flat, papillary, papillary and invasive, or simply invasive. Benign transitional cell papillomas are rare.

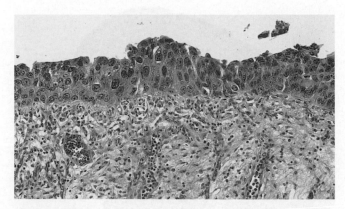

FIGURE 17-6. **Urothelial carcinoma in situ.** The urothelial mucosa shows nuclear pleomorphism and lack of polarity from the basal layer to the surface, without evidence of maturation.

TABLE 17–1
TNM Staging of Urothelial Carcinoma of the Urinary Bladder
T—Primary tumor
T0 = No grossly visible tumor
Ta = Noninvasive papillary carcinoma
Tis = Carcinoma in situ
T1 = Invasion of the lamina propria
T2 = Invasion of the muscularis propria
T2a = Superficial invasion of the muscularis (inner half)
T2b = Invasion of deep muscle (outer half)
T3 = Invasion of the perivesical tissue
T4 = Extravesical spread into adjacent organs or distant metastases
N—Regional lymph nodes
N0 = No lymph node involvement
N1 = Single lymph node metastasis
N2, N3 = More lymph nodes involved
M—Distant metastases
M0 = No metastases
M1 = Distant metastases

from carcinoma in situ rather than from papillary transitional cell cancers. When confined to the bladder, transitional cell carcinoma in situ is currently treated with intravesical chemotherapy agents or the bacillus Calmette-Guérin (BCG) vaccine. Patients are followed closely for signs of invasion, which requires radical surgery.

Urothelial Carcinoma Ranges from Superficial Papillary to Deeply Invasive

Bladder cancers vary from exophytic, without invasion to flat and deeply penetrating.

 PATHOLOGY: Papillary cancer arises most frequently from the lateral or posterior bladder walls. At cystoscopy, tumors may be small, delicate, low-grade papillary lesions limited to the mucosal surface or larger, higher-grade, solid invasive masses, which are often ulcerated (Fig. 17-7). Papillary and exophytic cancers tend to be better differentiated; infiltrating tumors are usually more anaplastic.

Bladder cancers are staged according to the TNM classification system (Table 17-1). Histologically, these tumors are classified as either **low- or high-grade papillary urothelial carcinomas**. (Fig. 17-8A–D). In about 10% of low-grade disease, there is invasion of the lamina propria or the muscle layer of the bladder (muscularis propria). About 80% of all high-grade tumors show invasion into the lamina propria and less often into the muscularis propria or through the entire thickness of the bladder wall. In order of decreasing frequency, metastases of bladder cancer occur in regional and periaortic lymph nodes, liver, lung, and bone.

 CLINICAL FEATURES: Urothelial carcinoma of the bladder typically manifests as sudden **hematuria** and less frequently as **dysuria**. Cystoscopy reveals single or multiple tumors. At the time of initial presentation, 85% of tumors are confined to the urinary bladder, and 15% have regional or distant metastases. Papillary lesions limited to the mucosa (stage T0) or lamina propria (stage T1) are commonly treated conservatively by transurethral resection. Radical cystectomy is done for patients whose tumors show muscle invasion and occasionally for advanced-stage tumors.

Nonurothelial Forms of Bladder Cancer are Rare

Squamous cell carcinoma of the bladder develops in foci of squamous metaplasia, usually due to schistosomiasis. Virtually all patients with this tumor demonstrate bladder wall invasion at the time of initial presentation and thus have a poor prognosis.

Adenocarcinoma accounts for only 1% of all malignant tumors of the bladder. It originates from foci of cystitis glandularis or intestinal metaplasia or from remnants of urachal epithelium in the bladder dome. Most bladder adenocarcinomas are deeply invasive at the time of initial presentation and are not curable.

PENIS, URETHRA, AND SCROTUM

Congenital Disorders of the Penis

HYPOSPADIAS: *This term refers to a congenital anomaly in which the urethra opens on the underside (ventral surface) of the penis, so that the meatus is proximal to its normal glandular location.* In 90% of cases, the meatus is located on the underside of the glans or the corona. Less often, it is found along the midshaft of the penis, in the scrotum, and even in the perineum. It results from incomplete closure of the urethral folds of the urogenital sinus. Hypospadias has a frequency of 1 in 350 male neonates. Most cases are sporadic, but a familial occurrence has been noted. It also shows an association with other urogenital anomalies and complex, multisystemic, developmental syndromes. Surgical repair is usually uncomplicated.

EPISPADIAS: *In this rare congenital anomaly, the urethra opens on the upper side (dorsal surface) of the penis.* In the most common form of epispadias, the entire penile urethra is open along the entire shaft. Severe epispadias may be associated with bladder exstrophy. In its mildest form, the defect is limited to the glandular

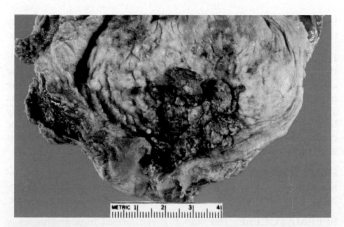

FIGURE 17-7. **Urothelial carcinoma of the urinary bladder.** A large exophytic tumor is situated above the bladder neck.

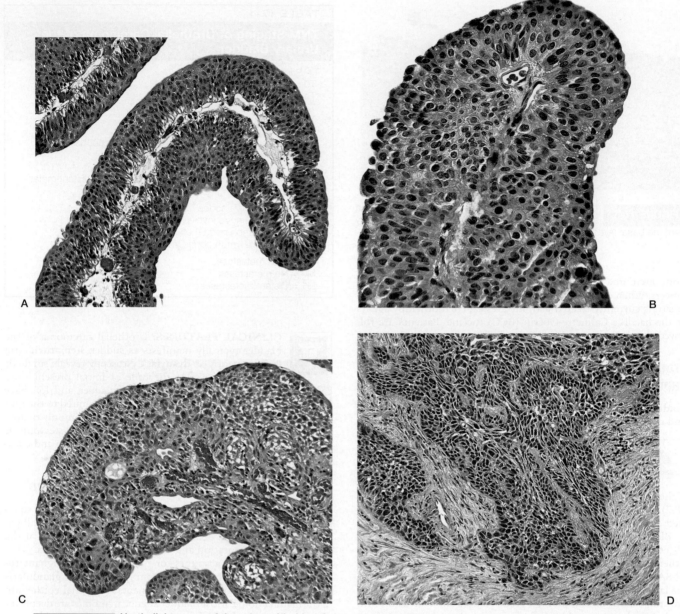

FIGURE 17-8. **Urothelial tumors of the urinary bladder. A.** Low-grade papillary urothelial carcinoma consists of exophytic papillae that have a central connective tissue core and are lined by slightly disorganized transitional epithelium. **B.** Low-grade papillary urothelial carcinoma at higher magnification shows mild architectural and cytologic atypia. **C.** High-grade papillary urothelial carcinoma shows prominent architectural disorganization of the epithelium, which contains cells with pleomorphic hyperchromatic nuclei. **D.** Invasive high-grade papillary urothelial carcinoma consists of irregular nests of hyperchromatic cells invading into the muscularis.

urethra. Surgical treatment of epispadias is more complicated than that of hypospadias.

PHIMOSIS: *The orifice of the prepuce may be too narrow to allow retraction over the glans penis.* Phimosis predisposes the penis to infections. If a narrow prepuce is forcefully retracted, it may strangulate the glans and impede the outflow of venous blood, a condition termed **paraphimosis**. Congenital phimosis must be distinguished from acquired phimosis, which is usually a consequence of recurrent infections or trauma of the prepuce in uncircumcised men. Circumcision cures both phimosis and paraphimosis.

Scrotal Masses

Scrotal masses and conditions that lead to scrotal swelling or enlargement often reflect abnormalities of testicular, epididymal, and scrotal development. Clinical problems related to these patho-

logic conditions are most often encountered in children but may be found in adults (Fig. 17-9A–D).

HYDROCELE: This term refers to a collection of serous fluid in the scrotal sac between the two layers of the tunica vaginalis. The cavity is lined by mesothelium. A hydrocele may be congenital (the most common cause of scrotal swelling in infants) or acquired as a result of infection, tumor, or trauma. Hydroceles are generally benign, but long-standing disease may cause testicular atrophy or compression of the epididymis, or the fluid may become infected and lead to **periorchitis**.

HEMATOCELE: *An accumulation of blood between the layers of the tunica vaginalis* may develop after trauma or hemorrhage into a hydrocele. Testicular tumors and infections may also lead to a hematocele.

SPERMATOCELE: *This mass is a cyst formed from protrusions of widened efferent ducts of the rete testis or epididymis.* It manifests as a hilar paratesticular nodule or a fluctuating mass filled with milky fluid. The cyst is lined by cuboidal epithelium that contains spermatozoa in various stages of degeneration.

VARICOCELE: Dilation of testicular veins appears as a nodularity on the lateral side of the scrotum. Most are asymptomatic and are discovered during physical examination of infertile men. A varicocele is considered a common cause of infertility and oligospermia. Testicular atrophy is found only rarely and only in long-standing disease. Surgical resection by ligation of the internal spermatic vein often improves reproductive function.

Inflammatory Disorders

The most important inflammatory conditions affecting the penis are (1) sexually transmitted diseases; (2) nonspecific infections; (3) diseases of unknown etiology, such as balanitis xerotica obliterans; (4) dermatoses (see Chapter 24); and (5) dermatitis involving the shaft of the penis and scrotum. Sexually transmitted diseases are reviewed in detail in Chapter 9.

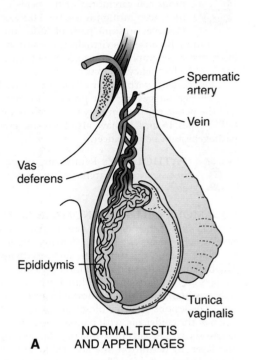

A NORMAL TESTIS AND APPENDAGES

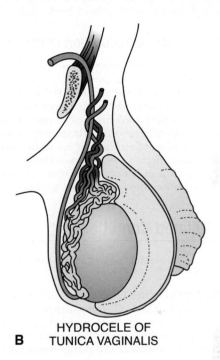

B HYDROCELE OF TUNICA VAGINALIS

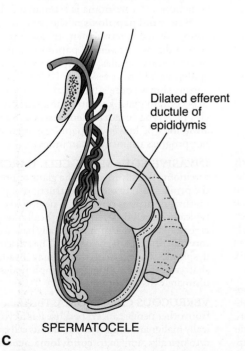

C SPERMATOCELE

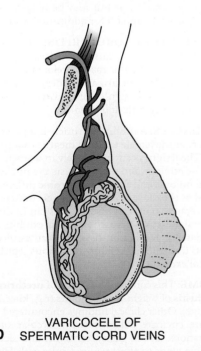

D VARICOCELE OF SPERMATIC CORD VEINS

FIGURE 17-9. Scrotal masses. **A.** Normal testis. **B.** Hydrocele. **C.** Spermatocele. **D.** Varicocele.

Balanitis is Inflammation of the Glans of the Penis

In uncircumcised men, balanitis usually extends from the glans to the foreskin and is called **balanoposthitis**. Most often, it is caused by bacteria, but in immunosuppressed individuals and in diabetics, it can also be caused by fungi. Balanitis is typically a result of poor hygiene. Significant complications of chronic balanoposthitis are meatal stricture, phimosis, and paraphimosis.

BALANITIS XEROTICA OBLITERANS: This chronic inflammatory condition of unknown origin is characterized by fibrosis and sclerosis of subepithelial connective tissue. The affected portion of the glans is white and indurated. Fibrosis may constrict the urethral meatus or cause phimosis. This condition is equivalent to lichen sclerosus et atrophicus of the vulva (see Chapter 18).

Peyronie Disease is a Fibrous Induration of the Penis

Peyronie disease is a malady of unknown etiology characterized by focal, asymmetric fibrosis of the penile shaft. Penile curvature (penile strabismus) results, accompanied by pain during erection. The penile shaft demonstrates an ill-defined induration of the shaft with no change in the overlying skin. On microscopic examination, dense fibrosis is associated with sparse, nonspecific, chronic inflammatory infiltration. Collagen focally replaces muscle in the septum of the corpus cavernosum. Peyronie disease affects 1% of men over the age of 40, but in most instances, it is mild and does not interfere with sexual function. This disorder is more common in chronic alcoholics.

Urethritis and Related Conditions

Urethritis is inflammation of the urethra, which may be either acute or chronic.

SEXUALLY TRANSMITTED URETHRITIS: Urethritis is the most common manifestation of sexually transmitted diseases in men, in whom it typically presents with urethral discharge. Women rarely notice distinct urethral discharge and usually complain of vaginal discharge. **Gonococcal and nongonococcal** urethritis have an acute onset and are related to recent sexual intercourse. Nongonococcal urethritis is mostly caused by *Chlamydia trachomatis* or *Ureaplasma urealyticum* but may be related to a variety of other pathogens. See Chapter 9 for additional details.

NONSPECIFIC INFECTIOUS URETHRITIS: Uropathogens such as *E. coli* and *Pseudomonas* can cause urethritis. Typically, infection is associated with cystitis but may be related to other diseases (e.g., prostatic hyperplasia or urinary stones). In men, infectious urethritis may be the only sign of prostatitis; in women, it may be a complication of vaginitis and vulvitis.

URETHRAL CARUNCLES: A urethral caruncle is a polypoid inflammatory lesions near the female urethral meatus that produces pain and bleeding. The lesions occur exclusively in women, mostly after menopause. The etiology and pathogenesis are unclear; prolapse of the urethral mucosa and associated chronic inflammation have been suggested as the cause. Urethral caruncle presents as an exophytic, often ulcerated, polypoid mass, 1 to 2 cm in diameter, at or near the urethral meatus. Microscopically, it exhibits acutely and chronically inflamed granulation tissue as well as ulceration and hyperplasia of transitional cell or squamous epithelium. Treatment is surgical excision.

REITER SYNDROME: This condition is a triad of **urethritis, conjunctivitis, and arthritis** of weight-bearing joints (e.g., knee, sacroiliac and vertebral joints). Other clinical findings encountered in variable proportions are circinate balanitis (with circular or linear plaque-like discolorations on the glans), cervicitis, and skin eruptions. Reiter syndrome tends to affect young adults with HLA-B27. Symptoms usually appear a few weeks after chlamydial urethritis or enteric infection with such pathogens as *Shigella, Salmonella,* or

Campylobacter. It is thus thought to represent an inappropriate immune reaction to unknown microbial antigen(s). Symptoms usually disappear spontaneously over 3 to 6 months, but arthritis recurs in half of patients (see also Chapter 26).

Cancer of the Penis

Cancer of the penis originates from the squamous mucosa of the glans and contiguous urethral meatus or the prepuce and skin covering the penile shaft.

 EPIDEMIOLOGY: In the United States, invasive squamous cell carcinoma of the penis is an uncommon tumor, accounting for less than 0.5% of all cancers in men. However, in some parts of Africa and Asia, it is 20 times as common. Because it is virtually unknown in men circumcised at birth, these geographic variations have been attributed to differences in the frequency of circumcision.

Most patients with cancer of the penis have had phimosis since an early age, suggesting that prolonged contact between smegma and the penile epithelium may play a role. Human papillomavirus (HPV) types 16 and 18 have also been suggested as factors in the pathogenesis of penile cancer.

 PATHOLOGY: Penile carcinoma occurs in a preinvasive form (carcinoma in situ) and an invasive variety.

SQUAMOUS CELL CARCINOMA IN SITU: Historically, carcinoma in situ of the penis was described in two forms: **Bowen disease**, which appears as a sharply demarcated, erythematous or grayish-white plaque on the shaft, and **erythroplasia of Queyrat**, which manifests as solitary or multiple, shiny, soft, erythematous plaques on the glans and foreskin. Both forms appear microscopically as **squamous cell carcinoma in situ**, similar to that in other sites. The lesions show cytologic atypia of the keratinocytes of all layers of the epidermis, with parakeratosis or hyperkeratosis; papillomatosis with broad epidermal papillae; and thinning of the granular layer. By definition, the atypical keratinocytes do not invade the underlying dermis. Chronic inflammation may be present in the subjacent dermis. The frequency of progression to invasive squamous cell carcinoma is estimated to be less than 10% of cases.

Bowenoid papulosis of the penis is caused by HPV and affects young, sexually active men. In contrast to the solitary lesion of Bowen disease, bowenoid papulosis appears as multiple brownish or violaceous papules, which are sharply demarcated from normal epidermis and thus resemble HPV-induced warts. The altered epidermis shows some superficial stratification and maturation and may contain giant keratinocytes with multinucleated atypical nuclei. HPV type 16 can be demonstrated in 80% of patients. Virtually all lesions of bowenoid papulosis regress spontaneously and do not progress to invasive carcinoma.

INVASIVE SQUAMOUS CELL CARCINOMA: Squamous cell carcinoma usually involves the glans or prepuce and less commonly, the penile shaft. Extensive destruction of penile tissue, including the urethral meatus, is observed in neglected cases. Microscopically, it is typically a well-differentiated, focally keratinizing, squamous cell carcinoma. Invasive tumors usually have a dense, chronic inflammatory cell infiltrate in the dermis. The adjacent epidermis often shows dysplastic changes. The tumor may invade deeply along the penile shaft and spread to inguinal lymph nodes, then to iliac nodes and ultimately distant organs.

VERRUCOUS CARCINOMA: This tumor deserves to be separated from other penile cancers because it is a cytologically benign but clinically malignant exophytic squamous cell carcinoma. It is grossly and cytologically similar to **condyloma acuminatum** (benign HPV-induced penile warts), but unlike such warts, verrucous carcinoma shows local invasion. This low-grade squamous cell carcinoma usually does not metastasize, and surgical removal is curative.

CLINICAL FEATURES: Most squamous cell cancers are confined to the penis at the time of initial presentation, but occult metastases to inguinal lymph nodes are not uncommon. Patients with superficially invasive cancer have a 90% 5-year survival rate; inguinal lymph node metastases reduce 5-year survival to 20% to 50%. Amputation of the penis is usually necessary

TESTIS, EPIDIDYMIS, AND VAS DEFERENS

Cryptorchidism

*Cryptorchidism, clinically known as **undescended testis**, is a congenital abnormality in which one or both testes are not found in their normal position in the scrotum.* In 5% of male infants born at term and 30% of those born prematurely, the testes are not in the scrotum or are easily retracted. In the large majority of these infants, testes descend into the scrotum during the first year of life. Cryptorchidism is usually unilateral but is bilateral in 30% of affected men.

 PATHOGENESIS: The causes of testicular maldescent are usually unknown, but theoretically the condition could be related to (1) developmental disorders of the gonad, (2) endocrine factors, or (3) mechanical factors that prevent passage of the fetal testis through the inguinal canal.

 PATHOLOGY: Testicular descent may be arrested at any point from the abdominal cavity to the upper scrotum (Fig. 17-10). Cryptorchid testes are smaller than normal even at an early age, and the difference between the affected and the normal testis becomes more prominent with age. Such testes appear firm, as a result of parenchymal fibrosis. The histology of cryptorchid testes varies with age. In infancy and early childhood, the seminiferous tubules in the affected testes are smaller and have fewer germ cells than normal. Postpubertal testes also contain fewer germ cells than normal, and spermatogenesis is limited to a minority of tubules. Hyaline thickening of tubular basement membranes and prominent stromal fibrosis are observed (Fig. 17-11). Eventually, tubules become devoid of spermatogenic cells and are entirely hyalinized. **Orchiopexy** (surgical placement of a testis into the scrotum) performed either in childhood or after puberty does not prevent the loss of seminiferous epithelium and tubules.

 CLINICAL FEATURES: The clinical significance is related to an increased incidence of **infertility** and **germ cell neoplasia**. All men with bilateral cryptorchid testes have **azoospermia** and are infertile. Unilateral cryptorchidism

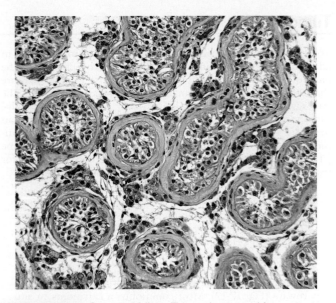

FIGURE 17-11. **Cryptorchidism.** This testis removed from a postpubertal man shows markedly thickened hyalinized basement membrane of seminiferous tubules, which show no signs of spermatogenesis.

is associated with **oligospermia**, defined as a sperm count below 20 million/mL, in 40% of cases. Most urologists recommend orchiopexy between the ages of 6 months and 1 year, but it is not clear whether this treatment improves the eventual sperm count.

Cryptorchidism is associated with a 20- to 40-fold greater-than-normal risk for testicular cancer. Intra-abdominal testes are at higher risk than those retained in the inguinal canal; in turn, inguinal testes are at higher risk than those high in the scrotum. The contralateral, normally descended testis is also at risk, but its incidence of cancer is only four times that in normal men. Unfortunately, orchiopexy does not reduce cancer risk.

Orchitis

Orchitis is acute or chronic inflammation of the testis. It may be part of epididymo-orchitis, usually caused by ascending infection, or it may occur as an isolated testicular inflammation. **Gram-negative bacterial orchitis** is the most common form of the disease. It is often secondary to urinary tract infection and is typically associated with epididymitis. Infection may also manifest as intratesticular abscess or peritesticular suppuration and fibrosis. Syphilis and mumps can produce orchitis, although immunization has reduced the frequency of the latter. **Granulomatous orchitis** of unknown cause is an infrequent disorder of middle-aged men that presents acutely as painful testicular enlargement or insidiously as testicular induration. It is characterized microscopically by noncaseating granulomas that fail to reveal either organisms or sperm remnants that might act as inciting agents.

Torsion of the Testis

Torsion of the spermatic cord, if complete, produces severe pain and infarction of the testicular germ cells within a few hours. Torsion often presents after vigorous physical activity and may be associated with a congenital abnormality that allows excess mobility of the testis. An abrupt onset of scrotal pain followed by swelling accompanies torsion. The swollen testis shows the gross and microscopic features of hemorrhagic infarction. Reduction of torsion within 6 hours usually leads to complete recovery, but delay in reduction by 12 to 24 hours may be associated with severe or total loss of testicular viability.

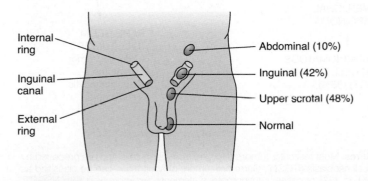

Internal ring
Inguinal canal
External ring

Abdominal (10%)
Inguinal (42%)
Upper scrotal (48%)
Normal

FIGURE 17-10. **Cryptorchidism.** In most instances, the testis has an upper scrotal location or is retained in the inguinal canal.

Tumors of the Testis

Tumors of the testis account for less than 1% of all malignancies in adult males. Testicular tumors are classified histogenetically on the basis of their cell of origin into several groups (Table 17-2).More than 90% of these tumors are malignant and of germ cell origin. The etiology of testicular tumors is unknown. Such tumors are five times more common among Americans of European descent than in blacks. The only consistent cytogenetic abnormality found in tumors is an additional fragment of chromosome 12 (isochromosome p12). As discussed previously, the only documented risk factors for testicular tumors are **cryptorchidism and gonadal dysgenesis**.

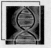 **PATHOGENESIS:** Malignant transformation of germ cells may occur as early as during fetal development. However, because germ cell tumors rarely occur before puberty, malignant transformation may present in the peripubertal period and involve spermatogonia that are stimulated hormonally to proliferate and differentiate into spermatocytes. Germ cell tumors progress through two pathways (Fig. 17-12). Most commonly, a carcinoma in situ

TABLE 17-2
Testicular Tumors
Germ cell tumors: 90%
Seminoma (40%)
Nonseminomatous germ cell tumors
Embryonal carcinoma (5%)
Teratocarcinoma (35%)
Choriocarcinoma (<1%)
Mixed germ cell tumors (15%)
Teratoma (1%)
Spermatocytic seminoma (1%)
Yolk sac tumor of infancy (2%)
Sex cord cell tumors: 5%
Leydig cell tumors (60%)
Sertoli cell tumors
Metastases: 5%

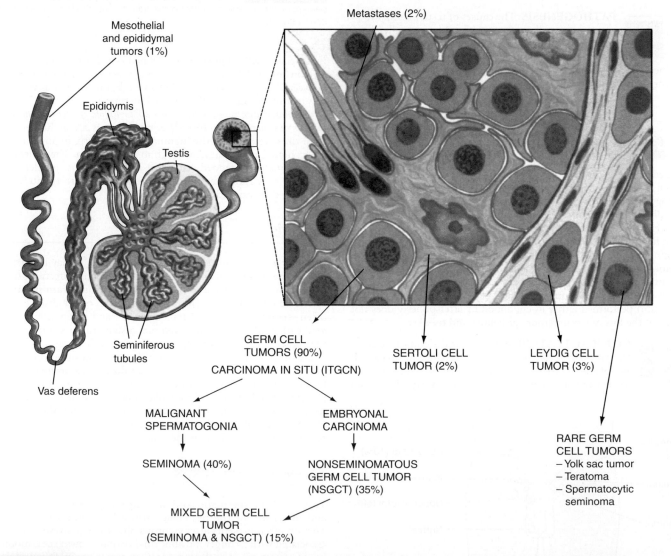

FIGURE 17-12. **Tumors of the testis, epididymis, and related structures.** Most testicular tumors originate from germ cells and are preceded by a carcinoma in situ stage known as intratubular germ cell neoplasia (ITGCN). Germ cell tumors of adult testis can be classified as seminomas (40%) or nonseminomatous germ cell tumors (NSGCTs) (35%). In 15% of cases, seminomatous elements are intermixed with NSGCT, forming mixed germ cell tumors. Some germ cell tumors (yolk sac tumor of childhood, childhood teratomas, and spermatocytic seminomas) develop without passing through a preinvasive ITGCN stage. Tumors originating from sex cord stromal cells (Leydig and Sertoli cell tumors), epididymal tumors, tumors of the mesothelial lining of the tunica vaginalis (adenomatoid tumors), and metastases are rare.

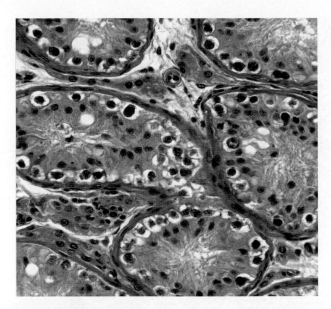

FIGURE 17-13. Intratubular germ cell neoplasia (ITGCN). The seminiferous tubules show no signs of spermatogenesis but instead contain large atypical cells corresponding to intratubular carcinoma in situ.

stage, also known as **intratubular testicular germ cell neoplasia** (ITGCN), precedes and progresses to invasive carcinoma (see below), accounting for most **adult** germ cell tumors.

Tumor cells of ITGCN resemble spermatogonia or fetal germ cells but have much larger polyploid nuclei (Fig.17-13). Like fetal germ cells, these cells express placental-like alkaline phosphatase on their surface. In infertile men with a history of cryptorchid testes, ITGCN can persist unchanged for 5 to 10 years before acquiring invasive properties and producing infiltrating malignant tumors. The malignant cells that retain the phenotypic features of spermatogonia give rise to **seminomas**. Alternatively, the neoplastic germ cells can differentiate into malignant embryonic cells (**embryonal carcinoma**).

In some cases, embryonal carcinoma cells proliferate in an undifferentiated form. In others, they differentiate into the three embryonic germ layers (ectoderm, mesoderm, endoderm) or extraembryonic tissues that form the fetal membranes and the placenta. The extraembryonic derivatives of embryonal carcinoma cells give rise to chorionic epithelium (cytotrophoblast and syncytiotrophoblast) and yolk sac-like epithelium. These complex tumors, composed of malignant, undifferentiated, embryonal carcinoma cells and their somatic and extraembryonic derivatives, are called **teratocarcinomas** or **malignant teratomas**. When embryonal carcinoma cells proliferate without further differentiating and exhibit a single histologic pattern, the tumor is labeled **embryonal carcinoma**. In rare instances, extraembryonic components of teratocarcinomas overgrow and destroy all other components. Such tumors are composed of a single tumor type and are classified as **yolk sac carcinoma** or **choriocarcinoma**. *For clinical purposes, all germ cell tumors with embryonal carcinoma as their malignant stem cells are termed **nonseminomatous germ cell tumors (NSGCTs)***, to distinguish them from seminomas. Pure yolk sac carcinomas of the adult testis and choriocarcinomas are also included in this group. In 15% of cases, germ cell tumors contain both seminoma and nonseminomatous elements. Such **mixed germ cell tumors** are treated clinically as nonseminomatous neoplasms.

Intratubular Germ Cell Neoplasia (ITGCN) Refers to Testicular Carcinoma In Situ

ITGCN is assumed to represent a preinvasive form of germ cell tumors because of the settings in which it occurs. ITGCN can be seen as (1) an iso-

lated focal histologic change in 2% of cryptorchid testes or testicular biopsies performed for infertility, (2) widespread carcinoma in situ adjacent to invasive germ cell tumors, and (3) lesions in 5% of contralateral testes in patients who had an orchiectomy for a testicular germ cell tumor.

 PATHOLOGY: ITGCN involves testes in a patchy manner, usually affecting less than 10% to 30% of the tubules. Seminiferous tubules harboring ITGCN have thick basement membranes and no sperm. The normal germ cells are replaced by neoplastic germ cells that are broadly attached to the basal lamina (see Fig. 17-13). The neoplastic cells appear larger than normal spermatogonia. Their nuclei are large, have finely dispersed chromatin, and display prominent nucleoli. The nuclei are centrally located and surrounded by abundant, clear cytoplasm that contains large amounts of glycogen. The nuclear DNA content is increased, suggesting that the cells are triploid. The plasma membrane is distinct and stains with antibodies to placental alkaline phosphatase (PLAP).

 CLINICAL FEATURES: ITGCN is a precursor of invasive carcinoma that develops at an unpredictable pace. Half of men with ITGCN will develop invasive cancer within 5 years, and 70% will develop it in 7 years. The diagnosis of ITGCN on testicular biopsy is an indication for prophylactic orchiectomy.

Seminoma Contains Monomorphous Cells that Resemble Spermatogonia

 EPIDEMIOLOGY: Seminoma, the most common testicular cancer, accounts for 40% of all germ cells tumors. The peak incidence is between 30 to 40 years of age. Seminomas are never found in prepubertal children, except in those who have dysgenetic gonads.

 PATHOLOGY: On gross examination, the tumors are solid, rubbery-firm, lumpy masses. Tumor tissue is usually sharply demarcated from normal testicular tissue, which may be compressed, atrophic, and fibrotic. On cross-section, seminomas appear lobulated and homogeneously tan or grayish-yellow (Fig. 17-14). Areas of necrosis or hemorrhage are usually inconspicuous but may be seen in larger tumors.

Microscopically, seminoma is equivalent to **ovarian dysgerminoma** (see Chapter 18). The tumor features a single population of uniform polygonal cells with centrally located vesicular nuclei. The ample cytoplasm may appear pale and eosinophilic or clear in standard histologic sections because it contains large amounts of glycogen and some lipid. Tumor cells are arranged as nests or sheets separated by fibrous septa infiltrated with lymphocytes, plasma cells, and macrophages. Occasionally, the septa contain granulomas with giant cells. Tumor cells invade the testicular parenchyma but also spread through the seminiferous tubules and into rete testis. Invasion of the epididymis is seen later in the disease, usually before spread to abdominal lymph nodes. Like fetal spermatogonia and primordial germ cells in the fetus, seminoma cells express PLAP on the plasma membrane. PLAP is shed into the blood in small amounts but cannot be used for diagnostic purposes.

 CLINICAL FEATURES: Seminoma manifests as a progressively growing scrotal mass and is usually diagnosed while it can still be cured by orchiectomy, with or without abdominal lymph node dissection. Seminomas are highly radiosensitive, and radiotherapy plays an important role in treating tumors that cannot be cured by surgery alone. Those in advanced stages of dissemination are treated with additional chemotherapy. *The cure rate for all histologic types of seminoma is greater than 90%.*

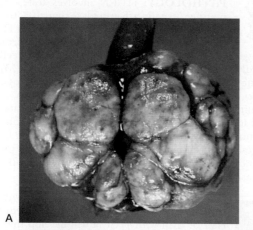

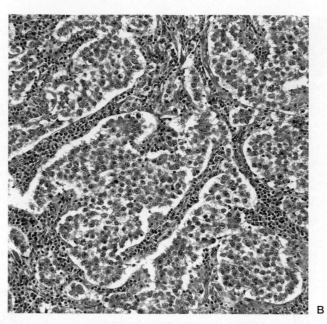

FIGURE 17-14. Seminoma. **A.** The cut surface of this nodular tumor is tan and bulging, suggesting that the tumor is firm and rubbery. **B.** Groups of tumor cells are surrounded by fibrous septa infiltrated with lymphocytes. Tumor cells have vesicular nuclei that are much larger than the small round nuclei of the lymphocytes.

Non-seminomatous Germ Cell Tumors (NSGCTs) are Derived from Embryonal Cells

NSGCTs of the testis include several additional pathologic entities, two of which account for most tumors: (1) pure embryonal carcinomas and (2) teratocarcinomas, also known as **malignant teratomas** or **mixed germ cell tumors**. Pure choriocarcinoma and pure yolk sac carcinoma of the adult testis are rare NSGCTs. Mixed germ cell tumors are NSGCTs combined with seminomas. NSGCTs constitute 55% of all testicular germ cell tumors, and teratocarcinomas account for two thirds of all NSGCTs Like seminomas, NSGCTs have peak incidence in the 25- to 40-year-old age group. At diagnosis, these patients are usually somewhat younger than those with seminomas.

 PATHOLOGY: Nonseminomatous tumors vary in size and shape and may be solid or partially cystic. Solid areas vary in color from white to yellow to red, indicating that they are composed of viable tumor cells, foci of necrosis, and hemorrhage, respectively (Fig. 17-15).

The histology of NSGCTs is highly variable. Pure embryonal carcinomas are composed exclusively of undifferentiated embryonal carcinoma cells similar to cells from preimplantation-stage embryos (Fig. 17-16). Because the tumor cells have little cytoplasm, their hyperchromatic, disproportionately large nuclei seem to overlap. Embryonal carcinoma cells may be arranged as broad solid sheets, cords, gland-like tubules and acini, and sometimes even papillary structures. Numerous mitoses and apoptotic cells are characteristic. Embryonal carcinoma invades the testis, epididymis, and blood vessels and metastasizes to abdominal lymph nodes, lungs, and other organs.

Embryonal carcinoma cells are the stem cells of **teratocarcinomas** (malignant teratomas), which feature differentiated somatic elements (i.e., tissues that are normally found in various organs

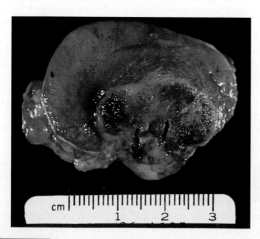

FIGURE 17-15. **Nonseminomatous germ cell tumor of the testis.** The cut surface of this small testicular tumor shows considerable heterogeneity, varying in color from white to dark red.

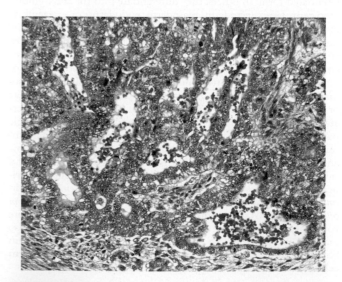

FIGURE 17-16. Embryonal carcinoma component of a NSGCT. Because these undifferentiated cells have scant cytoplasm, their hyperchromatic nuclei impart a bluish color to the tumor. The nuclei appear crowded and seem to overlap each other. The cells form cords and sheets surrounding dilated vascular channels filled with red blood cells.

and extraembryonic elements, including yolk sac cells and trophoblastic cells). Microscopically, such nonseminomatous tumors thus reveal foci of embryonal carcinoma and a variety of other tissues (Fig. 17-17). A similar tumor that also contains seminoma cells would, however, be called a **mixed germ cell tumor**.

NSGCTs can give rise to clones of highly malignant cytotrophoblastic and syncytiotrophoblastic cells, which overgrow other elements. Tumors composed exclusively of malignant chorionic epithelium are termed **choriocarcinomas**. Likewise, clones of malignant yolk sac epithelium produce **yolk sac carcinoma**.

Teratomas of the prepubertal testes are benign and are composed of mature somatic tissues. Orchiectomy, and even testis-sparing surgery, is curative. Some histologically benign teratomas of **postpubertal young men** may have a malignant clinical course, although they appear to be only mature, nonproliferating somatic tissues, without embryonal elements. These tumors are clinically known as the **growing teratoma syndrome**. In other cases, teratoma tissues remain undifferentiated and resemble embryonic organs or embryonic tumors such as neuroblastoma. These **immature teratomas** are also potentially malignant tumors.

 CLINICAL FEATURES: Most NSGCTs manifest as testicular masses. They tend to grow faster than seminomas and metastasize more readily and more widely. Hence, in some NSGCTs, metastases may be the first sign of the neoplastic disease.

In contrast to seminomas, NSGCTs often contain yolk sac components and syncytiotrophoblastic cells. Yolk sac cells secrete α-fetoprotein (AFP), a fetal plasma protein that is not normally found in the blood. Syncytiotrophoblastic cells release hCG, a hormone of pregnancy, that is also not found in males. *Elevated levels of serum AFP or hCG are found in 70% of patients harboring NSGCTs and are thus reliable tumor markers in postoperative follow-up.* Patients whose initially high levels of AFP and hCG normalize after treatment but subsequently rise again have recurrent metastatic disease.

Treatment of NSGCT includes an orchiectomy to remove the primary tumor, then platinum-based chemotherapy, and, if indicated, surgical dissection of abdominal lymph nodes. Chemotherapy usually eliminates metastatic embryonal carcinoma cells, but differentiated tissues originating from them are resistant. Such tissues do not grow and are not likely to endanger the patient. Only 3 decades ago, patients with NSGCTs had only a 35% chance for 5-year survival. *By contrast, complete cures are now recorded in more than 90% of cases.*

Gonadal Stromal/Sex Cord Tumors are Composed of Cells that Resemble Sertoli or Leydig Cells

Gonadal stroma/sex cord tumors constitute 5% of all testicular tumors.

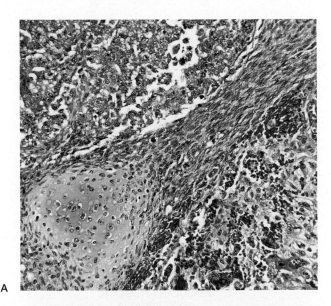

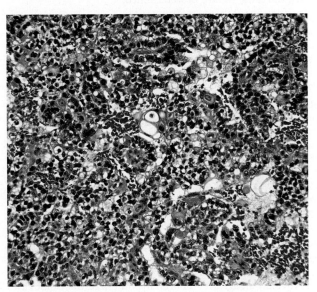

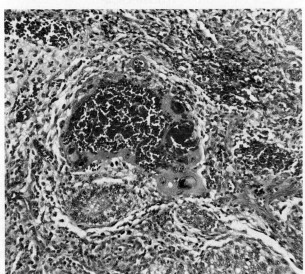

FIGURE 17-17. Nonseminomatous germ cell tumor (NSGCT). **A.** Somatic tissue of this tumor includes well-differentiated cartilage and nondescript connective tissue separating the embryonal carcinoma *(upper left corner)* from the hemorrhagic choriocarcinoma *(right lower corner)*. **B.** Yolk sac component consists of interlacing cord of epithelial cells surrounded by loose stroma resembling the early yolk sac. **C.** Choriocarcinoma component of the NSGCT consists of multinucleated syncytiotrophoblastic giant cells and mononuclear cytotrophoblastic cells. Invasive growth of trophoblasts is usually associated with hemorrhage.

LEYDIG CELL TUMORS: *Rare neoplasms are composed of cells resembling interstitial (Leydig) cells of the testis.* They can be hormonally active and secrete androgens, estrogens, or both. Leydig cell tumors can occur at any age, with two distinct peaks, one in childhood and one in adults from the third to the sixth decade. The androgenic effects of testicular Leydig cell tumors in prepubertal boys lead to precocious physical and sexual development. By contrast, feminization and gynecomastia are observed in some adults with this tumor. Although most (90%) of Leydig cell tumors are benign (only 10% are malignant), it is difficult to predict biological behavior on histologic grounds. All Leydig cell tumors in children and almost all tumors in adults are cured by orchiectomy.

SERTOLI CELL TUMORS: *Some testicular sex cord stromal cell tumors are composed of neoplastic Sertoli cells.* Most (90%) tumors are benign and produce few if any hormonal symptoms. The majority of patients with Sertoli cell tumors are under 40 years of age and come to medical attention because of a scrotal mass. Orchiectomy is curative.

PROSTATE

Prostatitis

Prostatitis refers to inflammation of the prostate, which can occur in acute and chronic forms. It is usually caused by coliform uropathogens, but often the cause cannot be determined.

ACUTE PROSTATITIS: *Typically a complication of other urinary tract infections, acute prostatitis results from reflux of infected urine into the prostate.* An acute inflammatory infiltrate is seen in prostatic acini and stroma. The disorder causes intense discomfort on urination and is often associated with fever, chills, and perineal pain. Most patients respond well to standard antibiotic treatment.

CHRONIC BACTERIAL PROSTATITIS: *This infection of longer duration may or may not be preceded by an episode of acute prostatitis.* Most patients with chronic prostatitis complain of dysuria and burning at the urethral meatus. Suprapubic, perineal, and low back pain, or discomfort and nocturia may also be present. The urine usually contains bacteria. In addition to reflux of urine, factors such as prostatic calculi and local prostatic duct obstruction may contribute to the development of chronic bacterial prostatitis. Microscopically, infiltrates of lymphocytes, plasma cells, and macrophages are the rule. Prolonged antibiotic therapy is often, but not necessarily, curative.

NONBACTERIAL PROSTATITIS: *There exists a form of chronic prostatitis in which no causative organism is identified.* Nonbacterial prostatitis typically affects men older than 50 years of age but has been seen at virtually all ages. It has been hypothesized that some cases may be due to *Chlamydia trachomatis, Mycoplasma, Ureaplasma, urealyticum,* or *Trichomonas vaginalis.* However, in practice, it is a diagnosis of exclusion. The most common histologic pattern consists of dilated glands filled with neutrophils and foamy macrophages and surrounded by chronic inflammatory cells. The condition may be asymptomatic or cause symptoms similar to those in chronic bacterial prostatitis. In most cases, no specific therapy is available.

CLINICAL FEATURES: As indicated above, the symptoms of chronic prostatitis are highly variable, and treatment may be quite frustrating. Most importantly, chronic prostatitis may cause elevated serum prostate-specific antigen (PSA), raising the specter of prostatic malignancy. The diagnosis is thus often made by biopsy done to exclude cancer.

Nodular Hyperplasia of the Prostate

Nodular prostatic hyperplasia, also termed **benign prostatic hyperplasia** (BPH), is a common disorder characterized clinically by enlargement of the prostate and urinary outflow tract obstruction, and pathologically by proliferation of glands and stroma.

EPIDEMIOLOGY: BPH is most frequent in Western Europe and the United States and least common in Asia. The prevalence of the disorder in the United States is higher among blacks than among whites. Clinical prostatism (i.e., BPH severe enough to interfere with urination) peaks in the seventh decade. In fact, 75% of men 80 years of age or older have some degree of prostatic hyperplasia. The disorder is rarely observed in men younger than 40.

PATHOGENESIS: Prepubertal castration prevents the subsequent development of BPH. However, exogenous testosterone has no effect on either the histologic appearance of the hyperplastic nodules or the areas of the prostate that show senile atrophy. Drugs that block 5α-reductase (e.g., finasteride) and inhibit dihydrotestosterone synthesis reduce the size of the prostate in men with BPH.

PATHOLOGY: Early nodular hyperplasia begins in the submucosa of the proximal urethra (**the transitional zone**). The enlarging nodules compress the centrally located urethral lumen and the more peripherally located normal prostate (Fig. 17-18). On cut section, an individ-

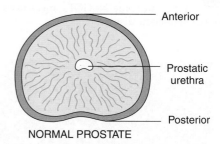
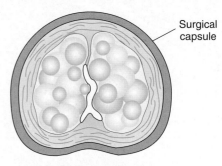
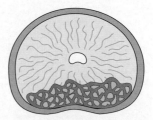

FIGURE 17-18. Normal prostate, nodular hyperplasia, and adenocarcinoma. In prostatic hyperplasia, which involves predominantly the periurethral part of the gland, the nodules compress and distort the urethra. The expansion of the central prostatic glands leads to compression of the peripheral parts and fibrosis, resulting in the formation of so-called surgical capsule. Prostatic carcinoma usually arises from the peripheral glands, and compression of the urethra is a late clinical event.

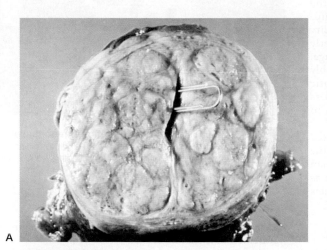

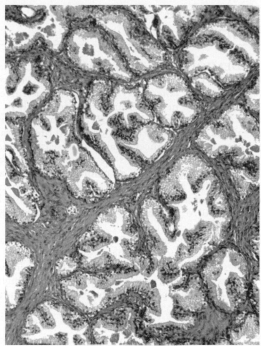

A   B

FIGURE 17-19. **Nodular hyperplasia of the prostate. A.** THE cut surface of a prostate enlarged by nodular hyperplasia shows numerous well-circumscribed nodules of prostatic tissue. The prostatic urethra *(paper clip)* has been compressed to a narrow slit. **B.** The columnar epithelium lining the acini is composed of two cell layers: polarized clear cuboidal cells lining the acinar lumen and flattened basal cells interposed between the cuboidal acinar cells and the stroma. Hyperplastic cells line papillary projections protruding into the lumina of the acini.

ual nodule is clearly demarcated by an enveloping fibrous pseudocapsule (Fig. 17-19). Secondary changes reflect bladder outlet obstruction (Fig. 17-20).

Histologically, BPH features proliferation of epithelial cells of acini and ductules, smooth muscle cells, and stromal fibroblasts, all in variable proportions. Accordingly, several types of nodules have been described, and fibromyoadenomatous nodules are the most common. In such nodules, variably sized hyperplastic prostatic acini are randomly scattered throughout the stroma. The epithelial (adenomatous) component is composed of a double layer of cells, with tall columnar cells overlying the basal layer (see Fig. 17-19B). Papillary hyperplasia of glandular epithelium is characteristic. Hyperplastic nodules often show signs of nonspecific prostatitis with acute and chronic inflammatory cells infiltrating between and within glands. Corpora amylacea (eosinophilic laminated concretions) are frequently seen within glandular acini. Areas of infarction may be present, especially in larger nodules. Immunoperoxidase staining of hyperplastic epithelium is consistently positive for PSA and prostatic acid phosphatase. Squamous metaplasia of ductal epithelium at the periphery of infarcts is typical. Incidental foci of prostatic adenocarcinoma are found in 10% of surgical specimens submitted with preoperative diagnoses of BPH.

 CLINICAL FEATURES: The clinical symptoms of nodular hyperplasia result from compression of the prostatic urethra and consequent bladder outlet obstruction. A history of decreased vigor of the urinary stream and increasing urinary frequency is typical. Rectal examination reveals a firm, enlarged, nodular prostate. If the duration of severe obstruction is prolonged, back-pressure results in hydroureter, hydronephrosis, and ultimately renal failure and death.

The classic treatment of BPH has been surgical. Currently, drugs that inhibit 5α-reductase are usually used to decrease prostate size. α-Adrenergic blockers reduce muscular tone in the prostate and ameliorate the symptoms of urinary obstruction.

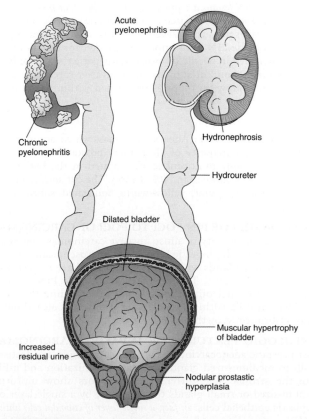

FIGURE 17-20. Complications of nodular prostatic hyperplasia.

In Situ and Invasive Adenocarcinoma of the Prostate

EPIDEMIOLOGY: *In 1990, prostatic adenocarcinoma became the cancer most frequently diagnosed in American men, surpassing lung cancer for the first time.* An estimated 230,000 new cases are diagnosed yearly in the United States. Approximately 27,000 American men die annually of this malignancy, a figure that is one-third the mortality from lung cancer. Prostate cancer is largely a disease of elderly men, and 75% of diagnosed patients are 60 to 80 years of age. The true frequency of prostatic carcinoma is considerably higher than its clinical incidence. The prevalence of prostatic carcinoma determined at autopsy increases with age, from less than 10% in men 40 to 50 years of age to more than 70% in those older than 80.

There is considerable geographic variation in the age-related death rates for adenocarcinoma of the prostate throughout the world; the highest is in the United States and the Scandinavian countries. American blacks, who exhibit a rate twice as high as white Americans, have the highest prostate carcinoma death rates in the world.

PATHOGENESIS: The cause of prostatic adenocarcinoma is unknown, but the principal focus of research interest is endocrine influences. Androgenic control of normal prostatic growth and the responsiveness of prostate cancer to castration and exogenous estrogens support a role for male hormones.

There is no evidence that prostatic adenocarcinoma originates from hyperplastic nodules. Current attention addresses intraductal dysplastic foci, termed **prostatic intraepithelial neoplasia** *(PIN). PIN refers to resident prostatic ducts lined by cytologically atypical luminal cells and a concomitant decrease in basal cells. Substantial evidence now supports the contention that PIN lesions are premalignant changes that progress to prostatic adenocarcinoma.* Such lesions precede invasive cancer by two decades, and their severity increases with increasing age. High-grade PIN is an important marker for carcinoma when identified in needle biopsies. Many patients with only high-grade PIN on initial biopsy have invasive carcinoma in subsequent follow-up biopsies performed within weeks to months.

PATHOLOGY: Adenocarcinomas, which account for the vast majority of all primary prostatic tumors, are commonly multicentric and located in the peripheral zones in more than 70% of cases. The cut surface of the prostate shows irregular, yellow-white, indurated subcapsular nodules.

RELATIONSHIP OF PIN FOCI TO FOCI OF CARCINOMA: Notably, in the vicinity of most invasive carcinomas, one may identify lesions of high-grade PIN, which microscopically are dilated branching glands with intraluminal papillary projections lined by atypical cells. The nuclei of high-grade PIN are enlarged, contain nucleoli, and show marked crowding (Fig. 17-21). Atypical cells within PIN-affected ducts may also show a flat or cribriform growth pattern.

HISTOLOGIC FEATURES OF INVASIVE CARCINOMA: Most prostatic adenocarcinomas are of acinar origin and feature small- to medium-sized glands that lack organization and infiltrate the stroma. Well-differentiated tumors show uniform medium-sized or small glands that are lined by a single layer of neoplastic epithelial cells. *In fact, a single layer of cuboidal cells lining neoplastic acini is the most frequently used criterion to diagnose prostatic*

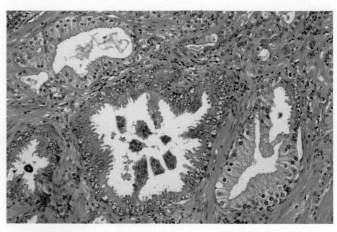

FIGURE 17-21. High-grade prostatic intraepithelial neoplasia (PIN). The large duct in the center is lined by atypical cells with enlarged nuclei and prominent nucleoli. Two normal ducts are located adjacent to the neoplastic one.

adenocarcinoma. Progressive loss of differentiation of prostatic adenocarcinomas is characterized by:

- Increasing variability of gland size and configuration
- Papillary and cribriform patterns
- Rudimentary (or no) gland formation, with only solid cords of infiltrating tumor cells

GRADING: Prostatic adenocarcinoma is most commonly classified according to the **Gleason grading system** (Fig. 17-22), which is based on five histologic patterns of tumor gland formation and infiltration. Recognizing the high frequency of mixed tumor patterns, the Gleason score is the sum of the grades (1 through 5) attributed to the most prominent pattern and that of the minority pattern. The best-differentiated tumors have a Gleason score of 2 (1 + 1), whereas very poorly differentiated cancers have scores of 10 (5 + 5). Most tumors score 4 to 7 (2 + 2, to 3 + 4 or 4 + 3). When combined with the tumor stage, the Gleason grading system has prognostic value: lower scores correlate with better prognoses.

INVASION AND METASTASIS: The high frequency of invasion of the prostatic capsule by adenocarcinoma relates to the subcapsular location of the tumor. Perineural tumor invasion within the prostate and adjacent tissues is usual. Because peripheral nerves are devoid of perineural lymphatic channels, this mode of invasion represents contiguous spread of the tumor along a tissue space that offers the plane of least resistance.

The seminal vesicles are almost always involved by direct extension of prostate cancer. The earliest metastases occur in the obturator lymph node, with subsequent dissemination to iliac and periaortic lymph nodes. Metastases to the lung reflect further lymphatic spread. Bony metastases, particularly to the vertebral column ribs and pelvic bones, are painful and present a common difficult clinical problem. Widespread tumor dissemination (carcinomatosis), frequently with terminal pneumonia or sepsis, is the most common cause of death.

CLINICAL FEATURES: The current widespread screening programs for prostate cancer that use digital rectal examination in combination with serum PSA levels detect this malignancy in most cases. Patients with elevated serum PSA levels are further evaluated by needle biopsies. Serum PSA is a useful screening test for the disease and an indicator of response to treatment. Serum prostatic alkaline

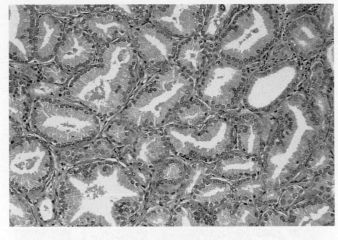

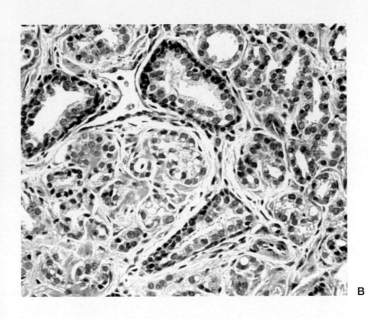

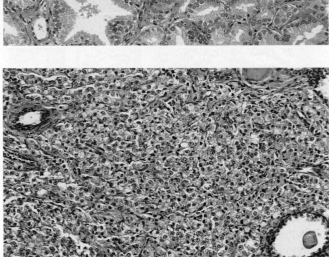

FIGURE 17-22. **Gleason grading system. A.** Gleason grade 1. **B.** Gleason grade 3. **C.** Gleason grade 5.

phosphatase levels are elevated in patients with osteoblastic bony metastases.

Therapy for prostate cancer depends on the stage of the tumor. Patients with cancer localized to the prostate are treated by radical prostatectomy or radiation therapy. In cases with microinvasive disease, radiation therapy is the treatment of choice, acknowledging that half of these patients have occult node metastases, which cannot be cured by surgical means. For patients whose tumors progress clinically and for all patients judged to have regional or distant metastases at initial presentation, the principal form of therapy is hormonal. This treatment involves orchiectomy or administration of pituitary LH or LH-releasing hormone antagonists. In either case, the goal is androgen deprivation. The 5-year survival rate in disease confined to the prostate is 90%; in cases of metastatic disease, this figure falls to 40% to 10% depending on disease stage.

18 The Female Reproductive System

Stanley J. Robboy
Maria J. Merino
George L. Mutter

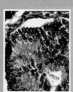
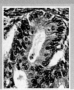
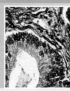

The broad scope of disease expressed in the female reproductive tract represents the complex functional anatomy of the system. As a portal of entry, it is the locus for venereal and other infectious agents. The menstrual cycle requires the interplay between the ovary and other endocrine organs for normal function. The organs of the female reproductive tract host an array of epithelial, mesenchymal, and germ cell-derived neoplasms, both benign and malignant. The understanding of the viral etiology and success in early detection of one such lesion, cervical cancer, represents a triumph in our understanding of disease pathogenesis, which is also of immense value to public health.

Genital Infections

Sexually Transmitted Genital Infections

Infectious diseases of the female genital tract are common and are caused by many pathogenic organisms (Table 18-1), which are also discussed in Chapter 9. Most of the important infectious diseases affecting the female genital tract are sexually transmitted.

Bacterial Infections

Gonorrhea

Gonorrhea is caused by *Neisseria gonorrhoeae,* a fastidious, gram-negative diplococcus. The infection is a frequent cause of acute salpingitis and pelvic inflammatory disease (PID) (Fig. 18-1).

 PATHOGENESIS AND PATHOLOGY: The organisms ascend through the cervix and the endometrial cavity, where they cause acute endometritis. The bacteria then attach to mucosal cells in the fallopian tube and elicit an acute inflammatory reaction, which is confined to the mucosal surface (**acute salpingitis**). From the tubal lumen, the infection spreads to involve the ovary, sometimes resulting in a **tuboovarian abscess**. It may also involve the pelvic and abdominal cavities, with formation of subdiaphragmatic and pelvic abscesses. The healing process distorts and destroys the plicae of the fallopian tube, often leading to sterility.

Syphilis

Syphilis, caused by the spirochete *Treponema pallidum,* is discussed in detail in Chapter 9.

TABLE 18–1

Infectious Diseases of the Female Genital Tract

Organism	Disease	Diagnostic Feature
Sexually Transmitted Diseases		
Gram-negative rods and cocci		
Calymmatobacterium granulomatis	Granuloma inguinale	Donovan body
Gardnerella vaginalis	*Gardnerella* infection	Clue cell
Haemophilus ducreyi	Chancroid (soft chancre)	
Neisseria gonorrhoeae	Gonorrhea	Gram-negative diplococcus
Spirochetes		
Treponema pallidum	Syphilis	Spirochete
Mycoplasmas		
Mycoplasma hominis	Nonspecific vaginitis	
Ureaplasma urealyticum	Nonspecific vaginitis	
Rickettsiae		
Chlamydia trachomatis type D-K	Various forms of PID	
Chlamydia trachomatis type L1–3	Lymphogranuloma venereum	
Viruses		
Human papillomavirus (HPV)	Condyloma acuminatum/planum	Koilocyte
	Neoplastic potential	
Types 6, 11, 40, 42, 43, 44, 57	Low risk	
Types 16, 18, 31, 33, 35, 39, 45, 51, 52, 56, 58, 66	High risk	
Herpes simplex, type 2	Herpes genitalis	Multinucleated giant cell with intranuclear homogenization and inclusion bodies
Cytomegalovirus (CMV)	Cytomegalic inclusion disease	Bulbous intranuclear inclusion body
Molluscum contagiosum	Molluscum infection	Molluscum body
Protozoa		
Trichomonas vaginalis	Trichomoniasis	Trichomonad
Selected Nonsexually Transmitted Diseases		
Actinomyces and related organisms		
Actinomyces israelii	PID (one of many organisms)	Sulphur granules
Mycobacterium tuberculosis	Tuberculosis	Necrotizing granulomas
Fungi		
Candida albicans	Candidiasis	Candida species

PID, pelvic inflammatory disease.

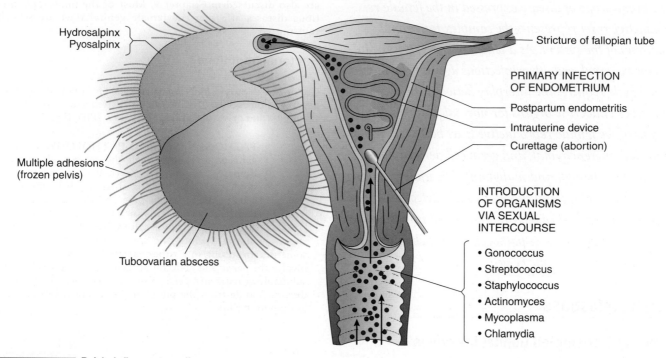

Hydrosalpinx
Pyosalpinx

Stricture of fallopian tube

PRIMARY INFECTION
OF ENDOMETRIUM

Postpartum endometritis

Intrauterine device

Curettage (abortion)

Multiple adhesions
(frozen pelvis)

INTRODUCTION
OF ORGANISMS
VIA SEXUAL
INTERCOURSE

Tuboovarian abscess

• Gonococcus
• Streptococcus
• Staphylococcus
• Actinomyces
• Mycoplasma
• Chlamydia

FIGURE 18-1. Pelvic inflammatory disease.

Chlamydia Infections

Chlamydia trachomatis is a common, venereally transmitted organism, which is a gram-negative intracellular parasite. This organism has been found in the genital tract of about 8% of asymptomatic women and 20% of women presenting with symptoms of lower genital tract infection. Chlamydial infection is easily confused with gonorrhea, as the symptoms of both diseases are similar (see also Chapter 9).

 PATHOLOGY: During infection, the cervical mucosa is severely inflamed, and endocervical and metaplastic squamous cells reveal small inclusion bodies. Cytologically, chlamydia infection manifests as perinuclear intracytoplasmic inclusions with distinct borders and intracytoplasmic **coccoid bodies**. Complications include ascending infection of the endometrium, fallopian tube, and ovary, which may result in tubal occlusion and infertility. Chlamydia also infects Bartholin glands and can cause acute urethritis.

Viral Infections

Human Papillomavirus

Human papillomavirus (HPV) is a DNA virus that infects a number of skin and mucosal surfaces to produce wart-like lesions, referred to as **verrucae** and **condylomata** (Fig. 18-2). More than 100 HPV serotypes are known, one-third of which cause genital tract lesions. In the United States, as many as two thirds of graduating college women have genital HPV infections, which result from sexual contact with an infected person. Approximately 20 million people are currently infected with HPV in this country. HPV types 6 and 11 are detected in more than 80% of macroscopically visible condylomata. Several strains of HPV are the major etiologic factors for squamous cell cancer in the female lower genital tract. Types 16 and 18 are associated with about 60% of cases; types 31, 33, 45, 52, and 58 account for most other occurrences of intraepithelial neoplasia and invasive cancer (see the section on the cervix below).

Most cases of HPV are diagnosed by cervical Pap smear. Tests that directly assay for HPV DNA are seeing increasing clinical use. Treatment for HPV infection has been inadequate, and most infections spontaneously disappear. A recently approved prophylactic vaccine directed against four common serotypes of HPV poten-

tially provides protection against the HPV strains responsible for 70% of cervical cancer and 90% of cervical warts and is recommended for all females between the ages of 9 and 26.

Herpesvirus

Herpes simplex type 2 is a double-stranded DNA virus that is a common cause of sexually transmitted genital infections. After an incubation period of 1 to 3 weeks, small vesicles develop on the vulva and erode into painful ulcers. Similar lesions occur in the vagina and cervix. Epithelial cells adjacent to intraepithelial vesicles show ballooning degeneration and many contain large nuclei with eosinophilic inclusions (see also Chapter 9).

Genital herpes tends to become latent, at which time the virus remains in the sacral ganglia. If the virus reactivates in pregnancy, the newborn may acquire fatal herpes infection during passage through the birth canal. For this reason, active herpetic lesions in the vagina at the time of delivery are an indication for Cesarean section.

Trichomoniasis

T. vaginalis is a large, pear-shaped, flagellated protozoan that commonly causes vaginitis. The disease is sexually transmitted, and 25% of infected women are asymptomatic carriers. Infection manifests as a heavy, yellow-gray, thick, foamy discharge accompanied by severe itching, dyspareunia (painful intercourse), and dysuria (painful urination). The diagnosis is confirmed by a wet mount preparation in which the motile trichomonads are seen. The organisms are also demonstrated in Pap smears.

Pelvic Inflammatory Disease (PID)

PID describes an infection of pelvic organs that follows extension of any of a variety of microorganisms beyond the uterine corpus (see Fig. 18-1). Ascent of the infection results in bilateral acute salpingitis, pyosalpinx, and tuboovarian abscesses. *N. gonorrhoeae* and chlamydia are the principal organisms causing PID, but most infections are polymicrobial. The incidence of PID is far greater in sexually promiscuous women than in those who are monogamous. Occasionally, PID is a sequel to postpartum endometritis or a complication of endometrial curettage.

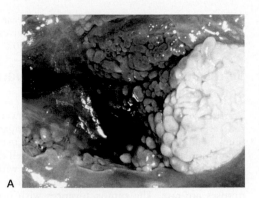

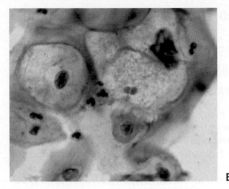

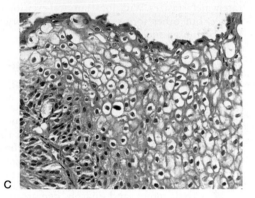

 FIGURE 18-2. Human papillomavirus-induced condylomatous infections. **A.** Condyloma acuminatum on the cervix, visible with the naked eye as cauliflower-like excrescences. **B.** A cervical smear contains characteristic koilocytes with a perinuclear halo and a wrinkled nucleus that contains viral particles. **C.** Biopsy of the condyloma shows koilocytes with perinuclear halos but lacking nuclear atypia.

Patients with PID typically present with lower abdominal pain. Complications of PID include (1) rupture of a tuboovarian abscess, which may result in life-threatening peritonitis; (2) infertility from scarring of the healed tubal plicae; (3) increased rates of ectopic pregnancy; and (4) intestinal obstruction from fibrous bands and adhesions.

Toxic Shock Syndrome is Associated with Vaginal Staphylococcal Infection

Toxic shock syndrome is an acute, sometimes fatal disorder characterized by fever, shock, and a desquamative erythematous rash. In addition, vomiting, diarrhea, myalgia, neurologic signs, and thrombocytopenia are common. Certain strains of *Staphylococcus aureus* release an exotoxin called **toxic shock syndrome toxin-1**. This toxin alters the function of mononuclear phagocytes, thus impairing clearance of other potentially toxic substances, such as endotoxin. In addition to the pathologic alterations characteristic of shock, the lesions of disseminated intravascular coagulation (DIC) are usually prominent (see Chapter 20). The occurrence of toxic shock syndrome has decreased markedly since the role of prolonged tampon placement in promoting *S. aureus* colonization of the vagina has been recognized.

VULVA

Cysts

BARTHOLIN GLAND CYSTS: The paired Bartholin glands located immediately posterolateral to the introitus produce a clear mucoid secretion that continuously lubricates the vestibular surface. The ducts are prone to obstruction and consequent cysts. In turn, cyst infection leads to abscess formation. Staphylococci,

chlamydia, and anaerobes are frequently the cause. Treatment consists of incision, drainage, marsupialization, and appropriate antibiotics.

FOLLICULAR CYSTS: The follicular cyst recapitulates the most distal portion of the hair follicle. Also termed **epithelial inclusion cysts** or **keratinous cysts**, follicular cysts frequently appear on the vulva, especially the labia majora. They contain a white cheesy material and typically are lined by stratified squamous epithelium.

MUCINOUS CYSTS: Mucinous glands of the vulva occasionally become obstructed and subsequently cystic. Mucinous columnar cells line the cyst and may become infected.

Dermatoses

Lichen Sclerosus is Associated with Autoimmune Disorders

Lichen sclerosus is an inflammatory disease of the vulva associated with autoimmune disorders such as vitiligo, pernicious anemia, and thyroiditis, and an increased risk of vulvar squamous cell carcinoma.

PATHOLOGY: The condition is represented by white plaques, atrophic skin, a parchment-like or crinkled appearance, and, occasionally, marked contracture of the vulvar tissues. Histological findings include hyperkeratosis, loss of rete ridges, epithelial thinning with flattening of rete pegs, cytoplasmic vacuolation of the basal layer, and a homogeneous, acellular zone in the upper dermis. A band of chronic inflammatory cells consisting of lymphocytes with few plasma cells typically lies beneath this layer. Itching is the most common symptom, and dyspareunia is frequent. The disease develops insidiously and is progressive. *Women with symptomatic lichen sclerosus have a 15% chance of developing squamous cell carcinoma.*

Malignant Tumors and Premalignant Conditions

Vulvar Intraepithelial Neoplasia (VIN) is a Precursor of Invasive Cancer

VIN reflects a spectrum of neoplastic changes that range from minimal cellular atypia to the most marked cellular changes short of invasive cancer. Between 1983 and 2000, there has been about a twofold increase in the frequency of VIN, much of which occurs in women under the age of 40 years. *As with comparable lesions in the cervix (cervical intraepithelial neoplasia [CIN]), VIN is a precursor of vulvar squamous cell carcinoma, of which at least 30% to 40% of cases are caused by HPV.*

 PATHOLOGY: The lesions of VIN may be single or multiple, and macular, papular, or plaque-like. Microscopically, the grades are labeled VIN I, II, and III, corresponding to mild, moderate, and severe dysplasia, respectively. Grade III also includes squamous cell carcinoma in situ (CIS). VIN, even if locally excised, often recurs (25%), in which case it may progress to invasive squamous cell carcinoma (6%). Women with VIN may have squamous neoplasms similar to VIN elsewhere in the lower genital tract.

Squamous Cell Carcinoma Follows VIN

Squamous cell carcinoma of the vulva (Fig. 18-3) is the end result of a multistep process that begins with VIN. This tumor accounts for 3% of all genital cancers in women and is the most common cancer of the vulva. In the past, it mainly affected older women, but like VIN, it now occurs with increasing frequency in younger women. Two thirds of larger tumors are exophytic; the others are ulcerative and endophytic. Pruritus of long duration is commonly the first symptom. Ulceration, bleeding, and secondary infection may develop. The tumors grow slowly and then extend to the contiguous skin, vagina, and rectum. They metastasize to superficial inguinal and then deep inguinal, femoral, and pelvic lymph nodes.

The outlook correlates with the stage of disease and lymph node status. The prognosis of patients with vulvar cancer is generally good, with an overall 5-year survival rate of 70%.

Verrucous Carcinoma is a Distinct Variety of Squamous Cell Carcinoma

Verrucous carcinoma of the vulva is a distinct variety of squamous cell carcinoma that manifests as a large fungating mass resembling a giant condyloma acuminatum. HPV, usually type 6 or 11, is commonly identified. The tumor is very well differentiated and is composed of large nests of squamous cells with abundant cytoplasm and small, bland nuclei. Squamous pearls are common, and mitoses are rare. The tumor advances with broad tongues but rarely metastasizes. Wide local surgical excision is the treatment of choice, but other forms of therapy (cryosurgery and retinoids) have been used successfully.

Extramammary Paget Disease Exhibits Intraepithelial Cells with Copious Pale Cytoplasm

Paget disease of the vulva is named after similar-appearing tumors in the nipple and extramammary sites such as the axilla and perianal region. The disorder usually occurs on the labia majora in older women. Women with Paget disease of the vulva complain of pruritus or a burning sensation for many years.

 PATHOLOGY: The lesion of Paget disease is large, red, moist, and sharply demarcated. The diagnostic cells (Paget cells) are thought to arise in the epidermis or epidermally derived adnexal structures. Paget cells have pale, vacuolated cytoplasm with abundant glycosaminoglycans; they stain with periodic acid-Schiff as well as mucicarmine and express carcinoembryonic antigen. Paget cells appear as large single cells or, less often, as clusters of cells that lack intercellular bridges and are usually confined to the epidermis. In contrast to Paget disease of the breast, which is almost always associated with underlying duct carcinoma, extramammary Paget disease is only rarely associated with carcinoma of the skin ad-

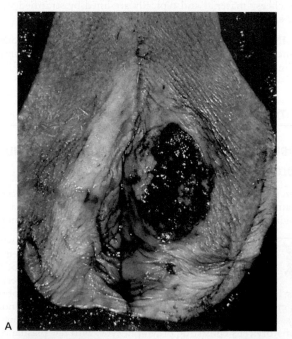

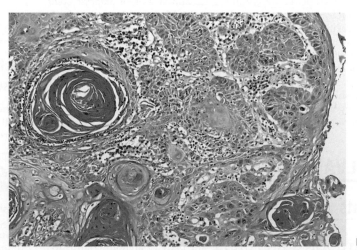

FIGURE 18-3. **Squamous cell carcinoma of the vulva. A.** The tumor is situated in an extensive area of lichen sclerosus *(white)*. **B.** Small nests of neoplastic squamous cells, some with keratin pearls, are evident in this well-differentiated tumor.

nexa. Metastases rarely occur, so treatment requires only wide local excision or simple vulvectomy.

VAGINA

Nonneoplastic Conditions and Benign Tumors

Vaginal Adenosis Occurs in Females Exposed to Diethylstilbestrol (DES) in Utero

Vaginal adenosis is the failure of the glandular epithelium that normally lines the embryonic vagina to be replaced during fetal life by squamous epithelium. In the 1970s, the use of DES to prevent miscarriages in women who were prone to repetitive abortions led to a substantial increase in the incidence of this disorder in young daughters of women who had taken DES during pregnancy. Adenosis manifests as red, granular patches on the vaginal mucosa, which microscopically are composed of mucinous columnar cells (resembling those lining the endocervix) and ciliated cells (similar to those lining the endometrium and fallopian tubes). Rare cases of **clear cell adenocarcinoma** of the vagina have occurred in the daughters of women treated with DES. These tumors are almost invariably curable when they are small and asymptomatic, but in more advanced stages, they may spread by hematogenous or lymphatic routes.

Malignant Tumors

Primary malignant tumors of the vagina are uncommon, constituting about 2% of all genital tract tumors. Most (80%) vaginal malignancies represent secondary spread. The most common symptoms are a vaginal discharge and bleeding during coitus, but advanced tumors may cause pelvic or abdominal pain and edema of the legs.

Squamous Cell Carcinoma Accounts for More than 90% of Primary Vaginal Malignancies

It is generally a disease of older women, with a peak incidence between the ages of 60 and 70 years. It appears most commonly in the anterior wall of the upper third of the vagina, where it usually manifests as an exophytic mass. **Vaginal intraepithelial neoplasia** often precedes invasive carcinoma. Commonly, squamous cell carcinoma of the vagina develops a few years after cervical or vulvar carcinoma. The 5-year survival rate for tumors confined to the vagina (stage I) is 80%, whereas it is only 20% for those with extensive spread (stages III/IV).

Embryonal Rhabdomyosarcoma (Sarcoma Botryoides) is a Malignant Childhood Tumor

Embryonal rhabdomyosarcoma is a rare vaginal tumor that appears as confluent polypoid masses resembling a bunch of grapes, hence the name sarcoma botryoides (from the Greek botrys, a cluster of grapes). It occurs almost exclusively in girls under 4 years of age. The tumor arises in the lamina propria of the vagina and consists of primitive spindle rhabdomyoblasts, some of which display cross-striations. It is usually detected because of spotting on the child's diaper. Tumors under 3 cm in greatest dimension tend to be localized and may be cured by wide excision and chemotherapy. Larger masses are likely to have invaded adjacent structures, metastasized to regional lymph nodes, and spread hematogenously to distant sites. Even in advanced cases, half of the patients survive with radical surgery and chemotherapy.

CERVIX

Cervicitis

Inflammation of the cervix is common and is related to constant exposure to bacterial flora in the vagina. Acute and chronic cervicitis result from infection with many microorganisms, particularly endogenous vaginal aerobes and anaerobes, *Streptococcus*, *Staphylococcus*, and *Enterococcus*. Other specific organisms include *Chlamydia trachomatis*, *Neisseria gonorrhoeae*, and occasionally herpes simplex, type 2.

 PATHOLOGY: In **acute cervicitis**, the cervix is grossly red, swollen, and edematous, with copious pus "dripping" from the external os. Microscopically, the tissues exhibit an extensive infiltrate of polymorphonuclear leukocytes and stromal edema.

In **chronic cervicitis**, which is more common, the cervical mucosa is hyperemic, and there may be true epithelial erosions. Microscopically, the stroma is infiltrated by mononuclear cells, principally lymphocytes and plasma cells. Metaplastic squamous epithelium of the transformation zone may extend into endocervical glands, forming clusters of squamous epithelium with slightly enlarged nuclei, which must be differentiated from carcinoma.

Endocervical Polyp

Endocervical polyps are the most common cervical growths. They appear as single smooth or lobulated masses, usually under 3 cm in greatest dimension. The polyps typically manifest as vaginal bleeding or discharge. The lining epithelium is mucinous, with varying degrees of squamous metaplasia but may feature erosions and granulation tissue in women with symptoms. Simple excision or curettage is curative. Cancer rarely arises in an endocervical polyp (0.2% of cases).

Squamous Cell Neoplasia

Fifty years ago, cervical cancer was the leading cause of cancer death in American women. In the United States, it is now the sixth most common type of cancer found in females, and the mortality rate has fallen by more than 70%. However, worldwide, cervical cancer remains the second most common cancer in women.

Cervical Intraepithelial Neoplasia (CIN) is the Precursor of Invasive Cancer

CIN is defined as a spectrum of intraepithelial changes that begins with minimal atypia and progresses through stages of more marked intraepithelial abnormalities to invasive squamous cell carcinoma (Fig. 18-4). **CIN, dysplasia, CIS, and squamous intraepithelial lesion (SIL)** are commonly used interchangeably. *Dysplasia in the cervical epithelium carries a risk for **malignant transformation*** (Figs. 18-4 and 18-5). The concept of CIN emphasizes that dysplasia and CIS are points on a disease spectrum rather than separate entities.

The grades of CIN are as follows:

- CIN-1: mild dysplasia
- CIN-2: moderate dysplasia
- CIN-3: severe dysplasia and CIS

The "Bethesda System for Reporting Cervical/Vaginal Cytologic Diagnoses" groups these lesions slightly differently (see Fig. 18-4). Low-grade SIL (LSIL) reflects conditions that should rarely progress in severity and commonly disappear (CIN-1, mild

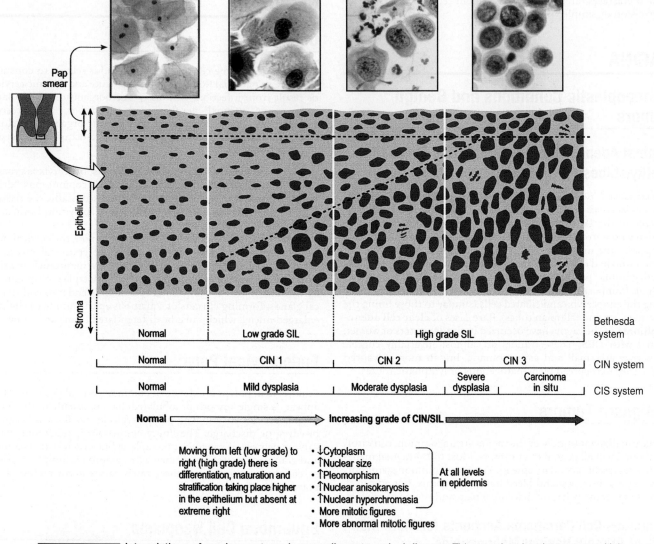

FIGURE 18-4. **Interrelations of naming systems in premalignant cervical disease.** This complex chart integrates multiple aspects of the disease complex. It lists the qualitative and quantitative features that become increasingly abnormal as the premalignant disease advances in severity. It also illustrates the changes in progressively more abnormal disease states and provides translation nomenclature for the dysplasia/carcinoma in situ (CIS) system, cervical intraepithelial neoplasia (CIN) system, and the Bethesda system. Finally, the scheme illustrates the corresponding cytologic smear resulting from exfoliation of the most superficial cells, indicating that even in the mildest disease state, abnormal cells reach the surface and are shed. SIL, squamous intraepithelial lesion.

dysplasia). High-grade SIL corresponds to more severe histologic lesions (CIN-2 and CIN-3), which tend to progress and require treatment.

EPIDEMIOLOGY AND PATHOGENESIS: Epidemiologic features of CIN and invasive cancer are similar. Cervical cancer usually manifests between 40 and 60 years of age (mean, 54), but CIN generally occurs under the age of 40. *The critical factor is HPV infection, which correlates with multiple sexual partners and early age at first coitus.* Thus CIN is essentially a **sexually transmitted disease**. Smoking seems to increase the incidence of cervical cancer, but the mechanism is obscure.

HPV infection leads to CIN and cervical cancer (see Fig. 18-5). There is accumulating evidence that early phases of infection by all HPV types show episomal viral replication, resulting in an LSIL cytology. Massive numbers of viral copies accumulate in the cell cytoplasm and can be seen microscopically as **koilocytes** (see Fig. 18-

2B). Lesions associated with nononcogenic types often progress no further than LSIL, as free viral replication results in cell death. Oncogenic types of HPV (such as HPV 16) integrate into the genome and lead to monoclonal outgrowth of those cells, with progression to high-grade SIL (see Chapter 5). After HPV integrates into host DNA, the viral capsid becomes superfluous. As a result, copies of the whole virus do not accumulate, and koilocytes are absent in many cases of high-grade dysplasia and all invasive cancers (see above for additional details).

PATHOLOGY: Hormonally induced eversion of the cervix and an acidic vaginal environment encourage the development of the transformation zone. Under physiologic conditions, benign squamous metaplasia is the eventual outcome. CIN is nearly always a disease of metaplastic squamous epithelium in the transformation zone or the endocervix. *The extent of the transformation zone determines the distribution of CIN, and hence cervical cancer, on the exposed portion of the cervix.*

The normal process by which cervical squamous epithelium matures is disturbed in CIN, as evidenced morphologically by changes in cellularity, differentiation, polarity, nuclear features,

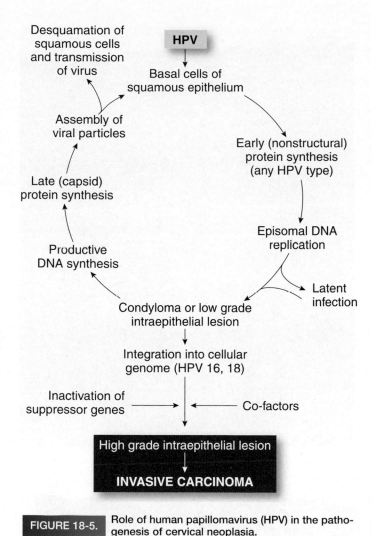

FIGURE 18-5. Role of human papillomavirus (HPV) in the pathogenesis of cervical neoplasia.

and mitotic activity. The sequence of histologic changes from CIN-1 to CIN-3 is illustrated in Figure 18-6.

CIN-1 (mild dysplasia): The most pronounced changes are seen in the basal third of the epithelium. Substantial cytoplasmic differentiation proceeds as abnormal cells migrate through the upper two thirds of the epithelium, but the nuclei in the upper levels are still morphologically abnormal. Thus, the sloughed cells can be detected as abnormal in Pap smears.

CIN-2 (moderate dysplasia): Abnormal cells are present throughout the entire thickness of the epithelium. However, most of the cellular abnormalities are in the lower and middle thirds. Cytodifferentiation occurs in cells in the upper third, but it is less than in CIN-1.

CIN-3 (severe dysplasia and CIS): The cells in the superficial (upper) epithelium disclose some, albeit minimal, differentiation, whereas CIS shows none at all.

The mean age at which women develop CIN is 24 to 27 years for CIN-1 and CIN-2, and 35 to 42 for CIN-3. Based on morphologic criteria, half of CIN-1 cases regress, 10% progress to CIN-3, and less than 2% become invasive cancer. The average time for all grades of dysplasia to progress to CIS is about 10 years. *At least 20% of CIN-3 cases progress to invasive carcinoma within that time.*

 CLINICAL FEATURES: Women with CIN-1 are often followed conservatively (i.e., repeated Pap smears plus close follow-up). High-grade lesions are treated according to the extent of disease. Loop electrosurgical excision procedure (a form of electrocautery), which can be performed on an outpatient basis, is commonly used. In certain situations, cervical conization (removal of a cone of tissue around the external os), cryosurgery, and (rarely) hysterectomy are performed. Follow-up smears and clinical examinations should continue for life, as vaginal or vulvar squamous cancer may develop later.

Microinvasive Squamous Cell Carcinoma is the Earliest Stage of Invasive Cervical Cancer

Microinvasive cancer features neoplastic cells that invade the stroma minimally (Fig. 18-7). About 7% of specimens removed for CIS show foci of microinvasive cancer. Small clusters of cells or solid lesions in the stroma have the following characteristics.

- Invasion to a depth of less than 3 mm (stage 1A1) or 5 mm (stage 1A2) below the basement membrane
- 7-mm maximum lateral extension
- Lack of vascular invasion
- No lymph node metastases

Conization or simple hysterectomy generally suffices to cure microinvasive cancers less than 3 mm deep.

Invasive Squamous Cell Carcinoma is Still Common Worldwide

 EPIDEMIOLOGY: Squamous cell carcinoma is by far the most common type of cervical cancer. Even in the United States, it still accounts for about 10,000 new cases annually. However, in developing countries, where cytologic screening is less available, squamous cell cervical cancer is still a major cause of cancer death. A **cervical cancer vaccine** has recently been approved and recommended for women between the ages of 9 and 26 (see above), which in clinical trials decreased the risk of cervical cancer by 97%. Vaccinated women developed neither HPV-associated precancer nor invasive cervical cancer.

 PATHOLOGY: Early stages of cervical cancer often manifest as poorly defined, granular, eroded lesions or nodular and exophytic masses (Fig. 18-8A). On microscopic examination, most tumors display a nonkeratinizing pattern, characterized by solid nests of large malignant squamous cells. Occasional cancers exhibit nests of keratinized cells organized in concentric whorls, so-called keratin pearls (see Fig. 18-8B). The least common pattern of squamous cell cancer is small cell carcinoma, which is the most aggressive type of cervical cancer and has the worst prognosis. It consists of infiltrating masses of small, cohesive, nonkeratinized, malignant cells.

Cervical cancer spreads by direct extension and through lymphatic vessels and only rarely by the hematogenous route. Local extension into surrounding tissues (parametrium) results in **ureteral compression** and ultimately renal failure, the most common cause of death (50% of patients). Bladder and rectal involvement may lead to fistula formation. Metastases to regional lymph nodes involve paracervical, hypogastric, and external iliac nodes.

CLINICAL FEATURES: The Pap smear remains the most reliable screening test for detecting cervical cancer. In the earliest stages of cervical cancer, patients complain most often of vaginal bleeding after intercourse or douching. The clinical stage of cervical cancer is the best prognostic index of survival. The overall 5-year survival rate is 60% and decreases to 10% in widely disseminated disease. Radical hysterectomy is favored for localized tumor, especially in younger women; radiation therapy or combinations of the two are used for more advanced tumors.

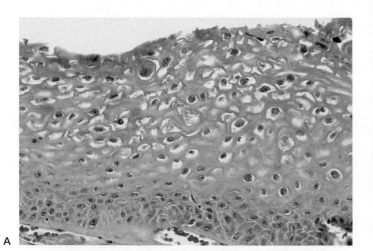

A

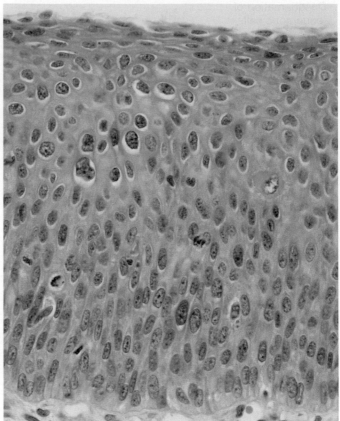

B

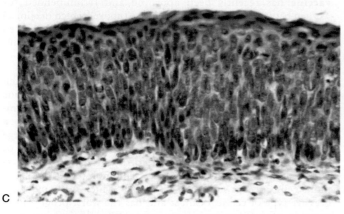

C

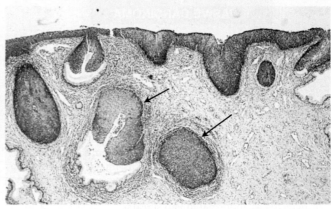

D

FIGURE 18-6. **Cervical intraepithelial neoplasia (CIN). A.** CIN-1: The cervical epithelium shows pronounced cellular atypia in the basal third. Some cells in the upper two thirds of the epithelium have abnormal nuclei, but all show cytoplasmic differentiation. **B.** CIN-2 to CIN-3: The lower two thirds of the epithelium displays pronounced cell atypia. Although cytodifferentiation occurs in the upper third of the epithelium, it is less pronounced than in CIN-1. **C.** CIN-3 (carcinoma in situ, CIS): Neoplastic cells are present throughout the entire epithelium. **D.** CIN-3: CIS partially or completely replaces the columnar epithelium of the endocervical glands.

Endocervical Adenocarcinoma Accounts for 20% of Malignant Cervical Tumors

An increased incidence of cervical adenocarcinoma has been reported recently, with a mean age at presentation of 56 years. Most tumors are of the endocervical cell (mucinous) type, but the various subtypes have little importance for overall survival. Adenocarcinoma shares epidemiologic factors with squamous cell carcinoma of the cervix and spreads similarly. The tumors are often associated with adenocarcinoma in situ and are frequently infected with HPV types 16 and 18.

UTERUS

The Menstrual Cycle

The normal endometrium undergoes a series of sequential changes that support the growth of implanted fertilized ova (zygotes) (Fig. 18-9). If conception does not occur, the endometrium is shed and then regenerated to support a fertilized ovum in the next cycle.

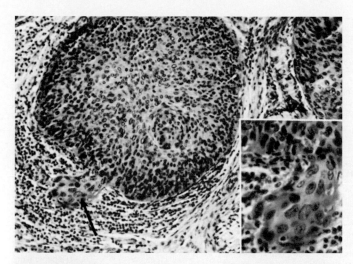

FIGURE 18-7. Microinvasive squamous cell carcinoma. This section of the cervix shows that carcinoma in situ in an endocervical gland has broken through the basement membrane *(arrow)* to invade the stroma. *(Inset)* A higher-power view of the microinvasive focus.

PROLIFERATIVE PHASE: During the first 14 days of the menstrual cycle, the endometrium is under estrogenic stimulation. The functional zone exhibits tubular to coiled glands, which are evenly distributed and supported by a cellular, monomorphic stroma (see Fig. 18-9A). As proliferation progresses, the columnar cells lining the glands increase from one layer in thickness to a pseudostratified epithelium that is mitotically active. The stroma is also mitotically active. Spiral arteries are narrow and mostly inconspicuous.

SECRETORY PHASE: Ovulation occurs about 14 days after the last menstrual period. Afterwards, the Graafian follicle that has discharged its ovum becomes a corpus luteum. The granulosa cells of the corpus luteum begin to secrete progesterone, the hormone that transforms the endometrium from a proliferative into a secretory state (see Fig. 18-9B,C).

- **Days 17 to 19:** Endometrial glands enlarge, dilate, and become more coiled. The lining cells develop abundant glycogen-rich, subnuclear vacuoles.

- **Days 20 to 22:** The endometrium displays prominent glandular secretions and stromal edema. The glands dilate and are more tortuous.
- **Days 23 to 27:** The stromal cells enlarge and exhibit large, round, vesicular nuclei and abundant eosinophilic cytoplasm. These cells, which normally appear first about the spiral arterioles, are the precursors of the decidual cells of pregnancy. By day 27, the full thickness of the stroma is "predecidualized." The tubular glands continue to dilate and develop serrated (sawtoothed) borders.

MENSTRUAL PHASE: In the absence of pregnancy (i.e., without a blastocyst to elaborate human chorionic gonadotropin [hCG]), granulosa and thecal cells of the corpus luteum degenerate. As the corpus luteum degenerates, progesterone levels fall, the endometrium becomes desiccated, the spiral arteries collapse, and the stroma disintegrates. Menses commence on day 28, last 3 to 7 days, and result in a flow of about 35 mL of blood. The denuded surface is re-epithelialized by extension of the residual glandular epithelium.

ATROPHIC ENDOMETRIUM: After menopause, the number of glands and quantity of stroma progressively decrease. Remaining glands are often oriented parallel to the surface, and the stroma contains abundant collagen. The glands of the atrophic endometrium are often conspicuously dilated, an appearance termed **senile cystic atrophy of the endometrium**.

ENDOMETRIUM OF PREGNANCY: Maintenance of the corpus luteum of pregnancy depends on continuous stimulation by hCG secreted by placental trophoblast of the developing embryo. The trophoblast begins to develop about day 23. Under the influence of hCG, the corpus luteum increases its output of progesterone, thereby stimulating secretion of fluid by endometrial glands. The hypersecretory endometrium of pregnancy shows widely dilated glands lined by cells with abundant glycogen. These features can persist for up to 8 weeks after delivery.

Endometritis

Endometritis, or an inflamed endometrium, is a diagnosis based on the finding of an abnormal inflammatory infiltrate in the endometrium. It must be distinguished from the normal presence of polymorphonuclear leukocytes

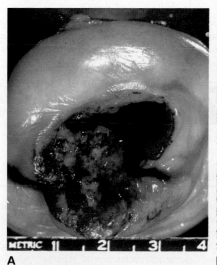
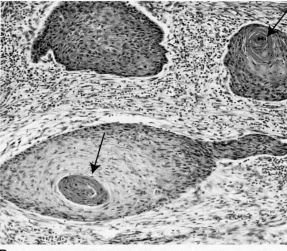

A   B

FIGURE 18-8. **Squamous cell cancer. A.** The cervix is distorted by the presence of an exophytic, ulcerated squamous cell carcinoma. **B.** The keratinizing pattern of the tumor is manifested as whorls of keratinized cells ("keratin pearls") *(arrows)*.

Day of Cycle		Before 14	15–16	17	18	19–22	23	24–25	26–27	28+
Post-ovulatory day			1–2	3	4	5–8	9	10–11	12–13	14+
Cycle phases		Proliferative	Interval	Early secretory		Mid-secretory			Late secretory	Menstrual
Key feature		Mitoses	Mitoses and subnuclear vacuoles	Maximum subnuclear vacuoles	Subnuclear vacuoles present	Stromal edema	Focal decidua around spiral arteries	Patchy decidua	Extensive decidua	Stromal crumbling
Microscopic features of functional zone	Stroma	Loose stroma. Mitoses	Same as proliferative	Loose stroma. Scanty mitoses	Loose stroma	Stromal edema	Focal decidua around spiral arteries. Edema prominent	Decidua throughout stroma. Some edema	Extensive decidua. Prominent granulated lymphocytes	Stromal crumbling. Hemorrhage
	Glands	Straight to tightly coiled tubules. Mitoses	Some subnuclear vacuoles, otherwise as proliferative	Extensive subnuclear vacuoles	Dilated glands. Some subnuclear vacuoles	Dilated glands with irregular outline. Luminal secretion		'Saw tooth' glands	Prominent 'saw tooth' glands	Disrupted glands. Secretory exhaustion. Regenerating epithelium
Appearances		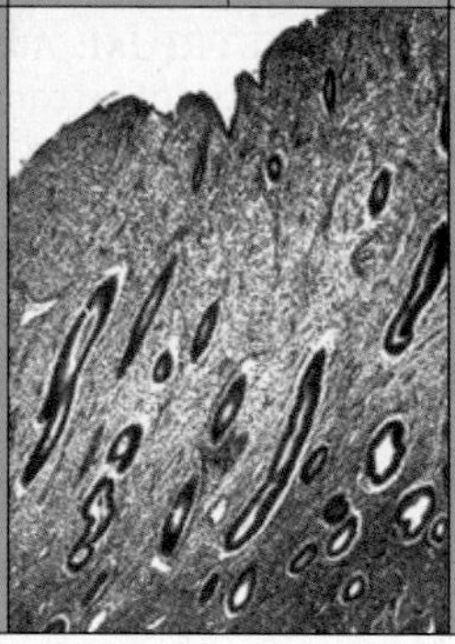				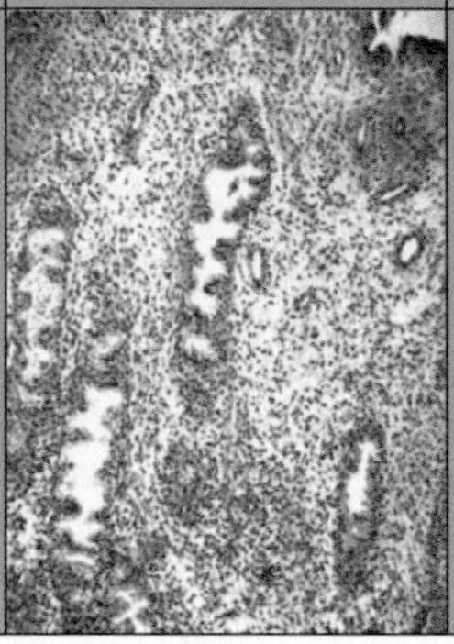			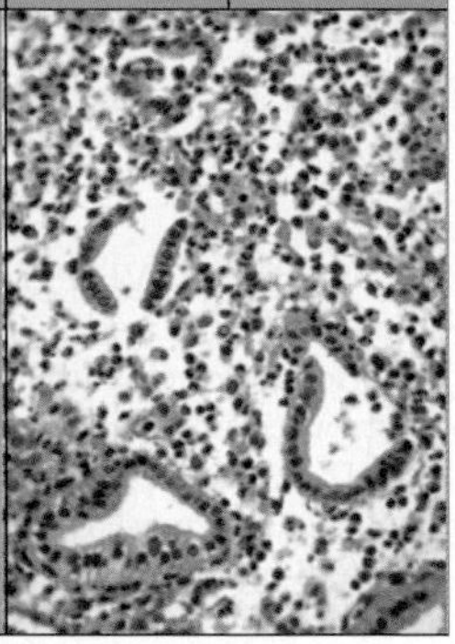	

A   **B**   **C**

FIGURE 18-9. **Main histologic features of the endometrial phases of the normal menstrual cycle. A.** Proliferative phase. Straight tubular glands are embedded in a cellular monomorphic stroma. **B.** Secretory phase, day 24. Dilated tortuous glands with serrated borders are situated in a predecidual stroma. **C.** Menstrual endometrium. Fragmented glands, dissolution of the stroma, and numerous neutrophils are evident.

during menstruation and a mild lymphocytic infiltrate at other times. The findings in most cases of endometritis are nonspecific and rarely point to a specific cause.

ACUTE ENDOMETRITIS: This condition is defined as the abnormal presence of polymorphonuclear leukocytes in the endometrium. Most cases result from an ascending infection from the cervix, for example, after the usually impervious cervical barrier is compromised by abortion, delivery, or medical instrumentation.

CHRONIC ENDOMETRITIS: Although lymphocytes and lymphoid follicles are occasionally scattered in a normal endometrium, plasma cells in the endometrium are diagnostic of chronic endometritis. The disorder is associated with intrauterine devices (IUDs), pelvic inflammatory disease, and retained products of conception after an abortion or delivery. The condition is generally self-limited.

Adenomyosis

Adenomyosis is the presence of endometrial glands and stroma within the myometrium. Adenomyosis is more likely to be symptomatic the more deeply it penetrates the myometrium. Pain occurs as foci of adenomyosis enlarge when blood is entrapped during menses. One fifth of all uteri removed at surgery show some degree of adenomyosis.

 PATHOLOGY: The uterus may be enlarged. The myometrium discloses small, soft, tan areas, some of which are cystic. Microscopic examination reveals glands lined by mildly proliferative to inactive endometrium and surrounded by endometrial stroma with varying degrees of fibrosis. Varying degrees of glandular hyperplasia may be seen, and occasionally hyperplastic surface endometrium extends into the foci of adenomyosis.

CLINICAL FEATURES: Many patients with adenomyosis are asymptomatic, but varying degrees of pelvic pain, dysfunctional uterine bleeding, dysmenorrhea, and dyspareunia are common. The cause of adenomyosis remains unknown.

Endometriosis

Endometriosis is the presence of benign endometrial glands and stroma outside the uterus. It afflicts 5% to 10% of women of reproductive age and regresses after natural or artificial menopause. Sites most frequently involved are the ovaries (>60%), other uterine adnexa (uterine ligaments, rectovaginal septum, pouch of Douglas) and the pelvic peritoneum covering the uterus, fallopian tubes, rectosigmoid colon, and bladder (Fig. 18-10). Endometriosis can be even more widespread and occasionally affects the cervix, vagina, perineum, bladder, and umbilicus.

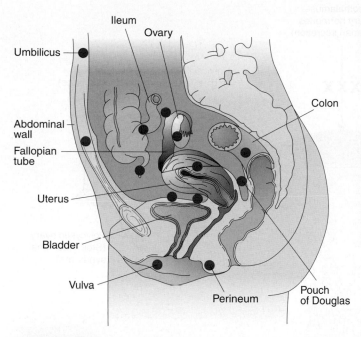

FIGURE 18-10. Sites of endometriosis.

PATHOGENESIS: There are three theories to explain the histogenesis of endometriosis that are not mutually exclusive: (1) **Transplantation** of menstrual endometrial fragments refluxed through the fallopian tubes to ectopic sites (the most widely accepted theory); (2) **Metaplasia** of the multipotential celomic peritoneum; and (3) **Induction** of undifferentiated mesenchyme in ectopic sites to form lesions after exposure to substances released from shed endometrium.

PATHOLOGY: On gross examination, the lesions of endometriosis vary in color. Yellow-red stains, when confined to the serosa, reflect the breakdown of blood products and are often the earliest detectable lesions. Red

lesions also reflect an early form of the disease, in which foci of endometriosis are actively growing. With repeated cycles of hemorrhage and the onset of fibrosis, the affected surface may show scarring and take on a grossly brown discoloration ("powder burns"). Sometimes, scarring leads to complications, such as intestinal obstruction. In the ovaries, repeated hemorrhage may cause endometriotic foci to form cysts up to 15 cm in diameter, which contain inspissated, chocolate-colored material ("chocolate cysts"). Microscopically, endometriosis shows ectopic endometrial glands and stroma (Fig. 18-11). Occasionally, healed foci of endometriosis may consist only of fibrous tissue and hemosiderin-laden macrophages, features that by themselves are not diagnostic.

CLINICAL FEATURES: The signs and symptoms of endometriosis depend on the location of the implants. The most common complaint is dysmenorrhea, owing to implants on the uterosacral ligaments. These lesions swell immediately before or during menstruation, producing pelvic pain. In fact, half of all women with dysmenorrhea have endometriosis. **Infertility is the primary complaint in one third of women with endometriosis** (Fig. 18-12). With conservative surgery to restore pelvic anatomy, many women who suffer from endometriosis may eventually become pregnant. Malignancy occurs in about 1% to 2% of cases of endometriosis. Clear cell and endometrioid tumors (see below) are the most frequent forms.

Hormonal Effects

Dysfunctional Uterine Bleeding Occurs During or Between Menstrual Periods

In dysfunctional bleeding, the cause lies outside the uterus. It is one of the most common gynecological disorders of women of reproductive age but is still poorly understood. Most cases are related to an endocrine disturbance that involves an aspect of the hypothalamic–pituitary-ovarian axis (Table 18-2). Ovarian dysfunction is usual, especially in the presence of anovulation. Some causes of menstrual irregularity are intrinsic to the uterus and are not considered dysfunctional. These causes include (1) growths (e.g., carcinoma, endometrial intraepithelial neoplasia [EIN], submucous leiomyomata, and polyps), (2) inflammation (e.g., endometritis), (3) pregnancy (e.g., complications of intrauterine or ectopic preg-

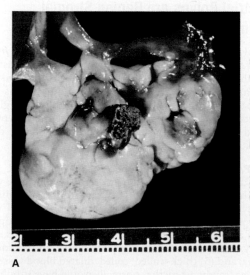

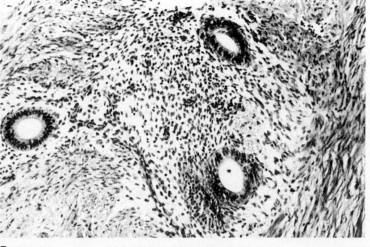

A   B

FIGURE 18-11. **Endometriosis. A.** Implants of endometriosis on the ovary appear as red-blue nodules. **B.** A microscopic section shows endometrial glands and stroma in the ovary.

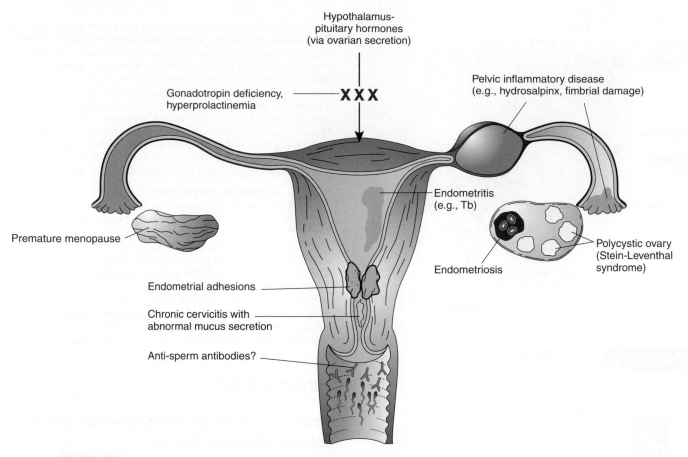

FIGURE 18-12. Causes of acquired infertility. Tb, Tuberculosis.

TABLE 18–2	
Causes of Abnormal Uterine Bleeding (Including Uterine and Extrauterine Causes)	
Newborn	Maternal estrogen

Childhood	Iatrogenic (trauma, foreign body, infection of vagina)
	    Vaginal neoplasms (sarcoma botryoides)
	    Ovarian tumors (functional)

Adolescence	Hypothalamic immaturity Psychogenic and nutritional problems Inadequate luteal function

Reproductive age	Anovulatory
	    Central: psychogenic, stress
	    Systemic: nutritional and endocrine
	    disease
	    Gonadal: functional tumors
	    End-organ: benign endometrial
	    hyperplasia
	Pregnancy: ectopic, retained placenta,
	abortion, mole
	Ovulatory
	    Organic: neoplasia, infections (PID),
	    leiomyomas
	    Polymenorrhea: short follicular or luteal
	    phases
	    Iatrogenic: anticoagulants, IUD
	    Irregular shedding

Menopause	Carcinoma, EIN, benign hyperplasias, polyps, leiomyomata
Postmenopause	Carcinoma, EIN, polyps, leiomyomata

EIN, endometrial intraepithelial neoplasia; IUD, intrauterine device; PID, pelvic inflammatory disease.

nancy), and (4) the effects of intrauterine devices. *Anovulatory bleeding is a complex syndrome of many causes that manifests as the absence of ovulation during the reproductive years.* It is most often noted at either end of reproductive life (i.e., menarche and menopause).

Tumors

Endometrial Polyps are Benign Stromal Neoplasms in the Endometrial Cavity

Endometrial polyps are benign localized overgrowths that project from the endometrial surface into the endometrial cavity. They occur most commonly in the perimenopausal period and are virtually unknown before menarche. Polyps arise as monoclonal outgrowths of endometrial stroma with secondary induction of polyclonal glandular elements. The stroma and glands of endometrial polyps have diminished hormonal responsiveness and do not slough during menstruation.

 PATHOLOGY: Most endometrial polyps arise in the fundus, although they may originate anywhere within the endometrial cavity. They vary from several millimeters to growths filling the entire endometrial cavity. Most polyps are solitary, but 20% are multiple. Microscopically, the core of a polyp is composed of (1) endometrial glands, which are often cystically dilated and hyperplastic; (2) a fibrous endometrial stroma; and (3) thick-walled, coiled, dilated blood vessels, derived from a straight artery that normally would have supplied the basal zone of the endometrium. A mantle of endometrial epithelium covers the polyp. The glandular epithelium is usually not at the same stage of the cycle as that of the adjacent, normal endometrium.

CLINICAL FEATURES: Endometrial polyps typically present with intermenstrual bleeding, due to surface ulceration or hemorrhagic infarction. Because bleeding in an older woman may be due to endometrial cancer, this sign must be thoroughly evaluated. Endometrial polyps are not ordinarily precancerous, but up to 0.5% harbor adenocarcinoma.

Benign Endometrial Hyperplasia is Caused by Excess Estrogenic Stimulation

Benign endometrial hyperplasia refers to a spectrum of endometrial-wide changes resulting from abnormal estrogenic stimulation, with randomly distributed architectural and cytologic changes. Estrogenic stimulation of the endometrium beyond the 2-week interval of a normal proliferative menstrual cycle causes progressive changes that have been associated with a 2- to 10-fold increased risk of endometrial cancer. Aside from women with coexisting endometrial intraepithelial neoplasia (EIN, see below), it is not possible on histopathologic grounds to stratify cancer risk within this group of patients by a single histologic examination. The earliest changes are often designated "persistent proliferative" or "disordered proliferative" endometrium and are characterized by isolated cystic expansion of scattered proliferative glands without a substantial change in gland density. There is a gradual transition to benign endometrial hyperplasia as gland density becomes irregular throughout, and some regions have more glands than stroma.

 PATHOLOGY: Benign endometrial hyperplasia affects the entire endometrial compartment, where remodeling of glands and stroma creates an irregular density of commingled cystic, slightly branching and tubular glands (Fig. 18-13). *The presence of cytologic atypia is the most important prognostic feature.*

- **Simple hyperplasia:** This proliferative lesion shows minimal glandular complexity and crowding and no cytologic atypia. The epithelial lining is usually one cell layer thick and the stroma between the glands is abundant. **One percent of cases of simple endometrial hyperplasia progress to adenocarcinoma.**
- **Complex hyperplasia:** This variant exhibits marked glandular complexity and crowding but no cytologic atypia (see Fig. 18-13). Glands are increased in number and may vary in size. The stroma between the glands is scanty. **Three percent of patients develop adenocarcinoma.**
- **Atypical hyperplasia:** *This lesion shows cytologic atypia and marked glandular crowding, often as back-to-back glands.* Glands may show complex architecture, with an intraluminal papillary arrangement or the appearance of budding glands in the stroma (Fig. 18-14). Epithelial cells are enlarged and hyperchromatic with prominent nucleoli and increased nuclear-to-cytoplasmic ratios. **One fourth of these cases progress to adenocarcinoma, which is almost always of the endometrioid type.**

 CLINICAL FEATURES: Benign endometrial hyperplasia may result from anovulatory cycles, polycystic ovary syndrome, an estrogen-producing tumor, therapeutic administration of estrogens, or obesity. In such cases, therapy aimed at the primary cause may alleviate estrogenic stimulation. The short-term risk for endometrial cancer remains low for women with benign endometrial hyperplasia, providing no EIN is seen. The long-term risk of refractory hyperplasia requires constant evaluation.

Endometrial Intraepithelial Neoplasia (EIN) and Adenocarcinoma are Separate from Benign Endometrial Hyperplasia

Endometrial hyperplasias of the several types mentioned above may be considered endometrial in situ neoplasia (EIN). *In this paradigm, EIN is recognized as monoclonal neoplastic growths of genetically*

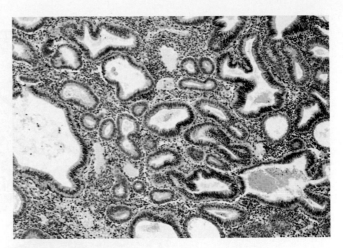

FIGURE 18-13. **Complex endometrial hyperplasia.** The endometrial glands, which are in the proliferative phase, are closely packed and display moderate architectural disarray (budding and branching). No cytologic atypia is present.

altered cells having a greatly increased clinical risk of conversion to the endometrioid type of endometrial adenocarcinoma. Benign endometrial hyperplasia, by contrast, is intrinsically normal endometrium that displays global morphologic changes due to the extrinsic influence of unopposed estrogens. EIN and benign endometrial hyperplasia coexist in many patients and may be distinguished. Systemic hormonal factors are relevant to both diseases, as they can act as positive or negative selection factors for mutated cells within an EIN lesion.

Endometrial Intraepithelial Neoplasia

EIN is a monoclonal neoplastic proliferation prone to malignant transformation. It shows a continuity of acquired genetic markers upon transformation into a malignant phase.

 PATHOGENESIS: EIN lesions are aggregates of neoplastic endometrial glands with altered cytology and architecture that allow differentiation from benign lesions. Unlike benign endometrial hyperplasia, which involves all the endometrium at inception, EIN lesions begin locally and only later overrun the endometrial compartment. *Loss of hormonally regulated PTEN tumor suppressor gene function occurs clonally in two thirds of EIN lesions and an increased fraction in subsequent endometrial carcinomas.* Cancers that develop in women with EIN are usually endometrioid adenocarcinoma. There is usually a relationship to estrogen exposure.

 PATHOLOGY: At emergence, EIN lesions extend outward from a central lesion by interposition of neoplastic glands between normal glands. They are composed of tight aggregates of individually recognizable glands that (1) differ cytologically from the background endometrium, (2) have a gland area that exceeds that of stroma, and (3) measure more than 1 mm in dimension in a single fragment. About 80% of atypical hyperplasias (as defined above) would be diagnosed as EIN using this newer classification scheme (see Fig. 18-14). *Malignant transformation of EIN is evident when the glands develop solid, cribriform, or maze-like patterns characteristic of adenocarcinoma.*

 CLINICAL FEATURES: Women newly diagnosed with EIN have a 40% chance of having endometrial cancer diagnosed within 1 year, suggesting that in most cases, the cancer was already present at the time of the initial biopsy. Excluding women with concurrent cancer (i.e., only looking at those with a cancer-free interval of 1 year), EIN-positive pa-

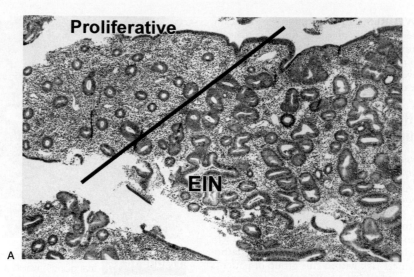

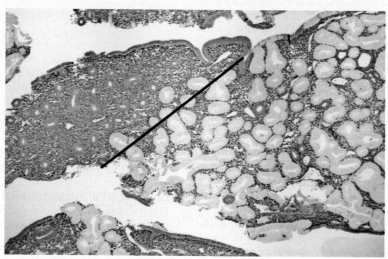

 FIGURE 18-14. **Endometrial intraepithelial neoplasia (EIN). A.** Tight clusters of cytologically altered neoplastic endometrial glands with abundant cytoplasm and rounded nuclei *(right)* are offset from the background endometrium *(left)* in this geographic focus of EIN. Measurement across the perimeter of this aggregate of individual tubular glands exceeds 1 mm, and features of adenocarcinoma such as cribriform, maze-like, or solid architecture are lacking. **B.** Glands affected by EIN show loss of PTEN expression by immunohistochemistry (loss of brown staining).

tients have a 45-fold increased risk of developing of endometrial cancer. Hysterectomy is usually considered the therapy of choice if a woman has decided not to have any more children.

Endometrial Adenocarcinoma

 EPIDEMIOLOGY: Endometrial carcinoma is the fourth most frequent type of cancer in American women and the most common gynecological cancer. It can be divided into (1) **endometrioid cancers**, which are associated with EIN precursors, prior estrogen exposure, and a slow clinical course, and (2) **nonendometrioid cancers**, which emerge without warning in older women and have much higher fatality rates. Endometrial carcinoma was responsible for an estimated 7,000 deaths in the United States in 2006 (3% of all cancer deaths in women). The use of estrogens for easing menopausal symptoms in the 1970s was initially associated with a marked increase in disease frequency, which was ameliorated by lowering the estrogen dose and incorporating progestins (estrogen antagonists) into treatment regimens. The occurrence of endometrial cancer varies with age. The incidence is 12 cases per 100,000 in women at age 40, but is seven-fold higher in 60-year-olds. Three quarters of women with endometrial cancer are postmenopausal. The median age at diagnosis is 63.

 PATHOGENESIS: *The major form of endometrial cancer, endometrioid adenocarcinoma, is linked to prolonged estrogenic stimulation of the endometrium and defects in the PTEN tumor suppressor pathway.* In addition to treatment with exogenous estrogens, the most common risk factors are obesity, diabetes, nulliparity, early menarche, and late menopause, all potentially associated with high exposure to estrogen.

Nonendometrioid cancers, especially **serous and clear cell adenocarcinoma**, are unrelated to estrogen exposure and usually occur in women in their 60s and 70s. The adjacent endometrium is generally atrophic, a sign of estrogen deficiency. Endometrial cancer also occurs in association with a higher incidence of both breast and ovarian cancers in closely related women, suggesting a genetic predisposition.

PATHOLOGY: Endometrial cancer grows in a diffuse or exophytic pattern. Regardless of its site of origin, the tumor often tends to involve multiple areas. Large tumors are usually hemorrhagic and necrotic.

ENDOMETRIOID ADENOCARCINOMA OF THE ENDOMETRIUM: This type of endometrial cancer is composed entirely of glandular cells and is the most common histologic variant (60%). The tumor is divided into three grades on the basis of the ratio of glandular to solid elements, the latter signifying poorer differentiation (Fig. 18-15).

The nuclei of endometrial adenocarcinoma range from bland to markedly pleomorphic, usually showing prominent nucleoli. Mitotic figures are abundant and may be abnormal in less differentiated tumors. Tumor cells that grow in solid sheets generally are poorly differentiated and considered as high grade.

ENDOMETRIOID ADENOCARCINOMA, WITH SQUAMOUS DIFFERENTIATION: One third of all endometrial carcinomas contain squamous cells in addition to glandular elements. If the squamous element is well differentiated, with no more than minimal atypia, the tumor is called **well-differentiated adenocarcinoma with squamous differentiation**. If the squamous element appears malignant, the tumor is **poorly differentiated adenocarcinoma with squamous differentiation** (also known as **adenosquamous carcinoma**). These two variants represent 22% and 7% of all endometrial cancers, respectively.

ENDOMETRIOID ADENOCARCINOMA, SECRETORY TYPE: This tumor is a variant of endometrioid adenocarcinoma, having cells with subnuclear glycogen-containing vacuoles, which usually occurs in premenopausal women. The tumor is extremely well differentiated and has the most favorable outcome of any type of adenocarcinoma.

OTHER TYPES (NONENDOMETRIOID) OF ENDOMETRIAL CARCINOMA: Nonendometrioid types of endometrial carcinoma are less common and are unassociated with estrogen exposure. Because they tend to be aggressive as a group, histologic grading is not of clinical value. These tumors include serous and clear cell adenocarcinomas and carcinosarcoma, which shows mixed epithelial and mesenchymal differentiation.

CLINICAL FEATURES: Endometrial carcinoma usually occurs in perimenopausal or postmenopausal women. The chief complaint is commonly abnormal uterine bleeding, especially if the tumor is in its early stages of growth (i.e., confined to the endometrium). Unfortunately, cervicovaginal cytological screening is unsuitable for early detection of endometrial cancer. Unlike cervical cancer, endometrial cancer may spread directly to para-aortic lymph nodes, thereby skipping pelvic nodes. Patients with advanced cancers may also develop pulmonary metastases (40% of cases with metastases). Women with well-differentiated cancers confined to the endometrium are usually treated by simple hysterectomy. Postoperative radiation is considered if (1) the tumor is poorly differentiated or nonendometrioid in type, (2) the myometrium is deeply invaded, (3) the cervix is involved, or (4) lymph nodes contain metastases.

Survival in endometrial carcinoma is related to multiple factors including (1) stage and grade, (2) age, and (3) other measurable risk factors, such as progesterone receptor activity. High levels of estrogen and progesterone receptors in the tumor and low levels of proliferative activity correlate with a better prognosis. Actuarial survival of all patients with endometrial cancer following treatment is 80% after the second year, decreasing to 65% after 10 years.

Leiomyoma is the Most Common Tumor of the Female Genital Tract

Leiomyoma, a benign tumor of smooth muscle origin, is colloquially known as a "myoma" or "fibroid." If minute tumors are included, uterine leiomyomas occur in 75% of women over 30 years of age. They are

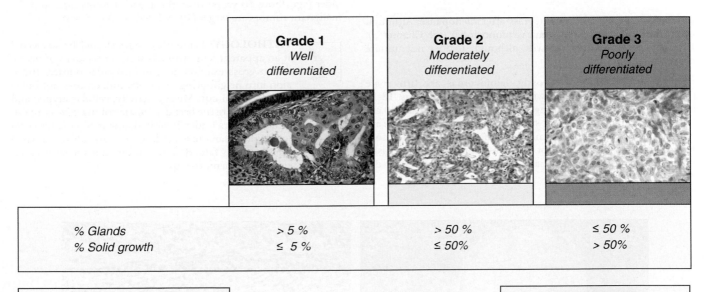

FIGURE 18-15. **Grading of endometrial adenocarcinoma.** The grade depends primarily on the architectural pattern, but significant nuclear atypia changes a grade 1 tumor to grade 2, and a grade 2 tumor to grade 3. Nuclear atypia is characterized by round nuclei; variation in shape, size, and staining; hyperchromasia; coarsely clumped chromating; prominent nucleoli; and frequent and abnormal mitoses. Significant nuclear atypia if present increases the tumor grade.

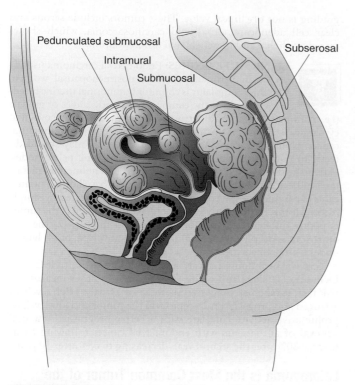

FIGURE 18-16. **Leiomyomas of the uterus.** The leiomyomas are intramural; submucosal (a pedunculated one appearing in the form of an endometrial polyp) and subserosal (one compressing the bladder and the other compressing the rectum).

rare before age 20, and most regress after menopause. Although often multiple, each leiomyoma is monoclonal (see Chapter 5). Estrogen promotes their growth, although it does not initiate them.

PATHOLOGY: Grossly, leiomyomas are firm, pale gray, whorled, and without encapsulation (Figs. 18-16 and 18-17). They range from 1 mm to more than 30 cm in diameter. The cut surface bulges, and the borders are smooth and distinct from neighboring myometrium. Most leiomyomas are intramural, but some are submucosal, subserosal, or pedunculated. Many, especially larger ones, show areas of de-

generative hyalinization that are sharply demarcated from adjacent normal myometrium. Leiomyomas that display low mitotic activity (≤4 mitoses per 10 high-power fields) lack nuclear atypia and geographical necrosis and have little or no malignant potential. "**Mitotically active leiomyomas**" show brisk mitotic activity but are small, sharply demarcated from the adjacent normal myometrium, and lack both geographical necrosis and significant cellular atypia. They are generally considered to be benign. Microscopically leiomyomas exhibit interlacing fascicles of uniform spindle cells, in which nuclei are elongated and have blunt ends (see Fig. 18-17B). The cytoplasm is abundant, eosinophilic, and fibrillar. The myocytes of leiomyomas and adjacent myometrium are cytologically identical.

CLINICAL FEATURES: Submucosal leiomyomas may cause bleeding, owing to ulceration of the thinned, overlying endometrium. Some submucosal leiomyomas become pedunculated and protrude through the cervical os, eliciting cramping pains. Many intramural leiomyomas are symptomatic because of sheer bulk, and large ones may interfere with bowel or bladder function or cause dystocia in labor. Leiomyomas usually grow slowly but occasionally enlarge rapidly during pregnancy. Large symptomatic leiomyomas are removed by myomectomy or hysterectomy.

Leiomyosarcoma is Rare in Comparison to Leiomyoma

Leiomyosarcoma is a malignancy of smooth muscle origin with an incidence of only 1/1,000 that of its benign counterpart. It accounts for 2% of uterine malignancies. Its pathogenesis is uncertain, but at least some appear to arise from within leiomyomas. Women with leiomyosarcomas are on average more than a decade older (age above 50 years) than those with leiomyomas, and the malignant tumors are larger (10 to 15 cm vs. 3 to 5 cm).

PATHOLOGY: Leiomyosarcoma should be suspected if an apparent leiomyoma is soft, shows areas of necrosis on gross examination, has irregular borders (invasion into neighboring myometrium), or does not bulge above the surface when cut. Mitotic activity, cellular atypia, and geographical necrosis are the best diagnostic criteria. Size is an important feature. Tumors under 5 cm in diameter almost never recur, but most leiomyosarcomas are large and are advanced when detected and are usually fatal despite combinations of surgery, radiation therapy, and chemotherapy.

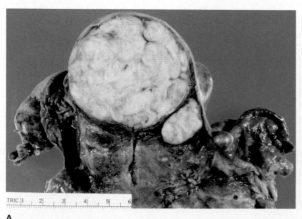

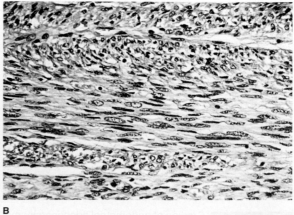

A

B

FIGURE 18-17. **Leiomyoma of the uterus. A.** A bisected uterus displays a prominent, sharply circumscribed fleshy tumor. **B.** Microscopically, smooth muscle cells intertwine in bundles, some of which are cut longitudinally (elongated nuclei) and others transversely.

FALLOPIAN TUBE

Salpingitis

Salpingitis is inflammation of the fallopian tubes, typically due to infections ascending from the lower genital tract. The most common causative organisms are *Neisseria gonorrhoeae, Escherichia coli, Chlamydia,* and *Mycoplasma.* Infection is typically polymicrobial. Acute episodes of salpingitis (particularly those associated with chlamydial infection) may be asymptomatic. A fallopian tube damaged by prior infection is particularly susceptible to reinfection. In most cases, chronic salpingitis develops only after repeated episodes of acute salpingitis.

PATHOLOGY AND CLINICAL FEATURES: In acute salpingitis, microscopic examination reveals marked infiltration by polymorphonuclear leukocytes, pronounced edema, and congestion of the mucosal folds (plicae). The inflammatory infiltrate in chronic salpingitis consists of lymphocytes and plasma cells. Edema and congestion tend to be minimal. In late stages, the fallopian tube may seal and become distended with pus (**pyosalpinx**) or a transudate (**hydrosalpinx**). The fallopian tube allows ascending microorganisms from the lower genital tract to reach the peritoneal cavity, leading to peritonitis and PID. The adjacent ovary may also be involved, sometimes giving rise to a **tubo-ovarian abscess**.

Complications also ensue from damage to the fallopian tube itself. Destruction of the epithelium or deposition of fibrin on the mucosa results in formation of fibrin bridges, which cause the plicae to adhere to one another The damage caused by chronic salpingitis may impair tubal motility and the passage of sperm, in which case **infertility** results. Chronic salpingitis is a common cause of **ectopic pregnancy**, because adherent mucosal plicae create pockets in which ova become entrapped.

Ectopic Pregnancy

Ectopic pregnancy refers to implantation of a fertilized ovum outside the endometrium. More than 95% of ectopic pregnancies occur in the fallopian tube, mostly in the distal and middle thirds.

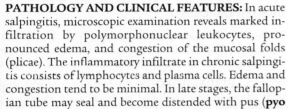

PATHOLOGY: Ectopic pregnancy results when passage of the conceptus along the fallopian tube is impeded, for example, by mucosal adhesions or abnormal tubal motility secondary to inflammatory disease or endometriosis. The trophoblast readily penetrates the mucosa and muscular tubal wall. Blood from the implantation site in the tube enters the peritoneal cavity, causing abdominal pain. The thin tubal wall usually ruptures by the 12th week of gestation. *Tubal rupture is life-threatening to the mother because it can result in rapid exsanguination.* Ectopic pregnancy must be treated promptly with surgical or chemotherapeutic intervention.

OVARY

Cystic Lesions of the Ovaries

Cysts are the most common cause of enlarged ovaries. Those that arise from the invaginated surface epithelium (serous cysts) are quite common. Almost all of the rest derive from ovarian follicles.

Follicle Cysts Tend to be Asymptomatic

Follicle cysts are thin-walled, fluid-filled structures that are lined internally by granulosa cells and externally by theca interna cells. They occur at any age up to menopause, are unilocular and may be single or multiple, unilateral, or bilateral. These cysts arise from ovarian follicles and are probably related to abnormalities in pituitary gonadotropin release.

PATHOLOGY: Follicle cysts rarely exceed 5 cm in the greatest dimension. In an unstimulated state, the granulosa cells of the cyst have uniform, round nuclei and little cytoplasm. Theca cells are small and spindle-shaped. Occasionally, the layers may be luteinized, in which case the lumen contains fluid high in estrogen or progesterone. If the cyst persists, hormonal output can cause precocious puberty in a child and menstrual irregularities in an adult. The only significant complication is mild intraperitoneal bleeding.

Corpus Luteum Cyst Can Bleed

A cyst results from delayed resolution of a corpus luteum's central cavity. Continued progesterone synthesis by the luteal cyst leads to menstrual irregularities. Rupture of a cyst can cause mild hemorrhage into the abdominal cavity. A corpus luteum cyst is typically unilocular, 3 to 5 cm in size, and possesses a yellow wall. The contents of the cyst vary from serosanguinous fluid to clotted blood. Microscopic examination shows numerous large, luteinized granulosa cells. The condition is self-limited.

Theca Lutein Cysts Relate to High Gonadotropin Levels

Theca lutein cysts, also known as hyperreactio luteinalis, are commonly multiple and bilateral. They are associated with high levels of circulating gonadotropins (e.g., in pregnancy, hydatidiform mole, choriocarcinoma, and exogenous gonadotropin therapy) or physical impediments to ovulation (dense adhesions, cortical fibrosis). The excessive gonadotropin levels lead to exaggerated stimulation of the theca interna and extensive cyst formation.

PATHOLOGY: Multiple thin-walled cysts filled with clear fluid replace both ovaries. Microscopically, cysts show a markedly luteinized layer of theca interna. Ovarian parenchyma shows edema and foci of luteinized stromal cells. Intra-abdominal hemorrhage secondary to torsion or rupture of the cyst may require surgical intervention.

Polycystic Ovary Syndrome

Polycystic ovary syndrome, also known as **Stein-Leventhal syndrome**, describes (1) clinical manifestations related to the secretion of excess androgenic hormones, (2) persistent anovulation, and (3) ovaries containing many small subcapsular cysts. It was described initially as a syndrome of **secondary amenorrhea, hirsutism, and obesity**. However, clinical presentations are now known to be far more variable and include amenorrheic women who appear otherwise normal and, even rarely, have ovaries lacking polycystic features. *Polycystic ovary syndrome is a common cause of infertility, and 7% of women experience the condition.*

PATHOGENESIS: The central abnormality in polycystic ovary syndrome is a state of functional ovarian hyperandrogenism with elevated levels of LH, although increased amounts of this hormone are probably a result, rather than a cause, of ovarian dysfunction (Fig. 18-18). Excess ovarian androgens act locally to cause (1) premature follicular atresia, (2) multiple follicular cysts, and (3) a persistent anovulatory state. Impaired follicular maturation causes decreased secretion of progesterone. Peripherally, hyperandrogenism leads to hirsutism, acne, and male-pattern (androgen-dependent) alopecia.

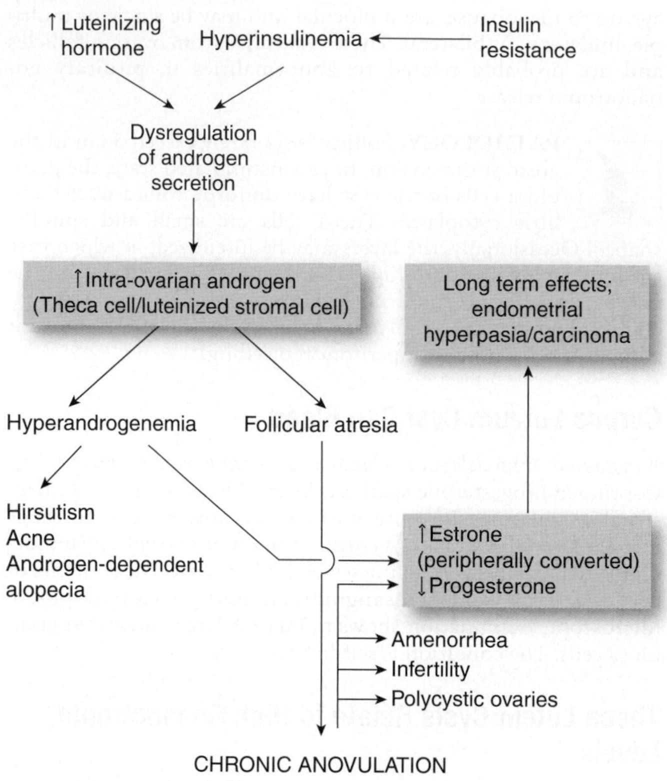

↑Luteinizing hormone → Hyperinsulinemia ← Insulin resistance

Dysregulation of androgen secretion

↑Intra-ovarian androgen (Theca cell/luteinized stromal cell)

Long term effects; endometrial hyperpasia/carcinoma

Hyperandrogenemia   Follicular atresia

Hirsutism
Acne
Androgen-dependent alopecia

↑Estrone (peripherally converted)
↓Progesterone

→ Amenorrhea
→ Infertility
→ Polycystic ovaries

CHRONIC ANOVULATION

FIGURE 18-18. Pathogenesis of the polycystic ovary syndrome.

PATHOLOGY: On gross examination, both ovaries are enlarged. The surface is smooth, reflecting the absence of ovulation. On cut section, the cortex is thickened and discloses numerous theca-lutein type cysts, typically 2 to 8 mm in diameter. These are arranged peripherally around a dense core of stroma or scattered throughout an increased amount of stroma. Microscopically, the following features are present: (1) numerous follicles in early stages of development; (2) follicular atresia; (3) increased stroma, occasionally with luteinized cells (hyperthecosis); and (4) morphologic signs of an absence of ovulation (thick, smooth capsule, and absence of corpora lutea and corpora albicantiae). Many subcapsular cysts show thick zones of theca interna, in which some cells may be luteinized.

CLINICAL FEATURES: Nearly three quarters of women in the United States with anovulatory infertility have polycystic ovary syndrome. Patients are typically in their 20s and report early obesity, menstrual problems, and hirsutism. Half of women with polycystic ovary syndrome are amenorrheic and most others have irregular menstrual periods. Only 75% of affected women are actually infertile, indicating that some do occasionally ovulate. Unopposed acyclic estrogen activity increases the incidence of endometrial hyperplasia and adenocarcinoma. Treatment of polycystic ovary syndrome is mostly hormonal and is directed toward interrupting the constant excess of androgens.

Ovarian Tumors

Ovarian cancer is the second most frequent gynecological malignancy after endometrial cancer. In the United States, it carries a higher mortality rate than all other female genital cancers combined. Approximately 20,000 new cases of ovarian cancer are diagnosed each year in the United States, and more than 15,000 women die from the disease. These tumors predominate in women older than 60 years, but may occur in younger women with a family history of the disease. Unfortunately, this cancer is difficult to detect early in its evolution, when it is still curable. More than three fourths of patients already have extragonadal tumor spread to the pelvis or abdomen at the time of diagnosis.

The broad range of histologic features in these tumors reflects the diverse anatomical structure of the ovary itself. The classification of ovarian tumors identifies them by the tissue of origin (Fig. 18-19). Most frequently encountered tumors arise from surface epithelium and are termed **common epithelial tumors**. Other important groups include germ cell tumors, sex cord/stromal tumors, steroid cell tumors, and tumors metastatic to the ovary.

Epithelial Tumors Account for More than 90% of Ovarian Cancers

Tumors of **common epithelial origin** can be broadly classified as (1) benign, (2) of borderline malignancy (also called **atypical proliferating** or **low malignant potential**), and (3) malignant.

EPIDEMIOLOGY: Epidemiologic studies suggest that common epithelial neoplasms are related to repeated disruption and repair of the epithelial surface, which is part of cyclic ovulation. Thus, tumors most commonly afflict women who are nulliparous and, conversely, occur least often in women in whom ovulation has been suppressed (e.g., by pregnancy or oral contraceptives).

A family history of ovarian carcinoma is occasionally elicited. Women with a first-degree relative with ovarian cancer have a 3.5-fold increased risk of developing the same disease. Women with a history of ovarian carcinoma are also at greater risk for breast cancer and vice versa. A gene implicated in many hereditary breast cancers, *BRCA-1* (17q12-q23), has been incriminated in familial ovarian cancers as well. Women who bear *BRCA-1* tend to develop ovarian cancer much earlier than those who have sporadic ovarian cancer, but their prognosis is considerably better.

PATHOGENESIS: Most common epithelial tumors, especially serous carcinomas, arise from the ovarian surface epithelium or serosa. As the ovary develops, the surface epithelium may extend into the ovarian stroma to form glands and cysts.

PATHOLOGY: In order of decreasing frequency, the **common epithelial tumors** are:

- **Serous tumors**, which resemble the epithelium of the fallopian tube
- **Mucinous tumors**, which mimic the mucosa of the endocervix
- **Endometrioid tumors**, which are similar to the glands of the endometrium
- **Clear cell tumors**, which display glycogen-rich cells that resemble endometrial glands in pregnancy
- **Transitional cell tumors**, which resemble the mucosa of the bladder
- **Mixed tumors**

Benign Epithelial Tumors

SEROUS OR MUCINOUS ADENOMAS: Benign common epithelial tumors are almost always serous or mucinous adenomas and generally arise in women between 20 and 60 years old. The neoplasms are frequently large, often 15 to 30 cm in diameter. Some, particularly the mucinous variety, reach massive proportions, exceeding 50 cm in diameter, in which case they may mimic the appearance of a term pregnancy. Benign epithelial tumors are typically cystic, hence the term **cystadenoma**. Serous cystadenomas are more commonly bilateral (15%) than mucinous cystadenomas and tend to be unilocular (Fig. 18-20). By contrast, **muci-**

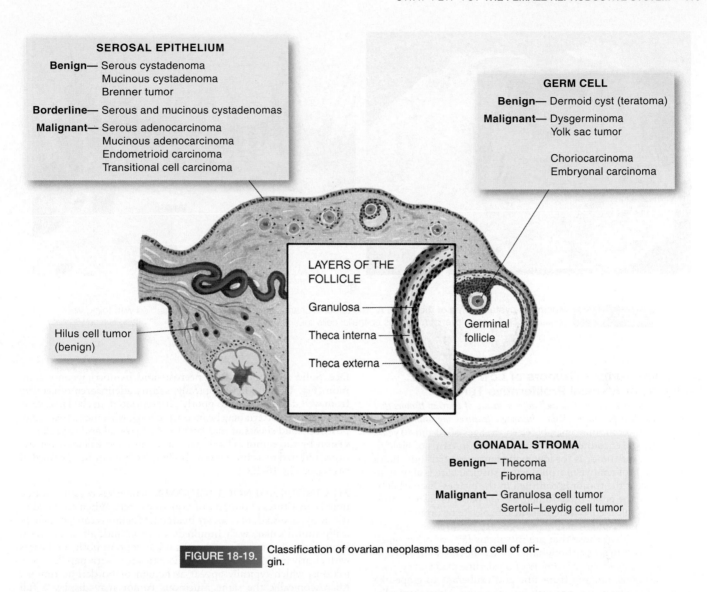

SEROSAL EPITHELIUM

Benign— Serous cystadenoma
Mucinous cystadenoma
Brenner tumor

Borderline— Serous and mucinous cystadenomas

Malignant— Serous adenocarcinoma
Mucinous adenocarcinoma
Endometrioid carcinoma
Transitional cell carcinoma

GERM CELL

Benign— Dermoid cyst (teratoma)

Malignant— Dysgerminoma
Yolk sac tumor

Choriocarcinoma
Embryonal carcinoma

LAYERS OF THE
FOLLICLE

Granulosa

Theca interna

Theca externa

Germinal
follicle

Hilus cell tumor
(benign)

GONADAL STROMA

Benign— Thecoma
Fibroma

Malignant— Granulosa cell tumor
Sertoli–Leydig cell tumor

FIGURE 18-19. Classification of ovarian neoplasms based on cell of origin.

nous tumors characteristically show hundreds of small cysts (locules) (Fig. 18-21). As opposed to their malignant counterparts, benign ovarian epithelial tumors tend to have thin walls and lack solid areas. Microscopically, one layer of tall columnar epithelium lines the cysts. Papillae, when present, consist of a fibrovascular core covered by a single layer of tall columnar epithelium identical to that of the cyst lining.

TRANSITIONAL CELL TUMOR (BRENNER TUMOR): The typical Brenner tumor is benign and occurs at all ages, with half of the cases presenting in women over the age of 50 years. Size varies from a microscopic focus to masses as large as 8 cm or more in diameter. Histologically, Brenner tumors show solid nests of transitional-like (urothelium-like) cells encased in a dense, fibrous stroma. The most superficial epithelial cells may exhibit mucinous differentiation.

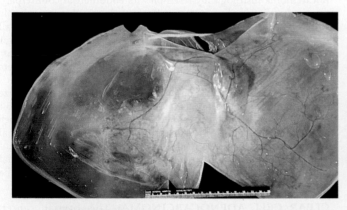

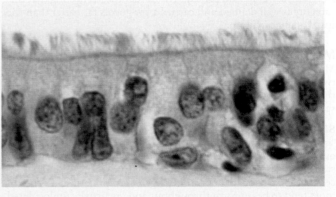

FIGURE 18-20. **Serous cystadenoma of the ovary.** The fluid has been removed from this huge unilocular serous cystadenoma. The wall is thin and translucent. On microscopic examination, the cyst is lined by a single layer of ciliated tubal-type epithelium.

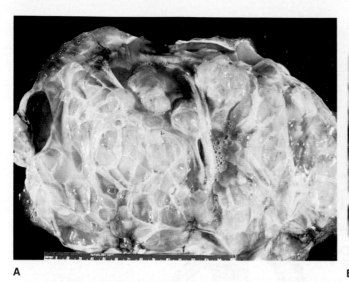

A

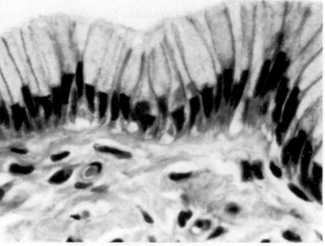

B

FIGURE 18-21. Mucinous cystadenoma of the ovary. **A.** The tumor is characterized by numerous cysts filled with thick, viscous fluid. **B.** A single layer of mucinous epithelial cells lines the cyst.

Borderline Tumors (Tumors of Low Malignant Potential) or Atypical Proliferative Tumors

"Borderline tumors" comprise a well-defined group of ovarian tumors that share an excellent prognosis, despite histologic features suggesting cancer. They generally occur in women between the ages of 20 and 40 years but may also be encountered in older women. In terms of biological behavior, the tumor is "of low malignant potential" but shows atypical and proliferative morphology. A surgical cure is almost always possible if the tumor is confined to the ovaries. Even when it has spread to the pelvis or abdomen, 80% of patients are alive after 5 years, although there is a significant rate of late recurrence.

Serous tumors of borderline malignancy are more commonly bilateral (35%) than those that are mucinous (5%) or other types. The tumors vary in size, although mucinous ones are sometimes gigantic (100+ kg). In serous tumors of borderline malignancy, papillary projections, ranging from fine and exuberant to grape-like clusters arising from the cyst wall, are common. Microscopically, these structures resemble papillary fronds in benign cystadenomas, but they are distinguished from them by (1) epithelial stratification, (2) nuclear atypism, and (3) mitotic activity. The same criteria apply to borderline mucinous tumors, although papillary projections are less conspicuous. *By definition, the presence of more than focal microinvasion (which is defined as discrete nests of epithelial cells that invade less than 3 mm into the ovarian stoma) identifies a tumor as frankly malignant, rather than borderline.* However, borderline tumors with lymph node metastases or implants in the peritoneum, whether noninvasive or invasive, are still considered "borderline," reflecting that this category is well defined and carries a prognosis far better than the usual adenocarcinoma.

Malignant Epithelial Tumors

Malignant epithelial tumors of the ovary are most common between 40 and 60 years of age and are rare under the age of 35. By the time an ovarian cancer has reached 10 to 15 cm, it has often spread beyond the ovary and seeded the peritoneum.

SEROUS ADENOCARCINOMA: This tumor (commonly called "cystadenocarcinoma") is the most common malignancy of the ovary, accounting for one third of all ovarian cancers. Advanced stage tumors tend to be bilateral, as are two thirds of serous cancers with extragonadal spread. On gross examination, serous tumors tend to be uniform throughout and are usually uniloculated or pauciloculated, with soft, delicate papillae lining the entire surface. Solid areas, often with necrosis and hemorrhage, are common (Fig. 18-22). Microscopically, serous adenocarcinomas vary from well differentiated to poorly differentiated. In the latter case, the papillary pattern may be inconspicuous, with most areas composed of solid sheets of malignant cells. Stromal and capsular invasion by the tumor cells is evident. Laminated calcified concretions, referred to as psammoma bodies, are present in one third of cases (see Fig. 18-22C).

MUCINOUS ADENOCARCINOMA: Mucinous cystadenocarcinoma constitutes about 10% of ovarian cancers. When confined to the ovary, one-sixth of cases are bilateral. Mucinous cancers are typically multilocular, with hundreds to thousands of small cysts. Primary ovarian mucinous tumors often contain both solid areas with clearly malignant features and cystic areas with papillary projections, which typically appear as benign or borderline tumors. Microscopically, the same mucinous tumor may display a full range of appearances from well to poorly differentiated. Well-differentiated mucinous tumors contain neoplastic glands lined by tall columnar, mucin-producing cells, usually with some solid or cribriform areas (Fig. 18-23). Poorly differentiated mucinous adenocarcinomas exhibit irregular nests and cords of tumor cells and numerous mitoses. Stromal invasion is the rule, and infiltration of the serosa is common.

ENDOMETRIOID ADENOCARCINOMA: Endometrioid adenocarcinoma histologically resembles its endometrial counterpart, may include areas of squamous differentiation, and is second only to serous adenocarcinoma in frequency, accounting for 20% of all ovarian cancers. The tumor occurs most commonly after menopause. In contrast to serous and mucinous neoplasms, most endometrioid tumors are malignant. Up to one half of these cancers are bilateral.

On gross examination, endometrioid carcinomas vary in size from 2 cm to more than 30 cm. Most are largely solid and exhibit necrotic areas, although they may be cystic. Microscopically, they are graded according to the same scheme used for endometrial adenocarcinomas. Between 15% and 50% of patients with endometrioid carcinoma of the ovary also harbor an endometrial cancer. As with all malignant epithelial tumors of the ovary, the prognosis depends on the stage at which it presents.

CLEAR CELL ADENOCARCINOMA: This ovarian cancer, which is closely related to endometrioid adenocarcinoma, often

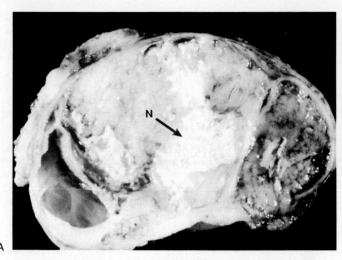

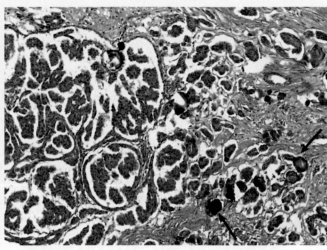

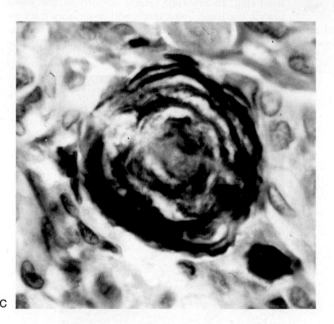

FIGURE 18-22. Serous cystadenocarcinoma. **A.** The ovary is enlarged by a solid tumor that exhibits extensive necrosis *(N)*. **B.** Microscopic examination shows a papillary cancer invading the ovarian stroma. Several psammoma bodies are present *(arrows)*. **C.** A higher-power view shows the laminated structure of a psammoma body.

occurs in association with endometriosis. It constitutes 5% to 10% of all ovarian cancers, usually occurring after menopause. The size ranges from 2 to 30 cm in diameter, and 40% are bilateral. Most of these tumors are partially cystic and exhibit necrosis and hemorrhage in the solid areas.

Microscopically, clear cell ovarian adenocarcinoma displays sheets or tubules of malignant cells with clear cytoplasm. In its tubular form, malignant cells often display bulbous nuclei that protrude into the lumen of the tubule ("hobnail cells"). The clinical course parallels that of endometrioid carcinoma.

 CLINICAL FEATURES: Most ovarian tumors do not secrete hormones. However, an antibody to the cancer antigen, CA-125, in the serum detects half of the epithelial tumors that are confined to the ovary and 90% that have already spread.

Ovarian masses rarely cause symptoms until they are large. When they distend the abdomen, they cause pain, pelvic pressure, or compression of regional organs. By the time ovarian cancers are diagnosed, many have metastasized (implanted) to the surfaces of the pelvis, abdominal organs, bladder, diaphragm, paracolic gutters, or omentum. Lymphatic dissemination carries malignant cells preferentially to para-aortic lymph nodes. In addition to spe-

cific symptoms, metastatic cancers are associated with ascites, weakness, weight loss, and cachexia. Survival for patients with malignant ovarian tumors is generally poor. Overall, the 5-year survival rate is only 35%, because more than half of the tumors have spread to the abdominal cavity or elsewhere by the time they are discovered. The cornerstone to managing ovarian cancer is surgery, which removes the primary tumor, establishes the diagnosis, and assesses the extent of spread. Adjuvant chemotherapy is used to treat distant occult sites of tumor spread.

Germ Cell Tumors Tend to be Benign in Adults and Malignant in Children

Tumors derived from germ cells constitute one fourth of all ovarian tumors. In adult females, germ cell tumors are virtually all benign (mature cystic teratoma, dermoid cyst), whereas in children and young adults, they are largely cancerous. In children, germ cell tumors are the most common type of ovarian cancer (60%); they are rare after menopause. The neoplastic germ cell may follow one of several lines of differentiation, giving rise to tumors analogous to those found in the male testes (Fig. 18-24; see also Chapter 17).

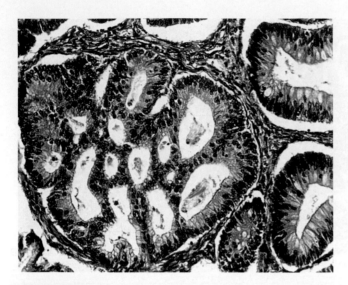

FIGURE 18-23. Mucinous cystadenocarcinoma. The malignant glands are arranged in a cribriform pattern and are composed of mucin-producing columnar cells.

Dysgerminoma

Dysgerminoma is the ovarian counterpart of testicular seminoma and is composed of primordial germ cells. It accounts for less than 2% of all ovarian cancers but constitutes 10% of these malignancies in women younger than 20 years of age. Most patients are between 10 and 30 years old. The tumors are bilateral in 15% of cases.

PATHOLOGY: Grossly, dysgerminomas are often large and firm and have a bosselated external surface. The cut surface is soft and fleshy. Microscopic examination reveals large nests of monotonously uniform tumor cells, which have a clear glycogen-filled cytoplasm and irregularly flattened central nuclei. Fibrous septa containing lymphocytes traverse the tumor.

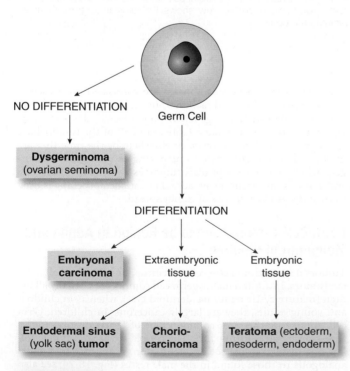

FIGURE 18-24. Classification of germ cell tumors of the ovary.

Dysgerminoma is treated surgically, and the 5-year survival rate for patients with stage I tumor approaches 100%. Because the tumor is highly radiosensitive and also responsive to chemotherapy, 5-year survival rates even for higher-stage tumors still exceed 80%.

Teratoma

Teratoma is a tumor of germ cell origin that differentiates toward somatic structures. Most teratomas contain tissues from at least two and usually all three embryonic layers.

MATURE TERATOMA (MATURE CYSTIC TERATOMA, DERMOID CYST): This benign neoplasm accounts for one fourth of all ovarian tumors, with a peak incidence in the third decade. Mature teratomas develop by parthenogenesis. Haploid (postmeiotic) germ cells endoreduplicate to give rise to diploid, genetically female, tumor cells (46,XX).

PATHOLOGY: Mature teratomas are cystic and more than 90% contain skin, sebaceous glands, and hair follicles (Fig. 18-25). Half exhibit smooth muscle, sweat glands, cartilage, bone, teeth, and respiratory tract epithelium. Tissues such as gut, thyroid, and brain are seen less frequently. **Struma ovarii** refers to a cystic lesion composed pre-

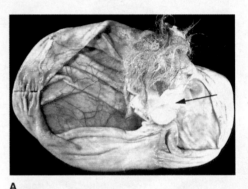

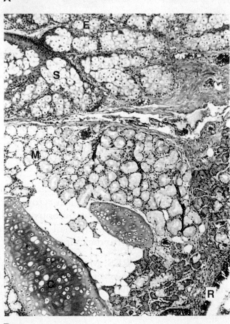

FIGURE 18-25. Mature cystic teratoma of the ovary. A. A mature cystic teratoma has been opened to reveal a solid knob *(arrow)* from which hair projects. B. A photomicrograph of the solid knob shows epidermal and respiratory components. Tissue resembling the skin exhibits an epidermis *(E)* with underlying sebaceous glands *(S)*. The respiratory tissue consists of mucous glands *(M)*, cartilage *(C)*, and respiratory epithelium *(R)*.

dominantly of thyroid tissue (5% to 20% of mature cystic teratomas). Rare cases of hyperthyroidism have been associated with struma ovarii.

Very few (1%) of dermoid cysts become malignant. These cancers usually occur in older women and correspond to the tumors that arise in other differentiated tissues of the body. Three fourths of all cancers that arise in dermoid cysts are squamous cell carcinomas. The remainder includes carcinoid tumors, basal cell carcinoma, thyroid cancer, adenocarcinoma, and others. The prognosis of patients with malignant transformation of mature cystic teratoma is related largely to stage of the cancer.

IMMATURE TERATOMA: Immature teratomas of the ovary are composed of elements derived from the three germ layers. However, unlike mature cystic teratoma, the immature variety contains embryonal tissues. Immature teratoma accounts for 20% of malignant tumors at all sites in women under the age of 20 years and becomes progressively less common in older women.

 PATHOLOGY: Immature teratoma is predominantly solid and lobulated, with numerous small cysts. Solid areas may contain grossly recognizable immature bone and cartilage. Microscopically, multiple tumor components are usually found, including those differentiating toward nerve (neuroepithelial rosettes and immature glia) glands and other structures found in mature cystic teratomas. Survival correlates with tumor grade. Well-differentiated immature teratomas generally have a favorable outcome, but high-grade tumors (predominantly embryonal tissue) have a poor prognosis.

Yolk Sac Tumor

Yolk sac tumor is a highly malignant tumor of women under the age of 30 years that histologically resembles the mesenchyme of the primitive yolk sac. It is the second most common malignant germ cell tumor and is almost always unilateral.

 PATHOLOGY: Typically, the neoplasm is large and displays extensive necrosis and hemorrhage. Microscopic examination reveals multiple patterns. The most common appearance is a reticular, honeycombed structure of communicating spaces lined by primitive cells. **Schiller-Duval bodies** are found sparingly in a few tumors but are characteristic. They consist of papillae that protrude into a space lined by tumor cells, resembling the glomerular Bowman's space. The papillae are covered by a mantle of embryonal cells and contain a fibrovascular core and a central blood vessel.

Yolk sack tumors secrete α-fetoprotein, which can be demonstrated histochemically within eosinophilic droplets. Detection of α-fetoprotein in the blood is useful for diagnosis and for monitoring the effectiveness of therapy. The neoplasm was previously nearly always fatal but with chemotherapy, the 5-year survival rate for stage I yolk sac tumors exceeds 80%.

Choriocarcinoma

Choriocarcinoma of the ovary is a rare tumor that mimics the epithelial covering of placental villi, namely, cytotrophoblast and syncytiotrophoblast. Derivation from ovarian germ cells is assumed if the tumor arises before puberty or in combination with another germ cell tumor. In women of reproductive age, however, ovarian choriocarcinoma may also be a metastasis from an intrauterine gestational tumor. Choriocarcinoma of germ cell origin manifests in young girls as precocious sexual development, menstrual irregularities, or rapid breast enlargement.

 PATHOLOGY: Choriocarcinoma is unilateral, solid, and widely hemorrhagic. Microscopically, it shows a mixture of malignant cytotrophoblast and syncytiotrophoblast (see placenta, choriocarcinoma, below). The syncytial cells secrete hCG, which accounts for the frequent finding of a positive pregnancy test result. Serial serum hCG determinations are useful both for diagnosis and follow-up. The tumor is highly aggressive but responds to chemotherapy.

Sex Cord/Stromal Tumors are Clinically Functional

Tumors of the sex cord and stroma originate from either primitive sex cords or from mesenchymal stroma of the developing gonad. They account for 10% of ovarian tumors. The tumors range from benign to low-grade malignant and may differentiate toward female (granulosa and theca cells) or male (Sertoli and Leydig cells) structures.

Ovarian Fibroma

Fibromas account for 75% of all stromal tumors and 7% of all ovarian tumors. They occur at all ages, with a peak in the perimenopausal period and are virtually always benign.

 PATHOLOGY: Fibromas are solid, firm, and white. Microscopically, the cells resemble the stroma of the normal ovarian cortex, appearing as well-differentiated spindle cells embedded in variable amounts of collagen. Half of the larger tumors are associated with ascites and, rarely, with ascites and pleural effusions (**Meigs syndrome**).

Thecoma

Thecomas are functional ovarian tumors that arise in postmenopausal women and are almost always benign. They are closely related to fibromas but additionally contain varying amounts of steroidogenic cells, which in many cases produce estrogens or androgen.

 PATHOLOGY: Thecomas are solid tumors, usually 5 to 10 cm in diameter. The cut section is yellow, due to the presence of many lipid-laden theca cells. Microscopically, the cells are large and oblong to round, with a vacuolated cytoplasm that contains lipid. Bands of hyalinized collagen separate nests of theca cells. Because of estrogen output by the tumor, thecomas in premenopausal women commonly cause irregularity in menstrual cycles and breast enlargement. Endometrial hyperplasia and cancer are well-recognized complications.

Granulosa Cell Tumor

Granulosa cell tumor is the prototypical functional neoplasm of the ovary associated with estrogen secretion. This tumor should be considered malignant because of its potential for local spread and the rare occurrence of distant metastases.

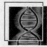 **PATHOGENESIS:** Most granulosa cell tumors occur after menopause (adult form) and are unusual before puberty. The juvenile form, which occurs in children and young women, has distinct clinical and pathologic features (hyperestrinism and precocious puberty).

 PATHOLOGY: Adult-type granulosa cell tumors, like most ovarian tumors, are large and focally cystic to solid. The cut surface shows yellow areas, representing lipid-laden luteinized granulosa cells and white zones of stroma and focal hemorrhages (Fig. 18-26). Microscopically, granulosa cell tumors display an array of growth patterns: (1) diffuse (sarcomatoid); (2) insular (islands of cells); or (3) trabecular (anastomotic bands of granulosa cells). Haphazard orientation of nuclei about a central degenerative space results in a characteristic follicular pattern (**Call-Exner bodies**) (see Fig. 18-26B). Tumor cells are typically spindle-shaped and commonly have a cleaved, elongated nucleus (coffee bean appearance).

 CLINICAL FEATURES: *Three fourths of granulosa cell tumors secrete estrogens.* Thus, benign endometrial hyperplasia is a common presenting sign. It predisposes to EIN or endometrial adenocarcinoma if the functioning

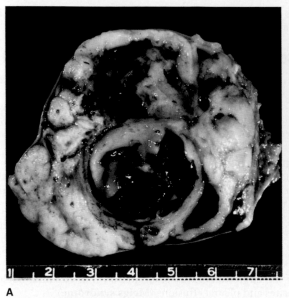

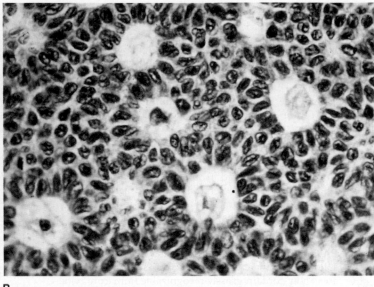

A　　　　　B

FIGURE 18-26. **Granulosa cell tumor of the ovary. A.** Cross-section of the enlarged ovary shows a variegated solid tumor with focal hemorrhages. The yellow areas represent collections of lipid-laden luteinized granulosa cells. **B.** The orientation of tumor cells about central spaces results in the characteristic follicular pattern (Call-Exner bodies).

granulosa cell tumor remains undetected. When detected clinically, 90% of granulosa cell tumors are confined to the ovary (stage I). The 10-year survival rate for these patients is greater than 90%. Tumors that have extended into the pelvis and lower abdomen have a poorer prognosis. Late recurrence after surgical removal is not uncommon after 5 to 10 years and is usually fatal.

Sertoli-Leydig Cell Tumors

Ovarian Sertoli-Leydig cell tumor (arrhenoblastoma or androblastoma) is a rare mesenchymal neoplasm of low malignant potential that resembles the embryonic testes. It is the prototypical androgen-secreting ovarian tumor. Sertoli-Leydig cell tumors occur at all ages but are most common in young women of childbearing age.

PATHOLOGY: Sertoli-Leydig cell tumors are unilateral, most measuring between 5 and 15 cm in diameter. They tend to be lobulated, solid, and brown to yellow. Microscopically, they vary from well differentiated to poorly differentiated and some exhibit heterologous elements (e.g., mucinous glands and, rarely, even cartilage). The most characteristic features are large Leydig cells, which have abundant eosinophilic cytoplasm and a central round-to-oval nucleus with a prominent nucleolus. The tumor cells are embedded in a sarcomatoid stroma, which often differentiates into immature solid tubules of embryonic Sertoli cells (Fig. 18-27).

CLINICAL FEATURES: Nearly half of all patients with Sertoli-Leydig cell tumors exhibit androgenic effects. Initially, these are expressed as defeminization (breast atrophy, amenorrhea, and loss of hip fat), followed by signs of virilization including hirsutism, male escutcheon, enlarged clitoris, and deepened voice. These signs lessen or disappear following tumor removal. Well-differentiated tumors are virtually always cured by surgical resection, but poorly differentiated tumors may metastasize.

Tumors Metastatic to the Ovary May Mimic a Primary Tumor

About 3% of ovarian cancers arise elsewhere. The most common primary sites are the breast, large intestine, endometrium, and stomach, in descending order. These tumors vary in size from microscopic lesions to large masses. Of those metastatic tumors large

enough to manifest clinically, the colon is the most frequent site of origin. The tumor cells usually stimulate the ovarian stroma to differentiate into hormonally active cells (luteinized stromal cells), thereby inducing androgenic and sometimes estrogenic symptoms. *Krukenberg tumors are ovarian metastases in which the tumor appears as nests of mucin-filled "signet-ring" cells within a cellular stroma derived from the ovary.* The stomach is the primary site in 75% of cases, and most of the other Krukenberg tumors are from the colon.

PLACENTA AND GESTATIONAL DISEASE

Infections

Chorioamnionitis Results from Ascending Infection

Chorioamnionitis is inflammation of the amnion, chorion, and extraplacental membranes. Infectious organisms ascend from the maternal birth canal, commonly after premature rupture of the membranes.

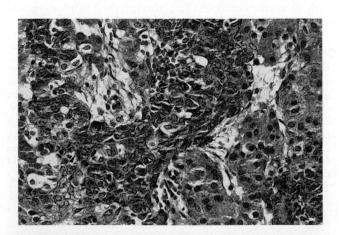

FIGURE 18-27. **Sertoli-Leydig cell tumor.** Immature solid tubules of embryonic Sertoli cells are adjacent to clusters of Leydig cells that exhibit abundant eosinophilic cytoplasm.

The inflammatory process affects primarily the membranes (chorioamnionitis) rather than the chorionic villi.

 PATHOLOGY: The amniotic fluid is usually cloudy. Membrane walls are slightly opaque, malodorous, and edematous. Microscopically, they show a neutrophilic infiltrate, often with fibrin deposition. With more extensive spread, the umbilical cord may become infected **(funisitis)**. Generally, chorionic villi remain free of inflammatory infiltrate. Microorganisms isolated from placentas with chorioamnionitis, in descending frequency, are (1) genital mycoplasmas (*Ureaplasma urealyticum, Mycoplasma hominis*), (2) anaerobic organisms of the *Bacteroides* group, and (3) aerobes (group *B* streptococci, *E. coli*, and *Gardnerella vaginalis*).

 CLINICAL FEATURES: Acute chorioamnionitis is found in 10% of placentas and is associated with preterm labor, fetal and neonatal infections, and intrauterine hypoxia. The risks of chorioamnionitis to the fetus include (1) pneumonia after inhalation of infected amniotic fluid, (2) skin or eye infections from direct contact with organisms in the fluid, and (3) neonatal gastritis, enteritis, or peritonitis from ingesting infected fluid. Major risks to the mother are intrapartum fever, postpartum endometritis, and pelvic sepsis with venous thrombosis.

Preeclampsia and Eclampsia

The hypertensive disorders of pregnancy, namely preeclampsia and eclampsia, define a syndrome of hypertension, proteinuria, and edema, and, most severely, convulsions. **Preeclampsia** occurs in 6% of pregnant women in their last trimester, especially with the first child. The disorder becomes **eclampsia** if convulsive seizures appear.

 PATHOGENESIS: The pathogenesis of preeclampsia and eclampsia is still not resolved. Immunologic and genetic factors have been invoked as well as altered vascular reactivity, endothelial injury, and coagulation abnormalities (Fig. 18-28). Regardless of the precise cause, certain features are characteristic:

- Preeclampsia occurs with hydatidiform mole (see below), which suggests that the trophoblast is the most likely responsible tissue and that preeclampsia is a trophoblastic disease.
- Maternal blood flow to the placenta is markedly reduced because the normal changes in the maternal spiral arteries of the placental bed do not take place.
- Renal involvement in preeclampsia contributes to hypertension and proteinuria.
- DIC is a prominent feature of preeclampsia. Treatment with antiplatelet agents, particularly low-dose aspirin, ameliorates or prevents DIC.
- The risk of preeclampsia in the first pregnancy is manyfold higher than in subsequent pregnancies. Findings suggest that previous exposure to paternal antigens may protect against the disease.
- Eclampsia is a cerebrovascular disorder characterized by seizures, worsening hypertension, and cerebral edema. It is often the first sign of preeclampsia but does not necessarily evolve from it.

The pathologic changes in the placenta reflect reduced maternal blood flow to the uteroplacental unit. *The key factor in preeclampsia resides in the spiral arteries of the uteroplacental bed, which never fully dilate.* These arteries are smaller than normal and retain their musculoelastic wall, which is ordinarily attenuated by infiltrative trophoblasts. Normally, extravillous trophoblast invades these arteries and destroys their vascular tone, thereby allowing the vessels to dilate. In preeclampsia, up to half of spiral arteries escape invasion by endovascular trophoblastic tissue, and thus dilation does not occur. In women with preeclampsia, the spiral arteries commonly exhibit **acute atherosis**, (fibrinoid necrosis with accumulation of lipid-laden macrophages), thrombosis and resultant focal placental infarctions, which contribute to inadequate blood flow and placental ischemia.

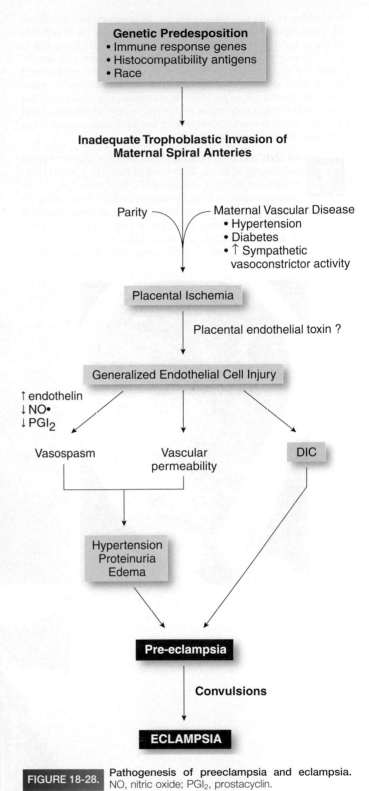

FIGURE 18-28. Pathogenesis of preeclampsia and eclampsia. NO, nitric oxide; PGI_2, prostacyclin.

 PATHOLOGY: The placenta and maternal organs of women with preeclampsia show conspicuous changes. Extensive placental infarction is seen in nearly one third of women with severe preeclampsia. Retroplacental hemorrhage occurs in 15% of patients. Microscopically, chorionic villi show signs of underperfusion. The cytotrophoblastic cells lining them are hyperplastic, and the basement membrane is thickened. *The kidneys always show glomerular changes.* Glomeruli are enlarged, and endothelial cells are swollen. Fibrin is present between the endothelial cells and the glomerular capillary basement membrane. Mesangial cell hyperplasia is common. The changes in the maternal kidneys are reversible with therapy or after delivery. Fatal cases of eclampsia often show cerebral hemorrhages, ranging from petechiae to large hematomas.

 CLINICAL FEATURES: Preeclampsia usually begins insidiously after the 20th week of pregnancy with (1) excessive weight gain occasioned by fluid retention, (2) increased maternal blood pressure, and (3) proteinuria. As preeclampsia progresses from mild to severe, diastolic pressure persistently exceeds 110 mm Hg, proteinuria is greater than 3 g/day, and renal function declines. DIC often supervenes. Preeclampsia is treated with antihypertensive and antiplatelet drugs, but definitive therapy requires removing the placenta, hopefully by normal delivery.

Gestational Trophoblastic Disease

The term **gestational trophoblastic disease** is a spectrum of disorders with abnormal trophoblast proliferation and maturation, as well as neoplasms derived from trophoblast.

Complete Hydatidiform Mole Does Not Contain an Embryo

Complete hydatidiform mole is a placenta with grossly swollen chorionic villi resembling bunches of grapes and showing varying degrees of trophoblastic proliferation. Villi are enlarged, often exceeding 5 mm in diameter (Fig. 18-29).

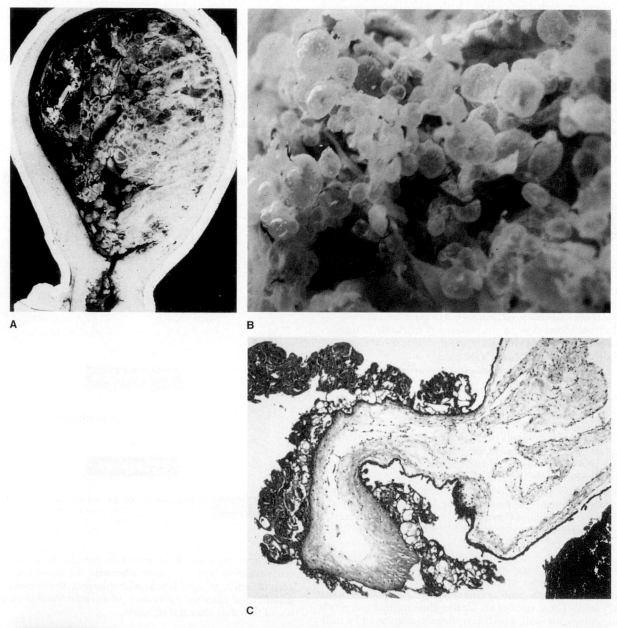

A

B

C

FIGURE 18-29. **Complete hydatidiform mole. A.** Complete mole in which the entire uterine cavity is filled with swollen villi. **B.** The villi are each 1 to 3 mm in diameter and appear grape-like. **C.** Individual molar villi, many of which have cavitated central cisterns, exhibit considerable trophoblastic hyperplasia and atypia. The blood vessels of the villi have atrophied and disappeared.

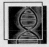

PATHOGENESIS: Complete mole results from fertilization of an empty ovum that lacks functional maternal DNA. Most commonly, a haploid (23,X) set of paternal chromosomes introduced by monospermy duplicates to 46,XX, but dispermic 46,XX and 46,XY moles also occur. Because the embryo dies at a very early stage, before placental circulation has developed, few chorionic villi develop blood vessels, and fetal parts are absent.

RISK FACTORS: The risk of hydatidiform mole relates to maternal age and has two peaks. Girls younger than 15 years of age have a 20-fold higher risk than women between 20 and 35 years. The risk increases progressively for women over 40 years of age. Women older than 50 years of age have 200 times the risk of those between 20 and 40. The incidence is manyfold higher in Asian women than among white women. Women who had a prior hydatidiform mole have a 20-fold greater risk of a subsequent molar pregnancy than does the general population.

PATHOLOGY: Molar tissue is voluminous and consists of macroscopically visible villi that are obviously swollen. Microscopically, many individual villi have cisternae, which are central, acellular, fluid-filled spaces devoid of mesenchymal cells. The trophoblast is hyperplastic and composed of syncytiotrophoblast, cytotrophoblast, and intermediate trophoblast. Considerable cellular atypia is present.

CLINICAL FEATURES: Patients with complete moles commonly present between the 11th and 25th weeks of pregnancy and complain of excessive uterine enlargement and often abnormal uterine bleeding. Passage of tissue fragments, which appear as small grape-like masses, is common. The serum hCG concentration is markedly elevated and increases with time

Complications of complete mole include uterine hemorrhage, DIC, uterine perforation, trophoblastic embolism, and infection. *The most important complication is the development of choriocarcinoma, which occurs in 2% of patients after the mole has been evacuated.*

Treatment consists of suction curettage of the uterus and subsequent monitoring of serum hCG levels. As many as 20% of patients require adjuvant chemotherapy for persistent disease, as

judged by stable or rising hCG levels. With such management, the survival rate approaches 100%.

Partial Hydatidiform Mole Features Triploid Cells

Partial hydatidiform mole is a distinct form of mole that almost never evolves into choriocarcinoma (see Table 18-3). These moles have 69 chromosomes (triploidy), of which one haploid set is maternal and two are paternal in origin. This abnormal chromosomal complement results from fertilization of a normal ovum (23,X) by two normal spermatozoa, each carrying 23 chromosomes, or a single spermatozoon that has not undergone meiotic reduction and bears 46 chromosomes. The fetus associated with a partial mole usually dies after 10 weeks' gestation, and the mole is aborted shortly thereafter. In contrast to a complete mole, fetal parts may be present.

PATHOLOGY: Partial moles have two populations of chorionic villi. Some are normal, whereas others are enlarged by hydropic swelling and show central cavitation. Trophoblastic proliferation is focal and less pronounced than in a complete mole. Blood vessels are typically found within chorionic villi and contain fetal (nucleated) erythrocytes.

Invasive Hydatidiform Mole Penetrates the Underlying Myometrium

PATHOLOGY: Villi of a hydatidiform mole may extend only superficially into the myometrium or may invade the uterus and even the broad ligament. The mole tends to enter dilated venous channels in the myometrium, and one third of them spread to distant sites, mostly the lungs. Unlike choriocarcinoma (see below), distant deposits of an invasive mole do not penetrate beyond the confines of the blood vessels in which they are lodged, and death from such spread is unusual. The clinical distinction between invasive mole and choriocarcinoma is often difficult.

Histologically, invasive moles show less hydropic change than complete moles. Trophoblastic proliferation is usually prominent. Uterine perforation is a major complication, but occurs in only a minority of cases. Theca lutein cysts, which may occur with any form of trophoblastic disease as a result of hCG stimulation, are prominent with invasive moles.

TABLE 18-3		
Comparative Features of Complete and Partial Hydatidiform Mole		
Features	**Complete Mole**	**Partial Mole**
Karyotype	46,XX	47,XXY or 47,XXX
Parental origin of haploid genome sets	Both paternal	1 maternal, 2 paternal
Preoperative diagnosis	Mole	Missed abortion
Marked vaginal bleeding	3+	1+
Uterus	Large	Small
Serum hCG	High	Less elevated
Hydropic villi	All	Some
Trophoblastic proliferation	Diffuse	Focal
Atypia	Diffuse	Minimal
hCG in tissue	3+	1+
Embryo present	No	Some
Blood vessels	No	Common
Nucleated erythrocytes	No	Sometimes
Persists after initial therapy	20%	7%
Choriocarcinoma	2% after mole	No choriocarcinoma

hCG, human chorionic gonadotropin.

Choriocarcinoma is a Tumor Allograft in the Host Mother

Gestational choriocarcinoma is a malignant tumor derived from tro- phoblast.

EPIDEMIOLOGY: Choriocarcinoma occurs in 1 in 30,000 pregnancies in the United States; in eastern Asia, the frequency is far greater. The incidence seems related to abnormalities of pregnancy. Thus, the tumor occurs in 1 of 160,000 normal gestations, 1 of 15,000 spontaneous abor- tions, 1 of 5,000 ectopic pregnancies, and 1 of 40 complete molar pregnancies. Although the risk that a complete hydatidiform mole will transform into choriocarcinoma is only 2%, it is still several or- ders of magnitude higher than if the pregnancy were normal.

PATHOLOGY: The uterine lesions of choriocarcinoma range from microscopic foci to huge necrotic and hem- orrhagic tumors. Viable tumor is usually confined to the rim of the neoplasm because, unlike most other cancers, choriocarcinoma lacks an intrinsic tumor vasculature. Histo- logically, the tumor contains a dimorphic population of cytotro- phoblast and syncytiotrophoblast, with varying degrees of inter- mediate trophoblast. *By definition, tumors containing any villous struc- tures, even if metastatic, are considered to be a hydatidiform mole and not choriocarcinoma.* Choriocarcinoma invades primarily through ve- nous sinuses in the myometrium. It metastasizes widely by the hematogenous route, especially to lungs (more than 90%), brain, gastrointestinal tract, liver, and vagina.

CLINICAL FEATURES: Abnormal uterine bleeding is the most frequent initial indication that heralds chorio- carcinoma. Occasionally, the first sign relates to metas- tases to the lungs or brain. In some cases, it may only be- come evident 10 or more years after the last pregnancy.

With currently available chemotherapy, recognition of risk fac- tors (high hCG levels and prolonged interval since antecedent pregnancy), and early treatment, most patients are cured. Survival rates exceed 70% for tumors that have metastasized and virtually 100% remission is expected if a tumor is localized. Serial serum hCG levels monitor the effectiveness of treatment.

19 The Breast

Ann D. Thor
Adeboye O. Osunkoya

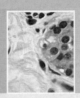
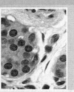
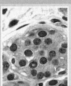
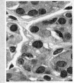

Diseases of the breast have been recognized throughout history, certainly because of their necessity for infant survival. An Egyptian surgical papyrus dating from 1600 BC, possibly the oldest medical text extant, describes a breast tumor which may have been cancer. The Greek physician Soranus detailed breast care during lactation to prevent nipple abscesses. Celsus recognized the breast as being particularly susceptible to "carcinoma." References to a female medica a mammis *suggests that specialists in breast disease were recognized in Roman medicine. Although it is now a matter of choice in deciding if the breast is to be used in its natural function, nursing, breast cancer remains one of the leading causes of death in women. It is, therefore, important to understand the biology of malignant tumors and of factors associated with an increased risk of cancer.*

Fibrocystic Change

Fibrocystic change is a constellation of morphologic features characterized by (1) cystic dilation of terminal ducts, (2) a relative increase in fibrous stroma, and (3) variable proliferation of terminal duct epithelial elements. It is most often diagnosed in women from their late 20s to the time of menopause. Fibrocystic change occurs to some degree in 75% of adult women in the United States. Symptomatic fibrocystic change, in which large, clinically detectable cysts are formed, may be seen in 10% of women between 35 and 55 years of age. The frequency of fibrocystic change decreases after menopause. Lesions demonstrating florid proliferation are designated **proliferative fibrocystic change**. Such lesions are more common in populations that have an increased risk of breast cancer, but progression to cancer has not been documented. Fibrocystic change without epithelial proliferation (**nonproliferative fibrocystic change**) does not involve an increased risk of breast cancer.

PATHOLOGY: Nonproliferative fibrocystic change is characterized by an increase in dense, fibrous stroma and some cystic dilation of the terminal ducts (Fig. 19-1B,C). Most often, cystic changes are minor and do not cause discrete masses. The large cysts, up to 5 cm in diameter, often contain dark, thin fluid that imparts a blue color to the unopened cysts (*blue-*

domed cysts of Bloodgood; see Fig. 19-1B). On microscopic examination, the epithelium lining the cysts varies from columnar to flattened or may even be entirely absent. **Apocrine metaplasia** is frequently seen in nonproliferative fibrocystic change (see Fig. 19-1D). The metaplastic cells are larger and more eosinophilic than the usual duct lining cells and resemble apocrine sweat gland epithelium.

The most common of several forms of **proliferative fibrocystic change** is an increase in the number of cells or layers lining the dilated terminal ducts, termed **ductal epithelial hyperplasia** (see Fig. 19-1E). Epithelial proliferation can at times become exuberant and widespread, forming intraductal epithelial papillary structures with central fibrovascular cores (**papillomatosis**). *Proliferative (hyperplastic) lesions may also demonstrate cytologic atypia.* These atypical lesions are subclassified by the degree of microscopic atypia and the extent of breast involvement (see below).

Proliferative Fibrocystic Change Increases the Risk of Cancer

- **Proliferative, nonatypical fibrocystic change** is associated with a minimal increased risk for the development of invasive cancer (1.5- to 2-fold).
- **Atypical hyperplasia** with fibrocystic change is associated with a 4- to 5-fold increased risk for developing invasive cancer

compared to the general population. This risk increases further if there is a strong family history of the disease. Atypical hyperplasia may be multifocal and bilateral. The risk of subsequent carcinoma is equal in both breasts.

Women at high risk may reduce their chances of developing breast cancer by chemical or surgical castration or the administration of anti-estrogenic agents (e.g., tamoxifen). Exogenous hormones (e.g., estrogens) may increase the risk of breast cancer, particularly in postmenopausal women or women at high risk for breast cancer, although the extent to which this might occur is controversial.

Sclerosing Adenosis is a Less Common Variant of Proliferative Fibrocystic Change

This lesion is characterized by proliferation of small ducts and myoepithelial cells with surrounding stromal fibrosis. Sclerosing adenosis is almost always associated with other forms of proliferative fibrocystic change. On mammogram, these lesions often demonstrate microcalcifications in patterns that resemble those seen in malignancies and may be difficult to distinguish clinically from cancer. Microscopically, lobular units may be deformed and enlarged, forming a mass of epithelial and stromal elements, which can be difficult to distinguish from invasive carcinoma.

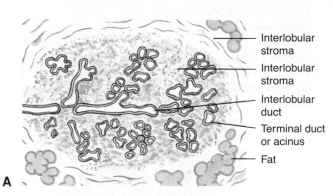

A — Interlobular stroma
— Interlobular stroma
— Interlobular duct
— Terminal duct or acinus
— Fat

Terminal duct lobular unit

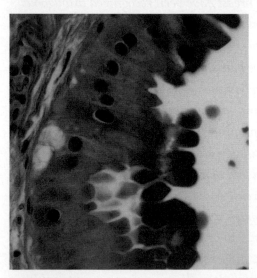

B

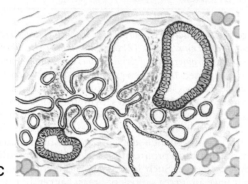

C

Nonproliferative fibrocystic change

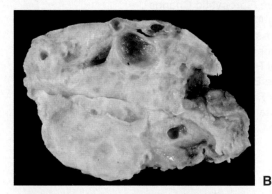

D

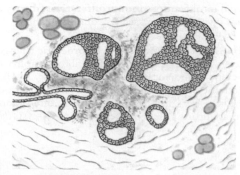

E

Proliferative fibrocystic change

FIGURE 19-1. **Fibrocystic change. A.** Normal terminal lobular unit. **B.** Surgical specimen: Cysts of various sizes are dispersed in dense, fibrous connective tissue. Some of the cysts are large and contain old blood-tinged proteinaceous debris. **C.** Nonproliferative fibrocystic change combines cystic dilation of the terminal ducts with varying degrees of apocrine metaplasia of the epithelium and increased fibrous stroma. **D.** Apocrine metaplasia: Epithelial cells have apocrine features with eosinophilic cytoplasm. **E.** Proliferative fibrocystic change: Terminal duct dilation and intraductal epithelial hyperplasia are present.

Benign Tumors

Fibroadenoma is the Most Common Benign Neoplasm of the Breast

These benign neoplasms are composed of epithelial and stromal elements that originate from the terminal ductal lobular unit. Fibroadenomas are usually solitary masses, although some women develop more than one during their lifetime. They are most often diagnosed in women between the ages of 20 and 35 years. Fibroadenomas commonly enlarge more rapidly during pregnancy (i.e., they are hormone-responsive) and cease to grow after menopause. Some fibroadenomas are associated with an increase in breast cancer risk, including (1) complex fibroadenomas (those associated with large cysts, sclerosing adenosis, calcifications or papillary apocrine change), (2) fibroadenoma with adjacent proliferative disease, or (3) fibroadenoma in patients with a first-degree family history of breast cancer.

 PATHOLOGY: Fibroadenomas vary in size, from a microscopic, incidental lesion to a large tumor, most often 2 to 4 cm in diameter. They are rubbery tumors that are sharply demarcated from the surrounding breast. These lesions can be identified on mammography or by palpation. Fibroadenomas are typically mobile and may be tender, particularly during the mid-to-late menstrual cycle. The cut surface appears glistening, gray-white, and sharply demarcated from the adjacent breast (Fig. 19-2A).

On microscopic examination, fibroadenomas are composed of a mixture of fibrous connective tissue and ducts (see Fig. 19-2B). The ducts may be either simple and round or elongate and branching and are dispersed within a characteristic fibrous stroma, which varies from loose and myxomatous to hyalinized collagen. This connective tissue, which forms most of the tumor, often compresses the proliferated ducts, reducing them to curvilinear slits. The epithelium's appearance ranges from the double layer of epithelium of normal lobules to varying degrees of hyperplasia.

Intraductal Papillomas Occur in the Lactiferous Ducts of Middle-Aged and Older Women

Intraductal papillomas typically arise from the surface of the large, subareolar ducts of middle-aged and older women and are often associated with a serous or bloody nipple discharge. A solitary intraductal papilloma is neither a premalignant lesion nor is it a marker of risk for breast cancer.

 PATHOLOGY: Intraductal papilloma is a single tumor, usually a few millimeters in diameter, which is attached to the wall of the duct by a fibrovascular stalk. The papillomatous portion consists of a double layer of epithelial cells, an outer layer of cuboidal or columnar cells, and an inner layer of more-rounded myoepithelial cells.

Cancer of the Breast

Breast cancer is the most common malignancy of women in the United States, and the mortality rate from this disease among women is second only to that of lung cancer.

 EPIDEMIOLOGY: The incidence of breast cancer has slowly increased over the past 20 years but now appears to have leveled off. Death rates have decreased during the last 25 years because of earlier detection and better therapy. Currently, one in eight American women may be expected to develop breast cancer, one quarter of whom will die of the disease. In Western industrialized countries with high rates of breast cancer, the incidence of this tumor continues to increase throughout life. The disease is uncommon before the age of 35 years. Breast cancer is four to five times more frequent in Western industrialized countries than in developing countries. It has been suggested that diet, in particular dietary fat, may in part explain differences in the geographical distribution of breast cancer, but this concept remains controversial. Breast cancer rarely develops in men, although when it does occur, it may be equally deadly (see below).

 PATHOGENESIS: The pathogenesis of breast cancer is poorly understood, but epidemiologic, molecular, and genetic studies outline complex risk factors. Breast cancers also exhibit diversity in histopathology, molecular features, and overall patient outcomes. Hence, the disease can be viewed as a multifaceted and complex epithelial malignancy.

Approximately 5% of Breast Cancers are Thought to Reflect Hereditary Factors

The strongest association with an increased risk for breast cancer is a family history, specifically breast cancer in first-degree relatives (mother, sister, daughter). The risk is greater when the relative is afflicted at a young age or with bilateral breast cancer.

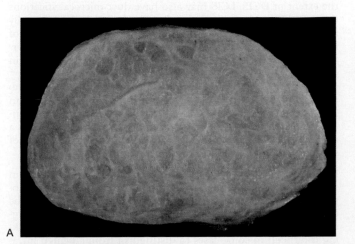

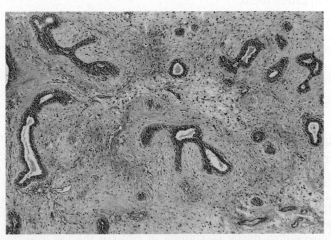

FIGURE 19-2. **Fibroadenoma. A.** Surgical specimen. This well-circumscribed tumor was easily enucleated from the surrounding tissue. The cut surface is characteristically glistening tannish-white and has a septate appearance. **B.** Microscopic section. Elongated epithelial duct structures are situated within a loose, myxoid stroma.

The **BRCA1 gene** (breast cancer 1), a tumor suppressor gene located on chromosome 17 (17q21), has been implicated in the pathogenesis of hereditary breast and ovarian cancers, and possibly prostate and colon cancer. Mutations in this tumor-suppressor gene are thought to be carried by 1 in 200 to 400 people in the United States. Germline point mutations and deletions in *BRCA1* confer a 60% to 85% lifetime risk for breast cancer, with more than half of the tumors developing before 50 years of age. It is currently suspected that mutated *BRCA1* is responsible for 20% of all cases of **inherited** breast cancer and is responsible for about 3% of all breast cancers. Somatic mutations in *BRCA1* are infrequently detected in **sporadic** breast cancers.

The **BRCA2** gene, located on chromosome 13q12, has been incriminated in approximately 20% of hereditary breast cancers. Women with one copy of a mutated *BRCA2* gene have a 30% to 40% lifetime chance of developing breast cancer. Like patients with *BRCA1,* these women have an increased risk of ovarian cancer. *BRCA2* mutations also put male carriers at increased risk of breast cancer. Mutations of *BRCA2* are particularly common among Ashkenazi Jewish women.

The **p53 gene** is mutated in the Li-Fraumeni syndrome (see Chapter 5). Breast cancer will develop in almost all young women with the disease. Germline (inherited) mutations in *p53* account for 1% of breast cancers among women under the age of 40 years. Somatic *p53* mutations are common in sporadic breast cancers.

Most Breast Cancers are Not Associated with Heritable Factors

HORMONAL STATUS: *A link between breast cancer and the hormonal status of women is strongly suggested by the association of (1) early menarche, (2) late menopause, and (3) older age at first-term pregnancy, with an increased the risk of disease.* Nulliparous women, or those who become pregnant for the first time after age 35, have a two- to threefold higher risk of breast cancer than women whose first pregnancy occurred before age 25.

RADIATION: The female breast is susceptible to radiation-induced neoplasia. The risk of breast cancer was increased in atomic bomb survivors and in women irradiated for postpartum mastitis and Hodgkin disease; the highest risk occurred when exposure took place in childhood and adolescence. Modern mammographic techniques use extremely low doses of radiation that are unlikely to pose a hazard.

PREVIOUS CANCER OF THE BREAST: Women who have previously had breast cancer have at least a 10-fold increased risk of developing a second primary breast cancer in the same or in the contralateral breast.

FIBROCYSTIC CHANGE: Women with proliferative fibrocystic change (and particularly those demonstrating atypical hyperplasia) are at increased risk for cancer (see above).

 PATHOLOGY: Breast cancers are almost entirely adenocarcinomas derived from progenitor cells of the glandular epithelium. They are classified based on a combination of histologic pattern and cytologic characteristics.

Carcinoma In Situ of the Breast is Often a Preinvasive Lesion

The term **carcinoma in situ** *refers to the presence of apparently malignant epithelial cells that have not penetrated the basement membrane.* Histologically, the various subtypes of carcinoma in situ have invasive counterparts. However, only 20% to 30% of women with biopsy-proven **ductal carcinoma in situ (DCIS)**, but who received no further therapy, subsequently developed invasive cancer. A strong family history for breast cancer elevates the risk for breast cancer in women with in situ disease.

The diagnosis of DCIS has risen significantly in the last three decades, with the advent of more sensitive mammographic techniques. Intraductal carcinomas arise within terminal ductal lobular units as dysplastic cells replace normal or hyperplastic cells and spread by luminal extension. Low- and moderate-grade lesions show little cell proliferation or necrosis. High-grade lesions have pronounced cytologic atypia, rapidly proliferating cells, and necrosis.

DCIS-COMEDOCARCINOMA (HIGH-GRADE) SUBTYPE: This subtype is composed of very large, pleomorphic epithelial cells with abundant cytoplasm, irregular nuclei, and often prominent, heterogeneous nucleoli. Cancer cells grow rapidly within ducts and frequently demonstrate intraductal necrosis (Fig. 19-3). Grossly, the lesion often shows distended duct-like structures containing white, necrotic material resembling comedos, which often undergoes dystrophic calcification; this results in multiple, microscopic calcified bodies, which can be visualized on a mammogram. These microcalcifications may assume a linear, branching appearance because of their intraductal location (see Fig. 19-3A). Although the malignant cells do not invade through the basement membrane, this form of carcinoma in situ may incite chronic inflammation, neovascularization, and a desmoplastic response (fibroblast proliferation and subsequent fibrosis) in a peritubular distribution (see Fig. 19-3B,C).

DCIS-NONCOMEDOCARCINOMA (LOW-TO-MODERATE-GRADE SUBTYPES): This tumor has multiple architectural patterns, which are often intermixed and exhibit a spectrum of cytologic atypia. The patterns are classified as micropapillary, cribriform (Fig. 19-4), and solid. The tumor cells and nuclei are smaller and more regular than those of the comedo type. Noncomedo DCIS is less likely than the comedo type to incite a desmoplastic response in the surrounding tissue. Necrosis is minimal or absent.

RISK OF INVASIVE DISEASE: DCIS, treated only by biopsy, carries a 30% risk of developing invasive carcinoma in the same breast over the ensuing 20 years. The risk of cancer in the contralateral breast is also increased but not to the same degree as with lobular carcinoma in situ (see below). The chance of local recurrence as either in situ or invasive cancer is substantially greater for the comedo than the noncomedo subtypes.

LOBULAR CARCINOMA IN SITU (LCIS): The second most common subtype of in situ breast carcinoma also arises in the terminal ductal lobular unit. In this tumor, cells tend to be smaller and more monotonous than in DCIS, with round, regular nuclei and minute nucleoli (Fig. 19-5). The malignant cells appear as solid clusters that pack and distend the terminal ducts but not to the extent of DCIS. LCIS may also have duct microcalcifications that are detectable radiographically. The lesion does not usually incite dense fibrosis and chronic inflammation so characteristic of DCIS and so is less likely to cause a detectable mass. Lobular carcinoma is associated with truncating mutations of the E-cadherin gene.

As with DCIS, 20% to 30% of women with LCIS receiving no further treatment after biopsy will develop invasive cancer within 20 years. About half of these invasive cancers will arise in the contralateral breast and may be either lobular or ductal cancers. As a result, LCIS, more than DCIS, is a harbinger of an increased risk of subsequent invasive cancer in both breasts.

PAPILLARY CARCINOMA IN SITU: Papillary carcinoma in situ is much less common than either DCIS or LCIS. This neoplasm originates in the larger branches of the ductal system. The tumor is usually well differentiated and exhibits a papillary configuration. The neoplastic cells are typically small and regular, making it difficult in some cases to distinguish from a benign intraductal papilloma. Papillary carcinoma in situ does not carry an increased risk of developing invasive cancer if it is completely resected.

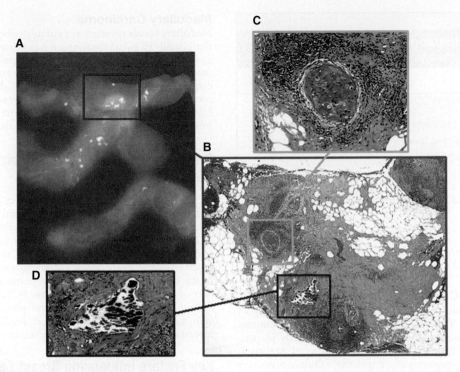

FIGURE 19-3. **Ductal carcinoma in situ. A.** Specimen radiograph of core biopsy shows linear and punctate atypical calcifications that are highly suspicious for cancer. **B.** Low-power photomicrograph showing high-grade in situ ductal carcinoma. **C.** High-power image of a duct expanded by in situ ductal carcinoma. **D.** High-power photomicrograph of tissue calcification.

Invasive Breast Carcinoma Exhibits an Array of Subtypes

Invasive carcinoma of the breast exhibits a morphologic spectrum, and different subtypes are associated with varying prognoses (Table 19-1).

Invasive Ductal Carcinoma (IDC)

Invasive (or infiltrating) ductal carcinoma is the most common histologic type of breast cancer. Invasion is defined by the presence of tumor cells outside of the duct-lobular units and extending into breast stroma. Invasion of the stroma incites a desmoplastic reaction, which may lead to a firm, palpable mass. The tumor may modify the contour of the breast or be visible as a dense mass lesion by mammography or ultrasonography (Fig. 19-6A). Invasive breast cancers are variably associated with calcifications.

On gross examination, IDC is typically firm and shows irregular margins. The cut surface is pale gray, gritty, and flecked with yellow, chalky streaks (see Fig. 19-6B). Microscopically, IDC is characterized by irregular nests and cords (tubules) of cytologically aberrant epithelial cells outside of the ductal-lobular units and located haphazardly within the stroma (see Fig. 19-6C).

Paget Disease of the Nipple

Paget disease is an uncommon variant of ductal carcinoma, either in situ or invasive, that extends to involve the epidermis of the nipple and areola. This condition usually comes to medical attention because of an eczematous change in the skin of the nipple and areola. Microscopically, large cells with clear cytoplasm (**Paget cells**) are

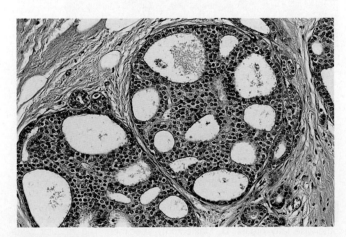

FIGURE 19-4. **Ductal carcinoma in situ–noncomedo type.** A cribriform arrangement of tumor cells is evident.

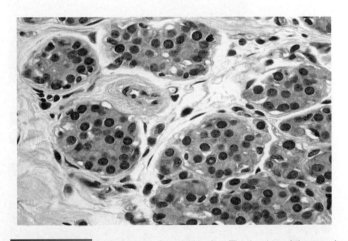

FIGURE 19-5. **Lobular carcinoma in situ.** The lumina of the terminal duct lobular units are distended by tumor cells, which exhibit round nuclei and small nucleoli. The cancer cells in the lobular form of carcinoma in situ are smaller and have less cytoplasm than those in the ductal type.

TABLE 19–1

Frequency of Histologic Subtypes of Invasive Breast Cancer

Subtype	Frequency (%)
Invasive ductal carcinoma	
Pure	55
Mixed with other types (including lobular)	25
Invasive lobular carcinoma (pure)	10
Medullary carcinoma (pure)	<5
Other pure types	4
Other mixed types	1

found singly or in groups within the epidermis. The prognosis of Paget disease is related to that of the underlying ductal cancer.

Invasive Lobular Carcinoma

Invasive lobular carcinoma is the second most common form of invasive breast cancer. The incidence of invasive lobular carcinoma has increased significantly since the mid-1980s, mostly in peri- and postmenopausal women. Because the amount of fibrosis is variable, the clinical presentation of invasive lobular carcinoma varies from a discrete firm mass, similar to ductal carcinoma, to a more subtle, diffuse, indurated area. Microscopically, the classic invasive lobular carcinoma consists of single strands of malignant cells infiltrating between stromal fibers, a feature termed **Indian filing** (Fig. 19-7). The small, regular cells are cytologically identical to those in LCIS (see Fig. 19-5), and mitotic activity is rare. Twenty-five percent of invasive carcinomas have features of both ductal and lobular carcinoma (see Table 19-1).

Medullary Carcinoma

Medullary cancer presents as a circumscribed, rapidly growing mass that usually lacks calcifications. It has a distinctive gross appearance and is well-circumscribed, fleshy, and pale gray. Microscopically, medullary carcinoma is composed of sheets of highly pleomorphic cancer cells, which have a distinct, rounded border and are surrounded by a chronic inflammatory infiltrate. Despite its highly malignant appearance, medullary carcinoma has a distinctly better prognosis than infiltrating ductal or lobular carcinomas.

Breast Cancer Usually Metastasizes First to Regional Lymph Nodes

Breast cancer spreads regionally by direct extension (e.g., to chest wall) or via lymphatic channels (to regional lymph nodes, including the axillary, internal mammary, and supraclavicular nodes). Small or low-grade invasive breast cancers may be localized to the breast and may be curable by complete surgical excision alone. *The axillary lymph nodes are the most common site of regional metastases.* Identification of the specific **sentinal nodes** is important in evaluating the presence of lymphatic spread (see Chapter 5). The most common sites of distant metastases are the lung and pleura, liver, bone, adrenals, skin, and brain. Unlike many tumors, breast cancers may recur and metastasize decades after a primary tumor has been removed.

Key Factors Influencing Breast Cancer Prognosis Include the Extent of Metastases, Histologic Grade, and Molecular Markers of Differentiation

STAGE: Breast cancer survival is most strongly influenced by the stage of the tumor at the time of diagnosis and in particular whether the tumor is confined to the breast, has metastasized to local (axillary) lymph nodes, has spread into local soft tissue, or

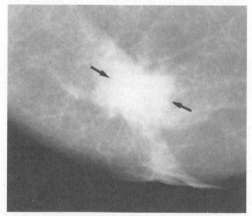

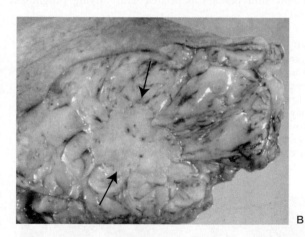

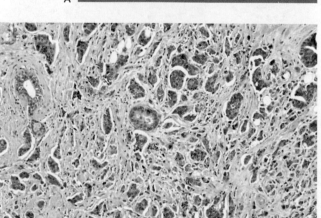

FIGURE 19-6. **Carcinoma of the breast. A.** Mammogram. An irregularly shaped, dense mass *(arrows)* is seen in this otherwise fatty breast. **B.** Mastectomy specimen. The irregular white, firm mass in the center is surrounded by fatty tissue. **C.** Photomicrograph showing irregular cords and nests of invasive ductal carcinoma cells invading stroma.

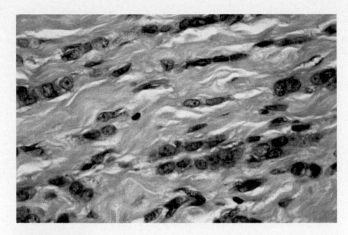

FIGURE 19-7. **Lobular carcinoma.** Invasive lobular carcinoma. In contrast to invasive ductal carcinoma, the cells of lobular carcinoma tend to form single strands that invade between collagen fibers in a single pattern. The tumor cells are similar to those seen in lobular carcinoma in situ.

has metastasized to distant sites. Small tumors that are confined to the breast have an excellent prognosis, with a 98% 5-year survival. However, the 5-year survival rate falls to 25% in cases where metastatic disease at sites distant from the breast occurs. Fortunately, with expanding use of screening mammography, more than half of breast cancers currently diagnosed in the United States are still confined to the breast.

GRADE: In addition to the histologic subtype and stage of the cancer, the histologic grade of the primary tumor is also a useful prognostic indicator. The histologic grade includes (1) the degree of glandular differentiation, (2) the degree of nuclear atypia, and (3) the mitotic index.

ESTROGEN AND PROGESTERONE RECEPTORS: Women whose cancers express hormone receptors are typically older and have lower-grade tumors and a better prognosis. The presence of these receptors also portends a greater probability of response to anti-estrogenic therapy.

PROLIFERATIVE CAPACITY AND PLOIDY: In general, increased proliferative capacity is associated with a poorer prognosis. Aneuploidy, which is found in two thirds of breast cancers, is also associated with a poorer prognosis.

HER2/neu (erB-2) ONCOGENE ALTERATIONS AND OTHER FACTORS: Overexpression of *HER2/neu* is identified in 10% to 35% of primary breast tumors and is mostly attributable to gene amplification. Patients whose tumors demonstrate *HER2/neu* gene amplification benefit from therapy with a monoclonal antibody (Herceptin™), which selectively binds to the extracellular domain of the protein. Gene expression profiling using microarray analysis has permitted separation of patients into prognostic groups, which are not otherwise defined either clinically or by histopathological analysis. Such technology remains in its early stages, but it is likely to have an important role in determining breast cancer prognosis in the near future.

Phyllodes Tumor

Phyllodes tumor of the breast is a proliferation of stromal elements accompanied by a benign growth of ductal structures. These tumors usually occur in women between 30 and 70 years of age, with a peak in the fifth decade. The original term for this tumor, **cystosarcoma**

phyllodes, implies malignant behavior, although only a minority of these tumors are capable of invasion and metastasis.

 PATHOLOGY: Phyllodes tumors resemble fibroadenomas in their overall architecture and the presence of glandular and stromal elements. Like fibroadenoma, a benign phyllodes tumor is sharply circumscribed, and the cut surface is firm, glistening, and grayish white. Benign and malignant phyllodes tumors are similar in gross appearance. Average sizes today are ≤5 cm in diameter. Microscopically, the stroma of a benign phyllodes tumor is hypercellular and has mitotic activity. Differentiation from fibroadenoma and distinction between benign and malignant forms is by the histologic and cytologic characteristics of the stromal component. Malignant phyllodes tumors have an obviously sarcomatous stroma with abundant mitotic activity, and the stromal component is increased out of proportion to the benign duct elements. They are usually poorly circumscribed and locally invasive. Malignant tumors may exhibit various sarcomatous tissue types, such as malignant fibrous histiocytoma, chondrosarcoma, and osteosarcoma.

 CLINICAL FEATURES: Benign phyllodes tumors are adequately treated by local excision. The initial treatment of a malignant phyllodes tumor is wide excision if the tumor is small or a simple mastectomy if the tumor is large. Malignant phyllodes tumors tend to recur locally, and 15% eventually metastasize to both distant sites and axillary lymph nodes.

The Male Breast

Gynecomastia is Most Often Related to Estrogen/Androgen Imbalance

Gynecomastia refers to an enlargement of the adult male breast. It is typically bilateral, is usually caused by hormones or certain medications, and is morphologically similar to juvenile hypertrophy of the female breast. Unilateral or focal male breast enlargement is not gynecomastia and is usually cause for a biopsy.

 PATHOGENESIS: Gynecomastia is caused by an absolute increase in circulating estrogens or by a relative increase in the estrogen/ androgen ratio, most commonly due to: (1) intake of exogenous estrogens or estrogen-like agents (e.g., digitalis, opiates); (2) hormone-secreting adrenal or testicular tumors; (3) paraneoplastic production of gonadotropins by cancers of the liver, lung, and other organs; and (4) metabolic disorders such as liver disease and hyperthyroidism. There is no evidence that gynecomastia is associated with an increased risk of cancer in males.

Cancer of the Male Breast is Distinctly Uncommon

Cancer in the male breast accounts for less than 1% of all cases of breast cancer. As in women, the most common subtype is infiltrating ductal carcinoma. Because there is less fat in the male breast, these tumors more often invade the musculature of the chest wall. For cancers of the same stage, however, the prognosis for males is similar to that of the female. Predisposing factors for the development of breast cancer in men are largely unknown. Mutations of the *BRCA2* gene have been associated with an increased risk of male breast cancer.c

20 Hematopathology

Roland Schwarting
Steven McKenzie
Raphael Rubin

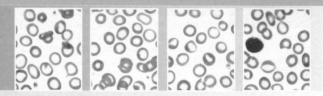

Cellular elements of the blood and lymphoid organs are responsible for a number of vital functions including transport of oxygen, defense against microorganisms and parasites, and the preservation of vascular integrity. These cells derive from a single pool of pluripotential stem cells in the bone marrow, which gives rise to two distinct types of multipotential stem cells, namely, lymphopoietic stem cells (lymphoid precursor cells of CFU-L), which migrate to lymphoid organs and multipotential hemopoietic stem cells (CFU-GEMM), which remain in the marrow and form three progenitor lines for the erythroid, granulocytic-monocytic, and megakaryocytic elements of the mature marrow (Fig. 20-1).

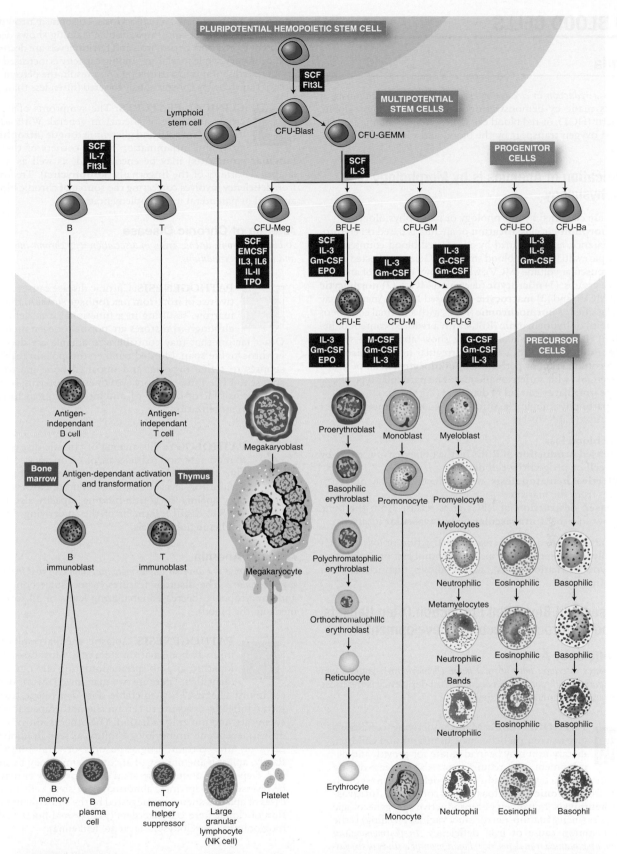

FIGURE 20-1. **Cellular differentiation and maturation of the lymphoid and myeloid components of the hematopoietic system.** Only the precursor cells (blasts and maturing cells) are identifiable by light microscopic evaluation of the bone marrow. BFU, burst-forming unit; CFU, colony-forming unit; Ba, basophils; E, erythroid; Eo, eosinophils; G, polymorphonuclear leukocytes; GM, granulocyte-monocyte; M, monocyte/macrophages; Meg, megakaryocytic; EPO, erythropoietin; GM-CSF, granulocyte-macrophage colony stimulating factor; IL, interleukin; NK, natural killer; SCF, stem cell factor; TPO, thrombopoietin.

RED BLOOD CELLS

Anemia

Anemia is a reduction in circulating erythrocyte mass. A diagnosis of anemia is made by demonstrating a reduction in hemoglobin, hematocrit (HCT), or red blood cell (RBC) count. Anemia leads to decreased oxygen transport by the blood and ultimately to tissue hypoxia.

Classification of Anemias is by Morphology or Pathophysiology

Anemias are classified by morphology or pathophysiology.

The **morphologic classification** of anemia is based on erythrocyte appearance, as determined by automated blood counters and microscopic evaluation of a blood smear. RBC size is reflected in the mean corpuscular volume (MCV), which allows division of anemias into three groups: (1) **microcytic** (decreased MCV), (2) **normocytic** (normal MCV), and (3) **macrocytic** (increased MCV). Anemias may also be classified as **normochromic** (RBCs with a normal content of hemoglobin) or **hypochromic** (RBCs with a reduced content of hemoglobin). Blood smear analysis may show abnormally shaped RBCs **(poikilocytosis)**, RBCs that are irregular in size **(anisocytosis)**, or a combination of both **(anisopoikilocytosis)**, all of which can be seen in a wide variety of anemias. The particular type of size and shape irregularity can aid in diagnosis (Fig. 20-2).

The pathophysiologic classification of anemia includes four major groups (Table 20-1):

1. **Acute blood loss**
2. **Decreased production** of RBCs by the bone marrow, either by **stem-cell or progenitor-cell defects**
3. **Ineffective hematopoiesis** with reduced release of erythrocytes from the marrow
4. **Increased destruction** of RBCs after release from the bone marrow, in either **intravascular** or **extravascular** locations

Anemias associated with increased destruction or loss of RBCs are usually characterized by increased numbers of circulating reticulocytes **(reticulocytosis)**, which allows distinction from other groups.

Decreased Red Blood Cell Production Often Reflects Impaired Erythrocyte Precursor Development

Iron Deficiency Anemia

Iron deficiency interferes with normal heme (hemoglobin) synthesis and leads to impaired erythropoiesis and anemia. Iron deficiency is the most common cause of anemia worldwide.

 PATHOGENESIS: Many underlying conditions give rise to iron deficiency. In infants and children, dietary iron may be inadequate for growth and development. Iron requirements also increase during pregnancy and lactation. In adults, iron deficiency most often results from **chronic blood loss** or, less commonly, **intravascular hemolysis**. In women of reproductive age, gynecologic blood loss (menstruation, parturition, vaginal bleeding) is the most common cause of iron deficiency. *In postmenopausal women, unexplained iron deficiency should prompt a study of the gastrointestinal tract for tumors or vascular lesions, as this is the most common site of chronic blood loss.*

 PATHOLOGY: Iron deficiency is characterized by a microcytic, hypochromic anemia (Fig. 20-3), which also shows variation in erythrocyte size and shape **(anisopoikilocytosis)**. Because of the production defect in the mar-

row, there is no associated reticulocytosis. The bone marrow displays erythroid hyperplasia, and Prussian blue staining shows decreased or absent stored iron. Serum iron and ferritin levels are decreased by iron deficiency, while total iron-binding capacity is increased (due to an increased serum transferrin level). As a result, the percent saturation of transferrin is conspicuously lowered (often less than 5%).

 CLINICAL FEATURES: The symptoms of iron deficiency are those of anemia in general. With advanced disease, a smooth and glistening tongue (**atrophic glossitis**) and inflammation at the corners of the mouth (**angular stomatitis**) may be encountered, as well as a spoon-shaped deformity of the fingernails (**koilonychia**). Treatment of iron deficiency involves correcting the source of chronic blood loss and oral or parenteral iron supplementation.

Anemia of Chronic Disease
Anemia of chronic disease arises in association with chronic inflammatory and malignant conditions.

 PATHOGENESIS: Chronic disease causes ineffective use of iron from macrophage stores in the bone marrow, resulting in a functional iron deficiency, although iron stores are normal or even increased. Other factors that may contribute to anemia are decreased erythrocyte life span, blunted renal erythropoietin (EPO) responses to tissue hypoxia, and impaired bone marrow response to EPO. Inflammatory cytokines (lactoferrin, IL-1, tumor necrosis factor-α [TNF-α], and interferon) may interfere with iron mobilization.

 PATHOLOGY: The anemia of chronic disease is mild to moderate, and red cells are often microcytic. Prussian blue staining shows normal or increased iron storage. Serum iron levels tend to be reduced. However, unlike iron-deficiency anemia, total iron-binding capacity also tends to be decreased. Successful treatment of the underlying disease restores normal hemoglobin levels.

Aplastic Anemia
Aplastic anemia is a disorder of pluripotential stem cells that leads to bone marrow failure. The disorder features hypocellular bone marrow and pancytopenia (decreased circulating levels of all formed elements in the blood).

 PATHOGENESIS: Aplastic anemia results from injury to bone marrow stem cells. Most cases are idiopathic, and no specific initiating etiology can be identified. There are two main mechanisms of stem cell injury. The first is a predictable, dose-dependent, toxic injury, typified by exposure to certain chemotherapeutic drugs, chemicals, and ionizing radiation. The other is idiosyncratic, dose-independent, immunologic injury, as seen in idiopathic cases or after certain drug exposures or viral infections. Rarely, aplastic anemia (e.g., Fanconi anemia) may be inherited. Depending on its cause, stem cell injury may or may not be reversible. An intrinsic abnormality of stem cells in some cases of aplastic anemia is suggested by the subsequent evolution of clonal stem cell disorders (paroxysmal nocturnal hemoglobinuria, myelodysplasia, acute leukemia).

 PATHOLOGY: The bone marrow in aplastic anemia shows variably reduced cellularity, depending on the clinical stage of the disease, with a corresponding increase in fat (Fig. 20-4). Myeloid, erythroid, and megakaryocytic lineage cells are decreased in number, with a relative increase in marrow lymphocytes and plasma cells. Hence, the disease is characterized by anemia, leukopenia (mainly gran-

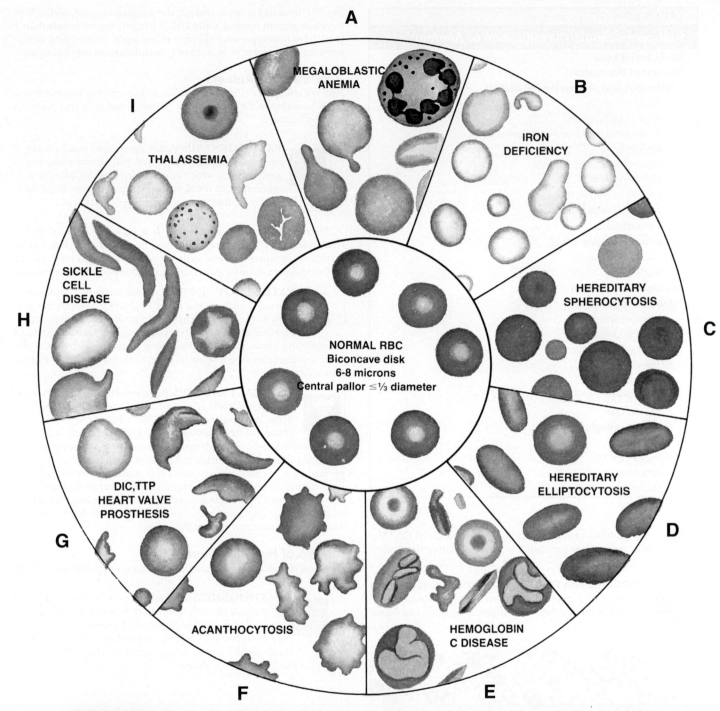

FIGURE 20-2. **Anemias.** The pathophysiology of characteristic morphologic features of various anemias are shown. The morphology of normal erythrocytes is contrasted in the central circle.

A. Megaloblastic anemia **(disturbance in DNA synthesis)**: Oval macrocytes, teardrop poikilocytosis, and hypersegmented neutrophils

B. Iron deficiency **(disturbance in hemoglobin synthesis; lack of iron)**: Hypochromic, microcytic erythrocytes

C. Hereditary spherocytosis **(membrane defect)**: Spherocytes

D. Hereditary elliptocytosis **(membrane defect)**: Elliptocytes

E. Hemoglobin C disease **(abnormal globin chain)**: Target cells, rhomboid crystals

F. Acanthocytosis **(membrane lipid defect, e.g., abetalipoproteinemia)**: Irregular spiculation

G. Disseminated intravascular coagulation (DIC), thrombocytic thrombocytopenic purpura (TTP), heart valve prosthesis sequela **(mechanical damage to erythrocytes)**: Schistocytes

H. Sickle cell disease **(abnormal globin chain)**: Sickle cells

I. Thalassemia **(disturbance in hemoglobin synthesis)**: Hypochromic, microcytic erythrocytes, poikilocytosis, basophilic stip-

TABLE 20–1

Pathophysiologic Classification of Anemia

Acute Blood Loss

Decreased Production

Stem cell and progenitor cell defects

Aplastic anemia

Pure red cell aplasia

Paroxysmal nocturnal hemoglobinuria

Leukemia

Myelodysplastic syndromes

Marrow infiltration

Anemia of chronic disease

Anemia of renal disease

Iron deficiency

Ineffective Hematopoiesis

Megaloblastic anemia

Thalassemia

Increased Destruction

Intracorpuscular

Membrane defect

Enzyme defect

Hemoglobinopathies

Extracorpuscular

Immunologic

Autoimmune

Alloimmune

Nonimmunologic

Mechanical

Hypersplenism

Infectious

Chemical

ulocytopenia), and thrombocytopenia. Despite elevated EPO levels, reticulocytosis is not present, which underscores the underlying stem cell defect.

 CLINICAL FEATURES: Patients with aplastic anemia present with signs and symptoms attributable to pancytopenia, namely weakness, fatigue, infection, and bleed-

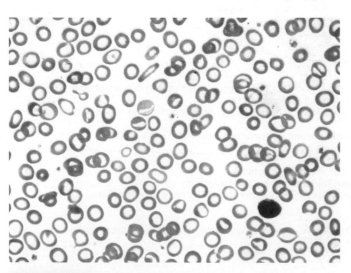

FIGURE 20-3. Microcytic hypochromic anemia caused by iron deficiency. Red blood cells are significantly smaller than the nucleus of a lymphocyte.

ing. For untreated aplastic anemia, the prognosis is grim, with a 3- to 6-month median survival. Only 20% of patients survive longer than 1 year. Immunosuppressive therapy often leads to transient remissions, and bone marrow or stem cell transplantation may be curative.

Pure Red Cell Aplasia

Pure red cell aplasia (PRCA) is a selective suppression of committed erythroid precursors in the bone marrow. White blood cells and platelets are unaffected.

 PATHOGENESIS: PRCA most often results from immune suppression of red cell production, the stimulus for which is unknown. On occasion, it is secondary to viral infection (parvovirus B19) or thymic lesions (e.g., thymoma, thymic hyperplasia).

Diamond-Blackfan syndrome is a heritable type of PRCA that appears in the first year of life and is associated with defective erythroid precursors. These cells show a diminished response to EPO and decreased erythroid burst and colony-forming capacities.

 PATHOLOGY: In PRCA, overall marrow cellularity is normal, but there is a selective absence of erythroid precursors or arrest of these cells at the erythroblast stage. Myeloid and megakaryocytic precursors are adequate in number and show normal maturation. Patients with PRCA develop moderate to severe anemia, often with macrocytosis and no reticulocytosis.

 CLINICAL FEATURES: Acquired PRCA manifests as an acute self-limited illness or a chronic relapsing process. **Acute self-limited PRCA** is often due to parvovirus B19. This condition may not be clinically apparent unless the patient suffers from an underlying chronic hemolytic anemia (e.g., hereditary spherocytosis, sickle cell anemia). Such cases may be complicated by a so-called aplastic crisis (i.e., sudden worsening of anemia). Immunocompro-mised patients cannot clear parvovirus infection, and anemia may be prolonged. **Chronic relapsing PRCA** may be idiopathic or associated with an underlying thymic lesion. In these cases, thymectomy may correct the anemia.

Anemia of Renal Disease

Anemia of chronic renal insufficiency reflects decreased production of EPO.

 PATHOGENESIS: Renal disease of varying causes is associated with decreased production of EPO and subsequent development of anemia. The severity of anemia is proportional to the underlying degree of renal insufficiency. Administration of recombinant EPO is the treatment of choice.

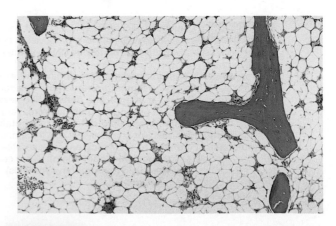

FIGURE 20-4. Aplastic anemia. The bone marrow consists largely of fat cells and lacks normal hematopoietic activity.

PATHOLOGY: The anemia of chronic renal disease is normocytic and normochromic. In some cases, erythrocytes with scalloped cell membranes can be seen (Burr cells). If renal insufficiency is secondary to malignant hypertension, red cell fragmentation with formation of schistocytes may be observed.

Anemia of Lead Poisoning

Lead poisoning results in anemia by interfering with several enzymes involved in heme synthesis (see Chapter 8).

Ineffective Red Cell Production is Characterized by Circulating Erythrocytes

Various anemias reflect abnormal erythrocyte production due to **ineffective hematopoiesis**. In contrast with stem cell or precursor cell disorders, the bone marrow erythrocyte precursor pool is expanded. Thus, sufficient erythrocyte precursors are formed in the bone marrow, but erythrocytes do not enter the circulation.

Megaloblastic Anemias

Megaloblastic anemias are caused by impaired DNA synthesis, usually because of a deficiency in vitamin B_{12} or folic acid.

 PATHOGENESIS: Impaired DNA synthesis results in abnormal nuclear development, which in turn, leads to ineffective erythrocyte maturation and anemia. Certain chemotherapeutic agents (methotrexate, hydroxyurea) or antiretroviral drugs (5-azacytidine) may also cause megaloblastic anemia. Less commonly, inherited defects in purine or pyrimidine metabolism may be involved.

Folate and vitamin B_{12} are critical for normal DNA synthesis. Tetrahydrofolate is converted from methyl tetrahydrofolate by methyl transferase and vitamin B_{12}, which serves as a cofactor. In the face of defective DNA synthesis, nuclear development is impaired, whereas the cytoplasm matures normally. This situation results in the formation of large nucleated erythrocyte precursors (**megaloblasts**), most of which do not mature enough to be released into the blood but rather undergo intramedullary destruction. Circulating erythrocytes are macrocytic.

Vitamin B_{12} (cyanocobalamin) is found in a variety of animal food sources and is synthesized by intestinal microorganisms. Proper vitamin B_{12} absorption from the distal ileum requires its binding to **intrinsic factor**, which is synthesized by gastric parietal cells and protects the vitamin from degradation by intestinal enzymes. Vitamin B_{12} deficiency arises from diverse causes. Inadequate dietary intake of vitamin B_{12} is rare and is usually encountered only in strict vegetarians (vegans). *Most commonly, lack of intrinsic factor leads to impaired absorption of vitamin B_{12}.* Intrinsic factor may be deficient as a result of previous gastric surgery that removes parietal cell mass of the stomach. **Pernicious anemia** is an autoimmune disorder in which patients develop antibodies against parietal cells and intrinsic factor. Anti-parietal cell antibodies also lead to atrophic gastritis with achlorhydria.

Folic acid is present in leafy vegetables, in meat, and eggs. The most common cause of folic acid deficiency is inadequate dietary intake, which occurs most often in patients with poorly balanced diets (alcoholics, recluses). Folate deficiency may also occur in pregnancy, lactation, periods of rapid growth, and chronic hemolytic processes. Primary intestinal diseases (inflammatory bowel disease, sprue) may interfere with absorption of folic acid. Various medications can also impair folic acid absorption (phenytoin) or metabolism (methotrexate).

 PATHOLOGY: The hematologic manifestations in bone marrow and blood are identical for either folic acid or vitamin B_{12} deficiency. Although the bone marrow tends to be hypercellular, the blood demonstrates pancytopenia

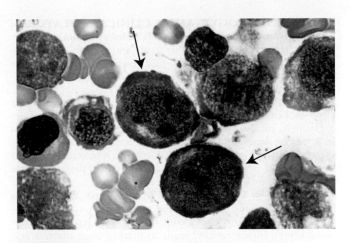

FIGURE 20-5. **Megaloblastic anemia.** A bone marrow aspirate from a patient with vitamin B12 deficiency (pernicious anemia) shows prominent megaloblastic erythroid precursors *(arrows)*.

because of **ineffective hemato-poiesis**. Megaloblastic maturation, characterized by cellular enlargement with asynchronous maturation between the nucleus and cytoplasm (Fig. 20-5), is noted in bone marrow precursors from all lineages. The degree of anemia varies but may be severe. Erythrocytes are macrocytic and may be oval. Anisopoikilocytosis is usually prominent, and teardrop cells may be seen. Circulating neutrophils often show nuclear hypersegmentation (more than five lobes). No increase in reticulocytes occurs.

 CLINICAL FEATURES: In general, folate deficiency develops more rapidly (months) than does vitamin B_{12} deficiency (years). Neurologic symptoms secondary to demyelination of the posterior and lateral columns of the spinal cord including both sensory and motor deficiencies, may occur with vitamin B_{12} deficiency. Without appropriate and prompt therapy, neurologic symptoms may be irreversible. Such findings are not encountered with folate deficiency.

Thalassemia

Thalassemias are anemias that result from defective globin chain synthesis. Ineffective hematopoiesis results from precipitation of abnormal hemoglobins within newly formed RBCs and increased erythrocyte fragility, features that lead to erythrocyte destruction in the marrow.

 EPIDEMIOLOGY: Although thalassemia is most common around the Mediterranean Sea, especially in Italy and Greece, it may be found in any area where malaria has been endemic (Middle East, India, Southeast Asia, and China). A heterozygous state for thalassemia may provide a protective effect against malaria, thereby explaining the persistence of thalassemic disorders.

 PATHOGENESIS Thalassemias are generally classified according to the affected globin chain. The two most clinically significant forms involve deficits of α and β chains. Thalassemias involving γ and δ globin chain synthesis have also been described but are not common.

β-Thalassemia

β-thalassemias are a heterogeneous group of disorders that are most often caused by point mutations in the β globin gene. Mutations may be in the gene's promoter region, a splice site or other coding regions, or may lead to the creation of an inappropriate stop codon. The result is that transcription of the gene is entirely (β°) or partly (β^{+}) suppressed. Occasionally, a mutation may also affect the adjacent δ globin gene, leading to a β-δ thalassemia.

PATHOLOGY AND CLINICAL FEATURES: **Homozygous β-thalassemia (Cooley's anemia)** is characterized by moderate-to-severe, microcytic, and hypochromic anemia (Fig. 20-6). There is a marked excess of α chains, which form unstable tetramers ($α_4$) that precipitate in the cytoplasm of developing erythroid precursors. In the β° type, fetal hemoglobin accounts for most of the hemoglobin, although increased levels (5% to 8%) of hemoglobin A_2 are also present. In the case of β+ type, some hemoglobin A may be detected (depending on the nature of the underlying defect), and hemoglobin A_2 is mildly increased. A modest increase in hemoglobin A_2 is characteristic of all forms of β-thalassemia, as δ-globin genes are upregulated in the disease.

In addition to microcytosis and hypochromia, blood smears demonstrate striking anisopoikilocytosis, with target cells, basophilic stippling, and circulating normoblasts (especially after splenectomy). Increased EPO leads to marked bone marrow erythroid hyperplasia. The marrow space is expanded, causing facial and cranial bone deformities. Extramedullary hematopoiesis contributes to hepatosplenomegaly and the formation of soft tissue masses. Excess erythropoiesis leads to increased iron absorption, which, together with repeated transfusions, creates iron overload. Excess iron deposition in tissues is a major cause of morbidity and mortality in thalassemic patients and often requires aggressive chelation therapy.

Heterozygous β-thalassemia is associated with microcytosis and hypochromia. The degree of microcytosis is disproportionate to the severity of the anemia, which is generally mild. There is often an accompanying erythrocytosis (increased RBC count) but minimal anisocytosis. Target cells, basophilic stippling, and a mild increase in hemoglobin A2 are present. Most patients are entirely asymptomatic.

α-Thalassemia

PATHOGENESIS: Unlike β-thalassemias, α-thalassemias are most frequently due to gene deletions. More syndromes are clinically observed because of the potential number (up to four) of α-globin genes that may be affected. α-thalassemia is associated with excess β or γ chains, which can then form the tetrameric hemoglobin H ($β_4$) and hemoglobin Bart ($γ_4$). Hemoglobins H and Bart are both unstable and precipitate in the cytoplasm. Further, they have high oxygen affinities and cause decreased tissue oxygen delivery. The relative amount

of these tetrameric hemoglobins depends on the number of α genes involved and the patient's age. Because of the underlying impairment in hemoglobin synthesis, circulating red cells are usually microcytic and hypochromic.

PATHOLOGY AND CLINICAL FEATURES:
- **Silent carrier α-thalassemia** (one gene affected) is difficult to diagnose, because the patients' only hematologic abnormality is small amounts of hemoglobin Bart, detectable only in infancy. There is no anemia, and patients are asymptomatic.
- **α-thalassemia trait** (two genes affected) is associated with a mild microcytic anemia. Up to 5% hemoglobin Bart can be seen during infancy.
- **Hemoglobin H disease** (three genes affected) is associated with moderate microcytic anemia. Increased hemoglobin Bart (up to 25% in infancy) and variable levels of hemoglobin H can be detected.
- **Homozygous** (four genes affected) **α-thalassemia,** also termed α hydrops fetalis, is incompatible with life. Affected infants die in utero or shortly after birth with severe anemia, marked variation in cell size and shape, and large amounts of hemoglobin Bart.

Hemolytic Anemias Feature Increased Red Cell Destruction

Premature elimination of circulating erythrocytes results in **hemolytic anemias**, which are classified by the site of red cell destruction. In **extravascular hemolysis**, the monocyte/macrophage system in the spleen and, to a lesser extent, the liver, are involved. In **intravascular hemolysis**, erythrocytes are destroyed in the circulation.

Erythrocyte Membrane Defects
Alterations in any portion of the red cell membrane can reduce its normal plasticity and render erythrocytes susceptible to hemolysis.

Hereditary Spherocytosis
Hereditary spherocytosis (HS) is a heterogeneous group of inherited disorders of the RBC cytoskeletons, characterized by a deficiency of spectrin or another cytoskeletal component (ankyrin, protein 4.2, band 3).

PATHOGENESIS: The deficiency of a cytoskeletal protein in HS leads to a **"vertical"** defect in the red cell membrane, with uncoupling of the lipid bilayer from the underlying cytoskeleton. The result is progressive loss of membrane surface area and **spherocyte** formation. These abnormal red cells are more rigid and cannot easily traverse the spleen, where they become "conditioned" and lose additional surface membrane before they ultimately undergo extravascular hemolysis. Most forms of HS are inherited as autosomal dominant traits. The rare recessive cases all involve the α subunit of spectrin.

PATHOLOGY: Patients with HS most commonly have moderate normocytic anemia. Conspicuous spherocytes that appear hyperchromic (have no central pallor) are typical, along with polychromasia and reticulocytosis (see Fig. 20-2). The bone marrow shows erythroid hyperplasia.

CLINICAL FEATURES: Most patients have splenomegaly due to chronic extravascular hemolysis. They may appear jaundiced, and up to 50% develop cholelithiasis, with pigmented (bilirubin) gallstones.

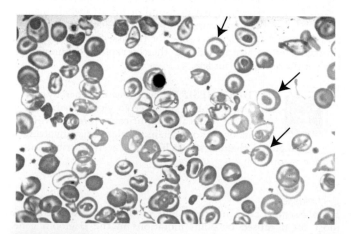

FIGURE 20-6. **Thalassemia.** The peripheral blood erythrocytes are hypochromic and microcytic and show anisocytosis, poikilocytosis, and target cells *(arrows)*.

Patients with HS can be managed effectively by splenectomy, although spherocytes still persist in the circulation.

Hereditary Elliptocytosis

Hereditary elliptocytosis (HE) is a heterogeneous group of inherited disorders involving the erythrocyte cytoskeleton.

 PATHOGENESIS: HE features a *"horizontal"* abnormality within the cytoskeleton. More commonly described variants of HE include defects in self-assembly of spectrin, spectrin–ankyrin binding, protein 4.1, and glycophorin C. Regardless of the underlying molecular abnormality, most circulating red cells are elliptical or oval. They still have an area of central pallor, because there is no loss of the lipid bilayer (as seen in HS). Most forms of HE are autosomal dominant.

 PATHOLOGY AND CLINICAL FEATURES: HE usually manifests with only mild normocytic anemia, and many patients are asymptomatic. Blood smears show numerous elliptocytes with only minimal reticulocytosis (see Fig. 20-2). Occasional patients with more severe hemolysis may require splenectomy.

Acanthocytosis

Acanthocytosis results from a defect within the lipid bilayer of the red cell membrane and features spiny projections of the surface, which may be associated with hemolysis.

The most common cause is chronic liver disease, in which increased free cholesterol is deposited within cell membranes. Acanthocytes (spur cells) are also a prominent feature in cases of abetalipoproteinemia, an autosomal recessive disorder associated with lipid membrane abnormalities. Such abnormalities cause erythrocytes to become deformed and develop irregular spiny surface projections and centrally dense cytoplasm (no central pallor) (Fig. 20-2). Hemolysis and anemia in acanthocytosis are mild.

Enzyme Defects: Glucose-6-Phosphate Deficiency

Glucose-6-phosphate deficiency is an X-linked disorder in which abnormal red cell sensitivity to oxidative stress manifests as hemolytic anemia. Inherited defects of enzymes in the glycolytic pathway can predispose circulating red cells to hemolysis. The most common enzyme defect involves glucose-6-phosphate dehydrogenase (G6PD), which catalyzes the conversion of glucose-6-phosphate to 6-phosphogluconate. Clinically, these defects cause variable degrees of anemia and are designated **hereditary nonspherocytic anemias.** G6PD deficiency is most prevalent in areas where malaria is historically endemic, notably Africa and the Mediterranean region since because mutations appear to provide some protective effect against malaria. The A variant of G6PD is seen in 10% to 15% of American blacks and is associated with reduced enzyme activity (10% of normal).

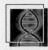 **PATHOGENESIS AND PATHOLOGY:** Because G6PD helps to recycle reduced glutathione, red cells deficient in this enzyme are susceptible to oxidative stress, which is accentuated by infections and some drugs. Ingestion of fava beans (a staple in the Mediterranean diet) may lead to fatal hemolysis (favism). Oxidation of hemoglobin causes its precipitation in the cytoplasm as Heinz bodies, increased cell rigidity, and ultimately, hemolysis. After passage through the spleen, circulating red cells may have part of their membrane removed, forming so-called **bite cells.**

Hemoglobinopathies

Most clinically relevant hemoglobinopathies are caused by point mutations in the β- globin chain gene.

Sickle Cell Disease

In sickle cell disease, an abnormal hemoglobin, namely hemoglobin S, transforms the erythrocyte into a sickle shape upon deoxygenation.

 EPIDEMIOLOGY: Hemoglobin S is most common in persons of African ancestry, although the mutation is also occasionally present in Mediterranean, Middle Eastern, and Indian populations. Ten percent of American blacks are heterozygous, and 1 in 650 is homozygous. Heterozygosity for hemoglobin S is thought to provide some protection against falciparum malaria. Infected erythrocytes selectively sickle and are removed from the circulation by splenic and hepatic macrophages, effectively destroying the parasite.

 PATHOGENESIS: In hemoglobin S, a point mutation in the gene for the β-globin chain gene substitutes valine for glutamic acid at the sixth amino acid. This single change generates a structurally abnormal molecule that polymerizes under conditions of deoxygenation. Polymerization of hemoglobin S transforms the cytoplasm into a rigid filamentous gel and leads to the formation of less-deformable sickled erythrocytes. This effect results in the primary manifestations of sickle cell disease in two ways: (1) obstruction of the microcirculation, with subsequent tissue hypoxia and ischemic injury in many organs and (2) increased susceptibility to destruction (hemolysis) during circulation through the spleen, which produces chronic extravascular hemolytic anemia.

 PATHOLOGY: Homozygous patients (hemoglobin SS) have severe normocytic or macrocytic anemia. The macrocytosis can be attributed to increased numbers of reticulocytes, secondary to chronic hemolysis. Blood smear examination reveals marked anisopoikilocytosis and polychromasia. Classic sickle cells and target cells, as well as a variety of other abnormally shaped erythrocytes, are observed (Fig. 20-7).

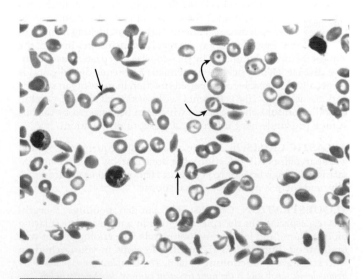

FIGURE 20-7. **Sickle cell anemia.** Sickled cells (*straight arrows*) and target cells (*curved arrows*) are evident.

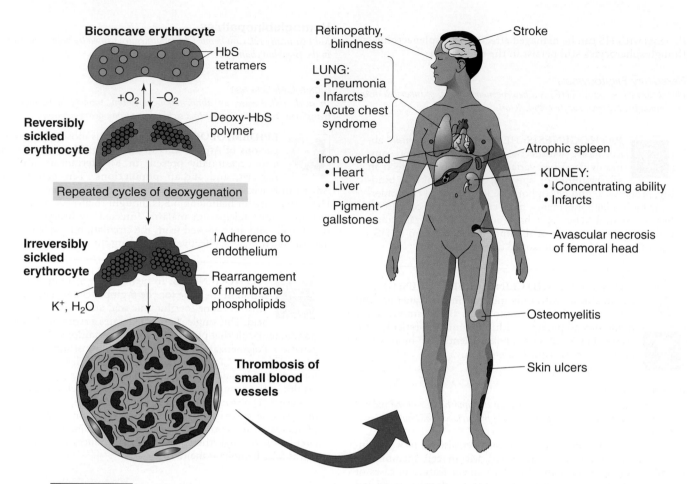

FIGURE 20-8. **Pathogenesis of the vascular complications of sickle cell anemia.** Substitution of valine for glutamic acid leads to an alteration in the surface charge of the hemoglobin molecule. Upon deoxygenation ($-O_2$), sickle hemoglobin (HbS) tetramers aggregate to form poorly soluble polymers. The erythrocytes change shape from a biconcave disk to a sickle form with the polymerization of HbS. This process is initially reversible upon reoxygenation ($+O_2$), but with repeated cycles of deoxygenation and reoxygenation, the erythrocytes become irreversibly sickled. Irreversibly sickled cells display a rearrangement of phospholipids between the outer and inner monolayers of the cell membrane, in particular an increase in aminophospholipids in the outer leaflet. Potassium (K^+) and water (H_2O) are lost from the cells. The erythrocytes are no longer deformable and are more adherent to endothelial cells, properties that predispose to thrombosis of small blood vessels. The resulting vascular occlusions lead to widespread ischemic complications.

CLINICAL FEATURES: People who are homozygous for hemoglobin S show the full clinical presentation of sickle cell disease. Patients suffer from lifelong hemolysis, but most do not require regular transfusions. Instead, the clinical picture is dominated by the sequelae of repeated **vasoocclusive disease**. Hence, sickle cell anemia is a systemic disorder and is eventually responsible for impaired function in most organ systems and tissues (Fig. 20-8). Patients with sickle cell disease develop episodic painful ischemic crises, which can be triggered by various stimuli (e.g. underlying infection, acidosis, or dehydration).

APLASTIC CRISIS: In aplastic crisis (most frequently associated with parvovirus B19 infection), the bone marrow fails to compensate for the high level of red cell loss. Hemoglobin levels drop rapidly, and there is no reticulocyte response.

SEQUESTRATION CRISIS: The sudden pooling of erythrocytes, especially in the spleen, results in a decreased circulating blood volume and low hemoglobin levels. The etiology is not well understood, but it most frequently develops in young children who still have a functioning spleen. *This complication is followed by hypovolemic shock and is the most frequent cause of death early in life.*

- **Heart:** Chronic demand for increased cardiac output may lead to cardiomegaly and congestive heart failure. Myocardial is-

chemia may result from obstruction of coronary microcirculation. Myocyte function may also be impaired by excess iron deposition, due to chronic hemolysis and repeated transfusions.

- **Lungs:** Up to one third of patients with sickle cell anemia show a rapid decrease in respiratory function, associated with pulmonary infiltrates on chest x-ray. This **acute chest syndrome** may be fatal. Pulmonary infarction may occur, and sickle cell patients are more susceptible to a variety of pulmonary infections.
- **Spleen:** Although splenomegaly is often found in childhood, repeated splenic infarction leads to a functional autosplenectomy. In most adults, only a small fibrous remnant of the spleen remains. *The asplenic state renders the patient prone to infections with encapsulated bacteria, especially pneumococcus.*
- **Brain:** Patients with sickle cell anemia develop neurologic complications related to vascular obstruction, including transient ischemic attacks, overt strokes, and cerebral hemorrhages.
- **Kidney:** Sickling commonly occurs in the renal medulla because of the hypoxic, acidotic, and hypertonic environment that normally exists there. Complications include inability to form concentrated urine, renal infarcts, and papillary necrosis.
- **Liver:** As in any form of chronic hemolytic anemia, patients with sickle cell anemia have increased levels of unconjugated (indirect) bilirubin, which predisposes to development of pigmented bilirubin gallstones.

- **Extremities:** Cutaneous ulcers over the lower extremities, especially near the ankles, are common and reflect obstruction of dermal capillaries. Sickle cell disease is also associated with an increased incidence of osteomyelitis, particularly with *Salmonella typhimurium*, possibly related to the underlying impairment in splenic function.

Heterozygotes for hemoglobin S (sickle cell trait) do not develop red cell sickling and are clinically normal.

Hemoglobin C Disease
Hemoglobin C disease results from homozygous inheritance of a structurally abnormal hemoglobin, which leads to increased erythrocyte rigidity and mild chronic hemolysis.

PATHOGENESIS: In hemoglobin C, lysine replaces glutamic acid at the sixth amino acid of β globin. In homozygous individuals, hemoglobin C precipitates in the erythrocyte cytoplasm and leads to cellular dehydration, decreased deformability, and increased splenic clearance. These effects result in mild normocytic anemia and splenomegaly. Hemoglobin C is found in the same populations as hemoglobin S, although its incidence is less frequent. Two to 3% of American blacks are heterozygous for hemoglobin C and are asymptomatic (hemoglobin C trait).

Other Hemoglobinopathies
Several hundred additional hemoglobin variants have been described that result from mutations in α- or β-globin genes. These mutations may lead to structural abnormalities or to a functional derangement of the hemoglobin molecule.

Immune Hemolytic Anemias
In immune hemolytic anemias, red cell destruction (hemolysis) is caused by antibodies against antigens at the erythrocyte surface that may be allo- or autoimmune in origin. The red cells themselves are intrinsically normal but are targets for an immune-mediated attack. The site of hemolysis may be extravascular or intravascular. Autoantibodies can be classified as either warm or cold antibodies.

Warm-Antibody Autoimmune Hemolytic Anemia (AIHA)

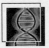

PATHOGENESIS: Warm autoantibodies have optimal reactivity at 37°C (98.6°F) and account for 80% of all cases of AIHA. They are usually IgG and directed against erythrocyte Rh determinants. *They do not bind complement, so extravascular hemolysis occurs, primarily in the spleen.* Splenic macrophages have Fc receptors that recognize the bound antibody resulting in erythrocyte membrane damage and eventual lysis. Warm-antibody AIHA affects women more often than men, and half of the cases are idiopathic. In the remaining cases, warm antibody reflects an underlying condition, such as infection, collagen vascular disease, lymphoproliferative disorders, and drug reactions. Drug-induced warm antibodies may arise by several different mechanisms.

- **Hapten mechanism:** A drug such as penicillin binds to the erythrocyte surface and elicits antibodies, some of which react with the cell-bound drug.
- **Immune complex mechanism:** A drug such as quinidine reacts with specific antibody to form circulating immune complexes, which are then bound to red cell membranes.
- **Autoantibody mechanism:** A drug (e.g., α-methyldopa) leads to the formation of antibodies that cross-react with components of the red cell membrane. Hemolysis can occur in the absence of the inciting drug.

PATHOLOGY AND CLINICAL FEATURES: Warm-antibody AIHA is associated with normocytic or occasionally macrocytic anemia, with spherocytes, and polychromasia. Treatment is with immunosuppressive agents or splenectomy.

Cold-Antibody Autoimmune Hemolytic Anemia (AIHA)
Cold antibodies have maximal reactivity at 4°C (39.2°F). Approximately 20% of cases of AIHA are caused by cold IgM or IgG antibodies.

PATHOGENESIS: Cold agglutinins are mostly IgM directed against the I/i antigen system on red cells. At cooler temperatures in the peripheral circulation, these antibodies bind to and agglutinate red cells and fix complement. Upon rewarming in the central circulation, the antibody dissociates, leaving unactivated complement attached. These complement-coated red cells may undergo extravascular hemolysis in the liver, because Kupffer cells have more complement receptors than do splenic macrophages. Occasionally, the thermal amplitude (thermal range of reactivity) of a cold agglutinin is high enough for the antibody to remain attached; complement becomes activated, and intravascular hemolysis occurs. Cold agglutinins may be idiopathic or develop secondary to an underlying condition, mostly infections (Epstein-Barr virus [EBV], *Mycoplasma*) or lymphoproliferative disorders.

PATHOLOGY AND CLINICAL FEATURES: Significant hemolysis is uncommon with cold agglutinins, and patients are more likely to develop peripheral vascular symptoms (Raynaud phenomenon) upon cold exposure because of red cell agglutination. Cold agglutinins are present in many healthy individuals; pathogenicity is associated with antibodies having either a very high titer or a wide thermal amplitude.

Cold Hemolysin Disease
Cold hemolysins (Donath-Landsteiner antibodies) are usually IgGs and directed against the P antigen system on red cells. Cold hemolysins have biphasic activity and are an uncommon cause of AIHA. The antibody binds to erythrocytes at low temperatures and fixes complement. Because the antibody is IgG, red cells do not agglutinate. Upon warming, the cold hemolysin remains attached, complement is activated, and intravascular hemolysis occurs. The clinical syndrome related to cold hemolysins is designated **paroxysmal cold hemoglobinuria** and most often follows a viral illness. Immunosuppressive therapy and splenectomy are usually ineffective, and supportive therapy is required.

Hemolytic Disease of the Newborn
Hemolytic disease of the newborn reflects incompatibility of blood types between a mother and her developing fetus; the mother lacks an antigen that is expressed by the fetus, which is a condition described in detail in Chapter 6.

Mechanical Red Cell Fragmentation Syndromes
In red cell fragmentation syndromes, intrinsically normal erythrocytes are subjected to mechanical disruption as they circulate in the blood (intravascular hemolysis).

PATHOGENESIS: *These disorders are classified as macroangiopathic (large vessels) or microangiopathic (capillaries), according to the site of hemolysis.* Mechanical fragmentation of red cells is due to alteration of the endothelial surface of blood vessels or disturbances in blood flow patterns that lead to turbulence and increased shear stress.

Macroangiopathic hemolytic anemia most often reflects direct red cell trauma from an abnormal vascular surface (e.g., prosthetic heart valve, synthetic vascular graft).

Microangiopathic hemolytic anemia more frequently results from abnormalities in the microcirculation. Classic examples of microangiopathic hemolysis are disseminated intravascular coagulation (DIC) and thrombotic thrombocytopenic purpura (TTP), both of which feature generalized capillary thrombosis (see Chapter 16 and below). Alterations in blood flow, as are encountered in malignant hypertension or vasculitis syndromes, may also lead to mechanical fragmentation of erythrocytes.

 PATHOLOGY: Laboratory findings are similar in macro- and microangiopathic hemolytic anemias. Anemia is mild to moderate, and an appropriate reticulocyte response is seen. Blood smears show fragmented erythrocytes (schistocytes) and polychromasia (Fig. 20-9). Abnormalities in coagulation and thrombocytopenia characterize DIC, whereas thrombocytopenia alone is seen in cases of TTP (see below).

Paroxysmal Nocturnal Hemoglobinuria

Paroxysmal nocturnal hemoglobinuria (PNH) is an acquired clonal stem cell disorder characterized by episodic intravascular hemolytic anemia due to increased sensitivity of erythrocytes to complement-mediated lysis.

 PATHOGENESIS: The underlying defect in cases of PNH involves somatic mutation of the *phosphatidylinositol glycan-class A (PIG-A)* gene, on the short arm of the X chromosome (Xp22.1) in hematopoietic stem cells. Mutation of the *PIG-A* gene leads to disrupted synthesis of glycosyl phosphatidylinositol (GPI), which normally anchors many proteins to red cell membranes, including **decay acceleration factor** (CD55) and, more importantly, **membrane inhibitor of reactive lysis** (CD59). Loss of these factors from erythrocyte surfaces renders the cells susceptible to complement-mediated hemolysis. Leukocytes and platelets derived from the abnormal stem cells also show loss of GPI-linked membrane proteins. PNH may develop as a primary disorder or evolve from pre-existing aplastic anemia. Because the defect is clonal, it may progress to myelodysplasia or overt acute leukemia (see below).

 PATHOLOGY: During hemolytic episodes, patients develop varyingly severe normocytic or macrocytic anemia, with an appropriate reticulocyte response. Because the hemolysis is intravascular, hemoglobin-uria is present, and iron deficiency may develop over time from recurrent iron loss in the urine. Leukopenia and thrombocytopenia are frequently detected, and sensitivity to complement may lead to inappropriate platelet activation.

 CLINICAL FEATURES: Patients develop intermittent intravascular hemolysis, although it is nocturnal in only a minority of cases. Venous and arterial thrombosis, notably Budd-Chiari syndrome (hepatic vein thrombosis), are increased in PNH because of complement-mediated platelet activation. Thrombocytopenia may lead to bleeding. Treatment has been supportive, and bone marrow transplantation is curative. A monoclonal antibody inhibiting the activation of complement component 5 (eculizumab, Soliris™) has recently been approved for therapy.

Polycythemia

Polycythemia (erythrocytosis) refers to an increase in the RBC mass.

 PATHOGENESIS: Polycythemia can be arbitrarily defined as a hematocrit (HCT) greater than 54% in men and 47% in women. At HCTs above 50%, blood viscosity increases exponentially, and cardiac function and peripheral blood flow may be impaired. With a HCT above 60%, blood flow may be so compromised as to lead to tissue hypoxia.

Polycythemia can be further divided on the basis of overall red cell mass into relative and absolute categories.

- **Relative polycythemia**, characteristic of dehydration, is characterized by decreased plasma volume and a normal red cell mass.
- **Absolute polycythemia** is a true increase in red cell mass and can be subclassified as primary and secondary.
  - **Primary polycythemia**, or **polycythemia vera (PV)**, is an autonomous, EPO-independent, proliferation of erythroid cells that is due to an acquired, clonal, hematopoietic stem cell disorder. PV is considered to be a chronic myeloproliferative disorder and is discussed below.
  - **Secondary polycythemia** arises from EPO-dependent stimulation of erythropoiesis, usually as a compensatory response to general tissue hypoxia. Renal cysts or hydronephrosis may exert direct pressure on the kidney, thereby leading to localized hypoxia and increased EPO production.

HEMOSTASIS

Hemostatic Disorders

Platelets, endothelium, and coagulation factors participate in hemostasis. Hemostasis is normally achieved by clot formation. Initially, platelets **adhere** to the vascular endothelium and subsequently form **aggregates** that are stabilized by fibrin after the coagulation cascade is activated. Clots can be dissolved by the **fibrinolytic system**.

Defects of the system for maintaining fluid blood passage through intact vessels fall into two categories: **hemostatic** disorders and **thrombotic** disorders. *Failure of the hemostatic system to restore the integrity of an injured vessel causes **bleeding**. Inability to maintain the fluidity of blood results in **thrombosis**.*

The clinical manifestations of hemorrhage associated with disorders of each component of the hemostatic system tend to be distinctive. Platelet abnormalities result in both petechiae and purpura in the skin and mucous membranes. Deficiencies of coagulation factors lead to hemorrhage into muscles, viscera, and joint spaces. Disorders of the blood vessels usually cause purpura.

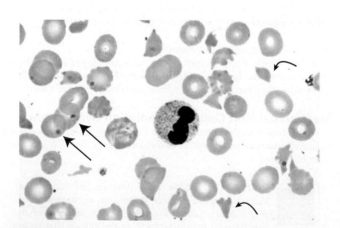

FIGURE 20-9. **Microangiopathic hemolytic anemia.** Irregular, fragmented erythrocytes (schistocytes, *curved arrows*) are seen in the blood smear of a patient with disseminated intravascular coagulation. Howell-Jolly bodies are also present (*straight arrows*).

Hemostatic Disorders of Blood Vessels Reflect Dysfunction of Extravascular or Vascular Tissues

Extravascular Dysfunction Resulting in Hemostatic Defects

Dysfunction of the extravascular tissues is of limited clinical significance. **Scurvy** associated with vitamin C deficiency is characterized by disturbed collagen synthesis and is commonly associated with purpura resulting from perifollicular hemorrhages in the skin (see Chapter 8). **Senile purpura** features superficial, sharply demarcated, persistent purpuric spots on the forearms and other sun-exposed areas. It results from age-associated atrophy of supporting connective tissue.

Vascular Dysfunction Resulting in Hemostatic Defects

Vascular dysfunction and associated hemostatic defects reflect:

- **Intrinsic genetic defects:** *Hereditary hemorrhagic telangiectasia (Rendu-Osler-Weber syndrome)* is an autosomal dominant disorder of blood vessel walls (venules and capillaries), which results in tortuous, dilated vessels (telangiectasias). Patients with hereditary hemorrhagic telangiectasia have recurrent hemorrhages that occur spontaneously or following trivial trauma. Recurrent bleeding may limit a patient's activities, but death from exsanguination is rare.
- **Vasculitis:** *Henoch-Schönlein purpura (allergic purpura)* is a vascular disease that results from immunological damage to blood vessel walls (see Chapter 16). In children, it often follows viral infections and is self-limited. In adults, it is associated with exposure to a variety of drugs and may be chronic.
- **Deposition of immunoglobulin fragments in the vessel wall:** *Amyloidosis, cryoglobulinemia, and paraproteinemias* may all result in damage to the vascular system (see Chapters 16 and 23).

Common Platelet Disorders Impair Hemostasis

Patients may have a history of easy bruising or life-threatening bleeding. Bleeding can occur in any damaged vascular bed, but a pattern of mucocutaneous bleeding, including gingival bleeding, epistaxis, and menorrhagia, is common. More severe manifestations are bleeding into the gastrointestinal tract, genitourinary tract, and brain. Petechiae, which are characteristic of platelet disorders, are nonblanching red lesions less than 2 mm in size. They usually occur in the lower extremities, in dependent regions of the body, on the buccal mucosal and soft palate, and at pressure points (waistband, wristwatch band). Petechiae may also occur in vascular disorders. *Platelet disorders reflect:*

- Decreased production
- Increased destruction
- Impaired function

Thrombocytopenia

Thrombocytopenia is defined as a platelet count under 150,000/μL. The lower the platelet count, the greater the risk of traumatic and perioperative bleeding. Patients with fewer than 10,000 platelets/μL are at an increased risk of spontaneous hemorrhage (Table 20-2).

Decreased platelet production *is caused by bone marrow infiltration with leukemic cells or metastatic cancer, which impair megakaryopoiesis.* Ineffective megakaryopoiesis in myelodysplasia also results in thrombocytopenia (see below). Bone marrow failure in patients with aplastic anemia or who received radiotherapy or chemotherapy produces pancytopenia, including thrombocytopenia. Certain viral infections, such as cytomegalovirus or any megaloblastic anemia, may cause severe thrombocytopenia.

Increased platelet destruction may reflect immune-mediated damage and removal of circulating platelets, as in idiopathic thrombocytopenic purpura and drug-induced thrombocytopenia.

Alternatively, intravascular platelet aggregation may produce thrombocytopenia (e.g., in TTP).

Immune Thrombocytopenic Purpura

Immune thrombocytopenic purpura (ITP) is a decrease in blood platelets caused by antibodies against platelet or megakaryocytic antigens. ITP occurs in two forms: an acute, self-limited, hemorrhagic syndrome in children and a chronic bleeding disorder in adolescents and adults.

 PATHOGENESIS: Like autoimmune hemolytic anemia, ITP reflects antibody-mediated destruction of platelets or their precursors. In most patients, these autoantibodies are of the IgG class, although IgM antiplatelet antibodies also occur.

Acute ITP typically appears in children of either gender after a viral illness and is likely caused by virus-induced changes in platelet antigens that elicit autoantibodies. Complement bound at the surface causes platelets to be lysed in the blood or phagocytosed and destroyed by splenic and hepatic macrophages.

Chronic ITP occurs mainly in adults and may be associated with collagen vascular diseases (e.g., systemic lupus erythematosus) or a malignant lymphoproliferative disease, especially chronic lymphocytic leukemia. It is also common in people infected with human immunodeficiency virus (HIV).

 PATHOLOGY: In acute ITP, the platelet count is typically less than 20,000/μL. In chronic adult ITP, platelet counts vary from a few thousand to 100,000/μL. Peripheral blood smears show numerous large platelets, which reflect accelerated release of young platelets by a bone marrow actively engaged in platelet production. Accordingly, bone marrow examination reveals compensatory increases in megakaryocytes.

 CLINICAL FEATURES: Children with acute ITP experience a sudden onset of petechiae and purpura but are otherwise asymptomatic. Spontaneous recovery occurs within 6 months in more than 80% of cases. Treatment is rarely necessary, but with serious disease, corticosteroids and intravenous immunoglobulin may be needed.

TABLE 20–2
Principal Causes of Thrombocytopenia
Decreased Production
Aplastic anemia
Bone marrow infiltration (neoplastic, fibrosis)
Bone marrow suppression by drugs or radiation
Ineffective Production
Megaloblastic anemia
Myelodysplasias
Increased Destruction
Immunologic (idiopathic, HIV, drugs, alloimmune, post transfusion purpura, neonatal)
Nonimmunologic (DIC, TTP, HUS, vascular malformations, drugs)
Increased Sequestration
Splenomegaly
Dilutional
Blood and plasma transfusions

DIC, disseminated intravascular coagulation; HIV, human immunodeficiency virus; HUS, hemolytic-uremic syndrome; TTP, thrombocytic thrombocytopenic purpura.

Chronic ITP in adults manifests as bleeding episodes, such as epistaxis, menorrhagia, or ecchymoses, but life-threatening hemorrhages are uncommon. Most adults with chronic ITP improve when given corticosteroids and intravenous γ-globulin. In the patients who do not respond adequately to drug therapy within 2 to 3 months, splenectomy produces complete or partial remission.

Drug-Induced Thrombocytopenia

Many drugs are known to cause immune-mediated platelet destruction: quinine, quinidine, heparin, sulfonamides, gold salts, antibiotics, sedatives, tranquilizers, and anticonvulsants. The drug often forms a complex with a platelet-related protein to make a neoepitope that elicits antibody production. By contrast, chemotherapeutic agents, ethanol, and thiazides cause thrombocytopenia by suppression of platelet production.

In **heparin-induced thrombocytopenia**, 25% of patients experience a mild, transient thrombocytopenia within the first 2 to 5 days of treatment initiation. However, 1% to 3% develop profound consumptive thrombocytopenia after 7 to 10 days of heparin therapy. These patients are predisposed to arterial and venous thromboembolic events that may be lethal.

TTP

TTP is a rare syndrome featuring thrombocytopenia, microangiopathic hemolytic anemia, neurologic symptoms, fever, and renal impairment. Platelet aggregation produces widespread microvascular deposition of platelets, which appear as hyaline thrombi.

PATHOGENESIS: The pathogenesis of TTP is obscure. *For unknown reasons, unusually large multimers of von Willebrand factor (vWF), possibly released from injured endothelial cells, are present in the plasma, where they are thought to mediate intravascular platelet aggregation.* A protease that cleaves vWF (ADAMTS13) is genetically absent or defective in familial TTP and is inactivated by autoantibodies in sporadic TTP. Although most cases arise in otherwise healthy persons, TTP may also complicate autoimmune collagen vascular disorders (systemic lupus erythematosus, rheumatoid arthritis, Sjögren syndrome) and drug-induced hypersensitivity reactions.

PATHOLOGY: The morphologic hallmark of TTP is the deposition of PAS-positive hyaline microthrombi in arterioles and capillaries throughout the body, mainly in the heart, brain, and kidneys. These microthrombi contain platelet aggregates, fibrin, and a few erythrocytes and leukocytes. Unlike immune-mediated vasculitis, there is no inflammation in TTP. Fragmented erythrocytes (schistocytes) are always evident in peripheral blood smears, as are numerous reticulocytes.

CLINICAL FEATURES: TTP occurs at virtually any age, but is most common in women in the fourth and fifth decades. It may be chronic and recurrent for years or, more frequently, occur as an acute, fulminant disease that is often fatal. Most patients present with neurologic symptoms, including seizures, focal weakness, aphasia, and alterations in the state of consciousness. Widespread purpura are often present, and vaginal bleeding may occur. Anemia is a constant feature, with hemoglobin levels often below 6 g/dL. Jaundice due to hemolysis may be severe. Renal dysfunction is often prominent, and half of these patients are azotemic.

More than half of patients with TTP have platelet counts below 20,000/μL. Despite the presence of aggregated platelets, activation of the coagulation cascade does not occur. Acute TTP was formerly fatal, but the cure rate is approximately 80% with plasma infusion and plasmapheresis.

Hemolytic–Uremic Syndrome

Hemolytic–uremic syndrome (HUS) resembles TTP, and its adult form is considered a variant of the latter. Classic HUS occurs in children, usually after an acute enteric infection. It appears to be a result of glomerular endothelial cell injury produced by verotoxins, usually elaborated by *Escherichia coli* or *Shigella dysenteriae* (see Chapter 16). Adult HUS is not related to enteric infection, and the pathogenesis of the endothelial injury is unknown.

Hereditary Disorders of Platelets

Hereditary disorders of platelets are uncommon and involve either quantitative or qualitative defects in membrane glycoprotein receptors or defects in platelet granules. The best characterized include:

- **Bernard-Soulier syndrome (giant platelet syndrome):** The syndrome is a rare autosomal recessive trait characterized by defects in the membrane glycoprotein complex (GPIb/IX [CD42]) that plays a prominent role in the adhesion of normal platelets to vWF in injured subendothelial tissues. Bernard-Soulier syndrome manifests in infancy or childhood with a bleeding pattern characteristic of abnormal platelet function, namely ecchymoses, epistaxis, and gingival bleeding. In adults, traumatic hemorrhage, gastrointestinal bleeding, and menorrhagia occur.
- **Glanzmann thrombasthenia:** The disorder is an autosomal recessive defect in platelet aggregation caused by a quantitative or qualitative abnormality in the glycoprotein IIb/IIIa complex (CD41/61). In normal platelets, this complex is activated during platelet adhesion and serves as a receptor for fibrinogen and vWF, mediating platelet aggregation, clot retraction, and the generation of a solid plug. The disease manifests shortly after birth, and older patients may suffer unexpected hemorrhage after trauma or surgery.
- **Alpha storage pool disease (grey platelet syndrome):** The disease is a rare inherited malady characterized by the absence of morphologically recognizable α granules in platelets. Thrombocytopenia is common, and platelets are large and pale. The bleeding diathesis tends to be mild.
- **Delta storage pool disease:** The disease is heterogeneous and affects the dense granules of platelets. Bleeding manifestations are mild to moderate.

Acquired Qualitative Disorders of Platelets

A variety of acquired disorders and drugs may adversely affect platelet function (see Table 20-2).

- **Drugs:** Various drugs can impair platelet function. Aspirin irreversibly acetylates cyclooxygenase, primarily COX-1, thereby blocking production of platelet thromboxane A_2, which is important in platelet aggregation. Platelets cannot synthesize cyclooxygenase, so the aspirin effect lasts for the life span of platelets (7 to 10 days). Nonsteroidal analgesics, such as indomethacin or ibuprofen, impair platelet function, but as their inhibition of cyclooxygenase is reversible, their effect on platelets is transient.
- **Renal failure:** End-stage kidney disease is often accompanied by a qualitative platelet defect that results in a prolonged bleeding time and a tendency toward hemorrhage. The platelet abnormality is heterogeneous and is aggravated by uremic anemia.
- **Cardiopulmonary bypass:** Platelet dysfunction due to platelet activation and fragmentation occurs in the extracorporeal circuit during bypass surgery.
- **Hematologic malignancies:** In chronic myeloproliferative disorders and myelodysplastic syndromes, platelet dysfunction is due to intrinsic platelet defects. In dysproteinemias, platelets are impaired because they are coated with plasma paraprotein.

Coagulopathies are Caused by Deficient or Abnormal Coagulation Factors

Quantitative and qualitative disorders of all of coagulation factors have been identified. These conditions may be hereditary or acquired. The hereditary deficiencies of factor VIII (hemophilia A), factor IX (hemophilia B), and vWF are the most common.

Hemophilia is an X-linked recessive disorder of blood clotting that results in spontaneous bleeding, particularly into joints, muscles, and internal organs. Classic hemophilia is actually two distinct diseases, resulting from mutations in the genes for factor VIII (hemophilia A) or factor IX (hemophilia B).

Hemophilia A (Factor VIII Deficiency)

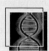 **PATHOGENESIS:** *Hemophilia A is the most common sex-linked inherited bleeding disorder (1 per 5,000 to 10,000 males).* Causative mutations in the very large factor VIII gene at the tip of the long arm of the X chromosome (Xq28) include deletions, inversions, point mutations, and insertions.

 CLINICAL FEATURES: Patients with hemophilia A have mild, moderate, or severe bleeding tendencies, generally paralleling factor VIII activity. Half of the patients have virtually no factor VIII activity and often suffer spontaneous bleeding. One-fifth have more than 10% of normal levels and bleed only after significant trauma or surgery. The most frequent complication of hemophilia A is a deforming arthritis caused by repeated bleeding into many joints. Although now uncommon, bleeding into the brain was formerly the most common cause of death. Treatment with factor VIII to maintain levels of this clotting factor generally controls the bleeding diathesis. Blood donor screening and the availability of human recombinant factor VIII now avoids the infectious complications of AIDS and viral hepatitis, which, in the past, ravaged the affected population.

Hemophilia B

 PATHOGENESIS: *Hemophilia B is an X-linked heritable disorder of factor IX deficiency.* At 1 in 20,000 male births, hemophilia B is four times less common than hemophilia A and accounts for 15% of all cases of hemophilia. Factor IX is a vitamin K-dependent protein that is made in the liver. Many different mutations, from single-base substitutions to gross deletions, have been linked to hemophilia B.

 CLINICAL FEATURES: The bleeding manifestations in hemophilia B are similar to those of hemophilia A. Treatment relies on the infusion of purified or recombinant protein.

von Willebrand Disease

von Willebrand disease (vWD) is a heterogeneous complex of hereditary bleeding disorders related to deficiency or abnormality of vWF. A simplified classification (see below) recognizes three major categories. It is likely that vWD is the most common inherited coagulopathy, affecting 1% to 2% of the population.

vWF is an adhesive molecule produced by endothelial cells and megakaryocytes as a 250-kd monomer that polymerizes to multimers with molecular weights in the millions. After endothelial injury, subendothelial vWF binds to platelet glycoprotein receptors (GPIb/IX or CD42), promoting platelet adherence and sealing the endothelial injury. In plasma, vWF binds to and protects factor VIII; its absence is associated with impaired factor VIII activity.

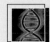 **PATHOGENESIS:** vWD is an autosomal disease, affecting men and women. The *vWF* gene on chromosome 12 is large and complex (180 kb with 52 exons). Three types of the disease are recognized, each of which is heterogeneous:

- **TYPE I** vWD: These variants constitute 75% of all cases of vWD and are inherited as autosomal dominant traits with variable penetrance and expressivity. Type I vWD is a **quantitative deficiency in vWF**, in which levels of **all** multimers are reduced, although their relative concentrations remain unchanged.
- **TYPE II** vWD: **Qualitative defects in vWF** characterize type II variants, which account for 20% of vWD. In type II disease, interactions of vWF and the blood vessel wall are defective.
- **TYPE III** vWD: This severe form of vWD is least common and may represent the presence of mutant alleles on each chromosome (either homozygous or compound heterozygous disease). vWF activity is absent, and plasma levels of factor VIII are less than 10% of normal.

 CLINICAL FEATURES: Most cases of vWD are associated with only a mild bleeding diathesis, with the exception of type III. Easy bruising, epistaxis, gastrointestinal bleeding, and menorrhagia are frequent. The presenting symptom is often excessive hemorrhage after trauma or surgery. Patients with type III vWD may have life-threatening hemorrhage from the gut; hemarthroses like those in hemophilia are not infrequent. The vasopressin analogue desmopressin (DDAVP) is the treatment of choice in types I and some forms of type II vWD because it increases the release of preformed vWF from endothelial storage pools. Intranasal sprays of DDAVP are now available.

Liver Disease

Many coagulation factors are produced in the liver. Severe liver disease may cause impaired secretion of these proteins as a manifestation of a general defect in protein synthesis. In this case, levels of *several* liver-synthesized coagulation factors may be low.

Vitamin K Deficiency

Liver-derived coagulation factors II, VII, IX, and X depend on vitamin K as an essential cofactor in γ-carboxylation of glutamic acid residues to Gla residues. The secreted proteins are functional only if Gla residues are present. Thus, in vitamin K deficiency, activities of all the above-mentioned factors are low. Warfarin-like anticoagulant drugs (e.g., Coumadin) inhibit the vitamin K-dependent modification reaction and also lead to low activity of these proteins.

 CLINICAL FEATURES: Levels of vitamin K are physiologically low in neonates, and it is standard practice to administer the vitamin to newborns to prevent hemorrhagic disease. In adults, vitamin K deficiency is uncommon and may reflect inadequate dietary intake. Because bacteria in the colon produce the form of vitamin K that is best absorbed, prolonged antibiotic intake or large colonic resections may lead to vitamin K deficiency.

Disseminated Intravascular Coagulation (DIC)

DIC refers to widespread ischemic changes secondary to the deposition of microvascular fibrin thrombi, which is accompanied by consumption of platelets, coagulation factors, and a hemorrhagic diathesis. It is a serious, often fatal, disorder that typically occurs as a complication of shock caused by massive trauma, sepsis from numerous organisms, and obstetric emergencies. It is also associated with metastatic cancer, hematopoietic malignancies, cardiovascular and liver disease, and many other conditions.

PATHOGENESIS: DIC begins with activation of the clotting cascades within the vascular compartment by tissue injury, endothelial damage, or both. *Subsequent generation of substantial amounts of thrombin (Fig. 20-10), combined with the initial failure of the natural inhibitory mechanisms to neutralize thrombin, triggers DIC.* With the consequent uncontrolled intravascular coagulation, the delicate balance between coagulation and fibrinolysis is disrupted. This leads to consumption of clotting factors, platelets, and fibrinogen as well as a consequent hemorrhagic diathesis.

Procoagulant Tissue Factor (TF) is released into the circulation after injury in a variety of circumstances, including direct trauma, brain injury, and obstetric accidents (e.g., premature separation of the placenta). **Bacterial endotoxin** also stimulates macrophages to release TF. **Certain tumor cells** cause DIC by releasing TF. With activation of the clotting cascade, intravascular fibrin microthrombi are deposited in the smallest blood vessels. Stimulation of the fibrinolytic system by fibrin generates fibrin split products, which possess anticoagulant properties and contribute to the bleeding diathesis.

Endothelial injury often plays an important role in the pathogenesis of DIC. The anticoagulant properties of the endothelium (Fig. 20-11) are impaired by widely varying injuries, including (1) TNF in gram-negative sepsis; (2) other inflammatory mediators, such as activated complement, IL-1, or neutrophil proteases; (3) viral or rickettsial infections; and (4) trauma (e.g., burns).

PATHOLOGY: Arterioles, capillaries, and venules throughout the body are occluded by **micro-thrombi** composed of fibrin and platelets. Micro-vascular obstruction is associated with widespread **ischemic changes**, particularly in the brain, kidneys, skin, lungs, and gastrointestinal tract. These organs are also sites of bleeding, which, in the case of the brain and gut, may be fatal.

Erythrocytes become fragmented (**schistocytes**) by passage through webs of intravascular fibrin, resulting in **microangiopathic hemolytic anemia**. Consumption of activated platelets leads to **thrombocytopenia**, while **depletion of clotting factors** such as plasma fibrinogen is reflected in a hemorrhagic state. Fibrinopeptide A and D-dimers are elevated (as markers of coagulation and fibrinolytic activation, respectively).

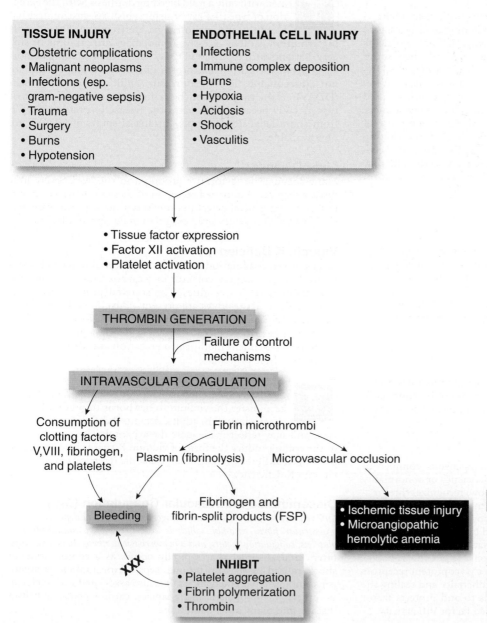

FIGURE 20-10. The pathophysiology of disseminated intravascular coagulation (DIC). The DIC syndrome is precipitated by tissue injury, endothelial cell injury, or a combination of the two. These injuries trigger increased expression of tissue factor on cell surfaces and activation of clotting factors (including XII and V) and platelets. With the failure of normal control mechanisms, generation of thrombin leads to intravascular coagulation.

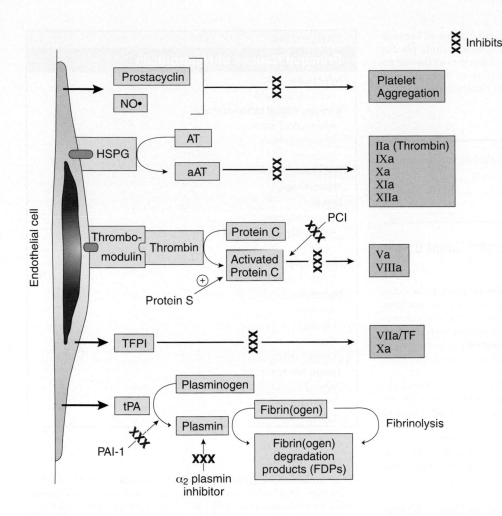

FIGURE 20-11. The role of endothelium in anticoagulation, platelet inhibition, and thrombolysis. The endothelial cell plays a central role in the inhibition of various components of the clotting mechanism. Heparan sulfate proteoglycan potentiates the activation of antithrombin (AT) 15-fold. Thrombomodulin stimulates the activation of protein C by thrombin 30-fold. NO, nitric oxide; HSPG, heparan sulfate proteoglycan; PCI, protein C inhibitor; tPA, tissue plasminogen activator; PAI-I, plasminogen activator inhibitor-I. *Arrows,* products secreted by the endothelial cell; *bars,* molecules bound to the cell surface; **+**, potentiation; XXX, inhibition.

 CLINICAL FEATURES: The symptoms of DIC reflect both microvascular thrombosis and a bleeding tendency. Ischemic changes in the brain lead to seizures and coma. Depending on the severity of DIC, renal symptoms range from mild azotemia to fulminant acute renal failure. The bleeding diathesis is evidenced by cerebral hemorrhage, ecchymoses, and hematuria. Patients with DIC are treated with (1) heparin anticoagulation to interrupt the cycle of intravascular coagulation and (2) replacement of platelets and clotting factors to control the bleeding.

Hypercoagulability May Cause Widespread Thrombosis

Hypercoagulability is defined as an increased risk of thrombosis in circumstances that would not cause thrombosis in a healthy person. The disorder may be inherited or acquired. Disorders that enhance thrombosis have also been considered elsewhere (Chapters 7, 10, and 11).

Inherited Hypercoagulability

Inherited hypercoagulable states are due to genetic mutations that affect one of the natural anticoagulant mechanisms. The hereditary tendency to develop thrombosis, regardless of its origin, is referred to as **thrombophilia**.

- **Activated protein C resistance—factor V Leiden:** A point mutation in the *factor V* gene (factor V Leiden) renders it resistant to proteolysis by activated protein C. *Resistance to activated protein C action is the most common genetic disorder associated with hypercoagulability, and its prevalence in patients with venous thrombosis*

has been reported to be as high as 65%. In the United States, the frequency of the factor V Leiden mutation is highest in whites (5%) and much less so in blacks (1%) and Asians (0.5%). Compared with healthy persons, the risk for deep venous thrombosis is increased sevenfold in heterozygotes and 80-fold in homozygotes.

- **Antithrombin deficiency:** This autosomal dominant disorder, which has incomplete penetrance, occurs in 0.2% to 0.4% of the general population and can result in either a quantitative or a qualitative effect on antithrombin. The risk of a thrombotic event (usually venous) ranges between 20% and 80% in different families.
- **Protein C and protein S deficiencies:** Homozygous protein C deficiency causes life-threatening neonatal thrombosis with **purpura fulminans**. Up to 0.5% of the general population has heterozygous protein C deficiency, but many of these persons are symptom free.

Acquired Hypercoagulability

Venous stasis contributes to the hypercoagulability associated with prolonged immobilization and congestive cardiac failure. Increased platelet activation probably accounts for the clotting tendency in patients with myeloproliferative disorders, heparin-induced thrombocytopenia, and TTP.

Antiphospholipid Antibody Syndrome

Antibodies directed against several negatively charged phospholipids are associated with the development of antiphospholipid antibody syndrome. This disorder features (1) thromboembolic events, (2) spontaneous abortions, and (3) thrombocytopenia. The antiphospholipid antibody syndrome is the leading acquired hematologic cause of thrombosis. Proposed mechanisms include platelet activation, endothelial cell activation, and alterations in the coagulation factor assembly on membranes. Interference with placental vascular function is the likely mechanism in recurrent fetal loss.

WHITE BLOOD CELLS

The reader is referred to Chapters 2 through 4 for discussions of white blood cell structure and function.

Nonmalignant Disorders

Neutropenia is an Absolute Neutrophil Count Below 1,800/μL

In most patients with neutropenia (**granulocytopenia**), the number of neutrophils is adequate to defend against microorganisms. When the number declines to 1,000/μL, patients become vulnerable to microbial infections, and serious risk ensues with absolute counts below 500/μL. The term **agranulocytosis** denotes virtual absence of neutrophils, caused by depletion of both the marginated pool and the bone marrow reserve.

Neutropenia reflects decreased production or increased destruction of neutrophils (Table 20-3). Most cases of neutropenia are asymptomatic and unexplained, and the term **chronic benign neutropenia** is used. In some cases, the total granulocyte pool is normal, but excessive neutrophils are stored in the marrow or marginated in blood vessels. Radiation or chemotherapeutic drugs interfere with the generation of neutrophils by suppressing marrow cell production.

Neutrophilia is an Absolute Neutrophil Count Above 7,000/μL

Neutrophilia has many causes (Table 20-4) and reflects (1) **increased mobilization** of neutrophils from bone marrow storage, (2) **enhanced release** from the peripheral blood marginal pool, or

TABLE 20-3
Principal Causes of Neutropenia
Decreased Production
Irradiation
Drug-induced (long- and short-term)
Viral infections
Congenital
Cyclic
Ineffective Production
Megaloblastic anemia
Myelodysplastic syndromes
Increased Destruction
Isoimmune neonatal
Autoimmune
Idiopathic
Drug-induced
Felty's syndrome
Systemic lupus erythematosus
Dialysis (induced by complement activation)
Splenic sequestration
Increased margination

TABLE 20-4
Principal Causes of Neutrophilia
Infections
Primarily bacterial
Immunological Inflammatory
Rheumatoid arthritis
Rheumatic fever
Vasculitis
Neoplasia
Hemorrhage
Drugs
Glucocorticoids
Colony-stimulating factors
Lithium
Hereditary
CD18 deficiency
Metabolic
Acidosis
Uremia
Gout
Thyroid storm
Tissue Necrosis
Infarction
Trauma
Burns

(3) **stimulation of granulopoiesis** in the bone marrow. In acute infections, neutrophilia may be so pronounced that it may be mistaken for leukemia, especially chronic myeloid leukemia (CML), in which case it is termed a **leukemoid reaction**.

Qualitative Disorders of Neutrophils are Associated with Impaired Function

If granulocyte function is impaired, resistance to infection may decrease despite a normal granulocyte count. A number of rare hereditary disorders of granulocytes have been described earlier (see Chapter 2), including chronic granulomatous disease, myeloperoxidase deficiency, and Chédiak-Higashi syndrome. The last is a rare autosomal recessive disease that is characterized by abnormal giant lysosomes in leukocytes and numerous other cells. Patients with Chédiak-Higashi syndrome suffer recurrent bacterial and fungal infections.

Langerhans Cell Histiocytosis is a Proliferative Disorder of Langerhans Cells

Langerhans cell histiocytosis (LCH) is a spectrum of uncommon clonal proliferations of Langerhans cells. The diseases range from asymptomatic involvement at a single site, such as bone or lymph nodes, to an aggressive, systemic, multiorgan disorder. Langerhans cells are mononuclear phagocytes derived from precursor cells in the bone marrow. They are found in the epidermis, lymph nodes, spleen, thymus, and mucosal tissues. Langerhans cells ingest, process and present antigens to T lymphocytes. In lymph nodes, Langerhans cells are termed **interdigitating reticulum cells**.

The etiology and pathogenesis of LCH are unknown. The disease may represent an atypical immunologic reaction, an unusual manifestation of an autoimmune disorder, or based on the clonal nature of the proliferation, a neoplastic disease. Infants, children, and young adults are most affected. The extent of disease and rate of progression correlate inversely with the age at presentation. Different presentations of LCH include the following:

- **Eosinophilic granuloma** is a localized, usually self-limited, disorder of older children (5 to 10 years old) and young adults (under 30 years). It accounts for almost 75% of all cases of LCH and afflicts males four times as frequently as females. The bones and lungs are the principal sites affected.
- **Hand-Schüller-Christian disease** is a multifocal and typically indolent disorder, usually in children 2 to 5 years of age, which represents about one fourth of all cases of LCH. Boys and girls are affected equally. Bony lesions tend to predominate, although involvement of endocrine glands may be prominent.
- **Letterer-Siwe disease** is a rare (less than 10% of cases), acute, disseminated variant of LCH in infants and children under 2 years of age. There is no gender predominance. Skin lesions and involvement of visceral organs and the hematopoietic system are characteristic.

 PATHOLOGY: Despite their clinical heterogeneity, LCHs share common histopathological findings. The cells that accumulate are large (15 to 25 μm in diameter), with round-to-indented nuclei, delicate vesicular chromatin, and small nucleoli. Electron microscopy discloses a distinctive rod-shaped or tubular cytoplasmic inclusion, with a dense core and a double outer sheath, termed the **Birbeck granule**. Frequently, one end of the granule is bulbous, in which case it resembles a tennis racket.

 CLINICAL FEATURES: The clinical manifestations of LCH reflect the sites involved. Skin involvement, principally in the Letterer-Siwe variant, takes the form of seborrheic or eczematoid dermatitis, most prominent on the scalp, face, and trunk. Otitis media is common. Painless localized or generalized lymphadenopathy and hepatosplenomegaly are frequent. Lytic lesions of bone cause pain or tenderness on palpation. Proptosis (protrusion of the eyeball) may be a complication of infiltration of the orbit. Diabetes insipidus occurs when the hypothalamic–pituitary axis is affected. *The classic triad of diabetes insipidus, proptosis, and defects in membranous bones occurs in only 15% of cases of Hand-Schüller-Christian disease.* The prognosis in LCH depends mainly on age at presentation. In general, the disorder is self-limited and benign in older persons (eosinophilic granuloma), whereas children younger than 2 years of age (Letterer-Siwe disease) tend to do poorly. The clinical course is rarely aggressive and indistinguishable from that of a malignant neoplasm.

Leukemias and Myelodysplastic Syndromes

*Malignant leukocytes originate from either myeloid cells or lymphoid cells. Malignant proliferations of myeloid cells are derived from bone marrow cells and manifest as **myelodysplastic syndromes, chronic myeloproliferative diseases, or acute myelogenous leukemias**. By contrast, malignant lymphocytes can arise in any compartment that contains lymphoid cells.*

Chronic Myeloproliferative Diseases are Clonal Stem Cell Disorders

Chronic myeloproliferative diseases involve increased proliferation of one or more myeloid lineages (granulocytes, erythrocytes, or megakaryocytes). Four types are usually distinguished: **chronic myelogenous leukemia, polycythemia vera, chronic idiopathic myelofibrosis, and essential thrombocythemia** (Table 20-5).

Chronic Myelogenous Leukemia (CML)

CML is derived from an abnormal pluripotent bone marrow stem cell and results in prominent neutrophilic leukocytosis over the full range of myeloid maturation. The presence of the **Philadelphia chromosome**, or molecular demonstration of the **BCR/ABL** *fusion gene*, is required to establish the diagnosis. CML is the most common myeloproliferative disease and accounts for 15% to 20% of all cases of leukemia.

 PATHOGENESIS: The cause in most cases of CML is unknown. Radiation exposure and myelotoxic agents such as benzene have been implicated in a small number of cases. Leukemic cells represent transformed pluripotent stem cells with predominantly granulocytic differentiation. In 95% of CML cases, the Philadelphia chromosome, which results from a t(9:22)(q34:q11) translocation, can be demonstrated by conventional cytogenetics and fluorescence in situ hybridization (Fig. 20-12). The *BCR* (break point cluster region) gene on chromosome 22 is fused to the *ABL* gene on chromosome 9. *The* BCR/ABL *gene encodes a fusion protein, p210, which is a constitutively activated tyrosine kinase.* A small number of cases involve additional chromosomal abnormalities.

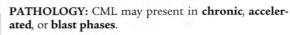

 PATHOLOGY: CML may present in **chronic, accelerated**, or **blast phases**.

- **Chronic phase of CML** features conspicuous leukocytosis, consisting mainly of maturing neutrophils. By definition, blasts are less than 10% of circulating leukocytes. Bone marrow biopsy shows hypercellularity, with total effacement of the marrow space by predominantly myeloid cells and their precursors (Fig. 20-13).
- **Accelerated phase of CML** often follows the chronic phase and may be associated with (1) 10% to 20% blasts in the blood or bone marrow, (2) more than 20% blood basophils, (3) persistent thrombocytopenia or thrombocytosis unresponsive to therapy, (4) splenomegaly, (5) increasing white blood cell count unresponsive to therapy, and (6) additional chromosomal abnormalities.
- **Blast phase of CML** is the ultimate outcome and features (1) at least 20% blasts in the bone marrow, (2) extramedullary proliferation of blasts (skin, lymph nodes, spleen, bone, brain), and (3) clusters of blasts in the bone marrow biopsy. Blast phase heralds a poor prognosis. In most cases (70%), the leukemic cells in the blast phase exhibit morphology and immunophenotype of myeloid lineage; in 30%, they resemble lymphoblasts, usually with a B-cell precursor immunophenotype.

 CLINICAL FEATURES: The peak incidence of CML is in the fifth and sixth decades of life, with a slight male predominance. Patients report fatigue, anorexia, weight loss, and vague abdominal discomfort due to hepatosplenomegaly. Peripheral granulocytes are markedly increased with a full maturation range. Clinical deterioration often heralds the blast phase.

CML is a paradigm for a malignancy with a well-defined cytogenetic abnormality that can be targeted by specific drug therapy. The drug imatinib blocks the ATP-binding site on the *BCR/ABL* tyrosine kinase, thereby inactivating it. A high level of sustained remissions has been achieved with imatinib, but up to 20% of patients eventually develop resistance. The newly introduced inhibitor dastinib is highly effective in such patients. Allogeneic bone marrow transplantation is also used with curative intent in patients with CML.

Polycythemia Vera (PV)

PV is a myeloproliferative disease that arises from a clonal hematopoietic stem cell and results in uncontrolled production of RBCs. The increase in

TABLE 20-5

Chronic Myeloproliferative Syndromes

	Chronic Myelogenous Leukemia	Polycythemia Vera	Chronic Idiopathic Myelofibrosis	Essential Thrombocythemia
Clinical Features				
Peak age range (years)	25–60	40–60	50–70	50–70
Splenomegaly	90%	75%	100%	30% (slight)
Hepatomegaly	50%	40%	80%	40% (slight)
Acute leukemic conversion	80%	5%–10%	5%–10%	2%–5%
Median survival (years)	3–4	13	5	>10
Bone Marrow				
Histopathology	Panhyperplasia (predominantly granulocytic)	Panhyperplasia (predominantly erythroid)	Panhyperplasia with fibrosis	Large megakaryocytes in clusters
M:E ratio	10:1 to 50:1	≤2:1	2:1 to 5:1	2:1 to 5:1
Fibrosis	<10%	15%–20%	90%–100%	<5%
Laboratory Findings				
Hemoglobin	Mild anemia	>20 g/dL	Mild anemia	Mild anemia
RBC morphology	Slight aniso- and poikilocytosis	Slight aniso- and poikilocytosis	Immature erythrocytes and marked aniso- and poikilocytosis	Hypochromic microcytes
Granulocytes	Moderate to markedly increased with spectrum of maturation	Normal to mildly increased; may show a few immature forms	Normal to moderately increased; some immature WBC	Normal to slightly increased
Platelets	Normal to moderately increased	Normal to moderately increased	Increased to decreased	Markedly increased with abnormal forms
Genetics	Philadelphia chromosome: BCR/ABL gene rearrangement	JAK2 activating mutation	JAK2 activating mutation	JAK2 activating mutation

M:E ratio, ratio of myeloid-to-erythroid.

erythrocytes in PV is autonomous and is not regulated by EPO serum levels, which are not elevated in the disease.

 PATHOGENESIS: PV derives from the malignant transformation of a single hematopoietic stem cell with primary commitment to the erythroid lineage. Proliferation of the neoplastic clone occurs mainly in the bone marrow but may involve such extramedullary sites as the spleen, lymph nodes, and liver (**myeloid metaplasia**).

No specific recurrent genetic defect has been identified in PV, although some cytogenetic abnormalities have been described. However, in bcr/abl-negative myeloproliferative diseases, including PV, essential thrombocythemia, and myelofibrosis, recent studies show an activating mutation in cytoplasmic Janus kinase 2 (JAK2; V617F), which has tyrosine kinase activity.

 PATHOLOGY: *The bone marrow in PV is hypercellular, with hyperplasia of all elements* (see Table 20-5). Unlike CML, erythroid precursor cells predominate, and the myeloid-to-erythroid ratio is less than 2:1. Erythroid

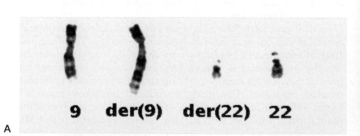

A

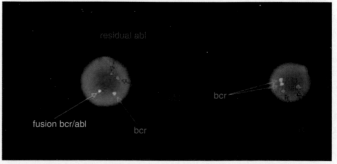

B

FIGURE 20-12. Chronic myelogenous leukemia. **A.** The Philadelphia chromosome der(22) is shown. **B.** Fluorescence in situ hybridization (FISH) in a patient with t(9;22) (Philadelphia chromosome)-positive chronic myeloid leukemia. A normal cell contains two separate bcr (chromosome 22) and abl (chromosome 9) genes (*right*). A leukemic cell with a fusion bcr/abl signal, residual abl signal, and two normal abl and bcr signals derived from normal chromosomes 9 and 22, respectively (*left*).

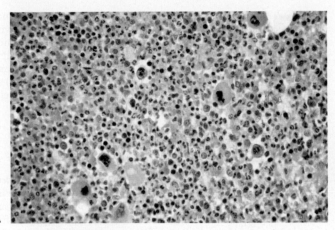
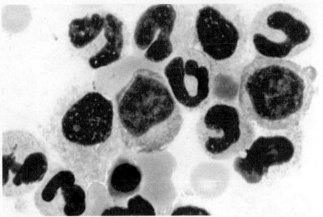

FIGURE 20-13. **Chronic myelogenous leukemia. A.** The bone marrow is conspicuously hypercellular, due to an increase in granulocyte precursors, mature granulocytes, and megakaryocytes. **B.** A smear of the bone marrow aspirate from the same patient reveals numerous granulocytes at various stages of development.

maturation is normal (normoblastic). The granulocyte series also shows normal maturation. Megakary-ocytes are typically increased in number and size and tend to cluster. The spleen is characteristically enlarged, with prominent accumulation of erythrocytes in the red pulp cords and sinuses. Myeloid metaplasia is common in the liver, lymph nodes, and spleen.

The peripheral blood smear reveals normal erythrocytes, although hypochromia and microcytosis are seen if there is iron deficiency. Iron deficiency anemia is common in PV, largely because storage iron is diverted to the increased red cell mass. Hyperuricemia and secondary gout may be present and are related to rapid cell turnover.

 CLINICAL FEATURES: In North America, 8 to 10 cases of PV per million are seen annually. The mean age at diagnosis is 60 years. The onset tends to be insidious, and symptoms are generally nonspecific, typically relating to the increased erythrocyte mass. Plethora (engorgement of vessels with cells) and splenomegaly are early findings. Headache, dizziness, and visual problems result from vascular disturbances in the brain and retina. Angina pectoris, secondary to slowing of coronary artery blood flow, and intermittent claudication caused by sluggish peripheral blood flow in the lower extremities may be observed. Major thrombotic complications occur in one third of cases, including stroke and myocardial infarction.

The clinical course of PV tends to proceed as a series of phases. The **proliferative phase** features erythroid proliferation and an increased erythrocyte mass. In one third of patients, the disease progresses to other stages. In 10% of cases of polycythemia overall, excessive proliferation of erythroid cells ceases, resulting in stable or decreased erythrocyte mass (**spent phase**). Another 10% of cases progress to myelofibrosis (**polycythemic myelofibrosis with myeloid metaplasia**, see below). **Acute myelogenous leukemia** eventually occurs in 5% to 10% of cases of PV.

The median survival rate of a patient with PV is 13 years. Specific causes of death related to the disease itself include thrombosis, hemorrhage, and acute myelogenous leukemia. Therapeutic reduction of erythrocyte mass by repeated phlebotomy or chemotherapy is effective management in most cases.

Chronic Idiopathic Myelofibrosis

Chronic idiopathic myelofibrosis is a clonal myeloproliferative disease in which marrow fibrosis is accompanied by prominent megakaryopoiesis and granulopoiesis.

 PATHOGENESIS: As in other types of myeloproliferative disease, exposure to benzene or radiation has occasionally been implicated in chronic idiopathic myelofibrosis. The malignant megakaryocytes produce PDGF and TGF-β, both of which are powerful fibroblast mitogens. Ultimately, the entire marrow space is displaced by connective tissue, although fibroblasts are not part of the clonal stem cell disorder. No genetic defect has been identified.

 PATHOLOGY: Most patients are diagnosed at the fibrotic stage, but 25% are first detected in a cellular phase. The **prefibrotic, cellular stage** features a hypercellular bone marrow, with predominant neutrophilic and megakaryocytic proliferation. The megakaryocytes are clustered and atypically lobated. In the **fibrotic stage**, the blood shows either leukopenia or marked leukocytosis, and myeloid precursors and nucleated RBCs (leukoerythroblastosis) are usually present. The red cells exhibit poikilocytosis and teardrop forms (Fig. 20-14A). Conspicuous fibrosis in the marrow defines this stage (see Fig. 20-14B). As in the cellular phase, many atypical megakaryocytes are present. Extramedullary hematopoiesis leads to splenomegaly, hepatomegaly, and lymphadenopathy, and may be seen in other organs (**myelofibrosis with myeloid metaplasia**).

 CLINICAL FEATURES: The annual incidence of idiopathic myelofibrosis is estimated at 0.5 to 1.5 per 100,000. It is a disease of the elderly, with a peak incidence in the seventh decade. One quarter of patients with idiopathic myelofibrosis are asymptomatic at diagnosis. Early clinical symptoms are nonspecific and include fatigue, low-grade fever, night sweats, and weight loss. Platelet function may be impaired, and patients display either increased platelet aggregation and thrombosis or decreased platelet aggregation with a bleeding diathesis. Transformation to acute myelogenous leukemia occurs in 15% of cases (see Table 20-5).

Essential Thrombocythemia

Essential thrombocythemia is an uncommon neoplastic disorder of hematopoietic stem cells, characterized by uncontrolled proliferation of megakaryocytes. A marked increase in circulating platelets ($>600,000/\mu L$) is accompanied by recurrent episodes of thrombosis and hemorrhage. The disease affects middle-aged persons, with a slight male predominance (see Table 20-5).

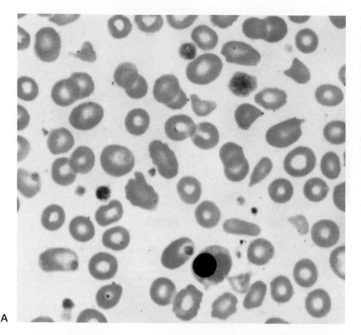

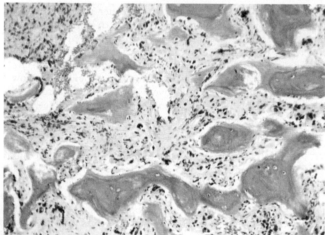

FIGURE 20-14. Chronic idiopathic myelofibrosis. **A.** Peripheral smear shows anisocytosis, poikilocytosis with teardrop forms, and nucleated erythrocytes. Giant platelets are also present. **B.** A section of bone marrow shows collagenous fibrosis, osteosclerosis, and numerous abnormal megakaryocytes.

 PATHOGENESIS: Essential thrombocythemia is a clonal disorder believed to derive from malignant transformation of a single hematopoietic stem cell with principal, but not exclusive, commitment to megakaryocytic lineage. The disease features marked proliferation of megakaryocytes, with up to a 15-fold or greater increase in platelet production. Chromosomal abnormalities are identified in fewer than 25% of patients.

 PATHOLOGY: Abnormalities of platelet function are common in primary thrombocythemia. Recurrent episodes of thrombosis in arteries or veins are attributed to severe thrombocytosis, and hemorrhage reflects defects in platelet function. The bone marrow is markedly hypercellular, with decreased fat cells and increased megakaryocytes, which form cohesive clusters or sheets. Reticulin fibers in the marrow are increased in one third of cases, but overt fibrosis is rare. Iron stores are normal or low.

 CLINICAL FEATURES: The clinical course of primary thrombocythemia is protracted, with a median survival rate of more than 10 years. In untreated cases, thrombosis of large arteries and veins is common, especially in the legs, heart, intestine, and kidneys. Hemorrhage is usually mild and not life-threatening. Acute myelogenous leukemia (AML) supervenes in up to 5% of cases. The disease is treated with platelet-pheresis and myelosuppressive chemotherapy.

Myelodysplastic Syndromes (MDS) are Clonal Disorders that Cause Ineffective Hematopoiesis

Dysplastic morphology in one or more hematopoietic lineages is characteristic of MDS. The disease is most common in the elderly. There is a discrepancy between the paucity of peripheral blood elements and the marked hyperplasia seen in the bone marrow, owing to ineffective hematopoiesis and increased apoptosis in the marrow. The classification of subtypes of MDS is complex and beyond the scope of this chapter. However, all types manifest refractory anemia or other cytopenias. Because MDS frequently converts to AML, it is also referred to as **preleukemic syndrome**.

Acute Myelogenous Leukemia (AML) is a Clonal Proliferation of Myeloblasts in the Marrow with Their Subsequent Appearance in Blood and Tissues

According to the World Health Organization (WHO) classification, a diagnosis of AML requires more than 20% myeloblasts in the bone marrow. Of all acute leukemias, 70% are myeloid leukemias. The rest are lymphoblastic leukemias (discussed below under lymphoid malignancies). AML is most common in adults, with a median age of 60 years at onset.

 PATHOGENESIS: Most cases of AML are of unknown etiology, but in a few instances, a causal relationship between radiation, cytotoxic chemotherapy, or benzene exposure has been documented. For example, an increase in AML was noted after the detonation of atomic bombs in Hiroshima and Nagasaki (see Chapter 8). Cigarette smoking doubles the risk for AML.

PATHOLOGY: Malignant myeloblasts of AML are detectable in the bone marrow and, in most instances, in the blood. Typically, the malignant cells pack the bone marrow and displace normal hematopoietic cells (Fig. 20-15). Myeloblasts are medium-sized to large cells with round or slightly irregular nuclei. Depending on the AML subtype, Auer rods may be present in the cytoplasm (Fig. 20-16). These inclusions are specific for the myeloid lineage and preclude a diagnosis of lymphoblastic leukemia.

Immunophenotyping by flow cytometry and cytogenetic studies is essential for correct classification of AML. Myeloid antigens frequently expressed include CD13, CD15, CD33, CD34, and CD117. AML with megakaryoblastic differentiation may show the platelet/megakaryocyte markers CD41 and CD61 (platelet GPIIb/IIIa complex). Important cytochemical markers include myeloperoxidase, Sudan black, and nonspecific esterase. Myeloperoxidase and Sudan black stain myeloid cells and their precursors with increased intensity in more mature forms. Nonspecific esterase labels monoblasts and promonocytes and is a marker for AML with monocytoid differentiation.

CLINICAL FEATURES: *The major problems associated with AML reflect the progressive accumulation in the marrow of immature myeloid cells that lack the potential for further differentiation and maturation, resulting in granulocytopenia, thrombocytopenia, and anemia.* Although leukemic myeloblasts replicate at a slower rate than do normal hematopoietic precur-

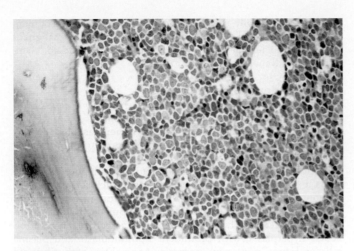

FIGURE 20-15. **Acute myelogenous leukemia.** A bone marrow section is hypercellular, due to effacement of the normal architecture by myeloblasts.

sor cells, the frequency of spontaneous cell death is also less than normal. The expanded pool of abnormal leukemic blasts encroaches on the marrow and suppresses normal hematopoiesis. Infections, particularly with opportunistic organisms (e.g., fungi), are common, as are cutaneous bleeding (petechiae and ecchymoses) and serosal hemorrhages over the viscera. Untreated AML carries a dismal prognosis. Chemotherapy leads to remission in more than 50% of patients, but the overall 5-year survival rate is less than 30%. Bone marrow transplantation is a common mode of treatment for high-risk forms of AML and for AML in relapse. The subclassification of AML is complex and of clinical and therapeutic importance but is beyond the scope of this text and presented only in summary. The current classification scheme is based on the WHO system and divides AML into four major subgroups (see Table 20-6). The French American British classification scheme has been subsumed into this system as **acute myeloid leukemia not otherwise classified**. Selected AML subtypes are considered:

ACUTE PROMYELOCYTIC LEUKEMIA (APL): Cate-gorized under "acute leukemia with recurrent genetic abnormalities," APL is defined by a chromosomal translocation involving the

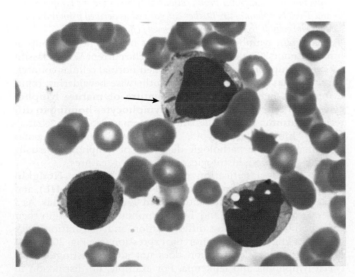

FIGURE 20-16. **Acute promyelocytic leukemia.** Auer rods are prominent (*arrow*).

TABLE 20-6

WHO Classification of AML

AML With Recurrent Genetic Abnormalities

AML with t(8;21)(q22;q22);(AML1/ETO)

AML with abnormal bone marrow eosinophils inv(16)(p13q22) or t(16;16)(p13;q22);(CBFβ/MY<H1>1)

Acute promyelocytic leukemia (AML with t(15;17)(q22;q12)(PML/RARα) and variants (M3)

AML with 11q23 (MLL) abnormalities

Acute Myelogenous Leukemia With Multilineage Dysplasia

Following a myelodysplastic syndrome or myelodysplastic syndrome/myeloproliferative disorder

Without antecedent myelodysplastic syndrome

Acute Myelogenous Leukemia and Myelodysplastic Syndromes, Therapy-Related

Alkylating agent—related

Topoisomerase type II inhibitor—related (some may be lymphoid)

Other types

Acute Myelogenous Leukemia Not Otherwise Categorized

AML minimally differentiated (M0)

AML without maturation (M1)

AML with maturation (M2)

AML (M4)

Acute monoblastic and monocytic leukemia (M5)

Acute erythroid leukemia (M6)

Acute megakaryoblastic leukemia (M7)

AML, acute myelogenous leukemia; MLL, myelomonocytic leukemia; PML, promyelocytic leukemia; RAR, retinoic acid receptor; WHO, World Health Organization.

PML1 gene and the retinoic acid receptor (RAR) gene, accounting for 5% to 10% of all cases of AML. APL is a paradigm for a molecularly defined disease in which the underlying genetic defect determines the type of treatment. The genetic abnormality in APL is a translocation involving the *PML* gene on chromosome 15 and the *RARα* gene on chromosome 17. The resulting *PML/RARα* fusion gene encodes a functional RAR. The receptor can be targeted by all-*trans*-retinoic acid, which mediates maturation of the tumor cells and is employed in the therapy of the disease.

THERAPY-INDUCED AML AND MYELODYSPLASTIC SYNDROMES: Treatment of solid tumors with chemotherapy or radiation therapy can induce later secondary malignancies, most commonly MDS and AML.

DISORDERS OF THE LYMPHOPOIETIC SYSTEM

Benign Disorders of the Lymphopoietic System

Lymphocytosis Denotes an Elevated Peripheral Blood Lymphocyte Count

The upper limits of normal for lymphocytes are 4,000/μL in adults, 7,000/μL in children, and 9,000/μL in infants. The principal causes of absolute peripheral blood lymphocytosis are (1) acute infections (infectious mononucleosis, whooping cough), (2) chronic bacterial infections (tuberculosis, brucellosis), and (3) lymphoproliferative diseases.

In addition to lymphocytosis, **variant lymphocytes** are a hallmark of viral infections, particularly infectious mononucleosis and some immunologic disorders, such as drug reactions and serum sickness. Most such cells are of the T-cell lineage (CD8+ cytotoxic/suppressor cells).

Lymphocytopenia Usually Reflects a Decrease in T-Helper Lymphocytes

Peripheral blood lymphocytopenia is defined as a decrease in blood lymphocytes to less than 1,500/μL in adults or less than 3,000/μL in children. Because the predominant lymphocytes in the blood are T-helper-inducer (CD4+) lymphocytes, lymphocytopenia generally indicates that these cells are decreased. Decreased production of lymphocytes as is seen in (1) congenital and acquired immunodeficiency syndromes, (2) increased destruction of lymphocytes (which may be drug or virally induced), and (3) loss of lymphocytes is most commonly associated with diseases that damage intestinal lymphatics.

Reactive Hyperplasia of Lymph Nodes is a Response to Infections, Inflammation, or Tumors

Lymph nodes may exhibit hyperplasia of all cellular components or any combination of B lymphocytes, T lymphocytes, and mononuclear phagocytic cells in response to a variety of infectious, inflammatory, and neoplastic disorders (Fig. 20-17).

The histopathology and degree of lymph node enlargement in reactive hyperplasias reflect (1) the patient's age (children tend to exhibit more pronounced immunoreactivity than adults), (2) the host's immunologic competence, and (3) the type of infectious agent or inflammatory disorder.

Acute suppurative or necrotizing lymphadenitis occurs in lymph nodes that drain a site of acute bacterial infection. Suppurative lymph nodes enlarge rapidly because of edema and hyperemia and are tender, due to distention of the capsule. Microscopically, infiltration of lymph node sinuses and stroma by polymorphonuclear leukocytes and prominent follicular hyperplasia are noted. The anatomical site of lymphadenopathy often provides a clue as to its cause, because the affected nodes are likely to drain the locus of infection. Generalized lymphadenopathy may occur in systemic infections, hyperthyroidism, drug reactions, and collagen vascular diseases.

Follicular Hyperplasia
Hyperplasia of secondary follicles (germinal centers) and plasmacytosis of medullary cords indicate B-lymphocyte immunoreactivity.

In **nonspecific reactive follicular hyperplasia**, which is a benign condition, prominent hyperplastic follicles occur principally in the cortex of the lymph node (see Figs. 20-17 and 20-18). Follicles are round or irregular and may be confluent. The activated B cells in the follicles range from small cells with irregular, cleaved nuclei to large immunoblasts. Numerous mitotic figures reflect the rapid proliferation of activated B lymphocytes. Scattered benign macrophages, with abundant pale cytoplasm containing pyknotic nuclear and cytoplasmic debris, impart the characteristic "starry sky" pattern of benign follicles. A well-defined mantle of normal small B lymphocytes surrounds the follicles, sharply separating them from the interfollicular regions. The cause of nonspecific reactive follicular hyperplasia is frequently not known, although a viral, drug, or inflammatory etiology is often suspected. The clinical course features rapid and complete resolution of the lymphadenopathy.

Lymphadenopathy, either localized or generalized, is common in rheumatoid arthritis. Follicular hyperplasia is also encountered

in AIDS. Additionally, the lymph nodes in AIDS show loss of mantle zones and have a high incidence of superimposed malignant neoplasms, including diffuse B-cell lymphomas, Hodgkin lymphoma, and Kaposi sarcoma.

Interfollicular Hyperplasia
Hyperplasia of the deep cortex or paracortex (interfollicular or diffuse hyperplasia) is characteristic of T-lymphocyte immunoreactivity.

Reactive nonspecific interfollicular hyperplasia (see Fig. 20-17) is most commonly due to viral infections or to immunologic reactions. Although the precise cause is often not determined, the condition resolves promptly. Interfollicular lymph node hyperplasia is a common finding in viral diseases, including infectious mononucleosis, varicella-herpes zoster infection, measles, and cytomegalovirus lymphadenitis. **Systemic lupus erythematosus** is often associated with lymphadenopathy characterized by interfollicular hyperplasia, with prominent immunoblasts and plasma cells and focal-to-massive necrosis. Arteriolitis, with fibrinoid necrosis of vessel walls, is frequently observed.

Mixed Patterns of Reactive Hyperplasia of Lymph Nodes
Some infectious diseases are associated with mixed patterns of lymph node hyperplasia, in which several different features are prominent. For example, in **toxoplasmosis**, one sees prominent follicular hyperplasia and small collections of epithelioid macrophages in interfollicular regions (see Fig. 20-17).

Sinus Histiocytosis Represents an Increase in Macrophages
Sinus histiocytosis is an increase in tissue macrophages (histiocytes) of the subcapsular and trabecular sinuses of the lymph nodes (see Fig. 20-17). Sinus histiocytes are derived from blood monocytes. The condition is common in lymph nodes draining sites of cancer and, less often, inflammatory and infectious foci. The nature of the phagocytic debris in the cytoplasm of the macrophages helps identify the origin of the sinus histiocytosis. For example, anthracotic pigment is frequently seen in macrophages of mediastinal lymph nodes that exhibit sinus histocytosis. Macrophages containing erythrocytes and hemosiderin pigment occur with autoimmune hemolytic anemia.

Malignant Lymphomas

Lymphomas are malignant proliferations of lymphocytes or lymphoblasts. B- and T-cell lymphomas are further categorized as derived from immature (precursor) cells or from mature (peripheral) effector cells.

Malignant lymphomas are the most heterogeneous group of human tumors (Tables 20-7 and 20-8). The current WHO classification of lymphomas is based upon their normal cellular counterparts and has helped to clarify an otherwise bewildering topic. Lymphomas may represent (1) **immature or mature lymphocytes**, (2) **B cells or T cells**, and (3) **lymphocytes homing to different anatomic sites**. Malignant lymphomas also exhibit characteristic immunophenotypic, cytogenetic, and molecular abnormalities. The pathologic diagnosis of lymphomas usually depends on clinical, histologic, and molecular features.

The WHO classification distinguishes between **Hodgkin Lymphoma (HL)** and **non-Hodgkin lymphoma (non-HL)**, and the latter is further divided into **B- and T-cell lymphomas**. As a general principle, the B- and T-cell lymphomas derive from their corresponding cell during differentiation and maturation, with corresponding immunophenotypic expression (see Fig. 20-19 and Fig. 20-20). This classification does not always distinguish between lymphoma and leukemia. For example, no distinction in principle is made between chronic lymphocytic leukemia (CLL)

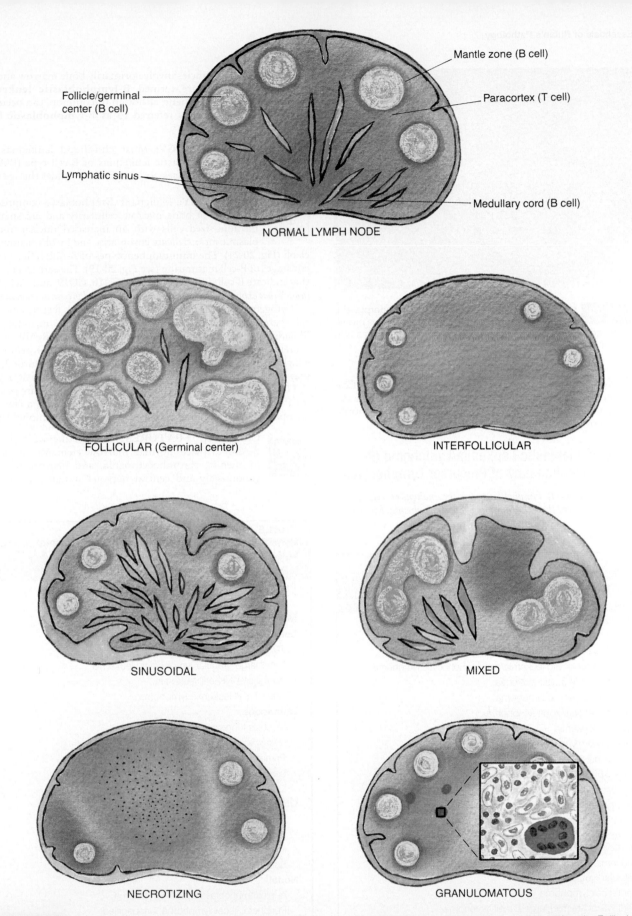

FIGURE 20-17. **Lymph nodes.** Patterns of benign reactive hyperplasia are contrasted with the structure of a normal lymphnode. Follicular hyperplasiawith prominent enlarged and irregular benign follicles, is characteristic of B cell immunoreactivity.Interfollicular hyperplasiais typical of T cell immunoreactivity. The sinusoidal patternwith expansion of sinuses by benignmacrophages is seen in reactive proliferations of the mononuclear–phagocyte system. Mixed patterns of follicular, interfollic-ular, and sinusoidal hyperplasia are common in a variety of complex immune reactions. In necrotizinglymphadenitis,variablenecrosis of the lymph node architecture with residual cell debris is present. In granulomatous inflammation,cohesive clustersof macrophages and occasional multinucleated giant cells are characteristic.

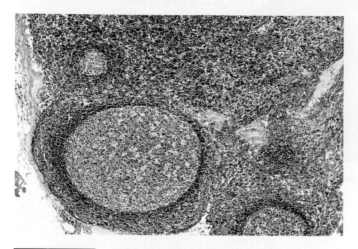

FIGURE 20-18. **Lymph node with reactive follicular hyperpla-sia.** A section of a hyperplastic lymph node shows prominent follicles (germinal centers) containing numerous macrophages with pale cytoplasm.

and small lymphocytic lymphoma (SLL). Although the classification of lymphocytic malignancies is clinically significant, the details are beyond the scope of this text. Hence, the following should be seen as an overview of a complex topic.

B-Acute Lymphoblastic Leukemia/Lymphoma (B-ALL/LBL) is a Malignancy of Precursor Lymphocytes

Immature (precursor) B lymphoblasts are the malignant cells in B-ALL/LBL and represent the most common childhood leukemia. Most pre-

cursor B-cell malignancies involve primarily bone marrow and peripheral blood and are termed **B-lymphoblastic leukemia**. However, nodal involvement, although uncommon, can occur, in which case the disease is referred to as **B-lymphoblastic lymphoma (LBL)**.

 EPIDEMIOLOGY: Most childhood leukemias are acute lymphoblastic leukemias of B-cell type (B-ALL). About 75% of cases occur in children under the age of 6.

 PATHOLOGY: Malignant lymphoblasts comprise at least 20% of bone marrow cellularity and are small to medium-sized cells with an increased nuclear-to-cytoplasmic ratio, delicate chromatin, and inconspicuous nucleoli (Fig. 20-21). The immunophenotypes of B-ALL reflect different stages of B-cell maturation (see Fig. 20-19). The earliest antigens that indicate B-cell differentiation are CD10, CD19, and TdT. *B-cell tumors that express cell surface Ig are not considered precursor leukemias.*

Cytogenetic abnormalities are involved. B-ALL features numerical aberrations and chromosomal translocations, including the Philadelphia chromosome. In childhood ALL, a BCR/ABL fusion protein, P190, is produced, in contrast to the fusion protein P210, which is seen in half of adult cases of ALL or CML. Progenitor B-ALL may present with the t(4;11) translocation involving the *MLL* gene at 11q23. About 25% of childhood pre—B-ALL patients are positive for the t(1;19) translocation, which involves *PBX/E2A*, a chimeric oncoprotein that serves to immortalize immature B lymphoblasts.

 CLINICAL FEATURES: The leukemic cells of B-ALL displace normal marrow elements, resulting in anemia, thrombocytopenia, and neutropenia. Organomegaly and central nervous system involvement

TABLE 20-7
WHO Histological Classification of B-Cell Neoplasms
Precursor B-Cell neoplasm
Precursor B-lymphoblastic leukemia/lymphoma
Mature B-Cell Neoplasms
Chronic lymphocytic leukemia/small lymphocytic lymphoma
B-cell prolymphocytic leukemia
Lymphoplasmacytic lymphoma
Splenic marginal zone lymphoma
Hairy cell leukemia
Plasma cell myeloma
Monoclonal gammopathy of undetermined significance
Solitary plasmacytoma of bone
Extraosseous plasmacytoma
Primary amyloidosis
Heavy-chain diseases
Extranodal marginal zone B-cell lymphoma of mucosa-associated lymphoid tissue (MALT lymphoma)
Nodal marginal zone B-cell lymphoma
Follicular lymphoma
Mantle cell lymphoma
Mediastinal (thymic) large B-cell lymphoma
Intravascular large B-cell lymphoma
Primary effusion lymphoma
Burkitt's lymphoma/leukemia

WHO, World Health Organization.

TABLE 20-8
WHO Histologic Classification of T-Cell and NK-Cell Neoplasms
Precursor T-Cell Neoplasm
Precursor T-lymphoblastic leukemia/lymphoma
Mature T-Cell Neoplasms
Leukemic/Disseminated
T-cell prolymphocytic leukemia
T-cell large granular lymphocytic leukemia
Aggressive NK-cell leukemia
Adult T-cell leukemia/lymphoma
Cutaneous
Mycosis fungoides
Sézary's syndrome
Primary cutaneous anaplastic lymphoma
Large cell lymphoma
Lymphomatoid papulosis
Other Extranodal
Extranodal NK-/T-cell lymphoma, nasal type
Enteropathy-type T-cell lymphoma
Hepatosplenic T-cell lymphoma
Subcutaneous panniculitis-like T-cell lymphoma
Nodal
Angioimmunoblastic T-cell lymphoma
Peripheral T-cell lymphoma, unspecified
Anaplastic large cell lymphoma
Neoplasm of Uncertain Lineage and Stage of Differentiation

NK, natural killer; WHO, World Health Organization.

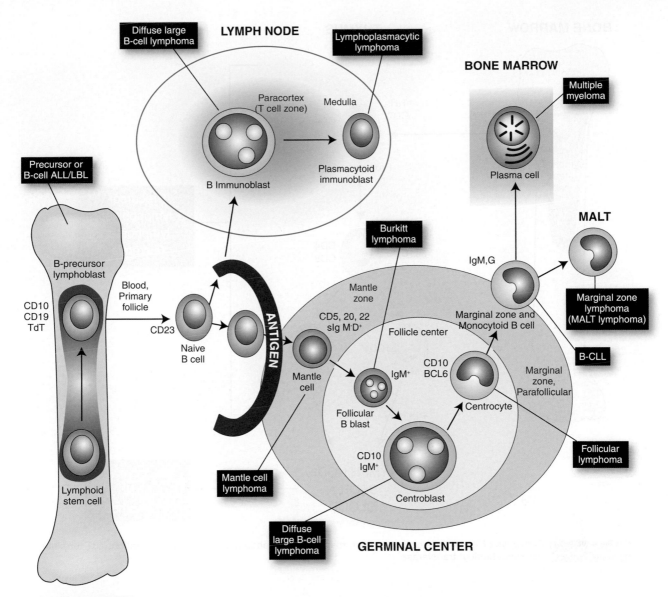

FIGURE 20-19. Pathway of B cell differentiation and corresponding B-cell lymphomas. Following the precursor status, B cells ma-ture into naive B lymphocytes. The germinal-center response represents an important turntable for immunoglobulin variable region gene mutations,Ig heavy-chain switch, and differentiation into plasma cells and memory cells. Cluster designation (CD) markers are shown. B immunoblasts andplasmacytoid immunoblasts reside in the T-cell-rich paracortex and medulla, respectively. Marginal zone B cells home to mucosa-associated lym-phoid tissue (MALT) sites and bone marrow. Neoplastic transformation occurs at all phases of B-cell differentiation. ALL/LBL acute lymphoblas-tic leukemia/lymphoma; B-CLLB-cell chronic lymphocytic leukemia; Ig immunoglobulin.

are common. The rapidly growing tumor cells in the marrow cause bone pain and arthralgias. In general, childhood B-ALL treated with chemotherapy has an excellent prognosis, with complete remission rates of better than 90%. However, age younger than 1 year or older than 12 years, several translocations, t(9;22), t(1;19), t(4;11), and any involving the MLL locus, indicate a poor prognosis.

Precursor T Cells Compose Most Lymphoblastic Lymphomas

Precursor T-acute lymphoblastic leukemia (T-ALL) and T-lymphoblastic lymphoma (T- LBL) are immature T-cell neoplasms. Whether the terms **leukemia** or **lymphoma** apply is often arbitrary, and the considerations are similar to those described for B-ALL.

 EPIDEMIOLOGY: Only 15% of childhood ALL originates from T cells. In adults, the percentage of T-lymphoblastic leukemia is higher. Lymphoblastic lymphoma, a tumor mass consisting of precursor lymphocytes, is 90% of T-cell origin.

 PATHOLOGY: The morphologic appearance of T lymphoblasts is like that of B lymphoblasts (see Fig. 20-21). Expression of antigens in T-ALL reflects normal T-cell differentiation and maturation in the bone marrow and thymus. The immunophenotypes in T-ALL reflect that sequence of antigen expression. As with B-ALL, T-ALL is positive for TdT (see Fig. 20-20). The genes encoding the four T-cell receptor chains (α, β, γ, δ chains) frequently participate in chromosomal translocations with transcription factor genes, often resulting in disturbed transcription regulation.

BONE MARROW   **THYMUS**

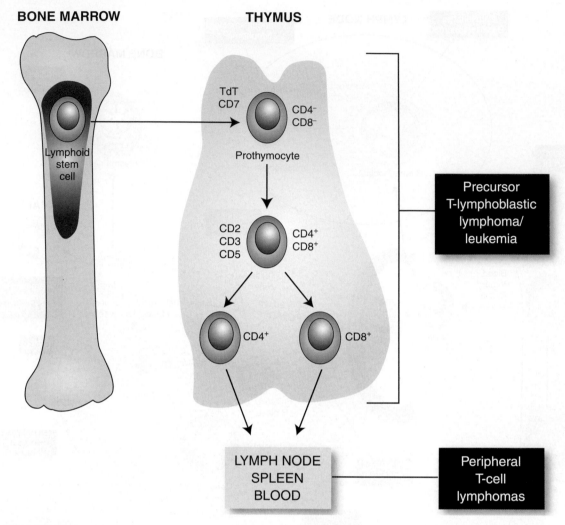

FIGURE 20-20. Pathways of T-cell development and corresponding lymphomas. CD cluster designation; TdT terminal deoxynucleotidyl transferase.

 CLINICAL FEATURES: Blood and bone marrow are most commonly involved in T-ALL. The leukemia frequently infiltrates peripheral lymph nodes, the brain, gonads, spleen, and liver. Precursor T-cell malignancies

that originate from thymic T cells most often present as a mediastinal mass. Like B-ALL, T-ALL has a poor prognosis after childhood.

Mature (Peripheral) B-Cell Lymphomas are the Most Common Type in the Western World

Mature B-cell malignancies are derived from the clonal proliferation of peripheral B cells. As B cells go through multiple steps of differentiation and maturation, from naïve B cells to mature plasma cells, lymphomas may arise at every step of the way (see Fig. 20-19).

 EPIDEMIOLOGY: The incidence of lymphomas in the United States is 15 per 100,000 annually. B-cell neoplasms by far outnumber T-cell malignancies, particularly in the Western world. *The most common B-cell lymphomas are follicular lymphoma (22.1%) and diffuse large cell lymphoma (30.6%)* (Table 20-9). Except for mediastinal B-cell and BL, most mature B-cell lymphomas occur in the sixth and seventh decades. Peripheral B-cell lymphomas are distinctly uncommon in children except for Burkitt lymphoma (BL) and large cell B-cell lymphoma.

 PATHOGENESIS: Most peripheral B-cell lymphomas occur without apparent cause. However, impairment of the immune system and certain infectious agents may give rise to malignant lymphomas.

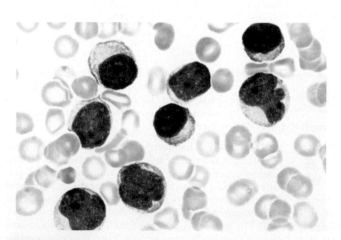

FIGURE 20-21. **Acute lymphoblastic leukemia.** The lymphoblasts in peripheral blood contain irregular and indented nuclei with prominent nucleoli and a moderate amount of cytoplasm.

TABLE 20-9

Frequency of B- and T-/NK-Cell Lymphomas

Diagnosis	Total Cases (%)
Diffuse large B-cell lymphoma	30.6
Follicular lymphoma	22.1
MALT lymphoma	7.6
Mature T-cell lymphomas (except ALCL)	7.6
Chronic lymphocytic leukemia/small lymphocytic lymphoma	6.7
Mantle cell lymphoma	6.0
Mediastinal large B-cell lymphoma	2.4
Anaplastic large cell lymphoma	2.4
Burkitt's lymphoma	2.5
Nodal marginal zone lymphoma	1.8
Precursor T-lymphoblastic lymphoma	1.7
Lymphoplasmacytic lymphoma	1.2
Other types	7.4

ALCL, anaplastic large cell lymphoma; MALT, mucosa-associated lymphoid tissue; NK, natural killer.

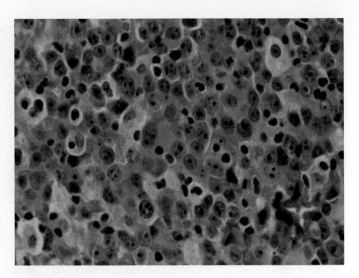

FIGURE 20-22. **Diffuse large B-cell lymphoma.** Tumor cells show prominent nucleoli

As discussed earlier, lymphomas are currently classified according to their respective normal lymphocytes during development and differentiation, as detailed in Figure 20-19. Ultimately, some B cells differentiate into plasma cells. These cells are the only B cells that secrete immunoglobulins, although they lack immunoglobulin expression on the cell surface. Plasma cells home to bone marrow, where they may give rise to **multiple myeloma**.

 CLINICAL FEATURES: Indolent lymphomas are distinguished from **aggressive** B-cell lymphomas. Typical indolent lymphomas are B-CLL and follicular lymphoma; aggressive B-cell lymphomas tend to be large B-cell lymphoma and Burkitt lymphoma. Ironically, although indolent lymphomas follow a prolonged clinical course, they are usually incurable. By contrast, aggressive lymphomas progress rapidly, but many of them are curable. Not all malignant lymphomas fall unequivocally into either category. MALT lymphomas, for example, are indolent lymphomas that can sometimes be cured by local irradiation or antibiotic treatment, as in some cases of gastric MALT lymphoma associated with *H. pylori* infection.

Our discussion of B-cell lymphomas will concentrate on several of the more common and important variants.

Diffuse Large B-Cell Lymphoma

Diffuse large B-cell lymphoma (DLBCL) is a heterogeneous group of aggressive, potentially curable B-cell neoplasms, which constitute 30% of all cases of B- and T-cell lymphomas. The disease occurs in all age groups but is most prevalent between the ages of 60 and 70 years. The cause of DLBCL is unknown, but it may be seen in association with EBV and HIV infections.

 PATHOLOGY: DLBCL may involve lymph nodes or extranodal sites. The tumor cells resemble **immunoblasts** or **centroblasts** (Fig. 20-22) or appear as anaplastic bizarre cells with marked nuclear irregularities. Immunoblasts are large B cells (see Fig. 20-19) with nuclei that exhibit prominent central nucleoli. The tumor cells of DLBCL express various B-cell antigens. As in follicular lymphoma (see below), clonal *BCL2* gene rearrangements are often seen, indicating a potential germinal center origin in some cases. DLBCL associated with immunodeficiency is usually positive for EBV.

 CLINICAL FEATURES: Rapidly evolving, multifocal, nodal, and extranodal tumor manifestations are typically seen at the time of presentation. DLBCL is potentially curable, but a high proliferation rate indicates an adverse prognosis.

Burkitt lymphoma (BL)

Burkitt lymphoma, one of the most rapidly growing malignancies, is defined by a chromosomal translocation involving 8q24, which harbors the MYC oncogene (see Chapter 5).

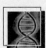 **EPIDEMIOLOGY: Endemic BL** is the most common childhood malignancy in Central Africa, with a peak incidence at ages 3 to 7 years. **Sporadic BL** affects mainly children and young adults in the Western world, where it accounts for 1% to 2% of all lymphomas. As in endemic BL, males are more often affected than females. **Immunodeficiency-associated BL** mainly occurs in HIV-infected individuals.

 PATHOGENESIS: EBV is present in virtually all cases of endemic BL but is seen in less than 30% of sporadic types. EBV-positive sporadic BL is associated with low socioeconomic status. Many patients experience a prodromal stage of polyclonal B-cell activation caused by bacterial, viral, or parasitic infections (malaria) (see Chapter 5).

PATHOLOGY: BL typically produces extranodal tumors rather than lymphadenopathy. All types of this lymphoma have a high risk for central nervous system involvement. The classic presentation for endemic BL is a destructive tumor in the jaws or other facial bones (Fig. 20-23A). Patients with sporadic BL typically present with abdominal masses. All types may involve ovaries, kidneys, and breasts.

Microscopically, BL cells are medium-sized and lack significant cytologic atypia. Tissue sections reveal a high number of mitotic figures, which attests to the extremely high proliferation rate in this tumor. The cellular debris of apoptotic tumor cells is cleared by macrophages, with a scattered appearance that termed "starry sky macrophage" (see Fig. 20-23B). Aspirate smears stained with Wright-Giemsa demonstrate numerous lipid vacuoles in the deeply basophilic cytoplasm of the tumor cells.

Burkitt cells express surface IgM and are positive for common B-cell antigens (CD19, CD20, CD22). They demonstrate CD10 and BCL-6 and are thus thought to be of germinal-center origin.

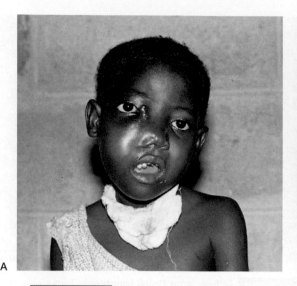
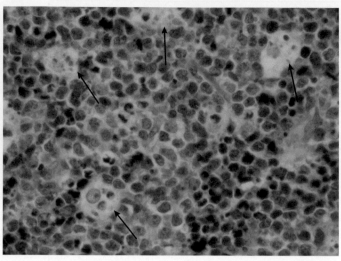

FIGURE 20-23. **Burkitt lymphoma. A.** A tumor of the jaw distorts the child's face. **B.** Lymph node is effaced by neoplastic lymphocytes with several "starry sky" macrophages (*arrows*).

Clonal *IgH* gene arrangement can be shown for heavy- and light-chain genes. Heavy-chain genes and *MYC* genes participate in a t(8;14) translocation. In endemic cases, the breakpoint on chromosome 14 occurs in the heavy-chain joining region, as seen in early B cells. In sporadic BL, the translocation occurs in the Ig switch region, which is more characteristic of mature B lymphocytes. In these cases, expression of the *MYC* gene is driven by the Ig heavy-chain promoter and leads to uncontrolled tumor cell growth (see Chapter 5).

 CLINICAL FEATURES: Most patients present with bulky extranodal tumors that emerge in a short time and respond to aggressive chemotherapy. Both endemic and sporadic BL are curable in up to 90% of patients.

Follicular Lymphoma

Follicular lymphoma (FL) is the malignant counterpart of lymphocytes derived from follicle centers. Follicle (germinal) centers consist of large round cells (centroblasts) and smaller cells with irregular or cleaved nuclei (centrocytes). *Unlike any other type of lymphoma, FL mimics an entire functional unit of lymphocytes (the follicle), including their ancillary cells. The opposite of FL is diffuse lymphoma.*

 EPIDEMIOLOGY: FL is a particularly common neoplasm in the United States, where it constitutes 35% of all adult malignant lymphomas. The disease shows a peak incidence at 60 years of age and is somewhat more common in women than in men.

 PATHOLOGY: FL (Fig. 20-24) predominantly involves lymph nodes and resembles benign follicular hyperplasia. However, FL is distinguished from the latter by extracapsular invasion into perinodal fat. FL usually displays surface Ig and is light-chain restricted. The tumor cells are positive for most B-cell antigens and CD10 but negative for CD5. *In contrast to benign germinal center B lymphocytes, FL expresses BCL-2 protein.* The most common cytogenetic translocation is t(14:18)(q32:q21), with *IgH* and *BCL-2* as partner genes. BCL-2 protein is an apoptosis inhibitor located in the mitochondrial membrane.

 CLINICAL FEATURES: FL predominantly affects lymph nodes. Other sites of involvement include the spleen, bone marrow, peripheral blood, head and neck region, gastrointestinal tract, soft tissue, and skin. Most patients have advanced disease at presentation. Low-grade FL is in-

dolent, but usually incurable, whereas high grade FL is more aggressive but is potentially curable. The prognosis worsens with the number of genetic abnormalities. One third of patients progress to (diffuse) large B-cell lymphoma.

Chronic lymphocytic leukemia/small lymphocytic lymphoma (CLL/SLL)

CLL/SLL is a malignant proliferation of small, mature-appearing, lymphocytes and a variable number of larger cells. A diagnosis of CLL is made if bone marrow and peripheral blood are primarily involved. If tumor cells predominantly give rise to lymphadenopathy or solid tumor masses, the term **small lymphocytic lymphoma** is more appropriate.

 EPIDEMIOLOGY: CLL/SLL is a typical indolent malignant lymphoma of the elderly (median age 65) and accounts for 7% of malignant lymphomas.

 PATHOLOGY: Lymph nodes infiltrated by CLL show complete effacement of architecture by small lymphocytes (Fig. 20-25). In the spleen, the white pulp is expanded, although tumor cells may also extend into the red pulp.

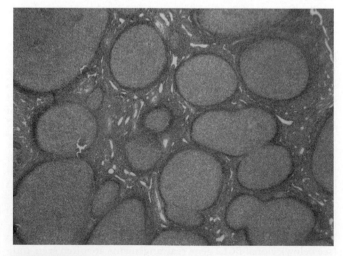

FIGURE 20-24. **Follicular lymphoma.** The normal lymph node architecture is replaced by malignant lymph follicles.

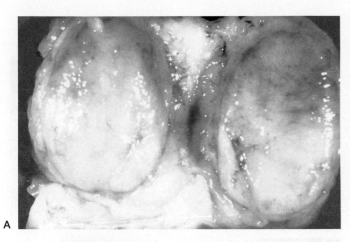
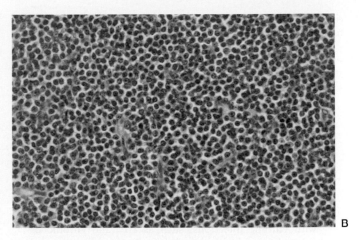

FIGURE 20-25. **Small lymphocytic lymphoma/leukemia. A.** A bisected, enlarged lymph node shows the characteristic uniform, glistening, gray color that imparts a fish-flesh appearance. **B.** On microscopic examination, the lymph nodal architecture is replaced by a diffuse infiltration of normal-appearing small lymphocytes.

Bone marrow involvement ranges from complete effacement of the marrow space to a more patchy distribution. In peripheral blood smears, some leukemic lymphocytes are destroyed and show ill-defined nuclear remnants ("smudge" cells). A variable number of larger cells with prominent nucleoli (prolymphocytes) can be seen.

SLL/CLL features a mature B-cell population that expresses CD19, CD20, CD22, and CD79. Half of the cases of B-CLL have not undergone somatic mutations in variable-region genes and thus reflect the genotype of naïve B cells. The other half has undergone *VH* gene mutations and resembles postgerminal center B cells.

 CLINICAL FEATURES: The diagnosis of CLL is established by demonstrating a sustained peripheral blood lymphocytosis, generally more than 15,000/μL and a bone marrow lymphocytosis exceeding 40% of marrow cells. A finding of monoclonality (light-chain restriction or clonal rearrangement of a light-chain gene) confirms the diagnosis of B-CLL.

Immunologic deficiencies, mainly of B cells but also of T cells, are common. Hypogammaglobulinemia occurs in 50% to 75% of cases at some time in the disease. The degree of hypogammaglobulinemia generally correlates with disease stage and is responsible for infectious complications. Patients with B-CLL also have increased peripheral blood T cells (>3,000/μL). There is an increase in CD8+ T cells and a corresponding decrease in CD4+ cells, with a resulting decrease in the CD4+/CD8+ cell ratio. The T cells often show impaired delayed-type hypersensitivity in vitro, which also contributes to the increased risk of infection.

The overall mean survival in B-CLL is 6 years. Initially, most patients with B-CLL are asymptomatic, and the diagnosis is suggested by finding lymphadenopathy and splenomegaly in a routine physical examination or lymphocytosis on a blood cell count. The subsequent clinical course is highly variable. In some cases, the disease progresses rapidly, and patients die within 2 to 3 years. Other patients remain asymptomatic for 10 to 20 years. The most common complications are bacterial infections and, less frequently, fungal and viral ones. Coombs-positive, autoimmune hemolytic anemia and hemorrhagic episodes secondary to thrombocytopenia are often observed.

Asymptomatic patients with B-CLL who have stable lymphocyte counts are ordinarily not treated. More advanced disease is treated with chemotherapeutic agents and antilymphocyte antibody. Splenectomy or splenic irradiation may be needed to manage refractory hypersplenism.

Lymphoplasmacytic Lymphoma (LPL)/Waldenström Macroglobulinemia

Lymphoplasmacytic lymphoma (LPL, also termed Waldenström disease, is a neoplastic proliferation of small lymphocytes and a variable number of IgM-

secreting plasma cells of the same malignant clone. Waldenström macroglobulinemia is not a variant of multiple myeloma, but rather an indolent malignant lymphoma that mainly affects the elderly.

 PATHOLOGY: Waldenström disease, or LPL, primarily involves the bone marrow but can also be seen in lymph nodes, spleen, and peripheral blood. In lymph nodes, LPL shows an interfollicular lymphocytic infiltrate with plasma cells. The leukemic bone marrow infiltrates are similar to those in CLL, although there may be more plasma cells. Transformation from LPL into a large cell lymphoma may occur. LPL expresses common B-cell antigens, and CD5 and CD23 are negative. The most common translocation is t(9;14). As in other lymphomas with plasma cell differentiation, rearrangement of the *PAX-5* gene, which encodes a B-cell-specific activator protein, is common.

 CLINICAL FEATURES: Eighty percent of patients present with a monoclonal IgM spike on serum electrophoresis (>3 g/dL). Many of the clinical symptoms result from **hyperviscosity syndrome**. Sludging and rouleaux formation of RBCs in the microvascular system may lead to visual disturbances and stroke. Complications of hyperviscosity are treated with plasmapheresis. Excess serum IgM may bind to clotting factors, platelets, and fibrin and thereby cause a coagulopathy. The clinical outcome of the disease is comparable to that of other indolent lymphomas, such as B-CLL.

Plasma Cell Neoplasia

Plasma cell neoplasia is a group of related malignant disorders of terminally differentiated B lymphocytes (plasma cells,) of which plasma cell myeloma or multiple myeloma is the most common (90% of cases). The condition is characterized by bone marrow multifocal infiltration by malignant plasma cells. There are typically multiple destructive (lytic) lesions or diffuse demineralization of bone. In most cases of plasma cell neoplasia, the tumor cells secrete a homogeneous, complete or partial, immunoglobulin molecule, an **M-component** or **paraprotein**, most commonly IgG or IgA.

 EPIDEMIOLOGY: Plasma cell neoplasia comprises 10% of all hematologic malignancies. About 7,500 cases are reported annually in the United States, with an overall incidence of 3 per 100,000 population. The disorder is more than twice as common in blacks (8 per 100,000 population) than in whites. The frequency of plasma cell neoplasia increases with age; the mean age at diagnosis of multiple myeloma is 65 years and that of solitary osseous myeloma and extramedullary plasmacytoma is a decade earlier. Plasma cell neoplasia is distinctly uncommon before age 40. There is a slight male predominance, and the male-to-female ratio is 1.5:1.

PATHOGENESIS: Several risk factors for plasma cell neoplasia have been identified.

- **A genetic predisposition** is suggested by an increased incidence of multiple myeloma in first-degree relatives of patients with plasma cell neoplasia and the higher frequency of multiple myeloma in blacks.
- **Ionizing radiation** has been incriminated in the etiology of plasma cell neoplasia. Long-term survivors of the bombing of Hiroshima and Nagasaki had a fivefold increased incidence of multiple myeloma.
- **Chronic antigenic stimulation** may constitute a risk factor. Some cases of multiple myeloma have been associated with chronic infections, such as HIV and chronic osteomyelitis, and with chronic inflammatory disorders (e.g., rheumatoid arthritis). A two-hit hypothesis is proposed by which (1) antigenic stimulation leads to reactive, polyclonal proliferation of B lymphocytes, and (2) a subsequent mutagenic event establishes a single malignant clone.

PATHOLOGY: On gross examination, the osseous and extraosseous plasma cell tumors are variably red, tan, or gray and have a consistency that ranges from fleshy to gelatinous. The bony lesions are well demarcated from the surrounding normal tissue. The cortical bone may be destroyed, with direct tumor extension into surrounding soft tissues. In multiple myeloma, moderate enlargement of the lymph nodes, spleen, and liver is occasionally observed, although the gross appearance of these organs is not distinctive. The kidneys are often contracted in size.

- **Bone marrow:** The microscopic hallmark of multiple myeloma in the bone marrow is diffuse sheets or nodular aggregates of plasma cells. Ultimately, normal hematopoietic tissues and fat cells are replaced by neoplastic plasma cells. In marrow aspirates, neoplastic plasma cells usually exceed 30% of all cells. The malignant cells may appear normal, but more often, they show atypical features including (1) prominent nucleoli, (2) irregular chromatin distribution, (3) binucleation and bizarre multinucleation, and (4) nuclear–cytoplasmic asynchrony, with immature nuclei and mature cytoplasm (Fig. 20-26).
- **Kidneys:** Renal abnormalities, including light-chain nephropathy and an M-component—related glomerulopathy, are seen in more than half of the cases. Additional renal findings in multiple myeloma include deposition of (1) amyloid in glomeruli and blood vessels, (2) calcium (nephrocalcinosis), and (3) uric acid crystals (urate nephropathy) (see Chapter 16).
- **Lymph nodes, spleen and liver:** These organs may be infiltrated by neoplastic plasma cells.

CLINICAL FEATURES: Lytic lesions of the skull and other flat bones, including the spine and ribs, are characteristic (but not diagnostic) radiographic findings. The most important disorder to consider in the differential diagnosis of multiple myeloma is the more common **monoclonal gammopathy of unknown significance (MGUS)** or **benign essential gammopathy.** The former term is preferred because the disorder is not necessarily benign. Of patients with MGUS, about 2% per year progress to a B-cell neoplasm (lymphoplasmacytic disorder or multiple myeloma). The strong link between MGUS and multiple myeloma suggests that a first oncogenic event produces MGUS and a second event results in multiple myeloma.

Bone destruction in multiple myeloma is due to both progressive tumor growth and secretion of osteoclast-activating factor by malignant plasma cells. Osteoclasts may also be activated by IL-6 (the activity of IL-6 is increased in patients with multiple

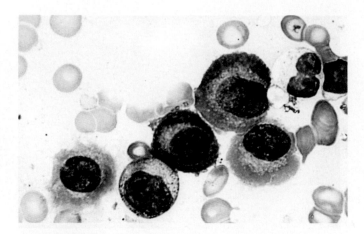

FIGURE 20-26. **Multiple myeloma.** A smear of a bone marrow aspirate shows a cluster of three neoplastic plasma cells.

myeloma). Common complications of bone destruction include pain, vertebral collapse, and pathologic fractures of long bones. Additionally, calcium released from the injured bone may precipitate in the kidneys and cause renal damage (nephrocalcinosis).

The hyperviscosity syndrome is particularly common in IgG and IgA myelomas, but it occurs far less often than in macroglobulinemia. Neurologic abnormalities and spontaneous bleeding episodes are observed.

Humoral immune deficiency, with decreased levels of normal serum Ig, is characteristic of multiple myeloma. This defect is due to (1) suppression of normal B lymphocytes by the neoplastic clone and (2) increased catabolism of normal IgG. Consequently, patients with multiple myeloma are susceptible to a variety of infectious complications, particularly pneumonia and pyelonephritis.

Multiple myeloma is an incurable disease, with a mean survival rate of 6 months in untreated patients and 3 years with chemotherapy. The clinical course tends to be biphasic. An initial chronic stable stage is followed by an aggressive or accelerated preterminal phase. Death is usually due to infection or renal failure.

Mature T-Cell and Natural Killer (NK)-Cell Lymphomas Have a Poor Prognosis

Mature (peripheral) T-cell and NK-cell malignancies originate from post-thymic T cells (see Fig. 20-20).

EPIDEMIOLOGY: Worldwide, T-cell malignancies account for 12% of non-Hodgkin lymphomas. T-cell and NK-cell lymphomas are more common in Asia than in the Western world. In Japan, many T-cell malignancies are attributed to infection with human T-cell leukemia virus.

PATHOLOGY: The immunophenotype of mature T-cell malignancies is uniformly characterized by expression of α,β or γ,δ pairs of T-cell receptors, both of which are linked to CD3. By definition, NK cells lack complete T-cell receptor gene expression. NK cells express CD2, CD7, and CD8. NK and cytotoxic T-cell malignancies both demonstrate the granule-associated proteins **perforin, granzyme B, and T-cell intracellular antigen.**

CLINICAL FEATURES: T-cell and NK-cell tumors are clinically grouped into leukemic or nodal, extranodal, and cutaneous malignancies. *These neoplasms and NK-cell lymphomas are generally more aggressive than most B-cell malignancies and Hodgkin lymphoma.* They are treated with standard chemotherapy for B-cell lymphomas. Many T-cell neoplasms respond poorly to treatment; the overall 5-year survival rate is 20% to 30%.

Mycosis Fungoides and Sézary Syndrome

Mycosis fungoides (MF) is a cutaneous T-cell lymphoma with epidermal tropism.

  EPIDEMIOLOGY: The disease occurs mainly in adults and the elderly. Men are more affected than women.

 PATHOLOGY: MF displays lymphocytic infiltrates at the dermal–epidermal junction, epidermis, and, in some cases, intraepidermal nests of tumor cells (Pautrier microabscesses). Most tumors show a mature T-helper cell immunophenotype (CD2+, CD3+, CD5+, CD4+, CD8⁻ and TCRα,β+). As with other peripheral T-cell lymphomas, CD7 is often absent. Clonal T-cell receptor gene rearrangements are common, which helps to distinguish subtle cases of mycosis fungoides from inflammatory infiltrates.

CLINICAL FEATURES: MF is an indolent lymphoma.

- The **premycotic or eczematous stage** lasts several years and is difficult to distinguish from many benign chronic dermatoses. A skin biopsy specimen is not diagnostic of lymphoma and shows a nonspecific perivascular and periadnexal lymphocytic infiltration with accompanying eosinophils and plasma cells.
- The **plaque stage** follows the premycotic stage. It is characterized by well-demarcated, raised cutaneous plaques. A definitive diagnosis of MF can usually be made in this stage. There is a dense subepidermal band-like infiltrate of lymphoid cells, with irregular nuclear contours and a spectrum of cell sizes. Distinctive medium-to-large lymphoid cells, with hyperchromatic nuclei and cerebriform nuclear contours, termed **mycosis cells**, are typical.
- The **tumor stage** features raised cutaneous tumors, mostly on the face and in body folds, which frequently ulcerate and become secondarily infected. The name **mycosis fungoides** derives from the raised, fungating, mushroom-like appearance of these tumors. Extracutaneous involvement, particularly of the lymph nodes, spleen, liver, bone marrow, and lungs, is common.

 PATHOLOGY: Spread of MF to other organs, including the lungs, spleen, liver, and peripheral blood, is termed **Sézary syndrome**. This disorder arises after extensive cutaneous lesions have existed for a long time. Small (**Lutzner**) cells or large (**Sézary**) tumor cells are found in the peripheral blood.

Hodgkin Lymphoma (HL) Features Hodgkin Cells and Reed-Sternberg Cells Against an Inflammatory Cell Background

Large atypical mononuclear or multinucleated tumor cells termed **Hodgkin and Reed-Sternberg cells,** *are the diagnostic hallmark of HL (Fig. 20-27). Most cases of HL are clonal neoplasms of B lymphocytes.* However, its unique clinicopathologic features warrant its recognition as a distinctive malignancy. Reed-Sternberg cells frequently constitute less than 1% of the total cell population. In fact, a salient feature of HL is the predominance in tumor tissue of reactive benign tissue components.

 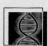 **EPIDEMIOLOGY AND PATHOGENESIS:** HL is the most common malignancy of Americans between the ages of 10 and 30 years. Approximately 8,000 cases are reported annually in the United States, for an incidence of 3 per 100,000 population. It is somewhat more common in men than in women (4:2.5) and in whites than in blacks (3.5:2). There is a distinctive bimodal age distribution

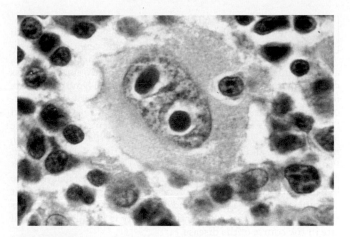

FIGURE 20-27. **Classic Reed-Sternberg cell.** Mirror-image nuclei contain large eosinophilic nucleoli.

in developed countries, with a peak in the late 20s, a decrease in frequency in the fourth and fifth decades, and a gradually increasing incidence after age 50.

A possible relationship between HL and infection with EBV has been suggested. Young adults who have had EBV infection (infectious mononucleosis) have a threefold increased risk of developing HL, and the EBV genome is frequently identified in the Reed-Sternberg cell. Mixed-cellularity HL is associated with EBV in 70% to 80% of cases. **Genetic factors** and **immune status** play a role in disease susceptibility. The frequency of certain HLA subtypes, particularly HLA-B18, is higher in patients with HL. Moreover, there is a sevenfold increased risk of HL in siblings of patients with this disorder and a 100-fold increased risk when the sibling is a monozygotic twin. HL is more frequent in patients with compromised immunity or with autoimmune diseases, such as rheumatoid arthritis.

 PATHOLOGY: Most patients with HL present with lymphadenopathy. After an initial diagnosis of HL, a comprehensive clinical and radiographic evaluation is commonly used to establish the extent, or stage, of disease. Abdominal exploratory surgery (staging laparotomy) may be performed to search for abdominal involvement. Bone marrow is also examined.

- **Lymph nodes:** On clinical examination, lymph nodes involved by HL are typically firm or rubbery, but they may be soft. If tumor tissue extends beyond the confines of individual lymph nodes, groups of nodes may be matted together.
- **Spleen:** The spleen is involved in one third of cases of HL at the time of diagnosis and in most patients at autopsy. HL occurs first in T-cell-dependent, periarteriolar lymphoid sheaths of the white pulp or in the marginal zone between the white pulp and the red pulp. As the disease progresses, single or multiple discrete tumor nodules or confluent multinodular tumor masses in the spleen are common.
- **Liver:** At autopsy, the liver is involved with HL in two thirds of patients with residual disease, although it is unusual at the time of presentation.
- **Bone marrow:** The bone marrow is only rarely involved initially. Early changes in the bone marrow are discrete foci of fibrotic tumor, without destruction of bony trabeculae. As the disease progresses, destruction of bone may produce an osteolytic appearance on radiologic examination.
- **Other systems:** Pulmonary involvement is seen at autopsy in more than half of patients with residual disease, and epidural spread of HL from paravertebral nodes through intervertebral foramina is a frequent neurological complication.

CLINICAL FEATURES: HL usually manifests as non-tender peripheral adenopathy involving a single lymph node or groups of lymph nodes. The cervical and mediastinal nodes are affected in more than half of cases, and the anterior mediastinum is also frequently involved. Less commonly, axillary, inguinal, and retroperitoneal lymph nodes are initially enlarged. Early HL spreads predictably between contiguous lymph node groups via efferent lymphatics. Constitutional ("B") symptoms are found in 40% of HL patients. These include low-grade fever, which is occasionally cyclical (Pel-Ebstein fever), night sweats, and weight loss exceeding 10% of body weight. Pruritus may occur as the disease progresses. Deficient T-lymphocyte function is characteristic of HL. Subtle defects of delayed-type hypersensitivity, which can be detected in most patients even at the time of initial diagnosis, tend to become more pronounced as the disease progresses. Humoral immunity is usually intact until late in the course of the disease.

The prognosis in HL depends mainly on the patient's age and the anatomic extent of the disease, that is, the stage and the histological classification (see below). A better prognosis is associated with (1) younger age, (2) lower clinical stage (localized disease), and (3) absence of B signs and symptoms. A comprehensive system, based on clinical evaluation and pathologic findings from a staging laparotomy, is used to assign stage (Ann Arbor system).

Complications of HL include compromise of vital organs by progressive tumor growth and secondary infections, owing to both the primary defect in delayed type hypersensitivity and the immunosuppressive effects of therapy. Development of second malignancies after therapy is of special concern, because more than 15% of treated patients may eventually suffer from this complication. AML develops in 5% of patients, and aggressive large cell lymphomas occur somewhat less frequently.

Histological Classification of Hodgkin Lymphoma (HL) is Important in Prognosis

Two major types of HL are distinguished, namely **nodular lymphocyte-predominant HL** (NLPHL) and **classical** HL (CHL). CHL is further subcategorized into four additional subtypes (see below).

Nodular Lymphocyte-Predominant HL (NLPHL)

NLPHL features Reed-Sternberg cell variants called "popcorn" or L&H (lymphohistiocytic) cells. NLPHL represents only a small proportion of all cases of HL and is clearly a neoplasm of B-lymphocyte origin. The Reed-Sternberg cells of this variant express specific B-cell lineage antigens and surface Ig and lack CD15 and CD30, which are usually (but not always) found on Reed-Sternberg cells of the other subtypes of HL. Nevertheless, classical types of HL are also considered to be B-lymphocyte neoplasms.

NLPHL is the most indolent type of HL. Men under 35 years of age are most often affected (male-to-female ratio, 4:1). At the time of diagnosis, the disease is usually localized (stage I), with the high cervical, axillary, or inguinal lymph nodes most commonly involved. B signs and symptoms are present in only 20% of cases. The overall survival rate is excellent, as more than 80% of patients at stages I and II survive for 10 years. However, lymphocyte-predominant HL has a high recurrence rate.

PATHOLOGY: The tumor completely effaces lymph node architecture in a vaguely nodular pattern. An inflammatory background of eosinophils and plasma cells is missing. The tumor cells in NLPHL are negative for EBV.

Classical HL (CHL)

CHL is characterized by clonal proliferation of typical mononuclear Hodgkin cells and multinucleated Reed-Sternberg cells (HRS cells). Expression of the lymphocytic activation antigen CD30 unites the different types of CHL. A variable inflammatory background of lymphocytes, eosinophils, macrophages, neutrophils, plasma cells, fibroblasts, and collagenous tissue determines the morphologic appearance of

the four different types of CHL. These categories are defined as lymphocyte-rich, nodular-sclerosis, mixed-cellularity, and lymphocyte-depleted variants.

PATHOLOGY: Typical mononuclear or multinucleated Reed-Sternberg cells with large nucleoli are immersed in a rich inflammatory background. These malignant cells produce several cytokines that elicit characteristic tissue effects. Eosinophils are attracted by the combined effects of IL-5 and eotaxin, and IL-6 can attract plasma cells. TGF-β activates fibroblasts and may account for nodular fibrosis.

Nodular-Sclerosis HL (NSHL)

NSHL features nodular architecture in which lymphoid tissue is surrounded by fibrosis (Fig. 20-28). Classical Reed-Sternberg cells with lacunar variants are typical. NSHL accounts for 70% of CHL, and most cases occur between 20 and 30 years of age. Mediastinal involvement is most common in this type of HL. NSHL is the most common form of HL and is often found in adolescent and young adult women between 15 and 35 years of age. The prognosis is good, with a cure rate of more than 80%.

Mixed-Cellularity HL (MCHL)

MCHL contains Reed-Sternberg cells against a mixed inflammatory background of eosinophils, neutrophils, macrophages, and plasma cells (Fig. 20-29). The histology is like that of the nodular sclerosis variety, but collagen bands are missing. People of any age may be affected, but

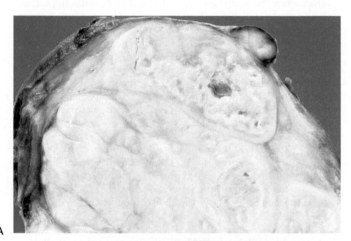

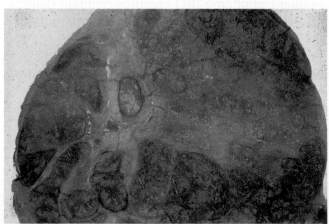

FIGURE 20-28. Hodgkin lymphoma; nodular sclerosis. **A.** A cut section of matted lymph nodes shows broad bands of fibrosis that divide the parenchyma into distinct nodules. Several foci of necrosis are evident. **B.** A low-power photomicrograph demonstrates broad bands of fibrosis.

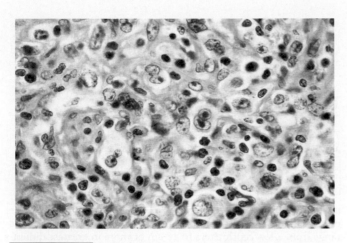

FIGURE 20-29. Hodgkin lymphoma; mixed cellularity. A photomicrograph of a lymph node shows classic, binucleated, and mononuclear Reed-Sternberg cells; lymphocytes; and mild diffuse fibrosis.

MCHL is most common in the fourth and fifth decades of life. The prognosis is intermediate, with a cure rate of 75%.

Lymphocyte-Rich HL (LRHL)
LRHL has recently been added to the list of HLs. It is characterized by classical Reed-Sternberg cells in an abundant background of small lymphocytes. Mixed inflammatory cells and collagen bands are missing. The prognosis is good, with a cure rate of about 85%.

Lymphocyte-Depleted HL (LDHL)
LDHL is the least common type of CHL. Histologically, it shows a predominance of tumor cells and a marked absence of background lymphocytes (Fig. 20-30). Without treatment, LDHL is the most clinically aggressive type and has the worst prognosis. Middle-aged to elderly men are most commonly affected. Retroperitoneal adenopathy is frequently prominent, and involvement of the spleen, liver, and bone marrow is common. Profound immunodeficiency develops, and death commonly results from inanition or secondary infections. The overall cure rate in both types of LDHL is 40% to 50%.

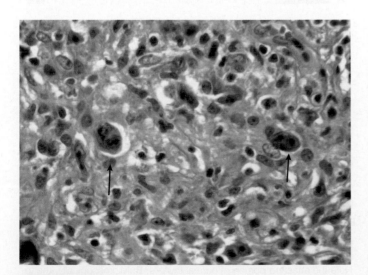

FIGURE 20-30. Hodgkin lymphoma; lymphocyte-depleted type. Two tumor cells are seen (arrows). The number of reactive lymphocytes in the fibrotic background is markedly reduced.

SPLEEN

Disorders of the Spleen: Splenomegaly

The spleen is a prominent member of the lymphopoietic and mononuclear phagocyte systems, and splenomegaly is common in a variety of unrelated functional, infectious, and infiltrative processes (Table 20-10).

Reactive Splenomegaly is Associated with Inflammatory Conditions

Reactive splenic hyperplasia occurs in a number of acute and chronic inflammatory conditions. It is probably caused by phagocytosis of blood-borne bacteria, which leads to the release of growth factors and other products of the inflammatory response. The spleen is moderately enlarged (up to 400 g), and macrophages and neutrophils abound in the red pulp.

In **chronic immunologic inflammatory disorders**, splenomegaly is caused by hyperplasia of the white pulp. Germinal centers are prominent, as in rheumatoid arthritis, and the red pulp displays an associated increase in mononuclear phagocytes, immunoblasts, plasma cells, and eosinophils.

Systemic lupus erythematosus is characterized by fibrinoid necrosis of capsular and trabecular collagen and concentric, or "onion skin," thickening of the penicilliary arteries and central arterioles of the white pulp.

In **infectious mononucleosis**, transformed lymphocytes (immunoblasts) prominently infiltrate the red pulp, whereas the

TABLE 20-10
Principal Causes of Splenomegaly
Infections
Acute
Subacute
Chronic
Immunologic Inflammatory Disorders
Felty's syndrome
Lupus erythematosus
Sarcoidosis
Amyloidosis
Thyroiditis
Hemolytic Anemias
Immune Thrombocytopenia
Splenic Vein Hypertension
Cirrhosis
Splenic or portal vein thrombosis or stenosis
Right-sided cardiac failure
Primary or metastatic neoplasm
Leukemia
Lymphoma
Hodgkin's disease
Myeloproliferative syndromes
Sarcoma
Carcinoma
Storage Diseases
Gaucher's
Niemann-Pick
Mucopolysaccharidoses

white pulp may no longer be evident. Infiltration of the capsular and trabecular systems and of blood vessels by lymphoid elements weakens the supporting structure of the spleen and accounts for **traumatic splenic rupture** in infectious mononucleosis.

Congestive Splenomegaly is Frequently Associated with Portal Hypertension

Chronic passive congestion of the spleen causes splenomegaly and hypersplenism. This condition is most common in patients with portal hypertension due to cirrhosis, thrombosis of the portal or splenic veins, or right-sided heart failure.

 PATHOLOGY: The spleen is modestly enlarged (300 to 700 g) and has a thickened, fibrotic capsule. The cut surface is firm, and the color varies from pink to deep red, depending on the extent of fibrosis. The parenchyma becomes fibrotic, and the red pulp is hypocellular. The white pulp tends to be atrophic.

Infiltrative Splenomegaly May be Related to Increase in Cellularity or Extracellular Material

The spleen may be enlarged by an increase in cellularity or by the deposition of extracellular material, as in amyloidosis. Splenic macrophages accumulate in chronic infections, hemolytic anemias, and a variety of storage diseases; Gaucher disease is the prototype (see Chapter 6). Splenomegaly is also caused by infiltration of malignant cells in hematologic proliferative disorders, such as leukemias and lymphomas.

THYMUS

Theories underlying the historical categorization of the thymus as an endocrine organ have long been discredited. Nevertheless, we know that the thymus elaborates a number of factors (thymic hormones) that play a key role in the maturation of the immune system and the development of immune tolerance. On this basis, we discuss certain entities associated with thymus abnormalities in this chapter.

Agenesis and Dysplasia

Alterations in the thymus vary from complete absence (**agenesis**) or severe **hypoplasia** to a situation in which the thymus is small but exhibits a normal architecture. Some small glands exhibit **thymic dysplasia**, characterized by an absence of thymocytes, few if any, Hassall corpuscles, and only epithelial components. Various developmental abnormalities are associated with immune deficiencies (see Chapter 4) and hematologic disorders.

Hyperplasia

Thymic hyperplasia denotes the presence of lymphoid follicles in the thymus regardless of the gland's size. The total weight of the thymus is usually within the normal range, although it may be increased. The follicles contain germinal centers and are composed largely of B lymphocytes that contain IgM and IgD. The follicles tend to occupy and distort the medullary zones.

The best known association of thymic hyperplasia is with **myasthenia gravis** (see Chapter 27), in which two thirds of patients exhibit this thymic abnormality. Interestingly, thymic epithelial and myoid cells contain nicotinic acetylcholine receptor protein, suggesting a potential source for the development of antibodies directed against this receptor. Thymic follicular hyperpla-

sia may also be found in other diseases in which autoimmunity is believed to play a role, including Graves disease, Addison disease, systemic lupus erythematosus, scleroderma, and rheumatoid arthritis.

Thymoma

Thymoma is a neoplasm of thymic epithelial cells. These tumors almost always occur in adult life and most (80%) are benign.

 PATHOLOGY: Most thymomas are located in the anterosuperior mediastinum, although a few have been described in other locations where thymic tissue is found, including the neck, middle and posterior mediastinum, and pulmonary hilus. Benign thymomas are irregularly shaped masses that range from a few centimeters to 15 cm or more in greatest dimension. They are encapsulated, firm, and gray-to-yellow tumors that are divided into lobules by fibrous septa (Fig. 20-31).

On microscopic examination, thymomas consist of a mixture of neoplastic epithelial cells and nontumorous lymphocytes. The proportions of these elements vary in individual cases and even among different lobules. The epithelial cells are plump or spindle-shaped and have vesicular nuclei. In cases in which epithelial cells predominate, they may exhibit an organoid differentiation, including perivascular spaces containing lymphocytes and macrophages, tumor cell rosettes and whorls, suggesting abortive Hassall corpuscle formation.

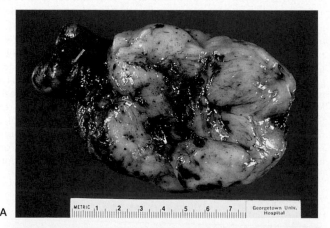

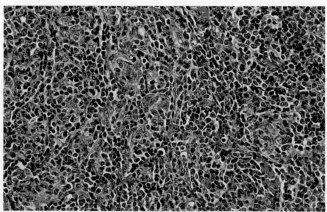

FIGURE 20-31. **Thymoma. A.** The tumor in cross-section is whitish and has a bulging surface with areas of hemorrhage. Note the attached portion of normal thymus. **B.** Microscopically, the tumor consists of a mixture of neoplastic epithelial cells and nontumorous lymphocytes.

MYASTHENIA GRAVIS: Fifteen percent of patients with myasthenia gravis have thymoma. Conversely, one third to one half of patients with thymoma develop myasthenia gravis. The occurrence of thymoma in persons with myasthenia gravis is more common in men over 50 years of age.

OTHER ASSOCIATED DISEASES: Thymoma is also associated with many other immune disorders. More than 10% of patients have hypogammaglobulinemia, and 5% have erythroid hypoplasia. Other associated diseases include myocarditis, dermatomyositis, rheumatoid arthritis, lupus erythematosus, scleroderma, and Sjögren syndrome. Certain malignant tumors have also been associated with thymoma, including T-cell leukemia, lymphoma, and multiple myeloma.

Malignant Thymoma Invades Locally and May Metastasize

One fourth of thymomas are not encapsulated and exhibit malignant features.

 PATHOLOGY: Type I malignant thymoma is the most common cancer of the thymus and is virtually indistinguishable histologically from encapsulated, benign thymoma. However, it penetrates the capsule, implants on pleural or pericardial surfaces, and metastasizes to lymph nodes, lung, liver, and bone.

Type II malignant thymoma is a very uncommon invasive tumor, which is also termed **thymic carcinoma**. Its morphology is highly variable and takes the form of squamous cell carcinoma, lymphoepithelioma-like carcinoma (identical to that found in the oropharynx), a sarcomatoid variant (carcinosarcoma), and a number of other rare patterns. These variants share a distinct epithelial appearance, and a mediastinal tumor that lacks this feature is probably not a thymic carcinoma.

 CLINICAL FEATURES: Malignant thymoma is treated by surgical excision and radiation therapy. Chemotherapy is added in cases with distant metastases. The prognosis for benign thymoma is excellent, and the presence or absence of myasthenic symptoms has little prognostic value. For type I malignant thymomas, prognosis correlates with the extent of disease. Most patients with type II thymomas die within 5 years of diagnosis.

Germ Cell Tumors of the Thymus Account for 20% of Mediastinal Tumors

Thymic germ cell tumors are likely to arise from cells left behind when germ cells migrate during embryogenesis. The histological appearance of mediastinal germ cell tumors is like those in the gonads (see Chapters 17 and 18). Mature cystic teratoma is most common. Seminoma, embryonal carcinoma, endodermal sinus tumor, teratocarcinoma, immature teratoma, and choriocarcinoma all occur. Mixed germ cell tumors are common. Mediastinal germ cell tumors may on occasion contain a somatic-type malignant component of sarcoma, carcinoma, or hematologic malignancies. Save for mature cystic teratoma, which affects both genders equally, the other tumors occur mostly in males, and thymic seminoma arises only in men. The prognosis is comparable to that of gonadal tumors, except that mediastinal nonseminomatous germ cell tumors are more aggressive.

21 The Endocrine System

Maria Merino
Martha Quezado
Raphael Rubin
Emanuel Rubin

The main function of the endocrine system is communication. Although there is some overlap between the nervous and endocrine systems in the soluble mediators and functions they serve, the key element of the endocrine system is its ability to communicate at a distance using soluble mediators. To qualify as a hormone, a chemical messenger must bind to a receptor, either on the surface of the cell or within it. Hormones act either on the final effector target or on other glands that in turn produce another hormone. Diseases of the endocrine system may lead to excessive or insufficient production of hormones. In addition, insensitivity of target tissues produces effects similar to those associated with the underproduction of hormones.

PITUITARY GLAND

Hypopituitarism

Hypopituitarism refers to deficient secretion of one or more of the pituitary hormones. It has many causes and various clinical presentations. Most commonly, only one or a few pituitary hormones are deficient. Occasionally, total failure of pituitary function, **panhypopituitarism**, occurs. The effects of hypopituitarism vary with (1) the extent of the loss, (2) the specific hormones involved, and (3) the patient's age. In general, symptoms relate to deficient function of the thyroid, adrenal glands, and the reproductive system. In children, growth retardation and delayed puberty are additional problems (Fig. 21-1).

PITUITARY TUMORS: More than half of all hypopituitarism in adults is caused by pituitary tumors, usually adenomas. The tumor itself may be functional, but symptoms of hypopituitarism often result from compression of adjacent tissue by the mass.

SHEEHAN SYNDROME: In this now rare condition, panhypopituitarism is caused by ischemic necrosis of the gland, often due to severe hypotension from postpartum hemorrhage. Agalactia, amenorrhea, hypothyroidism, and adrenocortical insufficiency are important consequences.

PITUITARY APOPLEXY: Hemorrhage and/or infarction can occur in a normal pituitary, but at least half of cases occur in association with endocrinologically inactive adenomas. Usually without endocrine effect, pituitary apoplexy may, on occasion, lead to hypopituitarism.

IATROGENIC HYPOPITUITARISM: Therapeutic radiation or neurosurgical procedures frequently cause neuroendocrine abnormalities, including hypopituitarism.

TRAUMA: Traumatic brain injury is associated with significant risk to the pituitary gland, with the potential development of diabetes, hypopituitarism, and other endocrinopathies.

GENETIC ABNORMALITIES OF PITUITARY DEVELOPMENT: Congenital growth hormone deficiency constitutes a unique group of disorders. It may occur in isolation, as so-called **isolated growth hormone deficiency**, which is related to mutations in the growth hormone (GH) gene or the growth hormone-releasing hormone receptor. The latter is the cause of **Laron dwarfism**, the condition that is responsible for the dwarfism of African pygmies. Because GH exerts its effects by promoting IGF-

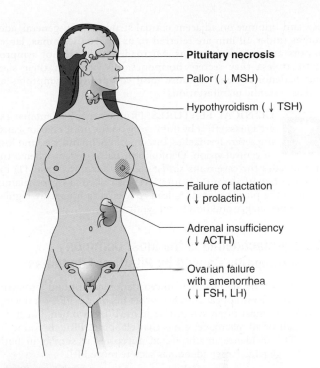

FIGURE 21-1. Major clinical manifestations of panhypopituitarism. ACTH, adrenocorticotropic hormone; FSH, follicle-stimulating hormone; LH, luteinizing hormone; MSH, melanocyte-stimulating hormone; TSH, thyroid-stimulating hormone.

I secretion, IGF-I is effective replacement therapy for Laron syndrome, mimicking most of the effects ascribed to GH itself. In addition, a number of mutations affecting transcription factors important in pituitary development have been identified. These mutations generally cause combined deficiencies of pituitary hormones.

EMPTY SELLA SYNDROME: This is primarily a radiologic term that describes an enlarged sella containing a thin, flattened pituitary at the base. It is secondary to a congenitally defective or absent diaphragma sella, which permits transmission of cerebrospinal fluid pressure into the sella. Endocrine disturbances are generally minor but may include hyperprolactinemia, oligomenorrhea or amenorrhea, frank hypopituitarism, acromegaly, diabetes insipidus, and Cushing syndrome.

Pituitary Adenomas

Pituitary adenomas are benign neoplasms of the anterior lobe of the pituitary and are often associated with excess secretion of pituitary hormones and corresponding endocrine hyperfunction. They occur in both genders, are more common in adults, and comprise only 2% of all adenomas in children. Small, apparently **nonfunctioning pituitary adenomas** are found incidentally in as many as 25% of adult autopsies.

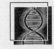 **PATHOGENESIS:** The etiology of pituitary adenomas is still obscure, but it is clear that its pathogenesis is related to hormonal and genetic factors.

 PATHOLOGY: Pituitary adenomas are now classified according to the hormone(s) they produce. Pituitary adenomas range from small lesions that do not enlarge the gland to expansive tumors that erode the sella turcica and impinge on adjacent cranial structures. In general, adenomas under 10 mm are referred to as **microadenomas**; larger tumors are **macroadenomas**. Microadenomas are not symptomatic unless they secrete hormones. By virtue of their size, macroadenomas tend to cause local compressive symptoms as well as systemic manifestations.

 CLINICAL FEATURES: Pituitary macroadenomas exert a mass effect by impinging on the optic chiasm, causing severe headaches, bitemporal hemianopsia, and loss of central vision. Oculomotor palsies occur when a tumor invades the cavernous sinuses. Large adenomas may (1) invade the hypothalamus; (2) interfere with normal hypothalamic input to the pituitary; and (3) lead to loss of temperature regulation, hyperphagia, and hormonal syndromes.

Hyperprolactinemia is the Most Common Endocrinopathy Caused by Pituitary Adenomas

Almost half of all pituitary microadenomas contain prolactin (PRL), but fewer appear to secrete this hormone. PRL-producing tumors are most often symptomatic in young women, but more than half of all macroadenomas that elaborate PRL are found in men. The incidence in unselected autopsies is similar in both sexes. In general, larger adenomas secrete more PRL.

 PATHOLOGY: Lactotroph adenomas tend to be chromophobic and contain spheroid nuclei with a prominent nucleolus. Endocrine amyloid (see Chapter 23) and psammoma bodies (calcospherites) are seen but are not pathognomonic.

 CLINICAL FEATURES: In women, functional lactotroph adenomas lead to amenorrhea, galactorrhea, and infertility. The consistently elevated blood PRL levels inhibit the surge of pituitary LH necessary for ovulation in women. Men tend to suffer from decreased libido and impotence. Functional lactotroph microadenomas are successfully treated with dopamine agonists (bromocriptine) to inhibit PRL secretion, whereas macroadenomas may require surgery.

Somatotroph Adenomas Secrete Growth Hormone (GH)

Dramatic changes result from excess secretion of GH. A somatotroph adenoma that arises in a child or adolescent before the epiphyses close results in **gigantism**. By contrast, after the epiphyses of the long bones have fused and adult height has been achieved, the same tumor produces **acromegaly**. Most tumors are macroadenomas and cause mass effects and tumor-induced adenohypophyseal hypofunction.

 PATHOLOGY: In patients with acromegaly, 75% have a somatotroph macroadenoma. Most of the rest have microadenomas. Variants of isolated GH-producing adenomas include the **densely granulated** composed of acidophilic cells (Fig. 21-2), and **sparsely granulated** composed of chromophobe cells.

 CLINICAL FEATURES: Acromegaly is uncommon, with an annual incidence of three cases per million. Over many years, patients with acro-megaly gradually develop coarse facial features (Fig. 21-3), with overgrowth of the mandible (prognathism) and maxilla, increased space between the upper incisor teeth, and a thickened nose. Hands and feet are often enlarged, and hat size increases. Acromegaly has serious complications including an increase in cardiovascular, cerebrovascular, and respiratory deaths.

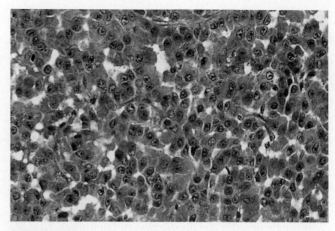

FIGURE 21-2. **Pituitary somatotrope adenoma from a man with acromegaly.** The tumor cells are arranged in thin cords and ribbons.

Treatment for somatotroph adenomas is usually transsphenoidal hypophysectomy, after which circulating GH levels may decline to normal levels within hours. Radiation therapy is an alternative when surgery is contraindicated. A long-acting analogue of somatostatin, an antagonist of GH, is a useful therapeutic adjunct.

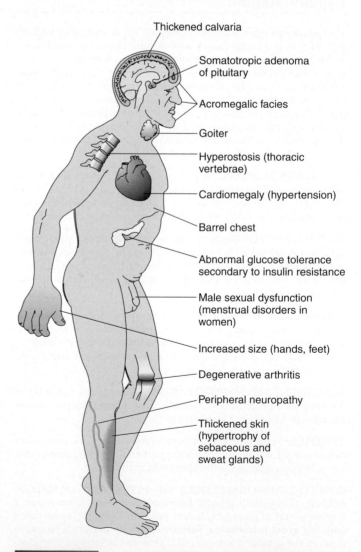

Thickened calvaria

Somatotropic adenoma of pituitary

Acromegalic facies

Goiter

Hyperostosis (thoracic vertebrae)

Cardiomegaly (hypertension)

Barrel chest

Abnormal glucose tolerance secondary to insulin resistance

Male sexual dysfunction (menstrual disorders in women)

Increased size (hands, feet)

Degenerative arthritis

Peripheral neuropathy

Thickened skin (hypertrophy of sebaceous and sweat glands)

FIGURE 21-3. Clinical manifestations of acromegaly.

Corticotroph Adenomas Produce ACTH (Adrenocorticotropic Hormone)

ACTH excess induces adrenal cortical hypersecretion to produce **Cushing disease** (see below). In most cases, the tumor is a microadenoma that is intensely basophilic and periodic acid–Schiff-positive. Immunohistochemistry demonstrates ACTH and related peptides, such as endorphins and lipotropin. A few functional corticotroph adenomas are chromophobic and more aggressive than their basophilic counterparts.

Gonadotroph Adenomas Secretes Luteinizing Hormone (LH) and Follicle Stimulating Hormone (FSH)

Most of these tumors are macroadenomas that are hormonally inactive and are detected either incidentally or due to compressive effects. Clinical presentations include headache, visual disturbance, and hypopituitarism. In general, gonadotroph adenomas are chromophobic and periodic acid–Schiff-negative. Tumor cells are strongly immunoreactive for FSH, LH, or both. Treatment is surgical resection.

Thyrotroph Adenomas Produce Thyroid Stimulating Hormone (TSH)

Thyrotrope adenomas are the most rare of all pituitary adenomas and come to medical attention when there are symptoms of hyperthyroidism, goiter, or a pituitary mass lesion. Circulating levels of TSH and thyroid hormone are usually elevated, a situation unique to this tumor. Thyrotroph adenomas are chromophobic, with polyhedral or columnar cells forming collars around blood vessels. They stain for α and β-TSH. In patients with long-standing hypothyroidism, hyperplasia of pituitary thyrotrophs (thyroid deficiency cells) is secondary to inadequate feedback inhibition by thyroid hormones.

Nonfunctional Pituitary Adenomas Do Not Cause Endocrinopathies

One quarter of pituitary tumors removed surgically do not secrete excess hormones. They are slowly growing macroadenomas diagnosed in older persons because of their mass effect.

Posterior Pituitary

Central diabetes insipidus (Fig. 21-4) is the only significant disease associated with the posterior pituitary. It is characterized by an inability to concentrate urine and consequent chronic water diuresis (polyuria), thirst, and polydipsia caused by a deficiency of ADH (arginine vasopressin). One third of cases of central diabetes insipidus are of unknown etiology or can be attributed to sporadic or familial mutations in the vasopressin–neurophysin II gene. Mutations or deletions in the vasopressin V2-receptor (Xq28) and the vasopressin-sensitive aquaporin-2 water channel genes have also been described in the context of **nephrogenic diabetes insipidus**.

One fourth of cases of central diabetes insipidus are associated with brain tumors, particularly **craniopharyngioma**. This tumor arises above the sella turcica from remnants of Rathke pouch and invades and compresses adjacent tissues. Trauma and hypophysectomy for anterior pituitary tumors account for most remaining cases of diabetes insipidus. Polyuria may be controlled by powdered posterior pituitary or vasopressin given as snuff.

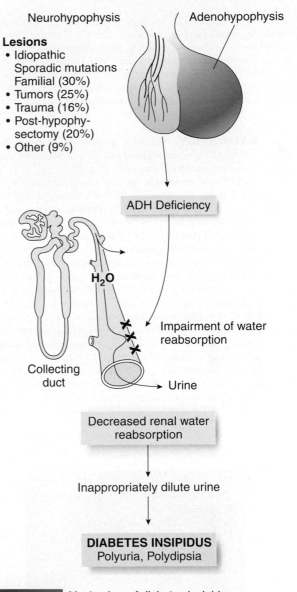

Neurohypophysis   Adenohypophysis

Lesions
- Idiopathic
  Sporadic mutations
  Familial (30%)
- Tumors (25%)
- Trauma (16%)
- Post-hypophy-
  sectomy (20%)
- Other (9%)

ADH Deficiency

H_2O

Impairment of water reabsorption

Collecting duct

Urine

Decreased renal water reabsorption

Inappropriately dilute urine

DIABETES INSIPIDUS
Polyuria, Polydipsia

FIGURE 21-4. Mechanism of diabetes insipidus.

THYROID GLAND

Nontoxic Goiter

Goiter refers to thyroid gland enlargement, either nodular or diffuse. It is classified according to its function.

Nontoxic goiter (from the Latin, guttur, *"throat"), also termed simple, colloid, or multinodular goiter, is enlargement of the thyroid without functional, inflammatory, or neoplastic alterations.* Thus, patients with nontoxic goiter are euthyroid and do not suffer from any form of thyroiditis (see below). The disease is far more common in women than in men (8:1). Diffuse goiter is frequent in adolescence and during pregnancy, whereas the multinodular type usually occurs in persons older than 50 years.

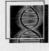 **PATHOGENESIS:** In nontoxic goiter, the capacity of the thyroid to produce thyroid hormone is impaired. The resulting increased secretion of TSH leads to enlargement of the gland, which maintains

the euthyroid state. The etiology of the decrease in thyroid hormone production is unknown. Simple nodular thyroid enlargement tends to be familial, suggesting a genetic factor in the disorder. Mutations in the thyroglobulin gene have been detected in a number of families affected by simple goiter. Goiters can develop in patients receiving a variety of medications, such as sulfonamides, or consuming excess iodine.

PATHOLOGY: Nontoxic goiters range from double the size of a normal gland (40 g) to a massive a thyroid weighing hundreds of grams (Fig. 21-5).

Diffuse nontoxic goiter characterizes the early stages of the disease. The gland is diffusely enlarged and microscopically exhibits hypertrophy and hyperplasia of the follicular epithelial cells. On occasion, the epithelium is papillary. At this stage, the amount of colloid in the follicles is decreased.

Multinodular nontoxic goiter reflects more chronic disease. The enlarged gland becomes increasingly nodular, and the cut surface is typically studded with numerous irregular nodules. When these nodules contain large amounts of colloid, the thyroid tends to be soft, glistening, and reddish. Microscopically, nodules vary considerably in size and shape. Some are distended with colloid; others are collapsed. Large colloid-containing follicles may fuse to form even larger "colloid cysts." The lining epithelial cells are flat to cuboidal and are occasionally arrayed as papillae that project into the follicular lumen. The individual follicles or groups of follicles are separated by dense fibrosis and dystrophic calcifications. Hemorrhage and chronic inflammation are common.

CLINICAL FEATURES: Patients with nontoxic goiter are typically asymptomatic with normal blood concentrations of thyroid hormones (T_4, T_3) and TSH; they come to medical attention because of a mass in the neck. Large goiters may cause dysphagia or inspiratory stridor by compressing the esophagus or trachea. Pressure on neck veins leads to venous congestion of the head and face. Hoarseness may result from recurrent laryngeal nerve compression. Occasionally, hemorrhage into a nodule or cyst leads to local pain. Nontoxic goiter is most commonly treated with thyroid hormone to reduce TSH levels and, thus, the stimulation to thyroid growth. Many patients with nontoxic goiter eventually develop hyperthyroidism, in which case the term **toxic multinodular goiter** is applied (see below).

Hypothyroidism

Hypothyroidism refers to the clinical manifestations of thyroid hormone deficiency. It can be the consequence of three general processes:

- **Defective thyroid hormone synthesis**, with compensatory goitrogenesis (goitrous hypothyroidism)
- **Inadequate thyroid parenchyma function**, usually due to thyroiditis, surgical resection of the gland, or therapeutic administration of radioiodine
- **Inadequate secretion of TSH** by the pituitary or of thyroid-releasing hormone (TRH) by the hypothalamus

Symptoms of hypothyroidism that develop insidiously reflect decreased circulating thyroid hormone (Fig. 21-6). Often, the first

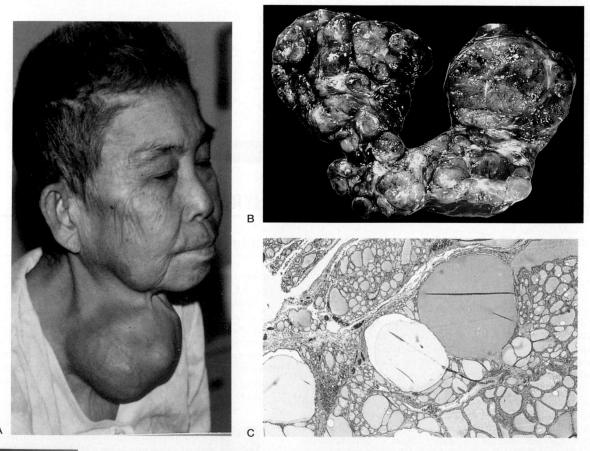

FIGURE 21-5. **Nontoxic goiter. A.** In a middle-aged woman with nontoxic goiter, the thyroid has enlarged to produce a conspicuous neck mass. **B.** Coronal section of the enlarged thyroid gland shows numerous irregular nodules, some with cystic degeneration and old hemorrhage. **C.** Microscopic view of one of the macroscopic nodules shows marked variation in follicle size.

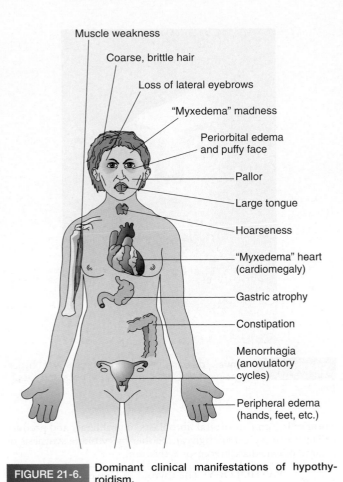

Muscle weakness

Coarse, brittle hair

Loss of lateral eyebrows

"Myxedema" madness

Periorbital edema and puffy face

Pallor

Large tongue

Hoarseness

"Myxedema" heart (cardiomegaly)

Gastric atrophy

Constipation

Menorrhagia (anovulatory cycles)

Peripheral edema (hands, feet, etc.)

FIGURE 21-6. Dominant clinical manifestations of hypothyroidism.

manifestations are tiredness, lethargy, sensitivity to cold, and inability to concentrate. Many organ systems are affected, and all are hypofunctional. Hypothy-roidism is treated effectively with thyroid hormone.

SKIN: Alterations in the skin are almost universal in patients with clinically apparent hypothyroidism. Proteogly-cans accumulate in the extracellular matrix and bind water, resulting in a peculiar form of edema termed **myxedema**. Myxedematous patients have boggy facies, puffy eyelids, edema of the hands and feet, and enlarged tongues. A pale, cool skin reflects cutaneous vasoconstriction. The skin is also dry and coarse, because sebaceous and sweat gland secretions are inadequate.

NERVOUS SYSTEM: Hypothyroidism in pregnancy has grave neurologic consequences for the fetus, expressed after birth as cretinism (see below). Hypothyroid adults are lethargic and somnolent and show memory loss and slowed mental processes. Psychiatric symptoms are prominent; paranoid ideation and depression are common. Severe agitation (**myxedema madness**) may develop.

HEART: In untreated hypothyroidism, so-called **myxedema heart** develops, which is characterized by a dilated heart and a pericardial effusion (see Chapter 11).

GASTROINTESTINAL TRACT: Constipation, due to decreased peristalsis, is common, and may be severe enough to lead to fecal impaction (**myxedema megacolon**).

REPRODUCTIVE SYSTEM: Women with hypothyroidism suffer ovulatory failure, progesterone deficiency, and irregular and excessive menstrual bleeding. In men, erectile dysfunction and oligospermia are common.

Primary (Idiopathic) Hypothyroidism is Often Autoimmune

Primary hypothyroidism is most common in the fifth and sixth decades and, like most thyroid disorders, is more common in women than in men. Three fourths of patients have circulating antibodies to thyroid antigens, suggesting that these cases represent the end stage of autoimmune thyroiditis (see below). Nongoitrous hypothyroidism may also result from antibodies that block TSH or TSH receptors without activating the thyroid. Some cases of primary hypothyroidism are part of multiglandular autoimmune syndrome (men), including insulin-dependent diabetes, pernicious anemia, hypoparathyroidism, adrenal atrophy, and hypogonadism (see below).

Goitrous Hypothyroidism Reflects Inadequate Secretion of Thyroid Hormone

There are a number of conditions in which thyroid enlargement (goiter) is associated with hypothyroidism. The etiology of goitrous hypothyroidism includes iodine deficiency, antithyroid agents (drugs or dietary goitrogens), long-term iodide intake, and a number of hereditary defects in thyroid hormone synthesis. *The evolution of the pathology of goitrous hypothyroidism is similar to that described earlier for nontoxic goiter.*

Endemic Goiter

Endemic goiter is goitrous hypothyroidism due to dietary iodine deficiency in locales with a high prevalence of the disease. The widespread availability of iodized salt has eliminated endemic goiter in many areas. Nevertheless, more than 200 million persons worldwide still have the disease. The pathologic evolution of endemic goiter is like that of nontoxic goiter (see above). However, unlike the latter, endemic goiter rarely causes hyperthyroidism. Administration of iodine may reverse the early, diffuse stage of endemic goiter but has little effect on a fully developed multinodular goiter. Replacement therapy with thyroid hormone is indicated, and local symptoms may necessitate surgical resection.

Goiter Induced by Antithyroid Agents and Iodide

A number of drugs and naturally occurring chemicals in foods suppress thyroid hormone synthesis and so are goitrogenic. Such goiters may or may not be associated with hypothyroidism. Common goitrogenic drugs include **lithium** (which is used to manage bipolar disorders), phenylbutazone, and *p*-aminosalicylic acid. Certain cruciferous vegetables (turnips, rutabaga, cassava) contain goitrogens, and their ingestion can potentiate an iodine-deficient diet to produce goitrous hypothyroidism. Goiter and hypothyroidism may also occur in persons who consume large amounts of iodide, either as a medicinal component (potassium iodide-containing expectorants) or in foods particularly rich in this halide (e.g., seaweed in Japan).

Congenital Hypothyroidism is also Termed Cretinism

Cretinism may be endemic, sporadic, or familial (see above) and is twice as frequent in girls as boys. In nonendemic regions, 90% of cases result from developmental defects of the thyroid (**thyroid dysgenesis**). The remainder principally has a variety of inherited metabolic defects, including mutations in the genes for thyroid releasing hormone (TRH) and its receptor, TSH and its receptor, sodium-iodide symporter, thyroglobulin, and thyroid oxidase.

 CLINICAL FEATURES: Symptoms of congenital hypothyroidism appear in the early weeks of life. Infants are apathetic and sluggish. Their abdomens are large and often show umbilical hernias. Body temperatures are often below 35°C (95°F), and the skin is pale and cold.

Refractory anemia and a dilated heart are frequent. By the age of 6 months, the clinical syndrome of congenital hypothyroidism is well developed. Mental retardation, stunted growth (due to defective osseous maturation), and characteristic facies are evident. Serum T_4 and T_3 levels are low, and TSH levels are high (unless the problem relates to a lack of TSH secretion itself). Prompt thyroid hormone replacement therapy is needed to prevent mental retardation and stunted growth. Although treatment may prevent dwarfism, its effects on mental development are more variable.

Hyperthyroidism

Hyperthyroidism refers to the clinical consequences of excessive circulating thyroid hormone. In general, signs and symptoms of hyperthyroidism reflect a hypermetabolic state of target tissues. Prolonged hypersecretion of thyroid hormone can result from (1) abnormal thyroid stimulator (Graves disease), (2) intrinsic disease of the thyroid gland (toxic multinodular goiter or functional adenoma), and (3) excess TSH production by a pituitary adenoma (rare).

Graves Disease is the Most Common Cause of Hyperthyroidism in Young Adults

Graves disease is an autoimmune disorder characterized by diffuse goiter, hyperthyroidism, exophthalmos (Fig. 21-7), and dermopathy. It is the most prevalent autoimmune disease in the United States, affecting 0.5% to 1% of the population under 40 years of age.

 PATHOGENESIS: The etiology of Graves disease is not fully understood and seems to involve an interplay between immune mechanisms, heredity, gender, and possibly emotional factors.

IMMUNE MECHANISMS: Patients have IgG antibodies that bind to the TSH receptor on the plasma membrane of thyrocytes. These antibodies act as agonists; that is, they stimulate the TSH receptor, thereby activating adenylyl cyclase and increasing thyroid hormone secretion. Under this continued stimulation, the thyroid becomes diffusely hyperplastic and excessively vascular.

GENETIC FACTORS: The strongest risk factor for Graves disease is a positive family history. No single gene is responsible, and the concordance rate in monozygotic twins is only 30% to 50%, whereas in dizygotic twins, it is merely 5%. Thus, both genetic and environmental factors are probably involved. Histocompatibility class II molecules (e.g., HLA-DR3, HLA-DQA1) increase the relative risk of Graves disease up to fourfold. Graves disease is also associated with polymorphism of cytotoxic T-lymphocyte antigen-4 (CTLA-4), which indicates the importance of autoreactive T cells. Patients with Graves disease and their relatives have a considerably higher incidence of other autoimmune diseases, including pernicious anemia and Hashimoto thyroiditis.

GENDER: Like other autoimmune diseases, Graves disease is far more common (7 to 10 times) in women than in men.

EMOTIONAL INFLUENCES: Endocrinologists have long observed that the onset of Graves disease often follows a period of emotional stress; however quantitative data are lacking.

SMOKING: Smoking is associated with an increased risk of Graves disease, and it increases the severity of the eye disease in patients who develop ophthalmopathy.

OPHTHALMOPATHY: Although exophthalmos (protrusion of eyeballs) is a common complication of Graves disease (see Fig. 21-7), its occurrence and severity correlate poorly with levels of thyroid hormone. Both T and B lymphocytes are sensitized to antigens shared by thyroid follicular cells and orbital fibroblasts.

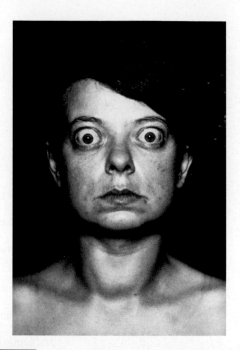

FIGURE 21-7. **Graves disease.** A young woman with hyperthyroidism displays a mass in the neck and exophthalmos.

These cells stimulate orbital fibroblasts to proliferate and produce collagen and glycosaminoglycans, either by cytokine synthesis or by antibody-mediated receptor activation.

 PATHOLOGY: The thyroid in Graves disease is symmetrically enlarged, usually 35 g to 100 g. The cut surfaces are firm and dark red. The tan translucence of normal thyroid, reflecting stored colloid, is notably absent. Microscopically, the gland is diffusely hyperplastic and highly vascular. The epithelial cells are tall and columnar and are often arranged as papillae that project into the lumen of the follicles. The colloid tends to be depleted and appears scalloped or "motheaten" where it abuts the epithelial cells (Fig. 21-8). Scattered B and T lymphocytes and plasma cells infiltrate the interstitial tissue and may even aggregate to form germinal follicles.

Exophthalmos is caused by enlargement of the orbital extraocular muscles that are swollen by mucinous edema, accumulation of fibroblasts, and lymphocyte infiltration. The increased orbital contents displace the eye forward (**proptosis**).

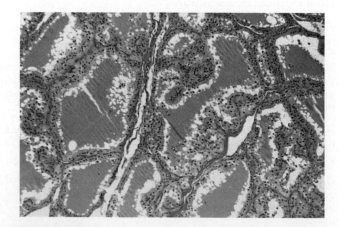

FIGURE 21-8. **Graves disease.** The follicles are lined by hyperplastic, tall columnar cells. Colloid is pink and scalloped at the periphery adjacent to the follicular cells.

CLINICAL FEATURES: Patients with Graves disease note a gradual onset of nonspecific symptoms, such as nervousness, emotional lability, tremor, weakness, and weight loss (Fig. 21-9). They are intolerant of heat, seek cooler environments, tend to sweat profusely, and may report palpitations. Excess thyroid hormone reduces systemic vascular resistance, enhances cardiac contractility, and increases the heart rate. In patients with pre-existing heart disease, congestive heart failure may ensue. Women develop oligomenorrhea, which may progress to amenorrhea.

Physical examination reveals a symmetrically enlarged thyroid, often with an audible bruit and a palpable thrill. Proptosis and retraction of the eyelids expose the sclera above the superior margin of the limbus. The skin is warm and moist, and some patients exhibit **Graves dermopathy**, a peculiar pretibial edema caused by fluid accumulation and glycosaminoglycans. The diagnosis is confirmed by increased thyroid radioactive iodine uptake, elevated serum levels of T_4 and T_3, and very low TSH.

The course of Graves disease is characterized by exacerbations and remissions. Treatment of the disorder includes the use of antithyroid medication such as thioisocyanate, destruction of thyroid tissue with radioactive iodine, and adjunctive therapy with corticosteroids and adrenergic antagonists. Surgical ablation is not often done. Unfortunately, despite successful relief of hyperthyroidism, exophthalmos often persists and may even worsen.

Toxic Multinodular Goiter Results from Functional Autonomy of Thyroid Nodules

Many patients with nontoxic multinodular goiter, usually over the age of 50, eventually develop a toxic form of the disease. Like its precursor disease, toxic goiter is 10 times more frequent in women than in men.

 PATHOGENESIS AND PATHOLOGY: The mechanisms by which nontoxic multinodular goiter assumes functional autonomy are not clear. In some patients, iodine uptake is diffuse and not affected by the administration of thyroid hormone. Microscopically, the thyroid shows groups of small hyperplastic follicles mixed with other nodules of varying size that appear to be inactive. A second pattern is characterized by focal accumulation of radiolabeled iodine in one or more nodules. Hyperfunction of these nodules suppresses the function of the rest of the thyroid. The functional nodules are clearly demarcated from the inactive areas histologically, contain large hyperplastic follicles, and thus resemble adenomas.

 CLINICAL FEATURES: Patients with toxic multinodular goiter usually have less severe symptoms of hyperthyroidism than those with Graves disease and never develop exophthalmos. Because patients with toxic goiter tend to be older, cardiac complications, including atrial fibrillation and congestive heart failure, may dominate the clinical presentation. Serum T_4 and T_3 levels are frequently only minimally elevated, and the uptake of radiolabeled iodine may be normal or only slightly elevated. Radiolabeled iodine following a course of antithyroid therapy is the most common treatment.

Toxic Adenoma is a Functional Neoplasm

Toxic adenoma is a benign, solitary, hyperfunctioning, follicular tumor in an otherwise normal thyroid. It is an infrequent cause of hyperthyroidism. Such tumors (1) display autonomous function, (2) are independent of TSH, and (3) are not suppressed if thyroid hormone is given. Hyperfunction of a toxic adenoma eventually

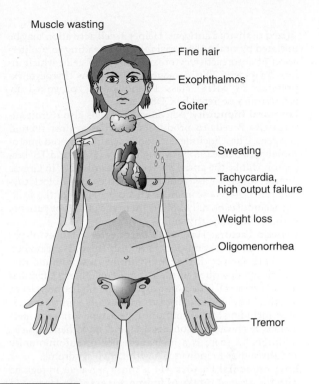

FIGURE 21-9. Major clinical manifestations of Graves disease.

suppresses the remainder of the thyroid, which then atrophies. Under these circumstances, a ^{131}I scintiscan shows a solitary focus of iodine uptake ("hot nodule") in a background of minimal uptake. Many, but not all, toxic adenomas exhibit a variety of somatic activating mutations of the TSH-receptor gene.

 CLINICAL FEATURES: Toxic thyroid adenoma is most common in the fourth and fifth decades of life. Because the normal thyroid tissue is suppressed, toxic adenoma is treated effectively with radiolabeled iodine. Large nodules may be excised surgically.

Thyroiditis

Thyroiditis describes a heterogeneous group of inflammatory disorders of the thyroid gland, including those that are caused by autoimmune mechanisms and infectious agents.

Chronic Autoimmune Thyroiditis (Hashimoto Thyroiditis) is the Most Common Cause of Goitrous Hypothyroidism in the United States

Hashimoto thyroiditis (HT) occurs predominantly in women between 30 and 50 years of age, although individuals of all ages can be affected. Patients present with diffuse thyroid enlargement accompanied by either mild hyperthyroidism or hypothyroidism. The disease can affect several family members, who often also suffer from other autoimmune conditions such as systemic lupus erythematosus, Graves disease, arteritis, and scleroderma.

 PATHOGENESIS: The pathogenesis of HT involves cellular and humoral immunity, genetic, and environmental factors.

- **Cellular Immunity:** The autoimmune process in HT arises from activation of CD4 (helper) T lymphocytes sensitized to thyroid antigens. Helper T-cell activation may be initiated by viral or bacterial infection, leading to proliferation of autoreactive cytotoxic (CD8+) T cells, which injure thyrocytes. This damage is followed by thyrocyte expression of MHC class II molecules, provoked by interferon-γ secreted by CD8+ cells

- **Humoral Immunity:** Activated CD4 cells also recruit autoreactive B cells to produce antibodies against thyroid antigens. These include antibodies against thyroid microsomal peroxidase (95%), thyroglobulin (60%), and TSH receptor. Unlike the anti-TSH receptor antibodies in Graves disease, which act as agonists, antibodies in HT block thyroid function. These immune effects account for the striking accumulation of lymphocytes in the glands of patients with autoimmune thyroiditis.

- **Genetic Factors:** Half of all first-degree relatives of patients with this condition have anti-thyroid antibodies, and both Graves disease and chronic autoimmune thyroiditis are described in these family members. A familial tendency for HT is demonstrated by the higher prevalence of other autoimmune diseases in patients and their relatives, including MEN syndrome type 2, type 1 diabetes, pernicious anemia, Addison disease, and myasthenia gravis. Additionally, there is a high incidence of autoimmunity and thyroiditis in individuals with Down syndrome.

- **Environmental Factors:** HT is most prevalent in regions with the greatest **intake of iodine,** for example, Japan and the United States. In iodine-deficient areas, iodine supplementation significantly increases the prevalence of chronic inflammation of the thyroid and the presence of thyroid autoantibodies.

 PATHOLOGY: On gross examination, the gland in patients with HT is diffusely enlarged and firm, weighing 60 to 200 g. The cut surface is pale tan and fleshy, with a vaguely nodular pattern (Fig. 21-10). The capsule is intact, and perithyroid tissues are not involved. Microscopically, the gland shows (1) a conspicuous infiltrate of lymphocytes and plasma cells, (2) destruction and atrophy of follicles, and (3) acidophilic metaplasia of follicular epithelial cells (**Hürthle** or **Askanazy cells**). Lymphoid follicles, often with germinal centers, are present.

 CLINICAL FEATURES: HT mainly affects women between 30 and 50 years of age, although no age group is spared. Patients present with diffuse thyroid enlargement and either mild hyperthyroidism or hypothyroidism. Eventually, one third to one half of all patients progress to an overt hypothyroid state, the risk of which is considerably greater among men than women. Many patients require no treatment. Thyroid hormone is given to alleviate hypothyroidism and to decrease the size of the gland. Surgery is reserved for patients who do not respond to suppressive hormone therapy or with troublesome pressure symptoms.

Subacute Thyroiditis (de Quervain, Granulomatous, or Giant Cell Thyroiditis) is Caused by a Viral Infection

Subacute thyroiditis, also known as granulomatous, de Quervain, or nonsuppurative thyroiditis, is an infrequent, self-limited disorder characterized by granulomatous inflammation. The disease typically occurs after upper respiratory viral infections, such as with influenza virus, adenovirus, echovirus, and coxsackievirus. Mumps virus has also been incriminated in some cases. de Quervain thyroiditis principally affects women between the ages of 30 and 50.

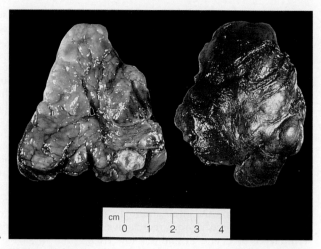

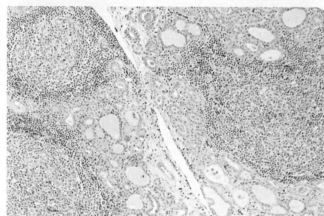

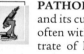 **FIGURE 21-10.** Chronic autoimmune (Hashimoto) thyroiditis. The thyroid gland is symmetrically enlarged and coarsely nodular. **A.** A coronal section of the right lobe shows irregular nodules and an intact capsule. **B.** A microscopic section of the thyroid reveals a conspicuous chronic inflammatory infiltrate and many atrophic thyroid follicles. The inflammatory cells form prominent lymphoid follicles with germinal centers.

 PATHOLOGY: The thyroid is enlarged to 40 to 60 g, and its cut surface is firm and pale. Acute inflammation, often with microabscesses, is followed by a patchy infiltrate of lymphocytes, plasma cells, and macrophages throughout the thyroid. Destruction of follicles allows the release of colloid, which elicits a conspicuous granulomatous reaction. Numerous foreign body-type, multinucleated giant cells, often containing colloid, are present. Although fibrosis of the thyroid may follow resolution of the inflammatory reaction, the normal thyroid architecture is usually restored.

CLINICAL FEATURES: Patients with subacute thyroiditis typically notice pain in the anterior neck, sometimes accompanied by fever, malaise, fatigue, and pain localized to the neck or radiating to the jaw. On physical examination, the thyroid is moderately enlarged and exquisitely tender. Subacute thyroiditis generally resolves within a few months without any clinical sequelae.

Riedel Thyroiditis Causes Fibrosis of the Thyroid

The "thyroiditis" in Riedel thyroiditis is something of a misnomer, as this rare disease also involves extrathyroidal soft tissues of the neck and is often associated with progressive fibrosis in other locations, including the retroperitoneum, mediastinum, and orbit.

Riedel thyroiditis is mainly a disease of middle age. The female-to-male ratio is 3:1. The etiology is unknown, but it does not appear to be related to other forms of thyroiditis. Patients with Riedel thyroiditis notice a gradual onset of painless goiter and present with a hard thyroid mass. Compression of the trachea (stridor), esophagus (dysphagia), and recurrent laryngeal nerve (hoarseness) may occur and are treated surgically

Follicular Adenoma of the Thyroid

Follicular adenoma is a benign clonal neoplasm showing follicular differentiation. It is the most common thyroid tumor and typically presents in euthyroid individuals as a solitary "cold" nodule, that is, a tumor that does not take up radiolabeled iodine. It is a solitary encapsulated neoplasm in which the cells are arranged in follicles resembling normal thyroid tissue or mimic stages in the embryonic development of the gland. Multiple adenomas may occur. Follicular adenoma is most common in the fourth and fifth decades, with a female-to-male ratio of 7:1.

 PATHOLOGY: Follicular adenoma appears as a solitary, circumscribed nodule 1 to 3 cm in diameter, which protrudes from the surface of the thyroid and is surrounded completely by a thin fibrous capsule. The cut surface of the tumor is soft and paler than the surrounding gland. Hemorrhage, fibrosis, and cystic change are common. There are several distinctive histologic patterns illustrated in Figure 21-11. Although these variants are of no particular clinical significance,

their recognition may be important in separating them from thyroid cancers. ***Atypical adenoma*** *is a follicular tumor that features mitoses, excessive cellularity, nuclear atypism, or equivocal capsular invasion, but for which a diagnosis of carcinoma cannot be established with certainty.*

Thyroid Cancer

Malignant thyroid neoplasms account for 0.4% of all cancer deaths in the United States. Approximately 25,000 new cases are diagnosed each year. The difficulty of distinguishing clinically between non-neoplastic lesions, benign tumors, and thyroid cancer is of major clinical and pathologic concern. Thyroid nodules are found in 1% to 10% of the population, but malignant tumors of the thyroid account for only about 1% of all cancers diagnosed. Most cases of thyroid carcinoma occur between the third and seventh decades, although children can also be affected. Tumors occur in women 2.5 times more often than in men.

Papillary Thyroid Carcinoma (PTC) is the Most Common Thyroid Cancer

PTC accounts for up to 90% of sporadic cases of thyroid cancer in the United States. It is most frequent between the ages of 20 and 50 years, with a female-to-male ratio of 3:1. However, it may arise at any age, and it is the most common thyroid tumor type in children and young adolescents. Elderly men have a worse prognosis with this type of thyroid cancer.

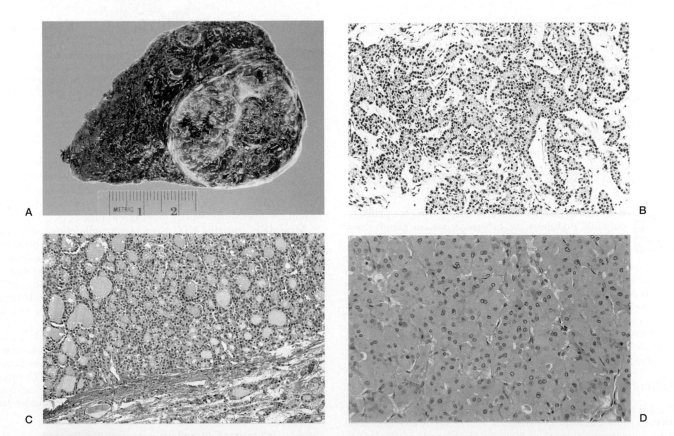

FIGURE 21-11. Follicular adenoma. **A.** Colloid adenoma. The cut surface of an encapsulated mass reveals hemorrhage, fibrosis, and cystic change. **B.** Embryonal adenoma. The tumor features a trabecular pattern with poorly formed follicles that contain little if any colloid. **C.** Fetal adenoma. A regular pattern of small follicles is noted. **D.** Hürthle cell adenoma. The tumor is composed of cells with small, regular nuclei and abundant eosinophilic cytoplasm.

PATHOGENESIS: Although the etiology of PTC remains to be established, a number of associations have been identified.

- **Iodine excess:** In endemic goiter regions, addition of iodine to the diet increased the proportion of thyroid cancers showing papillary, as compared with follicular, morphology.
- **Radiation:** External radiation to the neck of children and adults increases the incidence of later PTC.
- **Genetic factors:** Epidemiologic studies have reported a 4- to 10-fold higher risk for PTC in first-degree relatives of persons with that tumor. A concordance for PTC has been described in monozygotic twins. A familial form of PTC accounts for about 5% of all cases, but the genes responsible have not been identified.
- **Somatic mutations:** Somatic rearrangements of the *RET* protooncogene on chromosome 10 (10q11.2) are common in PTC, and 60% of such tumors in children exposed to radiation from the Chernobyl accident showed this mutation.

PATHOLOGY: PTCs vary from microscopic lesions to tumors larger than a normal gland. Serial sections of ostensibly normal thyroids obtained at autopsy have revealed a high proportion of papillary cancers that measure less than 1 mm across, but lymph node metastases in such cases are distinctly uncommon. Papillary cancers may be located anywhere in the gland, including the isthmus. PTCs are solid, and white-yellowish in color, with irregular and infiltrative borders. Lesions may be multiple and are occasionally encapsulated (Fig. 21-12A).

Microscopically, branching papillae are composed of a central fibrovascular core and a single or stratified lining of cuboidal to columnar cells (see Fig. 21-12B). Irregularly shaped or tubular neoplastic follicles are usually seen in the tumor, but the proportions of the papillary and follicular elements are highly variable. Nuclear atypism is an important diagnostic feature and includes clear (**ground-glass**) nuclei, eosinophilic pseudoinclusions (which represent invaginations of the cytoplasm into the nucleus), and nuclear grooves. Many papillary cancers show dense fibrosis. Calcospherites (**psammoma bodies**) are virtually diagnostic of papillary carcinoma and are seen in half of the cases. *PTC typically invades lymphatics and spreads to regional cervical lymph nodes.* Lymph node metastases vary from microscopic foci in otherwise normal lymph nodes to large masses that dwarf the primary lesion. Direct extension of PTC into soft tissues of the neck occurs in one fourth of cases. Hematogenous metastases are less common than in other varieties of thyroid cancer, but occur occasionally, mostly to the lungs.

CLINICAL FEATURES: PTC presents as (1) a painless, palpable nodule in an otherwise normal gland, (2) a nodule with enlarged cervical lymph nodes, or (3) cervical lymphadenopathy without a palpable thyroid nodule. Tumors larger than 0.5 cm can be detected as cold areas in a thyroid scintiscan. In general, the prognosis of PTC is excellent, and life expectancy for these patients differs little from that of the general population. In fatal cases of PTC, death is caused principally by metastases to the lungs or brain or by obstruction of the trachea or esophagus. Therapies include surgery (lobectomy or total thyroidectomy), with or without neck dissection, followed by the administration of radioiodine.

Follicular Thyroid Carcinoma (FTC) is Rarely Fatal

FTC is a purely follicular malignant tumor that contains no papillary or other elements. It includes approximately 15% to 30% of thyroid tumors. Most patients are older than 40 years of age, and the female-to-male ratio is 3:1. The incidence of follicular carcinoma is higher in endemic goiter areas among persons who do not receive iodine supplements. However, in regions where iodine is added to salt, such as the United States, FTC is uncommon, accounting for as few as 5% of all thyroid cancers.

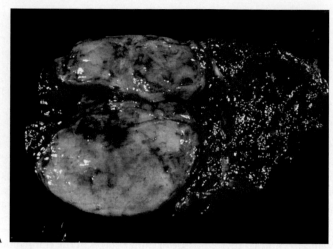

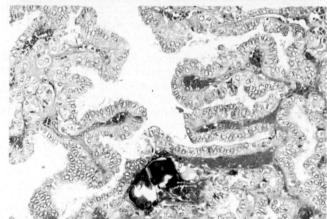

FIGURE 21-12. **Papillary carcinoma of the thyroid. A.** The cut surface of a surgically resected thyroid displays a circumscribed pale tan mass with foci of cystic change. **B.** Branching papillae are lined by neoplastic columnar epithelium with clear nuclei. A calcospherite, or psammoma body, is evident.

PATHOLOGY: Follicular cancer varies in size, has a yellow-tan color, and shows a thick white fibrous capsule. Areas of hemorrhage and necrosis are common, as are foci of cystic degeneration. FTCs are subdivided into minimally invasive and widely invasive variants.

Minimally invasive FTC is grossly a well-defined, encapsulated tumor. On cut section, it is soft and pale tan to pink and bulges from within its capsule. Microscopically, most lesions resemble follicular adenoma, although they tend more to exhibit a microfollicular or trabecular pattern. Mitoses are common, a feature that distinguishes follicular cancer from benign adenoma. Minimally invasive cancer is diagnosed when the tumor extends into, but not entirely through, the capsule.

Invasive FTC usually presents few diagnostic problems, because it extends through its capsule or shows vascular invasion (see Fig. 21-13), often within or adjacent to the capsule. The tumor may also extend into the surrounding soft tissues. FTC differs from PTC in that its metastases are blood-borne, rather than lymphatic, and are directed mainly to the bones of the shoulder and pelvic girdle, sternum, and skull.

CLINICAL FEATURES: Most follicular cancers are detected clinically as solitary palpable nodules or enlarged thyroids. Minimally invasive follicular tumors have a cure rate of at least 95%, compared with a survival rate of about 50% for the widely invasive form. FTC is treated with unilateral lobectomy. Metastases can be treated with radioiodine.

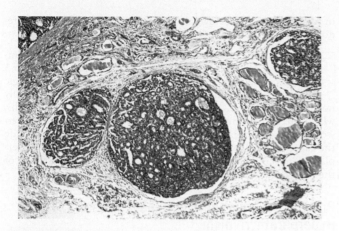

FIGURE 21-13. **Follicular carcinoma of the thyroid.** A microfollicular tumor has invaded veins in the thyroid parenchyma.

Medullary Thyroid Carcinoma (MTC) is Derived from C Cells of the Thyroid

Cells originate from the cells of the branchial pouches and secrete calcitonin as well as other peptides such as serotonin, ACTH, and somatostatin. MTC represents no more than 5% of all thyroid cancers. The disease occurs in sporadic and familial forms, the latter accounting for 20% of cases. Patients with the familial form of medullary carcinoma often have MEN type 2, which includes adrenal pheochromocytoma and parathyroid hyperplasia or adenoma. Somatic mutations in the *RET* protooncogene have been detected in 25% to 70% of cases of sporadic MTC. The mean age of patients with MTC is 50 years, but familial cases appear earlier (mean age, 20 years). There is a slight female predominance (1.5:1); in familial cases, the inheritance is autosomal dominant, and the gender distribution is equal.

 PATHOLOGY: On gross examination, MTCs tend to arise in the superior portion of the thyroid, the region richest in C cells. They are not encapsulated but are usually circumscribed. The cut surfaces are firm and grayish white. Characteristically, the tumor is solid, with polygonal, granular cells separated by a distinctly vascular stroma. However, the architectural patterns and appearances of the cells are highly variable. *A conspicuous feature is stromal amyloid, representing deposition of procalcitonin.* Nests of tumor cells are embedded in a hyalinized collagenous framework. Focal calcification is often present and may be extensive enough to be detected radiologically. In addition to amyloid, medullary carcinoma may contain mucin and melanin. Almost all of these tumors express carcinoembryonic antigen. Many are also positive for ACTH, serotonin, substance P, glucagon, insulin, and human chorionic gonadotropin.

MTC extends by direct invasion into soft tissues and metastasizes to regional lymph nodes, lung, liver, and bone. Sometimes, the initial presentation may be as metastatic disease. Metastases resemble primary tumors and also tend to contain amyloid.

The precursor lesion of the familial variety of MTC is C cell hyperplasia. Thus, patients with MEN types 2A and 2B (see section on adrenal medulla), are at risk for MTC and are monitored by periodic measurements of serum calcitonin, carcinoembryonic antigen, and sometimes chromogranin. When these levels are elevated, the patient is subjected to a total thyroidectomy.

 CLINICAL FEATURES: Patients with MTC often suffer symptoms related to endocrine secretion, including carcinoid syndrome (serotonin) and Cushing syndrome (ACTH). Watery diarrhea in one third of patients is caused by the secretion of vasoactive intestinal peptide, prostaglandins, and several kinins. In cases of familial MTC, patients may exhibit hyperparathyroidism, episodic hypertension, and other symptoms attributable to the secretion of catecholamines by pheochromocytoma.

The treatment of MTC is total thyroidectomy, but tumors recur locally in one third of patients. The prognosis depends on age (younger patients and women have better prognoses), as well as tumor size and stage. Other prognostic parameters include histologic type, mitotic count, necrosis, and amount of calcitonin present. The 5-year survival rate is 60% to 75%.

Anaplastic (Undifferentiated) Thyroid Carcinoma is Usually Fatal

Anaplastic thyroid cancer principally afflicts women (female-to-male ratio of 4:1) over the age of 60. The tumor constitutes 10% of thyroid cancers and is more common in areas of endemic goiter. In fact, at least half of patients suffer from long-standing goiter. In addition, many patients with anaplastic carcinoma have a history of a lower-grade thyroid cancer. Thus, it seems likely that the anaplastic variant often represents a transformation of a benign or low-grade thyroid neoplasm into a more poorly differentiated and more aggressive cancer. Mutations in the *p53* tumor suppressor gene are common in anaplastic cancers, but *RET* activation has not been observed.

 PATHOLOGY: Anaplastic carcinoma of the thyroid manifests as large, poorly circumscribed masses in the gland, which frequently extend into the soft tissues of the neck. The cut surface is hard and grayish white. The most common histologic pattern is a sarcoma-like proliferation of bizarre spindle and giant cells, with polyploid nuclei, many mitoses, necrosis, and stromal fibrosis (Fig. 21-14). The tumor tends to invade veins and arteries, often occluding the vessels and producing foci of infarction within the tumor.

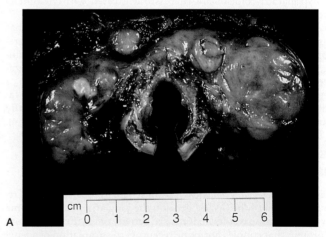

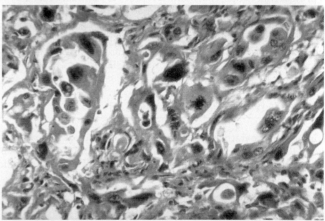

FIGURE 21-14. **Anaplastic carcinoma of the thyroid. A.** The tumor in transverse section partially surrounds the trachea and extends into the adjacent soft tissue. **B.** The tumor is composed of bizarre spindle and giant cells with polyploid nuclei and numerous mitoses.

CLINICAL FEATURES: Anaplastic tumors compress and destroy local structures. Accordingly, the tumor presents as a rapidly enlarging neck mass associated with symptoms such as dysphagia, hoarseness, dyspnea, and enlargement of cervical nodes. The prognosis is dismal, and widespread metastases are frequent. Less than 10% of patients survive for 5 years. Treatment with radiation and chemotherapy has had little success.

PARATHYROID GLANDS

Hypoparathyroidism

Hypoparathyroidism results from decreased secretion of PTH or end-organ insensitivity (pseudohypoparathyroidism) due to congenital or acquired conditions. The disease is clinically characterized by hypocalcemia and hyperphosphatemia.

Hypoparathyroidism is Most Often due to Surgical Removal of the Parathyroids at the Time of Thyroidectomy

The symptoms of hypoparathyroidism relate to hypocalcemia. Increased neuromuscular excitability may cause mild tingling in the hands and feet, severe muscle cramps, tetany, laryngeal stridor, and convulsions. Neuropsychiatric manifestations include depression, paranoia, and psychoses. High cerebrospinal fluid pressure and papilledema may mimic a brain tumor. Patients with all forms of hypoparathyroidism are successfully treated with vitamin D and calcium supplementation.

Familial isolated hypoparathyroidism is a rare disorder that has variable inheritance patterns and reflects deficient PTH secretion. **Familial hypoparathyroidism** may be part of a polyglandular syndrome that includes adrenal insufficiency and mucocutaneous candidiasis. **Idiopathic hypoparathyroidism** is a heterogeneous group of uncommon conditions, sporadic and familial, that share deficient secretion of PTH. **Agenesis of the parathyroid glands** is part of DiGeorge syndrome (see Chapter 4).

Pseudohypoparathyroidism Reflects Target Organ Insensitivity to PTH

This group of hereditary conditions is characterized by hypocalcemia and reflects mutation of the GNAS1 gene on the long arm of chromosome 20. The mutation results in decreased activity of G_s, the stimulatory G protein that couples hormone receptors to stimulation of adenyl cyclase. Consequently, in renal tubular epithelium, production of cAMP in response to PTH is impaired, and inadequate resorption of calcium from glomerular filtrate ensues. Patients with pseudohypoparathyroidism are also often resistant to other cAMP-coupled hormones, including TSH, glucagon, FSH, and LH.

Primary Hyperparathyroidism

Primary hyperparathyroidism may be caused by a parathyroid adenoma (80% to 90%), hyperplasia of all parathyroids (10% to 15%), or (rarely) parathyroid carcinoma (1% to 5%). PTH can be sporadic or part of familial syndromes such as MEN-1 and MEN-2A.

Parathyroid Adenoma Accounts for Most Cases of Hyperparathyroidism

Parathyroid adenoma is responsible for 85% of all primary hyperparathyroidism. These tumors arise sporadically or in the context of MEN-1 (20%, see below). Adenomas occur at any age but predominate after 50 years of age.

 PATHOLOGY: A parathyroid adenoma is a circumscribed, reddish-brown, solitary mass, measuring 1 to 3 cm in diameter and weighing 0.05 to 200 g. Hemorrhagic areas are common, and cystic changes are occasionally noted. Microscopically, they show sheets of neoplastic chief cells, which often show nuclear pleomorphism in a rich capillary network. A rim of normal parathyroid tissue is usually evident outside the capsule and distinguishes adenomas from parathyroid hyperplasia. Unaf-fected glands tend to be atrophic. Surgical resection of the tumor relieves the symptoms of hyperparathyroidism.

Primary Parathyroid Hyperplasia Causes 15% of Hyperparathyroidism

About 75% of cases occur in women. Of these, about 20% are associated with familial hyperparathyroidism or MEN syndromes (MEN types 1 and 2A). One third of cases of sporadic primary parathyroid hyperplasia are monoclonal, suggesting a neoplastic proliferation. In such instances, both chief cell hyperplasia and multiple small adenomas are seen in the same gland. Factors associated with sporadic primary hyperparathyroidism include external radiation and lithium ingestion.

 PATHOLOGY: Grossly, all four parathyroid glands are enlarged, combined weights ranging from under 1 g to 10 g. In half of the patients, one gland is noticeably larger than the others, which may make the distinction from adenoma difficult. Microscopically, the normal glandular adipose tissue is replaced by hyperplastic chief cells arranged in sheets or trabecular or follicular patterns. An important feature that distinguishes hyperplasia from adenoma is the lack of pleomorphism in the former.

Parathyroid Carcinoma Accounts for 1% of Hyperparathyroidism

Parathyroid carcinoma is rare, occurring in both genders principally between the ages of 30 and 60 years. It is usually a functioning tumor, and most patients present with symptoms of hyperparathyroidism. The etiology of this tumor is not known, but neck radiation and hereditary syndromes with a history of parathyroid adenoma are considered risk factors.

PATHOLOGY: Parathyroid carcinomas tend to be larger than adenomas and appear as lobulated, firm, tannish, unencapsulated masses, often adherent to surrounding soft tissues. Microscopically, most show a trabecular pattern, with significant mitotic activity and thick fibrous bands. Capsular or vascular invasion is occasionally noted. Importantly, the cell atypism often seen in parathyroid adenomas is rare in carcinomas.

After surgical removal, local recurrence is common; about one third of patients develop metastases to regional lymph nodes, lungs, liver, and bone. The 10-year survival rate is approximately 50%, with death most often attributed to hyperparathyroidism.

Clinical Features of Hyperparathyroidism are Highly Variable

Hypercalcemia and hypophosphatemia are characteristic of hyperparathyroidism, although some patients have asymptomatic disease detected only on routine blood analysis. Others show florid systemic, renal, and skeletal disease (Fig. 21-15). Excessive parathyroid hormone (PTH) leads to excessive loss of calcium from bones and enhanced calcium resorption by the renal tubules. The production of the activated form of vitamin D (1,25[OH]$_2$D) by renal tubules is

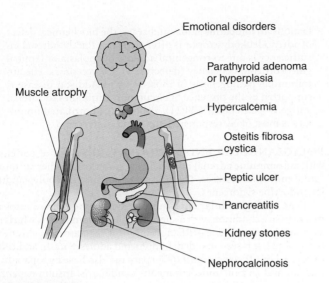

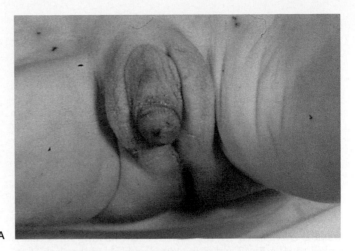

FIGURE 21-15. Major clinical features of hyperparathyroidism.

also stimulated by PTH, thereby increasing intestinal calcium absorption. The action of PTH on the kidney, together with hypercalcemia, leads to hypophosphatemia. Common symptoms include nausea, vomiting, fatigue, weight loss, anorexia, polyuria, and polydipsia. A neck mass is palpable in many patients. The classic bone lesions of hyperparathyroidism are known as **osteitis fibrosa cystica**, which occurs in a minority of patients who have an accelerated form of the disease. The kidney as well as nervous and gastrointestinal systems are also affected. See Chapter 26 for a detailed discussion.

Secondary Hyperparathyroidism

Secondary parathyroid hyperplasia is seen mainly in patients with chronic renal failure, but it also occurs in association with vitamin D deficiency, intestinal malabsorption, Fanconi syndrome, and renal tubular acidosis. Chronic hypocalcemia due to renal retention of phosphate, inadequate $1,25(OH)_2D$ production by diseased kidneys, and some skeletal resistance to PTH all lead to compensatory PTH hypersecretion. Secondary hyperplasia of all parathyroids produces excess levels of PTH, which cause the osseous manifestations of hyperparathyroidism, termed **renal osteodystrophy** (see Chapter 26).

ADRENAL CORTEX

Congenital Adrenal Hyperplasia (CAH)

Congenital adrenal hyperplasia (CAH) results from several autosomal recessive enzyme defects in the biosynthesis of cortisol from cholesterol. The extent of the defects varies from mild to complete deficiencies. In general, a deficiency in corticosteroid synthesis results in the unopposed action of ACTH and hence adrenal hyperplasia. CAH occurs equally in males and females and is the most common cause of ambiguous genitalia in newborn girls (Fig. 21-16A).

 PATHOLOGY: The adrenal glands are enlarged, weighing as much as 30 g (see Fig. 21-16B). The cut surface is soft, tan to brown, and either diffusely enlarged or nodular. Microscopically, the cortex is widened between the medulla and the zona glomerulosa (see Fig. 21-16C). The hyperplastic zone is filled by compact, granular, eosinophilic cells. In most cases, the zona glomerulosa is also hyperplastic, although not to the extent of the other zones, especially the zona fasciculata.

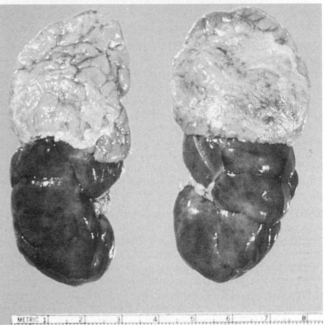

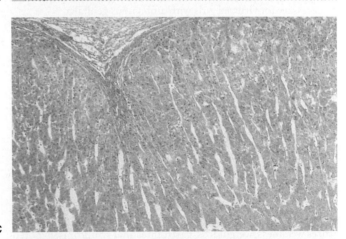

FIGURE 21-16. **Congenital adrenal hyperplasia. A.** A female infant is markedly virilized with hypertrophy of the clitoris and partial fusion of labioscrotal folds. **B.** A 7-week-old male died of severe salt-wasting congenital adrenal hyperplasia. At autopsy, both adrenal glands were markedly enlarged. **C.** A microscopic view shows a widened cortex containing compact eosinophilic cells.

21-Hydroxylase (P450$_{C21}$) Deficiency

The gene for P450$_{C21}$ (CYP21) is linked to the *MHC* locus on the short arm of chromosome 6 (6p21.3.) and is closely associated with *HLA-B* and the *C4A* and *C4B* complement genes. Mutations in this gene are responsible for more than 90% of cases of CAH. The incidence of this disease varies from about 1 in 10,000 among whites to 1 in 500 in Alaskan Eskimos. P450$_{C21}$ is a microsomal enzyme that converts 17-hydroxyprogesterone to 11-deoxycortisol. A deficiency in this enzymatic activity impairs cortisol biosynthesis, and accumulated precursors are instead converted to androgens.

 CLINICAL FEATURES: Classic CAH caused by P450$_{C21}$ deficiency manifests as several genetically distinct syndromes. Two variants affect newborns. One is **simple virilizing CAH**, in which there are low levels (about 2%) of residual enzyme activity; the other is a **salt-wasting form** that is linked to HLA-Bw47 and is associated with a complete lack of enzyme activity. There is also a less severe, late-onset (nonclassic) variant associated with somewhat higher levels of enzyme activity.

SIMPLE VIRILIZING CAH: Conversion of cortisol precursors into adrenal androgens is increased owing to the ACTH-dependent increase in the size of the gland. Female newborns exposed to a large excess of adrenal androgens in utero exhibit pseudohermaphroditism and are born with fused labia, an enlarged clitoris, and a urogenital sinus that may be mistaken for a penile urethra (see Fig. 21-16A). The sexual ambiguity may cause the infant to be mislabeled as male. Affected males exhibit no abnormalities of the sexual organs but experience sexual precocity. Eventually, the high levels of adrenal androgens lead to the premature closure of epiphyses and short stature. Adult women with CAH tend to be infertile, whereas men with CAH may or may not be fertile.

SALT-WASTING CAH: Aldosterone synthesis may be impaired because of 21-hydroxylase deficiency. As a result, hypoaldosteronism develops within the first few weeks of life in two thirds of newborns with the most severe form of CAH, manifested as hyponatremia, hyperkalemia, dehydration, hypotension, and increased renin secretion. These effects may be rapidly fatal if the disease is untreated (see Fig. 21-16B). Both variants of CAH caused by P450$_{C21}$ deficiency are treated with glucocorticoids and mineralocorticoids to suppress ACTH and replace steroids. Reconstructive surgery may be necessary for virilized girls with ambiguous genitalia.

Adrenal Cortical Insufficiency

Deficient production of adrenal cortical hormones can result from (1) adrenal gland destruction, (2) pituitary or hypothalamic dysfunction with decreased ACTH production, or (3) chronic corticosteroid therapy.

Primary Chronic Adrenal Insufficiency (Addison Disease) Often Reflects an Autoimmune Destruction of the Adrenal Glands

Addison disease is a fatal wasting disorder caused by failure of the adrenal glands to produce glucocorticoids, mineralocorticoids, and androgens. It causes weakness, weight loss, gastrointestinal symptoms, hypotension, electrolyte imbalance, and hyperpigmentation.

 PATHOGENESIS: In Western societies, autoimmunity is responsible for 75% of cases of chronic adrenal insufficiency although worldwide, tuberculosis is likely to be the most common cause. Autoimmune adrenalitis may be an isolated disorder or a part of two different polyglandular autoimmune syndromes. Other causes of adrenal destruction include metastatic carcinoma, amyloidosis, hemorrhage, sarcoidosis, and fungal in-fections. In idiopathic Addison disease, the biochemical defect of adreno-leukodystrophy is often detected. Rarely, adrenal insufficiency is due to congenital adrenal hypoplasia or familial glucocorticoid deficiency (defective ACTH receptor). The autoimmune pathogenesis of most cases of Addison disease is supported by the presence of circulating antibodies to adrenal antigens (particularly CYP21), although cell-mediated immunity is most likely responsible for gland destruction.

POLYGLANDULAR ENDOCRINOPATHIES: Half of patients with autoimmune adrenal insufficiency suffer from other autoimmune endocrine diseases. These are grouped into two polyglandular endocrine syndromes.

Type I polyglandular autoimmune syndrome is a rare autosomal recessive condition with a slight female predominance, which is associated with the gene *AIRE* (autoimmune regulator) on chromosome 21q22. It is seen in older children and adolescents. In addition to adrenal insufficiency, most (60%) patients also have hypoparathyroidism and chronic mucocutaneous candidiasis. Insulin-dependent diabetes (type I) is common. Premature ovarian failure, hypothyroidism, malabsorption syndromes, pernicious anemia, chronic hepatitis, alopecia totalis, and vitiligo are also encountered.

Type II polyglandular autoimmune syndrome (Schmidt syndrome) is more common than type I and always includes adrenal insufficiency. Women are affected twice as often as men. The disorder usually manifests between 20 and 40 years of age. Half of the cases are familial, but several modes of inheritance are known. Autoimmune thyroiditis and occasionally Graves disease occur in more than two thirds of cases. Insulin-dependent diabetes mellitus and premature ovarian failure are common. This condition is considered to be a polygenic disorder with linkage to genes associated with the MHC complex.

 PATHOLOGY: More than 90% of the adrenal gland must be destroyed before chronic adrenal insufficiency is symptomatic. Autoimmune adrenalitis leads to pale, irregular, shrunken glands, weighing 2 to 3 g or less. The medulla is intact but surrounded by fibrous tissue containing small islands of atrophic cortical cells (Fig. 21-17). Depending on the stage of the disease, lymphoid infiltrates, predominantly T cells, of varying density are encountered.

 CLINICAL FEATURES: Typically, the first symptom is an insidious onset of weakness, which may become so profound that a patient is bedridden. Anorexia and weight loss are invariably present. A diffuse tan pigmentation usually develops on the skin, and dark patches may appear on the mucous membranes. This hyperpigmentation is related to the skin melanocyte—stimulating hormone (MSH) activity derived from pituitary

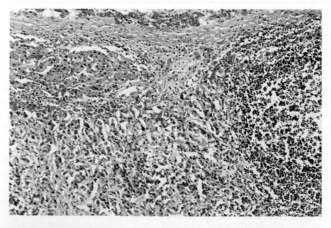

FIGURE 21-17. Autoimmune adrenalitis. A section of the adrenal gland from a patient with Addison disease shows chronic inflammation and fibrosis in the cortex, an island of residual atrophic cortical cells, and an intact medulla.

proopiomelanocortin. Hypotension, with blood pressures in the range of 80/50 mm Hg, is the rule. A variety of gastrointestinal symptoms, including vomiting, diarrhea, and abdominal pain, affects most patients and may be the presenting complaint. Patients with Addison disease often exhibit marked personality changes and even organic brain syndromes. With glucocorticoid and mineralocorticoid replacement, patients live normal lives.

Acute Adrenal Insufficiency is a Life-Threatening Emergency

Acute adrenal insufficiency, or adrenal crisis, reflects a sudden loss of adrenal cortical function. Symptoms are related more to mineralocorticoid deficiency than to inadequate glucocorticoids. Adrenal crisis occurs in three settings:

- Abrupt withdrawal of corticosteroid therapy in patients with adrenal atrophy is due to long-term administration of these steroids. This is the most common cause of acute adrenal insufficiency.
- Sudden, devastating worsening of chronic adrenal insufficiency may be precipitated by the stress of infection or surgery.

- *Waterhouse-Friderichsen syndrome is acute, bilateral, hemorrhagic infarction of the adrenal cortex, most commonly secondary to meningococca or* Pseudomonas *septicemia* (see Chapter 7).

 CLINICAL FEATURES: The initial manifestations of adrenal crisis are usually hypotension and shock. Nonspecific symptoms commonly include weakness, vomiting, abdominal pain, and lethargy, which may progress to coma. Typically in Waterhouse-Friderichsen syndrome, a young person suddenly develops hypotension and shock, together with abdominal or back pain, fever, and purpura. Adrenal crisis is almost invariably fatal unless the patient is promptly and aggressively treated with corticosteroids and supportive measures.

Adrenal Hyperfunction

Excess corticosteroid secretion occurs in adrenal hyperplasia or neoplasia (Fig. 21-18). Such hyperfunction may take one of two forms,

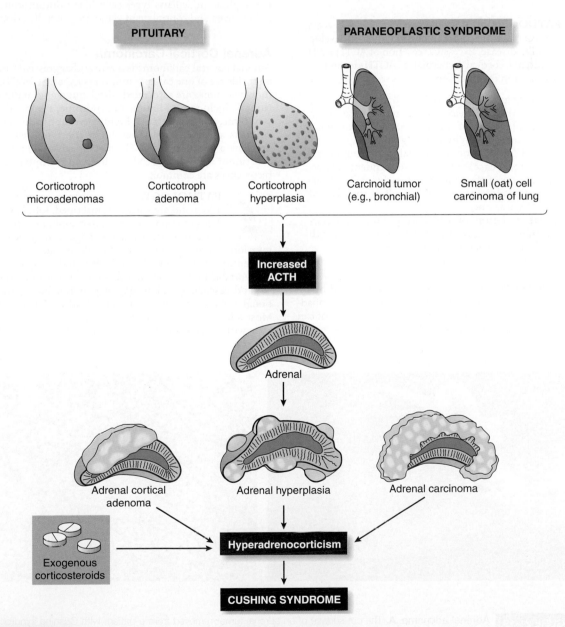

PITUITARY

Corticotroph microadenomas

Corticotroph adenoma

Corticotroph hyperplasia

PARANEOPLASTIC SYNDROME

Carcinoid tumor (e.g., bronchial)

Small (oat) cell carcinoma of lung

Increased ACTH

Adrenal

Adrenal cortical adenoma

Adrenal hyperplasia

Adrenal carcinoma

Exogenous corticosteroids

Hyperadrenocorticism

CUSHING SYNDROME

FIGURE 21-18. **The pathogenetic pathways of Cushing syndrome.** The ACTH-dependent pathway is referred to as Cushing disease. ACTH, adrenocorticotrophic hormone (corticotropin).

namely, **hypercortisolism** (Cushing syndrome) or **hyperaldosteronism** (Conn syndrome), disorders reflecting the two major classes of adrenal steroid hormones.

The constellation of clinical features (mainly obesity, hypertrichosis and amenorrhea, which reflects high glucocorticoid levels) can also result from pituitary hyperfunction, adrenal adenoma or carcinoma, ectopic production of ACTH or corticotropin-releasing hormone by a tumor, or exogenous administration of corticosteroids. Hypercorti-solism from any cause is now referred to as **Cushing syndrome**, and the term **Cushing disease** is reserved for excessive secretion of ACTH by pituitary corticotroph tumors. Excess secretion of ACTH by pituitary tumors is five times more common than hyperproduction of corticosteroids by adrenal tumors. The most common cause of Cushing syndrome in the United States is chronic corticosteroid administration to treat immune and inflammatory disorders. The second most common cause is a paraneoplastic effect associated with nonpituitary cancers that inappropriately produce ACTH.

ACTH-Dependent Adrenal Hyperfunction is of Pituitary or Ectopic Origin

 PATHOGENESIS: Women, usually 25 to 45 years old, are five times more likely than men to develop Cushing disease. Excessive secretion of ACTH leads to adrenal cortical hyperplasia. ACTH-dependent adrenal hyperfunction results from:

- Primary hypersecretion of ACTH by the pituitary (Cushing disease). The disease usually results from corticotroph microadenomas of the pituitary, or, in a few patients, diffuse corticotroph hyperplasia.
- Ectopic ACTH production by a malignant tumor accounts for most cases of ACTH-dependent hyperadrenalism. Cancer of the lung, particularly small cell carcinoma, is responsible for more than half of the cases of ectopic ACTH syndrome.
- Inappropriate secretion of corticotropin-releasing hormone by tumors arising outside the hypothalamus, with secondary pituitary hypersecretion of ACTH

 PATHOLOGY: Cushing disease is characterized by bilateral, diffuse (75%), or nodular (25%) hyperplasia of adrenal glands. Each gland usually weighs 8 to 10 g but can occasionally weigh as much as 20 g.

ACTH-Independent Adrenal Hyperfunction is Caused by Adrenal Tumors

In adults, the incidence of adrenal carcinoma peaks at 40 years of age and that of adenoma a decade later. In children, adrenal carcinoma accounts for one half of Cushing syndrome cases; 15% are caused by adenoma. At all ages, the female-to-male ratio is 4:1.

Adrenal Adenoma

 PATHOLOGY: Adenomas of the adrenal cortex are uncommon. A typical adenoma is encapsulated, firm, yellow, and slightly lobulated, measuring about 4 cm in diameter (Fig. 21-19). These tumors usually weigh 10 to 50 g, although weights up to 100 g have been recorded. The cut surface is mottled yellow and brown and occasionally black, owing to the deposition of lipofuscin pigment. A thin rim of compressed normal adrenal cortex surrounds the tumor. Necrosis and calcification may be present, even in small tumors. Microscopically, adenomas exhibit clear, lipid-laden (fasciculata type) cells arranged in sheets or nests, often with interspersed clusters of compact, lipid-depleted, eosinophilic (reticularis type) cells. The nontumorous cortexes of the involved and contralateral gland are generally atrophic.

Adrenal Cortical Carcinoma

Adrenal cortical carcinoma is a rare and aggressive tumor that has an incidence of one case per million per year. Several hereditary tumor syndromes are associated with benign and malignant adrenal tumors, including Li-Fraumeni syndrome, Beckwith-Wiedemann syndrome, and MEN type 1. Eighty percent of adrenal cortical carcinomas are functional. They occur more frequently in women and have a poor prognosis. The median survival rate is 30 months. The tumor metastasizes to lung, liver, and lymph nodes, and local recurrences are common.

 PATHOLOGY: The tumors weigh more than 100 g and are soft, circumscribed, lobulated, and bulky. The cut surface is variegated pink, brown, or yellow, often with necrosis, hemorrhage, and cystic change. Local invasion is common, and remnants of normal adrenal are difficult to identify. Microscopically, both clear and compact cells are present. Variable nuclear pleomorphism is seen. Mitotic figures, necrosis, and vascular invasion may or may not be apparent. In functional carcinomas, the contralateral adrenal cortex is atrophic. Most adrenal cortical carcinomas cannot be resected completely. Even with surgery, most patients survive for only 1 to 3 years.

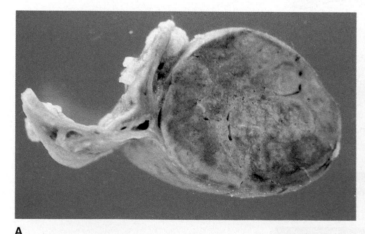

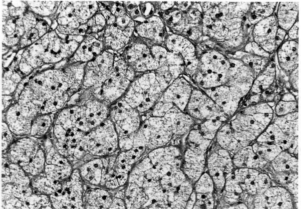

A   **B**

FIGURE 21-19. Adrenal adenoma. **A.** The cut surface of an adrenal tumor removed from a patient with Cushing syndrome is a mottled yellow with a rim of compressed normal adrenal tissue. **B.** A microscopic view reveals nests of clear, lipid-laden cells.

ACTH-Independent Cushing Syndrome May Result from Chronic Corticosteroid Administration

Many immunologic and inflammatory diseases are treated with glucocorticoids, constituting by far the most common cause of Cushing syndrome. The synthetic hormones ordinarily used (e.g., dexamethasone, prednisone) have only glucocorticoid activity and few or no mineralocorticoid or androgen effects. Thus, hypertension and hirsutism, features commonly seen in Cushing syndrome due to adrenal hyperplasia or neoplasia, are usually absent in this iatrogenic disorder.

Clinical Features of Cushing Syndrome are Seen in Many Organs

 CLINICAL FEATURES: The manifestations of Cushing syndrome (Fig. 21-20) depend on the degree and duration of excessive corticosteroid levels, as well as on the levels of adrenal androgens and mineralocorticoids.

OBESITY: Typically, the patient notes a gradual onset of obesity of the face (moon face), neck (buffalo hump), trunk, and abdomen. The extremities are characteristically unaffected or even wasted.

SKIN: The skin is atrophic, and subcutaneous fat is decreased. Enlargement of the abdomen and other areas of fat deposition stretches the thin skin and produces purplish striae, which represent venous channels that are visible through the attenuated dermis.

MUSCULOSKELETAL SYSTEM: Increased bone resorption causes osteoporosis. Back pain is common, and up to one fifth of patients with Cushing syndrome have radiologic evidence of vertebral compression fractures. Proximal muscle wasting (**steroid myopathy**) causes weakness, which may be so severe that the patient cannot rise from sitting or climb a flight of stairs.

CARDIOVASCULAR SYSTEM: Hypertension is common in Cushing syndrome, often reflecting excessive mineralocorticoid activity. In older patients, congestive heart failure is a frequent sequel.

SECONDARY SEX CHARACTERISTICS: Women with Cushing syndrome tend to be virilized, with increased facial hair, thinning of scalp hair, acne, and oligomenorrhea. Excess glucocorticoid levels in men cause erectile dysfunction, and both genders experience decreased libido.

GLUCOSE INTOLERANCE: Stimulation of gluconeogenesis by glucocorticoids leads to glucose intolerance and hyperinsulinemia. Diabetes mellitus develops in 15% of patients, usually in those with a family history of diabetes.

PSYCHOLOGICAL CHANGES: Most patients with Cushing syndrome, both endogenous and iatrogenic, suffer distinct personality changes. These include irritability, emotional lability, depression, and paranoia. The disturbance in mentation may be so severe that the patient becomes suicidal.

Cushing syndrome is treated by (1) extirpation (surgery or irradiation) of pituitary, adrenal, or ectopic ACTH-producing tumors; (2) discontinuation of corticosteroid therapy; or (3) administration of adrenal enzyme inhibitors (e.g., aminoglutethimide, ketoconazole, metapyrone). Cushing syndrome is highly curable when not associated with malignant neoplastic tumors.

Primary Aldosteronism (Conn Syndrome) Leads to Hypertension and Hypokalemia

Inappropriate secretion of aldosterone is caused by adrenal adenomas or hyperplasia. Aldosterone-secreting adenomas are more common in women than in men (3:1) and usually occur between the ages of 30 and 50 years.

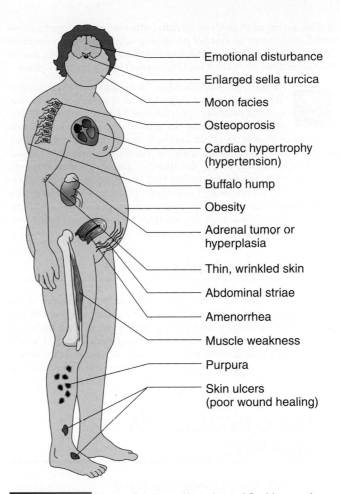

 FIGURE 21-20. Major clinical manifestations of Cushing syndrome.

- Emotional disturbance
- Enlarged sella turcica
- Moon facies
- Osteoporosis
- Cardiac hypertrophy (hypertension)
- Buffalo hump
- Obesity
- Adrenal tumor or hyperplasia
- Thin, wrinkled skin
- Abdominal striae
- Amenorrhea
- Muscle weakness
- Purpura
- Skin ulcers (poor wound healing)

 PATHOGENESIS: About 75% of cases of primary aldosteronism are caused by solitary adrenal adenomas (aldosteronoma). In one-quarter of cases, adrenal hyperplasia is involved. The remainder reflect bilateral hyperplasia of the adrenal zona glomerulosa. Only a few cases of primary aldosteronism are caused by adrenal carcinomas.

Two types of familial hyperaldosteronism are defined. **Type I (glucocorticoid-suppressible)** is an autosomal dominant disease in which the ACTH-responsive regulatory elements of the 11β-hydroxylase gene are fused to the aldosterone synthase gene, resulting in a hybrid aldosterone-producing gene. The fusion gene is ectopically and constitutively activated in the zona fasciculata, and bilateral hyperplasia of this zone results. By suppressing ACTH release, glucocorticoids ameliorate type I disease. By contrast, **type II familial hyperaldosteronism** is associated with adrenal cortical adenomas and is, therefore, not suppressible by glucocorticoids.

Aldosterone hypersecretion enhances renal tubular sodium reabsorption, thereby increasing body sodium. Hypertension is caused not only by retention of sodium and consequent volume expansion but also by increased peripheral vascular resistance. Hypokalemia reflects aldosterone-induced loss of potassium in the distal renal tubule.

PATHOLOGY: Most aldosterone-secreting adenomas measure less than 3 cm in diameter, weigh less than 6 g, and are yellow. However, the size varies, and tumors up to 50 g are reported. On microscopic examination, the dominant cells are clear and lipid-rich, resembling the zona fasciculata, and are arranged in cords or alveoli. Little nuclear pleomorphism is noted. In contrast to cortisol-producing adenomas, the nontumorous cortex in cases of hyperaldosteronism is not atrophic, because aldosterone does not inhibit ACTH secretion by the pituitary gland.

 CLINICAL FEATURES: Most patients with primary aldosteronism are diagnosed after detection of asymptomatic diastolic hypertension. Muscle weakness and fatigue are caused by the effects of potassium depletion on skeletal muscle. Polyuria and polydipsia result from a disturbance in the concentrating ability of the kidney, probably secondary to hypokalemia. Metabolic alkalosis and an alkaline urine are common. Primary aldosteronism that is caused by an adenoma is cured by surgical removal of the tumor. Bilateral adrenal hyperplasia in Conn syndrome is treated medically with aldosterone antagonists and sometimes with dexamethasone in the case of glucocorticoid-suppressible hyperaldosteronism.

Metastatic Carcinoma

Metastatic cancers to adrenal glands are commonly lung or breast carcinomas, or malignant melanomas. The glands may be unilaterally or bilaterally hugely enlarged, up to 20 to 45 g. They are largely replaced by tumor, often with necrosis and hemorrhage. Usually, enough functional adrenal cortex remains to ensure that Addison disease does not develop, particularly in view of the limited survival of these patients.

ADRENAL MEDULLA AND PARAGANGLIA

Pheochromocytomas are Rare Catecholamine-Secreting Tumors

Pheochromocytomas are catecholamine-secreting tumors of chromaffin cells of the adrenal medulla. If they arise in extra-adrenal sites, they are called **paragangliomas**. They are observed at any age, including infancy, but are uncommon after 60 years of age. *The presenting symptoms reflect sustained or episodic hypertension.* Other symptoms include pallor, anxiety, and cardiac arrhythmias. Although pheochromocytomas account for less than 0.1% of cases of hypertension, this tumor should be considered in evaluating any hypertensive patient. If detected early, pheochromocytomas are amenable to surgical resection, but when left untreated, patients can die from complications of prolonged hypertension.

 PATHOGENESIS: Pheochromocytomas are mostly sporadic. A minority are inherited, either alone or as part of hereditary syndromes, such as MEN types 2A and 2B, von Hippel-Lindau disease, neurofibromatosis type 1 (NF1), and McCune-Albright syndrome.

The features of the autosomal dominant MEN syndromes are:

- **MEN type 1** (**Wermer syndrome**) is **not** associated with pheochromocytomas but is most commonly associated with (1) pituitary adenoma, (2) parathyroid hyperplasia or adenoma, and (3) islet cell tumors of the pancreas (insulinoma, gastrinoma). The disease is caused by mutation of the MEN-1 tumor suppressor gene (chromosome 11q13), which encodes a protein termed **menin**.
- **MEN type 2 syndromes** feature MTC in virtually all patients and pheochromocytoma in about half.

MEN-2A (SIPPLE SYNDROME): Most (95%) MEN-2 patients are classified as 2A. In addition to medullary thyroid carcinoma

and pheochromocytoma, one third of patients show hyperparathyroidism due to parathyroid hyperplasia or adenoma. A variety of neural crest tumors may be seen with MEN type 2A, including gliomas, glioblastomas, and meningiomas.

MEN-2B: This disorder resembles MEN-2A, but it develops about 10 years earlier. Parathyroid disease is uncommon. The **mucosal neuroma syndrome** (ganglioneuromas of the conjunctiva, oral cavity, larynx, and gastrointestinal tract) is a feature of MEN-2B. Mucosal neuromas are always encountered, but only half of the patients express the full phenotype.

Adrenal medullary hyperplasia has been reported in some patients with both MEN-2A and 2B antedating the occurrence of pheochromocytoma. Grossly, an enlarged adrenal shows an expanded medulla. The chromaffin cells are larger than normal and are arranged in distinct nests or cords. Mutations in the **RET protooncogene** on chromosome 10q11.2 are responsible for the MEN-2 syndromes. *Identification of RET mutations is used to confirm the diagnosis of MEN-2 and identify asymptomatic family members.* People who carry *RET* mutations are screened for thyroid cancer, pheochromocytoma, and hyperparathyroidism. Somatic mutations in *RET* have been found in 10% to 20% of patients with sporadic pheochromocytomas. In addition, some sporadic pheochromocytomas exhibit mutations in the von Hippel-Lindau and *NF1* genes.

 PATHOLOGY: In sporadic pheochromocytomas, 80% of tumors are unilateral, 10% are bilateral, and 10% are in extraadrenal locations. Ten percent are malignant, and 10% occur in children. By contrast, two thirds of tumors occurring in the context of MEN are bilateral. Pheochromocytomas tend to be encapsulated, spongy, reddish masses, with prominent central scars, hemorrhage, and foci of cystic degeneration (Fig. 21-21A). Their histologic appearance is highly variable. Typically, circumscribed nests (**zellballen**) of neoplastic cells are present. Less commonly, trabecular or solid patterns are seen. Tumor cells range from polyhedral to fusiform, with granular, amphophilic, or basophilic cytoplasm and vesicular nuclei. Eosinophilic globules are usually seen in the cytoplasm. Cellular pleomorphism is often prominent and may include multinucleated tumor giant cells (see Fig. 21-21B). The tumor contains numerous capillaries. In 5% to 10% of cases, pheochromocytomas are malignant, although this figure may be higher for extraadrenal tumors. Malignancy is determined only by a pheochromocytoma's biological behavior (i.e., metastases) and cannot be judged from its histologic appearance. Both benign and malignant pheochromocytomas show mitoses, cellular pleomorphism, capsular or vascular invasion, and necrosis. Metastases are most common in the regional lymph nodes, bone, lung, and liver.

 CLINICAL FEATURES: Typically, episodic catecholamine release leads to a paroxysm or crisis of up to several hours, with severe throbbing headache, sweating, palpitations, tachycardia, abdominal pain, and vomiting. Blood pressure may be elevated, often to an extreme degree. A paroxysm can be precipitated by activities that place pressure on the abdominal contents (including the tumor), such as exercise, lifting, bending, or vigorous abdominal palpation. More than 90% of patients with pheochromocytoma show hypertension, which is sustained in two thirds of patients and resembles essential hypertension. In one third of patients, hypertension is episodic but may become sustained, and even evolve into malignant hypertension. Angina and myocardial infarction occur in the absence of coronary artery disease. The cardiac complications are attributed to myocardial necrosis caused by elevated catecholamine levels (*catecholamine cardiomyopathy*).

Pheochromocytoma is diagnosed by finding increased urinary levels of catecholamine metabolites, particularly vanillylmandelic acid. Treatment for pheochromocytoma is surgical removal. β-adrenergic blocking agents are used to control hypertensive crises, and β-adrenergic receptor antagonists are helpful adjuncts.

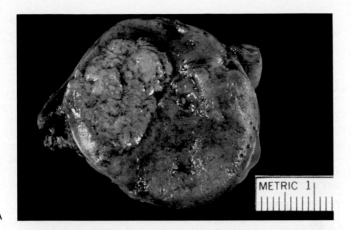

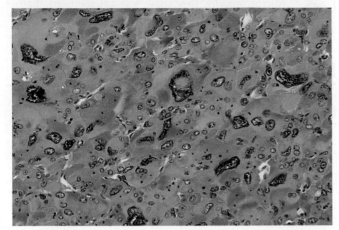

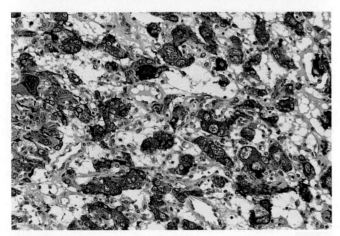

FIGURE 21-21. **Pheochromocytoma. A.** The cut surface of an adrenal tumor from a patient with episodic hypertension is reddish brown with a prominent area of fibrosis. Foci of hemorrhage and cystic degeneration are evident. **B.** A photomicrograph of the tumor shows polyhedral tumor cells with ample finely granular cytoplasm. Note the enlarged hyperchromatic nuclei. **C.** Many of the tumor cells show positive immunohistochemical staining for chromogranin A, a marker of neuroendocrine differentiation.

Paraganglioma is a Pheochromocytoma Arising at an Extra-Adrenal Site

Paragangliomas arise in paraganglia in any location, including the retroperitoneum, neck, posterior mediastinum, and urinary bladder. Bladder paragangliomas may present as a peculiar syndrome of headaches and paroxysmal hypertension on urination. The tumors may also arise in the base of the skull, in the neck, in vagal or aortic bodies, or in any organ that contains paraganglionic tissue, such as the larynx and small intestine. Most (90%) paragangliomas of the head and neck are benign but those in the retroperitoneum are more often malignant. *Carotid body tumor is a prototypic paraganglioma arising at the carotid bifurcation. It forms a palpable mass in the neck.* Interestingly, carotid body tumors are 10 times more frequent in persons living at a high altitude than those at sea level, suggesting that these tumors may represent a hyperplastic response to prolonged carotid body-sensing of hypoxia.

Neuroblastoma

Neuroblastoma (NB) is an embryonal malignant tumor of neural crest origin that is composed of neoplastic neuroblasts and originates in the adrenal medulla, paravertebral sympathetic ganglia, and sympathetic paraganglia. Neuroblastomas are the most common solid extracranial neoplasms of childhood, accounting for up to 10% of all childhood cancers and 15% of cancer deaths in children. The overall incidence is 1 in 7,000, and the peak incidence is in the first 3 years.

NB is congenital in some cases and has even been found in premature stillborns. In fact, NB accounts for half of all cancers diagnosed in the first month of life. Occasional cases are encountered in adolescents or adults. Although the occurrence of NB is sporadic, a few instances of familial tumors are recorded. NBs may occur with NF1, Beckwith-Wiedemann syndrome, and Hirschsprung disease.

 PATHOGENESIS: Embryogenesis of the adrenal medulla and presumably of other parts of the sympathetic nervous system continues during the first year of life. *Persistence and transformation of these embryonal structures may be related to the pathogenesis of NB.* The tumor is characterized by frequent deletions on chromosome 1 (1p35-36) and amplification of N-*myc*, the latter being key in determining the aggressiveness of neuroblastoma. It is thought that the locus on chromosome 1 encodes a gene that suppresses N-*myc* amplification.

 PATHOLOGY: NBs can arise at any site that contains neural crest-derived cells (i.e., from the posterior cranial fossa to the coccyx). One third of the tumors are in the adrenal, another third are elsewhere in the abdomen, and 20% are in the posterior mediastinum. NBs vary from minute, barely discernible nodules to tumors readily palpable through the abdominal wall. They are round, irregularly lobulated masses that may weigh 50 to 150 g or more (Fig. 21-22A). The cut surface is soft and friable, with a variegated maroon color. Areas of necrosis, hemorrhage, calcification, and cystic change are often present. NBs are composed of dense sheets of small, round-to-fusiform cells with hyperchromatic nuclei, scanty cytoplasm, and frequent mitoses. Characteristic Homer-Wright rosettes are defined by a rim of dark tumor cells in a circumferential arrangement around a central pale fibrillar core (see Fig. 21-22B). NBs readily infiltrate surrounding structures and metastasize to regional lymph nodes, liver, lungs, bones, and other sites.

 CLINICAL FEATURES: The presentation of NB is highly variable, a consequence of the many sites of the primary tumors and metastases. The first sign is often an enlarging abdomen in a young child. Physical examination discloses a firm, irregular, nontender mass. Hepatic metastases enlarge the liver and may cause ascites. Respiratory distress accompanies large masses in the thorax, and tumors in the pelvis obstruct the bowel or ureters. Severe diarrhea may be caused in tumors secreting vasoactive intestinal peptide. Urinary excretion of catecholamines and their metabolites is almost invariably elevated in patients with NB. The urine contains increased amounts of **norepinephrine**, **vanillylmandelic acid**, **homovanillic acid**, and **dopamine**.

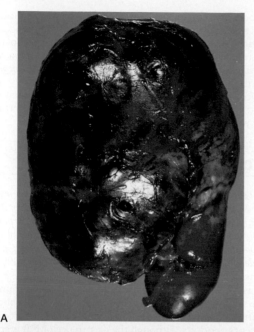

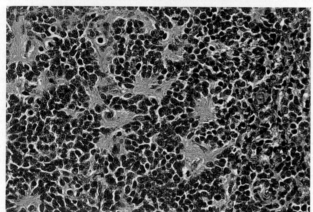

FIGURE 21-22. **Neuroblastoma. A.** A large, lobulated, hemorrhagic, and cystic tumor, adherent to the upper pole of the kidney, was removed from a child who presented with an abdominal mass. **B.** A photomicrograph illustrates the characteristic rosettes, formed by small, regular, dark tumor cells arranged around a central, pale fibrillar core.

Several factors are useful in predicting the outcome of NB:

- **Age:** Age at diagnosis is one of the most important indicators of survival. Children under 1 year have a better prognosis than do older patients with the same stage of the disease. Spontaneous tumor regression is common at this age.
- **Site:** Extra-adrenal tumors tend to be better differentiated and so less aggressive.
- **Stage:** The survival rate is 90% in stage I (tumor confined to the organ of origin) and decreases to less than 3% in stage IV (widespread metastases).
- **Other factors:** Low-grade tumors and lack of N-myc amplification suggest a better prognosis

Localized NBs are treated by surgical resection alone. Patients with disseminated tumors are given chemotherapy and sometimes irradiation.

Ganglioneuroma

Ganglioneuroma, like NB, is a tumor of neural crest origin. It is seen in older children and young adults. *Ganglio-neuroma is benign and arises in sympathetic ganglia, typically in the posterior mediastinum.* Up to 30% of these tumors occur in the adrenal medulla. Ganglioneuromas do not manifest the chromosomal abnormalities characteristic of NB.

 PATHOLOGY: Ganglioneuromas are well encapsulated and display a myxoid, glistening, cut surface. Microscopically, they show well-differentiated, mature ganglion cells, associated with spindle cells in a loose, abundant fibrillar stroma.

PINEAL GLAND

Neoplasms

 PATHOLOGY: Tumors of the pineal gland are rare, representing less than 1% of brain tumors. They include neoplasms originating from the pineal parenchyma, presumably from the pinealocyte, neoplasms located in the pineal gland region but not derived from the pinealocyte and, rarely, metastasis from other sites.

- **Germ cell tumors:** These are the most frequent pineal neoplasms and are apparently derived from misplaced germ cells. Germinomas, or dysgerminomas, account for about 60% of pineal tumors and are indistinguishable from their gonadal counterparts.
- **Pineocytoma:** This benign tumor is a solid, well-circumscribed mass that replaces the pineal body. Microscopically, small tumor cells with round nuclei and eosinophilic cytoplasm appear as nests separated by thin strands of connective tissue.
- **Pineoblastoma:** This highly malignant tumor is extremely rare and occurs in young adults. Soft masses, often showing hemorrhagic and necrotic areas, invade and infiltrate the surrounding structures. Microscopi-cally, pineoblastoma consists of small oval cells, with dark nuclei and scanty cytoplasm. Mitoses are generally numerous.

 CLINICAL FEATURES: Regardless of histologic type, pineal gland tumors present with signs and symptoms related to their impact on surrounding structures, including headaches and visual and behavioral disturbances. In children, these tumors are frequently associated with precocious puberty, predominantly in boys. The prognosis of pineal tumors is poor in the case of pineoblastoma but is also guarded in cases of pineocytoma. Even non-neoplastic pineal cysts pose a great threat to life because they are difficult to excise surgically.

22 Obesity, Diabetes Mellitus, and Metabolic Syndrome

Barry J. Goldstein
Serge Jabbour
Kevin Furlong

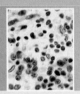
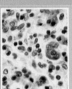
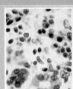
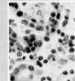

The genesis of obesity is indisputably complex but the fact remains that obesity develops because more calories are taken in than expended. *Obesity has reached epidemic proportions, with a prevalence that continues to increase globally. In the United States, 35% of adults are overweight, and another 30% are obese. The annual costs related to obesity have been estimated to exceed 100 billion dollars. More worrisome are the 15% of children and adolescents who are overweight or obese, one of the most rapidly increasing groups of overweight and obese people. Diabetes is strongly associated with obesity: more than 80% of cases of type 2 diabetes mellitus can be attributed to obesity.*

Obesity

Obesity is an Epidemic Disease Related to Both Genetic and Environmental Factors

Obesity is clearly associated with increased mortality. It is a multifactorial condition that involves complex interaction of genetic, metabolic, physiologic, social, and behavioral factors. Severe clinical obesity rarely has a monogenic cause.

More than 250 gene markers and chromosomal regions have been linked to human obesity in large population surveys. The clinical significance of most of these has yet to be determined, but in unusual cases, monogenic causes of obesity have been noted in humans.

GENETIC FACTORS: The most common single gene defect is mutations in the **melanocortin-4 receptor**, which occurs in about 5% of individuals with severe childhood-onset obesity. Rare homozygous mutations in the **leptin gene** and also in the **leptin receptor** are associated with hyperphagia and severe, early-onset obesity. *The increased leptin levels seen in the obese with normal leptin genes fail to prevent excessive fat accumulation.*

ENVIRONMENTAL FACTORS: The impact of environmental, sociologic, and psychologic factors on the development of obesity cannot be underestimated. A striking example of environmental influence on genetic predisposition is demonstrated by the Pima Native Americans in Arizona. The Pimas are now largely sedentary and eat a diet in which 50% of energy derives from fat, as opposed to their traditional low-fat diets. They have had dramatic increases in the incidence of obesity and diabetes. By contrast, the genetically related Pimas in the Sierra Madre Mountains of Northern Mexico are more physically active, have maintained more traditional low-fat diets, and have much lower rates of obesity and type 2 diabetes mellitus (T2DM).

 PATHOGENESIS: The pathologic lesion associated with these complications is hyperplasia and hypertrophy of fat cells. The excess from the imbalance between energy intake and energy expenditure is stored in adipocytes that enlarge or increase in number.

Determining how excess adiposity influences the regulation of glucose and lipid metabolism and contributes to cardiovascular risk is currently an area of active research, which has led to several hypotheses.

- **Portal/visceral hypothesis:** This theory proposes that increased central adiposity increases the delivery of free fatty acids to the liver, where they directly block insulin action. This hepatic insulin resistance has been implicated in the development of hyperglycemia in diabetes (see below).
- **Endocrine paradigm:** The hypothesis suggests that adipose tissue is an active secretory organ that releases many different types of hormones and cytokines into the blood. These include leptin, interleukin-6, and angiotensin II, among others, which have been shown to play a critical role in the development of insulin resistance in liver and skeletal muscle.
- **Ectopic fat storage hypothesis:** Excess lipid in obesity is stored in the liver, skeletal muscle, and pancreatic insulin-secreting β-cells. *This influences insulin signaling and secretion, contributing to development of T2DM.*

The Complications of Obesity Affect Most Organ Systems

Endocrine complications

- **T2DM:** Diabetes is strongly associated with obesity: more than 80% of cases of T2DM can be attributed to obesity (see below).
- **Dyslipidemia:** Obesity is associated with deleterious serum lipid abnormalities, including elevated triglycerides, reduced high-density lipoprotein, and increased small, dense, low-density lipoprotein particles, which are strongly associated with an increased risk of cardiovascular disease, particularly in persons with central adiposity.
- **Other:** Obesity is also associated with polycystic ovary syndrome, irregular menses, amenorrhea, infertility, and hypogonadism.

Cardiovascular complications

- **Hypertension:** Elevated blood pressure is strongly correlated with obesity and may be related to heightened sympathetic activity. Obesity makes hypertension more difficult to control by interfering with the action of antihypertensive agents. Even a small reduction in weight may decrease the average blood pressure in this population.
- **Coronary heart disease:** Body mass index has a modest and graded association with myocardial infarction, but body fat distribution, especially the waist-to-hip ratio, appears to be a stronger indicator of risk.
- **Congestive heart failure:** Obesity is associated with an increased risk of heart failure due to eccentric cardiac dilatation.
- **Thromboembolic disease:** The risks of deep venous thromboses and pulmonary embolism are increased in obesity.

Additional complications of obesity

- **Neurologic:** Obesity progressively increases the risk of fatal and nonfatal ischemic strokes as body mass index increases.
- **Pulmonary:** Obesity can interfere mechanically with lung function. Obesity is a major risk factor for development of **obstructive sleep apnea**, in which patients are prone to apnea and hypopnea during sleep. Obesity-hypoventilation syndrome in its most severe form is termed **Pickwickian syndrome**. It is characterized by extreme obesity, irregular breathing, cyanosis, secondary polycythemia, and right ventricular dysfunction, leading to fixed pulmonary hypertension.
- **Hepatobiliary**: Obese individuals, particularly women, have an increased incidence of gallstones. A diverse array of liver abnor-

malities may also complicate obesity. These represent a spectrum of disease known as **nonalcoholic fatty liver disease**, characterized by the accumulation of fat within hepatocytes (see Chapter 14).

The "Insulin Resistance/ Metabolic Syndrome"

The phenomenon of peripheral insulin resistance is a common consequence of obesity and a fundamental component in the pathogenesis of type 2 diabetes (see below). In obese persons, inhibitory mediators from adipose tissue (including free fatty acids and cytokines such as TNF-α and adiponectin are preferentially increased in the visceral-abdominal (upper body). These mediators interfere with insulin signaling by disrupting the propagation of protein-tyrosine phosphorylation.

Resistance to the action of insulin in target tissues and compensatory hyperinsulinemia are closely tied to a diverse set of cardiovascular risk factors that are prevalent in obese, sedentary persons and in patients with T2DM. These risk factors, together termed the **metabolic syndrome**, include (1) abdominal adiposity with increased waist circumference, (2) mild hypertension (perhaps related to a failure of endothelium-dependent vascular relaxation), and (3) dyslipidemia, characterized by reduced high-density lipoprotein cholesterol, increased circulating triglycerides, and small, dense, low-density lipoprotein particles.

DIABETES MELLITUS

Diabetes is a major health problem that affects increasing numbers of individuals in the developed world. Two major forms of diabetes mellitus are recognized, distinguished by their underlying pathophysiology. **Type 1 diabetes mellitus** (T1DM), formerly known as **insulin-dependent** or **juvenile-onset diabetes**, is caused by autoimmune destruction of the insulin-producing β-cells in the pancreatic islets of Langerhans and affects less than 10% of all patients with diabetes. By contrast, **type 2 diabetes mellitus**, formerly known as **non–insulin-dependent** or **maturity-onset diabetes**, is typically associated with obesity and results from a complex interrelationship between resistance to the metabolic action of insulin in its target tissues and inadequate secretion of insulin from the pancreas (Table 22-1).

Gestational diabetes develops in a small percentage of pregnant women, owing to the insulin resistance of pregnancy combined with a β-cell defect, but almost always abates after parturition. Diabetes can also occur secondary to other endocrine conditions or drug therapy, especially in patients with Cushing syndrome or during treatment with glucocorticoids.

Type 2 Diabetes Mellitus (T2DM)

T2DM is a disorder characterized by a combination of reduced tissue sensitivity to insulin and inadequate secretion of insulin from the pancreas. The disease usually develops in adults, with an increased prevalence in obese persons and in the elderly. Recently, T2DM has been appearing in increasing numbers in younger adults and adolescents, owing to worsening obesity and lack of exercise in this age group. *Hyperglycemia in T2DM is a failure of the β cells to meet an increased demand for insulin in the body.* T2DM affects more than 16 million Americans, almost half of whom are undiagnosed. Some 10% of persons older than 65 years of age are affected, and 80% of patients with T2DM are overweight. T2DM is most prevalent in all non-Caucasian ethnic minority groups in the United States, including Blacks, Hispanics, Asians, and Native Americans.

TABLE 22-1

Comparison of Type 1 and Type 2 Diabetes Mellitus

	Type 1 Diabetes	Type 2 Diabetes
Age at onset	Usually before 20	Usually after 30
Type of onset	Abrupt; symptomatic (polyuria, poly-dipsia, dehydration); often severe with ketoacidosis	Gradual; usually subtle; often asymptomatic
Usual body weight	Normal; recent weight loss is common	Overweight
Genetics (parents or siblings with diabetes)	<20%	>60%
Monozygotic twins	50% concordant	90% concordant
HLA associations	+	No
Antibodies to islet cell antigens (insulin, glutamic acid decarbo-xylase, IA-2)	+	No
Islet lesions	Early—inflammation Late—atrophy and fibrosis	Late—fibrosis, amyloid
β-cell mass	Markedly reduced	Normal or slightly reduced
Circulating insulin level	Markedly reduced	Elevated or normal
Clinical management	Insulin absolutely required	Lifestyle modification (diet, exercise); combinations of oral drugs; often insulin supplementation is needed

HLA, human leukocyte antigen; IA-2, islet cell antigen-512.

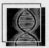 **PATHOGENESIS:** T2DM results from a complex interplay between underlying resistance to the action of insulin in its metabolic target tissues (liver, skeletal muscle, and adipose tissue) and a reduction in glucose-stimulated insulin secretion, which fails to compensate for the increased demand for insulin. Progression to overt diabetes in susceptible populations occurs most commonly in patients exhibiting both of these defects (Fig. 22-1).

GENETIC FACTORS: Multifactorial and multigenic inheritance is a key contributor to the development of T2DM. Sixty percent of patients have either a parent or a sibling with the disease. In some populations, notably Native Americans and some indigenous populations in Pacific Island nations, the adoption of a more affluent lifestyle has led to the occurrence of T2DM in 30% to 50% of the population. Among monozygotic twins, both are almost always affected. No association with genes of the major histocompatibility complex, as seen in T1DM, has been found. Despite the high familial prevalence of the disease, the inheritance pattern is complex and thought to be due to multiple interacting susceptibility genes. Constitutional factors such as obesity, hypertension, and the amount of exercise influence the phenotypic expression of the disorder and have complicated genetic analysis.

GLUCOSE METABOLISM: In a healthy person, the extracellular concentration of glucose in fed and fasting states is maintained in a tightly limited range. This rigid control is mediated by the opposing actions of insulin and glucagon. Following a carbohydrate-rich meal, the absorption of glucose from the gut leads to an increase in blood glucose, which stimulates insulin secretion by the pancreatic β cells and the consequent insulin-mediated increase in glucose uptake by skeletal muscle and adipose tissue. At the same time, insulin suppresses hepatic glucose production by (1) inhibiting gluconeogenesis, (2) enhancing glycogen synthesis, (3) blocking the effects of glucagon on the liver, and (4) antagonizing the release of glucagon from the pancreas.

β CELL FUNCTION: People with T2DM exhibit impaired β-cell insulin release in response to glucose stimulation, a defect that can

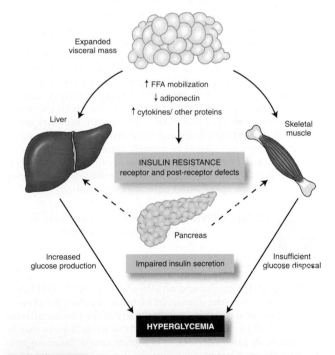

FIGURE 22-1. **Pathogenesis of obesity-related type 2 diabetes mellitus (T2DM).** The expanded visceral fat mass in upper-body obesity elaborates several factors that contribute to tissue insulin resistance. These include an increase in circulating free (nonesterified) fatty acids (FFAs) and other cytokines and proteins that inhibit insulin action, as well as a decrease in factors that enhance insulin signaling, such as adiponectin. These changes result in a block to insulin action in liver and skeletal muscle at the level of the insulin receptor and at postreceptor signaling sites, resulting in a failure of insulin to suppress hepatic glucose production and to promote glucose uptake into muscle. The resulting hyperglycemia is normally countered by increased insulin secretion by pancreatic β cells. In persons with T2DM, the combination of resistance to insulin action and a genetically determined impairment of the β-cell response to hyperglycemia results in hyperglycemia, and T2DM ensues.

appear early in the progression of the disease. This functional abnormality is specific for glucose, because the β cells retain the ability to respond to other secretagogues, such as amino acids. β-cell function may also be affected by the chronically elevated plasma levels of free fatty acids that occur in obese individuals. A variety of microscopic lesions are found in the islets of Langerhans of many, but not all, patients with T2DM. *Unlike T1DM, in T2DM, there is no consistent reduction in the number of β cells, and no morphologic lesions of these cells have been found by light or electron microscopy.*

In some islets, fibrous tissue accumulates, sometimes to such a degree that they are obliterated. Islet amyloid is often present (Fig. 22-2), particularly in patients over 60 years of age. This type of amyloid is composed of a polypeptide molecule known as **amylin**, which is secreted with insulin by the β cell. Importantly, as many as 20% of elderly nondiabetic persons also have amyloid deposits in their pancreas, a finding that has been attributed to the aging process itself.

Type 1 Diabetes Mellitus (T1DM)

T1DM is a lifelong disorder of glucose homeostasis that results from the autoimmune destruction of the β cells in the islets of Langerhans. The disease is characterized by few, if any, functional β cells and extremely limited or nonexistent insulin secretion. As a result, body fat rather than glucose is preferentially metabolized as a source of energy. In turn, oxidation of fat overproduces **ketone bodies** (acetoacetic acid and β-hydroxybutyric acid), which are released into the blood from the liver and lead to metabolic ketoacidosis. Hyperglycemia results from unsuppressed hepatic glucose output and reduced glucose disposal in skeletal muscle and adipose tissue, leading to glucosuria and dehydration from loss of body water into the urine. If uncorrected, the progressive acidosis and dehydration ultimately lead to coma and death (Fig. 22-3) The destruction of β-cells in T1DM generally develops slowly over years. Clinically apparent diabetes with hyperglycemia or ketoacidosis manifests only when at least 90% of the insulin-secreting cells have been eliminated and insulin deprivation becomes severe.

T1DM is most common among northern Europeans and their descendants and is not seen as frequently among Asians, Blacks, or Native Americans. For example, the incidence of T1DM in Finland is 20 to 40 times that in Japan. Although the disorder can develop at any age, the peak age of onset coincides with puberty.

 PATHOGENESIS: A variety of factors have been incriminated in the pathogenesis of T1DM.

GENETIC FACTORS: Fewer than 20% of those with T1DM have a parent or sibling with the disease. In identical (monozygotic) twins in which one twin is diabetic, both members of the pair are affected in less than half of cases. Disease occurrence in such pairs may be well separated in time. This lack of complete concordance suggests that environmental factors contribute in a major way to the development of the disease. However, certain genetic factors are important, especially major histocompatibility antigens. Approximately 95% of patients with T1DM have either HLA-DR3 orDR4, or both, compared with 20% of the general population. In addition, 96% of patients are homozygous for a single amino acid substitution in the DQ β-chain, compared with 19% of healthy unrelated individuals. Twenty other independent chromosomal regions have thus far also been associated with susceptibility to T1DM.

AUTOIMMUNITY: *Cell-mediated autoimmune mechanisms are fundamental to the pathogenesis of T1DM.* Cytotoxic T lymphocytes sensitized to β cells in T1DM persist indefinitely, possibly for a lifetime. This concept is supported by the observation that patients who die shortly after the onset of the disease often exhibit an infiltrate of

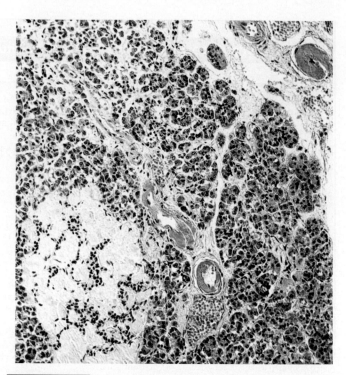

FIGURE 22-2. Amyloidosis (hyalinization) of an islet in the pancreas of a patient with T2DM *(lower left).* The blood vessel adjacent to the islet shows the advanced hyaline arteriolosclerosis characteristic of diabetes.

mononuclear cells in and around the islets of Langerhans, termed **insulitis** (Fig. 22-4). Among the inflammatory cells, CD8+ T lymphocytes predominate, although some CD4+ cells are also present. Circulating antibodies against components of the β cells (including insulin itself) are present in most newly diagnosed children with diabetes. Many patients develop islet cell antibodies months or years before insulin production decreases and clinical symptoms appear, a clinical state known as "pre-type 1 diabetes." However, these antibodies are regarded as a response to β-cell antigens released during destruction of β cells by cell-mediated immune mechanisms, rather than the cause of β-cell depletion. Nevertheless, detection of serum antibodies to islet β-cells remains a useful clinical tool for differentiating between type 1 and type 2 diabetes, which does not have an autoimmune basis. Ten percent of patients with T1DM manifest at least one other organ-specific autoimmune disease, including

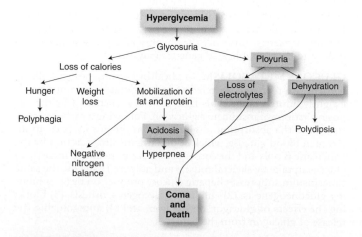

FIGURE 22-3. Symptoms and signs of uncontrolled hyperglycemia in diabetes mellitus.

Hashimoto thyroiditis, Graves disease, myasthenia gravis, Addison disease, and pernicious anemia. Interestingly, most patients with polyendocrine immune syndromes (see Chapter 21) also possess HLA DR3 and DR4 histocompatibility antigens.

ENVIRONMENTAL FACTORS: Viruses and chemicals have been implicated as causative factors in some cases of T1DM. For example, the disease occasionally develops after infection with mumps or group B coxsackie viruses. Children and young adults who were infected in utero with rubella also occasionally develop diabetes, presumably after viral injury of the fetal pancreas. Certain viral proteins may share antigenic epitopes with human cell-surface proteins and trigger the autoreactive disease process by "molecular mimicry." For example, a coxsackie B viral protein has close homology to the human GAD-65 islet protein. Geographical and seasonal differences in the incidence of T1DM further suggest that environmental factors are important in its pathogenesis.

 PATHOLOGY: The most characteristic early lesion in the pancreas of T1DM is a lymphocytic infiltrate in the islets (insulitis), sometimes accompanied by a few macrophages and neutrophils (see Fig. 22-4). *As the disease becomes chronic, the β cells of the islets are progressively depleted; eventually, insulin-producing cells are no longer discernible.* The loss of β cells results in variably sized islets, many of which appear as ribbon-like cords that are difficult to distinguish from the surrounding acinar tissue. Fibrosis of the islets is uncommon. In contrast to T2DM, deposition of amyloid in the islets of Langerhans is absent in T1DM. The exocrine pancreas in chronic T1DM often exhibits diffuse interlobular and interacinar fibrosis, accompanied by atrophy of the acinar cells.

 CLINICAL FEATURES: The clinical presentation of T1DM results from the loss of insulin, which has a unique role in energy metabolism in the body. The disease classically appears with acute metabolic decompensation characterized by ketoacidosis and hyperglycemia. Depending on the degree of absolute insulin deficiency, severe ketoacidosis may be preceded by weeks to months of increased urine output **(polyuria)** and increased thirst **(polydipsia)**. Excessive diuresis results from glucosuria. Weight loss despite increased appetite **(polyphagia)** is due to unregulated catabolism of body stores of fat, protein, and carbohydrate. The clinical onset of T1DM often coincides with another acute illness, such as a febrile viral or bacterial infection.

Complications of Diabetes

The discovery of insulin early in the 20th century promised to cure diabetes, but as diabetics lived longer, it became apparent that they were subject to numerous complications. *It is now clearly established that the severity and chronicity of hyperglycemia in both T1DM and T2DM are the major pathogenetic factors leading to the "microvascular" complications of diabetes. These factors include retinopathy, nephropathy, and neuropathy. Thus, control of blood glucose remains the major means by which the development of microvascular diabetic complications can be minimized.* It has been more difficult to demonstrate that glucose control can prevent atherosclerosis and its complications. These "macrovascular" complications are especially common in insulin-resistant patients with T2DM, because they tend to be older and frequently harbor additional vascular risk factors.

 PATHOGENESIS: A variety of biochemical mechanisms have been proposed to account for the development of pathological changes in diabetes.

EXCESSIVE REACTIVE OXYGEN SPECIES (ROS): In various cell types, hyperglycemia increases the production of reactive oxy-

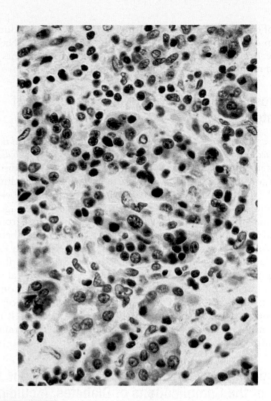

FIGURE 22-4. **Insulitis in type 1 diabetes mellitus.** A mononuclear inflammatory infiltrate is seen in and around the islet.

gen species as byproducts of mitochondrial oxidative phosphorylation. Reactive oxygen species are implicated in many types of cell injury (see Chapter 1).

PROTEIN GLYCOSYLATION: Glucose binds to an assortment of proteins nonenzymatically, via a process termed **glycosylation**. Glycosylation occurs roughly in proportion to the severity of hyperglycemia. Numerous cellular proteins are modified in this manner, including hemoglobin, components of the crystalline lens, and cellular basement membrane proteins. A specific fraction of the glycosylated hemoglobin in circulating red blood cells (hemoglobin A_{1c}) is measured routinely to monitor the overall degree of hyperglycemia that occurred during the preceding 6 to 8 weeks.

The initial glycosylation products are labile and can dissociate rapidly. With time, **advanced glycosylation products**, consisting of a glucose derivative covalently bound to the protein amino group, form. As a result, the structure of the protein is permanently altered, and its function may be affected. Unstable chemical bonds in proteins containing advanced glycosylation products can lead to physical cross-linking of nearby proteins, which may contribute to the characteristic thickening of vascular basement membranes in diabetes. Importantly, advanced glycosylation products can continue to cross-link proteins despite a return of blood glucose to normal levels.

THE ALDOSE REDUCTASE PATHWAY: By mass action, hyperglycemia also increases the uptake of glucose in tissues that do not depend on insulin. Some of the increased flux of glucose is metabolized by aldose reductase, leading to the accumulation of sorbitol. This sugar alcohol has been suspected to play a role in diabetic complications in a variety of tissues, including peripheral nerves, the retina, lens, and kidney.

PROTEIN KINASE C (PKC) ACTIVATION: In patients with hyperglycemia, specific PKC isoforms, mainly PKC-β and PKC-δ, are activated. PKC activation may lead to (1) increased production of extracellular matrix and cytokines, (2) enhanced microvascular contractility, (3) increased microvascular permeability, and (4) proliferation of endothelial and smooth muscle cells. PKC also induces activation of phospholipase A2 and inhibits the activity of Na^+/K^+-ATPase. Inhibition of PKC-β by a selective inhibitor prevents or reverses a number of vascular abnormalities in vitro and in vivo.

Atherosclerosis is a Frequent Complication of Diabetes

Cardiovascular disease, including atherosclerotic heart disease and ischemic stroke, account for more than half of all deaths among adults with diabetes. The extent and severity of atherosclerotic lesions in medium-sized and large arteries are increased in patients with long-standing diabetes. Diabetes eliminates the usual protective effect of being female, and coronary artery disease develops at a younger age than in nondiabetic individuals. Moreover, the mortality rate from myocardial infarction is higher in diabetic than in nondiabetic patients. As indicated above, patients with T2DM frequently exhibit multiple risk factors of the metabolic syndrome that contribute to development of atherosclerosis. Atherosclerotic peripheral vascular disease, particularly of the lower extremities, is a common complication of diabetes. Vascular insufficiency leads to ulcers and gangrene of the toes and feet, complications that ultimately necessitate amputation. Diabetes accounts for 40% of nontraumatic limb amputations in the United States.

Diabetic Microvascular Disease is Responsible for Many of the Complications of Diabetes, Including Renal Failure and Blindness

Arteriolosclerosis and capillary basement membrane thickening are characteristic vascular changes in diabetes. The frequent occurrence of hypertension contributes to the development of the arteriolar lesions. In addition, the deposition of basement membrane proteins, which may also become glycosylated, increases in diabetes. Aggregation of platelets in smaller blood vessels and impaired fibrinolytic mechanisms have also been suggested as playing a role in the pathogenesis of diabetic microvascular disease.

Whatever the pathogenetic processes, the effects of microvascular disease on tissue perfusion and wound healing are profound. For example, it is believed that blood flow to the heart, which is already compromised by coronary atherosclerosis, is reduced. Healing of chronic ulcers that develop from trauma and infection of the feet in diabetic patients is commonly defective, in part because of microvascular disease. The major complications of diabetic microvascular disease involve the kidney and the retina and are discussed in Chapters 16 and 29, respectively.

Diabetic Neuropathy Affects Sensory and Autonomic Innervation

Peripheral sensory impairment and autonomic nerve dysfunction are among the most common and distressing complications of diabetes. Changes in the nerves are complex, and abnormalities in axons, the myelin sheath, and Schwann cells have all been found. Microvasculopathy involving the small blood vessels of nerves contributes to the disorder. Evidence suggests that hyperglycemia increases the perception of pain, independent of any structural lesions in the nerves.

Peripheral neuropathy is initially characterized by pain and abnormal sensations in the extremities. Fine touch, pain detection, and proprioception are ultimately lost. As a result, diabetics tend to ignore irritation and minor trauma to feet, joints, and legs. Peripheral neuropathy can thus lead to foot ulcers, which often plague patients with severe diabetes. It also plays a role in the painless but destructive joint disease that occasionally occurs.

Abnormalities in neurogenic regulation of cardiovascular and gastrointestinal functions frequently result in postural hypotension and problems of gut motility, such as diarrhea. Erectile dysfunction and retrograde ejaculation are common complications of autonomic dysfunction, although vascular disease is also a contributing factor. Occasionally, hypotonic urinary bladder develops and results in urinary retention and predisposition to infection.

Bacterial and Fungal Infections Occur in Diabetic Patients Whose Hyperglycemia is Poorly Controlled

Multiple abnormalities in host responses to microbial invasion have been described in diabetic patients. Leukocyte function is compromised, and immune responses are blunted. Patients with well-controlled diabetes are much less susceptible to infections. However, urinary tract infections continue to be problematic because glucose in the urine provides an enriched culture medium. This problem is further complicated if patients have developed autonomic neuropathy leading to urinary retention from poor bladder emptying. Ascending infection from the bladder (pyelonephritis) is thus a constant concern. Renal papillary necrosis may be a devastating complication of bladder infection. A dreaded infectious complication of poorly controlled diabetes is mucormycosis. This often-fatal fungal infection tends to originate in the nasopharynx or paranasal sinuses and spreads rapidly to the orbit and brain.

Diabetes Occurring During Pregnancy May Put the Mother and Fetus at Risk

Gestational diabetes develops in a small percentage of seemingly healthy women during pregnancy and may continue after parturition in a small proportion. Pregnancy is ordinarily a state of insulin resistance, but only pregnant women with impaired β-cell insulin secretion become diabetic. Abnormalities in the amount and timing of pancreatic insulin secretion make these women highly susceptible to overt T2DM later in life.

Poor control of gestational diabetes may lead to the birth of large infants, make labor and delivery more difficult, and necessitate a cesarean section. The fetal pancreas tries to compensate for poor maternal control of diabetes during gestation. Such fetuses may develop β-cell hyperplasia, which may lead to hypoglycemia at birth and in the early postnatal period.

Infants of diabetic mothers have a 5% to 10% incidence of major developmental abnormalities, including anomalies of the heart and great vessels as well as neural tube defects, such as anencephaly and spina bifida. The frequency of these lesions is a function of the control of maternal diabetes during early gestation.

23 The Amyloidoses

Robert Kisilevsky

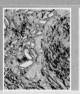

Amyloid refers to a group of diverse extracellular protein deposits that have (1) common morphologic properties, (2) affinities for specific dyes, and (3) when stained, a characteristic appearance under polarized light. Although they vary in amino acid sequence, all amyloid proteins are folded in such a way as to share common ultrastructural and physical properties. The symptomatology of amyloidosis is governed by both the underlying disease and the type and organ locations of the protein deposited. The diagnosis of amyloidosis ultimately rests on the histologic demonstration of amyloid deposition in biopsy specimens. Hence, the commonality of amyloidosis lies in the particular secondary structure of the many proteins involved rather than in specific mutation or organ system affected.

Constituents of Amyloid

Amyloid deposits are composed of two classes of constituents:

A DISEASE-SPECIFIC FIBRILLOGENIC PROTEIN: The nature of this protein varies with the underlying disease. The tertiary structure of the protein and the manner in which it interacts with other molecules are responsible for the characteristics of amyloid. *The specific fibrillogenic protein in various types of amyloid is now the determining factor in the classification of amyloid.*

A SET OF COMMON COMPONENTS FOUND IN ALL AMYLOIDS:

- The **amyloid P component** (AP) is a pentagonal, doughnut-shaped protein that is present in all types of amyloid. AP is identical with a normal circulating serum protein, termed *serum amyloid P (SAP)*. SAP is also a structural component of normal basement membranes.
- **Other molecular building blocks of basement membranes** are present in amyloid and include laminin, collagen type IV, and the proteoglycan perlecan. Heparan sulfate, the glycosaminoglycan side chain of perlecan is also crucial in altering the conformation of the disease-specific fibrillogenic proteins.
- **Apolipoprotein E** is a constituent of high-density lipoproteins and normally plays a role in cholesterol transport.

Not all amyloids are the same, and the disease-specific fibrillogenic proteins vary significantly. For example, in amyloids associated with multiple myeloma, the fibrillogenic component is a product of immunoglobulin light chains produced by myeloma cells. In amyloids associated with inflammatory diseases, the fibrillogenic component is derived from an acute phase protein that is produced by the liver and is unrelated to immunoglobulins. *In these two cases, amyloid is deposited systemically. In other situations, amyloid is deposited only locally.* Amyloid in medullary carcinoma of the thyroid is restricted to the tumor deposits, and its fibrillogenic component is derived from a polypeptide hormone related to calcitonin. In the pancreas, amyloid located either in an islet cell tumor or in the islets in type 2 diabetes is derived from a peptide hormone secreted with insulin (amylin, or islet amyloid polypeptide [IAPP]). In Alzheimer disease, the amyloid is restricted to the brain and its blood vessels; yet it is derived from a plasma membrane protein that is found not only in the central nervous system but distributed ubiquitously in the body.

Although the nature of amyloid deposits varies widely and the conditions under which they occur are disparate, a century of usage established the term **amyloidosis** as denoting a single disease. In current usage, however, amyloidosis refers to a group of diseases *characterized by proteinaceous tissue deposits with similar morphologic, structural, and staining properties, but with variable protein composition.*

Definition of Amyloid

The staining and structural properties of amyloid allow a general definition, based primarily on its morphologic characteristics.

- All forms of amyloid stain positively with Congo red (Fig. 23-1A) and show red–green birefringence when viewed under polarized light (Fig. 23-1B).
- Ultrastructurally, all forms of amyloid consist of interlacing bundles of parallel arrays of fibrils, which have a diameter of 7 to 13 nm (Fig. 23-2).
- The protein in the amyloid fibrils contains a large proportion of crossed β-pleated sheet structure.

Clinical Classification of the Amyloidoses

The classification of amyloidosis has undergone a major change (Table 23-1). Older classifications were based on the clinical presentation of the patient and did not account for the protein composition of deposited amyloid. Although newer groupings based on the protein type are now coming into general use, the older classification is still used in clinical medicine and will be reviewed

The older clinical classification categorizes amyloidosis as primary, secondary, familial, or isolated. Primary, secondary, and familial amyloidoses are usually, but not always, systemic diseases, in which patients frequently present with renal dysfunction or heart failure. The liver, spleen, gastrointestinal tract, tongue, and subcutaneous tissues are also frequent sites of amyloid deposition. Isolated amyloidosis is, by definition, restricted to a single organ.

Primary Amyloidosis Refers to the Presentation of Amyloid Without Any Preceding Disease

In one third of these cases, primary amyloidosis is an early sign of **plasma cell neoplasia**, such as multiple myeloma or other B-cell lymphomas. In this respect, primary amyloidosis forms part of the spectrum of amyloid disorders associated with B-cell dysfunction. *Whether the amyloidosis or the B-cell neoplasm presents first, the type of amyloid protein (AL amyloid) is the same.*

Secondary Amyloidosis Complicates Some Chronic Inflammatory Conditions

Secondary amyloidosis is associated with a previously existing, persistent inflammatory disorder, which may or may not have an immunologic basis. Patients with rheumatoid arthritis, ankylosing spondylitis, and occasionally systemic lupus erythematosus may develop secondary amyloidosis. Most other patients with secondary amyloidosis have long-standing inflammatory conditions (e.g., lung abscess, tuberculosis, or osteomyelitis). These disorders were the most common causes of systemic amyloidosis in the past, but the use of antibiotics and modern surgical techniques have drastically reduced the frequency of this complication. Secondary amyloidosis is also seen in patients with specific cancers, such as Hodgkin disease and renal cell carcinoma. The amyloid protein deposited secondary to these malignancies (**AA amyloid**) (see Table 23-1) is identical to that seen in rheumatoid arthritis, chronic infections, and other chronic inflammatory states discussed above.

The Incidence of Familial Amyloidoses May Vary with Ethnicity

Several geographical populations display genetically inherited forms of amyloidosis, of which Familial Mediterranean fever (FMF) is prototypical.

FMF: This autosomal recessive disease is found predominantly in the Mediterranean basin among Sephardic Jews, Turks, Armenians, and Arabs. FMF is characterized by polymorphonuclear leukocyte dysfunction and recurrent episodes of serositis, including peritonitis. Because there is recurrent inflammation, the type of amyloid protein deposited (AA amyloid) (see Table 23-1) is the same as that in secondary amyloidosis (above). The gene for Mediterranean fever *(MEFV)* has been mapped to the short arm of chromosome 16 and encodes a protein termed *pyrin* or more poetically, *marenostrin (from Mare Nostrum the Latin name for the Mediterranean Sea).* It is expressed in neutrophils and is

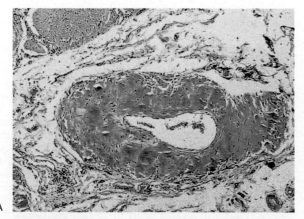
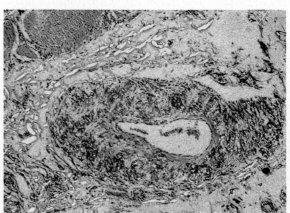

FIGURE 23-1. AL amyloid involving the wall of an artery stained with Congo red is shown under (A) ordinary light and (B) polarized light. Note the red-green birefringence of the amyloid. Collagen has a silvery appearance.

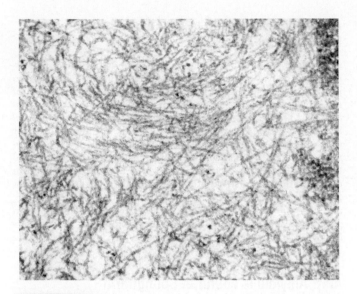

FIGURE 23-2. **Amyloid deposits in tissue.** Parallel and interlacing arrays of fibrils are evident in this electron micrograph.

thought to be a transcription factor that regulates other genes involved in the suppression of inflammation. Several other uncommon familial amyloidoses are summarized in Table 23-1. Additional current details are available by searching Online Mendelian Inheritance in Man (http://www.ncbi.nlm.nih.gov/entrez/query.fcgi?db5OMIM) for familial amyloidosis.

Isolated Amyloidosis Affects Individual Organs

Isolated amyloidosis has been described in the major arteries, lungs, heart, and various joints, and in association with endocrine tumors that secrete polypeptide hormones. In endocrine tumors, the amyloid is usually part of a hormone or a prohormone. By far, the most common organ-specific amyloids are those found in the aorta in atherosclerosis, in Alzheimer disease, and in type 2 diabetes.

Aortic Atherosclerosis and Arterial Inflammations

Amyloid has long been known to be present in the wall of the aorta at sites of atherosclerosis and in arteries with inflammation (e.g., giant cell arteritis) associated with elastic lamina. The amyloid peptide isolated in these conditions has been designated **medin** and has shown to be a 50-residue proteolytic fragment derived from **lactadherin**, previously described as a milk fat-globule membrane protein. Lactadherin is also synthesized by smooth muscle cells of the arterial media. The function of this protein, which has homology to coagulation factors V and VIII, is unknown.

Alzheimer Disease (Aβ amyloid)

In the most common form of dementia, Alzheimer disease (see Chapter 28), **Aβ amyloid** is restricted to the brain and its vessels. The deposited protein, a 4-kilodalton peptide called the Aβ protein, is a fragment of a larger **Aβ-protein precursor (Aβ-PP)**, which is a normal cell membrane constituent. Aβ PP is present not only in the cells of the central nervous system but also in most other tissues, although it is generally accepted that the source of Aβ amyloid is intracerebral. Aβ-protein is derived from Aβ-PP by proteolysis catalyzed by enzymes termed **secretases**.

TABLE 23–1

Classification of Human Amyloids

Amyloid Protein	Protein Precursor	Clinical Setting
AL	k or λ immunoglobulin light chain	Multiple myeloma, plasma cell dyscrasias, and primary amyloid
AH	γ immunoglobulin chain	Waldenström's macroglobulinemia
Aβ2M	β2-microglobulin	Hemodialysis-related
ATTR	Transthyretin	FAP, normal TTR in senile systemic amyloid
AA	Apo serum AA	Persistent acute inflammation; FMF; Certain malignancies
AApoAI	Apolipiprotein AI	FAP Iowa
AApoAII	ApolipoproteinAII	Familial
AApoAIV	ApolipoproteinAIV	Sporadic, age-associated
Aβ	β-protein precursor	Alzheimer's disease, Down syndrome, HCHWA, Dutch
ABri	ABriPP	Familial dementia, British
ADan	ADanPP	Familial dementia, Danish
APrP	Prion protein	CJD, scrapie, BSE, GSS, Kuru
ACys	Cystatin C	HCHWA, Icelandic
ALys	Lysozyme	Hereditary systemic amyloidosis, Ostertag-type
AFib	Fibrinogen	Hereditary renal amyloidosis
AGel	Gelsolin	Familial amyloidosis, Finnish
ACal	(Pro)calcitonin	Medullary carcinoma of the thyroid
AANF	Atrial natriuretic factor	Isolated atrial amyloid
AIAPP	Islet amyloid polypeptide	Type 2 diabetes, insulinomas
AIns	Insulin	Iatrogenic
APro	Prolactin	Pituitary, age associated
AMed	Lactadherin	Senile aortic, media
AKer	Keratoepithelin	Cornea, familial
ALac	Lactoferrin	Cornea

Apo, apolipoprotein; BSE, bovine spongiform encephalopathy; CJD, Creutzfeldt-Jakob disease; FAP, Familial amyloidotic polyneuropathy; FMF: familial Mediterranean fever; GSS, Gerstmann-Straussler-Sheinker syndrome; HCHWA, hereditary cerebral hemorrhage with amyloid; TTR, transthyretin.

Mutations adjacent to these cleavage sites (but not within Aβ-protein) are associated with several familial forms of Alzheimer disease, suggesting a pathogenetic role for amyloid in these situations. The gene for Aβ-PP is located on chromosome 21, which is likely to explain the observation that patients with **Down syndrome** (trisomy 21) all develop the morphologic lesions of Alzheimer disease by 35 years of age.

Diabetes (AIAPP Amyloid)

The amyloid deposited in the islets of Langerhans in type 2 diabetes (**AIAPP**) is also derived from a larger precursor, a peptide related to a variant of calcitonin, termed **islet amyloid polypeptide** (**IAPP**), or **amylin** (see Table 23-1). Like insulin, this novel hormone is produced by the β cells of the islets and has a profound effect on glucose uptake by the liver and striated muscle cells in pharmacological doses. IAPP's physiologic function has not yet been determined.

Senile Cardiac Amyloidosis

Isolated amyloid deposition may occur in the heart (**ATTR**), particularly in men, after the age of 70. This disorder is usually asymptomatic, but occasionally, extensive deposits in the myocardium may cause heart failure. The amyloid precursor responsible is **transthyretin** (see Table 23-1).

A General Scheme of Amyloidogenesis

The requirements for amyloidogenesis *in vivo* include (1) an adequate pool of an amyloidogenic protein, (2) a nidus or nucleus for fibrillogenesis, (3) conformational instability of the amyloidogenic protein (mutations, proteolysis, and protein interactions), and (4) amyloid turnover. These are schematically interrelated in Figure 23-3.

Biochemical Classification of Amyloidoses

The presence of amyloid deposits with identical proteins in seemingly distinct clinical entities implies that common pathologic processes occur. These various amyloid proteins are designated A (amyloid), followed by a letter or abbreviation that refers to the protein specific origin (see Table 23-1). The most common clinically related amyloids are (1) AMed and atherosclerosis, (2) Aβ and Alzheimer disease, and (3) AIAPP and type 2 diabetes.

AL Amyloid Derives from Immunoglobulin Light Chains

AL amyloid usually consists of the variable region of immunoglobulin light chains (L, light) and may be derived from either κ or λ chains. Occasionally, the AL amyloid subunit is larger than the variable end of light chains and may represent a complete immunoglobulin light chain. Within an individual patient, the sequence of AL amyloid protein is constant, regardless of the organ from which the amyloid is isolated, but the sequence differs between patients. *AL protein is common to primary amyloidosis and amyloidosis associated with multiple myeloma, B-cell lymphomas, or other plasma cell dyscrasias.* In some cases, the malignant disease presents first as multiple myeloma or lymphoma; in other circumstances, it is announced by AL deposits in various tissues. Only about 15% to 20 % of patients with multiple myeloma develop AL amyloid, probably because some κ or λ chains are more fibrillogenic than others (see Fig. 23-3).

AA Amyloid Occurs in a Variety of Chronic Inflammatory Processes

AA amyloid is common to a host of seemingly unrelated, persistent inflammatory, neoplastic, and hereditary disorders that lead to secondary amyloidosis. As with AL amyloid, there is a spectrum of AA peptides of differing sizes within AA deposits. *However, in contrast to AL protein, the amino-terminal sequence of AA proteins is identical in all patients, regardless of the underlying disorder.* The intact precursor of AA is **serum amyloid A** (**SAA**). The most prevalent size is a peptide of 76 amino acids, which corresponds to the amino-terminal two thirds of SAA. SAA is an acute-phase protein, and its serum concentration increases rapidly (up to 1,000-fold) during any inflammatory process under the influence of interleukin (IL)-1, IL-6, and tumor necrosis factor. The failure to degrade SAA is related in part to the appearance of a poorly defined substance termed *amyloid enhancing factor* in some individuals, which serves to promote the formation of amyloid fibrils (see Fig. 23-3).

APrP Amyloid is Found in Spongiform Encephalopathies

Prion proteins (**PrPs**) are natural plasma membrane constituents found in a variety of cells, including the central nervous system. Their physiologic function is not yet apparent. In the vast majority of people, the conformation of PrP is in a nonfibrillar, non-"infectious" state. In rare instances, a PrP protein, with or without a mutation, may experience an alteration in its conformational stability and then an altered susceptibility to proteolysis. Such altered PrP and its aggregates form fibrils with the characteristics of amyloid and are believed to play a role in a group of human and animal degenerative diseases of the brain such as **kuru, Creutzfeldt-Jakob disease, Gerstmann-Straussler-Sheinker disease, scrapie, and bovine spongiform encephalopathy (mad cow disease)** (see Chapters 9 and 28).

Deposition of ATTR Amyloid (Transthyretin Amyloid) Occurs in Several Different Types of Amyloidosis, Including Familial Amyloidotic Polyneuropathy

Transthyretin (**TTR**) is secreted by the liver into the plasma, where it serves as a carrier of thyroid hormone and of retinal binding protein. At least 80 mutants of TTR have been described, each responsible for a clinical variant of familial amyloidotic polyneuropathy (see Table 23-1). Interestingly, normal TTR is deposited in isolated cardiac amyloidosis and in a systemic form of amyloidosis associated with aging, indicating that an altered amino acid sequence is not an absolute requirement for the deposition of ATTR.

Other Amyloid Proteins May be Less Well Characterized

Other forms of amyloid are derived from normal pre-prohormones or from hormonal products secreted by endocrine tissues or tumors. Medullary thyroid carcinoma originates from thyroid C-type cells, which secrete calcitonin. Amyloid deposited in this tumor is a fragment of procalcitonin. In isolated atrial amyloid, the peptide is atrial natriuretic factor. Amyloid proteins related to keratin have been reported in the skin. In other isolated forms of human amyloidosis (e.g., amyloid in osteoarthritic joints associated with aging), the deposited materials are not yet characterized. Conformational instability of several other proteins with amyloid-like fibril formation is believed to play a role in several neurological diseases.

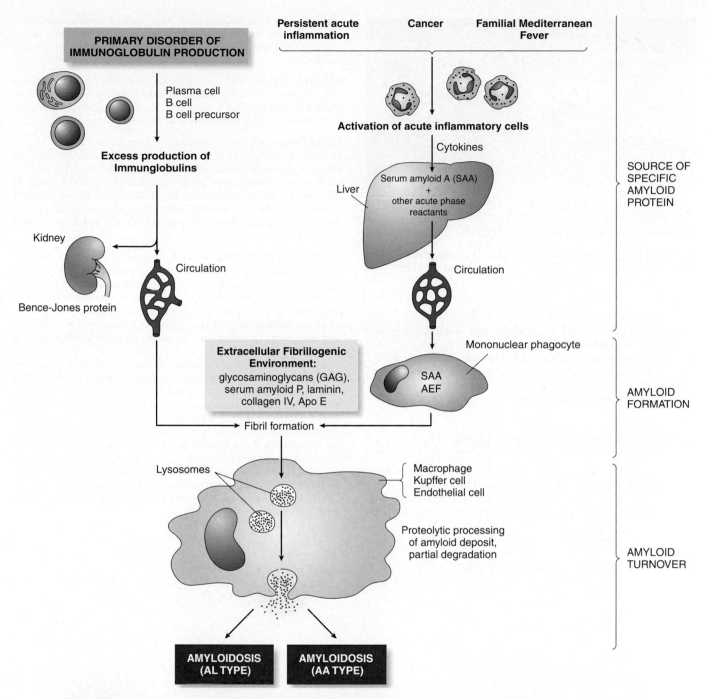

FIGURE 23-3. **The mechanisms of amyloid deposition.** For **AL amyloid:** Lymphocyte- and plasma cell-derived intact immunoglobulins light chains are amyloidogenic within a fibrillogenic environment. Macrophages are involved in amyloid turnover occurs by proteolytic processing. For **AA amyloid** deposition: A variety of diseases is associated with the activation of polymorphonuclear leukocytes and macrophages, which in turn leads to the synthesis and release of acute phase reactants by the liver, including serum amyloid A (SAA). SAA in the presence oTf amyloid-enhancing factor (AEF) is likely released substantially intact by macrophages. In a fibrillogenic environment, the released products complex with glycosaminoglycans and serum amyloid PV (SAP). Macrophages are involved in amyloid turnover occurs by proteolytic processing.

Morphologic Features of Amyloidoses

Amyloid fibrils are usually first deposited in close association with subendothelial basement membranes. *Because amyloid accumulates along stromal networks, the deposits take on the architectural framework of the organs involved.* The morphologic differences in amyloid deposition among organs simply reflect differences between tissues in stromal organization. Amyloid adds interstitial material to sites of deposition, thereby increasing the size of affected organs. This increase may be counterbalanced by the deposition of amyloid in blood vessels (Fig. 23-4), which impairs circulation and may lead to organ atrophy. Affected organs may thus increase or decrease in size. Compact amyloid deposits are essentially avascular, so the involved organs are commonly pale and firm. Regardless of whether amyloid is laid down in a systemic or local fashion, deposits tend

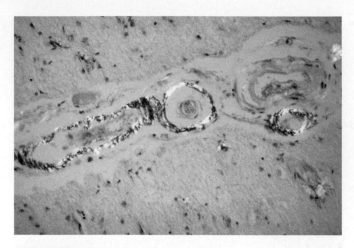

FIGURE 23-4. Cerebrovascular amyloid in a case of Alzheimer's disease. The section was stained with Congo red and examined under polarized light.

to occur between parenchymal cells and their blood supply, interfering with normal nutrition and gas exchange. Amyloid may eventually entrap parenchymal cells. Alternatively, it may have a direct toxic effect on these cells through the interaction of protofibrils and cell membranes. *In each case, amyloidosis leads to strangulation, atrophy, and death of cells.*

Clinical Features of Amyloidoses

No single set of symptoms points unequivocally to amyloidosis as a diagnosis. Amyloid is readily demonstrated in gingival and rectal biopsy specimens and in abdominal subcutaneous fat. Amyloidosis may also be diagnosed unexpectedly in the course of evaluation for an unrelated condition, with no clinical manifestations referable to the amyloidosis itself. In other cases, unexplained renal and cardiac complications may be the presenting conditions.

KIDNEY: Patients with multiple myeloma, chronic long-standing inflammatory disorders, or FMF who develop nephrotic syndrome should be suspected of having amyloidosis. Progressive glomerular obliteration may ultimately lead to renal failure and uremia.

HEART: Amyloid involvement of the myocardium should be suspected in systemic forms of amyloidosis in which congestive failure or cardiomegaly is associated with low voltage on the electrocardiogram. Entrapment of the conduction system leads to arrhythmias, which in turn can result in sudden death. Amyloid deposition in the myocardium may also impair ventricular pliancy and limit filling, an effect that appears clinically as a *restrictive form of cardiomyopathy.*

GASTROINTESTINAL TRACT: The ganglia, smooth muscle, vasculature, and submucosa of the gastrointestinal tract may all be affected by amyloid. Deposits in these locations alter gastrointestinal motility and absorption. Patients complain of either constipation or diarrhea, occasionally in association with malabsorption. Enlargement of the tongue is classic, and interference with its motor function may be severe enough to affect speech and swallowing.

In all systemic forms of amyloidosis, the patient's course is usually unremitting and ultimately fatal. Patients with multiple myeloma and AL amyloidosis generally die within 1 to 2 years, either from the malignancy itself or from cardiac or renal complications of amyloidosis. Patients with AA amyloidosis secondary to long-standing inflammatory disease have a more protracted course, but often die, usually from cardiac or renal failure within 5 years of diagnosis. Successful treatment of the underlying condition, such as multiple myeloma or an inflammatory disorder, may on occasion lead to resorption and resolution of amyloid deposits. These clinical observations indicate that amyloid does turn over, albeit slowly.

24 The Skin

Craig A. Storm
David E. Elder

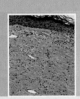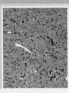

*The skin is our interface with the environment. It serves as
a critical protective barrier. Microorganisms find it almost
impossible to penetrate the epidermis from the outside,
and water loss from the inside is carefully controlled. The
skin is vital in regulating temperature and protecting
against ultraviolet light. A variety of sensory receptors
communicate details related to the immediate environment. The skin also plays a prominent role in immune
regulation through skin-associated lymphoid tissues, which
consist of lymphocytes and antigen-presenting cells that
travel between the skin and regional lymph nodes via the
lymphatics and bloodstream. Keratinocytes, Langerhans
cells, mast cells, lymphocytes, and macrophages all serve
functions related to immunity and reside in the skin.
Damage to a majority of the skin through congenital or
acquired disease, or from trauma such as burns will have
serious consequences for the individual and may well result in death from fluid loss and infections. Historically,
the skin was seen as the mirror of the soul. Visible lesions
were noted and ascribed to defects in character as well as
the body. The image of the leper and his bell still resonates.
Even today, visible lesions of the skin have a social significance that may equal or exceed the pathologic aspects.*

Diseases of the Epidermis

Ichthyoses Feature Epidermal Thickening and Scales

*Ichthyosiform dermatoses, many of which are heritable, comprise a hetero-
geneous group of diseases characterized by striking thickening of the stratum
corneum. The term **ichthyosis** reflects the similarity of the diseased*

skin to coarse, fish-like scales (Fig. 24-1). Several rare ichthyoses are associated with other abnormalities, such as abnormal lipid metabolism, neurologic disorders, bone diseases, and cancer.

 PATHOGENESIS: Three general defects are involved in the excessive epidermal cornification of the ichthyoses:

- **Increased cohesiveness** of the cells of the stratum corneum, possibly related to altered lipid metabolism
- **Abnormal keratinization** manifested as impaired tonofilament (intermediate keratin filament) formation, keratohyaline synthesis, and excessive cornification
- **Increased basal cell proliferation** associated with a decrease in the transit time of keratinocytes across the epidermis

 PATHOLOGY: All ichthyoses (with the possible exception of lamellar ichthyosis) have a stratum corneum that is disproportionately thick in comparison with the nucleated epidermal layers. Virtually all diseases characterized by thickening of the nucleated epidermal layers also exhibit hyperkeratosis; however, in ichthyosis, the stratum corneum may be five times thicker than normal, although it overlies a disproportionately thin nucleated epidermis.

Ichthyosis Vulgaris

Ichthyosis vulgaris is an autosomal dominant disorder responsible for 95% of cases of ichthyosis and is the prototype of disproportionate corneal thickening. The disease is associated with decreased or absent synthesis of **profilaggrin**, the major component of the keratohyaline granules in the stratum corneum. Degradation products of the molecule normally serve to maintain skin flexibility. Scaly skin results from increased cohesiveness of the stratum corneum. The stratum corneum is loose and has a basket-weave appearance, which differs from normal only in amount. The granular layer is greatly diminished and often appears absent (see Fig. 24-1B).

 CLINICAL FEATURES: Ichthyosis vulgaris begins in early childhood, and a family history of this condition is often obtained. Small white scales occur on the extensor surfaces of extremities and on the trunk and face. The disease is life-long, but most patients can be maintained free of scales with topical treatment.

Other Congenital Ichthyoses

Several other heritable ichthyotic conditions are associated with mutations of several genes. The diseases include:

- **X-linked ichthyosis** is characterized by a lack of steroid sulfatase and leads to delayed dissolution of desmosomal disks in the stratum corneum.
- **Epidermolytic hyperkeratosis** is an autosomal dominant condition characterized by hyperkeratosis and blistering, which results from mutations in several keratin genes that prevent normal development of the cytoskeleton. As a consequence, epidermal "lysis" and a tendency to form vesicles occur.
- **Lamellar ichthyosis** is an autosomal recessive congenital disorder of cornification characterized by severe and generalized ichthyosis. The disease is often caused by mutations in transglutaminase 1 (*TGM1;* chromosome 14q11). Children with the disorder are born covered in a "collodion" membrane, which is shed soon after birth and is accompanied by the development of disfiguring hyperkeratosis.

Acquired Ichthyosis

Clinical and histologic states similar to ichthyosis vulgaris are occasionally associated with other diseases or may follow the use of drugs. Lymphomas, especially Hodgkin disease, other neoplasms, systemic granulomatous disorders, and connective tissue diseases may be associated with ichthyosis. Drugs may produce ichthyosis by interfering with pathways of lipid metabolism.

Psoriasis is a Proliferative Skin Disease Characterized by Persistent Epidermal Hyperplasia

Psoriasis is a chronic, often familial, disorder that features large, erythematous, scaly plaques, commonly on extensor cutaneous surfaces. It affects 1% to 2% of the population worldwide and may arise at any age but shows a peak in late adolescence. Interestingly, psoriasis is not seen among American Indians and is infrequent among Asians.

 PATHOGENESIS: The pathogenesis of psoriasis is poorly understood and is likely multifactorial.

GENETIC FACTORS: Psoriasis unquestionably has a genetic component, although only one third of patients with psoriasis have a family history of the disease. The more severe the illness is, the greater the likelihood of a familial background. The genetic basis for psoriasis rests on a number of observations: (1) increased incidence among relatives and offspring of patients with

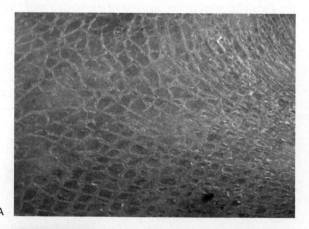 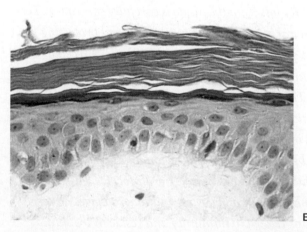

FIGURE 24-1. **Ichthyosis vulgaris. A.** Noninflammatory fish-like scales are evident on the thigh of a patient with a strong family history of ichthyosis vulgaris. **B.** There is disproportionate thickening of the stratum corneum relative to the normal thickness of the nucleated epidermal layer. The stratum granulosum is thin and focally absent.

psoriasis; (2) 65% concordance for psoriasis in monozygotic twins; and (3) increases in certain HLA haplotypes in affected persons, especially HLA-B13, HLA-B17, HLA-Bw57, and particularly HLA-Cw6. In fact, individuals with HLA-Cw6 are 10 to 15 times more likely to develop psoriasis than is the general population.

ENVIRONMENTAL FACTORS: Clinical lesions may occur anywhere on the skin. A variety of stimuli, such as physical injury ("Köbner phenomenon"), infection, certain drugs, and photosensitivity, may produce psoriatic lesions in apparently normal skin.

ABNORMAL CELLULAR PROLIFERATION: There is evidence to suggest that deregulation of epidermal proliferation and an abnormality in the dermal microcirculation produce psoriatic lesions (Fig. 24-2). Decreased adenylyl cyclase activity in the lower proliferative compartment of the epidermis has been attributed to faulty β-adrenergic receptors. The decrease in cyclic AMP alters cutaneous responses to trauma in complex ways that are not fully understood.

MICROCIRCULATORY CHANGES: In psoriatic skin, the capillary loops of the dermal papillae become venular, showing multiple layers of basal lamina material, wide lumina, and "bridged" fenestrations between endothelial cells. The vascular change, which occurs in concert with a striking increase in neutrophilic chemotactic factors, leads to diapedesis of many neutrophils at the tips of dermal papillae and subsequent migration into the epidermis (see Fig. 24-2). This unusual pattern of neutrophilic inflammation is responsible for the dense collections of neutrophils in the stratum corneum (**Munro microabscesses**), as well as for the scattering of neutrophils throughout the epidermis (**spongiform pustules**).

IMMUNOLOGIC FACTORS: T lymphocytes may be key to the pathogenesis of psoriatic lesions. The eruption of psoriatic lesions coincides with T-cell infiltration into the epidermis. By contrast, the resolution of psoriatic plaques, whether spontaneous or induced by treatment, follows disappearance of, or reduction in, epidermal T cells.

PATHOLOGY: The epidermis in patients with psoriasis is thickened and shows hyperkeratosis and parakeratosis (persistence of nuclei in the cells of the stratum corneum). Parakeratosis may be present as circumscribed, ellipsoidal foci, or it may be diffuse, in which case the granular layer is diminished or absent. The nucleated layers of the epidermis are thickened several-fold in the rete pegs and are frequently thinner over the dermal papillae (Fig. 24-3). In turn, the papillae are elongated and appear as sections of cones, with their apices toward the dermis. In chronic lesions, dermal papillae tend to appear as bulbous clubs with short handles (see Fig. 24-3). The rete ridges of the epidermis have a profile reciprocal to that of the dermal papillae, resulting in interlocked dermal and epidermal clubs, with alternatively reversed polarity. The capillaries of the papillae are dilated and tortuous.

Neutrophils may become localized in the epidermal spinous layer or in small Munro microabscesses in the stratum corneum and may be associated with circumscribed areas of parakeratosis. The dermis below the papillae contains a variable mononuclear inflammatory infiltrate, mostly lymphocytes, around the superficial vascular plexus. The inflammatory process does not extend into the subjacent reticular dermis.

CLINICAL FEATURES: The initial presentation of psoriasis is variable, and disease activity is intermittent. The severity of the disorder varies from annoying scaly lesions over the elbows to a serious debilitating disorder involving most of the skin, which is often associated with arthritis (see Fig. 24-3A). A typical plaque is 4 to 5 cm in diameter, is sharply demarcated at its margin, and is covered by a sur-

face of silvery scales. When the scales are detached, pinpoint foci of bleeding, originating from the dilated capillaries in the dermal papillae, dot the underlying glossy erythematous surface ("Auspitz sign").

Of all patients with psoriasis, 7% develop **seronegative arthritis** (see Chapter 26). The tendency to arthropathy is linked to several HLA haplotypes, particularly HLA-B27. Psoriatic arthritis closely resembles its rheumatoid counterpart, but it is usually milder and causes little disability.

Psoriasis has long been treated with coal tar or wood tar derivatives and anthralin, a strong reducing agent. Topical and systemic corticosteroids have also been used. Severe, generalized psoriasis justifies systemic treatment with methotrexate. Phototherapy ("PUVA") after administration of psoralens, ultraviolet-absorbing compounds that bind to DNA, is often effective. More recently, synthetic vitamin A and vitamin D derivatives have also been used.

Pemphigus Vulgaris (PV) is a Blistering Skin Disorder Caused by Antibodies to Keratinocytes

Dyshesive disorders are cutaneous maladies in which blister formation is secondary to diminished cohesiveness of the epidermal keratinocytes. PV (Greek, *pemphix*, "bubble"), the prototype of dyshesive diseases, is a chronic, blistering skin disorder, which is most common in people between 40 and 60 years of age, but is seen in all age groups, including children. All races are susceptible, but persons of Jewish or Mediterranean heritage are at greater risk.

PATHOGENESIS: PV is an autoimmune disease in which circulating IgG antibodies react with an epidermal surface antigen called **desmoglein 3**, a desmosomal protein. Antigen–antibody union results in dyshesion, which is augmented by the release of plasminogen activator and the generation of plasmin. This proteolytic enzyme acts on intercellular substance and may be the dominant factor in dyshesion. Internalization of the pemphigus antigen–antibody complex, disappearance of attachment plaques, and retraction of perinuclear tonofilaments may all act in concert with proteinases to cause dyshesion and vesiculation.

PATHOLOGY: The blister in PV forms because of the separation of the outer epidermal layers from the basal layer. This suprabasal dyshesion results in a blister that has an intact basal layer as a floor and the remaining epidermis as a roof (Fig. 24-4). Desmoglein 3 is concentrated in the lower epidermis, explaining the location of the blister. The blister contains moderate numbers of lymphocytes, macrophages, eosinophils, and neutrophils. Distinctive, rounded keratinocytes, termed acantholytic cells, are shed into the vesicle during dyshesion. The subjacent dermis shows a moderate infiltrate of lymphocytes, macrophages, eosinophils, and neutrophils, predominantly around the capillary venular bed.

CLINICAL FEATURES: The characteristic lesion of PV is a large, easily ruptured blister, which leaves extensive denuded or crusted areas. Lesions are most common on the scalp and mucous membranes and in periumbilical and intertriginous areas. Corticosteroid treatment is effective, but without it, PV is progressive and usually fatal, and much of the skin surface may become denuded. Immunosuppressive agents are also useful for maintenance therapy. With appropriate treatment, the 10-year mortality rate for PV is less than 10%.

Pemphigus may be associated with other autoimmune diseases, such as myasthenia gravis and lupus erythematosus, and may also be seen with benign thymomas.

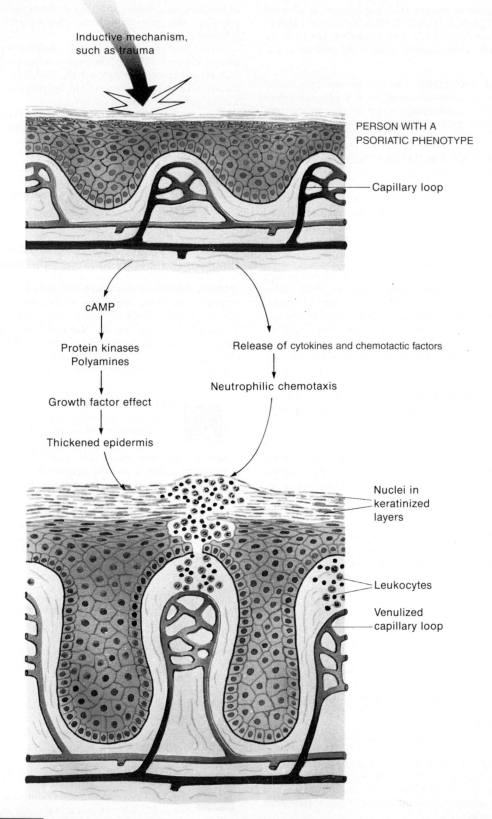

Inductive mechanism, such as trauma

PERSON WITH A PSORIATIC PHENOTYPE

Capillary loop

cAMP

Protein kinases
Polyamines

Release of cytokines and chemotactic factors

Growth factor effect

Neutrophilic chemotaxis

Thickened epidermis

Nuclei in keratinized layers

Leukocytes

Venulized capillary loop

FIGURE 24-2. **Pathogenetic mechanisms in psoriasis.** The drawing depicts the deregulation of epidermal growth, venulization of the capillary loop, and a unique form of neutrophilic inflammation. The altered epidermal growth is thought to be caused by defective epidermal cell surface receptors. This results in a decrease in cyclic adenosine monophosphate (cAMP), together with the effects indicated. The decrease in cAMP is also likely to be related to the increased production of arachidonic acid, which in turn leads to activation of leukotriene B4 (LTB-4). This potent neutrophilic chemotactic agent acts on a venulized capillary loop. Neutrophils then emerge from the tips of the capillary loop at the apex of the dermal papilla rather than from the postcapillary venule, as is the rule in most inflammatory skin diseases.

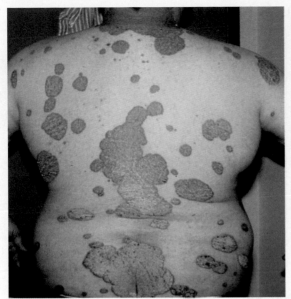
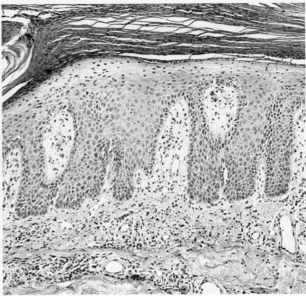

FIGURE 24-3. **Psoriasis.** This disorder is the prototype of psoriasiform epidermal hyperplasia. **A.** A patient with psoriasis shows large, confluent, sharply demarcated, erythematous plaques on the trunk. **B.** Microscopic examination of a lesion demonstrates that the rete ridges are uniformly elongated, as are the dermal papillae, giving an interlocking pattern of alternately reversed "clubs." The dermal papillae are edematous and reside beneath a thinned epidermis (suprapapillary thinning). There is striking parakeratosis, which is the scale observed clinically.

Diseases of the Basement Membrane Zone (BMZ) (Dermal–Epidermal Interface)

Epidermolysis Bullosa (EB) Features Blister Formation in the Basement Membrane Zone

EB comprises a heterogeneous group of disorders defined by their hereditary nature and by a tendency to form blisters at the sites of minor trauma. The clinical spectrum ranges from a minor annoyance to a widespread, life-threatening blistering disease. *EB blisters are almost always noted at birth or shortly thereafter.* The classification of these disorders is based on the site of blister formation in the BMZ. The different mechanisms of blister formation underlie each of the three major categories of EB (Fig. 24-5).

- **Epidermolytic EB** (**EB simplex**) is a group of autosomal dominant skin diseases in which blisters form as a result of disruption of basal keratinocytes. The condition has been attributed to mutations of genes encoding cytokeratin intermediate filaments. Cytolysis of basal keratinocytes results in blisters that develop in response to minor trauma but heal without scarring.

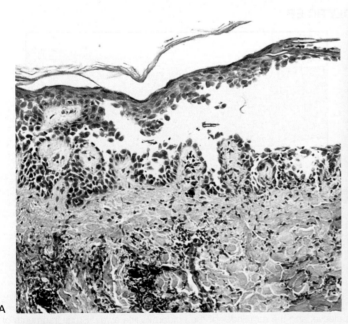
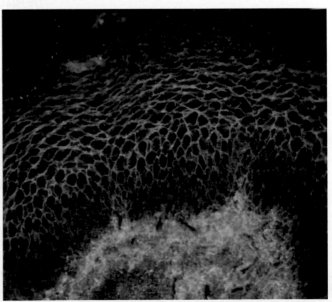

FIGURE 24-4. **Pemphigus vulgaris. A.** Suprabasal dyshesion leads to an intraepidermal blister containing acantholytic keratinocytes. The basal keratinocytes are slightly separated from each other and totally separated from the stratum spinosum. The basal keratinocytes are firmly attached to the epidermal basement membrane zone. **B.** Direct immunofluorescence examination of perilesional skin reveals antibodies, usually of the immunoglobulin G (IgG) type, deposited in the intercellular substance of the epidermis, yielding a lace-like pattern outlining the keratinocytes.

EPIDERMOLYTIC EB

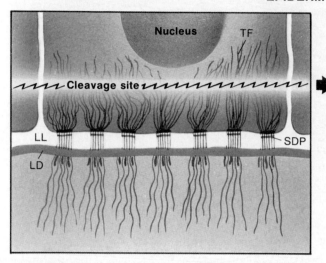
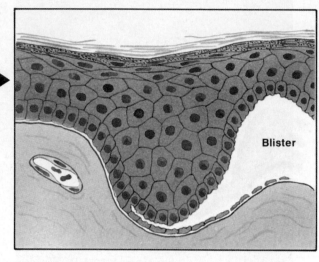

JUNCTIONAL EB

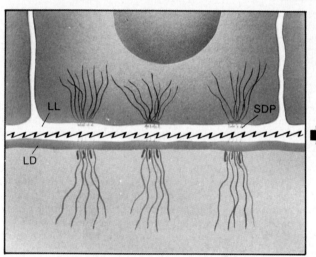
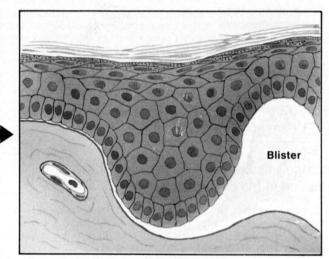

DERMOLYTIC EB

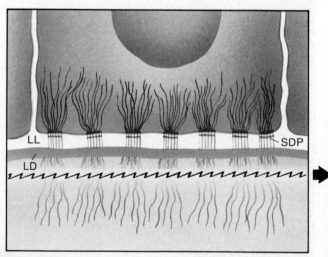
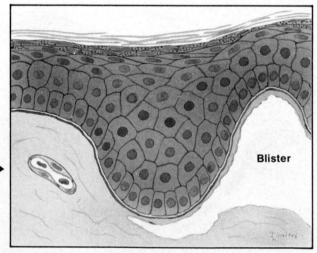

FIGURE 24-5. **Epidermolysis bullosa (EB).** Three distinct mechanisms of blister formation are shown. Electron microscopic images are diagrammed on the *left;* light microscopic images are on the *right.* Epidermolytic EB is caused by disintegration of the lowermost regions of the epidermal basal cells. The bottom portions of the basal cells cleave, and the remainder of the epidermis lifts away. Small fragments of basal cells remain attached to the basement membrane zone. Junctional EB is characterized by cleavage in the lamina lucida. Dermolytic EB is associated with rudimentary and fragmented anchoring fibrils. The entire basement membrane zone and epidermis split away from the dermis in relationship to these flawed anchoring fibrils. LL, lamina lucida; LD, lamina densa; SDP, subdesomosomal dense plate.

- **Junctional EB** is a heritable, autosomal recessive skin disease in which blisters form within the lamina lucida. The clinical expression ranges from a benign disease with no effect on life span (associated with mutations in the gene for type XVII collagen) to a severe condition that may be fatal within the first 2 years of life. The latter features mutations in the genes for some laminin isoforms and integrins.

- **Dermolytic (or dystrophic) EB** is a heritable skin condition in which blisters are located immediately deep to the lamina densa. Dermolytic disease may be either dominant or recessive, and the latter is more severe. In both variants, healed blisters are characterized by atrophic ("dystrophic") scarring. The basic lesion is a mutation in the gene encoding collagen type VII on chromosome 3 (3p21), which leads to a defect in the anchoring fibrils, a structure that helps to anchor the epidermis to the underlying dermis. Disruption of the anchoring fibers results in subepidermal bullae.

Bullous Pemphigoid (BP) is a Blistering Disease Caused by Autoantibodies Against Basement Membrane Proteins

BP is a common, autoimmune, blistering disease with clinical similarities to pemphigus vulgaris (thus, the term "pemphigoid") but in which acantholysis is absent. The disease is most common in the later decades of life, although it shows no predilection regarding race or gender.

 PATHOGENESIS: Like PV, BP is an autoimmune disease, but in this case, complement-fixing IgG antibodies are directed against two basement membrane proteins, BPAG1 and BPAG2. The antigen–antibody complex may injure the basal cell plasma membrane via the C5b-C9 membrane attack complex (see Chapter 4). The immune injury leads to the recruitment of eosinophils, granules of which contain tissue-damaging substances, including eosinophil peroxidase and major basic protein. These molecules, together with proteases of neutrophilic and mast cell origin, cause dermal–epidermal separation within the lamina lucida.

 PATHOLOGY: The blisters of BP are subepidermal; the roof is intact epidermis, and the base is the lamina densa of the BMZ (Fig. 24-6). The blisters contain numerous eosinophils, together with fibrin, lymphocytes, and neutrophils.

 CLINICAL FEATURES: The blisters of BP are large and tense and may appear on normal-appearing skin or on an erythematous base (see Fig. 24-6). The medial thighs and flexor aspects of the forearms are commonly affected, but the groin, axillae, and other cutaneous sites may also develop blisters. The disease is self-limited but chronic, and the patient's general health is usually unaffected. The course of the disease is greatly shortened by systemic administration of corticosteroids.

Erythema Multiforme (EM) is Often a Reaction to a Drug or Infection

EM is an acute, self-limited disorder that varies from a few erythematous macules and blisters (EM minor) to a life-threatening, widespread ulceration of the skin and mucous membranes (EM major, Stevens-Johnson syndrome). *This phenomenon is usually a reaction to a drug or an infectious agent, in particular, herpes simplex infection.*

 PATHOGENESIS: The list of agents that may provoke EM is long and includes Herpesvirus, *Mycoplasma,* and sulfonamides. However, a precipitating factor is found in only half of the cases. In postherpetic EM, viral antigens, IgM, and C3 are deposited in a perivascular location and at the epidermal BMZ. The combination of infiltrating lymphocytes and antigen–antibody complexes within the lesions suggests that both humoral and cellular hypersensitivity are involved.

 PATHOLOGY: The dermis in EM shows a sparse lymphocyte infiltrate about the superficial vascular bed and at the dermal–epidermal interface. The characteristic morphologic feature in the epidermis is the presence of apoptotic keratinocytes, which have a pyknotic nucleus and an

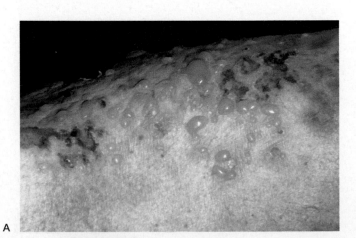

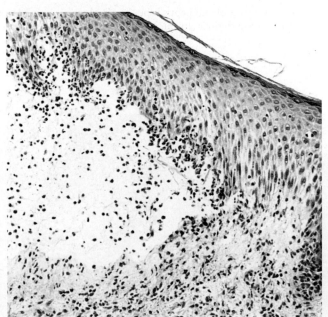

FIGURE 24-6. Bullous pemphigoid. A. The skin shows multiple tense bullae on an erythematous base and erosions, distributed primarily on the medial thighs and trunk. **B.** A subepidermal blister has an edematous papillary dermis as its base. The roof of the blister consists of the intact, entire epidermis, including the stratum basalis. Inflammatory cells, fibrin, and fluid fill the blister.

eosinophilic cytoplasm. Apoptosis may be extensive and associated with a subepidermal vesicle with a roof that is an almost completely necrotic epidermis.

CLINICAL FEATURES: The characteristic "target" or "iris" lesions of EM have a central, dark red zone, occasionally with a blister, surrounded by a paler area (Fig. 24-7). In turn, the latter is encompassed by a peripheral red rim. Urticarial plaques are common. The presence of vesicles and bullae usually predicts a more severe course. EM is a common condition, with a peak incidence in the second and third decades of life. **Stevens-Johnson syndrome** refers to an unusually severe form of EM that involves several mucosal surfaces, internal organs, and is frequently fatal.

Systemic Lupus Erythematosus (SLE) is an Immune Complex Disease

SLE, the paradigm of an immune complex disease, is characterized by a variety of autoantibodies and other immune abnormalities (see Chapters 4 and 16). Although cutaneous involvement may be severe and cosmetically devastating, by itself, it is not life-threatening.

PATHOGENESIS: Immune complexes are not likely to be solely responsible for the cutaneous lesions of SLE, because they are present in both lesional and normal-appearing skin. Deposition of immune reactants along the epidermal BMZ (positive lupus band test) of "normal" skin is important in the diagnosis of SLE (Fig. 24-8). Epidermal injury seems to be initiated by exogenous agents such as ultraviolet light and perpetuated by cell-mediated immune reactions. The manifestations of epidermal injury include (1) vacuolization of basal keratinocytes, hyperkeratosis, and diminished epidermal thickness; (2) release of DNA and other nuclear and cytoplasmic antigens to the circulation; and (3) deposition of DNA and other antigenic determinants in the epidermal BMZ (lamina densa and immediately subjacent dermis). Thus, epidermal injury, local immune-complex formation, deposition of circulating immune complexes, and lymphocyte-induced cellular injury all seem to act in concert.

The various forms of cutaneous lupus erythematosus have been classified according to their chronicity, but considerable overlap in features is possible. There is an inverse relationship between the prominence of skin lesions and the extent of systemic pathology.

CHRONIC CUTANEOUS (DISCOID) LUPUS ERYTHEMATOSUS: This form of lupus is usually limited to the skin. Disease generally manifests above the neck, on the face (especially the malar area), scalp, and ears. The lesions begin as slightly elevated violaceous papules with a rough scale of keratin. As they enlarge, they assume a disk shape, with a hyperkeratotic margin and a depigmented center. The cutaneous lesions may culminate in disfiguring scars. Elevation of circulating antinuclear antibodies (ANAs) is seen in fewer than 10% of patients.

SUBACUTE CUTANEOUS LUPUS ERYTHEMATOSUS: This disorder primarily afflicts young and middle-aged white women. In contrast to discoid lupus, subacute cutaneous lupus may also involve the musculoskeletal system and kidneys. Initially, scaly erythematous papules develop and then enlarge into psoriasiform or annular lesions, which may fuse. The skin changes are seen in the upper chest, upper back, and extensor surfaces of the arms, a distribution indicating that light exposure plays a role in the pathogenesis of the disorder. Significant scarring does not occur. About 70% of patients have circulating anti-Ro (ss-A) antibodies, and ANA levels are elevated in 70%.

ACUTE SLE: More than 80% of patients with SLE have acute cutaneous manifestations during their illness, in association with disease of the kidneys and joints. The rash is often the first manifestation of the disease and may precede the onset of systemic symptoms by a few months. The typical "butterfly" rash of SLE is a delicate erythema of the malar area of the face, which may pass in a few hours or a few days. Many patients exhibit a maculopapular eruption of the chest and extremities, often developing after sun exposure. Both rashes heal without scarring. Lesions indistinguishable from discoid lupus may occur. ANA levels are elevated in more than 90% of patients.

Lichen Planus is a Hypersensitivity Reaction with Lymphocytic Infiltrates at the Dermal–Epidermal Junction

"Lichenoid" tissue reactions are so named because the clinical lesions resemble certain lichens that form a scaly growth on rocks or tree trunks. Histologically, a lichenoid infiltrate is characterized by a band-like infiltrate of lymphocytes that obscures the dermal–epidermal

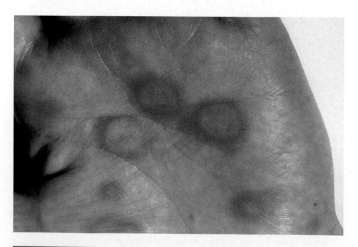

FIGURE 24-7.   Erythema multiforme. Steroid-responsive "target" papules, characterized by central bullae with surrounding erythema, appeared after antibiotic therapy.

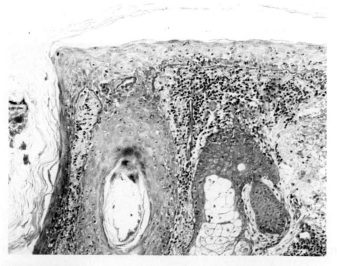

FIGURE 24-8.   Lupus erythematosus. A variably cell-rich to cell-poor, band-like, lymphocytic infiltrate is present in the papillary and adventitial dermis. There is epidermal atrophy arising from damage to the epidermis, which is mediated by infiltrating lymphocytes.

junction. The disease is characterized by reduced epidermal turnover and subsequent hyperkeratosis without parakeratosis (retention of nuclei in the cells of the stratum corneum). Lichen planus (LP) is the prototypic disorder of this group.

 PATHOGENESIS: The etiology of LP is unknown. It is occasionally familial and may also accompany a variety of autoimmune disorders. Drugs such as gold, chlorothiazide, and chloroquine and some external chemicals may induce lichenoid reactions. Evidence supports the notion that LP is a delayed type of hypersensitivity reaction, initiated and amplified by cytokines such as gamma interferon (IFN-γ) and IL-6, with expression that is due not only to infiltrating lymphocytes but also to stimulated keratinocytes. An association of LP with hepatitis B and C infections has been observed.

 PATHOLOGY: The distinctive pathological changes of LP are at the dermal–epidermal interface. The basal row of cuboidal cells is replaced by flattened or polygonal keratinocytes. The undulating interface between the dermal papillae and the rounded profiles of the rete ridges is obscured by a dense infiltrate of lymphocytes and macrophages, many of the latter containing melanin pigment (melanophages) (Fig. 24-9). Commonly admixed with the infiltrate (in the epidermis or dermis) are globular, fibrillary, eosinophilic bodies, 15 to 20 mm in diameter which represent apoptotic keratinocytes. These structures are variably termed *apoptotic, colloid, Civatte, or fibrillary bodies.*

 CLINICAL FEATURES: LP is a chronic eruption characterized by violaceous, flat-topped papules, usually on the flexor surfaces of the wrists (see Fig. 24-9A). White patches or streaks may also be present on the oral mucous membranes. In most patients, the pruritic lesions resolve in less than a year, but they occasionally persist for longer periods.

Inflammatory Diseases of the Superficial and Deep Vascular Bed

Urticaria and Angioedema are IgE-Dependent Hypersensitivity Reactions

These reactions are initiated by degranulation of mast cells sensitized to a specific antigen. **Urticaria** or hives are raised, pale, well-demarcated pruritic papules and plaques, which appear and disap-

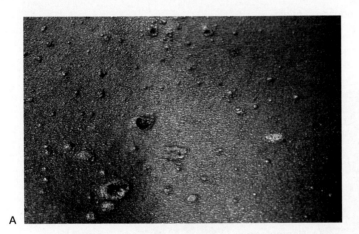

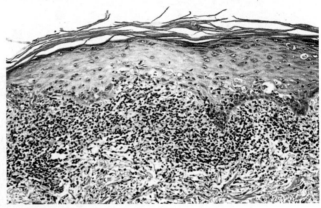

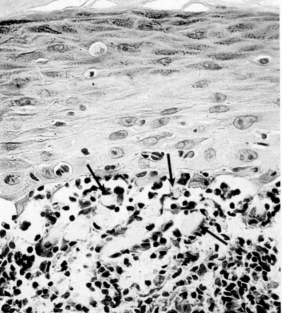

FIGURE 24-9. **Lichen planus. A.** The skin displays multiple flat-topped violaceous polygonal papules. **B.** A cell-rich, band-like, lymphocytic infiltrate disrupts the stratum basalis. Unlike lupus erythematosus, there is usually epidermal hyperplasia, hyperkeratosis, and wedge-like hypergranulosis. **C.** Hypergranulosis and loss of rete ridges are noted. The site of pathologic injury is at the dermal-epidermal junction where there is a striking infiltrate of lymphocytes, many of which surround apoptotic keratinocytes.

pear within a few hours. The lesions represent edema of the superficial portion of the dermis. **Angioedema** refers to a condition in which the edema involves the deeper dermis or subcutis, resulting in an egg-like swelling. Both entities have a rapid onset and range in severity from simply annoying lesions to life-threatening anaphylactic reactions. The mainstays of treatment are avoidance of the offending agent and prompt administration of antihistamines.

 PATHOGENESIS: Most cases of urticaria are IgE-dependent and reflect exaggerated venule permeability, owing to mast cell degranulation. An almost endless list of materials may react with IgE antibodies on the surface of the mast cell. Urticaria occurs in both atopic and nonatopic individuals.

Initially, cutaneous venules react to degranulation of mast cells and the release of their vasoactive mediators, with increased permeability resulting in rapidly forming edema. If the reaction persists, inflammatory cells are attracted to the area, and a persistent urticarial plaque (lasting more than a day) results.

 PATHOLOGY: In urticaria, collagen fibers and fibrils are splayed apart by excess fluid. Lymphatic vessels are dilated and venules show margination of neutrophils and eosinophils. Vessels are cuffed by a few lymphocytes. Persistent urticaria shows increased lymphocytes and eosinophils, but neutrophils are sparse.

Allergic Contact Dermatitis is Cell-Mediated Hypersensitivity to Exogenous Sensitizing Agents

Many of the most common sensitizing agents are members of the *Rhus* genus of plants. About 90% of the population of the United States is sensitive to these offenders: *Rhus radicans* (poison ivy), *Rhus diversiloba* (poison oak), and *Rhus vernix* (poison sumac). These plant dermatitides are so well known that the resultant disease is commonly labeled according to the offending plant.

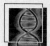 **PATHOGENESIS:** The plants contain low-molecular-weight oleoresins, which combine with a carrier protein in the affected person. Formation of this hapten-carrier complex requires about 1

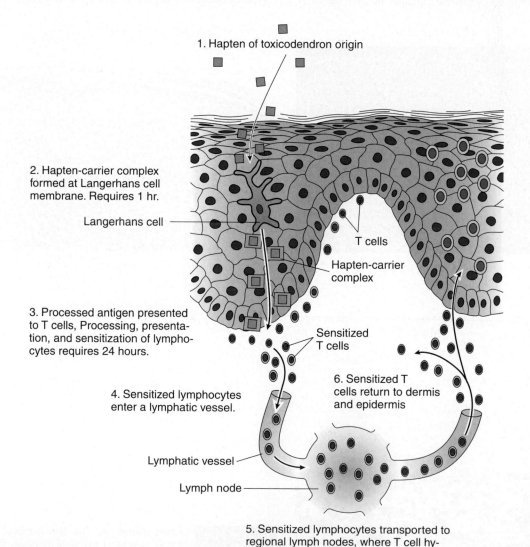

1. Hapten of toxicodendron origin

2. Hapten-carrier complex formed at Langerhans cell membrane. Requires 1 hr.

Langerhans cell

T cells

Hapten-carrier complex

3. Processed antigen presented to T cells, Processing, presentation, and sensitization of lymphocytes requires 24 hours.

Sensitized T cells

4. Sensitized lymphocytes enter a lymphatic vessel.

6. Sensitized T cells return to dermis and epidermis

Lymphatic vessel

Lymph node

5. Sensitized lymphocytes transported to regional lymph nodes, where T cell hyperplasia is induced

FIGURE 24-10. **Allergic contact dermatitis.** Pathogenetic mechanisms are shown.

hour, after which it is processed as an antigen by the Langerhans cells. These cells carry the antigen through the lymphatics to regional lymph nodes and present the antigen to CD4+ T lymphocytes (Fig. 24-10). After 5 to 7 days, some clones of these T lymphocytes become sensitized and circulate in the blood as memory cells. Others migrate to the skin, where they are ready to react with the antigen if they encounter it. IL-1 is produced by Langerhans cells and supports the proliferation of CD4+ Th1 lymphocytes, the effector cells of delayed hypersensitivity. Cytokine production leads to the accumulation of more T cells and macrophages, an inflammatory infiltrate that is responsible for epidermal cell injury.

PATHOLOGY: Allergic contact dermatitis is a model of **spongiotic dermatitis**. In the initial 24 hours following re-exposure to the offending plant, numerous lymphocytes and macrophages accumulate about the superficial venular bed and extend into the epidermis. The epidermal keratinocytes are partially separated by edema fluid, creating a sponge-like appearance (spongiosis) (Fig. 24-11). Later, numerous mononuclear inflammatory cells and eosinophils accumulate. Vesicles containing lymphocytes and macrophages are present, and large amounts of eosinophilic coagulated fluid accumulate in the stratum corneum.

CLINICAL FEATURES: Five to 7 days after the first exposure, the site of contact becomes intensely pruritic, after which erythema and small vesicles rapidly develop (see Fig. 24-11). Over the next few days, the area enlarges, becomes fiery red, develops numerous vesicles and exudes a large amount of clear proteinaceous fluid accompanied by intense pruritus. The entire process lasts about 3 weeks. Exudation gradually subsides, and the whole area is covered by an irregular crust that eventually falls off. Pruritus diminishes, and healing occurs without scarring. When a sensitized patient again comes into contact with poison ivy, the process is accelerated. Within 24 to 48 hours lesions appear, spread rapidly, and produce the same clinical appearance. However, the reaction is usually more intense. Again, the lesions clear in about 3 weeks. Allergic contact dermatitis responds to topical or systemic administration of corticosteroids.

Acne Vulgaris is a Disorder of the Pilosebaceous Unit

Acne vulgaris is a self-limited, inflammatory disorder of sebaceous follicles that typically afflicts adolescents, results in intermittent formation of discrete papular or pustular lesions, and may lead to scarring.

PATHOGENESIS AND PATHOLOGY: The development of acne is related to (1) excessive hormonally induced production of sebum, (2) abnormal cornification of portions of the follicular epithelium, (3) a response to the anaerobic diphtheroid *Propionibacterium acnes*, and (4) follicle rupture and subsequent inflammation. The change in hormonal status at puberty leads to sebum production in the follicle and altered cornification in the neck of the sebaceous follicle (infundibulum), effects that lead to dilation of the follicular canal. Desquamation of squamous cells and the accretion of keratinous debris provide a rich environment for P. acnes proliferation within the follicle. These combined changes produce a distended, plugged follicle, termed a **comedone**. Neutrophils attracted to the area by chemotactic factors released by P. acnes release hydrolytic enzymes to form a follicular abscess (**pustule**), which extends into the perifollicular tissue as a perifollicular abscess (Fig. 24-12). In addition, numerous macrophages, lymphocytes, and foreign body giant cells accumulate in response to the rupture of sebaceous follicles.

CLINICAL FEATURES: Acne vulgaris features a variety of skin lesions in different stages of development, including comedones, papules, pustules, nodules, cysts, and pitted scars. Comedones, the primary noninflammatory lesions of acne, are either open (**blackheads**) or closed (**whiteheads**). More advanced inflammatory lesions vary from small, erythematous papules to large, tender, purulent nodules and cysts.

Acne vulgaris is treated with topical cleansing, keratolytic, and antibacterial agents. Severe cases are managed with topical vitamin A, systemic antibiotics, and synthetic oral retinoids (isotretinoin).

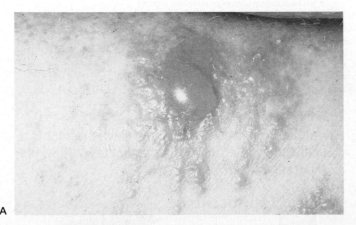

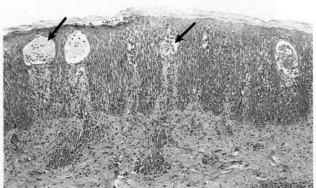

A   B

FIGURE 24-11. **Allergic contact dermatitis. A.** Vesicles and bullae developed on the volar forearm after application of perfume. **B.** Epidermal spongiosis and spongiotic vesicles *(arrows)* are present in this biopsy of "poison ivy." Infiltrating lymphocytes are apparent in the epidermis, where they effect the cell-mediated delayed hypersensitivity reaction.

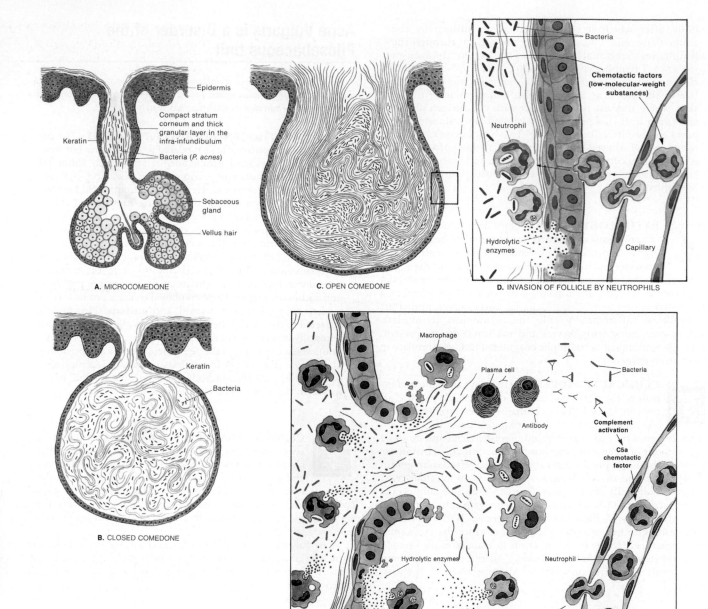

A. MICROCOMEDONE

C. OPEN COMEDONE

D. INVASION OF FOLLICLE BY NEUTROPHILS

B. CLOSED COMEDONE

E. INFLAMMATION AND RUPTURE OF SEBACEOUS FOLLICLE

FIGURE 24-12. **Acne vulgaris.** The pathogenesis of follicular distention, rupture, and inflammation is depicted. Acne is a disease of the follicular canal of a sebaceous follicle. A compact stratum corneum and a thickened granular layer in the infrainfundibulum are the beginning of the formation of a comedone. Microcomedones **(A)** and closed **(B)** and open **(C)** comedones form. Excessive sebum secretion occurs, and the bacterium *Propionibacterium acnes* proliferates. The organism produces chemotactic factors, leading to neutrophil migration into the intact comedone. Neutrophilic enzymes are released, and the comedone ruptures, inducing a cycle of chemotaxis and intense neutrophilic inflammation **(D,E)**.

Primary Neoplasms of the Skin: Melanocytic Neoplasia

The incidence of cutaneous tumors and malignant melanoma in particular, is increasing at an alarming rate. It is estimated that more than 1% of children born today will develop malignant melanoma. The prognosis of most melanomas is excellent if lesions are recognized and excised before entering a vertical growth phase. However, if the tumor exceeds a critical depth in the dermis, patients are likely to die of metastatic disease.

Common Acquired Melanocytic Nevus (Mole) is a Localized Proliferation of Melanocytes Within the Epidermis or Dermis

 PATHOGENESIS: There is an unequivocal causal relationship between ultraviolet light, melanocytic nevi, and malignant melanoma, but the relationship is complex. Some people with fair skin form relatively few nevi, whereas some with dark skin develop numerous ones. The ability to form nevi has been correlated with variants of the melanocortin receptor and with subsequent variation in the ratio of red pheomelanin to brown eumelanin skin pigments. Most people are exposed to a significant amount of light in the first 15 years of life and develop 10 to 50 nevi on their skin. Black skin can develop nevi, but less commonly, and such nevi do not progress to melanoma. However, if nevi are located on the palms of the hands, the soles of the feet, or on the genital skin, the risk of melanoma is the same in all races. Red-haired, blue-eyed persons with milk-white skin are notable exceptions, in that they are exquisitely sensitive to light and form freckles, but they do not develop a significant number of nevi.

Epidemiologic studies have shown melanocytic nevi to be potential precursor lesions for melanomas. A person with 100 or more nevi that are 2 to 5 mm in greatest dimension has a threefold greater risk of developing melanoma than a person with fewer than 25 similar nevi. Patients with clinically atypical or histologically proven dysplastic nevi are at even greater risk for melanoma, although the risk of progression of any one nevus is small. A majority of nevi have an activating mutation of the gene encoding the oncogene *B-RAF*, which can lead to growth stimulation through the mitogen-activated protein kinase pathway. Growth is ordinarily suppressed by the activity of p16, an inhibitor of the cyclin-mediated cell cycle mechanism encoded by the gene *CDKN2A* on chromosome 9p21, but the latter is commonly lost during melanoma progression.

Melanocytic nevi begin to appear between the first and second years of life and continue to emerge for the first 2 decades of life. A nevus first appears as a small tan dot no bigger than 1 to 2 mm in diameter. During the next 3 to 4 years, the dot enlarges to become a uniform tan to brown circular or oval area. The peripheral outline usually remains regular. When it reaches 4 to 5 mm in diameter, it is flat or slightly elevated, stops enlarging peripherally, and is sharply demarcated from the surrounding normal skin. Over the next 10 years, the lesion elevates, and its color pales to the point of becoming a tan tag-like protrusion. For the next decade or two, it gradually flattens, and the skin may approximate a normal appearance. In most people, the number of nevi gradually decreases over time. *Notably, many melanoma patients tend to retain increased numbers of nevi, including those that are atypical, in the later decades of life.*

 PATHOLOGY: At the inception of a melanocytic nevus, melanocytes are increased in the basal epidermis, with subsequent hyperpigmentation. The histologic classification of melanocytic nevi reflects the continuing evolution of the lesions:

- **Junctional nevus:** Melanocytes form nests at the tips of epidermal rete ridges.
- **Compound nevus:** Nests of melanocytes are seen in the epidermis, and some of the cells have migrated into the dermis (Fig. 24-13).
- **Dermal nevus:** Intraepidermal melanocytic growth has ceased.

Dysplastic (Atypical) Nevus is a Risk Marker for Melanoma

 PATHOGENESIS: Some common acquired nevi do not follow the pattern of growth, differentiation, and disappearance described above. Such lesions persist and are often more than 5 mm in greatest dimension. These nevi may show foci of aberrant melanocytic growth and become larger and more irregular peripherally. The irregular area is flat (macular) and extends asymmetrically from the parent nevus. Patients with dysplastic nevi are at in-

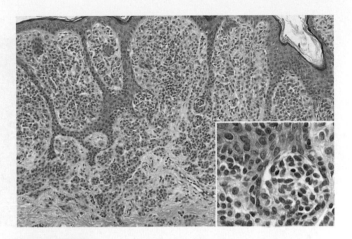

FIGURE 24-13. **Compound melanocytic nevus.** Melanocytes are present as nests within the epidermis and dermis. An intraepidermal nest of melanocytes is surrounded by keratinocytes *(inset)*.

creased risk of developing melanoma. The magnitude of this risk varies with the number of nevi and is especially high in patients with prior melanoma or a family history of melanoma. Germline mutations of the above-mentioned tumor suppressor gene, CDKN2A, occur in such families.

 PATHOLOGY: Initially, the basal epidermis is abnormal in architectural pattern, not in cytologic features. A band of eosinophilic connective tissue ("lamellar fibroplasia") is seen around the rete ridges, which contain aberrantly growing melanocytes. These aberrant melanocytes may grow to become continuous streams of melanocytes extending from rete to rete ("bridging"). As these architectural features become more prominent, melanocytes with large atypical nuclei that are reminiscent of malignant cells may also appear in the areas of architectural disorder. This combination of architectural disorder and cytologic atypia constitutes a dysplastic nevus (Fig. 24-14). Areas of dysplasia may also be associated with a subjacent lymphocytic infiltrate. *More than one third of malignant melanomas have a precursor nevus demonstrating melanocytic dysplasia. However, most dysplastic nevi are stable and will never progress to melanoma.*

The Prognosis of Malignant Melanoma is a Function of the Depth of Invasion

Radial Growth Phase Melanoma

The most frequently encountered form of melanoma is the **radial growth phase**, also termed **superficial spreading melanoma** (Fig. 24-15).

 PATHOLOGY: Large epithelioid melanocytes are dispersed in nests and as individual cells through the entire thickness of the epidermis. These melanocytes may be limited to the epidermis **(melanoma in situ)** or they may extend into the papillary dermis. *In the radial growth phase, no nest has growth preference (larger size) over the other nests (Fig. 24-16), so the cells grow in all directions: upward in the epidermis, peripherally in the epidermis, and downward into the dermis.* These lesions enlarge at the periphery, hence the term **radial**, but only rarely metastasize. Mitoses are not seen in dermal melanocytes. Melanocytes of the radial growth phase are typically associated with a brisk lymphocytic response.

 CLINICAL FEATURES: The "ABCD rule" is a convenient mnemonic that is commonly taught to patients to help them recognize changes in nevi that should prompt them to seek medical attention: **A**symmetry of

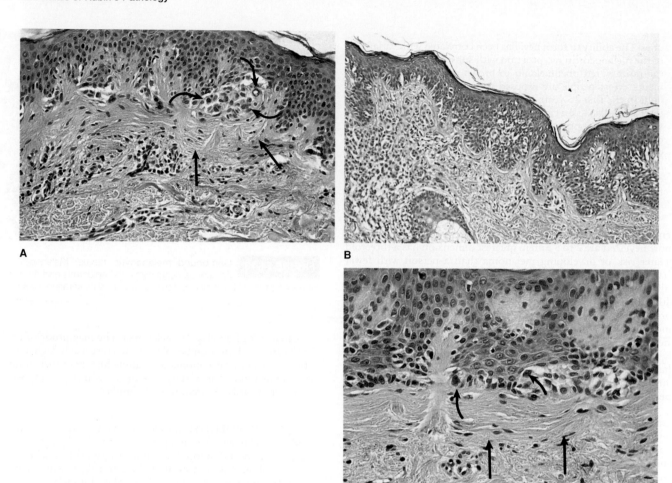

Dysplastic nevus. A. There is bridging of rete ridges by nests of melanocytes, melanocytes with cytological atypia *(curved arrows)*, lamellar fibroplasia *(straight arrows)*, and a scant perivascular lymphocytic infiltrate. **B.** To the *left* is a zone containing typical dermal nevic cells of a compound melanocytic nevus. In the epidermis on the *right* is a lentiginous proliferation of atypical melanocytes with lamellar fibroplasia. This photomicrograph is taken from the junction of the papular and macular components of this dysplastic nevus. Dysplasia usually develops in the macular portion, which takes up most of the field. **C.** These ellipsoid melanocytic nests resting above lamellar fibroplasia *(straight arrows)* exhibit large epithelioid melanocytes with atypia *(curved arrows)*.

shape, **B**order irregularity, **C**olor variation, and a **D**iameter more than 6 mm. However, not all early melanomas exhibit these attributes, and any changing lesion should be evaluated for excisional biopsy. Early melanomas in the radial growth phase have slightly elevated and palpable borders. The neoplasm is usually variably and haphazardly pigmented (see Figs. 24-15 and 24-17). Patients with documented melanoma frequently state that a change in the lesion, such as itching, increase in size, darkening, bleeding, or oozing prompted concern. *Even in the absence of such patient observations, any lesion that prompts clinical suspicion of melanoma warrants an excisional biopsy.*

Vertical Growth Phase Melanoma

 PATHOLOGY: After a variable time (usually 1 to 2 years), the character of growth begins to change. Melanocytes exhibit mitotic activity and grow as spheroid nodules of increased size that expand more rapidly than the rest of the tumor in the surrounding papillary dermis (Fig. 24-17). *The net direction of growth tends to be perpendicular to that of the radial growth phase, hence the term* **vertical** *(Figs. 24-18 and 24-19).* The dominant site of tumor growth shifts from the epidermis to the dermis. The melanocytes tend to differ in appearance from those of the radial growth phase. For example, they may now contain little pigment, whereas in the radial growth phase, they were melanotic.

Even when tumors enter the vertical growth phase, they may still lack the propensity to metastasize. Thus, vertical growth phase melanomas less than 1.7 mm thick that lack mitoses and exhibit a brisk infiltrate of lymphocytes rarely metastasize. *However vertical growth phase melanomas more than 3.6 mm thick, with*

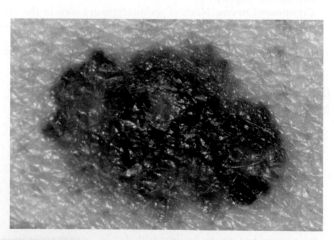

The clinical appearance of the radial growth phase in malignant melanoma of the superficial spreading type. The larger diameter is 1.8 cm.

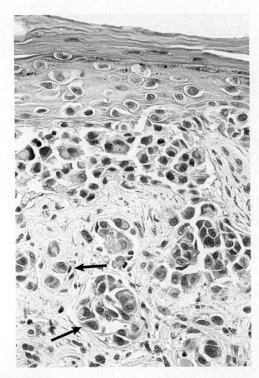

FIGURE 24-16. **Malignant melanoma, superficial spreading type, radial growth phase.** Melanocytes grow singly within the epidermis at all levels and as large, irregularly sized nests at the dermal–epidermal junction. Tumor cells are present in the papillary dermis *(arrows)*, but no nest shows preferential growth over the others.

more than 6 mitoses/mm², and without tumor-infiltrating lymphocytes frequently metastasize.

Metastatic Melanoma

Metastatic melanoma arises from the melanocytes of the vertical growth phase. Initial metastases usually involve regional lymph nodes, although hematogenous spread is also possible. When the latter occurs, metastases are unusually widespread in comparison with other neoplasms, and virtually any organ may be involved. Many metastatic melanomas remain dormant for long periods, only to reappear years after excision of the primary tumor.

Variant Forms of Melanoma

- **Nodular melanoma** is an uncommon form of the tumor (10%) that appears as a circumscribed, elevated, spheroidal nodule. The tumor does **not** develop through a radial growth phase and manifests all of the malignant characteristics of the initial vertical growth phase lesion when first observed (Fig. 24-20).
- **Lentigo maligna melanoma or (Hutchinson melanotic freckle)** is a large, pigmented macule that develops almost exclusively in fair-skinned elderly persons who are chronically exposed to solar ultraviolet light. In the radial growth phase, lentigo maligna melanoma is a flat, irregular, brown-to-black patch that may cover a large part of the face or dorsal hands (Fig. 24-21).
- **Acral lentiginous melanoma** is the most common form of melanoma in dark-skinned people and, as the name implies, is generally limited to the palms, soles, and subungual regions. In the radial growth phase, acral lentiginous melanoma forms an irregular, brown-to-black patch that covers a part of the palm or sole or arises under a nail, usually on a thumb or great toe (Fig. 24-22).

Staging and Prognosis of Melanoma

The prognosis of a patient with melanoma in the vertical growth phase is based on a number of attributes.

TUMOR THICKNESS: Tumor thickness is the strongest prognostic variable for melanomas that are apparently confined to their primary sites. The thickness of a melanoma is measured from the most superficial aspect of the stratum granulosum to the point of deepest penetration of the tumor into the dermis (see Fig. 24-19). The prognosis up to 10 years after removal of the primary lesion may then be estimated from Table 24-1.

DERMAL MITOTIC RATE: For tumor cells in the vertical growth phase, the mitotic rate is highly predictive of survival. Survival becomes progressively worse as the mitotic rate increases. The 5-year survival rate is 99% for patients with a mitotic rate of zero and 68% with a mitotic rate over 6 mitoses/mm².

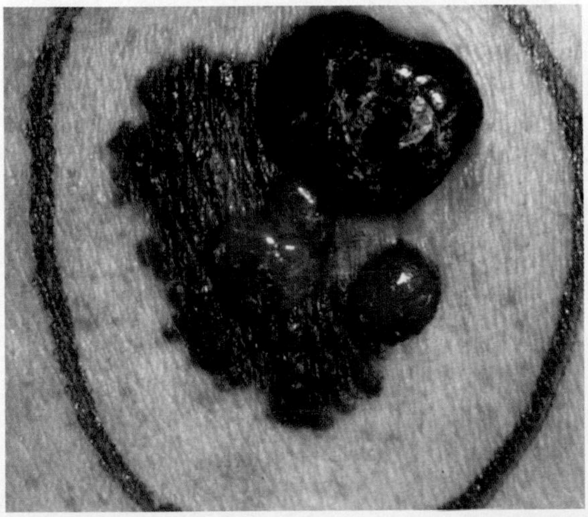

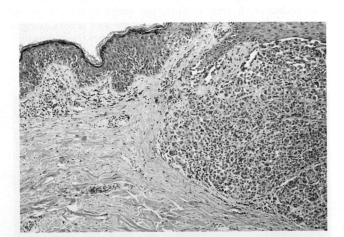

FIGURE 24-17. **Malignant melanoma.** The superficial spreading type is represented by the relatively flat, dark, brown-black portion of the tumor. Three areas in this lesion are characteristic of the vertical growth phase. All are nodular in configuration; two have a pink coloration, and the largest is a rich, ebony black.

FIGURE 24-18. **Malignant melanoma, superficial spreading type, vertical growth phase.** Vertical growth is manifested by the distinct spheroid tumor nodule to the *right*. A focus of melanocytes clearly has a growth advantage (larger size) over other nests in the radial growth phase *(left)*. The nodule distorts the papillary dermal-reticular dermal junction and therefore is level III.

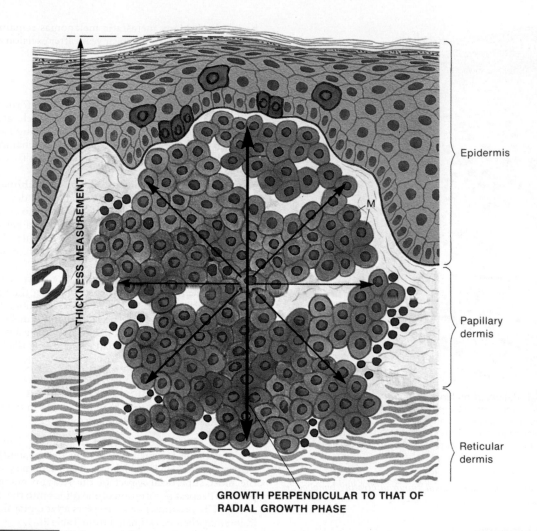

FIGURE 24-19. **Malignant melanoma.** The evolved vertical growth phase in malignant melanoma of the superficial spreading type is shown with an indication of how thickness is measured. In this illustration, the vertical growth phase has extended into the reticular dermis. Small nodules of tumor cells that clearly have a growth preference over other tumor cells may be a manifestation of the vertical growth phase. Thickness measurements *(arrows)* are taken from the outermost granular layer across the tumor in its thickest part.

LYMPHOCYTIC RESPONSE: The interaction of lymphocytes with tumor cells in the vertical growth phase is an important prognostic indicator. If tumor-infiltrating lymphocytes are present throughout the vertical growth phase or are seen across its entire base, the infiltrate is said to be "brisk." The higher the tumor-infiltrating lymphocyte grade is, the better the prognosis will be.

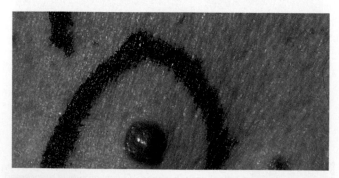

FIGURE 24-20. **Malignant melanoma of the nodular type.** The primary focus of growth of this 0.5-cm lesion is in the dermis.

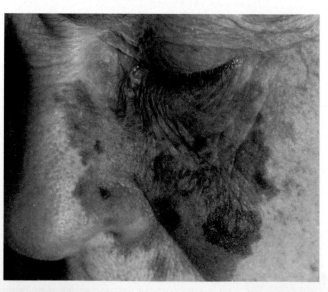

FIGURE 24-21. **Malignant melanoma of the lentigo maligna type,** radial growth phase.

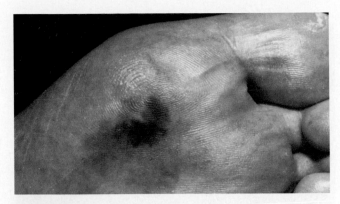

FIGURE 24-22. **Malignant melanoma, acral lentiginous type (radial growth phase).** The clinical appearance of the sole of the foot is depicted.

LOCATION: Melanomas on the extremities have a better prognosis than those on the head, neck, or trunk (axial). However, melanomas on the sole of the foot or the subungual region have a prognosis similar to, or worse than, axial lesions.

SEX: For every site and thickness, women have better prognoses than men.

REGRESSION: Many primary melanomas show some spontaneous regression in the radial growth phase component, indicated clinically by a color change to blue-white or white. Patients whose tumors show such changes have a somewhat worse prognosis than those in whom regression is absent.

ULCERATION: Ulceration in a primary melanoma is associated with decreased survival.

LEVELS OF INVASION: The Clark level system describes the degree of tumor penetration within the anatomical layers of the skin. For example, level I corresponds to tumor cells being entirely above the basement membrane (in situ); in level V disease, the tumor extends into subcutaneous fat. Clark levels predict the likelihood of metastasis, but not as accurately as tumor thickness.

STAGE: The stage of the disease is perhaps the most important single factor influencing a patient's survival. Metastasis to regional lymph nodes is associated with an estimated 40% decrease in 5-year survival, compared to patients with clinically localized tumors. The number of involved lymph nodes is also highly predictive of prognosis. Patients with 1 positive node have a 10-year survival rate of 40%, compared with 25% with 2 to 4 nodes, and 15% with 5 or more nodes involved.

The current recommendations regarding excision of confirmed melanomas state that (1) a 5-mm margin of uninvolved tissue should be obtained with in situ melanoma, (2) a 1-cm margin is proper for a tumor thickness of 1 mm or less, and (3) a 2-cm margin is suggested for a tumor thickness greater than 1 mm or with Clark level IV or greater.

TABLE 24–1	
Tumor Thickness as Sole Predictor of Outcome 10 Years After Definitive Therapy of Primary Melanoma	
Thickness (mm)	**Survival (%)**
≤1	83–88
1.01–2	64–79
2.01–4	51–64
>4	32–54

Benign Tumors of Melanocytes May Mimic Melanoma

A number of benign or "borderline" lesions may mimic melanoma.

CONGENITAL MELANOCYTIC NEVUS: About 1% of white children are born with some form of pigmented lesion on their skin. Rarely, the trunk or an extremity is covered by a large pigmented patch or plaque that is cosmetically deforming ("giant hairy" or "garment" nevus). Such lesions are associated with a striking increase in intraepidermal and dermal melanocytes, which may extend deep into the subcutaneous tissue. Malignant melanoma may develop in these large congenital melanocytic nevi.

SPITZ TUMOR: Spitz tumors (also known as spindle and epithelioid cell nevi) occur in children or adolescents and, less often, in adults as an elevated, spheroid, pink, smooth nodule, usually on the head or neck. The cells are so atypical that an incorrect diagnosis of melanoma may be made, although melanoma is exquisitely rare in childhood. Most Spitz tumors are benign, but a few may metastasize; hence the prognosis is uncertain, especially in adults (Fig. 24-23).

BLUE NEVUS: Blue nevi appear in childhood or late adolescence as dark blue, gray or black, firm, well-demarcated papules or nodules on the dorsum of the hands or feet or on the buttocks, scalp, or face. The clinical appearance may prompt an excisional biopsy to rule out nodular melanoma.

FRECKLE AND LENTIGO: Freckles, or **ephelides**, are small, brown macules that occur on sun-exposed skin, especially in people with fair skin. They usually appear at about age 5. The pigmentation of a freckle deepens with exposure to sunlight and fades when light exposure ceases. A **lentigo** is a discrete, brown macule that appears at any age and on any part of the body and does not depend on solar exposure (Fig. 24-24). Larger lentiginous lesions may need to be biopsied to rule out lentigo maligna melanoma.

Verrucae are Warts Caused by Human Papillomavirus (HPV)

Verrucae are cutaneous tumors caused by HPV infection. They are elevated, circumscribed, symmetric, epidermal proliferations that often appear papillary.

PATHOLOGY:

- **Verruca vulgaris**, also known as the **common wart**, is an elevated papule with a verrucous (papillomatous) surface. They may be single or multiple and are most frequent on the dorsal surfaces of the hands or on the face. Histologically, verruca vulgaris displays hyperkeratosis and papillary epidermal hyperplasia (Fig. 24-25). **Koilocytes** (i.e., enlarged keratinocytes with a pyknotic nucleus surrounded by a halo-like cleared area) are observed within the upper epidermis. HPV, especially serotypes 2 and 4, are commonly found in verruca vulgaris. There is no malignant potential.
- **Plantar warts** are benign, frequently painful, hyperkeratotic nodules on the soles of the feet. Occasionally, similar lesions appear on the palms of the hands (**palmar warts**). Histologically, plantar warts are endophytic or exophytic, papillary, squamous epithelial proliferations. The cells contain abundant cytoplasmic inclusions that are similar in appearance to the darker-staining keratohyaline granules. The nuclei of keratinocytes near the bases of these warts also contain pink nuclear inclusions. HPV type 1 is the etiologic agent.

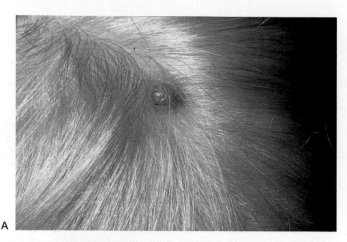

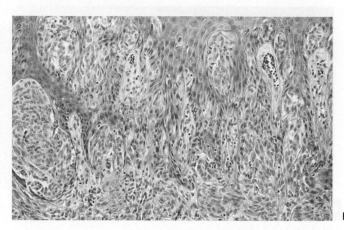

A   B

FIGURE 24-23. Spindle and epithelioid cell (Spitz) nevus. **A.** A symmetric pink nodule appeared suddenly in a child but then remained stable for several weeks until it was excised. **B.** Spitz tumors are composed of large melanocytes with prominent nuclei. Within a hyperplastic epidermis, the melanocytes are disposed in large nests. Although the cells are large and, at first glance, suggest melanoma, they are much more uniform than the cells of most malignant melanomas.

Keratosis is a Benign Horny Growth Composed of Keratinocytes

Seborrheic Keratosis

Seborrheic keratoses are scaly, frequently pigmented, elevated papules or plaques with scales that are easily rubbed off. Although they are among the most common keratoses, the etiology is unknown. The lesions generally occur in later life and tend to be familial. Clinically and microscopically, they appear "pasted on" and are composed of broad anastomosing cords of mature stratified squamous epithelium associated with small cysts of keratin (horn cysts). Seborrheic keratoses are innocuous but may be a cosmetic nuisance. The sudden appearance of numerous seborrheic keratoses has been associated with internal malignancies ("sign of Leser-Trélat"), especially gastric adenocarcinoma.

Actinic Keratosis

Actinic keratoses ("from the sun's rays") are keratinocytic neoplasms that develop in sun-damaged skin as circumscribed keratotic patches or plaques, commonly on the backs of the hands or the face. Microscopically, the stratum corneum is no longer loose and basket-weaved but is re-

placed by a dense parakeratotic scale. The underlying basal keratinocytes display significant atypia (Fig. 24-26). With time, actinic keratoses may evolve into squamous cell carcinoma in situ and finally into invasive squamous cell carcinoma. However, most are stable, and many regress.

Keratoacanthoma

Keratoacanthomas are rapidly growing keratotic papules on sun-exposed skin that develop over 3 to 6 weeks into crater-like nodules. They reach a maximum diameter of 2 to 3 cm. Spontaneous regression usually follows within 6 to 12 months, leaving an atrophic scar. Some lesions may cause considerable damage before they regress, and some fail to regress. Keratoacanthomas may be considered to be variants of squamous cell carcinoma, although this topic is controversial.

 PATHOLOGY: Histologically, keratoacanthomas are endophytic papillary proliferations of keratinocytes. The lesion is cup shaped, with a central, keratin-filled umbilication and overhanging ("buttressing") edges (Fig. 24-27). At the base of the keratin, keratinocytes are large and

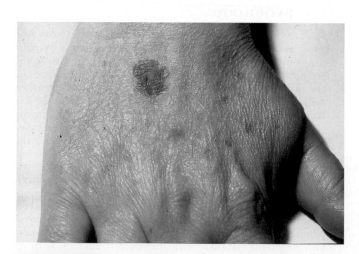

FIGURE 24-24. Lentigo. A 1-cm irregular patch of slightly variegated hyperpigmentation is present with a background of chronic solar damage.

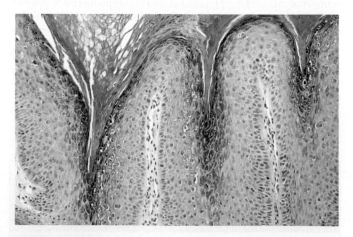

FIGURE 24-25. Verruca vulgaris. Verruca vulgaris is the prototype of papillary epidermal hyperplasia. Squamous epithelial-lined fronds have fibrovascular cores. The blood vessels within the cores extend close to the surface of verrucae, which makes them susceptible to traumatic hemorrhage and the resultant black "seeds" that patients observe.

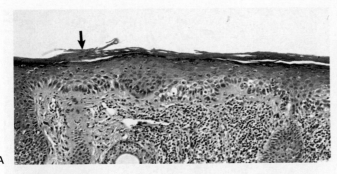
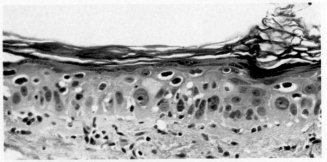

FIGURE 24-26. **Actinic keratosis. A.** A low-power view reveals cytologic atypia within the stratum basalis and lower stratum spinosum with loss of polarity. A lichenoid, band-like, lymphocytic infiltrate is frequently present. Parakeratosis is present here only in a small focus *(arrow)*. **B.** High-power examination of an actinic keratosis reveals striking cytologic atypia of the basal keratinocytes, the hallmark of actinic keratoses.

have abundant homogeneous, eosinophilic ("glassy") cytoplasm. At the lower aspect of the lesion, irregular tongues of squamous epithelium infiltrate the collagen of the reticular dermis. Older lesions show active fibroplasia in the dermis around these tongues. There may be focal lichenoid inflammation, and the dermis may be markedly infiltrated with neutrophils, lymphocytes, and eosinophils. Microabscesses of neutrophils and entrapped dermal elastic fibers may be present within the lesion.

Basal Cell Carcinoma (BCC) is a Locally Invasive Epidermal Neoplasm

BCC is the most common malignant tumor in persons with pale skin. Although it may be locally aggressive, metastases are exceedingly rare.

PATHOGENESIS: BCC usually develops on sun-damaged skin of people with fair skin and freckles. However, unlike squamous cell carcinoma, BCC also arises on areas not exposed to intense sunlight. It is unusual to find BCC on the fingers and dorsal surfaces of the hands. The tumor is thought to derive from pluripotential cells in the basal layer of the epidermis, more specifically, in the bulge region of the hair follicle. Somatic mutations in PTCH, a tumor suppressor gene on chromosome 9q22, have been implicated in up to 67% of sporadic BCC. Germline mutations of the gene are associated with **nevoid BCC syndrome**, which is characterized by the appearance of multiple BCCs at a young age, a predisposition to other neoplasms, and a number of developmental defects.

PATHOLOGY: BCC is composed of nests of deeply basophilic epithelial cells with narrow rims of cytoplasm that are attached to the epidermis and protrude into the subjacent papillary dermis (Fig. 24-28). The central part of each nest contains closely packed keratinocytes that are slightly smaller than the normal epidermal basal keratinocytes and show occasional apoptosis. The periphery of each nest shows an organized layer of polarized, columnar keratinocytes, with the long axis of each cell perpendicular to the surrounding BMZ ("peripheral palisading"). The tumor nests are often separated from adjacent stroma by thin clefts ("retraction artifact"), which may sometimes help distinguish BCC from other adnexal neoplasms displaying basaloid cell proliferation.

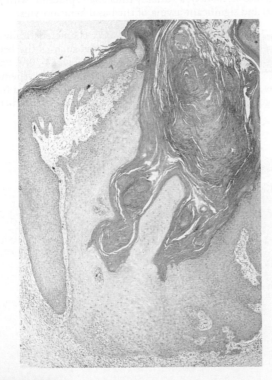

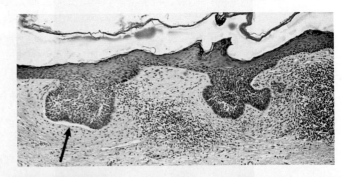

FIGURE 24-27. **Keratoacanthoma.** A keratin-filled crater (right) is lined by glassy proliferating keratinocytes that invade the dermis.

FIGURE 24-28. **Basal cell carcinoma, superficial type.** Buds of atypical basaloid keratinocytes extend from the overlying epidermis into the papillary dermis. The peripheral keratinocytes mimic the stratum basalis by palisading. The separation artifact *(arrow)* is present because of poorly formed basement membrane components and the hyaluronic acid-rich stroma that contains collagenase.

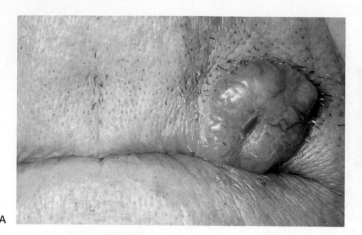

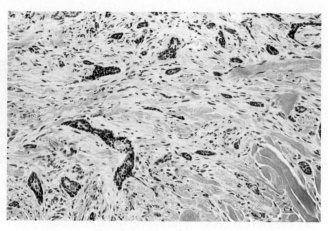

A

B

FIGURE 24-29. Basal cell carcinoma (BCC). **A.** Pearly papule: The tumor exhibits typical rolled pearly borders with telangiectases and central ulceration. **B.** Microscopic examination of morpheaform BCC shows a sclerosing and infiltrative lesion. Irregularly branching strands of tumor cells permeate the dermis, with induction of a cellular, fibroblastic, hyaluronic acid-rich stroma.

 CLINICAL FEATURES: A number of common forms of BCC are recognized.

- **Pearly papule** is the prototypic nodulocystic type of lesion, so named because it resembles a 2- to 3-mm pearl (Fig. 24-29). It is covered by tightly stretched epidermis and is laced with small, delicate, branching vessels (telangiectasia).
- **Rodent ulcer** is a small crater in the center of the pearl.
- **Superficial BCC** appears as a scaly, red, sharply demarcated plaque.

Although metastatic disease is exceedingly uncommon, the tumor can invade locally, can be difficult to eradicate, and can lead to disfiguring lesions. Thus, the tumor should be promptly treated by excision or other methods of eradication.

Squamous Cell Carcinoma (SCC) Typically Resembles Differentiated Keratinocytes

SCC is second only to BCC in incidence and may be caused by ultraviolet light, ionizing radiation, chemical carcinogens, and HPV. It is most common on sun-damaged skin of fair individuals with light hair and freckles and often originates in actinic keratoses. SCC is exceedingly rare on normal black skin.

 PATHOGENESIS: SCC has multiple causes, and ultraviolet light is the most common. SCC of the skin metastasizes only rarely (<2%). The tumor may also originate in chronic scarring processes, such as osteomyelitis sinus tracts, burn scars, and areas of radiation dermatitis. In these settings, SCC metastasizes more often. More than 90% of SCCs and many actinic keratoses have mutated p53 genes.

 PATHOLOGY: SCC is composed of tumor cells that mimic the epidermal stratum spinosum to varying degrees and extend into the subjacent dermis (Fig. 24-30). The edges of many tumors show changes typical of actinic keratosis, namely, a variably thickened epidermis with parakeratosis and significant atypia of the basal keratinocytes.

CLINICAL FEATURES: SCC characteristically arises in chronically sun-exposed areas such as the backs of the hands, face, lips, and ears (see Fig. 24-30A). Early lesions are small, scaly or ulcerated, erythematous papules, which may be pruritic. SCCs are usually treated by electrosurgery, topical chemotherapy, excision, or radiation therapy.

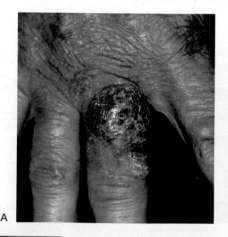

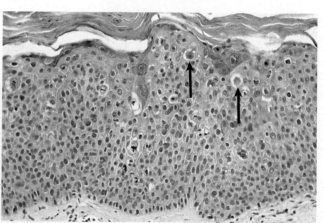

A

B

FIGURE 24-30. Squamous cell carcinoma. **A.** An ulcerated, encrusted, and infiltrating lesion is seen on the sun-exposed dorsal aspect of a finger. **B.** A microscopic view of the periphery of the lesion shows squamous cell carcinoma in situ. The entire epidermis is replaced by atypical keratinocytes. Mitoses (curved arrow) and multinucleation of keratinocytes are apparent, as is apoptosis (straight arrows).

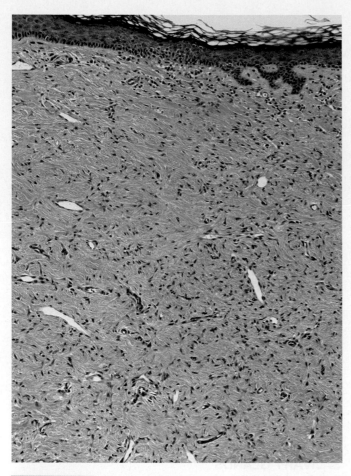

FIGURE 24-31. **Dermatofibroma.** Fibrous tissue replaces the dermis and forms ill-defined small cartwheels.

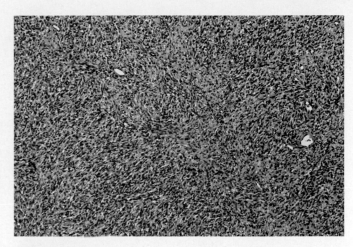

FIGURE 24-32. **Dermatofibrosarcoma protuberans.** Tumor cells form ill-defined small cartwheels with small central vascular spaces.

Merkel Cell Carcinoma is an Aggressive Tumor of Neurosecretory Cells that Shows Epithelial Differentiation

Merkel cell carcinoma is typically a solitary, dome-shaped, red-to-violaceous nodule or indurated plaque that arises on the skin of the head and neck in elderly white individuals. It is an aggressive tumor that causes death in 25% to 70% of patients within 5 years. The tumor is uncommon, with about 500 new cases diagnosed annually.

 PATHOLOGY: Merkel cell carcinomas consist mostly of large solid nests of undifferentiated cells that resemble small cell carcinoma of the lung. Nuclear chromatin is dense and evenly distributed, cytoplasm is scant, and mitotic figures and nuclear fragments are frequent. Tumor cells show evidence of both Merkel cell markers (cytokeratin 20) and neuroendocrine markers (such as chromogranin and synaptophysin).

Adnexal Tumors Differentiate Toward Skin Appendages

Adnexal tumors generally appear as elevated small skin nodules that often occur in people with a familial history of similar tumors. Frequently, the lesions appear at puberty. Although most are benign, malignant behavior is sometimes observed. These include:

- **Cylindroma:** Cylindromas are adnexal neoplasms with features of sweat gland differentiation. They may be solitary or multiple elevated nodules around the scalp. Microscopic examination shows sharply circumscribed nests of deeply basophilic cells surrounded by a hyalinized, thickened BMZ.
- **Syringoma:** Syringomas appear to derive from the intraepidermal portion of eccrine sweat glands and occur about the eyelid and upper cheek as small, elevated, flesh-colored papules.
- **Poroma:** Poroma is a common, solitary neoplasm that is histologically similar to seborrheic keratosis but exhibits narrow ductal lumina and occasional cystic spaces, which is believed to derive from eccrine sweat glands. Occasional malignant lesions with ductal differentiation are termed **porocarcinomas**.
- **Trichoepithelioma:** Trichoepithelioma is a neoplasm that differentiates toward hair structures. Lesions begin to appear at puberty, on the face, scalp, neck, and upper trunk. Microscopically, they resemble basal cell carcinomas but contain many "horn cysts," which display keratinized centers surrounded by basophilic epithelial cells.

Fibrohistiocytic Tumors of the Skin Show a Varied Spectrum of Differentiation

Dermatofibroma

Dermatofibroma is a common, benign tumor of neoplastic fibroblasts and macrophages. It occurs on the extremities as a dome-shaped, firm, rubbery nodule with ill-defined borders and pigmentation that ranges from pink to dark brown. They are rarely more than 3 to 5 mm in diameter. Microscopically, the papillary and reticular dermis are replaced by fibrous tissue that forms ill-defined small cartwheels with small central vascular spaces (Fig. 24-31).

Dermatofibrosarcoma Protuberans

Dermatofibrosarcoma protuberans is a slowly growing nodule or indurated plaque with intermediate malignant potential, which appears mostly on the trunk of young adults. Local recurrence after attempted complete excision is common, but metastases are rare. The most common histologic pattern is a poorly circumscribed, monotonous population of spindle cells arranged in a dense "storiform" (pinwheel-like) array (Fig. 24-32). As is not the case with dermatofibromas, tumor cells display CD34, a marker of endothelial cells, some neural tumor cells, as well as dermal fibroblast-like dendritic cells, the probable cells of origin.

25 The Head and Neck

Bruce M. Wenig

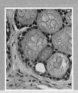
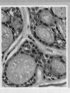
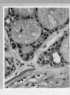
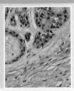

The pathology of the head and neck subsumes two major portals of entry into the body; hence, it is not surprising that the oral and nasal cavities and their connecting deeper anatomic structures are host to a multiplicity of common (and sometimes uncommon) infectious diseases. Lined with epithelia, containing salivary glands and elements of the host defense system, carcinomas and lymphomas are to be expected. As a specialized organ of sensation with access to the nasopharynx, the ear also suffers from infection, as well as more specialized defects of the sensory apparatus.

ORAL CAVITY

The oral cavity extends from the lips to the pharynx. The anatomic borders of the oral cavity include:

- The vermilion border of the lips (anterior)
- A line drawn from the junction of the hard and soft palate to the circumvallate papillae of the tongue (posterior)
- The hard palate until its junction with the soft palate (superior)
- The anterior two thirds of the tongue to the line of the circumvallate papillae (inferior)
- The buccal mucosa of the cheeks (lateral)

Infections of the Oral Cavity

Bacteria, spirochetes, viruses, fungi, and parasites are normal in the oral cavity and are usually harmless. If the mucosa is injured or immunity impaired, otherwise normal oral cavity organisms can become pathogenic (see Chapter 9 for further discussion).

The following terms are used to describe localized inflammation of the oral cavity:

- **Cheilitis** (lips)
- **Gingivitis** (gum)
- **Glossitis** (tongue)
- **Stomatitis** (oral mucosa)

Bacterial and Fungal Infections Commonly Affect the Oral Cavity

APHTHOUS STOMATITIS (CANKER SORES): *Aphthous stomatitis is a common disease characterized by painful, recurrent, solitary or multiple, small ulcers of oral mucosa.* The cause is unknown. Bacteria, mycoplasma, viruses, autoimmune reactions, and hypersensitivity have been implicated but are unproved. Microscopically, the lesion consists of a shallow ulcer covered by a fibrinopurulent exudate. The underlying inflammatory infiltrate is composed of mononuclear and polymorphonuclear leukocytes. The lesions heal without scar formation.

ACUTE NECROTIZING ULCERATIVE GINGIVITIS (VINCENT ANGINA): *Vincent angina is an infection by two symbiotic organisms, a fusiform bacillus and a spirochete (*Borrelia vincentii*).* The term **fusospirochetosis** is used to describe such an infection. These organisms are found in the mouth of many healthy people, suggesting that other factors such as decreased resistance to infection due to inadequate nutrition, immunodeficiency, or poor oral hygiene, are required for development of the disease. Vincent angina is characterized by punched-out erosions of the interdental papillae. The process tends to spread and eventually involve all gingival margins, which become covered by a necrotic pseudomembrane.

LUDWIG ANGINA: *Ludwig angina is a rapidly spreading cellulitis, which originates in the submaxillary or sublingual space but extends locally to involve both.* The responsible bacteria originate from oral flora, and a variety of aerobic or anaerobic microorganisms have been implicated. The disease is most often related to dental extraction or trauma to the floor of the mouth. After extraction of a tooth, hairline fractures may occur in the lingual cortex of the mandible, providing microorganisms ready access to the submaxillary space. This potentially life-threatening inflammatory process is uncommon in developed countries, except in patients with chronic illnesses associated with immunosuppression.

CANDIDIASIS: Also termed **thrush** or **moniliasis**, candidiasis is caused by *Candida albicans* (see Chapter 9), which is common on the surfaces of the oral cavity, gastrointestinal tract, and vagina. To cause disease, it must penetrate tissues, albeit superficially. Oral candidiasis is mostly seen in people with compromised immune systems and in diabetics. The incidence in patients with AIDS is 40% to 90%. The lesions are white, slightly elevated, soft patches (Fig. 25-1) that consist mainly of fungal hyphae.

Viral Infections Present as Vesicular or Ulcerative Lesions

HERPES SIMPLEX VIRUS TYPE 1 (HSV-1): Herpes labialis (cold sores, fever blisters) and herpetic stomatitis are caused by HSV-1 and are among the most common viral infections of the lips and oral mucosa in both children and young adults. Transmission occurs by droplet infection, and the virus can be recovered from the saliva of infected persons. Disease starts with painful inflammation of the affected mucosa, followed shortly by the formation of vesicles. These vesicles rupture and form shallow, painful ulcers, ranging from punctate size to a centimeter in diameter. Microscopically, herpetic vesicles form as a result of "ballooning degeneration" of epithelial cells. Some epithelial cells show intranuclear inclusion bodies. The ulcers heal spontaneously without scar formation. Once HSV-1 enters the body, it survives in a dormant state in the trigeminal ganglion. It can be reactivated to cause recurrent herpetic lesions in diverse ways, including trauma, allergy, menstruation, pregnancy, exposure to ultraviolet light, and by other viral infections. Recurrent oral cavity vesicles almost invariably develop on a mucosa that is tightly bound to periosteum, for example, the hard palate.

HUMAN PAPILLOMAVIRUS (HPV): The HPV family of viruses (see Chapter 9) causes epithelial proliferations including papillomas, for example, sinonasal (Schneiderian) papillomas and other mucosal papillomas, of various sites in the upper aerodigestive tract sites.

EPSTEIN-BARR VIRUS (EBV): EBV is the cause of infectious mononucleosis, oral hairy leukoplakia, and lymphoid malignancies. The list includes nasal-type natural killer (NK)/T-cell lymphoma and Hodgkin lymphoma (see Chapter 20). Certain cancers and epithelial malignancies (e.g., nasopharyngeal-type differentiated and undifferentiated carcinomas, salivary gland undifferentiated carcinoma) are also related to EBV infection.

OTHER VIRAL INFECTIONS: Coxsackievirus causes **herpangina**, an acute vesicular oropharyngitis. A brief course of infection confers lasting immunity. **Cytomegalovirus** infection typically presents with surface ulceration. Other viral infections that involve the oral mucosa include measles, rubella, chickenpox, and herpes zoster.

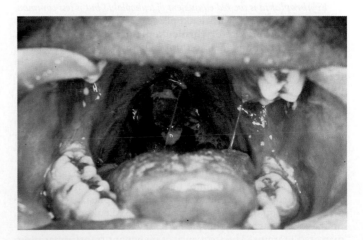

FIGURE 25-1. **Oral candidiasis.** White plaques coat mucous membranes of the oral cavity.

Benign Neoplasms

Benign tumors common elsewhere in the body are seen also in the oral cavity. These tumors include pigmented nevi, fibromas, hemangiomas, lymphangiomas, and squamous papillomas. Trauma may lead to ulceration of these lesions, in which case they may bleed or become infected.

PAPILLOMA: Squamous papilloma is a benign, exophytic epithelial neoplasm composed of branching fronds of squamous epithelium with fibrovascular cores. These are the most common benign oral cavity neoplasms and have been associated with HPV infection. They occur mainly in the third to fifth decades. The tongue, palate, buccal mucosa, tonsil, and uvula are most often involved.

LOBULAR CAPILLARY HEMANGIOMA (PYOGENIC GRANULOMA, PREGNANCY TUMOR): Lobular capillary hemangioma is a benign polypoid form of capillary hemangioma primarily occurring on skin and mucous membranes and most commonly on the gingiva. *The term* pyogenic granuloma *is a misnomer; it is neither infectious nor granulomatous.* In the oral cavity, the lesions range from a few millimeters to a centimeter and are elevated, soft, red or purple, with smooth, lobulated, ulcerated surfaces. Lobular capillary hemangioma is characterized by submucosal vascular proliferation arranged in lobules or clusters, with central capillaries and smaller ramifying tributaries (Fig. 25-2). In time, the lesions may become less vascular and may resemble a fibroma. In pregnant women, particularly near the end of the first trimester, a gingival lesion may develop that grossly and microscopically is identical to lobular capillary hemangioma. Termed **pregnancy tumor**, it may or may not regress after delivery.

Preneoplastic or Epithelial Precursor Lesions: Leukoplakia and Erythroplakia

Premalignant lesions of the upper aerodigestive tract include leukoplakia, erythroplakia, or speckled leukoplakia, the terms reflecting the presence of a white, red, or mixed white/red lesion, respectively. *Leukoplakia (from the Greek,* leukos, *"white" and* plax, *"plaque") is an asymptomatic white lesion on the surface of a mucous membrane.* Some of these lesions undergo transformation to squamous cell carcinoma. The disorders occur with equal frequency in both sexes, mostly after the third decade of life. A variety of diseases appear clinically as leukoplakia, including candidiasis, lichen planus, psoriasis, syphilis, various keratoses, hyperkeratosis, and squamous carcinoma in situ. *Thus, leukoplakia is not a histologic diagnosis but rather a descriptive clinical term that warrants further investigation.* As a preneoplastic lesion, the causes of leukoplakia are diverse and include use of tobacco products, alcoholism, and local irritation.

Erythroplakia is the red equivalent of leukoplakia but is less common. Red areas associated with leukoplakic lesions are referred to as **speckled leukoplakia (erythroleukoplakia, speckled mucosa)**. In contrast to leukoplakia, erythroplakia may represent moderate to severe dysplasia or carcinoma. Not all of these lesions herald dysplasia or carcinoma, as many red oral mucosal lesions may be inflammatory in nature.

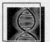 **PATHOLOGY:** Leukoplakia occurs most often on the buccal mucosa, tongue, and floor of the mouth. Plaques may be solitary or multiple and vary from small lesions to large patches. Erythroplakia is commonly associated with ominous histopathologic alterations, including severe dysplasia, carcinoma in situ, or invasive carcinoma. By contrast, leukoplakia may show a spectrum of histopathologic changes, from increased surface keratinization without dysplasia to invasive keratinizing squamous carcinoma (Fig. 25-3). Leukoplakic lesions, unlike those that are erythroplakic, tend to be well defined with demarcated margins. The frequency of malignant transformation in leukoplakia is about 10%, but the risk of an erythroplakic lesions being diagnosed as malignant is as high as 70% on initial biopsy.

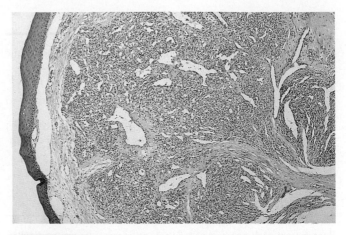

FIGURE 25-2. **Lobular capillary hemangioma (pyogenic granuloma).** Submucosal lesion characterized by the presence of cellular lobules consisting of dilated, irregularly shaped vascular spaces and surrounded by granulation tissue with a chronic inflammatory cell infiltrate.

Squamous Cell Carcinoma (SCC)

SCC is the most common malignant tumor of the oral mucosa and may occur at any site. It most frequently involves the tongue, followed in descending order by the floor of the mouth, alveolar mucosa, palate, and buccal mucosa. The male-to-female ratio is 2:1 for the gum but 10:1 for the lip. There are substantial variations in the geographic distribution of oral cancer; for example, it is the single most common cancer of men in India.

PATHOGENESIS: Predisposing factors in the pathogenesis of oral cancer include the use of tobacco products, alcoholism, Plummer-Vinson syndrome (esophageal webs, iron-deficiency anemia and dysphagia), physical and chemical irritants, chewing of betel nuts, ultraviolet light on the lips, and poor oral hygiene (craggy teeth and ill-fitting dentures). Some SCCs of the head and neck have been associated with HPV infection, but a direct causal relationship between HPV and the development of *oral* SCC is not definitively established.

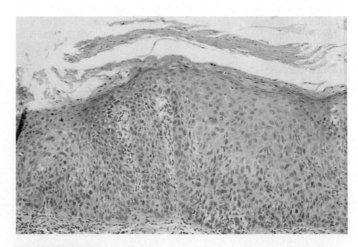

FIGURE 25-3. **Leukoplakia.** The lesion was seen as a white patch on the buccal mucosa of a heavy smoker. Histologically, epithelial hyperplasia, marked atypia, and parakeratosis are evident.

PATHOLOGY: Invasive SCC of the oral cavity is similar to the same tumor in other sites and is generally preceded by carcinoma in situ. Grade I carcinoma is well differentiated and frequently keratinizing. At the other end of the spectrum, grade IV tumors are so poorly differentiated that their origin is difficult to determine on morphologic grounds. Oral carcinoma metastasizes mainly to submandibular, superficial, and deep cervical lymph nodes. More than half of the patients who die of SCC of the head and neck have distant, blood-borne metastases, most commonly in lungs, liver, and bones.

Verrucous carcinoma (VC) is a highly differentiated variant of squamous cell carcinoma, which is locally destructive but does not metastasize. It generally occurs in the sixth and seventh decades of life. VCs may arise anywhere in this region but are most common on the buccal mucosa, gingiva, and larynx. The tumors are usually white, warty to fungating, or exophytic, and are generally attached by a broad base (Fig. 25-4A). Microscopically, they exhibit a benign-appearing squamous epithelium (without dysplasia), marked surface keratinization, and a pushing border of bulbous rete pegs (see Fig. 25-4B). VC carries a good prognosis if it is completely removed.

Dental Caries (Tooth Decay)

Caries is the most prevalent chronic disease of the calcified tissues of teeth. It affects both sexes and every age group throughout the world, and its incidence has markedly increased with modern civilization.

PATHOGENESIS: Dental caries results from the interactions of several factors.

BACTERIA: Dental caries is a chronic infectious disease of tooth enamel, dentin, and cementum; the organisms are part of the indigenous oral flora. Carious lesions result primarily from the leaching of mineral in dental tissues by acids produced from food residues by microorganisms. Tooth surfaces are normally colonized by many microorganisms, and unless the surface is cleaned thoroughly and frequently, bacterial colonies coalesce into a soft mass known as **dental plaque**. Numerous streptococci, lactobacilli, and actinomycetes are implicated in caries formation. Indirect evidence points strongly to *Streptococcus mutans* as the primary etiologic agent that initiates caries. Organisms other than *S. mutans* may be more capable of maintaining the destructive process deeper in the enamel and dentin.

SALIVA: Saliva has a high buffering capacity that helps neutralize microbially produced acids in the mouth. In addition, it contains several bacteriostatic factors, such as lysozyme, lactoferrin, the lactoperoxidase system, and secretory immunoglobulins. *Xerostomia (chronic dryness of the mouth from lack of saliva) results in rampant caries.*

DIETARY FACTORS: One of the most important factors in caries development is a high-carbohydrate diet. The roughage in raw and unrefined foods cleanses the teeth. Additionally, roughage necessitates more mastication, which further contributes to cleansing of the teeth. By contrast, soft and refined foods tend to stick to the teeth and also require less chewing.

FLUORIDE: Fluoride administration protects against dental caries. It is incorporated into the crystal lattice structure of enamel, where it forms fluoroapatite, a less acid-soluble compound than the apatite of enamel.

PATHOLOGY: Caries begins with disintegration of enamel prisms after decalcification of the interprismatic substance, events that lead to accumulation of debris and microorganisms (Fig. 25-5). These changes produce a small pit or fissure in the enamel. When the process reaches the dentinoenamel junction, it spreads laterally and also penetrates the dentin along the dentinal tubules. A substantial cavity then forms in the dentin, producing a flask-shaped lesion with a narrow orifice. Decalcification of dentin leads to focal coalescence of the destroyed dentinal tubules. Only when the vascular pulp of the tooth is invaded does an inflammatory reaction (**pulpitis**) appear, accompanied for the first time by pain.

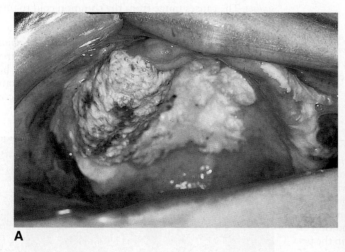

A

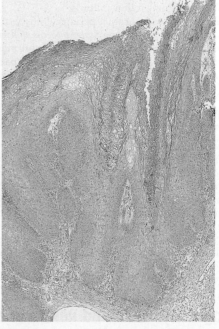

B

FIGURE 25-4. **Verrucous carcinoma. A.** The tumor is white with an exophytic appearance involving the alveolar ridge. Note the confluent white (leukoplakic) appearance of the palate. **B.** Microscopically, there is prominent surface keratinization ("church-spire" keratosis) composed of bland-appearing uniform squamous cells without dysplasia and broad or bulbous rete pegs with a pushing margin into the submucosa.

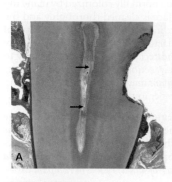
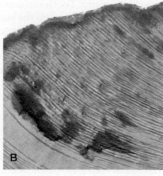

FIGURE 25-5. Dental caries. **A.** A large cavity close to the gingival margin is illustrated. Band of secondary dentin that lines the pulp chamber (arrows). This newly formed dentin is opposite the area of tooth destruction and was produced by the stimulated odontoblasts. **B.** Deposits of debris cover the surface. Bacterial colonies (dark purple) have extended into dentinal canals.

Diseases of the Pulp and Periapical Tissues

The dental pulp is delicate connective tissue enclosed within the calcified walls of dentin. The pulp chamber is lined by odontoblasts and has a minute apical foramen through which blood vessels, lymphatics, and small nerves penetrate.

- **Pulpitis** results from invasion by the oral bacteria involved in dental caries. Pain in acute pulpitis reflects increased pressure in the pulp chamber and is caused by edema and exudate.
- **Apical (or periapical granuloma),** the most common sequel of pulpitis, is chronically inflamed periapical granulation tissue. The inflammatory tissue gradually becomes surrounded by a fibrous capsule, and when the tooth is extracted, the encapsulated granuloma is found attached to the root.
- **Radicular cyst (apical periodontal cyst)** occurs when the squamous epithelium of an apical granuloma proliferates, forming a cavity or cyst.
- **Periapical abscess** may follow pulpitis.
- **Osteomyelitis** may complicate a periapical abscess, and usually involves *Staphylococcus aureus*, *Staphylococcus epidermidis*, various streptococci, or mixed organisms. Infection may traverse the cortical bone and spread to various tissue spaces of the head and neck, and rarely the mediastinum.

Periodontal Disease

Periodontal disease refers to acute and chronic disorders of the soft tissues surrounding teeth, which eventually lead to the loss of supporting bone. Chronic periodontal disease typically occurs in adults with poor oral hygiene or in individuals with a strong family history of the disease. Chronic periodontitis causes loss of more teeth in adults than does any other disease, including caries. The condition is caused by the accumulation of bacteria under the gingiva in the periodontal pocket. As the mass of bacteria adhering to the surface of tooth (**dental plaque**) ages, it mineralizes to form **calculus** (tartar). Adult periodontitis is mostly associated with *Bacteroides gingivalis*, *Bacteroides intermedius*, *Actinomyces* species, and *Haemophilus* species.

Hematologic Disorders and Periodontal Disease

Hematologic disorders may affect oral tissues and specifically, the gingiva. **Agranulocytosis** causes necrotizing ulcers anywhere in the oral and pharyngeal mucosa, but especially in the gingiva.

Infectious mononucleosis often results in gingivitis and stomatitis, with exudate and ulceration. **Acute and chronic leukemias** of all types cause oral lesions. The most common involvement of oral tissues is seen in **acute monocytic leukemia**, in which 80% of patients exhibit gingivitis, gingival hyperplasia, petechiae, and hemorrhage. Necrosis and ulceration of the gingiva lead to severe superimposed infection, which may cause loss of teeth and alveolar bone. A hemorrhagic diathesis may be reflected in gingival hemorrhage.

Odontogenic Tumors: Ameloblastoma

Ameloblastomas are tumors of odontogenic epithelia and are the most common clinically significant odontogenic tumor. They are slow-growing, locally invasive tumors that generally follow a benign clinical course. Most arise in the mandibular ramus or molar area, maxilla, or floor of the nasal cavity. The tumor tends to grow slowly as a central lesion of bone. Microscopically, ameloblastoma resembles the enamel organ in its various stages of differentiation, and a single tumor may show various histologic patterns. Accordingly, tumor cells resemble ameloblasts at the periphery of epithelial nests or cords, where columnar cells are oriented perpendicularly to the basement membrane (Fig. 25-6). Although incompletely excised tumors may recur, the tumor does not metastasize.

NASAL CAVITY AND PARANASAL SINUSES

Non-Neoplastic Diseases of the Nasal Cavity and Paranasal Sinuses

Rhinitis is Usually Viral or Allergic

Rhinitis is inflammation of the mucous membranes of the nasal cavity and sinuses. The causes range from the common cold to unusual infections, such as diphtheria, anthrax, and glanders.

VIRAL RHINITIS: *The most common cause of acute rhinitis is viral infection, especially the common cold (**acute coryza**).* The virus replicates in epithelial cells, causing the degenerating cells to be shed. The mucosa is edematous and engorged and is infiltrated by neutrophils as well as mononuclear cells. Clinically, mucosal swelling

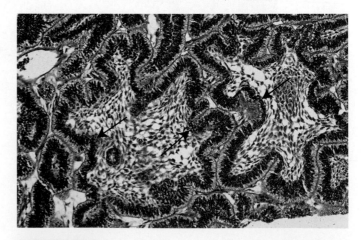

FIGURE 25-6. Ameloblastoma. A common histologic pattern is characterized by confluent islands of epithelium. The peripheral cells (arrows) form bands that separate the tumor from the stroma. Several microcysts are present.

is manifested as nasal stuffiness. Abundant mucus secretion and increased vascular permeability lead to **rhinorrhea** (free discharge of a thin nasal mucus). Viral rhinitis may be followed within a few days by secondary infection caused by normal nasal and pharyngeal flora. The abundant serous discharge then becomes mucopurulent, after which the surface epithelium is shed. The epithelial cells regenerate rapidly after the inflammation subsides.

CHRONIC RHINITIS: Repeated bouts of acute rhinitis may lead to chronic rhinitis. A deviated nasal septum is often a contributory factor. Chronic rhinitis is characterized by nasal mucosal thickening due to persistent hyperemia, mucous gland hyperplasia, and lymphocyte and plasma cell infiltration.

ALLERGIC RHINITIS: Numerous allergens are constantly present in our environment, and sensitivity to any one of them can cause allergic rhinitis. In this condition, airborne allergenic particles (e.g., pollens, molds, animal allergens) are deposited on the nasal mucosa. Often called **hay fever**, allergic rhinitis may be acute and seasonal or chronic and perennial (see Chapter 4).

Nasal Polyps are Focal Inflammatory Swellings

Sinonasal inflammatory polyps are non-neoplastic lesions of the mucosa. Most arise from the lateral nasal wall or ethmoid recess. They may be unilateral or bilateral, single or multiple. Symptoms include nasal obstruction, rhinorrhea, and headaches. The etiology involves multiple factors, including allergy, infections, diabetes mellitus, cystic fibrosis, and aspirin intolerance. Sinonasal allergic polyps are lined externally by respiratory epithelium and contain mucous glands within a loose mucoid stroma, which is infiltrated by plasma cells, lymphocytes, and many eosinophils.

Sinusitis is a Bacterial Infection

Sinusitis refers to inflammation of the mucous membranes of the paranasal sinuses.

 PATHOGENESIS: Any condition (inflammation, neoplasm, foreign body) that interferes with sinus drainage or aeration renders it liable to infection. If ostium of a sinus is blocked, secretions or exudate accumulate behind the obstruction. **Acute sinusitis** is a disorder of less than 3 weeks' duration, caused predominantly by extension of infection from the nasal mucosa. Most cases involve a rich bacterial flora; *Haemophilus influenzae* and *Branhamella catarrhalis* are the most common. Maxillary sinusitis may also be caused by odontogenic infections, in which case bacteria from the roots of the first and second molars penetrate the thin bony plate that separates them from the floor of the maxillary sinus. **Chronic sinusitis** is a sequel of acute inflammation, either as a result of incomplete resolution of infection or because of recurrent acute complications. In contrast to acute sinusitis, the purulent exudate in chronic sinusitis almost always includes anaerobic bacteria.

PATHOLOGY: Acute or chronic sinusitis may be followed by a number of complications, including mucocele (the accumulation of mucus) or pyocele (accumulation of mucopurulent exudate), osteomyelitis, septic thrombophlebitis and, ultimately, intracranial infections.

Rhinoscleroma is a Chronic Bacterial Infection of the Nose

*Rhinoscleroma (**scleroma**) is a chronic inflammatory process caused by a gram-negative diplobacillus,* Klebsiella rhinoscleromatis, *which usually begins in the nose and remains localized to that site, although it may extend slowly into the nasopharynx, larynx, and trachea.* Rhinoscleroma is endemic in some Mediterranean countries and in parts of Asia, Africa, and Latin America. Indigenous cases have also been recognized in the United States. It occurs in both sexes and at any age. Most patients have poor domestic and personal hygiene.

 PATHOLOGY: Infected tissues appear firm, greatly thickened, irregularly nodular, and often ulcerated. Microscopically, the granulation tissue is strikingly rich in plasma cells, lymphocytes, and foamy macrophages (Fig. 25-7). The characteristic large macrophages, referred to as *Mikulicz cells,* contain masses of phagocytosed bacilli. Serologic tests are valuable in establishing the diagnosis of rhinoscleroma, because specific antibodies are present in many patients. The disease is successfully treated with antibiotics.

Benign Neoplasms of the Nasal Cavity and Paranasal Sinuses

SQUAMOUS PAPILLOMA: The most frequent benign tumor of the nasal cavity is squamous papilloma, which almost always occurs in the nasal vestibule. The lesion is often indistinguishable from a wart (verruca vulgaris).

SCHNEIDERIAN PAPILLOMAS: These tumors are a group of benign neoplasms composed of a squamous or columnar epithelial proliferation with associated mucous cells. They arise from the sinonasal mucosa, the ectodermally derived lining of the sinonasal tract (Schneiderian membrane). Three morphologically distinct benign papillomas are recognized: **inverted**, **oncocytic** (cylindrical or columnar cell), and **fungiform** (exophytic, septal) papillomas. Collectively, Schneiderian papillomas represent less than 5% of all sinonasal tract tumors.

INVERTED PAPILLOMA: This tumor involves the lateral nasal wall and may spread into the paranasal sinuses. Inverted papillomas occur mainly in middle-aged individuals. As the name implies, they show characteristic inversions of the surface epithelium into the underlying stroma (Fig. 25-8). HPV types 6/11 and rarely other types (16/18, 33, 40, 57) have been found in inverted papillomas, but a cause-and-effect relationship is unproven. Although benign, these tumors may erode bone by pressure. Unless surgical resection extends beyond the boundaries of grossly visible lesions, they frequently recur. In 5% of cases, inverted papillomas give rise to squamous cell carcinoma.

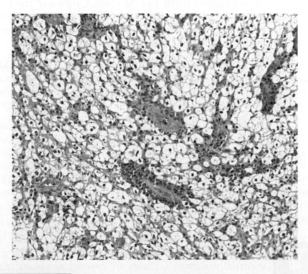

FIGURE 25-7. **Rhino scleroma.** Granulation tissue contains numerous foamy macrophages (Mikulicz cells).

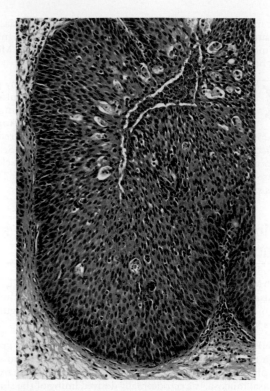

FIGURE 25-8. Sinonasal inverted papilloma. Epithelial nests are growing downward (inverted) into the submucosa. They are composed of a uniform cellular proliferation, which displays an inflammatory cell infiltrate and scattered microcysts.

Malignant Neoplasms of the Nasal Cavity and Paranasal Sinuses

SQUAMOUS CELL CARCINOMA: Most cancers of the nasal cavity and paranasal sinuses are squamous cell tumors (keratinizing and nonkeratinizing). Approximately 15% are adenocarcinomas or undifferentiated carcinomas. Several industrial chemicals including nickel, chromium, and aromatic hydrocarbons and occupations such as working with wood, leather, cutting oils, and textiles, increase the risk of cancer of the nose and sinuses. Squamous tumors in nickel workers usually arise from the middle turbinate, with latencies from 2 to 32 years. Cancers of the nasal cavity and sinuses grow relentlessly and invade adjacent structures. However, they typically do not give rise to distant metastases. Survival is usually only a few years.

NASAL-TYPE ANGIOCENTRIC NK/T-CELL LYMPH-OMA: *Nasal-type angiocentric NK/T-cell lymphoma has supplanted previous designations of lethal midline granuloma, midline malignant reticulosis, and polymorphic reticulosis.*

PATHOLOGY: This aggressive type of EBV-associated lymphoma manifests as necrotizing, ulcerating mucosal lesions of the upper respiratory tract. The tumor infiltrate is characteristically polymorphic and surrounds small-to-medium-sized blood vessels (angiocentric), infiltrates through vascular walls (angioinvasive), and often occludes vessel lumina like a thrombus, causing necrosis in adjacent tissues (ischemic-type) (Fig. 25-9).

CLINICAL FEATURES: After an insidious onset, the nasal mucosa becomes focally swollen, indurated, and eventually ulcerated. Ulcers are covered by a black crust, under which lesions progress to erode cartilage and bone, causing defects in the nasal septum, hard palate, and na-

sopharynx. The disease remains localized in half of the patients but disseminates widely in an equal proportion. Death is due to secondary bacterial infection, aspiration pneumonia, or hemorrhage from eroded large blood vessels. The infiltrates of nasal-type NK/T-cell lymphoma are, at least initially, radiosensitive, and remission with cytotoxic agents has also been reported.

NASOPHARYNX AND OROPHARYNX

Infections

Pharyngitis and tonsillitis are among the most common diseases of the head and neck. Nasopharyngeal inflammation occurs mainly in children, although it is also common in adolescents and young adults. Viral or bacterial infections may be limited to the palatine tonsils, but nasopharyngeal tonsils or adjacent pharyngeal mucosa may also be involved, often as part of a general upper respiratory tract infection. In the latter case, initial infecting agents are most often viruses spread by droplets or by direct contact. These viruses include influenza, parainfluenza, adenovirus, respiratory syncytial virus, and rhinovirus.

Acute tonsillitis is a bacterial infection, usually with *S. pyogenes* (group A β-hemolytic streptococci). Follicular tonsillitis is characterized by pinpoint exudates that can be extruded from the crypts.

Pseudomembranous tonsillitis refers to a necrotic mucosa covered by a coat of exudate, for instance, in diphtheria or in **Vincent angina** (see above).

Recurrent or chronic tonsillitis is not as common as once believed, and enlarged tonsils in children do not necessarily signify chronic tonsillitis. However, repeated infections can cause enlargement of tonsils and adenoids to a degree that obstructs air passages. In children, repeated bouts of streptococcal tonsillitis may lead to rheumatic fever or glomerulonephritis, and patients may benefit from tonsillectomy.

Peritonsillar abscess (quinsy) is a collection of purulent material behind the posterior capsule of the tonsil, usually due to infection with α- and β-hemolytic streptococci. One third of patients have a prior history of tonsillitis. Untreated, peritonsillar abscesses may lead to several life-threatening situations, such as rupture into the airway, weakening of the carotid artery wall or penetration into the mediastinum, the base of the skull, or the cranial vault.

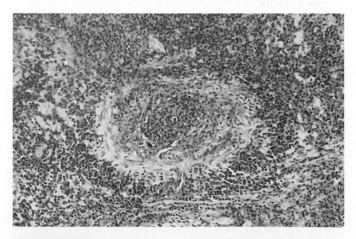

FIGURE 25-9. Angiocentric natural killer (NK)/T-cell lymphoma. A malignant cellular infiltrate growing around and into a medium-sized blood vessel with disruption of the external elastic membrane and occlusion of the vessel lumen.

Neoplasms

The Oropharynx is a Common Site for Squamous Cell Carcinomas

These tumors tend to be less differentiated and more biologically aggressive than their counterparts in the anterior oral cavity. At this site, they often metastasize early because of the rich lymphatic network in this region. The primary lymphatics drain into the superior deep jugular and submandibular lymph nodes and, to a somewhat lesser degree, into the retropharyngeal lymph nodes.

Nasopharyngeal Carcinoma (NPC) is Related to Epstein-Barr Virus (EBV)

NPC is a malignancy of the nasopharynx that is subclassified into keratinizing and nonkeratinizing subtypes. The latter are associated with EBV infection.

 EPIDEMIOLOGY: By far, the most common cancer of the nasopharynx, namely nasopharyngeal carcinoma, is the most frequent of all malignant tumors in the Chinese. In Hong Kong, nasopharyngeal undifferentiated carcinoma represents 18% of all cancers, compared with 0.25% worldwide. People of Chinese descent who are born in the United States have about a 20-fold greater mortality from nasopharyngeal carcinoma than do those of other ethnic backgrounds.

 PATHOGENESIS: Various environmental risk factors for NPC have been sought, but no association has been positively demonstrated. Recent studies point to a possible combined role for environmental and genetic factors in the pathogenesis of this tumor. There is an association with a specific HLA A2 allele (*0207), which is common in Chinese populations but not in whites, thereby supporting a genetic susceptibility in a particular ethnic group. EBV is present in the tumor cells and B lymphocytes of patients with NPC. Moreover, 85% of patients also have antibodies to EBV. EBV genomes are detected in almost all nonkeratinizing and undifferentiated types of NPC. In the keratinizing subtype, detection of EBV is variable. For more details on EBV infection and cancers, see Chapters 5 and 9.

 PATHOLOGY: *The epithelial nature of this tumor is underscored by the fact that tumor cells express cytokeratin but no hematologic or lymphoid markers.* Keratinizing tumors occur in older people and do not bear the same relation to EBV infection as do nonkeratinizing types. The latter are classified as differentiated or undifferentiated. *The undifferentiated subtype of nonkeratinizing carcinoma is particularly common in southeast Asia and parts of Africa.* Differentiated, nonkeratinizing, NPCs display a stratified appearance and distinct cell margins. By contrast, undifferentiated tumors exhibit clusters of poorly delimited or syncytial cells, bearing large oval nuclei and scant eosinophilic cytoplasm (Fig. 25-10).

 CLINICAL FEATURES: Because of their location, most NPCs remain asymptomatic for a long time. Palpable cervical lymph node metastases are the first sign of disease in about half of the cases, and even then, many patients have no complaints referable to the nasopharynx. The tumor infiltrates neighboring regions, such as the parapharyngeal space, orbit and cranial cavity, resulting in neurologic symptoms and hearing disturbances. Nasopharyngeal undifferentiated carcinoma is radiosensitive, and most patients whose tumors are restricted to the nasopharynx survive 5 or more years. Metastases to cervical lymph nodes reduce the prognosis considerably, and survival with cranial nerve involvement or distant metastases is dismal.

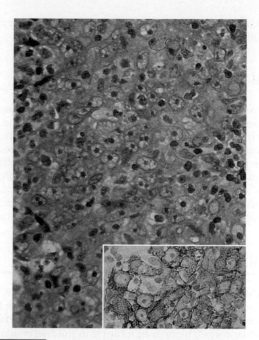

FIGURE 25-10. **Nasopharyngeal nonkeratinizing carcinoma, undifferentiated type.** The cells have large nuclei and prominent eosinophilic nucleoli. The cells are cytokeratin-positive (by immunohistochemistry, *inset*) indicating an epithelial cell proliferation.

Lymphomas of Waldeyer Ring are Mostly Diffuse B-Cell Tumors

Lymphomas comprise 5% of head and neck cancers. Waldeyer ring is by far the most common site of origin of lymphoma in this region. Enlargement of a single tonsil in any age group, or bilateral painless tonsillar enlargement in adults, should suggest the possibility of lymphoma. Nasopharyngeal lymphomas are histologically diffuse (90%), and more than half have been classified as large cell lymphomas. In the United States and Asia, the vast majority of lymphomas of Waldeyer ring are of B-cell origin.

Extramedullary Plasmacytomas Often Occur in the Head and Neck

Three fourths of extramedullary plasmacytomas occur in the head and neck, with a strong predilection for the nasopharynx, nasal cavity, and paranasal sinuses. Like extramedullary plasmacytomas in other body sites, these tumors are best considered as part of a spectrum of plasma cell disorders. The tumors may remain localized or may evolve into systemic plasma cell myeloma (see Chapter 20).

LARYNX AND HYPOPHARYNX

Infections

EPIGLOTTITIS: Inflammation of the epiglottis is a serious condition, most commonly caused by *Haemophilus influenzae*, type B. Occurring in infants and young children, this may be a life-threatening emergency, because swelling of the acutely inflamed epiglottis may obstruct airflow. Inspiratory stridor (a loud wheezing sound on inspiration) occurs, and the onset of cyanosis may indicate airway obstruction so severe as to require tracheostomy.

CROUP: Croup is a laryngotracheobronchitis in young children, with symptoms of inspiratory stridor, cough, and hoarseness that result from varying degrees of laryngeal obstruction. Croup is a complication of an upper respiratory infection and is marked by edema of the larynx.

Vocal Cord Nodule and Polyp

Vocal cord nodule/polyp is a stromal reactive process related to inflammation or trauma. Nodules/polyps may be seen in all age groups but are most common between the third and sixth decades. Symptoms related to vocal cord polyps and nodules are similar and include hoarseness or voice changes. Lesions occur after voice abuse, infection (laryngitis), alcohol consumption, smoking, or endocrine dysfunction (e.g., hypothyroidism). The histologic appearance varies from a myxoid, edematous, fibroblastic stroma in the early stages to a hyalinized, densely fibrotic stroma at a later time.

Neoplasms of the Larynx

SQUAMOUS PAPILLOMA AND PAPILLOMATOSIS: Squamous papillomas of the larynx are solitary or multiple papillary growths of mature squamous cells that line the surface of fibrovascular cores. They may be multiple in children or adolescents (juvenile laryngeal papillomatosis) and may extend into the trachea and bronchi. HPVs, especially types 6 and 11, are the principal causes. *The condition may cause life-threatening respiratory obstruction and, rarely, evolve into an overt squamous cell carcinoma, particularly in smokers or after radiation therapy.* Surgical excision may not be curative, because viral infection of the mucosa is often widespread, and the tumors tend to recur over many years.

SQUAMOUS CELL CARCINOMA: Almost all laryngeal cancers are squamous cell carcinomas, and virtually all of the patients are men, most of whom are cigarette smokers.

SALIVARY GLANDS

XEROSTOMIA: *Xerostomia is chronic mouth dryness due to lack of saliva and has many causes.* Diseases that involve the major salivary glands and produce xerostomia include mumps, Sjögren syndrome, sarcoidosis, radiation-induced atrophy, and drug sensitivity (antihistamines, tricyclic antidepressants, hypotensive drugs, phenothiazines).

ENLARGEMENT: Unilateral enlargement of major salivary glands is usually caused by cysts, inflammation, or neoplasms. Bilateral enlargement is due to inflammation (mumps, Sjögren syndrome; see below), granulomatous disease (sarcoidosis), or diffuse neoplastic involvement (leukemia or malignant lymphoma).

SIALOLITHIASIS: Calcific stones occur in salivary gland ducts, mostly in the submandibular gland. The most important consequence of stone formation is duct obstruction, often followed by inflammation distal to the occlusion.

PAROTITIS: Acute suppurative parotitis is caused by the ascent of bacteria (usually *Staphylococcus aureus*) from the oral cavity when salivary flow is reduced. It is most often seen in debilitated or postoperative patients. Acute and chronic parotitis is frequently associated with stricture of salivary ducts or obstruction by stones. The stagnant secretions serve as a medium for retrograde bacterial invasion.

Sjögren Syndrome

Sjögren syndrome is a chronic inflammatory disease of salivary and lacrimal glands; it may be limited to these sites or may be associated with a systemic collagen vascular disease. Salivary gland involvement leads to dry mouth (**xerostomia**). Lacrimal gland involvement results in dry eyes (**keratoconjunctivitis sicca**). The pathogenesis and clinical features of Sjögren syndrome are discussed in Chapter 4.

 PATHOLOGY: In Sjögren syndrome, parotid glands and sometimes submandibular glands are unilaterally or bilaterally enlarged, but their lobulation is preserved. Histologically, an initial periductal chronic inflammatory infiltrate gradually extends to the acini, until the glands are completely replaced by a sea of polyclonal lymphocytes, immunoblasts, germinal centers, and plasma cells. Proliferating myoepithelial cells surround remnants of damaged ducts and form so-called epimyoepithelial islands (Fig. 25-11). Late in the course of the disease, affected glands become atrophic with fibrosis and fatty infiltration of the parenchyma.

Benign Salivary Gland Neoplasms

Pleomorphic Adenoma (Mixed Tumor) is the Most Common Tumor of Salivary Glands

Pleomorphic adenoma is a benign neoplasm characterized by an admixture of epithelial and stromal elements. Two thirds of all tumors of the major salivary glands and about half of those in the minor ones are pleomorphic adenomas. The tumor usually arises in the superficial lobe of the parotid gland and is nine times more frequent in this gland than in the mandibular gland. It occurs most often in middle-aged people and shows a female preponderance.

 PATHOLOGY: Pleomorphic adenoma is a slowly growing, painless, movable, firm mass that has a smooth surface. Microscopically, the tumors show epithelial tissue intermingled with myxoid, mucoid, or chondroid areas (Fig. 25-12A), reflecting a mixture of epithelial and mesenchymal components. However, the neoplasm is now considered to be of epithelial origin. The epithelial component of pleomorphic adenoma consists of ductal and myoepithelial cells (Fig. 25-12B). The cells lining the ducts form tubules or small cystic structures and contain clear fluid or eosinophilic, periodic acid-Schiff-positive material. Around the ductal epithelial cells are smaller myoepithelial cells, which are the main cellular component. These cells form well-defined sheaths, cords, or nests and are often separated by a cellular ground substance that resembles cartilaginous, myxoid, or mucoid material.

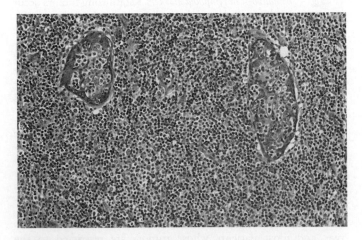

FIGURE 25-11. Sjögren syndrome. There is infiltration of the involved salivary gland by a mixed chronic inflammatory cell infiltrate. Extension of the infiltrate into epithelial (ductal) structures results in metaplasia and characteristic epimyoepithelial islands.

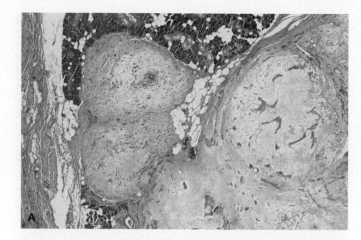

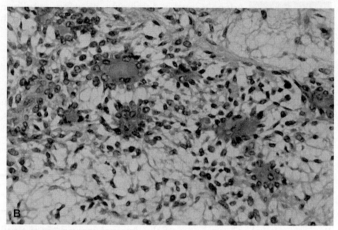

FIGURE 25-12. Pleomorphic adenoma of the parotid gland. **A.** The tumor contains characteristic myxoid and chondroid portions. The tumor is partly encapsulated, but a nodule protruding into the parotid gland lacks a capsule. If such nodules are not included in the resection, the tumor will recur. **B.** Cellular components of pleomorphic adenomas include an admixture of glands and myoepithelial cells within a chondromyxoid stroma.

CLINICAL FEATURES: Pleomorphic adenomas have fibrous capsules. As they grow, the surrounding fibrous tissue condenses around them. The tumors expand and tend to protrude focally into adjacent tissues, becoming nodular. Tumor cells implanted during surgery or tumor nodules left behind continue to grow as recurrences in the scar from the previous operation. Recurrence of pleomorphic adenomas represents local regrowth, not malignancy.

Carcinoma expleomorphic adenoma: Rarely, carcinomas may arise in pleomorphic adenomas that have been present for many years. Histologic examination reveals an unequivocal carcinoma in an otherwise benign pleomorphic adenoma. These tumors are usually high-grade malignancies, such as poorly differentiated or undifferentiated adenocarcinoma.

Warthin Tumor is the Most Common Monomorphic Adenoma

Monomorphic adenomas comprise 5% to 10% of benign salivary gland tumors. In such tumors, the epithelium is arranged in a regular, usually glandular pattern without a mesenchyme-like component. Monomorphic adenomas include a number of subtypes, of which Warthin tumor is the most common. *Warthin tumors are benign parotid gland neoplasms composed of cystic glandular spaces embedded in dense lymphoid tissue.* Although the neoplasm is clearly benign, it can be bilateral (15% of cases) or multifocal within the same

gland. Warthin tumor is the only tumor of salivary glands that is more common in men than in women. These tumors generally occur after the age of 30 years, with most arising after age 50.

 PATHOLOGY: Warthin tumors are composed of glandular spaces that tend to become cystic and show papillary projections. The cysts are lined by characteristic eosinophilic epithelial cells (oncocytes) and are embedded in dense lymphoid tissue with germinal centers (Fig. 25-13).

Malignant Salivary Gland Tumors

Salivary gland cancers account for about 5% of all head and neck neoplasms. Most (75%) arise in the parotid glands, 10% are in the submandibular glands, and 15% are located in minor salivary glands (mucoserous glands) of the upper aerodigestive tract. Less than 1% occur in the sublingual glands.

Mucoepidermoid Carcinoma Has Neoplastic Squamous, Glandular, and Intermediate Cells

Mucoepidermoid carcinoma is a malignant salivary gland tumor composed of a mixture of neoplastic epidermoid cells, mucus-secreting cells, and epithelial cells of an intermediate type. It originates from ductal epithelium, which has a considerable potential for metaplasia. This neoplasm accounts for 5% to 10% of major salivary gland tumors and 10% of those in the minor salivary glands. Within the major salivary glands, more than half of mucoepidermoid carcinomas arise in the parotid gland. In minor salivary glands, they develop most frequently in the palate. Although the tumor may occur in adolescents, most arise in adults and are more common in women.

 PATHOLOGY: Mucoepidermoid carcinoma grows slowly and presents as a firm painless mass. Microscopically, low-grade (well-differentiated) tumors form irregular solid, duct-like and cystic spaces, which

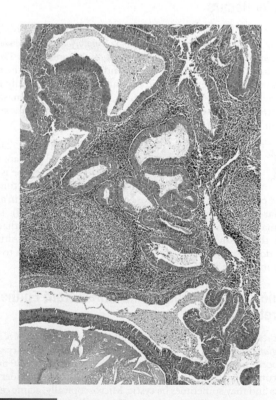

FIGURE 25-13. **Warthin tumor.** Cystic spaces and duct-like structures are lined by oncocytes. Follicular lymphoid tissue is present.

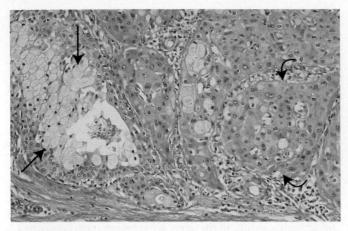

FIGURE 25-14. Mucoepidermoid carcinoma is characterized by an admixture of mucocytes, epidermoid cells, and intermediate cells. The mucocytes *(straight arrows)* are clustered and have a clear cytoplasm with eccentrically situated nuclei. Epidermoid cells *(curved arrows)* are squamous-like cells but lack keratinization and intercellular bridges. Intermediate cells (best seen at *lower left*) are smaller than epidermoid cells.

include squamous cells, mucus-secreting cells, and intermediate cells (Fig. 25-14). High-grade (poorly differentiated) carcinomas are pleomorphic, without evidence of differentiation except for scattered mucus-secreting cells.

 CLINICAL FEATURES: Even low-grade mucoepidermoid carcinomas can metastasize, but the 5-year survival rate is better than 90%, regardless of the primary site. High-grade mucoepidermoid carcinomas have a much lower survival rate (20% to 40%).

Adenoid Cystic Carcinoma Invades Locally and Usually Recurs

Adenoid cystic carcinoma, previously termed "cylindroma," is a slowly growing salivary gland malignancy, which is notorious for its tendency to invade locally and recur after surgical resection. It constitutes 5% of all tumors of the major salivary glands and 20% of those of the minor salivary glands. Adenoid cystic carcinoma occurs not only in the oral cavity but also in lacrimal glands, the nasopharynx, nasal cavity, paranasal sinuses, and lower respiratory tract and is most common in people 40 to 60 years of age.

 PATHOLOGY: Histologically, adenoid cystic carcinomas present varying patterns. The tumor cells are small, have scant cytoplasm, and grow in solid sheets or as small groups, strands, or columns. Within these structures, the tumor cells interconnect to enclose cystic spaces, resulting in a solid, tubular or cribriform (sieve-like) arrangement (Fig. 25-15). Tumor cells make a homogeneous basement membrane material that gives them the characteristic "cylindromatous" appearance. Although most do not metastasize for many years, they are difficult to eradicate completely, and the long-term prognosis is poor.

Acinic Cell Adenocarcinoma Arises from Epithelial Secretory Cells

Acinic cell adenocarcinomas are uncommon parotid tumors (10% of all salivary gland tumors). They arise occasionally in other salivary glands and occur principally in young men between the ages of 20 and 30. The tumors are encapsulated, round masses, usually under 3 cm across and may sometimes be cystic. Microscopically, acinic cell adenocarcinomas are composed of uniform cells with a small central nucleus and abundant basophilic cytoplasm, similar to the secretory (acinic) cells of the normal salivary glands. They may metastasize to

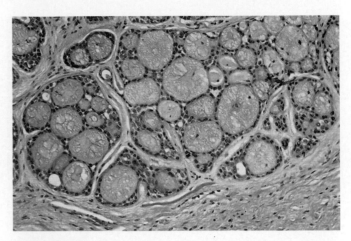

FIGURE 25-15. Adenoid cystic carcinoma showing cribriform growth in which cyst-like spaces are filled with basophilic material. The cystic spaces are really pseudocysts surrounded by myoepithelial cells.

the regional lymph nodes. After surgical resection, most (90%) patients survive for 5 years, but local recurrence may be expected in one third of patients. Only half of these patients survive for 20 years.

THE EAR

External Ear Neoplasms

Benign and malignant tumors of the external ear include the full gamut of skin-related neoplasms: squamous papillomas, seborrheic keratosis, basal cell carcinoma, squamous cell carcinoma, and benign and malignant adnexal tumors. Neoplasms arising from ceruminal glands are unique to this area. Benign tumors of these glands include ceruminoma (ceruminal gland adenoma) and salivary gland-type tumors arising from ceruminal glands (e.g., pleomorphic and monomorphic adenomas). Malignant tumors of ceruminal glands include adenocarcinoma and malignant salivary gland-type tumors (e.g., adenoid cystic carcinoma, mucoepidermoid carcinoma).

Middle Ear

Otitis Media Often Results from Obstruction of the Eustachian Tube

Otitis media is inflammation of the middle ear and usually results from an upper respiratory tract infection that extends from the nasopharynx.

 PATHOGENESIS: The infection almost invariably penetrates through the mastoid antrum into the mastoid cells. During an infection in the nasopharynx, microorganisms may reach the middle ear by ascending through the eustachian tube. Acute otitis media may be due to viral or bacterial infections or to obstruction of the eustachian tube without microorganisms. Viral otitis media may resolve without suppuration, or the middle ear may be secondarily invaded by pus-forming bacteria. *Obstruction of the eustachian tube is important in the production of middle ear effusion.* When the pharyngeal end of the eustachian tube is swollen, air cannot enter the tube. Air in the middle ear is then absorbed through the mucosa, and negative pressure causes transudation of plasma and occasionally bleeding. Antibiotics usually cure or suppress the condition.

- *Serous otitis media:* Obstruction of the eustachian tube may result from sudden changes in atmospheric pressure, particularly if there is an upper respiratory tract infection, acute allergic reaction, or viral or bacterial infection at the orifice of the tube. Inflammation may also occur without bacterial invasion of the middle ear. More than half of children in the United States have had at least one episode of serous otitis media before their third birthday. Repeated bouts of otitis media in early childhood often contribute to unsuspected hearing loss, which is due to residual (usually sterile) fluid in the middle ear. In chronic disease, mucus-producing (goblet) cell metaplasia may be seen in the mucosal lining of the middle ear. Cholesterol crystals derived from products of hemorrhage stimulate a foreign-body reaction and elicit a granulation tissue response, called a **cholesterol granuloma**.
- *Suppurative otitis media:* One of the most common infections of childhood, acute suppurative otitis media is caused by pyogenic bacteria that invade the middle ear, usually via the eustachian tube. *Streptococcus pneumoniae* (pneumococcus) is the most common causative agent in all age groups (30% to 40%). *Haemophilus influenzae* causes about 20% of cases but is less frequent with increasing age. If a purulent exudate accumulates in the middle ear, the eardrum ruptures and the pus is discharged. In most cases, the infection is self-limited and tends to heal even without therapy. Neglected or recurrent infection of the middle ear and mastoid process may eventually produce chronic inflammation of the mucosa or destruction of the periosteum covering the ossicles (Fig. 25-16).
- *ACUTE MASTOIDITIS:* This condition is now rare but is still seen in cases of inadequately treated otitis media.

Characteristically, mastoid air cells are filled with pus, and their thin osseous intercellular walls become destroyed. Extension of the infection from the mastoid bone to contiguous structures causes complications.
- **Cholesteatoma:** A cholesteatoma *is a mass of accumulated keratin and squamous mucosa that results from the growth of squamous epithelium from the external ear canal thorough the perforated eardrum into the middle ear.* In that location, it continues to produce keratin. Microscopically, cholesteatomas are surrounded by granulation tissue and fibrosis. The principal dangers of cholesteatoma arise from the erosion of bone, a process that may lead to destruction of important contiguous structures (e.g., auditory ossicles, facial nerve, labyrinth).
- *COMPLICATIONS OF ACUTE AND CHRONIC OTITIS MEDIA:* As a result of antibiotic treatment, complications of otitis media are now rare. However, there is potential for serious and even fatal complications. These include extension of the process through the mastoid bone with resulting meningitis and epidural, subdural, or cerebral abscess.

Jugulotympanic Paraganglioma Arises from Middle Ear Paraganglia

Jugulotympanic paraganglioma is the most common benign tumor of the middle ear. These tumors grow slowly, but over years, they may destroy the middle ear and extend into the internal ear and cranial cavity. Metastases are rare. Histologically, middle ear paragangliomas are identical to those arising elsewhere and show characteristic lobules of cells embedded in a richly vascular connective tissue (Fig. 25-17). The paraganglial cells are of neural crest origin and contain varying amounts of catecholamines, mostly epinephrine and norepinephrine.

Otosclerosis Results in Progressive Deafness

Otosclerosis is the formation of new spongy bone about the stapes and the oval window, resulting in progressive deafness. In some families, the defect demonstrates autosomal dominant inheritance. It is the most common cause of conductive hearing loss in young and middle-aged adults in the United States. Ten percent of white and 1% of black adult Americans have some otosclerosis, but 90% of cases are

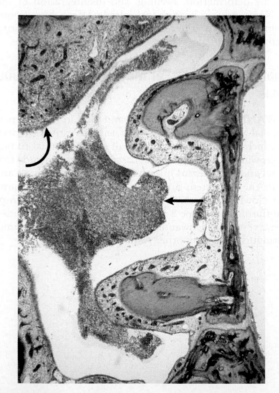

FIGURE 25-16. **Chronic suppurative otitis media.** A purulent exudate *(straight arrow)* is present in the middle ear cavity. The entire mucosa *(curved arrow)* is thickened by chronic inflammation and granulation tissue. The footplate and the crura of the stapes are shown *(right)*.

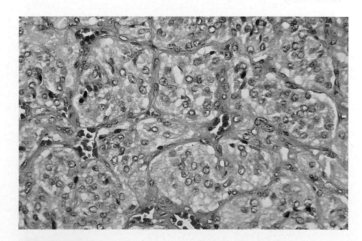

FIGURE 25-17. **Jugulotympanic paraganglioma.** Tumor cell nests are composed of cells with ill-defined cell borders and prominent eosinophilic cytoplasm (chief cells); difficult to identify by light microscopy are the peripherally situated sustentacular cells.

asymptomatic. The female-to-male ratio is 2:1. Both ears are usually affected. The pathogenesis of otosclerosis is obscure.

 PATHOLOGY: Although any part of the petrous bone may be affected, otosclerotic bone tends to form at particular points. The most frequent site (80% to 90%) is immediately anterior to the oval window. The focus of sclerotic bone extends posteriorly and may infiltrate and replace the stapes. This process progressively immobilizes the footplate of the stapes, and the developing bony ankylosis is functionally manifested as a slowly progressive conductive hearing loss.

Histologically, the initial lesion of otosclerosis is resorption of bone and formation of highly cellular fibrous tissue, with wide vascular spaces and osteoclasts. The focus of resorbed bone is later replaced by immature bone, which with repeated remodeling becomes mature bone. Otosclerosis is successfully treated by surgical mobilization of the auditory ossicles.

Ménière Disease is the Triad of Vertigo, Sensorineural Hearing Loss, and Tinnitus

A number of etiologic factors have been suggested, but the cause of **Ménière disease** is uncertain. Its pathologic correlate is hydropic distention of the endolymphatic system of the cochlea. **Ménière** disease is most common in the fourth and fifth decades and is bilateral in 15% of patients.

 PATHOLOGY: Microscopically, the earliest change is dilation of the cochlear duct and saccule. As the disease (**hydrops**) progresses, the entire endolymphatic system becomes dilated, and the membranous wall frequently tears. Ruptures are sometimes followed by collapse of the membranous labyrinth, but atrophy of sensory and neural structures is rare. It is thought that the symptoms of Ménière disease occur when endolymphatic hydrops causes rupture and the endolymph escapes into the perilymph.

 CLINICAL FEATURES: The attacks of vertigo, accompanied by often-incapacitating nausea and vomiting, last less than 24 hours. Weeks or months go by before another episode, and in time, the remissions become longer. The hearing loss recovers between attacks but later becomes permanent. Ménière disease seems to be improved by a low-salt diet and use of diuretics.

Labyrinthine Toxicity is a Drug-Induced Cause of Deafness

The best known drugs that have ototoxic side effects are aminoglycoside antibiotics, which can cause irreversible damage to vestibular or cochlear sensory cells. Other antibiotics, diuretics, antimalarial drugs, and salicylates may also produce transient or permanent sensorineural hearing loss. Among antineoplastic

agents, cisplatin causes temporary or permanent hearing loss. The labyrinth of the embryo is especially sensitive to some drugs (congenital deafness due to thalidomide, quinine, and chloroquine).

Viral Labyrinthitis Can Result in Congenital Deafness

Viral infections are becoming increasingly recognized as causes of inner ear disorders, particularly deafness. Most cases represent invasion of the labyrinth by the virus. Cytomegalovirus and rubella are the best-known prenatal viral infections that lead to congenital deafness through maternal-to-fetal transmission. Cytomegalovirus antigen has been demonstrated in the cells of the organ of Corti and neurons of the spiral ganglia. Among postnatal viral infections, mumps is the most common cause of deafness. The infection can cause rapid hearing loss, which is unilateral in 80% of cases.

Acoustic Trauma is Related to Mechanical Damage to the Inner Ear by High-Intensity Noise

Noise-induced hearing loss is a significant health problem in industrialized countries. Occupational or recreational exposure to loud tones or noises may cause temporary or permanent loss of hearing. **Acoustic trauma** specifically refers to hearing loss produced by brief exposure to high-level sounds (such as gunshots or explosions). Sound greater than 140 dB produce immediate hearing loss by mechanically disrupting the acoustic apparatus. Prolonged exposure to sounds of intermediate intensity (between 90 to –140 dB) cause "**noise-induced hearing loss**," which develops slowly with time and cumulative exposure. Sound levels produced at popular music concerts and by some home stereo systems can fall within this range. The earliest damage occurs in the external hair cells of the organ of Corti. Loss of sensory hairs is followed by deformation, swelling, and disintegration of the hair cells. Noise-induced hearing loss initially effects high frequencies and only gradually interferes with lower-frequency hearing and speech perception.

Tumors of the Inner Ear May Arise from Vestibular Nerves

SCHWANNOMA: Nearly all schwannomas in the internal auditory canal arise from the vestibular nerves. Vestibular schwannomas, which account for about 10% of all intracranial tumors, are slow growing and encapsulated. Larger tumors protrude from the internal auditory meatus into the cerebellopontine angle and may deform the brainstem and adjacent cerebellum. Schwannomas cause slowly progressive vestibular and auditory symptoms. Neurofibromatosis type 2 is characterized by a high incidence of bilateral vestibular schwannomas. Histologically, these tumors are indistinguishable from other vestibular schwannomas.

26 Bones and Joints

Benjamin L. Hoch
Michael J. Klein
Alan L. Schiller

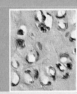

Bone functions in mechanical, mineral storage, and hematopoietic roles. Mechanical functions of bone include (1) protection for brain, spinal cord, and chest organs; (2) rigid internal support for limbs; and (3) deployment as lever arms in the skeletal muscle. Joints (articulations) serve as a union between bones and are necessary for the mechanical role of bone. Bone is the principal reservoir for calcium and stores other ions such as phosphate, sodium, and magnesium. The bones also serve as hosts for hematopoietic bone marrow. Joints also have specialized mechanical properties. Synovial (diarthrodial), movable joints are lined by a synovial membrane and articular cartilage, allowing for lubrication and reduction in friction of the apposed articulating surfaces. One third of the population of the United States older than 50 years of age develops clinically significant joint disease.

BONES

Anatomy of Bone

Macroscopically, two types of bone are recognized.

- **Cortical bone** is dense and compact, and its outer shell defines the shape of the bone. It comprises 80% of the skeleton. Because of its density, its functions are mainly biomechanical.
- **Coarse cancellous bone** (also termed **spongy, trabecular, or marrow bone**) is found at the ends of long bones within the medullary canal. Cancellous bone contains many more bone cells per unit volume than does cortical bone. Changes in the rate of bone turnover are manifested principally in cancellous bone.

The anatomy of bone is defined in relation to a transverse cartilage plate, which is present in the growing child. This structure is termed the **growth plate**, the **epiphyseal cartilage plate**, or **the physis** (Fig. 26-1).

- **The epiphysis** is the area of the bone that extends from the subarticular bone plate to the base of the growth plate.
- **The metaphysis** contains coarse cancellous bone and is the region from the side of the growth plate facing away from the joint to the area where the bone develops its fluted or funnel shape.
- **The diaphysis** corresponds to the body or shaft of the bone and is the zone between the two metaphyses in a long tubular bone.

The metaphysis blends into the diaphysis and is the area where coarse cancellous bone dissipates. *This area of bone is particularly important in hematogenous infections, tumors, and skeletal malformations.*

Two additional terms are essential to an understanding of bone organization:

- **Endochondral ossification** is the process by which bone tissue replaces cartilage.
- **Intramembranous ossification** refers to the mechanism by which bone tissue supplants membranous or fibrous tissue laid down by the periosteum.

The Bone Marrow Resides in the Marrow Space, also Termed the Medullary Canal

The marrow space is enclosed by the cortical bone. It is supported by a delicate connective tissue framework that enmeshes the marrow cells and the blood vessels (see Chapter 20).

Periosteum Covers All Bones and Can Form Bone

The internal layer of the periosteum, the **cambium layer**, is applied to the surface of the bone and consists of loosely arranged collagenous bundles, with spindle-shaped connective tissue cells and a network of thin elastic fibers. The outer **fibrous layer** is contiguous with soft tissue planes and fascia. It is composed of dense connective tissue containing blood vessels.

Bone Matrix is Organic and Mineralized

Bone tissue is composed of cells, an inorganic matrix (poorly crystalline hydroxyapatite), and an organic matrix. The **organic matrix** consists of 88% type I collagen, 10% other proteins, and 1% to 2% lipids and glycosaminoglycans. *Thus, type I collagen basically defines the organic matrix.*

Bone Cells Maintain the Structure of Bone

There are four types of cells in bone tissue, each of which has specific functions related to the formation, resorption, and remodeling of bone.

OSTEOPROGENITOR CELL: The osteoprogenitor cell, which ultimately differentiates into osteoblasts and osteocytes, is derived from a primitive stem cell. The stem cell can develop into adipocytes, myoblasts, fibroblasts, or osteoblasts. Osteoprogenitor cells are found in marrow, periosteum, and all supporting structures within the marrow cavity.

OSTEOBLAST: These protein-synthesizing cells produce and mineralize bone tissue. They are derived from mesenchymal progenitors that also give rise to chondrocytes, myocytes, adipocytes, and fibroblasts. These large mononuclear and polygonal cells are arrayed in a line along the bone surface (Fig. 26-2A). Underlying the layer of osteoblasts is a thin, eosinophilic zone of organic bone matrix that has not yet been mineralized, termed **osteoid**.

OSTEOCYTE: The osteocyte is an osteoblast that is completely embedded in bone matrix and is isolated in a lacuna (see Fig. 26-2B). Osteocytes deposit small quantities of bone around lacunae, but with time, they lose the capacity for protein synthesis. They have numerous processes that extend through bony canals, called **canaliculi**, and communicate with those from other osteocytes (see Fig. 26-2C). Evidence suggests that osteocytes may be the bone cell that recognizes and responds to mechanical forces.

OSTEOCLAST: Osteoclasts are the exclusive bone-resorptive cells. They are of hematopoietic origin and are members of the monocyte/macrophage family. Osteoclasts are multinucleated cells that contain many lysosomes and are rich in hydrolytic enzymes. They are found in small depressions, termed **Howship lacunae**, on bone surfaces.

Constant remodeling of bone is a normal part of skeletal maintenance. It is initiated by the activation of osteoclasts, which requires the interaction of a tumor necrosis factor (TNF) receptor-like molecule, RANK, found on the surface of osteoclasts, with a TNF-like ligand (RANKL) located on the surface of osteoblasts and stromal cells. RANKL is upregulated by parathyroid hormone (PTH), interleukin (IL)-6, $1,25(OH)_2D_3$ (see below), and other osteotropic stimulators. Macrophage colony stimulating factor is also required for osteoclast maturation. Soluble factors released during resorption and the above- mentioned osteotropic mole-

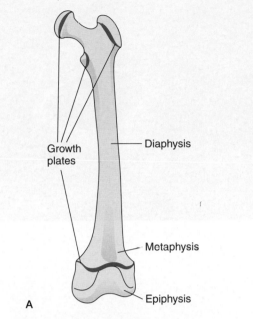

A

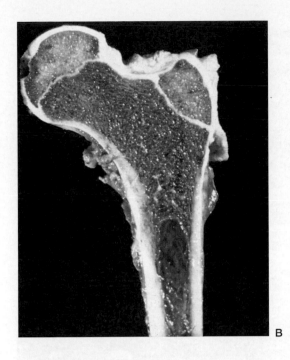

B

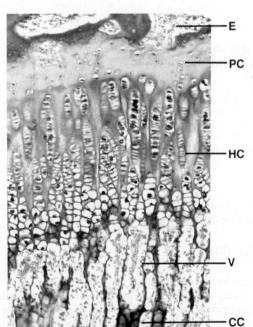

C

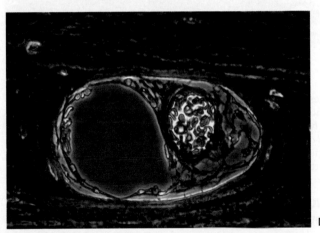

D

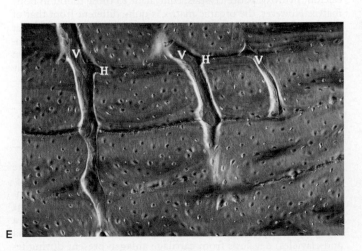

E

FIGURE 26-1. **Anatomy of a long bone. A.** Diagram of the femur illustrates the various compartments. **B.** Coronal section of the proximal femur illustrates the various anatomical parts of a long bone. The epiphysis of the femoral head and the apophysis of the greater trochanter are separated from the metaphysis by their respective growth plates. The cortex and the medullary cavity are well visualized. The medullary cavity contains cancellous bone until the metaphysis narrows into the diaphysis (shaft) of the bone, which is almost completely devoid of bone and filled with marrow. **C.** A section of the epiphysis with a zone of proliferating cartilage cells. Beneath this zone, the hypertrophic cartilage cells are arrayed in columns. At the *bottom*, the calcifying matrix is invaded by blood vessels. E, epiphysis; PC, proliferative cartilage; HC, hypertrophic cartilage; CC, calcified cartilage; V, vascular invasion. **D.** Haversian canal containing a venule (thin-walled wider vessel on *left*) and an arteriole (thicker-walled narrow vessel on the *right*.) **E.** Volkmann canals. In this photograph, three Volkmann canals are seen running parallel to each other *(v)* and perpendicular to the cortex. The openings of two haversian canals *(h)* are visible.

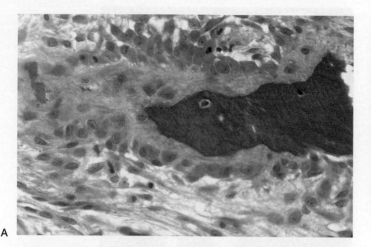

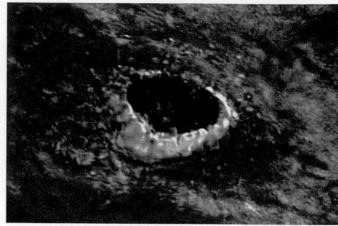

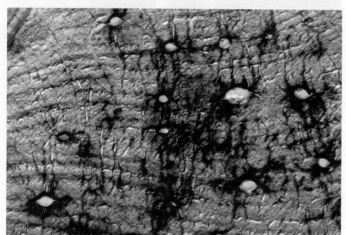

FIGURE 26-2. **A. The cells of bones.** A developing bone spicule demonstrates a prominent layer of plump osteoblasts lining the pink osteoid seam. The dark purple layer beneath the osteoid seam is mineralized bone. **B.** Osteocyte. Osteocytes represent trapped osteoblasts surrounded by bone matrix. The space surrounding the cell is called a *lacuna*. At this power, a few cytoplasmic extensions of the cell can be seen extending into narrow channels in the bone, called *canaliculi*. **C.** The extensive intercommunication of osteocyte processes via their canalicular network in cortical bone is visible in this section.

cules (e.g., PTH) aid in the recruitment of osteoblasts and their activation to form new bone. *Thus, bone remodeling involves replacing old bone with newly formed bone via the functional coupling of osteoclasts and osteoblasts, termed the **bone remodeling unit**.* This process enables bone to adapt to mechanical stress, maintain its strength, and regulate calcium homeostasis.

Two Types of Bone Tissue: Lamellar Bone and Woven Bone

Both types may be mineralized or unmineralized. Unmineralized bone is called **osteoid**.

Lamellar Bone

Lamellar bone is made slowly and is highly organized. As the stronger bone tissue, it forms the adult skeleton. *Anything other than lamellar bone in the adult skeleton is abnormal.* Lamellar bone is defined by (1) a parallel arrangement of type I collagen fibers, (2) few osteocytes in the matrix, and (3) uniform osteocytes in lacunae parallel to the long axis of the collagen fibers (Fig. 26-3).

Woven Bone

Woven bone is identified by (1) an irregular arrangement of type I collagen fibers, hence the term *woven*, (2) numerous osteocytes in the matrix, and (3) variation in osteocyte size and shape (see Fig. 26-4A,B). Woven bone is deposited more rapidly than lamellar bone, is haphazardly arranged and of low tensile strength, and serves as a temporary scaffolding for support. *Its presence in the adult*

skeleton is always abnormal and indicates that reactive tissue has been produced in response to some stress in the bone.

Cartilage

In contrast to bone, cartilage does not contain blood vessels, nerves, or lymphatics. It may be focally calcified to provide some internal strength in the appropriate areas. Like bone, cartilage may be viewed as an organic and inorganic biphasic material. The inorganic phase is composed of calcium hydroxyapatite crystals, equivalent to those found in bone matrix. However, the organic matrix is quite different from that of bone. Essentially, cartilage is a hyperhydrated structure, with water forming approximately 80% of its weight. The remaining 20% is composed principally of two types of macromolecules, type II collagen and proteoglycans (see Chapter 3). The water content is extremely important in the function of articular cartilage, as it enhances the resilience and lubrication of the joint.

Bone Formation and Growth

Bone tissue grows only by appositional growth, defined as the deposition of new matrix on the surface by adjacent surface cells. By contrast, virtually all other tissues, especially cartilage, increase by interstitial cell proliferation within the matrix as well as by appositional growth. Bone development in the fetus follows a stereotyped sequence. Most of the skeleton (except the calvaria and clavicles) develops from cartilage anlagen present during fetal development. In long bones, a **primary center of ossification**

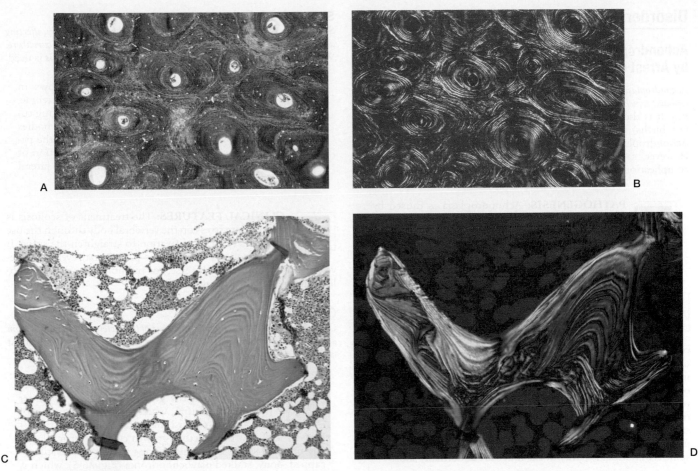

FIGURE 26-3. **Cortical lamellar bone. A.** Lamellae of the compacta (cortex) are arranged concentrically about haversian canals. **B.** The same field in polarized light shows the alternating light and dark layered arrangement of the collagen fibers. **C.** Lamellae of the spongiosa in a single mature trabecula are shown in a bright field view. **D.** Polarized light demonstrates that the lamellae are arranged in light and dark layers, but these layers are in long plates rather than in a concentric arrangement.

leads to the formation of a cartilaginous core, surrounded by woven bone, called **primary spongiosum** or **primary trabecula**. It is the first bone formed after the replacement of cartilage. **The secondary center of ossification**, also termed the **epiphyseal center of ossification**, forms at the ends of the bone as cartilage is resorbed. As the bony ends expand, a zone of cartilage is trapped between the end of the bone and the diaphysis. This car-

tilage is destined to be the **growth plate**, a layer of modified cartilage between the diaphysis and epiphysis. *The growth plate controls the longitudinal growth of bones and ultimately determines adult height.* Closure of the growth plate is induced by sex hormones and occurs earlier in girls than in boys. Renewal of chondrocytes slows and ultimately ceases, and the entire plate is eventually replaced by bone.

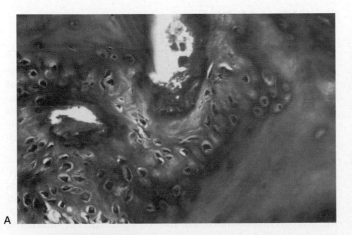
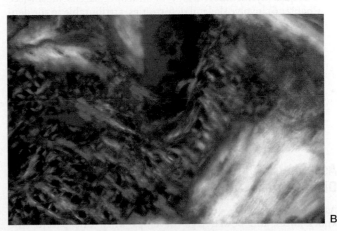

FIGURE 26-4. **Woven bone. A.** In this section, the woven bone constitutes early fracture repair. Note that in the area of new bone, there are many osteocytes that vary in size but are mainly large with prominent lacunae (compare with area of mature bone at *lower right*). **B.** This is the same section viewed in polarized light. Note that the collagen fibers are disposed in a pattern resembling the loose fiber pattern of coarsely woven burlap.

Disorders of the Growth Plate

Achondroplasia is an Inherited Dwarfism Caused by Arrest of the Growth Plate

Achondroplasia refers to a syndrome of short-limbed dwarfism and macrocephaly, which represents a failure of normal epiphyseal cartilage formation. It is the most common genetic form of dwarfism (1:15,000 live births) and is inherited as an autosomal dominant trait. Achondroplastic dwarfs have normal mentation and life spans. However, some patients develop severe kyphoscoliosis and its complications.

 PATHOGENESIS: Achondroplasia is caused by an activating mutation in the FGF receptor on chromosome 16 (4p16.3). The mutation constitutively inhibits chondrocyte differentiation and proliferation, which retards growth plate development.

 PATHOLOGY: The growth plate in achondroplasia is greatly thinned, and the zone of proliferative cartilage is either absent or extensively attenuated. The zone of provisional calcification, if present, undergoes endochondral ossification, but at a greatly reduced rate. A transverse bar of bone often seals off the growth plate, thereby preventing further bone formation and causing dwarfism. Interestingly, the secondary centers of ossification and the articular cartilage are normal. Because intramembranous ossification is undisturbed, the periosteum functions normally, and the bones become very short and thick. For the same reasons, the head of the dwarf appears unusually large, compared with the bones formed from the cartilage of the face. The spine is of normal length, but the limbs are abnormally short.

Several Other Conditions are Related to Growth Plate Disorders

- **Cretinism:** Cretinism results from maternal iodine deficiency (see Chapter 21) and has profound effects on the skeleton. Thyroid hormone plays a role in regulating chondrocytes, osteoblasts, and osteoclasts through the production of cytokines and other factors involved in bone development and growth. Linear growth is severely impaired in cretinism, resulting in dwarfism, with limbs disproportionately short in relation to the trunk.
- **Morquio Syndrome:** Many of mucopolysaccharidoses (see Chapter 6) involve skeletal deformities, attributable to the deposition of mucopolysaccharides (glycosaminoglycans) in developing bones. An example is Morquio syndrome (mucopolysaccharidosis type IV), which leads to a particularly severe form of dwarfism, in addition to dental defects, mental retardation, and corneal opacities.
- **Scurvy:** Today, scurvy (vitamin C deficiency) is a rare disease (see Chapter 8). The skeletal changes of scurvy reflect the lack of osteoblastic function. Woven bone is not formed because osteoblasts cannot produce and normally cross-link collagen.

Asymmetric Cartilage Growth Causes Spinal Disorders and Tumors

Asymmetric cartilage growth, such as occurs in patients with knock-knees and bowed legs, develops when one part of the growth plate, either medial or lateral, grows faster than the other. Most cases are hereditary, but mechanical forces such as trauma near the growth plate may stimulate one side to grow faster or in an asymmetric fashion.

Scoliosis and Kyphosis

Scoliosis is an abnormal lateral curvature of the spine, usually affecting adolescent girls. **Kyphosis** *refers to an abnormal anteroposterior curvature.* When both conditions are present, the term **kyphoscoliosis** is used.

 PATHOGENESIS: A vertebral body grows in length (height) from the endplates of the vertebrae, which correspond to the growth plates of long tubular bones. As in tubular bones, vertebral bodies increase in width by appositional bone growth from the periosteum. In scoliosis, for unknown reasons, one portion of the endplate grows faster than the other, producing lateral curvature of the spine.

 CLINICAL FEATURES: The treatment of scoliosis is appropriate stress on the vertebral body through the use of braces or internal fixation to straighten the spine. If kyphoscoliosis is severe, the patient may eventually develop chronic pulmonary disease, cor pulmonale, and joint problems, particularly involving the hip.

Osteochondroma

Osteochondroma is a developmental defect of the skeleton, which arises from a defect of the growth plate. Solitary osteochondroma is the most common form of the lesion.

 PATHOGENESIS: The ring of Ranvier is a peripheral area of the growth plate directly under the perichondrium, which guides the growth of the cartilage toward the metaphysis. If the ring of Ranvier is absent or defective, growth cartilage grows laterally into the soft tissue. This process results in a cartilage-capped, bony, stalked osteochondroma (Fig. 26-5), which is in direct continuity with the marrow cavity of the parent bone.

 PATHOLOGY: Osteochondromas tend to grow away from the joint. In radiographs, the cartilaginous mass is in direct continuity with the parent bone and lacks an underlying cortex. Histologically, a cartilage-capped, bony mass is surrounded by a surface fibrous membrane, which is the perichondrium. Active endochondral ossification deep to the cartilage cap allows the bony protuberance to lengthen.

Hereditary Multiple Osteochondromatosis (HMO)

HMO is a common autosomal dominant musculoskeletal disorder that is characterized by numerous osteochondromas. Loss of *EXT1* or *EXT2* gene function, which is important for normal chondrocyte proliferation, is the most common cause of HMO. This disorder occurs predominantly in men, but because of its variable expression, a seemingly unaffected woman from an affected family may transmit the condition.

 PATHOLOGY: Each individual lesion in HMO is identical to a solitary osteochondroma. In severe cases, dwarfism may result because of lateral displacement of the longitudinal growth plate by the osteochondroma. Metacarpals may be shortened, and fixed pronation or supination may develop if the lesions occur in the forearm and interfere with wrist function. Further difficulties may be caused by unequal leg length and disturbed joint function because of encroaching osteochondromas. Chondrosarcoma is a rare complication.

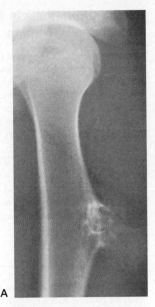
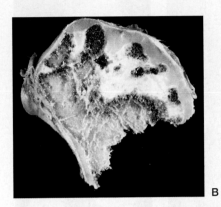

FIGURE 26-5. **Osteochondroma. A.** A radiograph of an osteochondroma of the humerus shows a lesion that is directly contiguous with the marrow space. **B.** The cross-section of an osteochondroma shows the cap of calcified cartilage overlying poorly organized cancellous bone.

Modeling Abnormalities: Osteopetrosis

*Osteopetrosis, also known as **marble bone disease** or **Albers-Schönberg disease**, is a heterogeneous group of rare inherited disorders characterized by increased skeletal mass due to abnormally dense bone.* The most common autosomal recessive form is a severe, sometimes fatal disease affecting infants and children. The death of infants with this variant is attributable to marked anemia, cranial nerve entrapment, hydrocephalus, and infection. A more benign form, transmitted as an autosomal dominant trait and seen in adulthood or adolescence, is associated with mild anemia or no symptoms at all.

PATHOGENESIS: *The sclerotic skeleton of osteopetrosis is the result of failed osteoclastic bone resorption.* The disease is caused by mutations in genes that govern osteoclast formation or function the most common of which cause defects in the ability of osteoclasts to acidify, a process that is necessary for osteoclastic bone resorption. Other mutations that cause osteopetrosis involve transcription factors or cytokines necessary for the osteoclast differentiation. Because osteoclast function is arrested, osteopetrosis is characterized by block-like, radiodense bones; hence the term **marble bone disease** (Fig. 26-6). These bones are extremely radiopaque and weigh two to three times more than normal bone. They fracture easily because their structure is disorganized and cannot remodel along lines of stress. The mineralized cartilage is also weak and friable.

PATHOLOGY AND CLINICAL FEATURES: Grossly, bones in osteopetrosis are widened in the metaphysis and diaphysis, resulting in the characteristic "Erlenmeyer flask" deformity. Histologically, the bone tissue is extremely irregular, and almost all areas contain a cartilage core. Depending on the mutation, osteoclasts may be absent, present in normal numbers, or even abundant. Suppression of hematopoiesis in osteopetrosis, which may to lead to severe anemia or pancytopenia is due to marrow replacement by sheets of abnormal osteoclasts or extensive fibrosis. To compensate for loss of marrow, extramedullary hematopoiesis occurs in the liver, spleen, and lymph node. Osteopetrosis is treated by bone marrow transplantation, which gives rise to a new clone of functional osteoclasts.

Delayed Maturation of Bone

Osteogenesis Imperfecta (OI) Relates to Abnormal Type I Collagen

Osteogenesis imperfecta (OI), or brittle bone disease, is a group of inherited disorders in which a generalized abnormality of connective tissue is expressed principally as fragility of bone. OI is inherited in an autosomal dominant pattern, although there are rare cases that are autosomal recessive.

PATHOGENESIS: *The genetic defects in OI are heterogeneous, but all affect type I collagen synthesis.* The pathogenesis of OI involves mutations of *COL1A1* and *COL1A2* genes, which encode the α1 and α2 chains of type I procollagen, the major structural protein of bone. These genes are located in chromosomes 17 (17q21.3-q22) and 7 (7q21.3-q22), respectively. Typically, mutations cause substitution of other amino acids for the obligate glycine at every third residue.

PATHOLOGY AND CLINICAL FEATURES: Type I OI is characterized by a normal appearance at birth, but fractures of many bones occur during infancy and at the time the child learns to walk. Children with type I OI typically have blue sclerae because the deficiency in collagen fibers imparts translucence to the structure. A high incidence of hearing loss occurs because fractures and fusion of the bones of the middle ear restrict their mobility. There may be hundreds of fractures a year with minor movement or trauma. On radiologic examination, the bones are extremely thin, delicate, and abnormally curved. Bone collagen has reduced tensile strength, and mineralization is abnormal.

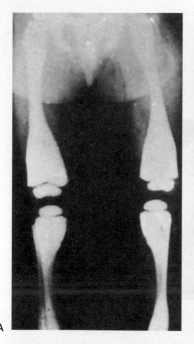
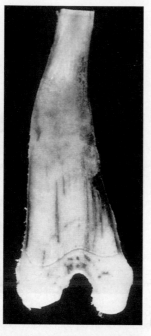

A

B

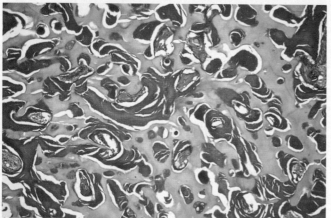

C

FIGURE 26-6. **Osteopetrosis. A.** A radiograph of a child shows markedly misshapen and dense bones of the lower extremities, characteristic of "marble bone disease." **B.** A gross specimen of the femur shows obliteration of the marrow space by dense bone. **C.** A photomicrograph of a child's bone with autosomal recessive osteopetrosis demonstrates disorganization of bony trabeculae by retention of primary spongiosa (mixed spicules) and further obliteration of the marrow space by secondary spongiosa. The result is complete disorganization of the trabeculae and absence of marrow.

Type II OI is usually fatal in utero or shortly after birth. The infants have a characteristic facial appearance and skeletal abnormalities. Those who are born alive usually die of respiratory failure within the first month of life.

Type III OI is the progressively deforming variant, which is ordinarily detected at birth by the presence of short stature and deformities caused by fractures in utero. Dental defects and hearing loss are common. Unlike other types of OI, type III is rarely inherited as an autosomal recessive trait.

Type IV OI is similar to type I, except that sclerae are normal, and the phenotype is more variable.

There is no single treatment for OI. Osteoprogenitor cells for bone marrow transplantation, growth factors, bisphosphonates, and gene therapy to improve collagen synthesis have been undergoing clinical trials in an attempt to modify the course and severity of the disease.

Enchondromatosis is Marked by Multiple Cartilaginous Tumors

*Enchondromatosis, also termed **Ollier disease**, is characterized by the development of numerous cartilaginous masses that lead to bony deformities.* The condition is not strictly a disease of delayed maturation of bone, but one in which residual hyaline cartilage, anlage cartilage, or cartilage from the growth plate does not undergo endochondral ossification and remains in the bones. As a consequence, bones show multiple, tumor-like masses of abnormally arranged hyaline cartilage (enchondromas), with zones of proliferative and hypertrophied cartilage (Fig. 26-7). These tumors tend to be located in the metaphyses. As growth continues, the enchondromas settle in the diaphysis of adolescents and adults. Whether enchondromas represent true neoplasms is debated, but they exhibit a strong tendency to undergo malignant change into chondrosarcomas in adult life.

Fracture

The most common bone lesion is a fracture, which is defined as a discontinuity of the bone. A force perpendicular to the long axis of the bone results in a **transverse fracture**. A force along the long axis of the bone yields a **compression fracture**. Torsional force results in **spiral fractures**, and combined tension and compression shear forces cause angulation and displacement of the fractured ends.

Fracture Healing is Divided into Inflammatory, Reparative, and Remodeling Phases

The duration of each phase (Fig. 26-8) depends on the patient's age, the site of fracture, the patient's overall health and nutritional status, and the extent of soft tissue injury. *In the repair of a bone fracture, anything other than the formation of bone tissue at the fracture site represents incomplete healing.*

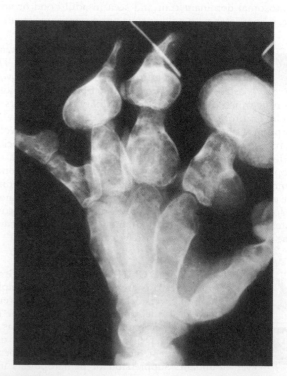

FIGURE 26-7. **Multiple enchondromatosis (Ollier disease).** A radiograph of the hand shows bulbous swellings that represent cartilage masses composed of hyaline cartilage, which is sometimes admixed with more primitive myxoid cartilage.

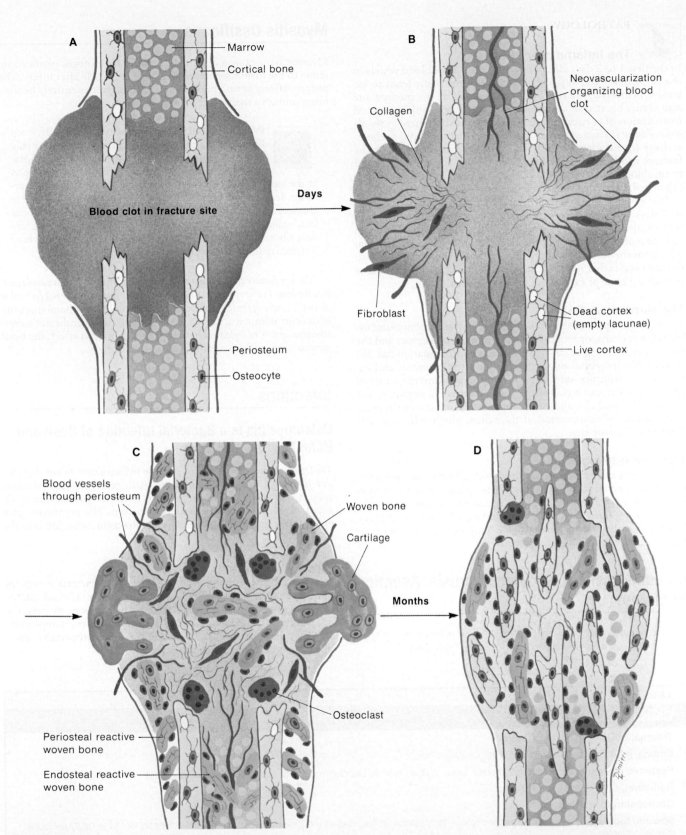

FIGURE 26-8. **Healing of a fracture. A.** Soon after a fracture is sustained, an extensive blood clot forms in the subperiosteal and soft tissue, as well as in the marrow cavity. The bone at the fracture site is jagged. **B.** The inflammatory phase of fracture healing is characterized by neovascularization and beginning organization of the blood clot. Because the osteocytes in the fracture site are dead, the lacunae are empty. The osteocytes of the cortex are necrotic well beyond the fracture site, due to the traumatic interruption of the perforating arteries from the periosteum. **C.** The reparative phase of fracture healing is characterized by the formation of a callus of cartilage and woven bone near the fracture site. The jagged edges of the original cortex have been remodeled and eroded by osteoclasts. The marrow space has been revascularized and contains reactive woven bone, as does the periosteal area. **D.** In the remodeling phase during which the cortex is revitalized, the reactive bone may be lamellar or woven. The new bone is organized along stress lines and mechanical forces. Extensive osteoclastic and osteoblastic cellular activity is maintained.

PATHOLOGY:

The Inflammatory Phase

In the first 1 to 2 days after a fracture, rupture of blood vessels in the periosteum and adjacent muscle and soft tissue leads to extensive hemorrhage. Extensive bone necrosis at the fracture site also occurs because of disruption of large vessels in the bone and interruption of cortical vessels. *Dead bone is characterized by the absence of osteocytes and empty osteocyte lacunae.* In 2 to 5 days, the hemorrhage forms a large clot, which must be resorbed so that the fracture can heal. Neovascularization begins to occur peripheral to this blood clot. By the end of the first week, most of the clot is organized by the invasion of blood vessels and early fibrosis.

The earliest bone, which is invariably woven bone, is formed after 7 days. *This corresponds to the "scar" of bone.* Because bone formation requires a good blood supply, the woven bone spicules begin to appear at the periphery of the clot. Pluripotential mesenchymal cells from the soft tissue and within the bone marrow give rise to the osteoblasts that synthesize the woven bone. Granulation tissue containing bone or cartilage is termed a **callus.**

The Reparative Phase

The reparative phase follows the first week after a fracture and extends for months, depending on the degree of movement and the fixation of the fracture. By this time, acute inflammation has dissipated. Pluripotential cells differentiate into fibroblasts and osteoblasts. Repair proceeds from the periphery toward the center of the fracture site and accomplishes two objectives: it organizes and resorbs the blood clot and, more importantly, it furnishes neovascularization for construction of the callus, which will eventually bridge the fracture site.

The Remodeling Phase

Several weeks after a fracture, the ingrowth of callus has sealed the bone ends, and remodeling begins. In this phase, the bone is reorganized so that the original cortex is restored. Occasionally, the bone is strong enough to qualify as a clinically healed fracture, but biologically, the fracture may not be truly healed and may continue to undergo remodeling for years.

Osteonecrosis (Avascular Necrosis, Aseptic Necrosis)

Osteonecrosis refers to the death of bone and marrow in the absence of infection. The causes of osteonecrosis are listed in Table 26-1.

Myositis Ossificans

Myositis ossificans, a distinctive form of heterotopic ossification, refers to the formation of reactive bone in muscle after injury. The process affects young persons and, although it is entirely benign, often mimics a malignant neoplasm.

PATHOGENESIS: The lesion typically results from blunt trauma to the muscle and soft tissues, usually of the lower limb; however, some cases occur spontaneously. Peripheral neovascularization and fibrosis at the site of damaged tissue, together with associated hemorrhage, lead in a short time to bone spicule formation. These changes are similar to those that occur at the initial hematoma in a healing fracture. Because myositis ossificans often occurs near a bone (such as the femur or tibia), on radiography, it may be misdiagnosed as a malignant bone-forming tumor.

The key feature that distinguishes myositis ossificans from a neoplasm is that the bone matures peripherally, whereas it is immature or not formed at all in the center of the lesion. The phenomenon of peripheral maturity with central immaturity, the *zonation effect,* clearly indicates a reactive process. A neoplasm has an opposite zonation effect: the most mature tissue of the tumor is located centrally.

Infections

Osteomyelitis is a Bacterial Infection of Bone and Bone Marrow

The term osteomyelitis most often describes inflammation caused by bacterial infection. The most common pathogens are *Staphylococcus* species, but other organisms, such as *E. coli, N. gonorrhoeae, H. influenza,* and *Salmonella* species, are also seen. The organisms gain entry either via the bloodstream or by direct introduction into the bone.

Direct Penetration

Infection by direct penetration or extension of bacteria is now the most common cause of osteomyelitis in the United States. Bacterial organisms are introduced directly into bone by penetrating wounds, fractures, or surgery. Staphylococci and streptococci are commonly incriminated, but in 25% of postoperative infections, anaerobic organisms are detected.

TABLE 26–1
Causes of Osteonecrosis
Trauma, including fracture and surgery
Emboli, producing focal bone infarction
Systemic diseases, such as polycythemia, lupus erythematosus, Gaucher's disease, sickle cell disease, and gout
Radiation, either internal or external
Corticosteroid administration
Specific focal bone necrosis at various sites—for instance, in the head of the femur (Legg-Calvé-Perthes disease) or in the navicular bone (Köhler's disease)
Organ transplantation, particularly renal, in patients with persistent hyperparathyroidism
Osteochondritis dissecans, a condition of unknown etiology in which a piece of articular cartilage and subchondral bone breaks off into a joint. It is thought that a focal area of bone necrosis occurs and eventually detaches.
Autografts and allografts
Thrombosis of local vessels secondary to the pressure of adjacent tumors or other space-occupying lesions
Idiopathic factors, as in the high incidence of osteonecrosis of the head and the femur in alcoholics. Necrotic bone heals differently in the cortex and in the underlying coarse cancellous bone.

Hematogenous Osteomyelitis

Infectious organisms may reach the bone from a focus elsewhere in the body through the bloodstream. Often the focus itself, (e.g., a skin pustule or infected teeth and gums) poses little threat. Even the mere brushing of teeth may create a temporary bacteremia, which may allow organisms to reach the bone. *The most common sites affected by hematogenous osteomyelitis are the metaphyses of the long bones, such as in the knee, ankle, and hip.* The infection principally affects boys aged 5 to 15 years, but it is occasionally seen in older age groups as well. Drug addicts may develop hematogenous osteomyelitis from infected needles.

PATHOGENESIS AND PATHOLOGY: Hematogenous osteomyelitis primarily affects the metaphyseal area because of the unique vascular supply in this region (Fig. 26-9). If the organism is virulent and continues to proliferate, it creates increased pressure on the adjacent thin-walled vessels because they lie in a closed space, the marrow cavity. Such pressure further compromises the vascular supply in this region and produces bone necrosis. The necrotic areas coalesce into an avascular zone, thereby allowing further bacterial proliferation.

If infection is not contained, pus and bacteria extend into the endosteal vascular channels that supply the cortex and spread throughout the Volkmann and haversian canals of the cortex. Eventually, pus forms underneath the periosteum, shearing off the perforating arteries of the periosteum and further devitalizing the cortex. The pus flows between the periosteum and the cortex, isolating more bone from its blood supply, and it may even invade the joint. Eventually, the pus penetrates the periosteum and the skin to form a draining sinus (Fig. 26-10). A sinus tract that extends to the skin may become epithelialized by epidermis that grows into the sinus tract. When this occurs, the sinus tract invariably remains open, continually draining pus, necrotic bone, and bacteria.

Vertebral Osteomyelitis

In adults, osteomyelitis frequently involves vertebral bodies. The intervertebral disk is not a barrier to bacterial osteomyelitis, particularly staphylococcal infection. Infections directly traverse the disk and travel from one vertebra to the next. The disk expands with pus and is eventually destroyed as the pus bores into the adjacent vertebral bodies. Half or more of cases of vertebral osteomyelitis are caused by *Staphylococcus aureus*. Twenty percent involve *E. coli* and other enteric organisms, many of which originate from the urinary

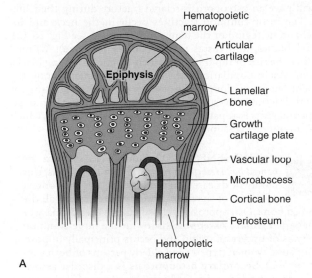

A

Hematopoietic marrow

Articular cartilage

Epiphysis

Lamellar bone

Growth cartilage plate

Vascular loop

Microabscess

Cortical bone

Periosteum

Hemopoietic marrow

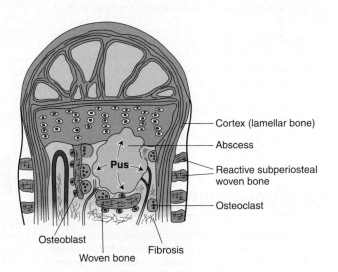

B

Cortex (lamellar bone)

Abscess

Pus

Reactive subperiosteal woven bone

Osteoclast

Osteoblast

Woven bone

Fibrosis

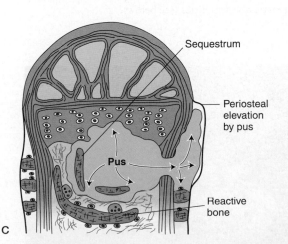

C

Sequestrum

Periosteal elevation by pus

Pus

Reactive bone

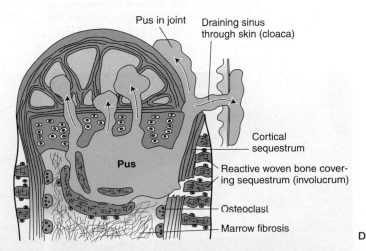

D

Pus in joint

Draining sinus through skin (cloaca)

Cortical sequestrum

Pus

Reactive woven bone covering sequestrum (involucrum)

Osteoclast

Marrow fibrosis

FIGURE 26-9. **Pathogenesis of hematogenous osteomyelitis. A.** The epiphysis, metaphysis, and growth plate are normal. A small, septic microabscess is forming at the capillary loop. **B.** Expansion of the septic focus stimulates resorption of adjacent bony trabeculae. Woven bone begins to surround this focus. The abscess expands into the cartilage and stimulates reactive bone formation by the periosteum. **C.** The abscess, which continues to expand through the cortex into the subperiosteal tissue, shears off the perforating arteries that supply the cortex with blood, thereby leading to necrosis of the cortex. **D.** The extension of this process into the joint space, the epiphysis, and the skin produces a draining sinus. The necrotic bone is called a sequestrum. The viable bone surrounding a sequestrum is termed the involucrum.

tract. Predisposing factors are intravenous drug abuse, upper urinary tract infections, urological procedures, and hematogenous spread of organisms from other sites. Vertebral osteomyelitis may lead to compression fractures of the vertebral body and to neurologic deficits.

The complications of osteomyelitis include septicemia, acute bacterial arthritis, pathologic fractures, and chronic infection. Chronic osteomyelitis may be associated with amyloidosis and the development of squamous cell carcinoma in long-standing, epithelialized sinus tracts (see Fig. 26-10). Treatment depends on the stage of the infection. Early osteomyelitis is treated with intravenous antibiotics for 6 or more weeks. Surgery is used to drain and decompress the infection within the bone or to drain abscesses that do not respond to antibiotic therapy.

Tuberculous Spondylitis (Pott Disease) Reflects a Primary Focus Elsewhere

Tuberculosis of bone invariably originates at other foci, usually the lungs or lymph nodes (see Chapter 9). The mycobacteria disseminate to the bone hematogenously, and only rarely by direct spread from a lung or lymph node, resulting in tuberculous spondylitis, arthritis, and osteomyelitis of the long bones. *Tuberculous spondylitis is a feared complication of childhood tuberculosis.* The disease affects vertebral bodies, sparing the lamina and spines and adjacent vertebrae. With antibiotic treatment, Pott disease is rare.

 PATHOLOGY: The pathology in tuberculous spondylitis is similar to tuberculosis at other sites. The granulomas first produce caseous necrosis of the bone marrow, which leads to slow resorption of bony trabeculae and, occasionally, to cystic spaces in the bone. *Because there is little or no reactive bone formation, affected vertebrae usually collapse, leading to kyphosis and scoliosis.* The intervertebral disk is crushed and destroyed by the compression fracture, rather than by invasion of organisms. The typical "hunchback" of bygone days was often the victim of Pott disease.

METABOLIC BONE DISEASES

Metabolic bone diseases are defined as disorders of metabolism that result in secondary structural effects on the skeleton, including diminished bone mass (due to decreased synthesis or increased destruction), reduced bone mineralization, or both. Because metabolic bone diseases are systemic, a biopsy of any bone should reveal the abnormality, although the severity may differ in various parts of the skeleton (Fig. 26-11).

Osteoporosis

Osteoporosis is a metabolic bone disease characterized by diffuse skeletal lesions, in which the mass of normally mineralized bone is decreased to the point that it no longer provides adequate mechanical support. The remaining bone has a normal ratio of mineralized to nonmineralized (i.e., osteoid) matrix. Bone loss and eventually fractures are the hallmarks of osteoporosis, regardless of the underlying causes (Fig. 26-12). The etiology of bone loss is diverse but includes smoking, vitamin D deficiency, low body mass index, hypogonadism, a sedentary lifestyle, and glucocorticoid therapy.

 EPIDEMIOLOGY: Osteoporosis and its complications are major public health problems that will expand as life expectancy increases. In healthy individuals of both genders, bone mass peaks between the ages of 25 and 35 and begins to decline in the fifth or sixth decade. Bone loss with age occurs in all races, but because of higher peak bone mass, blacks are less prone to osteoporosis than are Asians and whites. Bone loss in women has been divided into two phases: one due to menopause and one due to aging. The latter affects men as well as women. At a certain point, the loss of bone suffices to justify the label **osteoporosis** and renders weight-bearing bones susceptible to fractures. One out of two women and one out of four men will have an osteoporosis-related fracture during their lifetimes. The most common fractures occur in the neck and intertrochanteric region of the femur (hip fracture, see Fig. 26-12), vertebral bodies, and distal radius **(Colles fracture)**. Women have twice the risk of hip fracture as men, although among blacks and some Asian populations, the incidence is equal among the sexes. The female predominance of 8:1 is particularly striking for vertebral fractures. A subset of women in their early postmenopausal years is at particular risk of vertebral fractures, which are rare in middle-aged men.

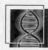 **PATHOGENESIS:** *Osteoporosis always reflects enhanced bone resorption relative to formation.* Thus, this family of diseases should be viewed in the context of failure of the remodeling cycle to replace all the resorbed bone. Osteoporosis is classified as either primary or secondary. **Primary osteoporosis**, by far the more common variety, is of uncertain origin and occurs principally in postmenopausal women (type 1) and elderly persons of both genders (type 2). **Secondary osteoporosis** is a disorder associated with a defined cause, including a variety of endocrine and genetic abnormalities (see below).

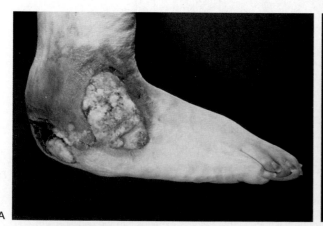
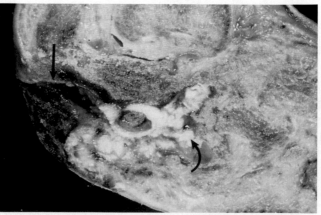

FIGURE 26-10. **Chronic osteomyelitis. A.** In this patient with chronic osteomyelitis, the skin overlying the infected bone is ulcerated, and a draining sinus *(dark area)* is evident over the heel. **B.** After amputation of the foot, a sagittal section shows a draining sinus *(straight arrow)* that connects the infected bone with the surface of the ulcerated skin. The white tissue *(curved arrow)* is invasive squamous cell carcinoma, which arose in the skin.

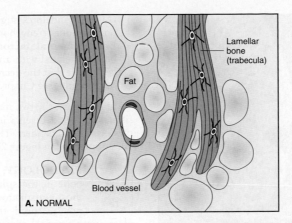

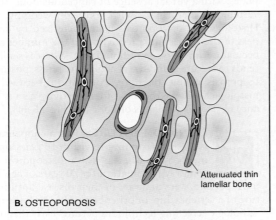

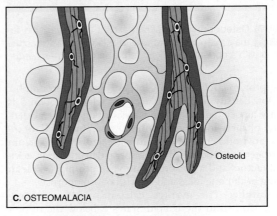

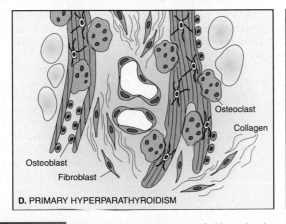

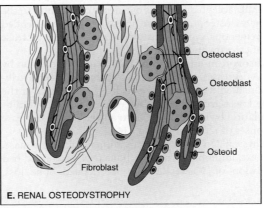

FIGURE 26-11. **Metabolic bone diseases. A.** Normal trabecular bone and fatty marrow. The trabecular bone is lamellar and contains evenly distributed osteocytes. **B.** Osteoporosis. The lamellar bone exhibits discontinuous, thin trabeculae. **C.** Osteomalacia. The trabeculae of the lamellar bone have abnormal amounts of nonmineralized bone (osteoid). These osteoid seams are thickened and cover a larger than normal area of the trabecular bone surface. **D.** Primary hyperparathyroidism. The lamellar bone trabeculae are actively resorbed by numerous osteoclasts that bore into each trabecula. The appearance of osteoclasts dissecting into the trabeculae, a process termed **dissecting osteitis**, is diagnostic of hyperparathyroidism. Osteoblastic activity also is pronounced. The marrow is replaced by fibrous tissue adjacent to the trabeculae. **E.** Renal osteodystrophy. The morphologic appearance is similar to that of primary hyperparathyroidism, except that prominent osteoid covers the trabeculae. Osteoclasts do not resorb osteoid, and wherever an osteoid seam is lacking, osteoclasts bore into the trabeculae. Osteoblastic activity in association with osteoclasts is again prominent.

Type 1 primary osteoporosis is due to an absolute increase in osteoclast activity. In the early postmenopausal period, estrogen withdrawal leads to the secretion of cytokines by cells derived from the marrow stroma, which recruit and activate osteoclasts. These cytokines, which are believed to be estrogen sensitive, include IL-1 and IL-6, TNF, and macrophage colony-stimulating factor (see Fig. 26-13).

Type 2 primary osteoporosis, also called **senile osteoporosis**, has a more complex pathogenesis than does type 1. Type 2 osteoporosis generally appears after age 70 and reflects decreased os-

teoblast function rather than increased osteoclast activity. Primary osteoporosis has been linked to a number of factors that influence peak bone mass and the rate of bone loss:

- **Genetic factors:** The development of clinically significant osteoporosis is related, in largest part, to the maximal amount of bone in a given person, referred to as the **peak bone mass**. In general, peak bone mass is greater in men than in women and in blacks than in whites or Asians. The formation of peak bone mass is, to a large degree, genetic. Sequence variance in the vita-

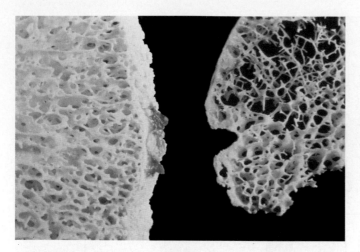

FIGURE 26-12. Osteoporosis. Femoral head of an 82-year-old female with osteoporosis and a femoral neck fracture *(right)* compared with a normal control cut to the same thickness *(left)*.

min D receptor, *Col1A1* collagen gene, estrogen receptor alpha, IL-6, and low-density lipoprotein receptor-related protein 5 is significantly associated with differences in bone mineral density. Several of these loci (e.g., vitamin D receptor and IL-6) interact with environmental and hormonal factors (e.g., calcium intake, estrogen) to modulate bone mineral density. Thus, environmental factors and a person's genotype both play a role in determining peak bone mass and the risk of osteoporosis.

- **Calcium intake:** The average calcium intake of postmenopausal women in the United States is below the recommended value of 1,200 mg/day for adults over the age of 50. It is now generally accepted that this deficiency contributes to the development of osteoporosis, and it has been recommended that both premenopausal and postmenopausal women increase the intake of calcium and vitamin D.
- **Calcium absorption and vitamin D:** Calcium absorption by the intestine decreases with age, an effect that has been attributed to age-related decreases in 1α-hydroxylase activity in the kidney. The lower activity of this enzyme is related to diminished stimulation by PTH, as well as to an age-related decrease in the responses of renal tubules to PTH.
- **Exercise:** Physical activity is necessary to maintain bone mass. In this context, immobilization of a bone (e.g., prolonged bed rest, application of a cast) leads to accelerated bone loss.

Current guidelines suggest exercise as being helpful in maintaining bone strength in the elderly.
- **Environmental factors:** Cigarette smoking in women has been correlated with an increased incidence of osteoporosis. It is possible that the decreased level of active estrogens produced by smoking (see Chapter 8) is responsible for this effect.

In summary, the two major determinants of primary osteoporosis are estrogen deficiency in postmenopausal women and the aging process in both genders. The possible mechanisms for these effects are summarized in Figure 26-13.

 PATHOLOGY: Because of the abundance of cancellous bone in the spine, osteoporotic changes are generally most conspicuous in that area. If the vertebral body is not fractured, there is a general outline of both endplates, with a virtual absence of cancellous bone. If fractured, the vertebra is deformed, with anterior wedging and collapse. Histologically, osteoporosis is characterized by decreased thickness of the cortex and a reduction in the number and size of trabeculae of the coarse cancellous bone. Whereas senile osteoporosis tends to feature reduced trabecular thickness, postmenopausal osteoporosis exhibits disrupted connections between trabeculae. In histologic sections, the loss of connectivity results in the appearance of "isolated" islands of bone (see Fig. 26-11).

CLINICAL FEATURES: Postmenopausal osteoporosis is usually recognizable within 10 years after onset of the menopause, whereas senile osteoporosis generally becomes symptomatic after 70 years of age. Until recently, most patients were unaware of their disease until they had a fracture of a vertebra, hip, or other bone. However, the use of sensitive radiologic screening techniques permits early diagnosis. Vertebral body compression fractures often occur after trivial trauma or may even follow lifting a heavy object. With each compression fracture, the patient becomes shorter and develops kyphosis **(dowager's hump)**. Serum calcium and phosphorus levels remain normal.

Estrogen therapy is an effective, if controversial, means of preventing postmenopausal osteoporosis. Because hormone treatment carries with it slightly increased risks of breast and endometrial cancers, other bone-specific antiosteoporotic drugs have been developed. A new class of inorganic compounds, known as **bisphosphonates**, is useful. All successful antiosteoporosis agents thus far developed block or slow the rate of bone resorption but do not stimulate bone formation. As a result, the drugs may prevent disease progression but cannot cure a patient who already has

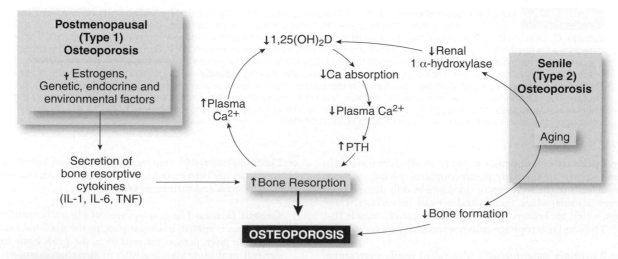
FIGURE 26-13. Pathogenesis of primary osteoporosis. Ca 2+, calcium; IL, interleukin; PTH, parathyroid hormone; TNF, tumor necrosis factor.

osteoporosis. Dietary calcium supplementation in elderly patients reduces the risk of osteoporotic fractures by half.

Secondary Osteoporosis Reflects Extraosseous Metabolic Disorders

Osteoporosis develops in association with many other conditions. Causes of secondary osteoporosis include adverse effects of drug therapy, endocrine diseases, eating disorders, immobilization, marrow-related conditions, gastrointestinal, biliary tract or renal disease, and cancer.

- **Endocrine disorders:** The most common form of secondary osteoporosis is iatrogenic and results from corticosteroid administration. Bone loss may also result from excess endogenous glucocorticoids, as in Cushing disease. Estrogen is a key hormone for maintaining bone mass. Estrogen deficiency is the major cause of age-related bone loss in both genders; estrogen deficiency or a low level of bioavailable estrogen decreases bone mass in elderly men. Hyperparathyroidism and hyperthyroidism are both associated with accelerated osteoclastic activity.
- **Hematologic malignancies:** A variety of hematologic cancers, particularly multiple myeloma, are accompanied by significant bone loss. The malignant plasma cells of multiple myeloma secrete osteoclast-activating factor, which is presumably responsible for secondary osteoporosis. Some leukemias and lymphomas are also associated with osteoporosis.
- **Malabsorption:** Gastrointestinal and hepatic diseases that cause malabsorption often contribute to osteoporosis, probably because of impaired absorption of calcium, phosphate, and vitamin D.
- **Alcoholism:** Chronic alcohol abuse has also been linked to development of osteoporosis. Alcohol is a direct inhibitor of osteoblasts and may also interfere with calcium absorption.

Osteomalacia and Rickets

Osteomalacia (soft bones) is a disorder of adults characterized by inadequate mineralization of newly formed bone matrix. Rickets refers to a similar disorder in children, in whom the growth plates (physes) are open. Thus, children with rickets manifest defective mineralization not only of bone (osteomalacia) but also of the cartilaginous matrix of the growth plate. Diverse conditions associated with osteomalacia and rickets include abnormalities in vitamin D metabolism, phosphate-deficiency states, and defects in the mineralization process itself.

Vitamin D Metabolism Influences Bone Mineralization

Vitamin D is ingested in food or synthesized in the skin from 7-dehydrocholesterol under the influence of ultraviolet light (Fig. 26-14). The vitamin is first hydroxylated in the liver to form its major circulating metabolite, 25-hydroxyvitamin D. It is again hydroxylated in the proximal renal tubules to produce the active hormone $1,25(OH)_2D$. Exposure to sunlight provides sufficient vitamin D for bone growth and mineralization, even if dietary sources are inadequate.

Receptors for $1,25(OH)_2D$ are not only present in classic targets, such as intestine, bone, and the kidney but are expressed in many cells. This steroid is a general inducer of differentiation, for example, influencing the maturation of hematopoietic and dermal cells, as well as that of many cancers. In the intestine, $1,25(OH)_2D$ stimulates calcium and phosphate absorption. It is also essential for osteoclast maturation. $1,25(OH)_2D$, in concert with PTH, maintains blood calcium and phosphate at levels that are required for proper mineralization of bone. *The key determinant of the formation of $1,25(OH)_2D$ is the blood calcium concentration.* Decreases in

blood calcium stimulate the release of PTH, which augments the renal synthesis of $1,25(OH)_2D$.

Hypovitaminosis D Can Result from a Variety of Causes

Hypovitaminosis D can result from (1) inadequate exposure to sunlight, (2) deficient dietary intake, or (3) defective intestinal absorption. In addition, there are hereditary and acquired disorders of vitamin D metabolism.

- **Rickets:** Dietary deficiency of vitamin D and inadequate sunlight exposure can result in rickets in children. The use of vitamin D-rich cod liver oil and later the fortification of milk and other foods with vitamin D effectively ended widespread rickets in Western countries.
- **Intestinal malabsorption:** Intrinsic diseases of the small intestine, cholestatic disorders of the liver, biliary obstruction, and chronic pancreatic insufficiency are the most frequent causes of osteomalacia in the United States.
- **Inherited disorders of vitamin D metabolism:** Vitamin D metabolism can be disturbed either by defective 1α-hydroxylation of vitamin D in the kidney (**vitamin D-dependent rickets type I**) or by insensitivity of the target organ to $1,25(OH)_2D$ (**vitamin D-dependent rickets type II**). Both are autosomal recessive diseases that usually manifest early in life.
- **Acquired alterations in vitamin D metabolism:** These include defective renal 1α-hydroxylation and end-organ insensitivity. Some of the causes of impaired α-hydroxylation are hypoparathyroidism, tumor-induced osteomalacia, chronic renal diseases, and old age. Osteomalacia occasionally complicates the treatment of epilepsy as a result of anticonvulsant drug therapy.

Renal Disorders of Phosphate Metabolism Interfere with Vitamin D Metabolism

Both rickets and osteomalacia may result from impaired reabsorption of phosphate by the proximal renal tubules, with resulting hypophosphatemia.

X-LINKED HYPOPHOSPHATEMIA: This condition, also termed **vitamin D-resistant rickets** or **phosphate diabetes**, is the most common type of hereditary rickets and is inherited as a dominant trait. Mutations in the *PHEX* (phosphate-regulating) gene on the X chromosome (Xp22) impair the transport of phosphate across the luminal membrane of proximal renal tubular cells. Although renal phosphate wasting is central to the disease, osteoblast function is also impaired. In boys, florid rickets appears during childhood, but girls often suffer only from hypophosphatemia. Microscopically, the bones of patients show severe osteomalacia and wide osteoid seams.

FANCONI SYNDROMES: *These inborn errors of metabolism are characterized by renal wastage of phosphate, glucose, bicarbonate, and amino acids.* They are all characterized by renal tubular acidosis and lead to rickets and osteomalacia. Fanconi syndromes include Wilson disease, tyrosinemia, galactosemia, glycogen-storage disease, and cystinosis. Renal tubular damage that leads to phosphate wastage may also be acquired, as in lead or mercury intoxication, amyloidosis, and Bence-Jones proteinuria.

TUMOR-ASSOCIATED OSTEOMALACIA: This disorder is a phosphate-wasting syndrome that is associated with predominantly benign and occasionally malignant tumors of soft tissue and bone, which secrete paraneoplastic phosphaturic factors known as **phosphatonins**. The typical laboratory features are hypophosphatemia, hyperphosphaturia, low serum concentrations of $1,25(OH)_2D$, and elevated serum alkaline phosphatase. Removal of the primary tumor is often curative.

PATHOLOGY:

OSTEOMALACIA: Osteomalacia, like osteoporosis, causes an osteopenic radiologic pattern. The only findings may be vertebral compression fractures and decreased bone thickness, as in osteoporosis. A specific finding that may be seen in osteomalacia is pseudofractures of **Milkman-Looser syndrome**. These are radiolucent transverse defects that are most common on the concave side of a long bone, medial side of the femoral neck, ischial and pubic rami, ribs, and scapula. Microscopically, defective mineralization in osteomalacia results in **exaggeration of osteoid seams**, both in thickness and in the proportion of trabecular surface covered (see Fig. 26-11). Areas of pseudofracture display abundant osteoid and may function as stress points for true fractures. These areas do not evoke formation of callus and do not extend through the entire diameter of the bone.

RICKETS: Rickets is a disease of children and thus causes extensive changes at the physeal plate (Fig. 26-15), which does not become adequately mineralized. The calcified cartilage and zones of hypertrophy and proliferative cartilage continue to grow because osteoclastic activity does not resorb the cartilage growth plate. As a consequence, the growth plate is conspicuously thickened, irregular, and lobulated. Endochondral ossification proceeds very slowly and preferentially at the peripheral portions of the metaphysis, resulting in a flared, cup-shaped epiphysis. The largest part of the primary spongiosum is composed of lamellar or woven bone, which importantly, remains unmineralized.

Microscopically, the growth plate exhibits striking changes. The resting zone is normal, but the zones of proliferating cartilage are greatly distorted. There is a disorderly profusion of chondrocytes separated by small amounts of matrix. The resulting lobulated masses of proliferating and hypertrophied carti-

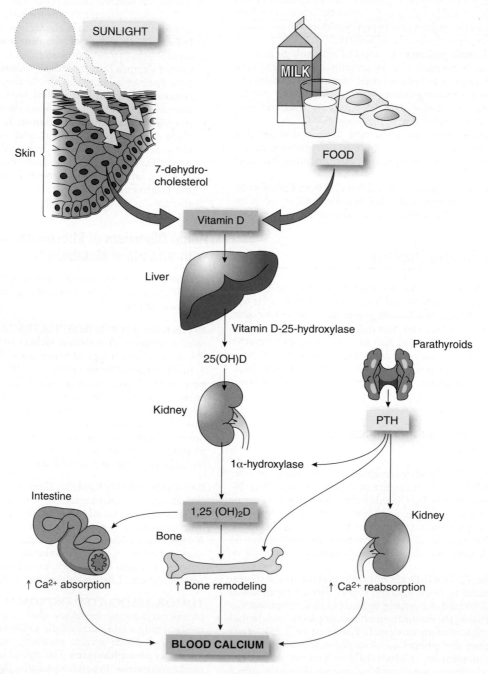

FIGURE 26-14.   Metabolism of vitamin D and the regulation of blood calcium. Ca $^{2+}$, calcium; PTH, parathyroid hormone.

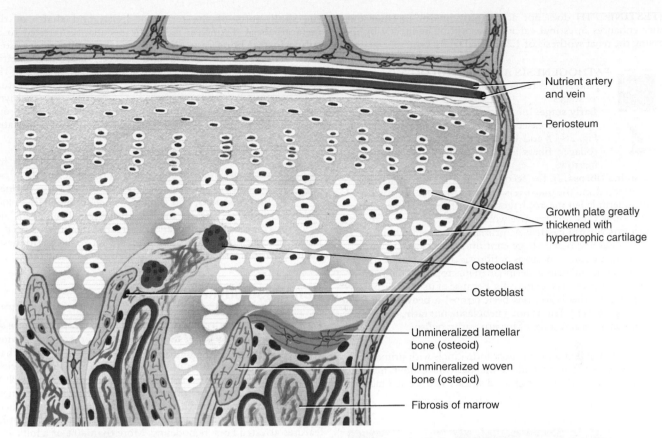

Nutrient artery and vein

Periosteum

Growth plate greatly thickened with hypertrophic cartilage

Osteoclast

Osteoblast

Unmineralized lamellar bone (osteoid)

Unmineralized woven bone (osteoid)

Fibrosis of marrow

FIGURE 26-15. **The growth plate in rickets.** The growth plate is thickened and disorganized, with a large zone of hypertrophic cartilage cells. Irregular perforation of the cartilage plate by osteoclasts occurs because there is little calcified cartilage. The woven bone on the surface of some of the primary trabeculae is unmineralized and therefore easily fractured. Such microfractures often lead to hemorrhage at the interface between the plate and the metaphysis.

lage are associated with increasing width of the growth plate, which may be 5 to 15 times the normal width. The zone of provisional calcification is poorly defined, and only a minimal amount of primary spongiosum is formed. Masses of proliferating cartilage extend into the metaphyseal region, without any apparent vascular invasion and with little osteoclastic activity.

CLINICAL FEATURES:

OSTEOMALACIA: The clinical diagnosis of osteomalacia is often difficult. Patients have nonspecific complaints, such as muscle weakness or diffuse aches and pains. In mild forms of the disease, only slowly progressive changes in bone are seen, and many patients are totally asymptomatic for years. In advanced cases, poorly localized bone pain and tenderness are common, especially in the spine, pelvis, and proximal parts of the extremities. Muscular weakness and hypotonia lead to a waddling gait in severe cases, and some patients are unable to walk.

RICKETS: Children with rickets are apathetic, irritable, and have short attention spans. They are content to be sedentary, assuming a Buddha-like posture. They are short, with characteristic changes of bones and teeth. Flattening of the skull, prominent frontal bones **(frontal bossing)**, and conspicuous suture lines are typical. Delayed dentition is associated with severe dental caries and enamel defects. The chest has the classic **rachitic rosary** (a grossly beaded appearance of the costochondral junctions due to enlargement of the costal cartilages) and indentations of the lower ribs at the insertion of the diaphragm. **Pectus carinatum** ("pigeon breast") reflects an outward curvature of the sternum. The overall musculature is weak, and abdominal weakness leads to a "potbelly." The limbs are shortened and deformed, with severe bowing of the arms and forearm as well as frequent fractures.

Primary Hyperparathyroidism

Primary hyperparathyroidism is a metabolic bone disease characterized by generalized bone resorption due to inappropriate secretion of parathyroid hormone (PTH). Owing to screening of hospitalized patients for abnormalities of serum calcium, severe primary hyperparathyroidism is rarely encountered, and clinically significant bone disease is unusual. The histologic changes of primary hyperparathyroidism are known as **osteitis fibrosa.** This term applies to all circumstances of markedly accelerated remodeling and may be seen in Paget disease and hyperthyroidism, and even in some patients with postmenopausal osteoporosis. Almost all (90%) cases of primary hyperparathyroidism are caused by one or more parathyroid adenomas (see Chapter 21). Because PTH promotes phosphate excretion in the urine and stimulates osteoclastic bone resorption, low serum phosphate and high serum calcium levels are characteristic.

PTH regulates extracellular calcium and hence affects bone, the kidneys, and (indirectly) intestine.

BONE: PTH mobilizes calcium from bone, the major reservoir of calcium in the body. It increases bone resorption in the context of accelerated remodeling. Thus, enhanced bone formation is also seen in hyperparathyroidism. Depending on the relative increase in bone resorption and formation, the secretion of excess PTH may result in decreased, normal, or increased bone mass.

KIDNEY: PTH stimulates reabsorption of calcium by the thick ascending and granular portions of the distal renal tubules. It also enhances phosphate excretion in proximal and distal convoluted tubules and augments the activity of 1α-hydroxylase in the proximal tubules, thereby stimulating the production of 1,25 $(OH)_2D$.

INTESTINE: PTH does not act directly on the intestine but rather enhances intestinal calcium absorption indirectly by increasing the renal synthesis of 1,25(OH)$_2$D.

PATHOGENESIS AND PATHOLOGY: The histogenesis of osteitis fibrosa may be classified into three stages.

- **Early stage:** Initially, osteoclasts are stimulated by the increased PTH levels to resorb bone (see Fig. 26-11 and Fig. 26-16A). At the same time, collagen fibers are laid down in the endosteal marrow.
- **Osteitis fibrosa:** In the second stage, the trabecular bone is resorbed and the marrow is replaced by loose fibrosis, hemosiderin-laden macrophages, areas of hemorrhage from microfractures, and reactive woven bone.
- **Osteitis fibrosa cystica:** As primary hyperparathyroidism progresses and hemorrhage continues, cystic degeneration ultimately occurs. The areas of fibrosis that contain reactive woven bone and hemosiderin-laden macrophages often display many osteoclast giant cells. Because of its macroscopic appearance, this lesion has been termed a **brown tumor** (see Fig. 26-16B). This is not a neoplasm, but rather a repair reaction as an end stage of hyperparathyroidism.

The skeletal radiographs of most individuals with primary hyperparathyroidism are normal. Some patients exhibit mottled bone cortices, with an irregular frayed surface in the outer table of the skull, tufts of the terminal digits, and shafts of the metacarpals. A distinctive radiologic peculiarity, referred to as **subperiosteal bone resorption**, is evident in the subperiosteal outer surface of the cortex and reflects dissecting osteitis. Resorption around tooth sockets causes the lamina dura of the teeth to disappear, a well-known finding on x-ray. A classic feature of osteitis fibrosa cystica is the presence of multiple, localized, lytic lesions, which represent hemorrhagic cysts or masses of fibrous tissue. These eccentric and well-demarcated lesions are separated from the soft tissue by a periosteal shell of bone.

CLINICAL FEATURES: The symptoms of primary hyperparathyroidism are related to the abnormality of calcium homeostasis and have been summarized as **"stones, bones, moans, and groans."** The "stones" refer to kidney stones and the "bones" to the skeletal changes. The "moans" describe psychiatric depression and other abnormalities associated with hypercalcemia, and the "groans" characterize the gastrointestinal irregularities associated with a high serum calcium level.

Renal Osteodystrophy

Renal osteodystrophy is a complex metabolic bone disease that occurs in the context of chronic renal failure. Severe renal osteodystrophy is most common in patients maintained on long-term dialysis and is characterized by (1) changes similar to those seen in nutritional rickets, (2) changes related to secondary hyperparathyroidism (such as osteitis fibrosa cystica, see above), and (3) osteosclerotic changes demonstrated by increased bone density, which is most prominent in the vertebrae. **The adynamic variant of renal osteodystrophy** features arrested bone remodeling. More than 40% of adults who are treated with hemodialysis exhibit evidence of the adynamic variant of renal osteodystrophy in a bone biopsy.

PATHOLOGY AND CLINICAL FEATURES: Renal osteodystrophy is characterized by varying degrees of osteomalacia, osteitis fibrosa, osteomalacia, osteosclerosis, and adynamic bone disease. Hyperphosphatemic patients with terminal chronic renal disease may display metastatic calcification at various sites, including the eyes, skin, muscular coats of arteries and arterioles, and periarticular soft tissues.

Paget Disease of Bone

Paget disease of bone results from disordered remodeling, in which excessive bone resorption initially results in lytic lesions and is followed by disorganized and excessive bone formation.

EPIDEMIOLOGY: Paget disease is common and generally affects men and women older than 60 years of age. In the United States, about 1% of elderly persons manifest the disease. The disorder has an unusual worldwide distribution, afflicting populations of the British Isles and following their migrations throughout the world. The disorder is almost nonexistent in Asia and in the indigenous populations of Africa and South America. For unknown reasons, the incidence of Paget disease appears to have decreased worldwide over the last several decades.

PATHOGENESIS: Overall, Paget disease is characterized by localized increases in osteoclast formation, which leads to bone resorption and associated osteoblastic activity. This situation is mediated by increases in IL-6 and the RANK signaling pathway. In some families, Paget disease is transmitted as an autosomal dominant trait with incomplete penetrance that increases with age. Hereditary forms of Paget disease and related bone disorders are caused by mutations in the gene encoding RANK (TN-

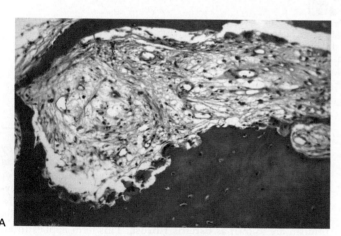

A

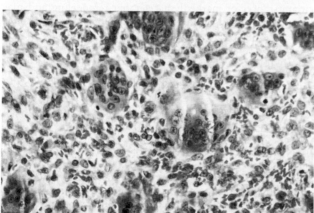

B

FIGURE 26-16. **A. Primary hyperparathyroidism.** Section through compact bone shows tunneling reabsorption of a haversian canal. Numerous osteoclasts and stromal fibrosis are evident. **B.** A section of tissue obtained from a "brown tumor" reveals numerous giant cells in a cellular, fibrous stroma. Scattered erythrocytes are present throughout the tissue.

FRS11A 18q22, see above) and other genes in the RANK pathway such as *Sequestosome 1* (SQSTM1 P62). Some evidence indicates that Paget disease is associated with viral infections, although the issue remains controversial.

 PATHOLOGY: The lesions of Paget disease may be solitary or may occur at multiple sites. They tend to localize to the bones of the axial skeleton, including the spine, skull, and pelvis. The proximal femur and tibia

may also be involved in the polyostotic form of the disease. Solitary Paget disease rarely involves the humerus, but in polyostotic disease, lesions involving this bone are common. Paget disease is an example of bone remodeling gone awry. The disease is triphasic:

1. **"Hot" or osteoclastic resorptive stage:** Radiologically, there is a characteristic, sharply defined, flame-shaped or wedge-shaped lysis of the cortex, which may mimic a tumor (Fig. 26-17A). Histologically, there is widespread osteolysis, with marrow fibrosis and dilation of marrow sinusoids.

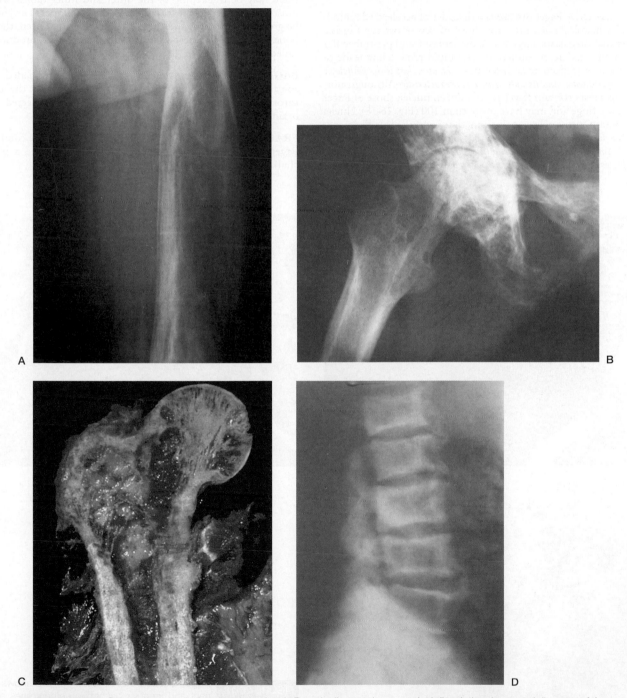

FIGURE 26-17. **Paget disease. A.** A radiograph of early Paget's disease shows cortical dissolution, increased diameter of the diaphysis, and an advancing, wedge-shaped area of cortical reabsorption ("flame sign"). Proximal to the edge of this wedge, the femur appears entirely normal. **B.** Later, Paget disease of the proximal femur and pelvis shows cortical disorganization and irregular coarse trabeculations. **C.** Gross specimen of proximal femur showing cortical thickening and coarse trabeculations of the femoral head and neck. **D.** Paget disease of the spine shows shortening and widening of the lumbar vertebral bodies. Their cortices and endplates are thickened and have a "picture-frame" appearance.

2. **Mixed stage of osteoblastic and osteoclastic activity:** By x-ray, the bones are larger than normal. In fact, Paget disease is one of only two diseases that produce **larger than normal bones** (the other is fibrous dysplasia, discussed below). The cortex in the mixed phase is thickened, and the accentuation of the coarse cancellous bone makes the bone look heavy and enlarged (see Fig. 26-17B,C). Involvement of vertebral bodies leads to a "picture frame" appearance (see Fig. 26-17D). Histologically, there is evidence of both irregular osteoclast activity and osteoblast activity.

3. **"Cold" or burnt-out stage:** This period is characterized histologically by little cellular activity and radiologically by thickened and disordered bones.

Because active Paget disease is a disorder of accelerated remodeling, its histologic features are those of severe osteitis fibrosa. Numerous osteoclasts, large active osteoblasts, and peritrabecular marrow fibrosis are encountered. The rapid remodeling leads to disruption of trabecular architecture. *The osteoclast is the pathologic cell of Paget disease, and its appearance is characteristic.* Although normal osteoclasts contain fewer than a dozen nuclei, those of Paget disease are huge and may have more than 100 (Fig. 26-18). Nuclei may contain intranuclear inclusions that contain virus-like particles. *The diagnostic hallmark of the "cold" stage is the abnormal arrangement of lamellar bone, in which islands of irregular bone formation, resembling pieces of a jigsaw puzzle, are separated by prominent **cement lines**.*

The result is a **mosaic pattern** in the bone, which can be seen particularly well under polarized light.

CLINICAL FEATURES: The most common focal symptom of Paget disease is pain in the affected bone, which may be related to microfractures, stimulation of free nerve endings by dilated blood vessels adjacent to the bones, or weight bearing in weaker bones. The diagnosis is primarily made by radiologic findings.

SKULL: Involvement of the skull is particularly common. The skull exhibits localized lysis, generally in the frontal and parietal bones, which is termed **osteoporosis circumscripta**. Alternatively, there may be thickening of the outer and inner tables, which is most pronounced in the frontal and occipital bones. The jaws may be grossly misshapen, and the teeth may fall out. Often, the facial bones increase in size, especially the maxillary bones, producing so-called **leontiasis ossea** (lion-like face).

PAGETIC STEAL: Occasionally, patients feel lightheaded, due to so-called pagetic steal, in which blood is shunted from the internal carotid system to the bones rather than being directed to the brain.

FRACTURES AND ARTHRITIS: Bone fractures are common in Paget disease, and the bones snap transversely like a piece of chalk.

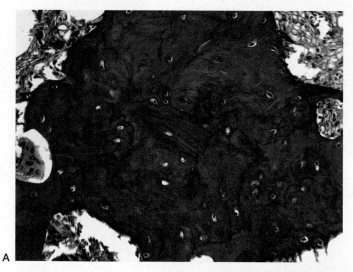

A

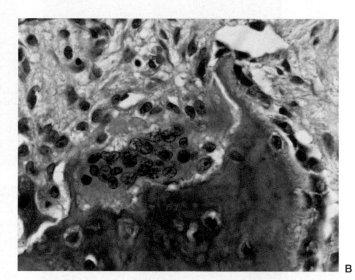

B

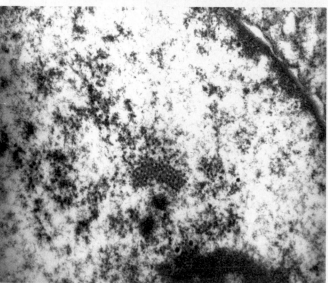

C

FIGURE 26-18. **Paget disease. A.** A section of bone shows prominent and irregular basophilic cement lines and numerous lining osteoclasts and osteoblasts. **B.** An osteoclast in pagetic bone contains many more nuclei than a usual osteoclast. A few of the nuclei contain eosinophilic intranuclear inclusion-like particles. **C.** On electron microscopy, the nuclei of the osteoclasts contain particles that resemble paramyxovirus in their shape and orientation.

HIGH-OUTPUT CARDIAC FAILURE: With extensive Paget disease, blood flow to the bones and subcutaneous tissue increases remarkably, requiring increased cardiac output. In the presence of underlying cardiac disease, it may be severe enough to result in cardiac failure.

SARCOMATOUS CHANGE: Neoplastic transformation may occur in a focus of Paget disease, usually in the femur, humerus, or pelvis. Although this complication occurs in less than 1% of all cases (usually the most severe), the risk of bone sarcoma is 1,000 times higher than that in the general population.

GIANT CELL TUMOR: This is not a neoplasm but rather a reactive phenomenon, similar to the "brown tumor" of hyperparathyroidism. Giant cell tumor is an overshoot of osteoclastic activity and an associated fibroblastic response. Radiation therapy to the giant cell tumor is curative in many cases.

Fortunately, most patients with Paget disease are asymptomatic and require no treatment. Fractures, osteoarthritis, and other orthopedic complications are treated symptomatically. Drugs directed at abnormal osteoclast function, including calcitonin, bisphosphonates, and mithramycin, may be useful.

Fibrous Dysplasia

Fibrous dysplasia is a developmental abnormality characterized by a disorganized mixture of fibrous and osseous elements in the medullary region of affected bones. It occurs in children or adults and may affect one (monostotic) or multiple bones (polyostotic) as well as other systems (McCune-Albright syndrome).

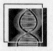

PATHOGENESIS: Activating mutations in the *GNAS1* gene (20q13) encoding the a subunit of the stimulatory guanine nucleotide-binding protein ($G_S\alpha$), which is linked to adenylyl cyclase, have been described in bone cells from patients with fibrous dysplasia and McCune-Albright syndrome. The result is constitutive activation of adenylyl cyclase and increased levels of cAMP, thereby enhancing certain functions of the affected cells (e.g., *c-fos* protooncogene, *c-jun*, IL-6, and IL-11).

PATHOLOGY AND CLINICAL FEATURES:

MONOSTOTIC FIBROUS DYSPLASIA: Monostotic fibrous dysplasia is the most common form of the disease and is most often seen in the second and third decades, with no predilection for either gender. The bones commonly involved are the proximal femur, tibia, ribs, and facial bones, although any bone may be affected. The disease may be asymptomatic, or it may lead to a pathologic fracture.

POLYOSTOTIC FIBROUS DYSPLASIA: One fourth of patients with polyostotic fibrous dysplasia exhibit disease in more than half of the skeleton, including the facial bones. Symptoms usually are seen in childhood, and almost all patients have pathologic fractures, limb deformities, or limb-length discrepancies. Polyostotic fibrous dysplasia is more common in females. Sometimes, the disease becomes quiescent at puberty, whereas pregnancy may stimulate the growth of lesions.

MCCUNE-ALBRIGHT SYNDROME: This condition is characterized by endocrine dysfunction, including acromegaly, Cushing syndrome, hyperthyroidism, vitamin D-resistant rickets, and characteristic skin lesions. The most common endocrine abnormality is precocious puberty in girls (boys rarely have McCune-Albright syndrome). As a result, premature closure of the growth plates may lead to abnormally short stature.

PATHOLOGY: The radiographic features of fibrous dysplasia are distinctive. The bone lesion has a lucent ground-glass appearance with well-marginated borders and a thin cortex. The bone may be ballooned, deformed or enlarged, and involvement may be focal or may encompass the entire bone (Fig. 26-19A). All forms of fibrous dysplasia have an identical histological pattern (see Fig. 26-19B,C). Benign fibroblastic tissue is arranged in a loose, whorled pattern. Irregularly arranged, purposeless spicules of woven bone that lack osteoblastic rimming are embedded in the fibrous tissue. In 10% of cases, irregular islands of hyaline cartilage are also present. Occasionally, cystic degeneration occurs, with hemosiderin-laden macrophages, hemorrhage, and osteoclasts congregated about the cyst. Treatment of fibrous dysplasia consists of curettage, fracture repair, and prevention of deformities.

NEOPLASMS OF BONE

Bone tumors of all kinds are uncommon, but are nevertheless important neoplasms because many occur in children as well as young persons and are potentially lethal. A primary bone tumor may arise from any of the cellular elements of bone. Most neoplasms of bone occur near the metaphyseal area, and more than 80% of primary tumors occur in the distal femur or proximal tibia (Fig. 26-20). In a growing child, these areas are characterized by conspicuous growth activity.

Benign Tumors of Bone

Osteoma is Composed of Compact Cortical Bone

Osteoma is a benign slow-growing tumor composed of cortical type bone. These lesions can be divided into four major clinicopathologic subtypes including (1) calvarial and mandibular osteomas, (2) osteomas of the sinonasal and orbital bones, (3) bone islands occurring in medullary bone, and (4) surface osteomas of long bones. Some osteomas are likely developmental or hamartomatous in nature. However, sinonasal osteomas may be benign osteoblastic neoplasms and may occur in the Gardner form of familial adenomatous polyposis in association with mutations in the APC gene (see Chapter 13).

Nonossifying Fibroma is a Solitary Lesion of Childhood

*Nonossifying fibroma, also termed **fibrous cortical defect**, is a benign tumor that occurs in the metaphysis of a long bone—most commonly, the tibia or femur.* It is very common and may be present in as many as 25% of all children between ages 4 and 10 years, after which it characteristically regresses. Whether nonossifying fibroma is a neoplasm or developmental lesion remains controversial. Most cases are asymptomatic, although pain or fracture through the thin cortex overlying the lesion occasionally calls attention to the condition.

PATHOLOGY: Radiologically, nonossifying fibromas are identified by a cortical, eccentric position and by well-demarcated, central lucent zones surrounded by scalloped, sclerotic margins. On gross examination, the lesion is granular and dark red to brown. Microscopically, bland spindle cells are arranged in an interlacing, whorled pattern in which multinuclear giant cells and foamy macrophages may be seen. The rare symptomatic or expanded lesions are treated with curettage and bone grafting.

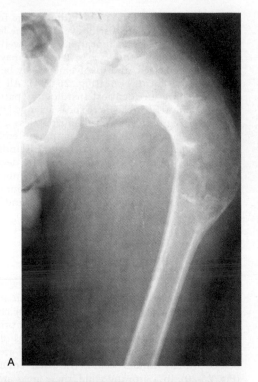

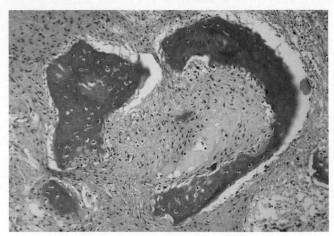

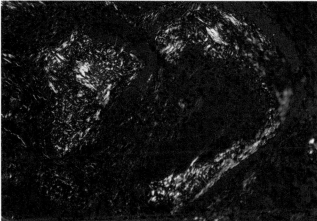

FIGURE 26-19. **Fibrous dysplasia. A.** A radiograph of the proximal femur shows a "shepherd's crook" deformity caused by fractures sustained over the years. Irregular, marginated, ground-glass lucencies are surrounded by reactive bone. The shaft has an appearance that has been likened to a soap bubble. **B.** Histologically, fibrous dysplasia consists of moderately cellular fibrous tissue in which irregular, curved spicules of woven bone develop without discernible appositional osteoblast activity. **C.** The same section in polarized light demonstrates not only that the spicules are woven, but also that their fiber pattern extends imperceptibly into the fiber pattern of the surrounding stroma.

Osteoid Osteoma is a Benign, Painful Lesion

Osteoid osteoma is composed of osseous tissue (the nidus) and surrounded by a halo of reactive bone formation. The typical patient is between 5 and 25 years old. Boys are affected more often than girls (3:1). Osteoid osteoma frequently arises in the cortex of the diaphysis of the tubular bones of the leg.

 PATHOGENESIS: Osteoid osteomas have limited tumor growth potential and do not metastasize. Chromosomal analysis of a few osteoid osteomas has disclosed abnormalities of chromosome 22q13 and loss of part of 17q, which suggests that osteoid osteomas are neoplasms.

 PATHOLOGY: Osteoid osteoma is a spherical, hyperemic tumor, about 1 cm in diameter, which is considerably softer than the surrounding bone (Fig. 26-21) and is easily enucleated at surgery. Microscopically, the tumor is composed of thin, irregular, trabeculae within a cellular granulation tissue containing osteoblasts and osteoclasts.

Trabeculae are more mature in the center, which is often partially calcified. Reactive, sclerotic bone surrounds the nidus.

CLINICAL FEATURES: Pain, typically nocturnal, is out of proportion to the size of the lesion. It is often exacerbated by drinking alcohol and is promptly relieved by aspirin, possibly because of the high prostaglandin content of the tumor and nerve fibers within the tumor. Surgical excision is curative.

Solitary Chondroma Features Hyaline Cartilage

Solitary chondroma (enchondroma) is a benign, intraosseous tumor composed of well-differentiated hyaline cartilage. Although its neoplastic nature has been questioned, cytogenetic analyses show chromosomal abnormalities in some chondromas, suggesting that they are, in fact, neoplasms. The diagnosis is made at any age, and many cases are entirely asymptomatic.

PATHOLOGY: Most solitary chondromas occur in the metacarpals and phalanges of the hands, and the remainder is in almost any other tubular bone. The tumor is small and grows slowly. On gross examination,

BENIGN TUMORS

EPIPHYSIS

Chondroblastoma,
Giant cell tumor

METAPHYSIS

Osteoblastoma
Osteochondroma
Non-ossifying fibroma
Osteoid osteoma
Chondromyxoid fibroma
Giant cell tumor

DIAPHYSIS

Enchondroma
Fibrous dysplasia

MALIGNANT TUMORS

DIAPHYSIS

Ewing sarcoma
Chondrosarcoma

METAPHYSIS

Osteosarcoma
Juxtacortical osteosarcoma

FIGURE 26-20. Location of primary bone tumors in long tubular bones.

solitary chondromas have the semitranslucent appearance of hyaline cartilage, often with a few calcified areas. Microscopically, the cartilaginous tissue is well differentiated with sparse chondrocytes. Asymptomatic chondromas are best left untreated. When pain intervenes, curettage and bone grafting are the treatment of choice.

Malignant Tumors of Bone

Osteosarcoma is the Most Common Primary Malignant Bone Tumor

*Osteosarcoma, also termed **osteogenic sarcoma**, is a highly malignant bone tumor characterized by the formation of bone tissue by tumor cells.* It represents one fifth of all bone cancers and is most frequent in adolescents between 10 and 20 years old, affecting boys more often than girls (2:1).

PATHOGENESIS: Osteosarcomas are associated with mutations in tumor suppressor genes: almost two thirds show mutations in the retinoblastoma gene (see Chapter 5) and many also have mutations in the p53 gene. Osteosarcoma can develop in adults and children previously subjected to external, therapeutic radiation for another tumor such as lymphoma. When osteosarcoma arise in older patients, they almost always occur in the context of Paget disease or radiation exposure. Several pre-existing benign bone lesions are associated with an increased risk of developing osteosarcoma, including fibrous dysplasia, osteomyelitis, and bone marrow infarcts. Although trauma may call attention to an existing osteosarcoma, there is no evidence that it ever causes the tumor.

PATHOLOGY: Osteosarcoma often arises near the knee in the lower femur (Fig. 26-22A), upper tibia, or fibula, although any metaphyseal area of a long bone may be affected. The proximal humerus is the second most common site. Radiologic evidence of bone destruction and bone formation is characteristic, the latter representing neoplastic bone. Often, the periosteum produces an incomplete rim of reactive bone adjacent to the site where it is lifted from the cortical surface by the tumor. A "sunburst" periosteal reaction is also often superimposed. The cut surface may show any combination of hemorrhagic, cystic soft, and bony areas. The neoplastic tissue may invade and break through the cortex, spread into the marrow cavity, or grow into the epiphysis, even reaching the joint space.

Histologic examination reveals malignant cells with osteoblastic differentiation producing woven bone (see Fig. 26-22B). The malignant cells stain prominently for alkaline phosphatase and osteonectin. The tumorous bone is laid down haphazardly and not aligned along stress lines. Often, foci of malignant cartilage cells or pleomorphic giant cells are intermixed. In areas of osteolysis, nonneoplastic osteoclasts are found at the advancing front of

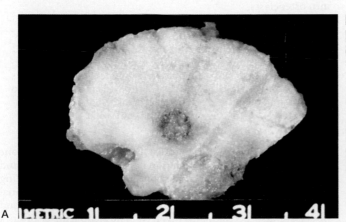

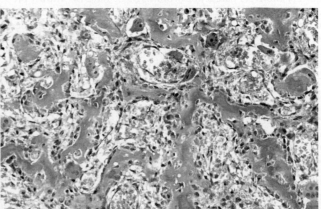

FIGURE 26-21. **Osteoid osteoma. A.** A gross specimen of an osteoid osteoma shows the central nidus, which is embedded in dense bone. **B.** A photomicrograph of the nidus reveals irregular trabeculae of woven bone surrounded by osteoblasts, osteoclasts, and fibrovascular marrow.

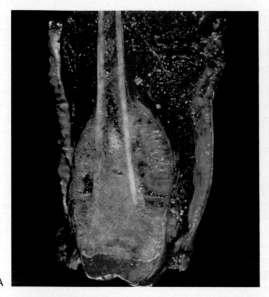
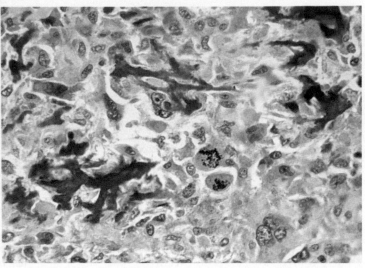

A   B

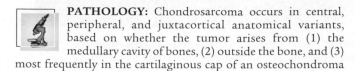

FIGURE 26-22. **Osteosarcoma. A.** The distal femur contains a dense osteoblastic malignant tumor that extends through the cortex into the soft tissue and the epiphysis. **B.** A photomicrograph reveals pleomorphic malignant cells, tumor giant cells, and mitoses. The tumor produces woven bone that is focally calcified.

the tumor. Almost all patients (98%) who die from this disease have lung metastases. Less commonly, the tumor metastasizes to other bones (35%), the pleura (33%), and the heart (20%).

 CLINICAL FEATURES: Osteosarcoma presents with mild or intermittent pain around the knee or other involved areas. As pain intensifies, the area becomes swollen and tender, and the adjacent joint becomes functionally limited. Serum alkaline phosphatase is increased in half of the patients and may decrease after amputation, only to increase again with recurrence or metastasis. Metastatic disease heralds rapid clinical deterioration and death. Today, chemotherapy and limb-sparing surgery give 5-year disease-free rates of 60% to 80%. Resection of isolated pulmonary metastases may prolong survival.

Chondrosarcoma is a Cartilaginous Malignancy, and Its Grade Determines Prognosis

Chondrosarcoma is a malignant tumor of cartilage that arises from pre-existing cartilage rests or enchondroma. Some patients have a history of enchondromas, solitary osteochondroma, or hereditary multiple osteochondromas. Most have no known pre-existing lesion. Chondrosarcoma is the second most common primary malignant bone tumor, occurring more commonly in men than in women (2:1). It is most frequently seen in the fourth to sixth decades (average age, 45 years).

 PATHOGENESIS: Numerous nonrandom chromosomal abnormalities have been discovered in chondrosarcoma. There probably is a different molecular mechanism resulting in tumor development between central chondrosarcoma and secondary peripheral chondrosarcoma (tumors arising in the cartilaginous cap of an osteochondroma) (see below).

PATHOLOGY: Chondrosarcoma occurs in central, peripheral, and juxtacortical anatomical variants, based on whether the tumor arises from (1) the medullary cavity of bones, (2) outside the bone, and (3) most frequently in the cartilaginous cap of an osteochondroma

or lying on the outer surface of the cortex of the metaphysis of long bones (see Fig. 26-23).

 CLINICAL FEATURES: Patients generally present with pain at the affected site. Chondrosarcoma is one of the few tumors in which microscopic grading has a significant prognostic value. The 5-year survival rate for low-grade chondrosarcomas is 80%, for moderate-grade tumors 50%, and for high-grade tumors, it is only 20%. Wide excision is the usual treatment.

Giant Cell Tumor (GCT) of Bone Occasionally Metastasizes

GCT of bone is a locally aggressive, potentially malignant neoplasm characterized by the presence of osteoclastic, multinucleated, giant cells. It usually occurs in the third and fourth decades, has a slight predilection for women, and seems to be more common in Asia than in Western countries. GCTs in the elderly may be secondary to irradiation. Paget disease may produce a giant cell reactive lesion that closely resembles a true GCT. The neoplasms are thought to arise from primitive stromal cells that can modulate into osteoclasts.

 PATHOGENESIS: GCT is composed of osteoclastic giant cells and two lineages of mononuclear cells. One population of mononuclear cells is believed to be of macrophage-monocyte origin and is likely non-neoplastic. The other mononuclear cells appear to represent a neoplastic primitive stromal cell of osteoclast lineage and are likely the origin of the giant cells.

 PATHOLOGY: In most cases (90%), GCT of bone originates at the junction between the metaphysis and the epiphysis of a long bone, with more than half being situated in the knee area (distal femur and proximal tibia; Fig. 26-24A). The lower end of the radius, humerus, and fibula are also occasionally involved. The neoplasm is often a lytic lesion that grows slowly enough to allow a periosteal reaction. On gross examination, GCT is clearly circumscribed, and its cut surface is soft and light brown, without bone or calcification.

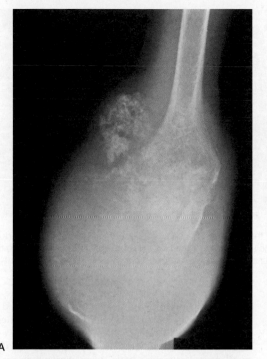

A

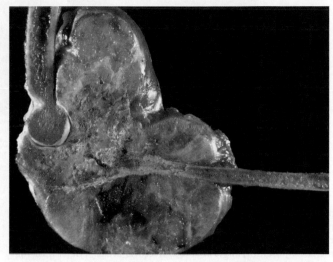

B

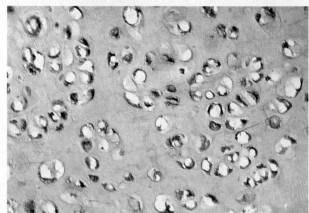

C

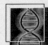**FIGURE 26-23.** **Chondrosarcoma. A.** Radiograph demonstrates a large, destructive mass replacing the proximal ulna. There is a huge soft tissue mass containing aggregates of ring-shaped and popcorn-like calcifications. **B.** Resected gross specimen demonstrates lobulated hyaline cartilage with calcifications, ossification, and focal liquefaction. **C.** A photomicrograph of a chondrosarcoma shows malignant chondrocytes with pronounced atypia.

Numerous hemorrhagic areas result in the appearance of a sponge full of blood.

Microscopically, GCT exhibits two types of cells (see Fig. 26-24B). The mononuclear ("stromal") cells are plump and oval, with large nuclei and scanty cytoplasm. Large osteoclastic giant cells, some with more than 100 nuclei, are scattered throughout the richly vascularized stroma. It is thought that the mononuclear cells are the neoplastic and proliferative components of GCT (mitotic activity is common in the mononuclear cells, but is not observed in the giant cells). The diagnosis of malignancy in a GCT depends on the morphology of the mononuclear cells rather than that of the multinucleated cells.

CLINICAL FEATURES: GCTs manifest with pain, usually in the joint adjacent to the tumor. Microfractures and pathologic fractures are frequent, due to thinning of the cortex. The tumor is usually treated with thorough curettage and bone grafting, although more aggressive management, including en bloc resection or even amputation, may be necessary. Local recurrence after simple curettage has been reported in one third to one half of the cases, and 5% to 10% metastasize. Most of these patients may enjoy an essentially normal life span, especially if the metastatic deposits are few and can be surgically removed.

Ewing Sarcoma (EWS) is a Primitive Neuroectodermal Tumor of Childhood

EWS is an uncommon malignant bone tumor composed of small, uniform, round cells. It represents only 5% of all bone tumors and is found in children and adolescents, with two thirds of cases occurring in patients younger than 20 years. Boys are affected more often than girls (2:1). EWS is very rare in blacks.

PATHOGENESIS: EWS is thought to arise from primitive marrow elements or immature mesenchymal cells. Virtually all (90%) of these tumors have a reciprocal translocation between chromosomes 11 and 22 [t(11;22)p(13;q12)], which results in the fusion of the amino terminus of the *EWS1* gene to the carboxy terminus of the *FLI-1* gene, which encodes a transcription factor. The resulting fusion protein, *EWS/FLI-1*, is an aberrant transcription factor with target genes that are not yet fully identified.

PATHOLOGY: EWS is primarily a tumor of the long bones in childhood, especially the humerus, tibia, and femur, where it occurs as a midshaft or metaphyseal lesion. It tends to parallel the distribution of red marrow,

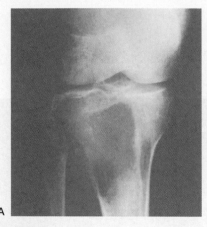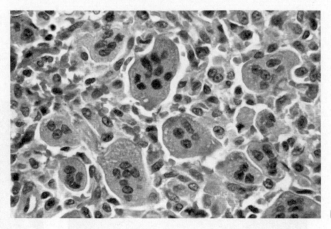

FIGURE 26-24. **Giant cell tumor of bone. A.** Radiograph of the proximal tibia shows an eccentric lytic lesion with virtually no new bone formation. The tumor extends to the subchondral bone plate and breaks through cortex into the soft tissue. **B.** Photomicrograph shows osteoclast-type giant cells and plump, oval, mononuclear cells. The nuclei of both types of cells are identical.

so when it arises in the third decade or later, it affects the pelvis and spine. However, no bone is immune from involvement. On gross examination, EWS is typically soft and grayish white, often studded by hemorrhagic foci and necrotic areas. The tumor may infiltrate the medullary spaces without destroying the bony trabeculae. It may also diffusely infiltrate the cortical bone or form

nodules in which the bone is completely resorbed. In many cases, the tumor mass penetrates the periosteum and extends into the soft tissues (see Fig. 26-25A).

Microscopically, EWS cells appear as sheets of closely packed, small, round cells with little cytoplasm, which are up to twice the size of a lymphocyte (see Fig. 26-25B). Fibrous strands separate the

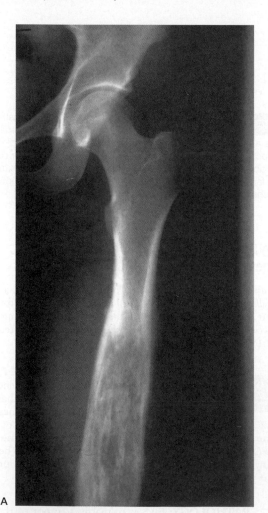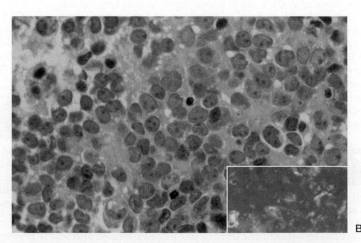

FIGURE 26-25. **Ewing sarcoma. A.** A clinical x-ray demonstrates expansile cortical destruction with poor circumscription and a delicate interrupted periosteal reaction. **B.** A biopsy specimen shows fairly uniform small cells with round, dark blue nuclei, a paucity of mitotic activity, and poorly defined cytoplasm. A periodic acid-Schiff (PAS) stain demonstrates abundant intracellular glycogen (inset).

sheets of cells into irregular nests. There is little or no interstitial stroma, and mitoses are infrequent. In some areas, the neoplastic cells tend to form rosettes. *An important diagnostic feature is the presence of substantial amounts of glycogen in the cytoplasm of the tumor cells, which is well visualized with the PA stain* (see Fig. 26-25B, *inset*). EWS metastasizes to many organs, including the lungs and brain. Other bones, especially the skull, are common sites for metastases (50% to 75% of cases).

 CLINICAL FEATURES: Patients with EWS initially present with mild pain, which becomes more intense and is followed by swelling of the affected area. Nonspecific symptoms, including fever and leukocytosis, commonly follow. In some cases, a soft tissue mass is encountered. In the past, the prognosis of EWS was dismal, with 5-year survival rates of only 5% after surgery or radiation therapy. Today, with the use of chemotherapy combined with radiation or surgery, the 5-year disease-free survival rate is 60% to 75%.

Metastatic Tumors are the Most Common Malignant Tumors in Bone

Most metastatic lesions to bone are carcinomas, particularly of the breast, prostate, lung, thyroid, and kidney. It is estimated that hematogenous skeletal metastases are found in at least 85% of cancer cases that have run their full clinical course. The vertebral column is, by far, the most common site. Some tumors (thyroid, gastrointestinal tract, kidney, neuroblastoma) produce mostly lytic lesions by stimulating osteoclasts. A few neoplasms (prostate, breast, lung, stomach) stimulate osteoblastic components to make bone, creating dense foci on radiographs. However, most deposits of metastatic cancer in the bones have mixtures of both lytic and blastic elements.

JOINTS

Osteoarthritis

Arthritis is joint inflammation, usually accompanied by pain, swelling, and changes in structure. Arthritis can generally be divided into two major forms: (1) **inflammatory arthritis**, usually involving the synovium and mediated by inflammatory cells (e.g., rheumatoid arthritis) and (2) **noninflammatory arthritis**, as exemplified by primary osteoarthritis. *Osteoarthritis is a slowly progressive destruction of articular cartilage that affects weight-bearing joints and fingers of older persons, or the joints of younger individuals subjected to trauma.* Osteoarthritis is the single most common form of joint disease and the major form of noninflammatory arthritis. It is a group of conditions that have in common the mechanical destruction of a joint.

In **primary osteoarthritis**, the destruction of joints results from intrinsic defects in the joint cartilage. The prevalence and severity of primary osteoarthritis increases with age. Of 18- to 24-year-olds, 4% are affected versus 85% of those 75 to 79 years of age. Before the age of 45, the disease mainly affects men. After age 55, osteoarthritis is more common in women. Many cases of primary osteoarthritis exhibit a familial clustering, suggesting a hereditary predisposition.

Primary osteoarthritis has variously been called **wear and tear arthritis** and **degenerative joint disease**. Progressive degradation of articular cartilage leads to joint narrowing, subchondral bone thickening, and eventually a nonfunctioning, painful joint. Although osteoarthritis is not primarily an inflammatory process, a mild inflammatory reaction may occur within the synovium.

Secondary osteoarthritis has a known underlying cause, including congenital or acquired defects of joints, trauma, crystal deposits, infection, metabolic diseases, endocrinopathies, inflammatory diseases, osteonecrosis, and hemarthrosis.

 PATHOGENESIS: Many factors play etiologic roles in osteoarthritis.

INCREASED UNIT LOAD: Abnormal force on the cartilage may have many causes, but it is often attributable to incongruities of the joint. When the critical unit load is exceeded, chondrocyte death causes degradation of articular cartilage.

RESILIENCE OF THE ARTICULAR CARTILAGE: Because articular cartilage binds extensive amounts of water, it normally has a swelling pressure of at least 3 atm. Disruption in water bonding leads to decreased resilience.

STIFFNESS OF SUBCHONDRAL COARSE CANCELLOUS BONE: The structure of bone adjacent to a joint is important in maintaining articular cartilage. Damage to the coarse cancellous bone results in an increased unit load on the cartilage because of an increase in the stiffness of subchondral bone, for example, in Paget disease.

BIOCHEMICAL ABNORMALITIES: The biochemical changes of osteoarthritis mainly involve proteoglycans. Proteoglycan content and aggregation decrease, and glycosaminoglycan chain length is reduced. The reduction in proteoglycans allows more water to be bound to collagen. Thus, osteoarthritic cartilage, or any cartilage that is fibrillated, swells more than normal cartilage.

GENETIC FACTORS: Studies of identical twins have demonstrated genetic contributions to the prevalence of osteoarthritis. Genetic analysis of patients with a type of familial, early-onset osteoarthritis has revealed a variety of mutations in the gene for type II collagen (COL2A1), the major collagen species of articular cartilage.

 PATHOLOGY: Joints commonly affected by osteoarthritis are the proximal and distal interphalangeal joints of the arm, knees, hips, as well as the cervical and lumbar segments of the spine. Radiologically, osteoarthritis is characterized by (1) narrowing of the joint space, which represents the loss of articular cartilage, (2) increased thickness of the subchondral bone, (3) subchondral bone cysts, and (4) large peripheral growths of bone and cartilage, called **osteophytes**. Histologic changes follow a well-described sequence.

1. The earliest changes of osteoarthritis are the loss of proteoglycans from the surface of the articular cartilage, which is seen histologically as decreased metachromatic staining accompanied by empty lacunae, indicating that chondrocytes have died (Fig. 26-26).
2. Osteoarthritis may arrest at this stage for many years before progressing to the next stage, which is characterized by **fibrillation** (i.e., development of surface cracks parallel to the long axis of the articular surface).
3. As fibrillations propagate, synovial fluid begins to flow into the defects. Eventually, pieces of articular cartilage break off and lodge in the synovium, inducing inflammation and a foreign-body giant cell reaction. The result is a hyperemic and hypertrophied synovium.
4. As the crack extends downward, neovascularization from the epiphysis and subchondral bone extends into the area of the crack, inducing subchondral osteoclastic bone resorption. Adjacent osteoblastic activity also occurs and results in a thickening of the subchondral bone plate in the area of the crack. As neovascularization progressively extends into the area of the crack, mesenchymal cells invade, and fibrocartilage forms as a poor substitute for the articular hyaline cartilage (Fig. 26-27A). These fibrocartilaginous plugs may persist, or they may be swept into the joint. The subchondral bone becomes exposed and burnished as it grinds against the opposite joint surface, which is undergoing the same process. These thick, shiny,

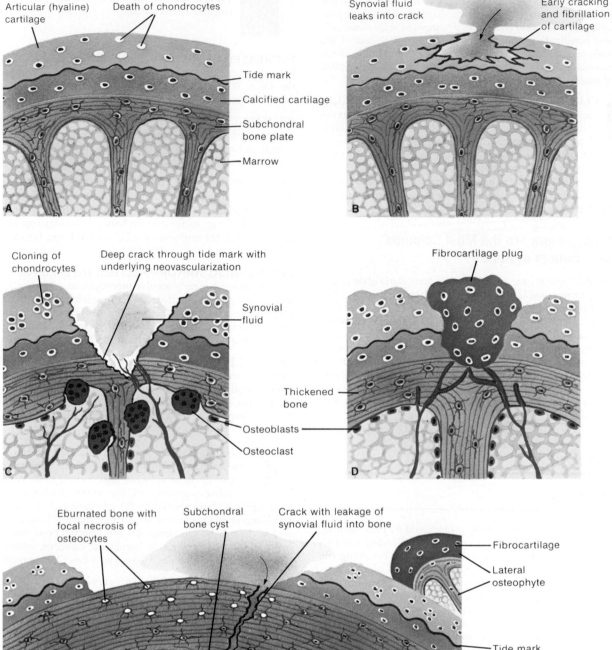

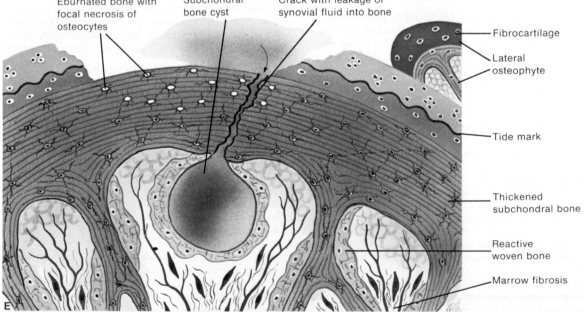

FIGURE 26-26. **Histogenesis of osteoarthritis. A.,B.** The death of chondrocytes leads to a crack in the articular cartilage that is followed by an influx of synovial fluid and further loss and degeneration of cartilage. **C.** As a result of this process, cartilage is gradually worn away. Below the tidemark, new vessels grow in from the epiphysis and fibrocartilage **(D)** is deposited. **E.** The fibrocartilage plug is not mechanically sufficient and may be worn away, thus exposing the subchondral bone plate, which becomes thickened and eburnated. If there is a crack in this region, synovial fluid leaks into the marrow space and produces a subchondral bone cyst. Focal regrowth of the articular surface leads to the formation of osteophytes.

smooth areas of subchondral bone are referred to as **eburnated** (ivory-like) bone.

5. In some areas, the eburnated bone cracks, allowing synovial fluid to extend from the joint surface into the subchondral bone marrow, where it eventually produces a **subchondral bone cyst** (see Fig. 26-27B).

6. An osteophyte develops, usually in the lateral portions of the joint, when the mesenchymal tissue of the synovium differentiates into osteoblasts and chondroblasts to form a mass of cartilage and bone. Osteophytes are pearly grayish bone nodules on the periphery of the joint surface. They may occur at lateral edges of intervertebral disks, where they produce the "lipping" pattern seen on radiographs as osteoarthritis of the spine. In the fingers, osteophytes at the distal interphalangeal joints are termed **Heberden nodes**.

CLINICAL FEATURES: The signs and symptoms of osteoarthritis are functions of the location of the involved joints and the severity and duration of the joint deterioration. The involved joints may be enlarged, tender, and boggy and may demonstrate crepitus. Deep, achy joint pain that follows activity and is relieved by rest is the clinical hallmark of osteoarthritis. Pain is usually a sign of significant joint destruction and arises in the periarticular structures, because articular cartilage lacks a nerve supply. Discomfort is also caused by short periods of stiffness, which is frequently experienced in the morning or after periods of minimal activity. Restricted joint motion indicates severe disease and may result from joint or muscle contractures, intra-articular loose bodies, large osteophytes, and loss of the joint surface congruity.

At present, osteoarthritis cannot be prevented or arrested. Therapy is directed at specific orthopedic conditions and includes exercise, weight loss, and other supportive measures. In disabling osteoarthritis, joint replacement may be necessary.

Rheumatoid Arthritis (RA)

RA is a systemic, chronic inflammatory disease in which chronic polyarthritis involves diarthrodial (synovial, moveable) joints. The proximal interphalangeal and metacarpophalangeal joints, elbows, knees, ankles, and spine are most commonly affected. RA may occur at any age but usually begins in the third or fourth decade, and the prevalence increases until age 70. The disease afflicts 1% to 2% of the adult population and its incidence is greater in women than in men (3:1). Commonly, joints of the extremities are simultaneously

affected, often symmetrically. The course of the disease varies and is often punctuated by remissions and exacerbations. The broad spectrum of clinical manifestations ranges from barely discernible to severe, destructive, mutilating disease.

It is now thought that classic RA comprises a heterogeneous group of disorders. Patients who are persistently seronegative for rheumatoid factor (RF) (see below) probably have disease of a different etiology than those who are seropositive. There are also rheumatoid-like diseases associated with underlying conditions, such as inflammatory bowel disease and cirrhosis.

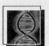

PATHOGENESIS: A number of interacting factors have been implicated in the development of RA.

GENETIC FACTORS: It has been estimated that 60% of the variation in the occurrence of RA in populations is genetic in nature. An important genetic polymorphism that predisposes to RA is present in the HLA II locus. A specific set of HLA-DRB1 alleles containing a pentapeptide sequence motif (shared epitope or SE region), which forms a potential antigen-binding pocket is strongly associated with RA. Evidence suggests that the antigen bound in this pocket is a citrullinated self-peptide produced by postsynthetic modification of protein in the joint space. The presence of RF (see below), antibodies to citrullinated peptide (anti-CP), and severe progressive disease are associated with certain alleles that have lysine (as opposed to arginine) at a specific residue within the SE region. Several non-HLA loci have also been associated with RA, including that of the enzyme responsible for the above-mentioned postsynthetic conversion of arginine residues to citrulline.

HUMORAL IMMUNITY: Immunologic mechanisms are important in the pathogenesis of RA. The SE region is an immune response allele likely to control the response to an as yet unidentified citrullinated peptide. Anti-CP is a highly specific and sensitive indicator of RA. Lymphocytes and plasma cells accumulate in the synovium, where they produce immunoglobulins. In addition, immune-complex deposits are present in the articular cartilage and the synovium. Increased serum levels of IgM, IgA, and IgG are also seen. Approximately 80% of patients with classic RA are positive for RF. RF represents multiple antibodies, mostly IgM, but sometimes IgG or IgA, directed against the Fc fragment of IgG. Significant titers of RF are also found in (1) patients with related collagen vascular diseases, (2) in many nonrheumatic disorders that are associated with chronic inflammation, and also (3) in otherwise healthy elderly persons. Although patients with classic RA

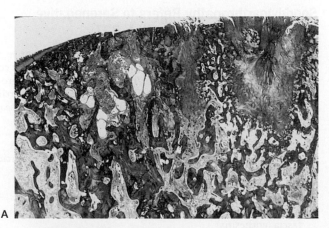

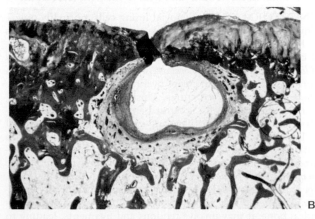

FIGURE 26-27. **Osteoarthritis. A.** A femoral head with osteoarthritis shows a fibrocartilaginous plug *(far right)* extending from the marrow onto the joint surface. Eburnated bone is present over the remaining surface. **B.** A section through the articular surface of an osteoarthritic joint demonstrates focal absence of the articular cartilage, thickening of subchondral bone *(left)*, and a subchondral bone cyst.

may be seronegative, the presence of RF in high titer is associated with severe and unremitting disease, many systemic complications, and a serious prognosis.

CELLULAR IMMUNITY: It has also been postulated that cell-mediated immunity contributes to RA, a contention strongly supported by the role of the HLA class II SE region. T cells may directly or indirectly interact with macrophages through the production of cytokines that inhibit migration and proliferation of the latter. Such cytokines have been found in rheumatoid synovial fluid and in supernatants from rheumatoid tissue explants. These studies provide strong evidence that the joint destruction in RA reflects local production of cytokines, especially TNF and IL-1. In this context, using TNF-blocking agents is useful in the treatment of RA.

INFECTIOUS AGENTS: Infectious bacteria and viruses are not detected in joints of patients with RA, although structures resembling viruses have been reported early in the disease. Most patients with RA develop antibodies against a nuclear antigen (RANA) found in B cells infected with Epstein-Barr virus. Moreover, Epstein-Barr virus is a polyclonal B-cell activator that stimulates production of RF. Interestingly, the blood of many patients with RA has increased numbers of EBV -infected B cells.

LOCAL FACTORS: Synovial cells cultured from rheumatic joints exhibit a decreased response to glucocorticoids and increased production of hyaluronate. These cells release a peptide (connective tissue-activating peptide) that may influence the function of other cells, producing increased amounts of prostaglandins, particularly PGE_2.

SMOKING: Cigarette smoking is a clear risk factor for RF in persons who carry SE1 positive alleles. This appears to be mediated by furthering the production of anti-CP.

Anti-CP and RF have occurred in individuals years before the onset of clinically apparent RA, suggesting that genetic susceptibility factors (such as SE) for the formation of antibodies to CP (and potentially RF) are necessary but not sufficient for RA. Interaction with an environmental agent such as tobacco smoke enhances the production of anti-CP and RF, thereby promoting inflammation within the joint and subsequent T-cell activation, macrophage stimulation, and the intra-articular production of destructive cytokines. Still to be determined is the exact nature of the citrullinated intra-articular antigen, the role of additional factors (such as infective agents), and the pathogenesis of seronegative RA.

PATHOLOGY: The early synovial changes of RA are edema and accumulation of plasma cells, lymphocytes, and macrophages (Fig. 26-28). Vascularity increases, with exudation of fibrin into the joint space, which may result in small fibrin nodules that float in the joint **(rice bodies)**.

PANNUS FORMATION: Synovial lining cells, normally only 1 to 3 layers thick, undergo hyperplasia and form layers 8 to 10 cells deep. Multinucleated giant cells are often found among the synovial cells. *The synovial lining is thus thrown into numerous villi and frond-like folds that fill the peripheral recesses of the joint* (Fig. 26-29A). In this process, the synovium creeps over the surface of the articular cartilage and adjacent structures. This inflammatory synovium, now containing mast cells, is termed a **pannus** (cloak). The pannus covers the articular cartilage and isolates it from the synovial fluid. Lymphocytes aggregate into masses and eventually develop follicular centers (*Allison–Ghormley bodies;* see Fig. 26-29B). *The pannus erodes the articular cartilage and adjacent bone, probably through the action of collagenase produced by the pannus* (see Fig. 26-29C).

The characteristic bone loss of RA is juxta-articular, that is, it is immediately adjacent to both sides of the joint. The pannus penetrates the subchondral bone; it may involve tendons and ligaments, leading to deformities and instabilities. Eventually, the joint is destroyed and undergoes fibrous fusion, termed ankylosis. Long-standing cases may lead to bony bridging of the joint **(bony ankylosis)**.

Rheumatoid Arthritis (RA) is a Systemic Disease Not Confined to Joints

RA is a systemic disease that also involves tissues other than joints and tendons. A characteristic lesion, termed the **rheumatoid nodule**, is found in extra-articular locations. It has a central core of fibrinoid necrosis, which is a mixture of fibrin and other proteins, such as degraded collagen. A surrounding rim of macrophages is arranged in a radial, or palisading, fashion. Beyond the macrophages is a circle of lymphocytes, plasma cells, and other mononuclear cells. The overall appearance resembles a peculiar granuloma surrounding a core of fibrinoid necrosis. Rheumatoid nodules, which are usually found in areas of pressure (e.g., the skin of elbows and legs), are movable, firm, rubbery, occasionally tender, and often recur after surgical removal. A large nodule may ulcerate. These nodules are sometimes found in visceral organs, such as the heart, lungs, and intestinal tract, and even the dura.

CLINICAL FEATURES: The clinical diagnosis of RA is imprecise and is based on a number of criteria, such as the number and types of joints involved, the presence of rheumatoid nodules, RF, anti-CP, and radiographic features characteristic of the disease. The onset of RA may be acute, slowly progressing, or insidious. Most patients describe slowly developing fatigue, weight loss, weakness, and vague musculoskeletal discomfort, which eventually localizes to the involved joints. Diseased joints tend to be warm, swollen, and painful. Unabated disease causes progressive destruction of the joint surfaces and periarticular structures. Eventually, patients manifest severe flexion and extension deformities associated with joint subluxation, which may terminate in joint ankylosis.

The natural history of RA is variable. In most patients, disease activity waxes and wanes. One fourth of patients seem to recover completely. Another fourth remain for many years with only slight functional impairment, whereas half have serious progressive and disabling joint disease. There is increased mortality from infection, gastrointestinal hemorrhage and perforation, vasculitis, heart and lung involvement, amyloidosis, and subluxation of the cervical spine. In fact, survival of patients with active RA is comparable to that observed in Hodgkin disease and diabetes.

Treatment of RA is complex, and the value of early aggressive therapy with disease-modifying drugs such as biological TNF-blocking agents (e.g., infliximab and adalimumab) to minimize joint destruction is being investigated. Anti-inflammatory agents, and in particular glucocorticoids, immunosuppressive drugs (the above-mentioned anti-TNF agents and methotrexate), and so-called remission-inducing drugs (gold salts, penicillamine, and chloroquine) remain the mainstays for therapy.

Spondyloarthropathy Refers to Seronegative Arthritis Mostly Linked to HLA-B27

Spondyloarthropathies include a number of seronegative inflammatory rheumatic diseases for which the strongest single contributing factor is positivity for the HLA B-27 antigen. The group includes ankylosing spondylitis, Reiter syndrome, psoriatic arthritis, and arthritis associated with inflammatory bowel disease. Shared features include:

- Seronegativity for RF and other serological markers of RA
- Association with class I histocompatibility antigens, particularly HLA-B27
- Sacroiliac and vertebral involvement
- Asymmetric involvement of only few peripheral joints
- A tendency toward inflammation of periarticular tendons and fascia (enthesitis)
- Systemic involvement of other organs, especially uveitis, carditis, and aortitis
- Preferential onset in young men

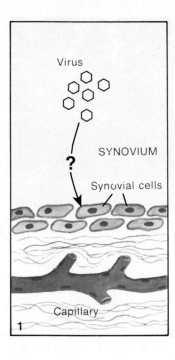

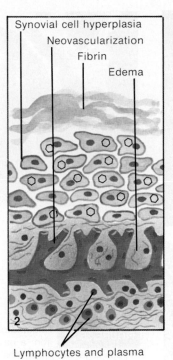

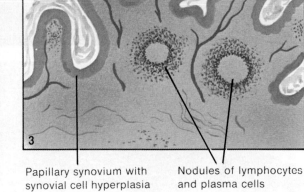

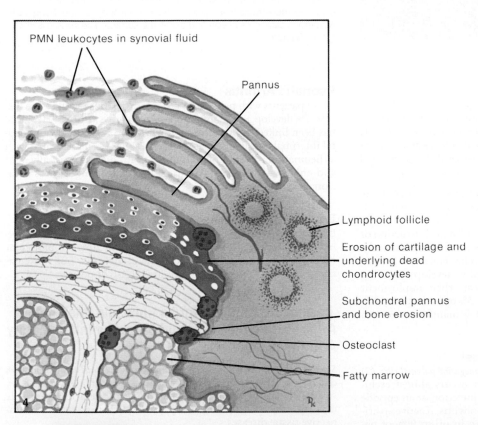

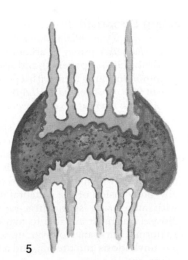

FIGURE 26-28. **Histogenesis of rheumatoid arthritis. 1.** A virus or an unknown stress may stimulate the synovial cells to proliferate. **2.** The influx of lymphocytes, plasma cells, and mast cells, together with neovascularization and edema, leads to hypertrophy and hyperplasia of the synovium. **3.** Lymphoid nodules are prominent. **4.** Proliferating synovium extends into the joint space, burrows into the bone beneath the articular cartilage, and covers the cartilage as a pannus. The articular cartilage is eventually destroyed by direct resorption or deprivation of its nutrient synovial fluid. The synovial tissue continues to proliferate in the subchondral region, as well as in the joint. **5.** Eventually, the joint is destroyed and becomes fused, a condition termed **ankylosis**.

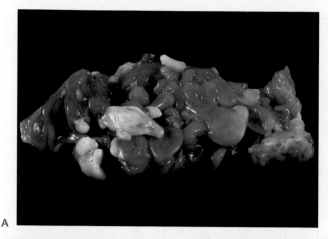

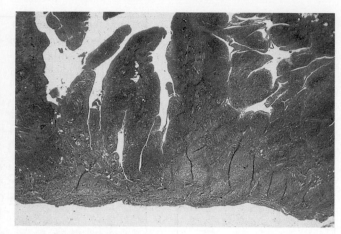

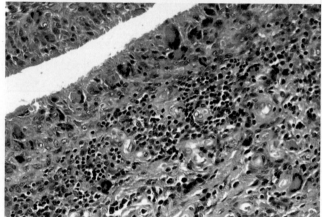

FIGURE 26-29. **Rheumatoid arthritis. A.** Hyperplastic synovium from a patient with rheumatoid arthritis shows numerous finger-like projections with focal pale areas of fibrin deposition. The brownish color of the synovium reflects hemosiderin accumulation derived from old hemorrhage. **B.** A microscopic view reveals prominent lymphoid follicles (Allison-Ghormley bodies), synovial hyperplasia and hypertrophy, villous folds, and thickening of the synovial membrane by fibrosis and inflammation. **C.** A higher-power view of the inflamed synovium demonstrates hyperplasia and hypertrophy of the lining cells. Numerous giant cells are on and below the surface. The stroma is chronically inflamed.

Ankylosing Spondylitis

Ankylosing spondylitis is an inflammatory arthropathy of the vertebral column and sacroiliac joints. It may be accompanied by asymmetric, peripheral arthritis (30% of patients), and systemic manifestations. It is most common in young men, with a peak incidence at about age 20. *More than 90% of patients have HLA-B27 (normal, 4% to 8%), and the disorder affects as many as 5% of individuals with this haplotype.*

 PATHOLOGY: Ankylosing spondylitis begins at the sacroiliac joints bilaterally, then ascends the spinal column by involving the small joints of the posterior elements of the spine. The result is ultimate destruction of these joints, after which the spine becomes fused posteriorly. Eventually, bony fusion of the vertebral bodies ensues. A few patients with ankylosing spondylitis rapidly develop crippling spinal disease, but most are able to maintain their employment and live a normal life span. However, up to 5% of patients develop amyloid A amyloidosis and uremia, and a few manifest severe cardiac involvement.

Reactive Arthritis (Reiter Syndrome)

Reactive arthritis is a triad that includes (1) seronegative polyarthritis, (2) conjunctivitis, and (3) nonspecific urethritis. It occurs almost exclusively in men and usually follows venereal infection or an episode of bacillary dysentery. As in ankylosing spondylitis, reactive arthritis is associated with the HLA-B27 antigen in up to 90% of patients. In fact, after an attack of dysentery, 20% of HLA-B27–positive men develop the disease. The pathologic features of reactive arthritis are comparable to those of RA. More than half of the patients develop mucocutaneous lesions similar to those of pustular psoriasis. In most patients, the disease remits within a year, but in 20%, progressive arthritis develops, including ankylosing spondylitis.

Psoriatic Arthritis

Of all patients with psoriasis, particularly in those with severe disease, 7% develop an inflammatory seronegative arthritis. HLA-B27 has been linked to psoriatic spondylitis and inflammation of distal interphalangeal joints, and HLA-DR4 has been associated with a rheumatoid pattern of involvement. Joint disease is usually mild and only slowly progressive, although a mutilating form is occasionally encountered.

Enteropathic Arthritis

Ulcerative colitis and Crohn disease are accompanied by seronegative peripheral arthritis in 20% of cases and spondylitis in 10%. No particular tissue type is associated with peripheral arthritis, but most patients with ankylosing spondylitis are HLA-B27 positive.

Juvenile Idiopathic Arthritis (Juvenile Rheumatoid Arthritis, Still Disease) Applies to Any Inflammatory Arthritis in Children

Several different chronic arthritic conditions of uncertain etiology occur in children younger than 16 years of age and are included in this designation. In addition to RA, some children with juvenile arthritis eventually develop ankylosing spondylitis, psoriatic arthritis, and other connective tissue diseases.

- **Polyarthritis (RF Positive):** Fewer than 10% of children with arthritis are positive for RF and have a polyarticular presentation. Females predominate (80%), and in most cases (75%), antinuclear antibodies are present. There is an association with HLA-D4, and more than half of the children eventually develop severe arthritis.

- **Polyarthritis (RF Negative):** One fourth of juvenile arthritis patients (90% girls) have disease of several joints, are seronegative, and do not manifest systemic symptoms. Fewer than 15% of these patients eventually develop severe arthritis.
- **Systemic Arthritis:** Twenty percent of children with polyarticular arthritis have prominent systemic symptoms, which include high fever, rash, hepatosplenomegaly, lymphadenopathy, pleuritis, pericarditis, anemia, and leukocytosis but are negative for RF. Most (60%) are boys, and one fourth of all of these children are left with severe arthritis.
- **Oligoarthritis:** Children with involvement of only a few large joints such as the knee, ankle, elbow, or hip girdle account for half of all juvenile arthritis cases and fall into two general groups. The larger group (80%) is mainly girls who are negative for RF but exhibit antinuclear antibodies and are positive for HLA-DR5, HLA-DRw6, or HLA-DRw8. Of these patients, one third have ocular disease, characterized by chronic iridocyclitis (inflammation of the iris and ciliary body). Only a small minority of these children has residual polyarthritis or ocular damage.
- **Spondyloarthropathy:** A small group of children with a pauciarticular presentation is composed almost exclusively of boys, is negative for both RF and antinuclear bodies, and is positive for HLA-B27 (75%). A few patients have acute iridocyclitis, which resolves spontaneously. Some of these boys subsequently develop ankylosing spondylitis.

Gout

Gout is a heterogeneous group of diseases in which the common denominator is an increased serum uric acid level and urate crystal deposition in joints and kidneys. All patients with gout have hyperuricemia, but fewer than 15% of people with hyperuricemia have gout. Gout is characterized by acute and chronic arthritis and is classified as primary or secondary, depending on the etiology of the hyperuricemia. In **primary gout**, hyperuricemia is present without any other disease, whereas **secondary gout** occurs in association with another illness. Of all cases of hyperuricemia, one third are primary, and the remainder are secondary.

 EPIDEMIOLOGY: Primary gout is a disease of adult men; only 5% of cases occur in women. It is rare in children before puberty (other than in uncommon inherited diseases) and in women during the reproductive years. The peak incidence is in the fifth decade. Positive correlations exist between the prevalence of hyperuricemia in a population and mean weight, protein intake, alcohol consumption, and other social variables. Thus, gout is a disease that exemplifies the interplay between genetic predisposition and environmental influences.

 PATHOGENESIS: Uric acid results from purine catabolism. There is a tight balance between uric acid production and the tissue deposition of urates. Uric acid is only eliminated in the urine. Gout can result from (1) overproduction of purines, (2) increased catabolism of nucleic acids due to greater cell turnover, (3) decreased salvage of free purine bases, or (4) decreased urinary uric acid excretion (Fig. 26-30). *A high dietary intake of purine-rich foods, particularly meat, by an otherwise healthy person does not lead to hyperuricemia and gout.*

PRIMARY GOUT most commonly (85%) *results from an as-yet-unexplained impairment of renal uric acid excretion.* In the remainder of patients, there is an overproduction of uric acid, but the underlying abnormality been identified in only a minority of cases. A familial tendency to gout has been recognized since the time of Galen. The consensus today is that multiple genes control the level of serum uric acid and can be associated with gout. Several rare inherited diseases result in gout. Defects in hypoxanthine phospho-

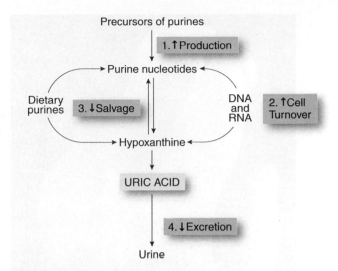

FIGURE 26-30. **Pathogenesis of hyperuricemia and gout.** Purine nucleotides are synthesized de novo from nonpurine precursors or derived from preformed purines in the diet. Purine nucleotides are catabolized to hypoxanthine or incorporated into nucleic acids. The degradation of nucleic acids and dietary purines also produces hypoxanthine. Hypoxanthine is converted to uric acid, which in turn is excreted into the urine. Hyperuricemia and gout result from (1) increased de novo purine synthesis, (2) increased cell turnover, (3) decreased salvage of dietary purines and hypoxanthine, and (4) decreased uric acid excretion by the kidneys.

ribosyl transferase (HPRT, Xq26-27) part of the purine base salvage system, lead to enhanced levels of purine synthesis. **Lesch-Nyhan syndrome**, a rare sex-linked disease, represents a total lack of HPRT and is associated with neurologic dysfunction, self-mutilation and hyperuricemia, with subsequent development of gouty arthritis and obstructive nephropathy. **Kelley-Seegmiller syndrome** is associated with reduced HPRT activity and demonstrates the metabolic effects of hyperuricemia, such as gout and urolithiasis, without the neurological impairment.

SECONDARY GOUT is associated with a number of conditions that result in hyperuricemia. As in primary gout, secondary hyperuricemia may reflect overproduction or decreased urinary excretion of uric acid. Increased production is most often associated with increased nucleic acid turnover, as seen in leukemias and lymphomas as well as after chemotherapy. Ethanol intake leads to secondary hyperuricemia, in part due to accelerated ATP catabolism and (to a lesser degree) decreased renal excretion of uric acid. Reduced urate excretion may result from primary renal disease. Dehydration and diuretics increase tubular reabsorption of uric acid and can lead to hyperuricemia. In fact, various drugs are implicated in 20% of patients with hyperuricemia.

 PATHOLOGY: When sodium urate crystals precipitate from supersaturated body fluids, they absorb fibronectin, complement, and a number of other proteins on their surfaces. Neutrophils that have ingested urate crystals release activated oxygen species and lysosomal enzymes, which mediate tissue injury and promote an inflammatory response. The presence of long, needle-shaped urate crystals that are negatively birefringent under polarized light is diagnostic of gout (Fig. 26-31). A tophus is an extracellular soft-tissue deposit of urate crystals surrounded by foreign-body giant cells and an associated inflammatory response of mononuclear cells. These granuloma-like areas are found in cartilage, in any of the soft tissues around joints, and even in the subchondral bone marrow adjacent to joints. Renal urate deposits may be observed in the kidney between the tubules, especially at the apices of the medulla. These deposits are grossly visible as golden-yellow streaks in the medulla.

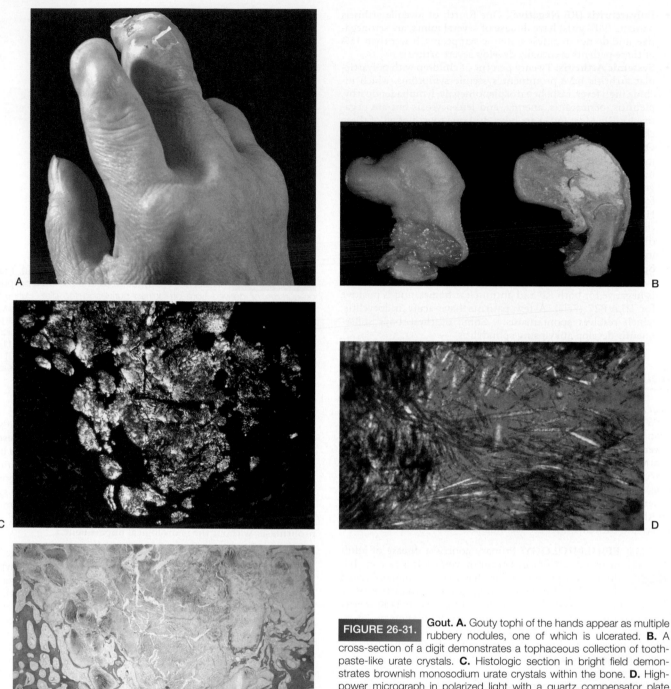

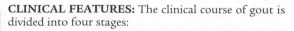

FIGURE 26-31. **Gout. A.** Gouty tophi of the hands appear as multiple rubbery nodules, one of which is ulcerated. **B.** A cross-section of a digit demonstrates a tophaceous collection of toothpaste-like urate crystals. **C.** Histologic section in bright field demonstrates brownish monosodium urate crystals within the bone. **D.** High-power micrograph in polarized light with a quartz compensator plate demonstrates negative birefringence of the crystals (those having their long axes parallel to the slow compensator axis are yellow). **E.** A section through the tophus (if usual aqueous processing is used) demonstrates a foreign body reaction around a pink, amorphous lesion from which the urate crystals have been dissolved in processing.

CLINICAL FEATURES: The clinical course of gout is divided into four stages:

- **Asymptomatic hyperuricemia** often precedes clinically evident gout by many years.
- **Acute gouty arthritis** is a painful condition that usually involves one joint, without constitutional symptoms. Later in the course of the disease, polyarticular involvement with fever is common. At least half of the patients are first seen with an exquisitely painful and red first metatarsophalangeal joint (great toe), designated **podagra**. Eventually, 90% of all patients have such an attack. Even when untreated, acute attacks of gout are self-limited.

- **The intercritical period** is the asymptomatic interval between the initial acute attack and subsequent episodes. These periods may last up to 10 years, but later attacks tend to be increasingly severe, prolonged, and polyarticular.
- **Tophaceous gout** eventually appears in the untreated patient in the form of tophi in the cartilage, synovial membranes, tendons, and soft tissues.

Renal failure is responsible for 10% of deaths in individuals with gout. **Urate stones** are 10% of all renal calculi in the United States and affect up to 25% of gout patients.

Treatment of gout is designed to (1) decrease the severity of acute attacks, (2) reduce serum urate, (3) prevent future attacks, (4) promote dissolution of urate deposits, and (5) alkalinize the urine to prevent stone formation. The main drugs used to interrupt the inflammatory process are nonsteroidal anti-inflammatory agents. Colchicine has been used for hundreds of years and has been administered prophylactically during the intervals between gouty attacks to prevent recurrent episodes. Allopurinol is a competitive inhibitor of xanthine oxidase, the enzyme that converts xanthine and hypoxanthine to uric acid. This drug causes a prompt decrease in uricosemia as well as uricosuria and is used in people with renal insufficiency or those who are resistant to other uricosuric drugs.

Tumors and Tumor-Like Lesions of Joints

True neoplasms of the joints are rare.

Pigmented villonodular synovitis (PVS) is an uncommon benign, but often locally aggressive neoplasm, characterized by exuberant proliferation of synovial lining cells with extension into the subsynovial tissue. The most common site (80%) is the knee, although PVS also occurs in the hip, ankles, calcaneocuboid joint, elbow, and tendon sheaths of the fingers and toes. The lesions of PVS invade the joint and erode the bone. They may insinuate through joint capsules into soft tissue and encompass nerves and arteries, sometimes necessitating radical surgical excision. The synovium develops enlarged folds and nodular excrescences. Microscopically, the tumor is composed of bland mononuclear cells with scattered multinucleated giant cells, in which the nuclei are arrayed peripherally. Hemosiderin-laden macrophages reflect previous hemorrhage. Treatment for PVS is surgical. Radiation therapy produces fibrosis of the proliferating synovial tissue, but amputation is occasionally necessary.

Malignant lesions of the synovium are most commonly metastatic carcinomas, particularly adenocarcinoma of the colon, breast, and lung. Lymphoproliferative diseases (e.g., leukemia) may also involve the synovium, mimicking other conditions, such as rheumatoid arthritis. It is unusual for primary malignant bone tumors to extend into the joint, although they may invade the joint capsule from the soft tissues.

SOFT TISSUE TUMORS

Soft tissue tumors are neoplasms that arise in certain extraskeletal mesodermal tissues of the body, including skeletal muscle, fat, fibrous tissue, blood vessels, and lymphatics. Tumors of peripheral nerves may be included in the category of soft tissue tumors, despite their derivation from the neuroectoderm (see Chapter 28). Soft tissue tumors are rare, accounting for less than 1% of all malignancies in the United States. Benign soft tissue neoplasms are 100 times more common than those that are malignant.

A few important general principles relate to soft tissue tumors:

- Deep, large and rapidly growing lesions are most often malignant.
- Calcification may exist in both benign and malignant tumors.
- Some soft tissue tumors are classified on the basis of genetic or molecular findings.

Tumors and Tumor-Like Conditions of Fibrous Origin

Nodular Fasciitis May be Mistaken for Sarcoma

Nodular fasciitis is a benign but rapidly growing reactive lesion that probably results from trauma and commonly affects the superficial tissues of the forearm, trunk, and back (Fig. 26-32). Most cases occur in adults,

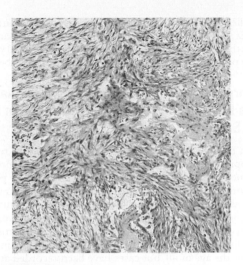

FIGURE 26-32. **Nodular fasciitis.** Swirls of tightly woven uniform spindle cells and collagen are admixed with a few lymphoid cells and vascular channels.

and the lesion's rapid growth usually prompts a patient to seek medical attention. Histologically, nodular fasciitis may be mistaken for a sarcoma, because it is hypercellular and has abundant mitoses and numerous, pleomorphic, spindle-shaped cells. Its true nature is revealed when it is recognized that the entire "mass" is the counterpart of granulation tissue or an exuberant scar in response to trauma. Cytogenetic abnormalities involving an area of chromosome 15 that codes for proteins involved in tissue repair (e.g., FGF-7) and oncogenic proteins have been reported. Nodular fasciitis is self-limited and is cured by surgical excision.

Fibrosarcoma is a Malignant Tumor of Fibroblasts

This tumor typically occurs in adults, although it may be seen in any age group and may even be congenital. Congenital (infantile) fibrosarcoma is associated with a chromosomal translocation, t(12;15)(p13;q26). Fibrosarcomas arise from connective tissue, such as fascia, scar tissue, periosteum, and tendons and are most common in the thigh, particularly around the knee. Macroscopically, the tumors are sharply demarcated and frequently exhibit necrosis and hemorrhage. They are characterized histologically by malignant-appearing fibroblasts (Fig. 26-33), which often form densely interlac-

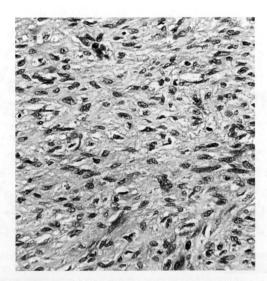

FIGURE 26-33. **Fibrosarcoma.** A photomicrograph demonstrates irregularly arranged malignant fibroblasts characterized by dark, irregular, and elongated nuclei of varying sizes.

ing bundles and fascicles, producing a "herringbone" pattern. The prognosis for high-grade conventional adult fibrosarcoma is guarded; the survival rate at 5 years is only 40% and at 10 years, it is 30%. The prognosis for the congenital form is distinctly better.

Pleomorphic Spindle Cell Sarcoma ("Malignant Fibrous Histiocytoma") is the Most Common Soft Tissue Sarcoma

The term malignant fibrous histiocytoma (MFH) now refers to a microscopic appearance that actually represents a phenotypically heterogeneous group of sarcomas generically termed **pleomorphic spindle cell sarcomas**. The histologic pattern of malignant fibrous histiocytoma/pleomorphic spindle cell sarcoma can be seen in pleomorphic variants of liposarcoma, leiomyosarcoma, rhabdomyosarcoma, myofibroblastic sarcoma, and fibrosarcoma. Collectively, these tumors are the most common sarcomas in patients over the age of 40, but cases have been recorded at all ages. In half of the cases, the tumors arise in the deep fascia or within skeletal muscle and have been reported in association with surgical scars, foreign bodies, and radiation treatment. In general, these tumors have complex cytogenetic abnormalities.

 PATHOLOGY: Adult pleomorphic spindle cell sarcomas are usually unencapsulated gray-white or tan tumors that may have areas of hemorrhage and necrosis. Microscopically, malignant fibrous histiocytoma-like tumors display a highly variable morphologic pattern, with areas of spindle-shaped tumor cells arrayed in an irregularly whorled (storiform) pattern adjacent to fields with bizarre pleomorphic cells (Fig. 26-34). The spindle cells tend to be better differentiated and may resemble fibroblasts. The extent of collagen deposition varies and sometimes dominates the microscopic pattern. The prognosis of adult pleomorphic spindle cell sarcomas depends on the degree of cytologic atypia, the extent of mitotic activity, and the degree of necrosis. Almost half of the patients develop a local recurrence after surgery, and a comparable proportion later manifest metastatic disease, particularly in the lungs. The overall 5-year survival rate is about 50%.

Tumors of Adipose Tissue

Lipoma Closely Resembles Normal Fat

Lipoma is composed of well-differentiated adipocytes and is the most common soft tissue mass. This benign, circumscribed tumor

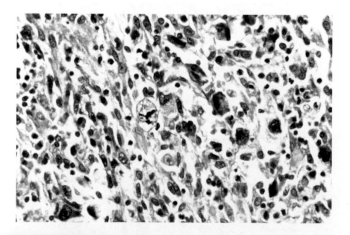

FIGURE 26-34. **Pleomorphic spindle cell sarcoma ("malignant fibrous histiocytoma").** An anaplastic tumor exhibits spindle cells, plump polygonal cells, bizarre tumor giant cells, an abnormal mitosis (*center*), and scattered chronic inflammatory cells. This appearance can be seen in pleomorphic fibrosarcomas as well as pleomorphic sarcomas with other lines of differentiation.

can originate at any site in the body that contains adipose tissue. Most of these tumors occur in the subcutaneous tissues of the upper half of the body, especially the trunk and neck. Lipomas are seen mainly in adults, and patients with multiple tumors often have relatives with a similar history.

 PATHOGENESIS: Numerous cytogenetic abnormalities have been documented in lipomas, but the molecular mechanism is unknown. Some lipomas have no cytogenetic abnormalities and may represent localized adipocyte hyperplasia.

 PATHOLOGY: On gross examination, lipomas are encapsulated, soft, yellow lesions that vary in size and may become very large. Deeper tumors are often poorly circumscribed. Histologically, a lipoma is often indistinguishable from normal adipose tissue. Lipomas are adequately treated by simple local excision. An **angiolipoma** is a small, well-circumscribed, subcutaneous lipoma with extensive vascular proliferation, which usually appears shortly after puberty. Angiolipomas are often multiple and painful.

Liposarcomas are the Second Most Common Sarcoma in Adults

Liposarcomas comprise 20% of all malignant soft tissue tumors. The neoplasm arises after 50 years of age and is most common in the deep thigh and retroperitoneum. Liposarcomas tend to grow slowly but may become extremely large and occur in several subtypes.

 PATHOGENESIS: In the myxoid variant of liposarcoma, most tumors exhibit a translocation between chromosomes 12 and 16 [t(12;16)(q13;p11)], in which the *TLS/FUS* gene on chromosome 16 is fused with the *CHOP* gene on chromosome 12. Well-differentiated liposarcomas are defined by a supernumerary circular or ring chromosome with amplification of the 12q14-15 region, which includes the *MDM2* gene. This gene is involved in the regulation of growth and survival signaling, in part through inhibition of p53 (see Chapter 5).

 PATHOLOGY: Liposarcomas typically measure 5 to 10 cm in diameter, although some measuring 40 cm in diameter and weighing in excess of 20 kg have been encountered. The gross appearance varies, depending on the proportions of adipose, mucinous, and fibrous tissue. Poorly differentiated liposarcomas are grossly similar to brain tissue and display necrosis, hemorrhage, and cysts. Microscopically, myxoid/round cell liposarcoma consists of variably differentiated "signet ring" lipoblasts and variable amounts of primitive round cells embedded in a vascularized myxoid stroma. Well-differentiated liposarcomas are often composed of large amounts of mature fat, and therefore can be confused with lipomas.

Local recurrence and metastases after surgery are common for round cell and pleomorphic liposarcomas, and the 5-year survival rate for these tumors is less than 20%. By contrast, the 5-year survival rate for patients with well-differentiated and myxoid tumors exceeds 70%.

Rhabdomyosarcoma

Rhabdomyosarcoma is a malignant tumor that displays features of striated muscle differentiation. It is uncommon in mature adults but is the most frequent soft tissue sarcoma of children and young adults.

PATHOLOGY: Most cases of rhabdomyosarcoma can be classified in one of four subtypes. Tumors may express nonspecific myoid markers such as actin and desmin, or more specific markers such as the skeletal muscle-specific transcription factors myogenin and MyoD1.

EMBRYONAL RHABDOMYOSARCOMA: This form is most common in children between 3 and 12 years old and frequently involves the head and neck, genitourinary tract, and retroperitoneum. Its appearance varies from that of a highly differentiated tumor containing rhabdomyoblasts with large eosinophilic cytoplasm and cross-striations (Fig. 26-35A), to that of a poorly differentiated neoplasm.

BOTRYOID EMBRYONAL RHABDOMYOSARCOMA: This tumor, also known as **sarcoma botryoides**, is distinguished by the formation of polypoid, grape-like tumor masses. Microscopically, the malignant cells are scattered in an abundant myxoid stroma. Botryoid foci may occur in any type of embryonal rhabdomyosarcoma, but they are most common in tumors of hollow visceral organs, including the vagina (see Chapter 18) and bladder.

ALVEOLAR RHABDOMYOSARCOMA: This neoplasm occurs less frequently than the embryonal type and principally affects individuals between ages 10 and 25; rarely, it may be seen in elderly patients. It is most common in the upper and lower extremities, but it can also be distributed in the same sites as the embryonal type. Typically, club-shaped tumor cells are arranged in clumps that are outlined by fibrous septa. The loose arrangement of the

cells in the center of the clusters leads to the "alveolar" pattern (see Fig. 26-35B). The tumor cells exhibit intense eosinophilia, and occasional multinucleated giant cells are identified. Malignant rhabdomyoblasts, recognizable by their cross-striations, occur less commonly in the alveolar variant than in embryonal rhabdomyosarcoma and are present in only 25% of cases. Most alveolar rhabdomyosarcomas express *PAX3-FKHR* or *PAX7-FKHR* gene fusions, resulting from t(2;13)(q35;q14) or t(1;13)(p36;q14) translocations, respectively.

PLEOMORPHIC RHABDOMYOSARCOMA: The least common form of rhabdomyosarcoma is found in the skeletal muscles of older patients, often in the thigh. This tumor differs from the other types of rhabdomyosarcoma in the pleomorphism of its irregularly arranged cells and can be categorized as one type of adult pleomorphic spindle cell sarcoma. Large, granular, eosinophilic rhabdomyoblasts, together with multinucleated giant cells, are common. Cross-striations are virtually nonexistent.

The historically dismal prognosis associated with most rhabdomyosarcomas has improved in the past 2 decades as a result of the introduction of combined therapeutic modalities, including surgery, radiation therapy, and chemotherapy. Today, more than 80% of patients with localized or regional disease are cured.

Smooth Muscle Tumors

LEIOMYOMA: This benign soft tissue tumor usually arises in subcutaneous tissues or from blood vessel walls. Leiomyomas are painful lesions that appear as firm, yellow, circumscribed nodules. Microscopically, intersecting fascicles of regular smooth cells are evident. Simple excision is curative.

LEIOMYOSARCOMA: This malignant soft tissue neoplasm is an uncommon tumor of adults that typically arises from the wall of blood vessels in the extremities. Macroscopically, leiomyosarcomas tend to be well circumscribed. They are larger and softer than leiomyomas and often exhibit necrosis, hemorrhage, and cystic degeneration. Histologically, the tumor cells are arranged in fascicles, often with palisaded nuclei. Well-differentiated tumor cells have elongated nuclei and eosinophilic cytoplasm and those that are poorly differentiated show increased cellularity and severe cytologic atypia (pleomorphic spindle cell sarcoma pattern). Leiomyosarcoma is differentiated from leiomyoma mainly by a high mitotic activity, which also indicates the prognosis. Most leiomyosarcomas eventually metastasize, although dissemination may occur as late as 15 or more years after primary tumor resection.

Synovial Sarcoma

Synovial sarcoma is a highly malignant soft tissue tumor that arises in the region of a joint, usually in association with tendon sheaths, bursae, and joint capsules. Fewer than 10% of synovial sarcomas are intra-articular. This tumor may also arise in other soft tissue sites as well as in other organs. Although the tumor bears a microscopic resemblance to synovium, its origin from this tissue has not been established. Thus, it is currently considered to be a malignant soft tissue tumor with both epithelial and mesenchymal differentiation. Synovial sarcoma occurs principally in adolescents and young adults as a painful or tender mass, usually in the vicinity of a large joint, particularly the knee.

 PATHOGENESIS: Synovial sarcomas display a specific, balanced chromosomal translocation involving chromosomes X and 18 [t(x;18)(p11.2;q11.2)]. This translocation results in fusion of the SYT (synteny) gene on chromosome 18 to the SSX gene (a transcriptional re-

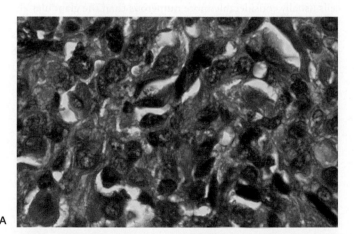
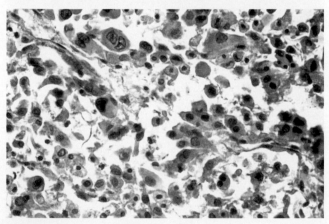

FIGURE 26-35. Rhabdomyosarcoma. A. The tumor contains polyhedral and spindle-shaped tumor cells with enlarged, hyperchromatic nuclei and deeply eosinophilic cytoplasm. A few cells have clearly visible cross striations. **B.** Alveolar rhabdomyosarcoma. The neoplastic cells are arranged in clusters that display an alveolar pattern.

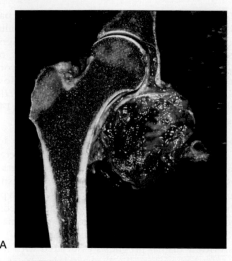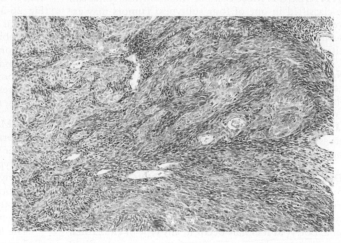

A   B

> **FIGURE 26-36.** **Synovial sarcoma. A.** Section of the upper femur and acetabulum reveals a tumor adjacent to the hip joint and the neck of the femur. **B.** A microscopic view demonstrates the biphasic appearance of a synovial sarcoma. Irregular glandular spaces are lined by plump, epithelial-like neoplastic cells. The intervening tissue contains smaller and darker-staining spindle cells.

pressor) on the X chromosome, leading to production of a hybrid protein, SYT-SSX1 or SYT-SSX2. The **SYT-SSX2** protein is associated with a better prognosis if the disease is localized.

PATHOLOGY: On gross examination, synovial sarcomas are usually circumscribed, round or multilobular masses attached to tendons, tendon sheaths, or the exterior wall of the joint capsule (Fig. 26-36A). The tumors tend to be surrounded by a glistening pseudocapsule and in many instances are cystic. They range from small nodules to masses of 15 cm or more in diameter, and the average size is 3 to 5 cm.

Microscopically, synovial sarcoma is classically described as having a **biphasic pattern** (see Fig. 26-36B). Fluid-filled glandular spaces lined by epithelial-like tumor cells are embedded in a sarcomatous, spindle cell background. These elements vary in proportion, distribution, and cellular differentiation, with the spindle cells usually considerably more numerous than the glandular elements. The recurrence rate of synovial sarcoma is high, and metastases occur in more than 60% of cases. The 5-year survival rate is about 50%, and patients who die usually have extensive lung metastases.

27 Skeletal Muscle

Lawrence C. Kenyon
Mark T. Curtis

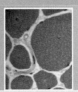
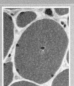
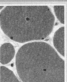
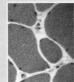

As the skin is our interface with the environment, skeletal muscle is the machine by which we interact with it. Making up about 40% of our weight, skeletal muscle provides the visible conformation of our body. When muscle fails, volitional movement fails, as do other functions critical for life. Respiratory distress and death are a common endpoint for many global diseases of skeletal muscle. Muscle is a molecular transducer that converts metabolic energy into molecular movement and contractile force with a power output per pound that is similar to an electric motor (and not that different from an automobile engine). Hence, many structural and biochemical defects of myocytes at the molecular level result in myopathies.

During development, a characteristic metabolic profile develops for different muscle fibers. Type I fibers (red or slow twitch) are responsible for slower and more prolonged contraction, resist fatigue, and depend on oxidative metabolism. Type II fibers (white, fast twitch) elicit faster and more powerful contractions of brief duration and depend on anaerobic glycolysis for energy. Fiber types in muscle can be distinguished using the alkaline histochemical reaction for myosin ATPase. Type I fibers remain almost unstained at high (alkaline) pH, whereas type II fibers stain darkly (see Fig. 27-1). *In humans, no muscles are composed exclusively of one fiber type.* However, the proportion of fiber types does vary from muscle to muscle. The pattern of fiber types in a given muscle varies between persons, a difference that is apparently genetically determined.

General Pathologic Reactions

Necrosis is a common response of myofibers to injury in primary muscle diseases (**myopathies**). Widespread acute necrosis of skeletal muscle fibers (**rhabdomyolysis**) releases cytosolic proteins, including myoglobin, into the circulation, which may result in myoglobinuria and acute renal failure. In many human myopathies, necrosis occurs in a segment along the length of the fiber, leaving two intact portions that flank the site of damage (Fig. 27-2). The injury quickly elicits two responses: an influx of blood-borne macrophages into the necrotic cytoplasm and activation of satellite cells, a population of dormant myoblasts located in close proximity to each fiber, which will proliferate and become active myoblasts. Within 2 days, they begin to fuse to each other and to the ends of the intact fiber remnants. This regenerating fiber is smaller in diameter than the parent fiber and has basophilic cytoplasm and large, vesicular nuclei with prominent nucleoli.

Regeneration can restore normal structure and function of muscle fibers within a few weeks after a single episode of injury. With subacute or chronic disorders, fiber necrosis proceeds concurrently with fiber regeneration, gradually leading to atrophy of muscle fibers and fibrosis.

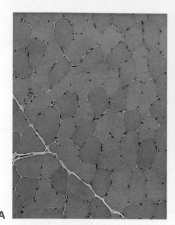
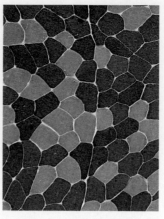

A

B

FIGURE 27-1. **Normal muscle. A.** Hematoxylin and eosin stain. In this transverse frozen section of the vastus lateralis, the polygonal myofibers are separated from each other by an indistinct, thin layer of connective tissue, the endomysium. The thicker band of connective tissue, the perimysium, demarcates a bundle or fascicle of fibers. All of the nuclei in this field are located at the periphery of the cells. Occasional nuclei are contained within satellite cells but cannot be distinguished from those of the myofibers by light microscopy. **B.** Myofibrillar (myosin) ATPase. Type I fibers are pale, at high (alkaline) pH; type II fibers are dark. Note the intermixture of fiber types.

Muscular Dystrophy

Muscular dystrophy is the name applied to primary muscular degeneration, which is frequently hereditary and relentlessly progressive. Muscle tissue from these patients shows necrosis of muscle fibers, regenerative activity, progressive fibrosis, infiltration of the muscle with fatty tissue, and little or no inflammation (Fig. 27-3). Numerous variants of this type of muscle disease have been described, and a classification of hereditary, progressive, noninflammatory degenerative conditions of muscle has evolved.

Duchenne and Becker Muscular Dystrophies are Inherited Noninflammatory Myopathies

Duchenne muscular dystrophy is a severe, progressive, X-linked inherited condition characterized by progressive degeneration of muscles, particularly those of the pelvic and shoulder girdles. It is the most common noninflammatory myopathy in children. A milder form of the disease is known as **Becker muscular dystrophy** (see Chapter 6 for the molecular genetics of both diseases). The serum creatine kinase activity is greatly increased in both conditions.

PATHOGENESIS: Duchenne muscular dystrophy is caused by mutations of a large gene on the short arm of the X chromosome (Xp21) that result in a decrease or absence of **dystrophin**, a protein localized on the inner surface of the sarcolemma. Dystrophin links the subsarcolemmal cytoskeleton to the exterior of the cell through a transmembrane complex of proteins and glycoproteins that binds to extracellular laminin (Fig. 27-4). Dystrophin-deficient muscle fibers thus lack the normal interaction between the sarcolemma and the extracellular matrix.

Becker muscular dystrophy is allelic to Duchenne dystrophy. Mutated dystrophin genes produce an altered, usually truncated, dystrophin molecule, which retains sufficient function to yield a less severe phenotype. *Other dystrophic diseases closely resemble the above dystrophies but are inherited in a recessive autosomal fashion.* Some of these patients have mutations that affect the expression of transmembrane proteins or glycoproteins and interrupt the link

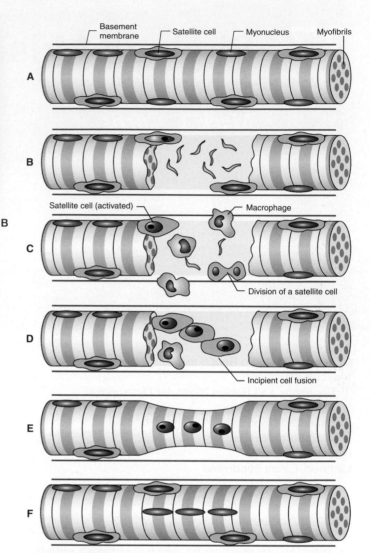

FIGURE 27-2. **Segmental necrosis and regeneration of a muscle fiber. A.** A normal muscle fiber contains myofibrils and subsarcolemmal nuclei and is covered by a basement membrane. Scattered satellite cells are situated on the surface of the sarcolemma, inside the basement membrane. These cells are dormant myoblasts, capable of proliferating and fusing to form differentiated fibers. They constitute 3% to 5% of the nuclei, as observed in a cross-section of skeletal muscle. **B.** In many muscle diseases (e.g., Duchenne muscular dystrophy or polymyositis), injury to the muscle fiber causes segmental necrosis with disintegration of the sarcoplasm, leaving a preserved basement membrane and nerve supply (not shown). **C.** The damaged segment attracts circulating macrophages that penetrate the basement membrane and begin to digest and engulf the sarcoplasmic contents (myophagocytosis). Regenerative processes begin with the activation and proliferation of the satellite cells, forming myoblasts within the basement membrane. Macrophages gradually leave the site of injury with their load of debris. **D.** At a later stage, the myoblasts are aligned in close proximity to each other in the center of the fiber and begin to fuse. **E.** Regeneration of the fiber segment is prominent, as indicated by the large, pale, vesicular, centrally located nuclei. **F.** The fiber is nearly normal except for a few persistent central nuclei. Eventually, the normal state **(A)** is restored.

between the cytoskeleton and extracellular matrix (Table 27-1 and see Fig. 27-4).

PATHOLOGY: The disease process in Duchenne dystrophy consists of (1) relentless necrosis of muscle fibers, (2) a continuous effort at repair and regeneration, and (3) progressive fibrosis.

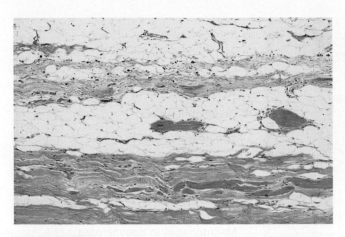

FIGURE 27-3. **End-stage neuromuscular disease.** In this section of the deltoid muscle stained by hematoxylin and eosin, skeletal muscle has been largely replaced by fibrofatty connective tissue. The few surviving muscle fibers have a deeper eosinophilia than does the abundant collagenous component.

TABLE 27-1	
Muscular Dystrophies and Congenital Myopathies Caused by Abnormalities in the Sarcolemma or Extracellular Matrix	
Muscle Disease	**Defective Proteins**
Sarcoglycanopathies	Sarcoglycans α-ε (muscle fiber plasma membrane proteins)
Dysferlinopathies (limb girdle and Miyoshi myopathy)	Dysferlin (muscle fiber plasma membrane protein)
Caveolinopathies (hereditary rippling muscle disorder)	Caveolin-3 (muscle fiber plasma membrane protein)

In the early stage of the disease, necrotic fibers and regenerating fibers tend to occur in small groups, together with scattered, large, hyalinized dark fibers. The latter are overly contracted and are thought to precede fiber necrosis (Fig. 27-5). Macrophages invade necrotic fibers and reflect a scavenging function rather than an inflammatory process. The end stage is characterized by almost complete loss of skeletal muscle fibers (see Fig. 27-3) but relative sparing of muscle spindle fibers (intrafusal fibers).

The diagnosis of Duchenne dystrophy can be established by polymerase chain reaction analysis of genomic DNA in cases where there are large gene deletions. About 30% of patients have small rearrangements or point mutations and can be evaluated by muscle biopsy, which shows little or no detectable dystrophin by immunocytochemistry.

 CLINICAL FEATURES: Boys with Duchenne muscular dystrophy have markedly increased serum creatine kinase levels from birth and morphologically abnormal muscle even in utero. Clinical weakness is not detectable during the first year but usually becomes evident by the third or fourth year, mainly around pelvic and shoulder girdles (proximal muscle weakness). "Pseudohypertro-phy," which refers to enlargement of a muscle by fibroadipose tissue eventually develops in the calf muscles. Patients are usually wheelchair bound by the age of 10 and bedridden by 15. Death most often results from complications of respiratory insufficiency caused by muscular weakness or cardiac arrhythmia due to myocardial involvement.

Myotonic Dystrophy is Characterized by Impaired Muscle Relaxation

Myotonic dystrophy, the most common form of adult muscular dystrophy, is an autosomal dominant disorder characterized by slowing muscle relax-

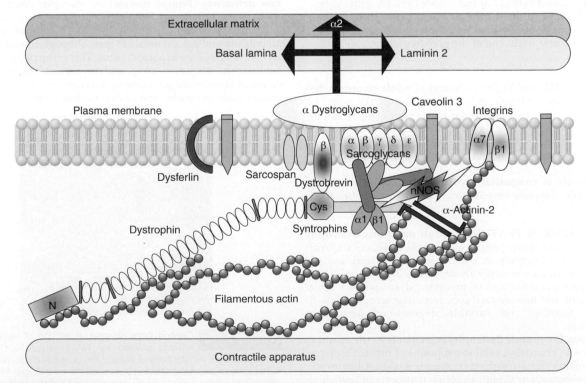

FIGURE 27-4. **Diagrammatic representation of proteins linking dystrophin to the plasma membrane and the contractile apparatus.** Several of these linking proteins are associated with known myopathies (see Table 27-1).

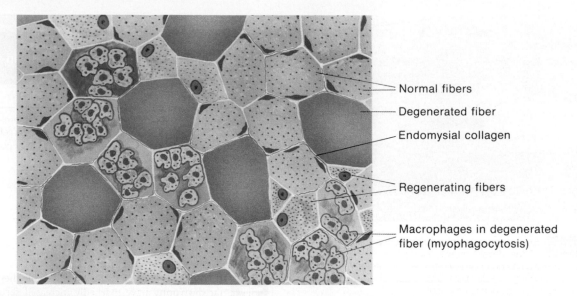

Normal fibers

Degenerated fiber

Endomysial collagen

Regenerating fibers

Macrophages in degenerated fiber (myophagocytosis)

FIGURE 27-5. **Duchenne muscular dystrophy.** The pathologic changes in skeletal muscle are illustrated by staining with the modified Gomori trichrome stain. Some fibers are slightly larger and darker than normal. These represent overcontracted segments of sarcoplasm situated between degenerated segments. Other fibers are packed with macrophages (myophagocytosis), which remove degenerated sarcoplasm. Other fibers are smaller than normal and have granular sarcoplasm. These fibers have enlarged, vesicular nuclei with prominent nucleoli and represent regenerating fibers. Developing endomysial fibrosis is represented by the deposition of collagen around individual muscle fibers. The changes are those of a chronic, active noninflammatory myopathy.

ation (myotonia) and progressive muscle weakness and wasting. The prevalence of the condition has been estimated to be as high as 14 per 100,000. Age at onset and severity of symptoms are extremely variable. Myotonic dystrophy is classified as either adult onset or congenital.

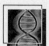

PATHOGENESIS: The gene for myotonic dystrophy has been localized to the long arm of chromosome 19 (19q13.3) and encodes a novel serine–threonine protein kinase. Most cases seem to be descended from one original mutation, the expansion of a CTG repeat near the 3′ end of the gene (see Chapter 6).

PATHOLOGY: The pathology of **adult myotonic dystrophy** is variable, even in muscles from the same person. Most patients display type I fiber atrophy and hypertrophy of type II fibers. Internally situated nuclei are a constant feature. Although occasionally present, necrosis and regeneration are not as prominent as they are in Duchenne muscular dystrophy.

The muscle of **congenital myotonic dystrophy** shows myofiber atrophy, frequent central nuclei, and failure of fiber differentiation.

CLINICAL FEATURES: Adult myotonic dystrophy features slowly progressive muscle weakness and stiffness, principally in the distal limbs. Facial and jaw muscles are virtually always affected; ptosis can be severe. Extramuscular features of myotonic dystrophy are sometimes present and include cataracts, testicular atrophy with diminished fertility, and variable degrees of personality deterioration.

Congenital myotonic dystrophy is seen only in the offspring of women who themselves exhibit symptoms of myotonic dystrophy. The infants are born with severe muscle weakness, but myotonia is inconspicuous or absent, although it appears in later childhood. A significant number of these patients suffer mental retardation.

Congenital Myopathies

Occasionally, a newborn manifests generalized hypotonia, with decreased deep tendon reflexes and muscle bulk. Many of these children have a difficult perinatal period because of weak respiration and consequent pulmonary complications. Some have "malignant" hypotonia, which is progressive and results in death within the first 12 months of life. **Werdnig-Hoffman disease** and **infantile acid maltase deficiency** (**Pompe disease**) are examples discussed below. Other infants have a relatively "benign" course, which persists throughout life but shows little or no progression. Patients become ambulatory and live a normal life span, although secondary skeletal complications of the hypotonia occur. This group of patients is subsumed in the category of "congenital myopathies." Three of the most common forms of congenital myopathies are central core disease, nemaline (rod) myopathy, and central nuclear myopathy (Figs. 27-6,

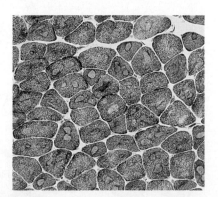

FIGURE 27-6. **Central core disease.** A section of vastus lateralis muscle stained for NADH-tetrazolium reductase shows a distinct circular zone of pallor in the center of most muscle fibers. A thin zone of excessive staining surrounds the core lesion. All of the myofibers in this case were type I, as demonstrated by the myofibrillar ATPase stain (not shown). Note the close resemblance of the core lesions to the target formations found in the muscle fibers of neurogenic disorders.

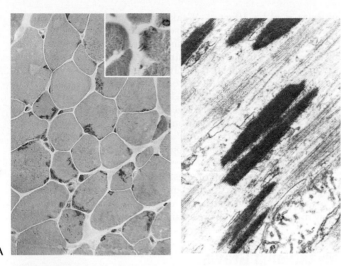

A

B

FIGURE 27-7. **Rod (nemaline) myopathy. A.** Muscle fibers contain dark aggregates of rods and granules (modified Gomori trichrome stain). As shown in the inset, these rods tend to be located at the fiber periphery near nuclei. **B.** An electron micrograph of the same biopsy shows that the structures are rod-shaped and are derived from the Z-disc.

27-7, and 27-8, respectively). Some generalizations can be made about these conditions: (1) they all show congenital hypotonia, decreased deep tendon reflexes, decreased muscle bulk, and delayed motor milestones; (2) in all three conditions, the morphologic abnormality is usually limited to type I (red) fibers. The patients often have an abnormal predominance of type I fibers or possibly a failure to develop type II (white) fibers; (3) the muscle does not show active myofiber necrosis or fibrosis, and patients have normal serum creatine kinase levels.

- **Central core disease:** This autosomal dominant disease results from mutations in the ryanodine receptor gene (19q13.1), the calcium-release channel of the sarcoplasmic reticulum. The disease is characterized by congenital hypotonia and proximal muscle weakness. Muscle biopsy reveals striking predominance of type I fibers, which show a central zone of degeneration (Fig.

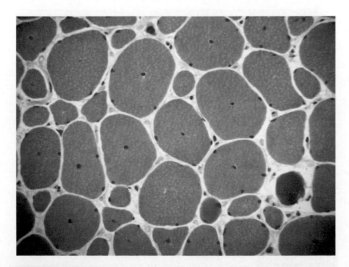

FIGURE 27-8. **Central nuclear (myotubular) myopathy.** Hematoxylin and eosin stain. Many muscle fibers contain a single central nucleus, and most of the affected muscle fibers are abnormally small. In addition, there are radiating spokes emanating from the central nuclei. These fibers resemble the late myotube stage of fetal development of skeletal muscle.

27-6). This central core abnormality extends the entire length of the fiber. Mutations of the ryanodine receptor gene also cause one form of **malignant hyperthermia**, a potentially fatal disorder triggered by surgical anesthesia.

- **Rod (nemaline) myopathy:** Rod myopathy includes a group of diseases that have in common the accumulation of rod-like inclusions within the sarcoplasm of skeletal muscle. (Nemaline derives from *nema*, Greek for thread.) The disease is highly heterogeneous and is caused by mutations in at least five genes (the most common of which is nebulin, a large protein involved in actin polymerization). The classic congenital form of rod myopathy is characterized by congenital hypotonia and delayed motor milestones. Later-onset forms (childhood and adult) tend to be associated with some muscle degeneration, increased serum creatine kinase levels, and a slowly progressive course. The findings on muscle biopsy are variable predominance of type I fibers and the accumulation of rod-shaped structures within their sarcoplasm. The aggregates of these inclusions are often located in subsarcolemmal regions near nuclei (see Fig. 27-7).

- **Central nuclear myopathy (myotubular myopathy):** Central nuclear myopathy (myotubular myopathy) is a group of clinically and genetically heterogeneous inherited conditions that have in common the presence of a centrally located nucleus in skeletal muscle cells. Autosomal recessive, autosomal dominant, and X-linked recessive (Xq28) varieties have been recognized. In X-linked inheritance, newborns are strikingly weak and hypotonic and may die of respiratory insufficiency during the neonatal period. The autosomal dominant form manifests later and is associated with a modest increase in serum creatine kinase levels. The disease progresses slowly. Biopsy specimens show type I fiber predominance (see Fig. 27-8). Many of these fibers are small and round, with a single central nucleus, accounting for the disease's name. In this respect, they resemble the myotubular stage in skeletal muscle embryogenesis.

Inflammatory Myopathies

The inflammatory myopathies are a heterogeneous group of acquired disorders, all of which feature symmetric proximal muscle weakness, increased serum levels of muscle-derived enzymes, and nonsuppurative inflammation of skeletal muscle. Inflammatory myopathies are uncommon, as the annual incidence is 1 in 100,000. Dermatomyositis affects children and adults, whereas polymyositis almost always occurs after the age of 20 years. Both disorders are more frequent in females than males. By contrast, inclusion body myositis usually occurs after the age of 50 years and is three times more common in men than women.

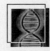 **PATHOGENESIS AND PATHOLOGY:** Although the inflammatory myopathies are thought to have an autoimmune origin, no specific target autoantigens in muscle or blood vessels have been identified. Antinuclear and anticytoplasmic antibodies exist in all of these diseases. The most common morphologic characteristics in the inflammatory myopathies are (1) the presence of inflammatory cells, (2) necrosis and phagocytosis of muscle fibers, (3) a mixture of regenerating and atrophic fibers, and (4) fibrosis.

DERMATOMYOSITIS: Muscle injury in dermatomyositis occurs primarily by complement-mediated cytotoxic antibodies directed against the microvasculature of skeletal muscle tissues. In fact, complement is detectable in the capillaries before inflammation or damage to muscle fibers and is the most specific finding of dermatomyositis. This microangiopathy leads to ischemic injury of individual muscle fibers and eventually to fiber atrophy. True infarcts may result from involvement of larger intramuscular arteries. The rash, which clinically distinguishes dermatomyositis from the other inflammatory myopathies, is presumably related to the same microangiopathy. The combination of perifascicular atrophy and immune complexes in capillary walls is virtually diagnostic of dermatomyositis, even in the absence of inflammation (see Fig. 27-9).

POLYMYOSITIS: In polymyositis, there is no evidence of microangiopathy like that found in dermatomyositis (see above). Rather, healthy muscle fibers are initially surrounded by CD8+ T lymphocytes (Fig. 27-10) and macrophages, after which the muscle fibers degenerate. Unlike normal muscle, muscles affected in polymyositis express MHC-I antigen on the sarcolemma. These findings support an immunopathologic basis for this disorder. The pathogenetic role of autoantibodies present in the disease remains unclear. Inflammatory cells infiltrate connective tissue mostly within the fascicles (endomysial inflammation) and invade apparently healthy muscle fibers (see Fig. 27-10). Isolated degenerating or regenerating fibers are scattered throughout fascicles. Perifascicular atrophy is not present in polymyositis.

Inclusion body myositis: The pathologic features of inclusion body myositis resemble those of polymyositis and consist of single-fiber necrosis and regeneration, with predominantly endomysial cytotoxic T cells. In addition, basophilic granular material is seen at the edge of slit-like vacuoles (rimmed vacuoles) within muscle fibers. The fibers also have small eosinophilic cytoplasmic inclusions, often near the rimmed vacuoles. (Fig. 27-11A,B). The inclusions are pathognomic for the disease and represent a form of intracellular amyloid (see Fig. 27-11C,D) that is immunoreactive for β-amyloid protein, the same type of amyloid present in the senile plaques of Alzheimer disease.

CLINICAL FEATURES: All inflammatory myopathies manifest as insidious proximal and symmetric muscle weakness, gradually increasing over a period of weeks to months. Patients have problems with simple activities that require the use of proximal muscles, including lifting objects, climbing steps, or combing hair. Dysphagia and difficulty in holding up the head reflect involvement of pharyngeal and neck-flexor muscles. Some patients with inclusion body myositis have distal muscle weakness of the limbs that equals or exceeds that of proximal muscles. In advanced cases, respiratory

muscles may be affected. Weakness progresses over weeks or months and leads to severe muscular wasting.

Dermatomyositis is distinguished from the other myopathies by a characteristic rash on the upper eyelids, face, trunk, and occasionally other body surfaces. It may occur alone or in association with scleroderma, mixed connective tissue disease, or other autoimmune conditions. When dermatomyositis occurs in a middle-aged man, it is associated with an increased risk of epithelial cancer, most commonly carcinoma of the lung. Poly-myositis and inclusion body myositis are not associated with malignancy.

Patients with inflammatory myopathies have increased serum creatine kinase and other muscle enzyme levels. Antinuclear and anticytoplasmic antibodies exist in all of these diseases, with specificity to several different antigens. Treatment of polymyositis and dermatomyositis with corticosteroids is usually successful, but inclusion body myositis is generally resistant to all therapy.

Myasthenia Gravis

Myasthenia gravis is an acquired autoimmune disease characterized by abnormal muscular fatigability caused by circulating antibodies to the acetylcholine (Ach) receptor at the myoneural junction. It occurs in all races

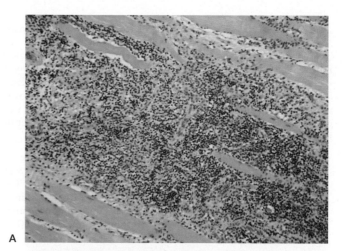

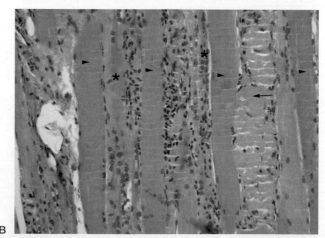

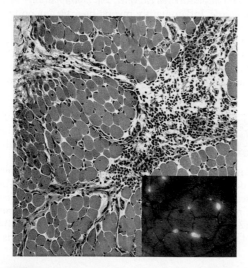

FIGURE 27-9. **Dermatomyositis.** Hematoxylin and eosin stain. The inflammatory cells infiltrate predominantly the perimysium rather than the endomysium. The periphery of muscle fascicles shows most of the muscle fiber atrophy and damage, resulting in a pattern of injury characteristic of dermatomyositis, termed *perifascicular atrophy.* Immunofluorescence *(inset)* reveals that the walls of many capillaries display C5b-9 (membrane attack complex), reflecting the altered microvasculature typical of dermatomyositis. A few small regenerating fibers are also stained by this method.

FIGURE 27-10. **Polymyositis. A.** Hematoxylin and eosin stain. A section of affected muscle shows an inflammatory myopathy. Mononuclear inflammatory cells infiltrate chiefly the endomysium. The field includes single-fiber necrosis. **B.** Region of healing inflammatory myopathy demonstrates intact fibers *(arrowheads)*, necrotic fibers *(arrow)*, and regenerating fibers characterized by enlarged nuclei and basophilic cytoplasm *(asterisk)*.

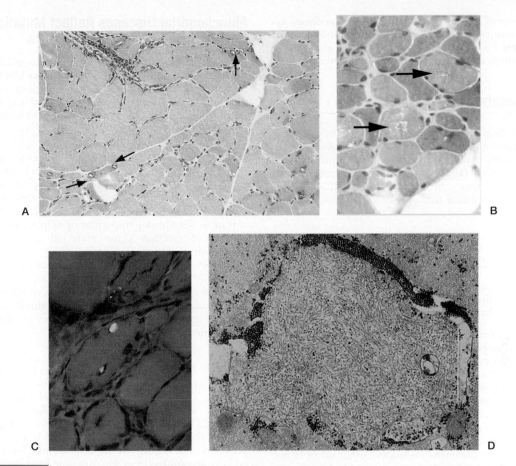

FIGURE 27-11. **Inclusion body myositis (IBM). A.** Hematoxylin and eosin stain. The features in IBM resemble those of polymyositis, but the muscle fibers also exhibit rimmed vacuoles *(arrows)* corresponding to enlarged lysosomes. The hyaline inclusions are sparse and difficult to visualize with this stain. **B.** Modified Gomori trichrome stain shows granular basophilic rimming of vacuoles. **C.** Congo red stain. The inclusion has weak congophilia, but the color signal is strong because it has been enhanced by fluorescence excitation. **D.** An electron micrograph shows the characteristic filaments of the amyloid inclusions.

and is twice as common in women as in men. The disease typically begins in young adults, but cases in children and the very old have also been described.

PATHOGENESIS: Myasthenia gravis is mediated by immunologic attack on the Ach receptor of the motor endplate. Antibodies attach to various receptor protein epitopes, thereby reducing the number of receptors. This antigen-antibody complex binds complement and leads to shedding of the Ach receptor-rich terminal portions of the folds of the neuromuscular junction. Antibody cross-linking leads to a net loss of Ach receptors via endocytosis. The combination of factors impairs signal transmission and causes muscle weakness and abnormal fatigability. The antireceptor antibodies do not, however, directly block binding of Ach.

About 40% of patients with myasthenia gravis have an associated thymoma, and 45% of the remaining patients have thymic hyperplasia. In such cases, thymectomy is often an effective treatment. Ach receptors have been demonstrated on the surface of some thymic cells in both thymoma and thymic hyperplasia. Thus, thymic T lymphocytes may activate B lymphocytes to produce antireceptor antibodies.

PATHOLOGY: The pathologic changes of myasthenia gravis are not marked. A muscle biopsy may reveal atrophy of type II muscle fibers and focal collections of lym-

phocytes within the fascicles. By electron microscopy, most muscle endplates are abnormal, even in muscles that are not weakened.

CLINICAL FEATURES: The clinical severity of the condition is very variable, and symptoms tend to wax and wane as in other autoimmune diseases. Weakness of the extraocular muscles is typically severe and causes ptosis and diplopia. In some cases, the disease may be confined to these muscles. More frequently, it progresses to muscles associated with swallowing, the trunk, and extremities. Patients with myasthenia gravis also have a high incidence of other autoimmune diseases.

The overall mortality rate of myasthenia gravis is about 10%, often because muscle weakness leads to respiratory insufficiency. In addition to thymectomy, corticosteroid therapy, methotrexate, and anticholinesterase drugs are used alone or in combination. Plasmapheresis reduces the titers of anti-Ach receptor antibodies and can ameliorate symptoms, but such clinical improvements are short-lived.

Lambert-Eaton Syndrome

Lambert-Eaton syndrome is a paraneoplastic disorder that manifests as muscular weakness, wasting, and fatigability of the proximal limbs and trunk. Also termed **myasthenic–myopathic syndrome**, the disease is usually associated with small cell lung cancer, although it may also occur in patients with other malignant diseases and rarely in the absence of an underlying malignancy. The disease appears to be autoimmune and results from IgG autoantibodies that target voltage-sensitive calcium channels, which are expressed in motor nerve terminals and in the cells of the lung cancer.

Inherited Metabolic Diseases

Skeletal muscle is dramatically affected by a variety of endocrine and metabolic diseases, such as Cushing syndrome, Addison disease, hypothyroidism, hyperthyroidism, and conditions associated with hepatic or renal failure. The following discussion, however, is limited to primary hereditary abnormalities in the metabolism of skeletal muscle that result in abnormal muscular function.

Glycogen-Storage Diseases are Genetic Disorders that Produce Variable Effects on Muscle

Glycogen-storage diseases (glycogenoses) are autosomal recessive, inherited, metabolic disorders characterized by an inability to degrade glycogen (see Chapter 6).

- **Type II glycogenosis (acid maltase deficiency, α-1,4-glucosidase deficiency, Pompe disease):** Various mutations affect muscle acid maltase activity and lead to distinctly different clinical syndromes, of which Pompe disease is the most severe. It occurs in neonates or young infants who suffer severe hypotonia and areflexia and die of cardiac failure by 2 years of age. Late infantile, juvenile, and adult-onset forms of type II glycogenosis are milder but result in a relentlessly progressive myopathy. In severe cases, muscles show massive accumulation of membrane-bound glycogen, and the myofilaments and other sarcoplasmic organelles disappear with little regeneration. Milder forms of the disease show varying degrees of vacuolar myopathy.
- **Type III glycogenosis (debranching enzyme deficiency, Cori disease, limit dextrinosis, amylo-1,6-glucosidase deficiency):** Type III glycogenosis is a rare, autosomal recessive disease that affects children or adults. The muscle symptoms vary, and the most severe and consistent involvement is related to liver dysfunction in children.
- **Type V glycogenosis (McArdle disease, myophosphorylase deficiency):** Type V glycogenosis is a more common metabolic myopathy, which is usually not progressive or severely debilitating. The deficient enzyme, myophosphorylase, is specific for skeletal muscle, and its lack causes muscles to cramp with exercise. Patients also cannot produce lactate during ischemic exercise, the basis for a metabolic test for the condition. Myocyte changes are subtle if present at all. If patients avoid strenuous exercise, myophosphorylase deficiency does not seriously interfere with their lives, although prolonged vigorous exercise can lead to myocyte necrosis, myoglobinuria, and renal failure.
- **Type VII glycogenosis (phosphofructokinase deficiency):** Phosphofructokinase deficiency is less common than McArdle disease (above) but causes an identical syndrome.

Lipid Myopathies are Caused by Defective Fat Metabolism

Occasionally, a muscle biopsy specimen from a patient with exercise intolerance or muscle weakness shows excess neutral lipids. This occurs in several metabolic disorders that affect lipid metabolism, more than a dozen of which have been identified. In brief, lipid myopathies may involve deficiencies in (1) fatty acid transport into mitochondria (carnitine-deficiency syndromes, carnitine palmityl transferase deficiency), (2) a variety of enzymes that mediate β-oxidation of fatty acids, (3) respiratory chain enzymes, and (4) triglyceride use.

Mitochondrial Diseases Reflect Mutations in Nuclear DNA or Mitochondrial DNA

Inherited diseases of mitochondria are classified genetically into two broad groups, defects of either **nuclear DNA** (nDNA) or **mitochondrial DNA** (mtDNA). Point mutations, deletions, and duplications of mtDNA have been identified and linked to several mitochondrial encephalomyopathies, diseases that affect both the central nervous system and muscle.

 PATHOGENESIS: Genes for most mitochondrial proteins are in nDNA, but mtDNA encodes 13 of the approximately 80 polypeptide subunits of the respiratory chain complexes. Defects in these proteins lead to the mitochondrial encephalomyopathies. In contrast to the Mendelian pattern of nDNA mutations, the diseases of mtDNA show maternal inheritance. Clinical expression of a disease produced by a given mutation of mtDNA depends on the proportion of the total content of mitochondrial genomes that is mutant (see Chapter 6). *The fraction of mutant mtDNA must exceed a critical value for a mitochondrial disease to be symptomatic.* This threshold varies in different organs and is presumably related to cellular energy requirements.

 PATHOLOGY: In skeletal muscle, the pathologic signature of an mtDNA defect is accumulation of mitochondria, excessive numbers of which may manifest as aggregates of reddish granular material in the sarcoplasm. The abnormality has been termed a **ragged red fiber** because of the irregular contour of the reddish deposits at the fiber periphery. The mitochondrial defects cause atrophy of myofibers and the accumulation of sarcoplasmic lipid and glycogen. Death of nerve cells and reactive astrocytosis occurs in the central nervous system.

 CLINICAL FEATURES: Clinical manifestations of the encephalomyopathies vary, but usually begin in childhood. Some patients start with muscle weakness and then develop a brain disorder. Others present with central nervous system disease with or without overt muscle weakness, although muscle biopsy indicates a mitochondrial disorder. Other organs, such as the heart, are often affected as part of a multisystem disorder.

Rhabdomyolysis

Rhabdomyolysis is the dissolution of skeletal muscle fibers and release of myoglobin into the circulation, an event that may result in myoglobinuria and acute renal failure. The disorder may be acute, subacute, or chronic. During acute rhabdomyolysis, muscles are swollen, tender, and profoundly weak.

Occasionally, an episode of rhabdomyolysis may complicate or follow influenza. Some patients develop rhabdomyolysis with apparently mild exercise and probably have some form of metabolic myopathy. After recovery, a subsequent biopsy may reveal muscle that is morphologically normal. Rhabdomyolysis may also complicate heat stroke or be associated with malignant hyperthermia after administration of an anesthetic such as halothane. Alcoholism is occasionally associated with either acute or chronic rhabdomyolysis.

Pathologic changes in rhabdomyolysis are those of an active, noninflammatory myopathy, with scattered necrosis of muscle fibers and varying degrees of degeneration and regeneration. Clusters of macrophages are seen in and around muscle fibers, but these are not accompanied by lymphocytes or inflammatory cells.

Denervation

The pathology of denervation reflects lesions of the lower motor neuron. When a skeletal muscle fiber becomes separated from contact with its lower motor neuron, it invariably atrophies, due to a progressive loss of myofibrils. On cross-section, atrophic fibers have characteristic angular configurations, seemingly compressed by surrounding normal muscle fibers (Fig. 27-12). The early phase of denervating disease is characterized by irregularly scattered, angular, atrophic fibers. As the disease progresses, these fibers are seen in groups, at first in small clusters of several fibers, and later in progressively larger groups (see Fig. 27-12B). Denervated fibers are a mixture of type I and type II fibers: *denervating conditions are not selective for only one type of motor neuron.* If a fiber is not reinnervated, atrophy progresses to complete loss of myofibrils, with nuclei condensing into aggregates. In the end stage, the muscle fibers disappear and are replaced chiefly by adipose tissue.

In a chronic denervating condition, reinnervation of each surviving motor unit gradually becomes larger. As a specific type of lower motor neuron takes over innervation of a given

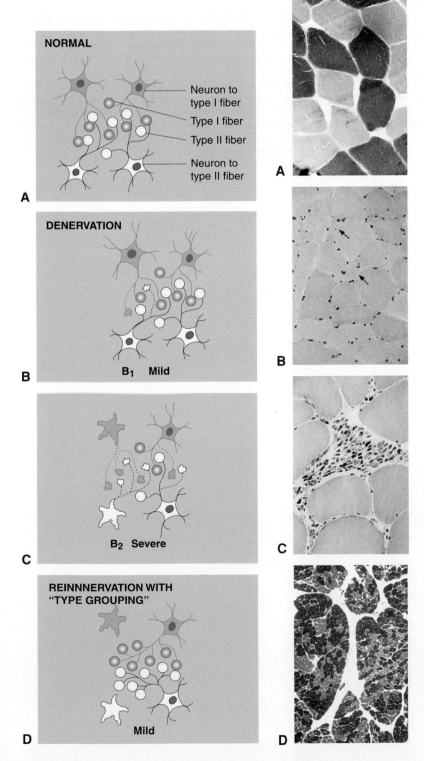

FIGURE 27-12. **Denervation/reinnervation. A.** As shown in the photomicrograph, the normal intermixed distribution of type I (*pale*) and type II (*dark*) muscle fibers is shown by staining for ATPase. In the drawing, two neurons (*red*) innervate type I muscle fibers, and two neurons (*yellow*) supply type II fibers. **B.** Denervation; hematoxylin and eosin stain. With early (mild) denervation (*B1*), portions of the axonal tree degenerate, resulting in angular atrophy of scattered type I and II muscle fibers. With more advanced (severe) denervation (*B2*), entire lower motor neurons or numerous axonal processes degenerate, causing small groups of angular atrophic fibers to appear as illustrated in the photomicrograph. **C.** Reinnervation; myofibrillar ATPase. As neurons degenerate, surviving neurons sprout more nerve endings and reinnervate some of the denervated fibers. These reinnervated fibers become either type I or type II, according to the type of neuron that reinnervates them. This process results in fewer, but larger, motor units and the appearance of clusters of fibers of one type adjacent to clusters of the other type, a pattern called "type grouping." The photomicrograph demonstrates type grouping. This field would appear normal except for a few atrophic fibers if it were stained with hematoxylin and eosin.

field of fibers, fiber groups of one type are seen adjacent to groups of another type. This pattern, called **type grouping**, is pathognomonic of denervation followed by reinnervation (see Fig. 27-12C). Patients with striking type grouping often have symptoms of muscle cramping, in addition to progressive muscular weakness. After a single episode of denervation, such as in poliomyelitis, reinnervation often leads to a remarkable recovery of strength. Years later, a biopsy shows a conspicuous pattern of type grouping, with scattered pyknotic nuclear clumps. In such cases, there are neither angular atrophic fibers nor target fibers.

Spinal Muscular Atrophy (SMA) Reflects Progressive Degeneration of Anterior Horn Cells

SMA is the second most common lethal autosomal recessive disorder after cystic fibrosis. Childhood SMA is classified into type I (**Werdnig-Hoffman disease**), type II (intermediate), and type III (**Kugelberg-Welander disease**). The survival motor neuron gene (5q11.2-13.3) is absent in virtually all (99%) cases of SMA.

WERDNIG-HOFFMAN DISEASE (INFANTILE SMA): *Werdnig-Hoffman disease results in progressive and severe weakness in early infancy, and infants seldom survive beyond 1 year of life.* The denervation seems to begin in utero after the establishment of motor units. The histologic pattern is virtually pathognomonic.

Groups of minute, rounded, atrophic fibers are still identifiable as either type I or type II. There are also fascicles of normal muscle fibers and almost invariably clusters of hypertrophied type I fibers.

KUGELBERG-WELANDER DISEASE (JUVENILE SMA): *This variant is a later-onset form of SMA and is not necessarily progressive.* Muscle biopsies show type grouping and other evidence of a neurogenic disorder but can resemble a myopathy in a small sample because of coexisting necrotic fibers and regenerating fibers.

Type II Fiber Atrophy Resembles Denervation Myopathy

A commonly misinterpreted pathologic pattern in muscle biopsy specimens is atrophy resulting from disuse, wasting, upper motor neuron disease, and corticosteroid toxicity. Pathologically, this diffuse, nonspecific atrophy appears as selective angular atrophy of type II fibers. Type II atrophy is a common condition that is often related to a chronic problem. For example, corticosteroid therapy can cause muscle weakness, and the muscle biopsy shows type II atrophy. In weakness caused by corticosteroid toxicity, patients do not show increased serum creatine kinase levels and histologically manifest selective atrophy of type II fibers, without muscle fiber degeneration and inflammation.

28 The Nervous System

Donna E. Hansel and Renee Z. Dintzis
John Q. Trojanowski and Lawrence Kenyon
(The Central Nervous System)
Thomas W. Bouldin (The Peripheral Nervous System)

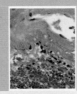

The nervous system is subdivided into central and peripheral elements which together comprise the brain, spinal cord, peripheral nerves, and ganglia. Although both the central and peripheral nervous systems rapidly transmit information, the basic components are somewhat different, as are the diseases and reaction to injury. Hence, the two elements will be discussed separately. Although cognitive, sensory, motor, and autonomic functions correlate with distinct anatomic regions, a defect in any one region may well affect the function of others. The nervous system forms an interconnected network, whose neurons may have axonal extensions that reach for a meter or more. Thus, damage to the body of the neuron may result in a functional deficit at a distant site.

THE CENTRAL NERVOUS SYSTEM (CNS)

Anatomy and Histology

The CNS is composed of five major components, which include neurons, astrocytes, oligodendroglia, ependymal cells, and microglia (Fig. 28-1).

Neurons Relay Information by Forming Networks

Neurons are large cells with a centrally located round nucleus and a prominent nucleolus. The cytoplasm is abundant and demonstrates prominent basophilic granules, termed *Nissl bodies*, which represent ribosome-laden endoplasmic reticulum. Neurons of the substantia nigra and locus ceruleus contain neuromelanin and, therefore, demonstrate a brown appearance (Fig. 28-2).

Signals originate in the cell body of a neuron and are then transmitted along axons to the dendrites of neighboring neurons. Myelination of neurons by **oligodendroglia** (see below) allows a rapid transmission of signals along the length of the axon. Only a small number of neurons are created during adult life, and their numbers decrease with age. This loss may have consequences beyond the cognitive. For example, the propensity for the elderly to suffer subdural hematomas after an injury is likely related to cerebral atrophy and the susceptibility of bridging veins to damage.

Neurons are exquisitely sensitive to injury, with a limited ability to regenerate axons following injury and very little capacity to recover after demyelination. Neuronal injury may manifest in the following ways:

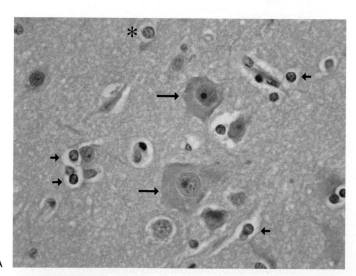

A

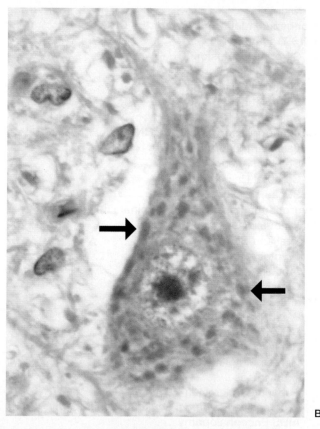

B

FIGURE 28-1. **Brain Cortex. A.** Neurons (*long arrows*) cells are typically pyramidal with a round nucleus and prominent nucleus. Oligodendrocytes (*short arrows*) and astrocytes (*asterisk*) are present. **B.** Motor neuron with abundant Nissl bodies (*arrows*). The granularity of the cytoplasm is imparted by rough endoplasmic reticulum (Nissl substance), but over 95% of the volume of large neurons is invested in its processes (axons and dendrites) which extend for very long distances (~1 m for some motor neurons). Neurons are the most highly asymmetric cells in humans and other mammals.

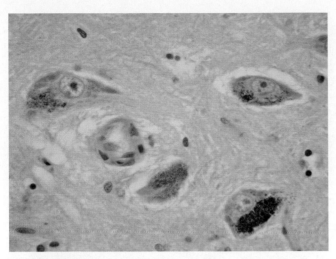

FIGURE 28-2. **Pigmented neurons.** Neurons of the substantia nigra and locus ceruleus are heavily pigmented with neuromelanin.

- **Chromatolysis:** a reversible process that involves neuronal swelling, cytoplasmic expansion, and eccentric positioning of the nucleus (Fig. 28-3).
- **Atrophy:** a reduction in brain volume or weight, evidenced microscopically by hyperchromatic neurons and a decrease in neuronal size
- **Neuronophagia:** phagocytosis of neuronal debris by brain macrophages or microglia
- **Intraneuronal inclusions:** cytoplasmic and nuclear inclusions that occur in certain infectious or neurodegenerative diseases

Astrocytes Function in the Response of the CNS to Injury

Astrocytes are glial cells of the CNS that serve a supportive and signaling role and function in the CNS response to injury (Fig. 28-4). These cells have a star-shaped appearance and contain a round nucleus with homogenous chromatin. Some astrocytes terminate their foot processes on blood vessels and may assist in the maintenance of the blood-brain barrier. Astrocytes can be identified with

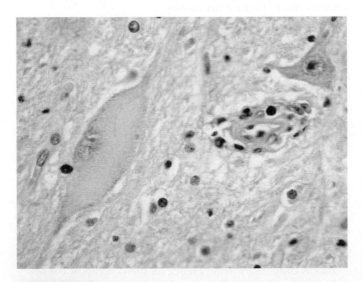

FIGURE 28-3. **Chromatolysis.** An injured neuron (*left*) appears swollen with pale cytoplasm, eccentric nucleus, and marginated Nissl substance near the plasma membrane. Compare to normal neuron at upper right.

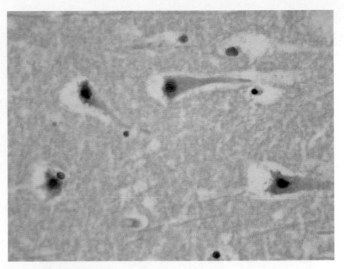

FIGURE 28-4. **Acute neuronal injury.** Injured neurons are pyknotic with hypereosinophilic cytoplasm.

a stain for glial fibrillary acidic protein (GFAP; Fig. 28-5A). Following injury, astrocytes proliferate locally and increase cytoplasmic GFAP synthesis. The cells are characterized by an eosinophilic cytoplasm and are termed **gemistocytic astrocytes** (Fig. 28-5B). Local proliferation and enhancement of the function of astrocytes leads to *gliosis* (the formation of a glial scar). Astrocytes are also responsible for the formation of amorphous, basophilic, rounded structures called **corpora amylacea**, which are aggregates of carbohydrates and proteins accumulated with normal aging. Finally, astrocytes may undergo neoplastic transformation to form **astrocytomas** (see below).

Oligodendroglia are Glial Cells Responsible for Myelin Formation

Oligodendroglia are glial cells that synthesize the myelin that surrounds axons. These cells have a small, dark, round nucleus and a thin rim of cytoplasm (see Fig. 28-1A), and are situated as satellites around neurons in the gray matter and longitudinally between myelinated fibers in the white matter. They can undergo neoplastic transformation to form **oligodendrogliomas** and are involved in **demyelinating disease** (see below).

Ependymal Cells Regulate Cerebrospinal Fluid (CSF) Transfer

Ependymal cells are glial cells that regulate the fluid transfer between the CSF and the CNS. These cells which form a single layer of cuboidal or flat cells, line the ventricular system, including the ventricular chambers, aqueduct of Sylvius, the central canal of the spinal cord, and the filium terminale. Ependymal cells can undergo malignant transformation to form **ependymomas** (see below).

Microglia are the Phagocytic Cells of the CNS

Microglia contain hyperchromatic, elongated nuclei and a thin rim of cytoplasm elaborated into fine processes, which are similar in appearance to antigen presenting dendritic cells (see Chapter 4). Following injury, the proliferation of microglia results in diffuse **gliosis** and in the formation of **microglial nodules** (aggregates of microglia and astrocytes seen predominantly in protozoal, rickettsial, and viral disease and near necrotic neurons) (Fig. 28-6). The intracellular accumulation of cellular debris and lipids (such as myelin) by microglia and other macrophage-like cells

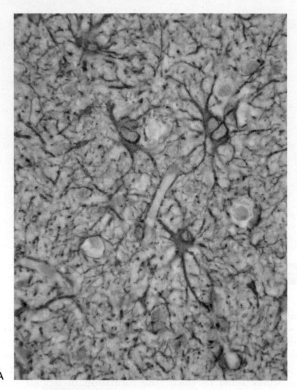

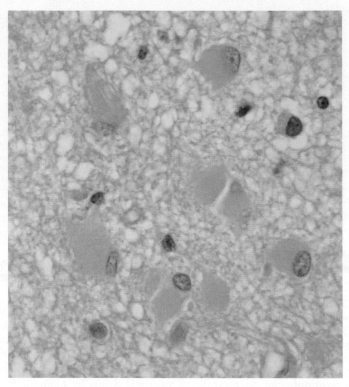

A

B

FIGURE 28-5. **Astrocytes. A.** The glial processes of astrocytes stain intensely for glial fibrillary acidic protein (GFAP). **B.** Hematoxylin and eosin (H&E)-stained reactive astrocytes are plump with pink cytoplasm (gemistocytic astrocytes).

leads to the formation of **gitter cells**, which are similar to the foamy macrophages seen outside of the CNS.

Congenital Malformations of the CNS

Specific congenital malformations may often have multiple potential causes, and an identical insult may result in different malformations, depending on the developmental stage of the fetus. The pathogenesis and clinical aspects of congenital malformations involving the neural tube and spinal cord are presented in Table 28-1. **Dysraphic defects** that feature delayed or defective closure

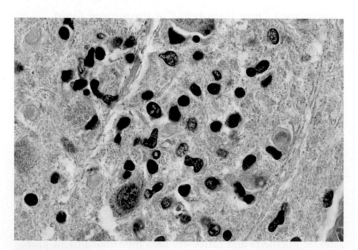

FIGURE 28-6. **Microglial nodule.** Microglia and astrocytes create cellular nodules in response to viral, protozoan, or rickettsial infections.

of the dorsal aspect of the neural tube are summarized in Figure 28-7.

*Epilepsy is defined as paroxysmal, transient disturbances in brain function, which are termed **seizures**.* It may occur in association with underlying congenital abnormalities or in association with a variety of other CNS disorders, such as intracranial tumors or arteriovenous malformations. Epilepsy has a prevalence of 6 per 1,000 people, and the majority of cases are idiopathic. Microscopically, the brains of patients with epilepsy often demonstrate focal gliosis (glial scarring), although it is unclear whether this represents a cause or effect of the seizure activity.

CNS Trauma

Trauma may result in a variety of intracranial hemorrhages, direct damage (penetrating trauma), or paralysis (spinal cord injuries). Table 28-2 compares the different types of intracranial hemorrhages.

Cerebral Contusion Results from Brain Trauma

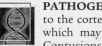 **PATHOGENESIS:** A contusion describes damage to the cortex in the form of a bruise or laceration, which may be associated with the hemorrhage. Contusions occur when a rapid anteroposterior displacement of the brain occurs, such as when the skull strikes an object and is subjected to rapid, sudden deceleration. A **coup** injury (from French for blow) occurs at the site of impact, whereas a **contrecoup** injury is contralateral to the site of initial injury (Fig. 28-8). The velocity of the acceleration and the abruptness of the deceleration of the head medi-

Table 28–1

Congenital Malformations of the Central Nervous System

Malformation	Pathogenesis	Findings
Neural tube defects		
Spina bifida	Failure of dorsal neural tube closure, hypervitaminosis A or folic acid deficiency	Most common congenital malformation and most frequently affects the dorsal lumbosacral region of the vertebral column. Severe forms of spina bifida may show sensory loss, lower limb paralysis, and incontinence.
Spina bifida occulta		Vertebral arch defect with external dimple or tuft of hair
Meningocele		Protrusion of meninges as fluid-filled sac; apical ulceration
Meningomyelocele		Exposed spinal canal; nerve roots trapped in scar tissue
Rachischisis		Spinal column appears as gaping canal often without recognizable spinal cord
Anencephaly	Possible failure of anterior neuropore closure or abnormal angiogenesis	Congenital absence of all or part of the brain and cranial vault; cerebrum is a highly vascularized, poorly differentiated structure; hypoplastic upper spinal cord
Spinal cord malformations		
Hydromyelia		Dilation of the central canal of the spinal cord
Syringomyelia	Occasionally trauma, ischemia, tumors	Tubular cavitation extends along the length of the spinal cord; may not communicate with central canal; filled with clear fluid; may cause sensory/motor deficits
Arnold-Chiari malformation	Increased intracranial pressure or possible tethering of cord by meningomyelocele	Caudal aspect of cerebellar vermis herniates through wide foramen magnum to level C3 to C5; beaking of quadrigeminal plate, inferior colliculus; caudally displaced brainstem; hydrocephalus
Congenital hydrocephalus	Congenital atresia of the aqueduct of Sylvius; viruses; many others	Ventricular enlargement
Cerebral gyri disorders		
Polymicrogyria		Small and excessive gyri; MR
Pachygyria		Reduced number of gyri; very broad gyri; MR
Lissencephaly	Neuronal migration defect	Smooth cortical surface; MR
Heterotopias	Neuronal migration defect	Ectopic nerve and glia, often in white matter, MR
Chromosomal abnormalities		
Down syndrome	Trisomy 21	MR, distinctive facial features, reduced brain weight; slender superior temporal gyri
Trisomy 13-15	Trisomy 13-15	Holoprosencephaly (absent interhemispheric fissure), arrhinencephaly (absence of olfactory tracts), absence of corpus callosum; cyclopia, cleft palate, plydactyly, "rocker bottom" feet

MR, mental retardation.

From Hansel DE, Dintzis RZ. Lippincott's Pocket Pathology. Baltimore: Lippincott Williams & Wilkins, 2006:844.

ate the severity of a contusion. Mild contusions result in cortical bruising (local hemorrhage), whereas severe contusions may cause deep cavitary lesions within the brain that extend into the white matter and product a mass effect (see below). Contusions may be life-threatening if complicated by edema and hemorrhage, which predispose to transtentorial herniation. *A **concussion** is a transient loss of consciousness due to trauma that causes a rapid torque on the brainstem, leading to a paralysis of neurons of the reticular formation.* The term concussion should not be confused with cerebral contusions.

 PATHOLOGY: The foci of necrotic brain tissue and extravasated red blood cells formed by a contusion are phagocytosed by macrophages. Hemosiderin laden macrophages and reactive astrocytes persist indefinitely

as a glial scar. In addition, diffuse axonal shearing injuries, which occur in the context of a contusion, are identified microscopically by **axonal spheroids** (ends of severed axons that retract) and multiple small hemorrhages.

Epidural Hematoma Results from Bleeding Between the Skull and Dura

PATHOGENESIS: Trauma to the temporal bone may result in transection of the middle meningeal artery, which is situated between the calvaria and dura. Damage to this artery causes a progressive accumulation of blood within the epidural space, termed an *epidural hematoma* (Fig. 28-9).

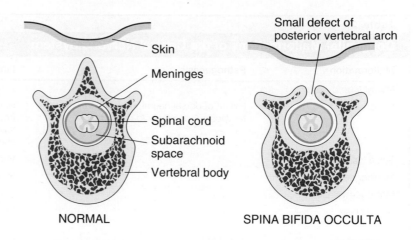

Skin

Menges

Spinal cord

Subarachnoid space

Vertebral body

NORMAL

Small defect of posterior vertebral arch

SPINA BIFIDA OCCULTA

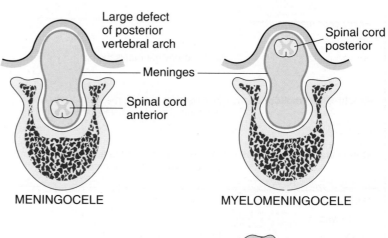

Large defect of posterior vertebral arch

Meninges

Spinal cord anterior

MENINGOCELE

Spinal cord posterior

Meninges

MYELOMENINGOCELE

Neural groove (no meninges)

SPINA BIFIDA

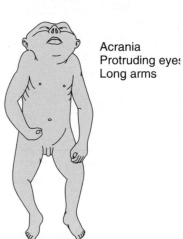

Acrania
Protruding eyes
Long arms

ANENCEPHALY

FIGURE 28-7. **Dysraphic defects of the neural tube.** Incomplete fusion of the neural tube and overlying bone, soft tissues, or skin leads to several defects, varying from mild anomalies (e.g., spina bifida occulta) to severe anomalies (e.g., anencephaly).

PATHOLOGY AND CLINICAL COURSE: Within the first 4 to 8 hours, patients are often asymptomatic; however, when a critical volume of 30 to 50 mL collects within the epidural space, patients demonstrate symptoms of a space-occupying lesion. As the hematoma enlarges, the large venous sinuses are compressed, leading to global cerebral hypoxia, ischemia, and confusion. In response to such injury, patients may demonstrate a *Cushing reflex*, which is an attempt to increase cerebral blood flow and oxygen delivery by slowing the heart rate (increased ventricular filling), increasing myocardial contraction, and increasing blood pressure. If epidural hematomas are left untreated, they can cause **transtentor-ial herniation**, defined as displacement of the midbrain through the tentorial opening (Fig. 28-10). This effect is evidenced by a fixed and dilated pupil on the side of the lesion and unconsciousness, as well as midbrain ischemia and necrosis. If untreated, an epidural hematoma is likely to be fatal within 24 to 48 hours.

Subdural Hematoma Occurs in the Context of Frontal or Occipital Trauma

Subdural hematoma *refers to hemorrhage in the frontal or occipital regions of the head that causes a rapid displacement of the cerebral hemispheres against the inner aspect of the skull, such as in falls, assaults, or car accidents.*

Table 28-2

Comparison of Intracranial Hemorrhages

	Epidural	Subdural	Subarachnoid
Vessel	Middle meningeal artery	Bridging vein	Arterial aneurysm
Injury	Temporal	Frontal/occipital	Variable/none
Time course	Rapid	Moderate/slow	Rapid
Bilateral	Rare	Common	Rare
Blood in CSF	No	No	Yes
Early symptom	None	Headache	Severe headache

From Hansel DE, Dintzis RZ. Lippincott's Pocket Pathology. Baltimore: Lippincott Williams & Wilkins, 2006:846.

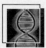 **PATHOGENESIS:** Trauma can cause a shearing effect on the bridging veins within the subdural space, leading to the formation of a subdural hematoma (see Fig. 28-9). Although the subdural space can expand, most commonly blood accumulates to a volume of 25 to 50 mL, resulting in a tamponade effect on the ruptured bridging veins (Fig. 28-11). However, in some cases, venous thrombosis and ischemia may develop in the bridging veins. Subdural hematomas may be bilateral, owing to the nature of the injury.

  PATHOLOGY AND CLINICAL COURSE: Patients with subdural hematomas may demonstrate headaches, contralateral weakness, seizures, or lack demonstrable symptoms. Bilateral hematomas may result in impaired cognitive function. The outcome of subdural hematomas is variable. During the first several weeks, subdural hematomas develop overlying granulation tissue, secondary to irritation between the hematoma and dura. Over time, the hematoma may resolve, remain static, or enlarge. Lesions that resolve contain only microscopic foci of hemosiderin-ladin macrophages. Hematomas that remain static

demonstrate a residual hematoma and occasionally calcification. Lesions that expand do so sporadically, often within 6 months of initial injury.

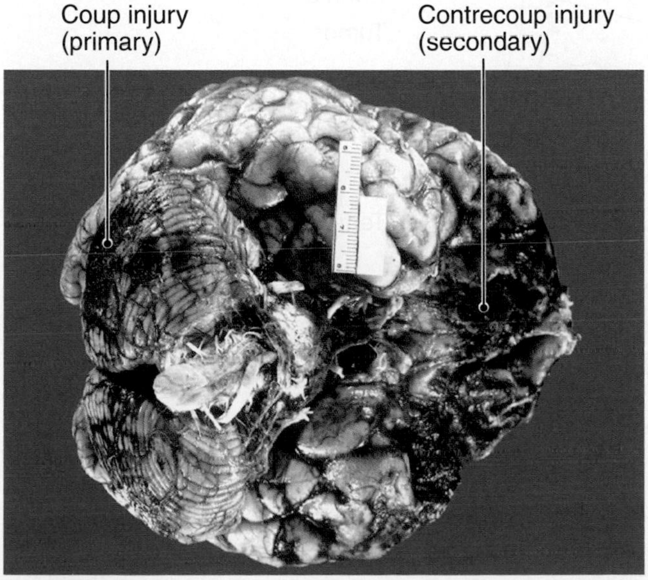

Subarachnoid Hemorrhage Often Occurs in the Circle of Willis

Subarachnoid hemorrhage may occur following trauma or rupture of a berry aneurysm in the Circle of Willis, as well as in instances of vasculitis and tumors (Fig. 28-12). It produces a sudden severe headache and photophobia, owing to meningeal irritation, which may be followed by coma. Often, patients experience a progressive decline in consciousness if they survive the initial hemorrhage. A subarachnoid bleed may be diagnosed by the presence of blood within the CSF when performing a lumbar puncture.

Spinal Cord Injuries Often Result from Trauma

The spinal cord may be injured by penetrating wounds, fractures of the vertebrae, hyperextension, or hyperflexion. Damage to the spinal cord often extends to levels above and below the point of original injury.

- **Hyperextension injury:** rapid posterior displacement of the head tears the anterior spinal ligament, an event that displaces the posterior spinal cord against the posterior process of the vertebral body.
- **Hyperflexion injury:** the head is driven forcefully forward and downward, resulting in a fracture of the underlying vertebral body and injury to the anterior spinal cord.

Injury to the spinal cord may result in concussion, contusion, or transection of the spinal cord, which can lead to **paraplegia** (paralysis of the lower body and extremities) or **quadriplegia** (paralysis of all four limbs).

Circulatory Disorders of the CNS

Vascular Malformations are Congenital Lesions Present in the CNS

Vascular malformations vary in location and histology. They may be asymptomatic or present with a variety of symptoms, including seizures and death when associated with bleeding. Specific malformations include the following:

- **Arteriovenous malformation:** most common congenital malformation, composed of anastomosing, abnormally thick-walled arteries and veins, which can enlarge over time; arteriovenous malformations increase the risk of seizures and intracranial hemorrhage (Fig. 28-13).

Coup injury (primary)   Contrecoup injury (secondary)

FIGURE 28-8. **Coup and contrecoup injuries.** This patient received a primary blow (the *coup injury*) to the back of the head (occiput). At the opposite (frontal) side of the skull is a more severe contusion in the frontal lobes (the *contrecoup* injury).

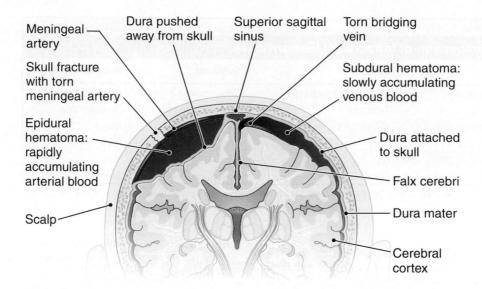

FIGURE 28-9. **Epidural and subdural hematomas.** Bleeding in epidural hematoma is rapid because of skull fracture and severance of a meningeal artery. Bleeding in subdural hematoma is slow and results from tearing of veins that extend across the subdural (subarachnoid) space.

- **Cavernous angioma:** large, irregular, thin-walled vascular channels, which are often asymptomatic
- **Telangiectasia:** focal aggregates of uniformly small vessels which may cause seizures
- **Venous angioma:** a focus of a few enlarged veins, which is often asymptomatic

Cerebral Aneurysms Result from Congenital Lesions and Intravascular Pressure

Cerebral aneurysms may be caused by developmental defects of the arterial wall, hypertension, atherosclerosis, bacterial infection, or trauma.

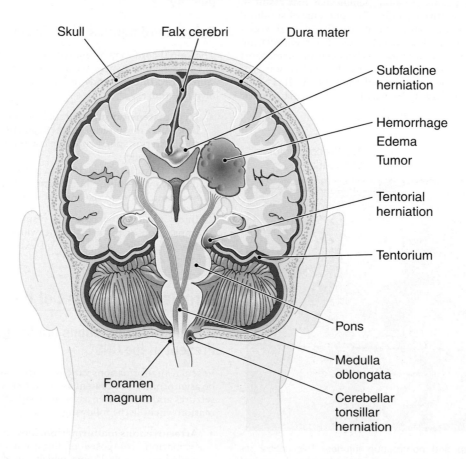

FIGURE 28-10. **Brain herniations.** Brain edema and intracranial tumor or hemorrhage are the usual causes.

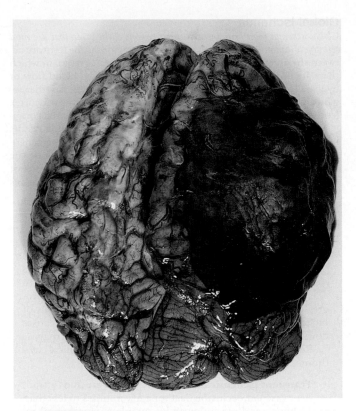

FIGURE 28-11. **Subdural hematoma.** The right hemisphere exhibits a large collection of blood in the subdural space, owing to rupture of the bridging veins.

Berry Aneurysms

PATHOGENESIS AND PATHOLOGY: Berry (saccular) aneurysms are most likely caused by a developmental defect in the arterial muscle at points of bifurcation, resulting in an arterial wall composed only of endothelium, an internal elastic lamina and an adventitia. Intravascular pressure at this site leads to expansion and potential rupture of the aneurysm. The most common sites of berry aneurysms are demonstrated in Figure 28-14. In 20% of cases, multiple berry aneurysms occur. These aneurysms may be associated with other inherited disease, most notably adult polycystic kidney disease (see Chapter 16).

CLINICAL FEATURES: Rupture of a berry aneurysm results in life-threatening subarachnoid hemorrhage and occasionally intracerebral or intraventricular hemorrhage as well. The initial rupture is lethal in about one third of patients. Those who survive the initial event may develop a progressive decline in consciousness secondary to arterial spasm and ischemia or aneurysmal rebleeding.

Atherosclerotic Aneurysms and Mycotic Aneurysms

Atherosclerotic aneurysms are situated primarily in large cerebral arteries (usually internal carotid and vertebral) and are caused by fibrous replacement of the media and destruction of the internal elastic membrane of the arterial wall, as detailed in Chapter 10. *These aneurysms most commonly result in thrombosis rather than rupture.* **Mycotic aneurysms** result from septic emboli that originate in infected cardiac valves and can cause arterial rupture, cerebral abscess, or meningitis.

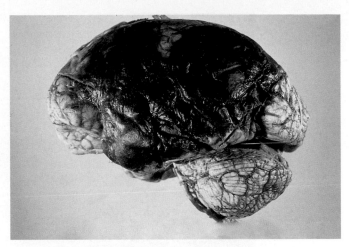

FIGURE 28-12. **Subarachnoid hemorrhage.** The subarachnoid space contains a large amount of blood secondary to rupture of an aneurysm.

Cerebral Hemorrhage is Most Often Associated with Hypertension

Spontaneous cerebral hemorrhage generally occurs as a consequence of longstanding hypertension. With persistent hypertension, the walls of arterioles undergo lipid deposition and hyaline change (lipohyalinosis), followed by fibrinoid necrosis, which weakens the wall and leads to so-called **Charcot-Bouchard** aneurysms. Formation and rupture of these aneurysms occurs most commonly along the trunk of the vessel, rather than at points of bifurcation, and most commonly affects the following:

- Basal ganglia-thalamus (65%)
- Pons (15%)
- Cerebellum (8%)

Rupture of a Charcot-Bouchard aneurysm leads to **cerebral hemorrhage (hemorrhagic stroke)** that can cause progressive neurological symptoms, especially weakness and possibly death. Occasionally, hemorrhage may extend into the ventricular system **(intraventricular hemorrhage)**, which may produce distention of the fourth ventricle and compression of the medulla. **Pontine hemorrhage** may damage the reticular system, leading to loss of consciousness. **Cerebellar hemorrhage** may produce abrupt ataxia, occipital headache, and vomiting; an expanding hemor-

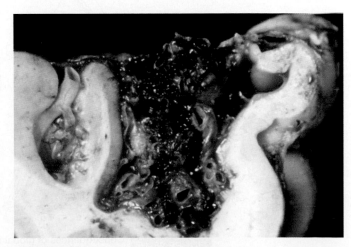

FIGURE 28-13. **Arteriovenous malformation.** A disorganized collection of arteries and veins is seen within the substance of the brain.

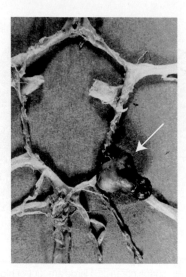

FIGURE 28-14. **Berry aneurysm.** A saccular aneurysm (*arrow*) arises from the posterior cerebral artery.

rhage may encroach on the medulla or produce cerebellar herniation through the foramen magnum by mass effect.

Stroke is Most Often Associated with Cerebral Ischemia and Infarction

Globally decreased oxygenation of the brain caused by hypoxia (near-drowning, carbon-monoxide poisoning, suffocation) or generalized decreased blood flow (cardiac arrest, external hemorrhage) may lead to diffuse (global) ischemia of the brain. By contrast, regional ischemia results from occlusive cerebrovascular disease (cerebral artery thrombosis), which is localized to a specific vascular distribution.

Global Ischemia

Global ischemia most prominently affects regions of the brain that are most sensitive to diminished blood flow. One of these regions is the territory between the anterior, middle, and posterior cerebral arteries, in which there are no anastomoses between vessels. Decreased blood flow or hypoxia to these regions results in **watershed infarcts**. Another region affected by global ischemia is the deeper layers of the neocortex (cortical layers V and VI), where short penetrator vessels that originate from pial vessels enter the gray matter; global ischemia results in *laminar necrosis* of this region of the cortex. Finally, certain neuronal types are more sensitive to decreased oxygen and include the Purkinje neurons of the cerebellum and the pyramidal neurons of the Sommer sector of the hippocampus. Figure 28-15 summarizes neuronal regions most sensitive to global ischemia.

Regional Ischemia

 PATHOGENESIS: Regional ischemia, which affects a single vascular distribution, often results from arterial thrombosis or embolism secondary to atherosclerosis. Whereas thrombotic disease progresses slowly over time and deprives downstream vessels of blood flow, embolic disease occurs suddenly and often causes downstream vascular necrosis and subsequent hemorrhage.

Regional ischemia produces three distinct clinical syndromes:

- **Transient ischemic attacks** (TIAs): TIAs are due to transient vascular occlusion, last for a few minutes to less than 24 hours, and are followed by complete neurological recovery.
- **Stroke in evolution:** This condition is usually caused by a propagation of a thrombus or embolus through a vessel and features progression of neurological symptoms while the patient is observed.
- **Completed stroke:** This term refers to a stable neurological deficit caused by an infarction.

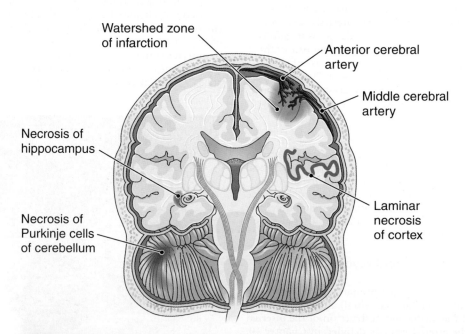

FIGURE 28-15. **Consequences of global ischemia.** Patients with global hypoxia (ischemia) may develop laminar cortical necrosis, necrosis of the hippocampus and cerebellar Purkinje neurons, and watershed infarcts of the cerebrum.

PATHOLOGY AND CLINICAL FEATURES: Regional occlusive cerebrovascular disease may be divided into subtypes based on the size and nature of the vessel involved:

- **Large extracranial and intracranial vessel occlusion (carotid, vertebral, and basilar arteries):** The carotid arteries are commonly affected by atherosclerosis, and their occlusion may present with ipsilateral hemisphere impairment or middle cerebral artery damage.
- **Circle of Willis vessel occlusion:** Often the middle cerebral artery is occluded by atherosclerosis, and emboli lodge in the trifurcation of the middle cerebral artery.
- **Parenchymal artery and arteriolar occlusion:** These vessels are often damaged by hypertension, resulting in lacunar infarcts that are typically small. *Impairment of cognition by multiple lacunar infarcts is termed **multiple infarct dementia**; hypertensive encephalopathy manifests as headache and vomiting that can progress to coma and death.*
- **Capillary bed occlusion:** Small emboli consisting of fat (following long bone trauma) or air (following rapid ascent from deep sea diving, **Caisson disease**, see Chapter 8) often cause multiple white matter infarcts and petechiae.
- **Cerebral vein occlusion:** Abrupt thrombosis secondary to systemic dehydration, phlebitis, neoplastic obstruction, or sickle cell disease, may cause bilateral frontal lobe hemorrhage, owing to blood stagnation in the sagittal sinus.

Microscopically, an acute infarction initially consists of necrotic brain tissue, which subsequently undergoes phagocytosis by macrophages and revascularization by capillary ingrowth. After many months, an infarct appears as a gliosis-lined cystic cavity. If the infracted region was large, the cavity may be bridged by atretic cobwebs of blood vessels (Fig. 28-16).

The clinical findings associated with regional ischemia reflect the underlying function of the region of the brain affected. For example, damage to the internal capsule results in hemiparesis or hemiplegia, whereas ischemia of the parietal cortex produces motor and sensory defects.

Hydrocephalus and Cerebrospinal Fluid (CSF)

Cerebrospinal fluid (CSF) is produced by the choroid plexus, which is located in the third ventricle, the foramen of Monro, and the lateral ventricles. Following production, the CSF circulates throughout the ventricular system and is ultimately absorbed by the arachnoid villi. An adult has approximately 150 mL of CSF, which serve to transport nutrients to cells of the nervous system, remove metabolic waste, and cushion structures.

PATHOLOGY AND CLINICAL FEATURES: Hydrocephalus reflects a dilation of the ventricular system secondary to increased CSF volume behind a region of obstruction. The sulci of the brain are compressed and the white matter is reduced in volume. During infancy, hydrocephalus results in expansion of the cranium (due to open suture lines) and may present with seizures, optic atrophy, weakness, or spasticity, although cognition is often spared. In adults, increased intracranial pressure causes headache, vomiting, papilledema, and, if advanced, mental deterioration. The obstruction may be relieved by surgical CSF drainage or shunting.

Noncommunicating hydrocephalus occurs when an obstruction to CSF flow resides within the ventricular system. It may occur with congenital malformations (aqueduct of Sylvius malfor-

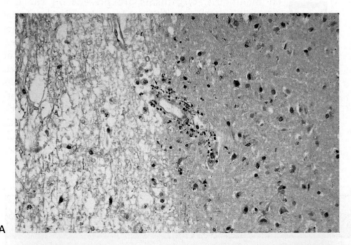

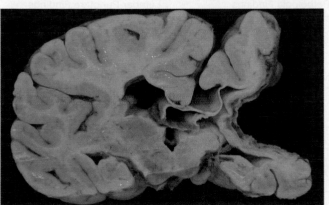

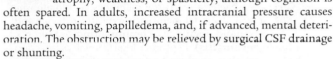

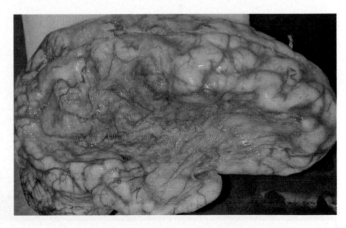

FIGURE 28-16. **Cerebral infarcts. A.** An 18-hour-old cerebral infarct (left) shows edema, hypereosinophilic neurons, and perivascular polymorphonuclear leukocytes. **B.** Remote right middle cerebral artery infarct. **C.** Remote right middle cerebral artery infarct in cross section with complete cavitation.

mations), neoplasms (ependymomas), inflammation (viral ependymitis), or hemorrhage.

Communicating hydrocephalus occurs when CSF cannot be reabsorbed by the arachnoid villi and may follow subarachnoid hemorrhage, meningitis, and tumor spread.

Infectious Diseases of the CNS

The CNS is prone to infection by bacteria, viruses, parasites, and prion diseases. The specific clinical findings associated with each infection are often distinct. Inflammation of the meninges is termed **meningitis**, that of the cortex is called **encephalitis**, and inflammation of the spinal cord is named **myelitis**. A number of potential portals of entry exist for infectious organisms including the skull and ear (see Chapter 25), and meningeal vessels.

Meningitis is Most Frequently Bacterial or Viral in Origin

Selected forms of meningitis are listed in Table 28-3.

Bacterial Meningitis

PATHOGENESIS: Bacterial meningitis occurs when bacteria reach the meninges via bloodborne spread. Bacterial meningitis may affect the pia and arachnoid meninges **(leptomeningitis)** or the dura **(pachymeningitis)**. Leptomeningitis involves infection of the CSF, which is a rich culture medium for many organisms (Fig. 28-17). By contrast, pachymeningitis commonly occurs when chronic sinusitis or mastoiditis extends into the external layer of the dura, often without additional spread within the CNS.

The most common bacteria that cause meningitis include the following:

- *Escherichia coli:* This organism affects newborns, in whom a lack of transplacental maternal IgM protection against gram-negative bacteria produces a high mortality rate.
- *Haemophilus influenzae:* This gram-negative organism affects infants between the age of 3 months and 3 years.
- *Streptococcus pneumoniae:* Also known as pneumococcus, this infection occurs in adulthood and has a high incidence following basilar skull fractures.

- *Neisseria meningitidis:* This microorganism affects persons in crowded places, such as schools or barracks. It resides in the nasopharynx and early symptoms of infection include fever, malaise, and petechial rash. Severe infections may result in adrenal hemorrhages **(Waterhouse-Friderichsen syndrome)** or acute fulminant meningitis.

PATHOLOGY: Macroscopic examination of the brain in patients that have succumbed to bacterial meningitis reveals an opacification of the meninges the result of purulent exudate, which is most evident over the cerebral hemispheres and the base of the brain. Occasionally, infection may spread to subarachnoid spaces. Although the pia is a strong barrier to the spread of infection, cerebral abscesses may occur in rare instances. Purulent exudates characteristic of the acute inflammatory reaction to bacteria are often grossly visible on the cerebral surface (see Fig. 28-17).

CLINICAL FEATURES: Most patients with meningitis present with headache, vomiting, and fever. Children may also have convulsions. Classic findings include cervical rigidity, inability to straighten the knee following hip flexion, owing to pain (Kernig sign), and knee and hip flexion following neck flexion secondary to pain (Brudzinski sign). Lumbar puncture often reveals polymorphonuclear leukocytes, increased protein, and decreased glucose level of the CSF.

Tuberculous Meningitis

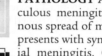

PATHOLOGY AND CLINICAL FEATURES: Tuberculous meningitis often occurs following hematogenous spread of mycobacteria to the leptomeninges and presents with symptoms comparable to those of bacterial meningitis. Organisms are present on the leptomeninges and in the CSF, and are identified by special stains for acid-fast bacilli. The meninges demonstrate granulomas composed of epithelioid histiocytes, Langerhans giant cells, and lymphocytes, which surround foci of caseous necrosis. Lumbar puncture often demonstrates increased numbers of lymphocytes in the CSF. If not properly treated, tuberculous meningitis may result in meningeal fibrosis, communicating hydrocephalus, and arteritis that may cause infarcts. Untreated tuberculous meningitis is usually fatal in 4 to 6 weeks. **Pott disease** refers to tuberculous infection of the spine, in which an epidural granulomatous mass destroys the spine and causes spinal cord compression.

Table 28-3

Forms of Meningitis

Disease	Organism(s)	Pathologic Findings	Lumbar Puncture Findings
Bacterial meningitis	*Escherichia coli, Haemophilus influenzae, Streptococcus pneumoniae, Neisseria meningitidis*	Opacified meninges; purulent exudates	Neutrophils, ↓ glucose, ↑ protein, organism by stain
Tuberculosus meningitis	*Mycobacterium tuberculosis*	Meningeal granulomas; organisms by acid fast stain	Lymphocytes, ↓ glucose, ↑ protein, organism by acid fast stain
Viral meningitis	Enterovirus (e.g., echovirus)	Often no findings	Lymphocytes, normal glucose, slight ↑ protein
Cryptococcal meningitis	*Cryptococcus neoformans*	1-mm white nodules containing organisms; minimal inflammation	Spheres with a halo by special stain; lymphocytes
Syphilitic meningitis	*Treponema pallidum*	Meningeal and perivascular lymphocytic infiltrate; + / - spirochetes	↑ lymphocytes, elevated protein, normal glucose

From Hansel DE, Dintzis RZ. Lippincott's Pocket Pathology. Baltimore: Lippincott Williams & Wilkins, 2006, p. 857.

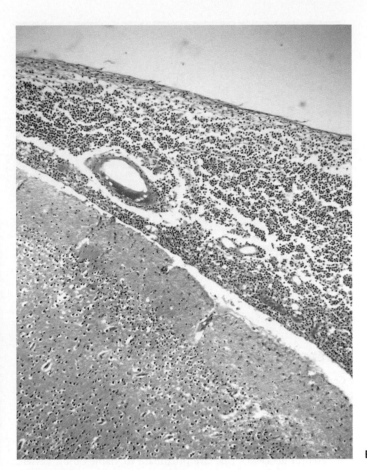

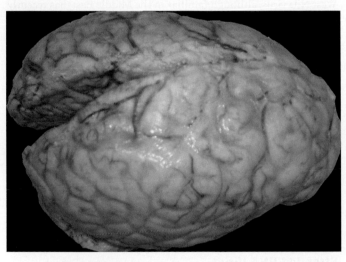

FIGURE 28-17. **Purulent meningitis. A.** A creamy exudate opacifies the leptomeninges. **B.** A microscopic section shows the accumulation of numerous neutrophils in the subarachnoid space.

Syphilitic Meningitis

The spirochete *Treponema pallidum* may affect the CNS following hematogenous spread. Often, the organisms are rapidly cleared from the meninges, and only a minor inflammatory reaction involving lymphocytes and plasma cells is present. However, three severe manifestations of tertiary syphilis may occur (see also Chapter 9).

- **Meningovascular syphilis:** Thickened meninges are caused by a fibroblastic response and obliterative endarteritis, resulting in multiple small infarcts. Microscopically the lesions show plasma cells surrounding cortical arterioles
- **Tabes dorsalis:** Transient infection around the dorsal nerve roots of the spinal cord causes wallerian degeneration of axons (see peripheral nerve system below), which extends to the posterior fasciculi and causes loss of position sense in the lower extremities.
- **Dementia paralytica (luetic dementia):** This condition occurs many years after infection and features dementia. Microscopically, there is focal loss of cortical neurons, astrogliosis, reactive microglia, and ependymal granulations

Viral Meningitis

Viral meningitis affects children and young adults and is often caused by infection with enterovirus (coxsackie B virus, echovirus) and rarely by herpes simplex virus and several others (see Chapter 9). Symptoms include a sudden fever and severe headache. Lumbar puncture demonstrates lymphocytes and increased protein in the CSF, but normal glucose. Most cases resolve without sequelae.

Cryptococcal Meningitis Occurs Most Frequently in Immunocompromised Persons

Cryptococcus neoformans causes meningitis primarily in immunocompromised hosts. Infection is often initiated by the inhalation of contaminated bird excreta. Lumbar puncture reveals large (5 to 15 μm) encapsulated spherical organisms that demonstrate a halo (capsule). Macroscopically, 1 mm white nodules are widely disseminated on the meninges, ependyma, and choroid plexus. Microscopically, organisms may be identified, although the surrounding inflammation may be minimal, with rare multinucleated giant cells and lymphocytes (Fig. 28-18).

Amebic Meningoencephalitis May be Water-Borne

Amebic meningoencephalitis is usually caused by the amoeba *Naegleria* and *Acanthamoeba*. Infection with *Acanthamoeba* produces a more protracted meningitis, as well as parenchymal abscesses and a granulomatous reaction. *Naegleria* infection occurs following swimming in infested waters and results in fulminant, often fatal, meningitis. *Naegleria* and *Acanthamoeba* can penetrate the cribriform plate and enter the cranial compartment by way of the olfactory nerves. Microscopically, these amoebae bear a striking resemblance to macrophages.

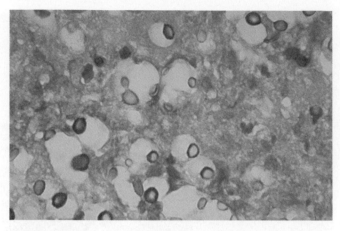

FIGURE 28-18. **Cryptococcal meningitis.** The cryptococcal organisms vary in size (5 to 15 Îm in diameter) (mucicarmine stain). They reproduce by budding.

Cerebral Abscess is the Result of Cerebritis

Cerebral abscesses originate when bloodborne microorganisms lodge within the capillary network of the cortex (Fig. 28-19). These organisms incite an acute inflammatory reaction (cerebritis), with neutrophil influx, edema, and liquefactive necrosis. The components of the abscess consist of inflammation, gliosis, and fibrosis. Collagen, although rare in the CNS, may be prominent in the wall of cerebral abscesses that are proximate to viable blood vessels. Expansion of the abscess may result in compression of blood vessels, leading to ischemia or mass effect. The latter may produce transtentorial herniation or rupture into a ventricle.

Viral Encephalomyelitis

Viruses that infect the CNS typically localize to specific sites within the brain and spinal cord and, therefore, demonstrate distinct clinicopathologic findings.

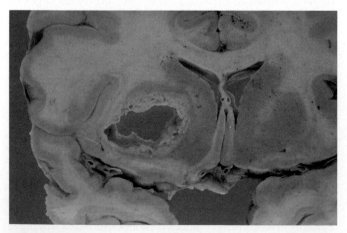

FIGURE 28-19. **Cerebral abscess.** A young man with bacterial endocarditis developed an abscess in the left basal ganglia.

 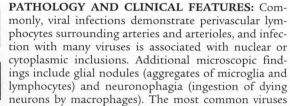

PATHOLOGY AND CLINICAL FEATURES: Commonly, viral infections demonstrate perivascular lymphocytes surrounding arteries and arterioles, and infection with many viruses is associated with nuclear or cytoplasmic inclusions. Additional microscopic findings include glial nodules (aggregates of microglia and lymphocytes) and neuronophagia (ingestion of dying neurons by macrophages). The most common viruses that affect the CNS are listed in Table 28-4. Typically, the onset of encephalitis is abrupt, but the duration of disease may vary from weeks to years.

West Nile Virus is a Recently Emergent Pathogen

West Nile virus, although familiar in the Middle East, has recently emerged as a public health concern in the United States and Canada, where it is now widespread. *This arbovirus is a zoonosis, with birds serving as a reservoir and mosquitos being the common vector for human disease.*

PATHOLOGY AND CLINICAL FEATURES: West Nile virus is associated with nonspecific signs of CNS injection, including variable meningitis, encephalitis, poliomyelitis (inflammation of the gray matter, from the Greek polios, gray) and occasional severe involvement of the cerebellum and medulla. Perivascular cuffing, and occasional microglial nodules are seen in some cases. Weakness may correlate with infection of anterior horn cells. Symptoms tend to be systemic and nonspecific, including fever, headache, myalgia and the like. The disease may be fatal in the elderly and those with concurrent systemic disease.

Poliomyelitis Refers to CNS Infection by a Single-Stranded RNA Virus

Poliomyelitis is caused by a nonenveloped, single-stranded RNA enterovirus that preferentially infects the anterior horn cells and bulbar motor nuclei of the spinal cord. Transmission occurs via the fecal-oral route, and the disease may spread rapidly among children in close quarters, although the development of effective vaccines has dramatically decreased the incidence of this disease.

PATHOGENESIS: Poliovirus binds to and enters motor neurons. Following infection, neurons undergo chromatolysis and subsequent ingestion by macrophages (neuronophagia) (see Fig. 28-3).

PATHOLOGY AND CLINICAL FEATURES: Microscopically, lymphocytes surround blood vessels in the spinal cord and brainstem, and inflammation may spread to the meninges. The cortex may demonstrate glial nodules, but viral inclusions are not present. Patients with poliomyelitis initially experience fever, headache, and malaise, followed by meningitis and variable paralysis. Death can result from respiratory failure following paralysis of the respiratory muscles.

Rabies is a Fatal Infection Transmitted by Animal Saliva

Rabies is caused by an enveloped, single-stranded RNA rhabdovirus. The infection is transmitted by contaminated saliva from animal bites (dogs, wolves, foxes, skunks, bats etc.) that serve as a reservoir for the virus.

PATHOGENESIS: The virus infects peripheral nerves at the site of a bite and is transported to the spinal cord and brain by retrograde axoplasmic flow. The onset of disease varies from 10 days to 3 months or longer following infection, perhaps depending on axonal length.

PATHOLOGY AND CLINICAL FEATURES: Infection with the rabies virus demonstrates a specific cytoplasmic inclusion, termed a *Negri body*, and other nonspecific signs of viral infection of the CNS, such as perivascular cuffing. Patients initially demonstrate painful throat spasms, difficulty swallowing (hence the term "hydrophobia"), and a tendency to aspirate fluids early in the course of the disease. Ultimately, a generalized encephalopathy, characterized by irritability, agitation, seizures, and delirium ensues, and death occurs within weeks prompt postexposure vaccination is effective in preventing disease.

Herpes Simplex Virus is the Most Common Cause of Nonepidemic Encephalitis

- Herpes simplex virus type 1 (HSV-1) causes cold sores on the lips and can retrogradely infect the gasserian ganglion via the mandibular nerve trunk. Infection of the CNS primarily affects the temporal lobes and results in swollen, hemorrhagic, necrotic brain parenchyma, with perivascular lymphocytic cuffing. Infected neurons and glial cells contain small, eosinophilic, nuclear inclusions, which can be specifically identified by immunostains for HSV-1 (Fig. 28-20).

- Herpes simplex virus type 2 (HSV-2) is a sexually transmitted disease that causes vesicular lesions of the vagina and penis (genital herpes). Transmission of HSV-2 to newborns during passage through the birth canal results in severe neonatal encephalitis, with liquefactive necrosis of the cerebrum and cerebellum.

Arboviruses are Transmitted to Humans by Infected Mosquitos or Tick Bites

Arboviruses (togavirus, bunyavirus) are transmitted to humans by the bite of infected mosquitos or ticks. The insect-borne viral encephalitides includes St. Louis encephalitis, Western equine encephalitis, and tickborne encephalitis, among others. The diseases are zoonoses, with a variety of animals serving as reservoirs/hosts. Patients demonstrate a range of presentations, from flulike symptoms to meningoencephalitis associated with severe inflammation of the gray matter, necrosis, and vessel thrombosis. In severe cases, patients die within days. Chronic long-term sequelae include mental retardation and neurological deficits, particularly in young children.

Subacute Sclerosing Panencephalitis (SSPE) is Caused by the Measles Virus

SSPE is caused by latent infection with a mutated form of the measles virus, which persists in the CNS for years and results in a chronic neurodegenerative process. It is rare in adults and found mainly in unvaccinated children. The virus primarily affects the

Table 28–4

Viral Encephalomyelitis

Disease	Virus Type	Location of Infection	Viral Inclusions	Clinical Features
Poliomyelitis	Noneveloped, SS RNA (enterovirus)	Anterior horn cells and bulbar motor nuclei of spinal cord	None	Fever, malaise followed by meningitis and paralysis
Rabies	Enveloped, SS RNA (rhabdovirus)	Brainstem and cerebellum; originally, peripheral nerve	Eosinophilic Negri body in cytoplasm	Throat spasm, difficulty with swallowing, encephalopathy
Herpes simplex virus-1 (HSV-1)	DS DNA	Temporal lobes; hemorrhagic necrotic parenchyma	Small, eosinophilic intra nuclear inclusion	Often children and young adults; changes in mood, behavior, memory
Herpes simplex virus-2 (HSV-2)	DS DNA	Cerebrum and cerebellum of newborns; obtained from birth canal	Small, eosinophilic intra-nuclear inclusion	Neonates; may cause severe hemorrhagic, necrotizing encephalomyelitis
Varicella zoster virus (VZV)	DS DNA	Severe meningitis	Glia and neurons	Often immunocompromised patients; well-delineated lesions with demyelination and necrosis
Cytomegalovirus	DS DNA	Transplacental spread to periventricular areas in utero; immunocompromised hosts	Large cytoplasmic and nuclear inclusions in neurons and astrocytes	Severe hemorrhagic, necrotic encephalomyelitis
Arthropod-borne	Togavirus, Bunyavirus	Mild meningitis to diffuse encephalitis	None	Flulike symptoms to severe meningoencephalitis
Subacute sclerosing panencephalitis (SSPE)	Measles virus (SS RNA)	Gray and white matter of cortex	Prominent basophilic nuclear inclusions with halo	Cognitive and behavioral deficits; motor/sensory deficits
Progressive mutifocal leukoencephalopathy (PML)	JC virus (DS DNA)	White matter of cortex; widespread demyelination	Nuclear ground-glass oligodendroglial inclusions	Dementia, weakness, visual loss, ataxia, death within 6 months

From Hansel DE, Dintzis RZ. Lippincott's Pocket Pathology. Baltimore: Lippincott Williams & Wilkins, 2006:860.

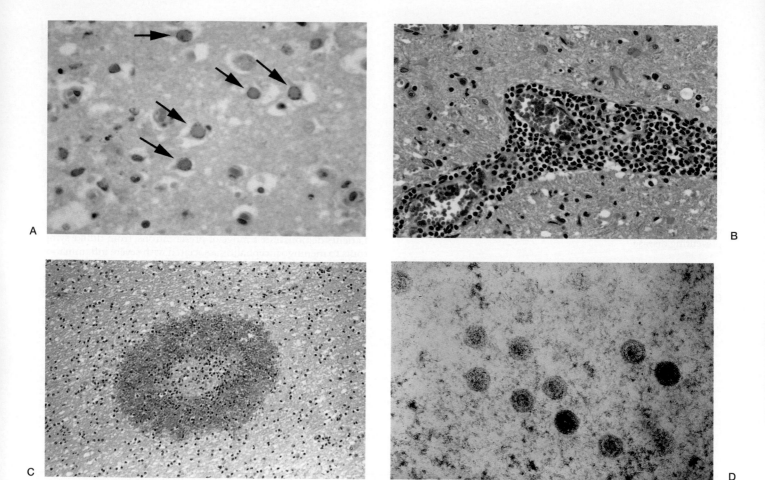

FIGURE 28-20. **Herpes simplex encephalitis. A.** The infected neurons display small, intranuclear, eosinophilic inclusions that lack halos *(arrows)*. **B.** Another area of the specimen exhibits pronounced perivascular chronic inflammation. **C.** A focus of parenchymal necrosis with surrounding hemorrhage is seen. **D.** Electron microscopy demonstrates herpes virus particles.

cortex, with marked gliosis in the gray and white matter, patchy loss of myelin, ubiquitous perivascular lymphocytes and macrophages, prominent basophilic nuclear inclusions rimmed by a prominent halo, and occasionally neurofibrillary tangles. Over time, SSPE causes behavioral changes, cognitive defects, motor and sensory impairments, and seizures.

Progressive Multifocal Leukoencephalopathy (PML) Most Often Affects Immunocompromised Patients

 PATHOGENESIS: PML is caused by infection with JC virus and rarely with Simian Virus 40 (SV40), both DNA papovaviruses. The disease occurs most often in immunocompromised individuals (most commonly AIDS patients and those treated for a lymphoproliferative disease).

 PATHOLOGY AND CLINICAL FEATURES: The virus primarily affects the white matter of the brain. PML infection demonstrates multiple discrete foci of demyelination near the gray-white junction in the cerebral hemispheres and brainstem. Typically, lesions measure several millimeters in diameter, demonstrate a central area devoid of myelin with residual axons and few oligodendrocytes, and macrophage infiltration. The

oligodendrocytes within the lesion appear enlarged and contain hyperchromatic intranuclear inclusion with a ground-glass appearance. Astrocytes appear pleomorphic and show multiple irregular nuclei and dense chromatin. Typically, PML affects immunocompromised patients and manifests with dementia, weakness, visual loss, and ataxia. Death often occurs within 6 months.

AIDS Encephalopathy is Often a Primary Manifestation of HIV Infection of the CNS

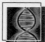 **PATHOGENESIS:** *AIDS encephalopathy occurs as a direct effect of macrophage and microglial infection by the HIV-1 retrovirus.* The disease may manifest as (a) a primary encephalopathy, (b) A leukoencephalopathy presenting as diffuse damage to the white matter, and (c) a lymphocytic meningitis.

  PATHOLOGY AND CLINICAL FEATURES: Macroscopically, the brains of these patients demonstrate mild cerebral atrophy. Microscopically, diffuse demyelination, astrogliosis, neuronal loss, microglial nodules, and multinucleated giant cells (which can be demonstrated to harbor HIV markers) are present. In the presence of microglial nodules, giant cells are considered as pathognomonic for primary HIV encephalitis (Fig. 28-

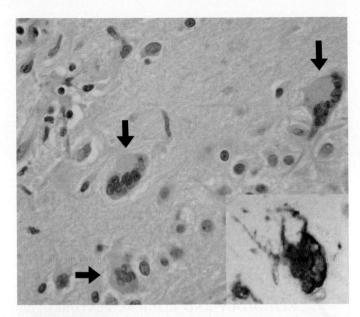

FIGURE 28-21. **Human immunodeficiency virus (HIV) encephalitis.** Multinucleated giant cells (*arrows*), often in a perivascular location, are characteristic of HIV encephalitis. *Inset*: Immunohistochemical stain for HIV anti-p24.

21). Patients classically present with encephalopathy **(AIDS dementia complex)**, which includes mild to severe cognitive impairment, paralysis, and loss of sensory function.

Prion Disease

Prion diseases comprise a group of neurodegenerative conditions characterized clinically by slowly progressive ataxia and dementia and pathologically by accumulations of fibrillar or insoluble prion proteins, degeneration of neurons, and vacuolization, termed **spongiform degeneration** (Fig. 28-22). The classic spongiform encephalopathies include several syndromes, including kuru, Creutzfeldt-Jakob disease (CJD), Gerstmann-Straussler-Scheinker syndrome (GSS), and fatal familial insomnia. In addition, similar diseases occur in animals, including scrapie in sheep and goats, bovine spongiform encephalopathy (BSE; mad cow disease), transmissible mink en-

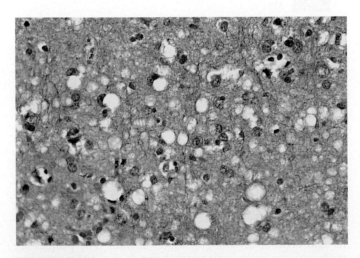

FIGURE 28-22. **Creutzfeldt-Jakob disease.** Spongiform degeneration of the gray matter is characterized by individual and clustered vacuoles, with no evidence of inflammation.

TABLE 28-5
Prion Diseases

I. Human
A. Creutzfeldt-Jakob disease (CJD)
  1. Sporadic (85% of all CJD cases; incidence 1 per million worldwide)
  2. Inherited mutation of the prion gene, autosomal dominant transmission (15% of all CJD cases)
  3. Iatrogenic
    a. Hormone injection
      Human growth hormone (55 cases)
      Human pituitary gonadotropin (5 cases)
    b. Tissue grafts
      Dura mater (11 cases)
      Cornea (1 case)
      Pericardium (1 case)
    c. Medical devices (inadequate sterilization)
      Depth electrodes (2 cases)
      Surgical instruments (not definitely proven)
  4. New variant CJD (vCJD)
B. Gerstmann-Straussler-Scheinker disease (GSS; inherited prion gene mutation, autosomal dominant transmission)
C. Fatal familial insomnia (FFI; inherited prion gene mutation, autosomal dominant transmission)
D. Kuru (confined to the Fore people of Papua New Guinea, formerly transmitted by cannibalistic ritual)

II. Animal
A. Scrapie (sheep and goats)
B. Bovine spongiform encephalopathy (BSE; "mad cow disease")
C. Transmissible mink encephalopathy
D. Feline spongiform encephalopathy
E. Captive exotic ungulate spongiform encephalopathy (nyala, gemsbok, eland, Arabian oryx, greater kudu)
F. Chronic wasting disease of deer and elk
G. Experimental transmission to many species, including primates and transgenic mice

cephalopathy, and chronic wasting disease in mule deer and elk. Prion diseases encompass infectious and autosomal dominant (due to prion gene mutations) forms but, in most cases, the mode of acquisition is uncertain. Recent data indicate a link between BSE ("mad cow disease") and a new variant of human CJD. (See also Chapter 9.) Prion diseases are listed in Table 28-5.

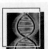 **PATHOGENESIS:** All spongiform encephalopathies are transmissible, and inadvertent human transmission of CJD has followed the administration of contaminated human pituitary growth hormone, corneal transplantation from a diseased donor, insufficiently sterilized neurosurgical instruments, and surgical implantation of contaminated dura. The infectious agent is a protein termed the **prion (proteinaceous infectious particles)**.

The human prion gene (*PRNP*) is located on the short arm of chromosome 20. The normal prion gene product, prion protein (PrP), is a constitutively expressed cell-surface glycoprotein that is bound to the plasmalemma by a glycolipid anchor. The high-est levels of PrP messenger RNA (mRNA) are found in CNS neurons, but the function of the protein is unknown. *Remarkably, the normal cellular prion protein, termed PrP^C, and the pathogenic (infectious) prion protein, PrP^SC, do not differ in amino acid sequence but rather in their three-dimensional conformation.* Specifically, PrP^C is rich in α-helix configuration, whereas the β-pleated sheet content of PrP^SC is predominant. This conformational change is presumed to (1) render PrP^SC resistant to proteinase digestion, (2) convert host

PrP^C to PrP^{SC}, *resulting in an autocatalytic, exponentially expanding accrual of abnormal PrP^{SC}*, and (3) compromise cell function and result in neurodegeneration by mechanisms that remain to be elucidated.

 PATHOLOGY: The cardinal morphologic features of prion diseases are neuronal degeneration and loss, gliosis, spongiform degeneration (small microcysts), and accumulations of insoluble prions with properties of amyloid (Fig. 28-23). These lesions are most prevalent in the cortical gray matter, but they also involve the deeper nuclei of the basal ganglia, hypothalamus, and cerebellum. All prion diseases are lethal over a span of months to years. Additional details of Creutzfeldt-Jakob disease and its variants are found in Chapter 9.

Demyelinating Diseases of the CNS

Demyelinating diseases refer to disorders in which a selective loss of myelin occurs. Hence, disorders in which there is a loss of myelin secondary to other injury to neural tissue (such as ischemic injury, trauma, infection and the like) are not considered as such.

Leukodystrophies are Inherited Disorders of Myelin Formation or Preservation

Metachromatic Leukodystrophy (MLD)

The most common leukodystrophy MLD, is an autosomal recessive disease caused by a deficiency in the activity of arylsulfatase.

 PATHOGENESIS: Arylsulfatase A is a lysosomal enzyme involved in the degradation of myelin sulfatides; deficiencies result in an accumulation of sulfatides in Schwann cells and oligodendrocytes (white matter). This results in a progressive loss of neural, cognitive and motor function.

 PATHOLOGY AND CLINICAL FEATURES: The most common form of the disease is manifested in infancy and results in progressive loss of motor and neurological function. Several less frequent late onset forms of the disease occur. Disease progression is relatively slow, and personality changes and dementia occur. The brain demonstrates diffuse myelin loss and accumulation of characteristic 15 to 20 μm cytoplasmic granules that stain metachromatically with cresyl violet and toluidine blue. Death intervenes within about 5 years. There is no specific therapy, but hematopoietic cell transplant may slow the course of the disease in patients with late onset.

Krabbe disease

Krabbe disease, or globoid cell leukodystrophy, is an autosomal recessive disorder caused by a deficiency of galactocerebroside β-galactosidase.

 PATHOGENESIS: The presence of abnormal sphingolipid metabolites leads to the toxic destruction of oligodendroglia and consequent demyelination.

 PATHOLOGY AND CLINICAL FEATURES: The disease is manifested in early infancy with severe motor, sensory, and cognitive deficits; it progresses to death within 1 to 2 years. The brain is small, with regions of partial and total demyelination and prominent astrogliosis, and there is almost a complete loss of oligodendroglia and myelin. *A characteristic feature is* the presence of perivascular, large (50 μm) mononuclear and multinucleated "globoid cells," which are macrophages that contain undigested galactocerebroside. Bone marrow or cord blood transplantation prior to onset of neurological symptoms may be of benefit.

Adrenoleukodystrophy (ALD)

ALD refers to an inherited demyelinating disease and impairment of adrenal function.

 PATHOGENESIS: ALD manifests between the ages of 3 and 10 years. This X-linked (Xq28) inherited disorder is associated with high levels of saturated very-long-chain fatty acids (VLFCAs). The defective gene (ABCD1) appears to function as a membrane transporter, and its role in the VLCFA degradation pathway remains unclear. Defects in the peroxisomal membrane prevent degradation of VLFCAs, and increased levels and accumulation of these fatty acids results in the loss of myelinated axons and oligodendroglia.

 PATHOLOGY AND CLINICAL FEATURES: The brain demonstrates confluent, bilaterally symmetrical demyelination, especially of the subcortical white matter of the parietooccipital region. Diffuse gliosis is common and perivascular lymphocytic cuffing may occur. The adrenals are atrophic, and electron microscopy reveals membrane-bound curvilinear inclusions of VLFCAs in the adrenal, Schwann cells, and CNS macrophages. Patients demonstrate neurologic symptoms that progress to a vegetative state. Treatment with a mixture of oleic and erucic acids (Lorenzo's Oil) may reduce or delay disease symptoms. Bone marrow transplantation is beneficial before the onset of severe symptoms.

Multiple Sclerosis is a Chronic Demyelinating Disease of Young Adults

Multiple sclerosis (MS) is a chronic demyelinating disease that most commonly affects young adults, with a 2:1 female to male predominance and a prevalence of 1 in 1,000. *MS is commonly characterized by a relapsing-remitting disease course over many years.*

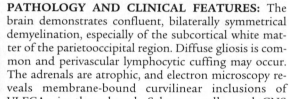 **PATHOGENESIS:** A number of mechanisms have been proposed to play a role in the pathogenesis of MS:

- **Genetic factors:** There is a 25% concordance for MS in monozygotic twins, familial aggregation, and linkage to a number of MHC alleles.
- **Immune factors:** Injection of myelin basic protein induces a similar disease in mice. Identification of oligoclonal T cells are identified in the CSF, together with perivascular lymphocyte and macrophage accumulation.
- **Infectious agents:** MS is a disease of temperate climates, and the risk varies with the age of relocation to various climates.

 PATHOLOGY: The classic pathologic feature of MS is the demyelinated plaque, which is a discrete region of demyelination and usually less than 2 cm in diameter (Fig. 28-24). These plaques occur in the white matter and occasionally the gray-white junction. The plaques are most common in the optic nerves, optic chiasm, and periventricular white matter. Microscopically, active plaques are well-demarcated and demonstrate prominent macrophage infiltration and selective loss of myelin in a region of axonal preservation. In

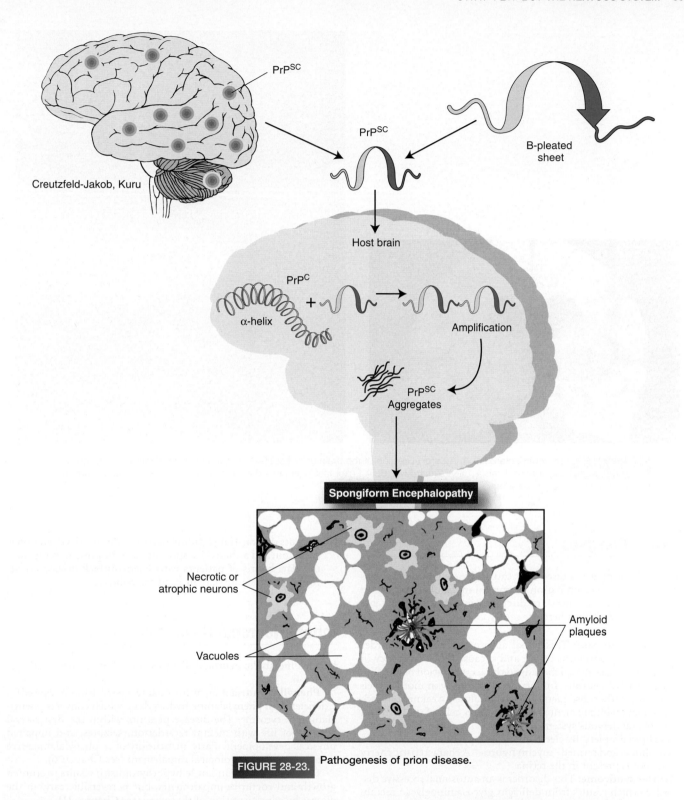

FIGURE 28-23. Pathogenesis of prion disease.

addition, lymphocytes often surround small veins and arteries, and edema may be prominent. The neuronal cell body is unaffected by the disease process, whereas the axon may undergo degeneration. Inactive MS plaques demonstrate gliosis and minimal to no inflammation.

 CLINICAL FEATURES: *The classical clinical feature associated with MS is the accumulation of demyelinating lesions in different regions of the brain at different periods (lesions separated in time and space).* This feature underlies the common relapsing-remitting course of MS, although some patients may demonstrate a relentless, progressive course of the disease. Early symptoms include loss of vision in one eye, blurred vision, vertigo, and weakness or numbness of one or both legs. These symptoms may resolve, but the development of additional lesions results in permanent defects

Over time, the degree of functional impairment varies from minor to severe, with many patients developing paralysis, dysarthria, severe visual defects, incontinence, and dementia. Most patients survive 20 to 30 years following the onset of disease and may ultimately die of respiratory failure or urinary tract infection. Some patients benefit from treatment with interferon-β.

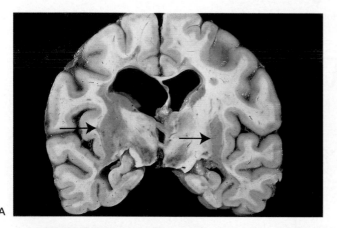

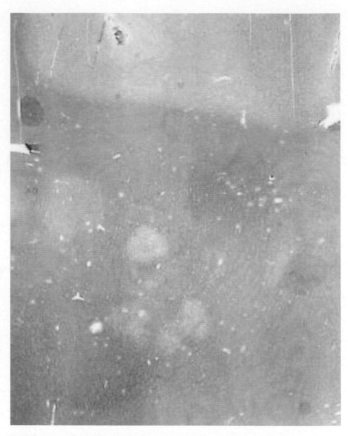

A

B

FIGURE 28-24. **Multiple sclerosis. A.** A coronal section of the brain demonstrates a prominent demyelinated plaque involving the left internal capsule (*arrows*). **B.** A Luxol fast blue stain demonstrates multiple small demyelinating plaques involving subcortical white matter.

Storage Diseases

This group of inherited diseases is caused by enzyme deficiencies that result in the accumulation of normal metabolic products in lysosomes. These disorders are discussed in detail in Chapter 6 and are briefly described here.

- **Tay-Sachs disease:** This lethal autosomal recessive disorder manifests by 6 months of age and is caused by a deficiency in hexosaminidase A, which leads to the accumulation of gangliosides in CNS neurons. Infants develop a delay in motor development, with subsequent flaccid paralysis, weakness, blindness, mental impairment and death. Nerve cells of the CNS and peripheral nervous system are distended and contain cytoplasmic lipid droplets. By electron microscopy, lysosomes are filled with lipids and termed "myelin figures." A characteristic cherry red spot is present in the retina.
- **Hurler syndrome:** This disorder is an autosomal recessive disorder, which results from deficient glycosaminoglycan metabolism and leads to intraneuronal accumulation of mucopolysaccharides. Involvement of the CNS is variable.
- **Gaucher disease:** This autosomal recessive disorder is caused by a deficiency in glucocerebrosidase and the accumulation of glucocerebroside in macrophages. The CNS is most severely involved in the infantile, or type II, form of the disease. Infants demonstrate severe neuronal loss and failure to thrive, with death at an early age.
- **Niemann-Pick disease:** An autosomal recessive disorder caused by a deficiency of sphingomyelinase, NiemannPick disease results in intraneuronal storage of sphingomyelin.

Patients demonstrate a failure to thrive. Retinal degeneration is common, and a cherry-red spot may also be present in the macula. The brains of patients with NiemannPick disease are atrophic and demonstrate marked astrogliosis.

Inborn Neuronal Disorders

Various metabolic neuronal diseases contribute to neuronal dysfunction.

Phenylketonuria is an autosomal recessive disorder caused by a deficiency in phenylalanine hydroxylase, which converts phenylalanine to tyrosine. The disease presents within the first several months of life with mental retardation, seizures, and impaired physical development. Early institution of a phenylalanine-free diet can prevent neurological impairment (see Chapter 6).

Cretinism (severe infantile hypothyroidism) results in stunted growth and cognitive impairments, but is reversible early in the disease by administration of thyroxine (see Chapter 21).

Wilson disease is an autosomal recessive disorder caused by mutations in the *WD* gene that lead to defective copper metabolism. Impaired biliary copper excretion results in deposition of copper in the brain and liver, causing the development of athetoid movements and insidious cirrhosis. In addition, the limbus of the cornea demonstrates a visible, golden-brown band, termed the Kayser-Fleischer ring. Grossly, the lenticular nuclei of the brain show a light golden discoloration, and often small cysts or clefts are present in the putamen or deep layers of the neocortex. Microscopically, mild neuronal loss and gliosis are present (see Chapter 14).

Metabolic Disorders

Chronic Alcohol Abuse Results in Direct Toxic Injury

Disorders caused by chronic alcohol use reflect direct toxic injury to neurons as well as injury occurring secondary to nutritional deficits. CNS lesions that occur with alcoholism include the following:

- **Wernicke syndrome:** Thiamine (vitamin B1) deficiency in alcoholics is associated with the rapid onset of thermal regulatory disturbances, altered consciousness, ophthalmoplegia and nystagmus. The brain shows lesions in the hypothalamus, mamillary bodies, periaqueductal region of the midbrain, and the pons. The disorder is rapidly reversed by thiamine administration (see Chapter 8.)
- **Korsakoff syndrome:** Disordered recent memory is compensated for by confabulation, reflected in the degeneration of neurons in the medial-dorsal nucleus of the thalamus.
- **Cerebral atrophy**
- **Atrophy of the superior aspect of the vermis of the cerebellum:** Atrophy of Purkinje and granular cells result in truncal ataxia.
- **Central pontine myelinolysis:** Demyelination of the pons is caused by overly rapid correction of hyponatremia consequent to abuse associated disease.

Hepatic Encephalopathy is a Result of Liver Failure

Hepatic encephalopathy occurs with liver failure and manifests as delirium, seizures, and coma. The only CNS findings are altered astroglia in the thalamus (Alzheimer type II astrocytes), which demonstrate enlarged nuclei and marginated chromatin (see Chapter 14).

Subacute Combined Degeneration of the Spinal Cord Reflects Vitamin B12 Deficiency

This disease is a result of vitamin B$_{12}$ deficiency, and it may occur in pernicious anemia, extensive gastric resection, malabsorption syndromes, or in strict vegetarians. Initially, the posterolateral columns of the spinal cord demonstrate symmetric myelin and axonal loss at the thoracic level. Often, burning sensations on the soles of the feet or other paresthesias are the earliest signs. Over time, gliosis and atrophy of the posterolateral columns occurs and results in weakness, defective postural sensation, and ataxia. This disease is rapidly progressive and poorly reversible (see Chapters 8 and 20.)

Neurodegenerative Diseases

This heterogeneous group of disorders includes Parkinson disease, amyotrophic lateral sclerosis, Huntington disease, the spinocerebellar ataxias, Alzheimer disease, and several other less common disorders. Some of these degenerative conditions primarily involve specific neuroanatomic systems (Parkinson and Huntington disease, amyotrophic lateral sclerosis), whereas others affect a wider regions of the nervous system (Alzheimer disease). Emerging data now implicate a number of different abnormal proteins that form aggregates with the properties of amyloid (congophilic and fibrillar, with a β-pleated sheet structure). *The deposition of amyloid is a common factor in the onset and progression of many sporadic and hereditary neurodegenerative disorders.* Thus, growing evidence provides a mechanistic link between the filamentous aggregates of amyloid deposits in the CNS and the degeneration of affected brain regions in neurodegenerative disorders. However, it is not clear how filamentous protein aggregates cause disease (Fig. 28-25).

Almost all of the neurodegenerative disorders occur as (1) a rare, early onset and highly aggressive familial disorder associated with missense mutations in the gene encoding the disease protein, and (2) as a more common sporadic form of the disorder in which the corresponding wild-type protein is found. However, both sporadic and inherited forms of the disease demonstrate the same hallmark brain lesions. Selected neurodegenerative diseases are presented in Table 28-6.

Parkinson Disease (PD) is Characterized by Movement Disorders

Parkinson Disease (PD) is a common neurologic condition that features loss of neurons in the substantia nigra and intracellular aggregates of α-synuclein, termed Lewy bodies.

 PATHOGENESIS: PD occurs in the sixth to eighth decades and affects 2% of the population of North America. The majority of cases are sporadic and of unknown origin, but rare cases of early onset, autosomal dominant, familial PD occur. The disease has also been reported to occur following viral encephalitis and the intake of the drug MPTP, a byproduct found in illicitly produced meperidine.

 PATHOLOGY: *Macroscopically, PD is characterized by a loss of pigmented, dopaminergic neurons in the substantia nigra and locus ceruleus (Fig. 28-26).* Microscopically, **Lewy bodies** (spherical, eosinophilic cytoplasmic inclusions) are present throughout the brain and represent aggregates of **α-synuclein** (a synaptic protein of unknown function) (Fig. 28-27). Lewy bodies have been hypothesized to reflect oxidative stress produced by the autooxidation of catecholamines during melanin formation by neurons in the substantia nigra and locus ceruleus.

 CLINICAL FEATURES: Damage to the extrapyramidal system results in the classic symptoms of PD, which include (1) a slowness of voluntary movements, (2) muscular rigidity through the entire range of movement, and (3) a coarse tremor of the distal extremities, which is present at rest and disappears with voluntary movement. Additional findings include an expressionless (masklike) facies and a reduced rate of swallowing, which leads to drooling. Late stages may be characterized by depression and dementia.

Treatment of PD includes levodopa administration, which becomes ineffective following several years. Newer treatments potentially include electrical deep-brain stimulation and possibly dopaminergic cell transplants.

Two diseases that are clinically very similar to PD are **striatonigral degeneration** and **progressive supranuclear palsy.**

- **Striatonigral degeneration:** This disease is clinically identical to PD and demonstrates atrophy of the corpus striatum and less atrophy of substantia nigra and locus ceruleus. It may be a component of multiple system atrophy (also associated with Shy-Drager disease and olivopontocerebellar atrophy). α-Synuclein inclusions are also noted.
- **Progressive supranuclear palsy:** Clinically similar to PD, this disorder features additional progressive paralysis of vertical eye movements, more widespread neuronal loss in the globus pallidus and dentate nuclei, and neurofibrillary tangles.

Amyotrophic Lateral Sclerosis (ALS) is Characterized by Progressive Weakness and Death

ALS features degeneration of motor neurons and results in progressive deterioration of the extremities and eventually the muscles of respiration.

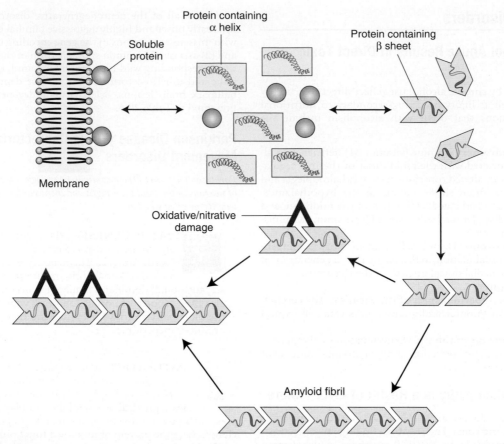

Protein containing
α helix

Soluble
protein

Protein containing
β sheet

Membrane

Oxidative/nitrative
damage

Amyloid fibril

FIGURE 28-25. **Filamentous protein aggregates: Targets of novel therapies for CNS neurodegenerative diseases.** The schematic depicts the stepwise conversion of normal soluble proteins that either lack secondary structure *(orange balls)* or have an α-helical secondary structure *(blue boxes)*. They may interact normally with other structures such as organelle membranes *(box at the upper left)*. Spontaneously or due to mutations, the proteins can adopt a β-sheet structure *(unconnected arrowheads)*, which is reversible. However, if the proteins go on to form dimers, trimers, tetramers, and so forth, then they assemble into amyloid fibrils *(connected arrowheads)*. This process also may be driven by posttranslational modifications such as oxidative/nitrative damage *(red carats)*. These changes may act in several ways to promote fibrillogenesis, including cross-linking proteins or inducing conformational changes that stabilize the protein polymers into fibrils, thereby promoting formation of amyloid deposits, senile plaques, neurofibrillary tangles, Lewy bodies, glial cytoplasmic inclusions, and prion amyloid lesions.

 PATHOGENESIS: ALS most commonly occurs in the fifth decade and demonstrates a male predominance. Some 5% of cases show autosomal dominant inheritance and are caused by a mutation in the superoxide dismutase 1 *(SOD1)* gene on chromosome 21q. Interestingly familial ALS caused by *SOD1* mutations is not due to deficient SOD activity but rather represents a gain of function mutation, with toxic results. Aggregation of SOD1 and other proteins, such as neurofilament subunits, presumably impairs the survival of motor neurons. Familial forms of ALS may be also be associated with mutations at several additional loci.

 PATHOLOGY: *ALS is characterized pathologically by a loss of motor neurons in the brain and spinal cord, specifically the anterior horn cells of the spinal cord, the motor nuclei of the brainstem (especially the hypoglossal nuclei), and the upper motor neurons of the cerebral cortex.* Loss of neurons is accompanied by a mild gliosis and often aggregations of neurofilaments within the axons to form spheroids. Myelin stains demonstrate a striking pallor of the lateral corticospinal tracts of the spinal cord. The muscles innervated by injured spinal areas become atrophic.

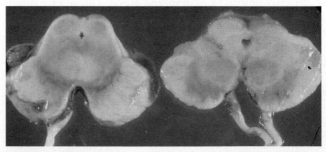

FIGURE 28-26. **Parkinson disease.** The affected substantia nigra (right) is depigmented, compared to a normal brain (left).

 CLINICAL FEATURES: ALS begins as weakness and wasting of the muscles of the hand, often accompanied by painful cramps of the arm. Fasciculations (irregular rapid contractions of the muscles that do not result in limb movements) are characteristic. ALS is progressive and results in weakness of the limbs, leading to total disability, unintelligible speech, and respiratory weakness. Dementia is uncommon in ALS. Patients often succumb within 10 years.

TABLE 28–6

Representative Neurodegenerative Diseases with Filamentous Amyloid Lesions

Disease	Lesion	Components	Location
Alzheimer disease	Senile plaques Neurofibrillary tangles	β-Amyloid tau	Extracellular Intracytoplasmic
Amyotrophic lateral sclerosis	Spheroids	Neurofilament subunits/super-oxide dismutase (SOD-1)	Intracytoplasmic
Dementia with Lewy bodies	Lewy bodies	α-Synuclein	Intracytoplasmic
Frontotemporal dementias	Neurofibrillary tangles	tau	Intracytoplasmic
Multiple system atrophy	Glial inclusions	tau	Intracytoplasmic
Parkinson disease	Lewy bodies	α-Synuclein	Intracytoplasmic
Prion diseases	Prion deposits	Prions	Extracellular
Trinucleotide repeat	Inclusions	Polyglutamine tracts	Intranuclear and cytoplasmic

Trinucleotide Repeat Expansion Syndromes are Associated with Neurodegenerative Diseases

A large number of diseases can be classified under triplet repeat expansion syndromes. *Triplet repeats are normal components of many genes and represent three nucleotides that repeat in sequence. The expansion of triplet repeats to certain critical lengths can lead to disease states.* Triplet repeat diseases may be inherited in an X-linked, autosomal dominant or in an autosomal recessive manner. An increase in triplet repeat length with each subsequent generation can lead to an earlier onset of disease, termed *anticipation*. Triplet repeats may occur within a coding region of a gene, leading to abnormal protein formation, or in a noncoding region of a gene, producing transcriptional interference (see Chapter 6).

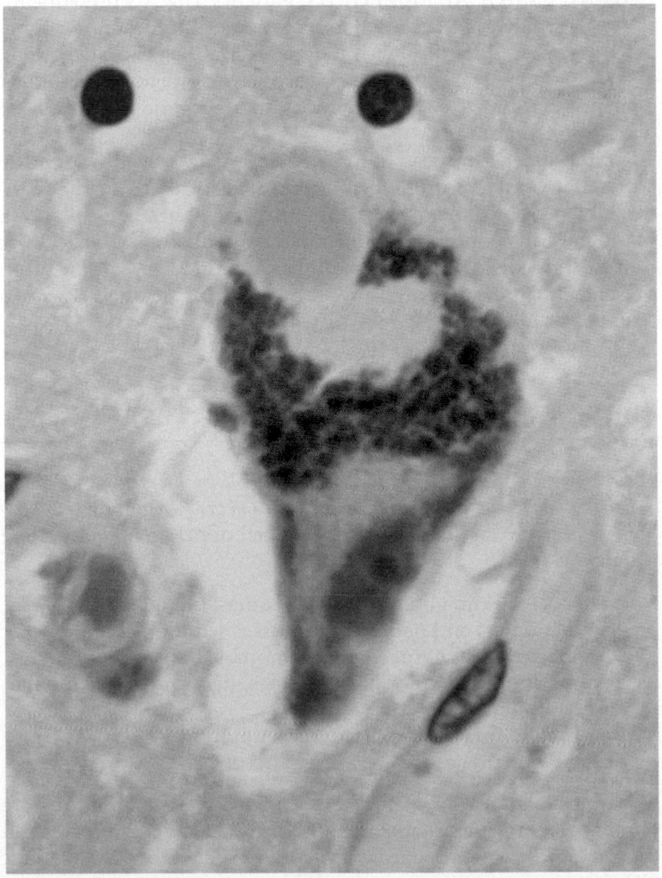

Huntington Disease (HD)

HD is a fatal inherited malady characterized by involuntary movements and cognitive deterioration.

 PATHOGENESIS: HD is caused by expansion of CAG repeats in the coding region of the *HD* gene on chromosome 4p16.3. The disease demonstrates an autosomal dominant inheritance pattern, although sporadic forms have been identified *The HD gene product, namely huntingtin, is expressed widely throughout the body, including in neurons and glia. Although the function of the protein is unknown, expansion of triplet repeats in this gene most likely leads to a toxic gain of function.* Aggregates of huntingtin may serve to impede critical gene functions. This disease commonly affects whites of northwestern European ancestry and has an incidence of 1 in 20,000.

 PATHOLOGY: At autopsy, the frontal cortex is symmetrically and moderately atrophied. In addition, the caudate nuclei undergo symmetric atrophy with an expansion of the lateral ventricles. Microscopically, a loss of small neurons with associated microgliosis is identified. Accumulation of abnormal huntingtin protein occurs in neuronal nuclei and processes, although its role in pathogenesis is unclear.

 CLINICAL FEATURES: The average age of onset is 40 years, and patients present initially with cognitive and emotional disturbances. These symptoms are followed in several years by the development of choreoathetoid movements. Affected persons ultimately develop severe intellectual deterioration, often accompanied by paranoia and delusions, as well as a severe, debilitating, movement disorder. Death commonly occurs about 15 years after HD has been diagnosed.

Inherited Spinocerebellar Ataxias: Friedreich Ataxia

The inherited spinocerebellar ataxias include a heterogeneous group of disorders that share features of a broad, but system-based, topography, a genetic contribution, and a precocious loss of neurons in the cerebellum, brainstem, and spinal cord. A subset of these

FIGURE 28-27. **Parkinson disease.** A pigmented neuron in the substantia nigra contains a Lewy body (the large eosinophilic cytoplasmic inclusion at the top with a surrounding halo).

diseases demonstrates expanded trinucleotide repeats. The most common inherited spinocerebellar ataxia is **Friedreich Ataxia (FA),** which is inherited in an autosomal recessive manner and demonstrates a prevalence in European populations of 1 in 50,000. FA may also occur sporadically. The onset of disease typically occurs before 25 years of age and progresses until death, which occurs some 30 years following diagnosis. FA is caused by expansion of a GAA repeat in the *frataxin* gene located at 9q13.3-21.1, which functions in iron transport into the mitochondria. Frataxin is most highly expressed in the heart and spinal cord, and disease occurs by loss of function of the frataxin protein. Patients demonstrate a combined ataxia of the upper and lower limbs, and frequently dysarthria, lower-limb areflexia, extensor plantar reflexes, and sensory loss. In addition, many patients also suffer skeletal deformities, hypertrophic cardiomyopathy, and diabetes mellitus. At autopsy, degeneration of the posterior columns (sensory loss), distal corticospinal tracts, and spinocerebellar tracts (ataxia) is evident.

Alzheimer Disease (AD) is the Most Common Cause of Dementia in the Elderly

AD is the most common cause of dementia in the elderly and demonstrates an increasing prevalence with age, with 10% of persons older than 85 years of age demonstrating features of the disease. The majority of AD cases are sporadic, although a familial form is recognized.

 PATHOGENESIS: A variety of genetic factors appear to contribute to the development of AD, including the following:

- **Apolipoprotein E:** The ε4 allele (chromosome 19q13.2) is associated with an increased risk and earlier onset of AD. The ε2 allele may be protective.
- **Presenilin-1:** Mutations on chromosome 14 are associated with early-onset familial AD.
- **Presenilin-2:** Mutations on chromosome 1 are associated with Volga German familial AD.

AD is characterized by the formation of senile (neuritic) plaques and neurofibrillary tangles (NFTs). Senile plaques are spherical aggregates of Aβ up to several hundred μm in diameter. Aβ is formed by altered cleavage of the **amyloid precursor protein** (APP), which is a transmembrane protein located on neurons and glia, the gene for which is found on chromosome 21. Normal degradation of APP results in proteolytic cleavage in the center of the Aβ region, located on the extracellular aspect of APP. By contrast, abnormal cleavage at either end of the Aβ portion of the molecule (in patients with mutated APP) results in the production of a 42-amino-acid, highly amyloidogenic, insoluble Aβ peptide that accumulates in **senile plaques** (Fig. 28-28). *Extensive senile plaque formation and early AD onset is characteristic of patients with Down syndrome, who have an extra copy of chromosome 21, thereby supporting the role of the Aβ peptide in the development of dementia.* Yet, many cognitively intact elderly persons have extensive plaque formation without clinical cognitive impairment, raising questions about the pathogenic significance of senile plaque.

Neurofibrillary tangles (NFTs) are a second prominent pathologic feature of AD (Fig. 28-29). NFTs are formed by an abnormal form of a microtubule-associated protein (MAP) termed *tau*. In AD, tau undergoes aberrant phosphorylation, which results in dissociation of the protein from microtubules and aggregation of paired helical filaments within the neuronal cytoplasm. Neuronal transport is, therefore, interrupted and contributes to compromised neuronal function.

 PATHOLOGY: On gross examination, the brain of patients with AD appears atrophic, evidenced by an average weight loss of 200 grams, narrow gyri and widened

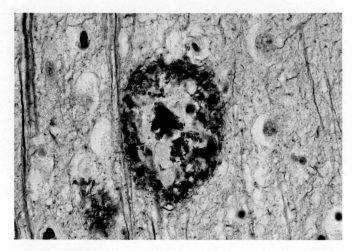

FIGURE 28-28. **Alzheimer disease.** A silver stain illustrates a senile plaque, with dystrophic neurites on the periphery and a central core of amyloid.

sulci (Fig. 28-30). The atrophy is symmetrical and predominantly in the frontal and hippocampal cortex. Microscopically, neuronal loss, gliosis, and the formation of senile plaques and NFTs are identified. Senile plaques are immunopositive for Aβ at the core and periphery, and are also positive for Congo red, thioflavin S, and silver stains. NFTs appear as irregular bundles of fibrils in the neuronal cytoplasm that are immunoreactive for tau. The mechanisms underlying AD are presented in Figure 28-31.

 CLINICAL FEATURES: Patients with AD present clinically with a gradual loss of memory and cognitive function, difficulty with language, and behavioral changes. The disease progresses, with development to full-blown dementia within 5 to 10 years. Most patients die as a result of bronchopneumonia.

Pick disease appears clinically similar to AD, although the cortical atrophy is initially unilateral and localized to the frontotemporal lobe; however, atrophy ultimately becomes bilateral. Many neurons contain cytoplasmic tau inclusions termed **Pick bodies.** Pick disease is commonly a sporadic disease that often presents in mid adult life and progresses to death in 3 to 10 years.

Tumors of the CNS

The majority of neoplasms within the CNS are actually metastatic lesions, although a variety of primary neoplasms can occur. Primary CNS neoplasms may be classified according to cell of origin, including the following:

- **Neuroectoderm:** gliomas (astrocytomas, oligodendrogliomas, ependymomas) and neuronal tumors (medulloblastoma)
- **Mesenchymal structures:** meningiomas, schwannomas
- **Ectopic tissues:** craniopharyngiomas, dermoid cysts, lipomas, dysgerminomas
- **Retained embryonic structures:** paraphyseal cysts
- **Metastases:** predominantly lung and breast

Approximately 40% of primary CNS neoplasms in adults are gliomas, 30% are meningiomas or other mesenchymal tumors, and the remainder is composed of various other neoplasms. About 30% of primary CNS tumors in children are astrocytomas of the posterior fossa. Neuronal tumors are uncommon. When they occur in childhood, they are often primitive, rapidly growing lesions that involve the cerebellum (medulloblastomas). Typically, the be-

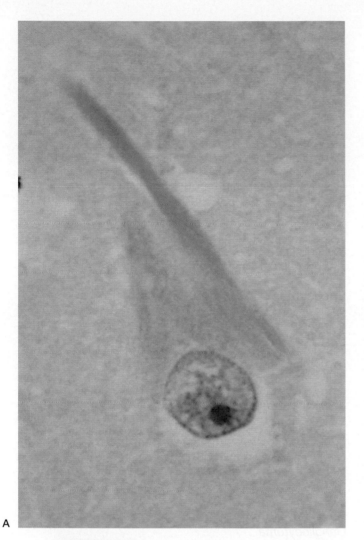

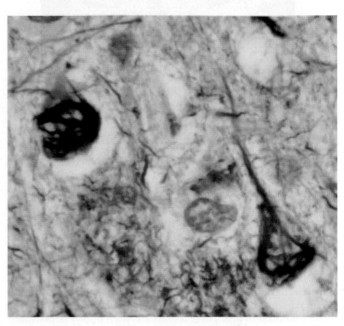

A

B

FIGURE 28-29. **Alzheimer disease. A.** A neuron exhibits a basophilic, cytoplasmic neurofibrillary tangle. **B.** A silver stain illustrates the intracellular structure of a neurofibrillary tangle.

havior of CNS neoplasms cannot be readily categorized into benign versus malignant, because (1) many lesions may demonstrate indolent growth and cause death only years following diagnosis, and (2) the vast majority of CNS neoplasms do not metastasize outside of the CNS but still exert ultimately lethal mass effects within the cerebral vault. The majority of CNS neoplasms also demonstrate specific intracranial locations and relatively well-defined age of onsets. Classical locations of CNS neoplasms are presented in Figure 28-32.

Intracranial tumors may lead to similar symptoms that are primarily caused by local infiltration and mass effect. Infiltration causes motor or sensory deficits, with general sparing of cognitive function. Irritation of neuronal regions results in the development of seizures. A mass effect caused directly by the tumor or by surrounding edema increases the risk of hydrocephalus and herniation. Various types of herniation include the following:

- **Transtentorial herniation:** The medial aspect of the hippocampus herniates through the tentorium and results in third nerve palsy and midbrain necrosis.
- **Foramen magnum herniation:** The cerebellar tonsils herniate into the foramen magnum and compress the cardiac and respiratory centers in the brainstem.
- **Subfalcine herniation:** The cingulate gyrus herniates beneath the falx.

Gliomas Include a Variety of Neurectodermally Derived Neoplasms

Astrocytomas

Astrocytomas range greatly in levels of differentiation, with the degree of malignancy often correlating with increased age of the patient. Generally, these tumors demonstrate expression of glial fibrillary acidic protein (GFAP), reflecting their origin from glial astrocytes, although poorly differentiated lesions may demonstrate some loss of this molecule. Astrocytomas are subclassified into four grades (WHO Criteria), based on the pathological findings.

Grade I Astrocytoma (Pilocytic Astrocytoma)

Grade I astrocytomas often occur in children and young adults and demonstrate the most favorable prognosis of all astrocytomas. They may be circumscribed and potentially respectable. Pilocytic astrocytomas often occur in the posterior fossa (the most common site for pediatric brain neoplasms), although the third ventricle, hypothalamus, and thalamus may be involved. The outcome is dependent on the extent of resection, with completely resected tumors having a nearly 100% 10-year survival. Pilocytic astrocytomas are often microcystic and demonstrate regions of parallel bundles of fibrillar ("piloid" or "hairlike") processes that are positive for GFAP. In addition, Rosenthal fibers, which are highly eosinophilic, irregular, "shattered appearing" aggregations

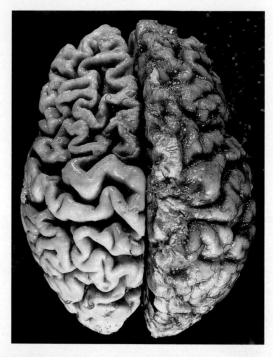

FIGURE 28-30. **Alzheimer disease.** The brain of an elderly patient is afflicted by severe atrophy of the cerebral cortex.

within glial processes, and eosinophilic intracellular or extracellular protein droplets (eosinophilic granular bodies) may be identified.

Grade II Astrocytoma (Diffuse Astrocytoma)

Grade II astrocytomas (diffuse astrocytomas) account for 20% of all CNS neoplasms and affect the spinal cord, optic nerve, third ventricle, midbrain, pons, and cerebellum in young adults, and the cerebral hemispheres in adults. The average age of onset is between 20 and 40 years of age. These lesions are often poorly demarcated, with tumor cells intermingling with normal parenchymal elements and presenting no distinct margin (Fig. 28-33). The neoplasm consists of a hypercellular cortex containing infiltrating, small, hyperchromatic, single glial cells, which demonstrate pleomorphic nuclei and rare to no mitotic figures. Patients with grade II astrocytomas demonstrate an average life expectancy of 5 years, and transformation to a higher grade astrocytoma may occur.

Grade III Astrocytoma (Anaplastic Astrocytoma)

Grade III astrocytomas (anaplastic astrocytoma) often occur in patients between ages 30 to 40 years and most commonly affect the cerebral hemispheres. Microscopically, these tumors are characterized by pleomorphic cells, greater cellularity, and modest mitotic activity. They do not demonstrate microvascular proliferation or coagulative necrosis (distinguishing them from grade IV tumors). The rapid growth of this lesion results in a life expectancy of 2 to 3 years.

Grade IV Astrocytoma

Grade IV astrocytomas, also termed **glioblastoma multiforme**, account for 40% of all primary CNS neoplasms and most commonly occur in patients over the age of 40 years. These lesions may affect any region of the brain and can cross the midline of the brain via the corpus callosum to give a butterflylike effect on radiographic imaging. Microscopically, this lesion is characterized by markedly pleomorphic cells, mitoses, palisading necrosis, and glomeruloid vascular proliferation (endothelial proliferation within the vascular lumen) (Fig. 28-34). These lesions are highly aggressive and life expectancy is only 18 months.

Oligodendroglioma

Oligodendrogliomas represent approximately 15% of all gliomas and most commonly occur in adults. These tumors are typically located in the white matter of the cerebral hemispheres. Grossly, oligodendrogliomas appear gelatinous or soft and often obscure the gray-white junction of the cortex. Microscopically, they are composed of uniform cells with small round nuclei with a perinuclear halo (clearing) caused by fixation ("fried egg cells") (Fig. 28-35). The tumor cells often surround large cortical neurons, a process termed *satellitosis*. Mitotic figures and necrosis are typically absent, although they may occur in higher grade lesions. The neoplastic cells are often surrounded by delicate small vessels. Oligodendrogliomas infiltrate the surrounding brain and are positive for GFAP. Loss of heterozygosity for chromosomes 1p and 19q tend to occur in these lesions and serves as a useful molecular marker. In some instances, oligodendrogliomas may undergo anaplastic transformation. The average life expectancy following diagnosis is 5 to 10 years. Oligodendrogliomas are particularly sensitive to PCV chemotherapy.

Ependymoma

Ependymomas most commonly occur during the first 2 decades of life and are often located in or adjacent to the fourth ventricle. Growth within the fourth ventricle may give rise to hydrocephalus. In contrast to other gliomas, ependymomas demonstrate a more discrete border with the surrounding brain and appear grossly as soft, fleshy lesions (Fig. 28-36). A common microscopic feature of ependymomas is the formation of *true rosettes* and *pseudorosettes* (Fig. 28-37). True rosettes appear similar to tire spokes, in which a circular arrangement of cells rims central fibrillar processes. When these structures surround blood vessels, they are termed pseudorosettes. Ependymomas stain positively for GFAP and may be subdivided into a number of types based on morphology. The outcome is related to the extent of surgical resection possible.

Neuronal Tumors

Gangliocytoma

Gangliocytomas are tumors formed of large neurons that have the morphologic appearance of ganglion cells. When admixed with neoplastic glial cells, they are termed **gangliogliomas**. These tumors are most common in children and young adults and preferentially affect the temporal lobes, although any site of the brain may be affected. Radiographically and macroscopically, they are well-circumscribed and most commonly demonstrate a cystic structure containing a mural nodule. Microscopically, gangliocytomas are formed of large, disordered neurons in a background of fibrillary stroma (neuronal processes), with little to no intervening brain tissue. Additional microscopic findings include cytoplasmic eosinophilic granular bodies, microcalcifications, and perivascular lymphocytic infiltrates. Patients often present with seizures.

Central neurocytoma

Central neurocytomas are tumors that often occur in young adults and appear grossly and radiographically as well-circumscribed, intraventricular lesions. They occur within the ventricular system near the foramen of Monro and, therefore, may present with obstruction of CSF flow and manifestations of hydrocephalus. Microscopically, these lesions are formed by uniform, small, round neurons, with finely speckled chromatin in a background fibrillar stroma formed by neuronal processes.

Medulloblastoma

Medulloblastomas occur within the first two decades of life and represent the most common neuroblastic tumor in the CNS. In addition to sporadic forms, these tumors may arise in association with Turcot or Gorlin syndromes. The lesions most likely arise

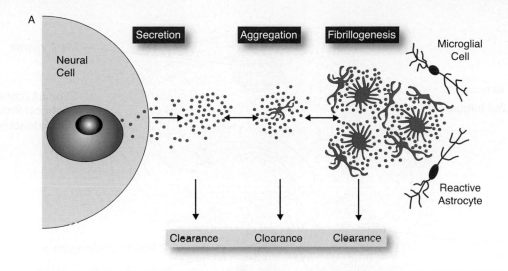

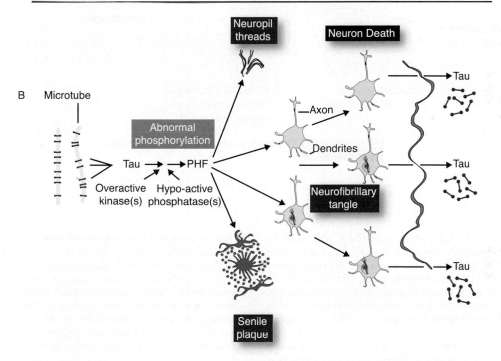

FIGURE 28-31. **Mechanisms of amyloidosis and brain degeneration in Alzheimer disease. A.** This schematic illustrates a hypothetical mechanism for the formation of senile plaques (SPs) from soluble Aβ peptides produced inside cells and secreted into the extracellular space. Amyloidogenic Aβ may encounter fibril-inducing cofactors and go on to form A fibrils to deposit in SPs (far right). SPs are surrounded by reactive astrocytes and microglial cells, which secrete cytokines that may contribute to the toxicity of the SPs. These steps may be reversible. Increasing Aβ clearance or reducing its production, as well as modulating the inflammatory response, may be effective therapeutic interventions for Alzheimer disease, in combination with therapies that target brain degeneration caused by NFTs. **B.** This schematic illustrates a hypothetical mechanism leading to the conversion of normal human central nervous system (CNS) tau overlying 2 microtubules into paired helical filaments (PHFs). PHFs are generated in neuronal perikarya and their processes. Overactive kinase(s) or hypoactive phosphatase(s) may contribute to this effect. Abnormally phosphorylated tau forms PHFs in neuronal processes (neuropil threads) and neuronal perikarya (neurofibrillary tangles, NFTs). Tau in PHFs loses the ability to bind microtubules, thus causing their depolymerization, disruption of axonal transport, and degeneration of neurons. Accumulation of PHFs in neurons could exacerbate this process by physically blocking transport in neurons. The death of affected neurons would release tau and increase the levels of tau in the cerebrospinal fluid (CSF) of patients with Alzheimer disease. NFT formation may be reversible, and drugs that block NFT formation, reverse it, or stabilize microtubules may be effective therapeutic interventions for Alzheimer disease.

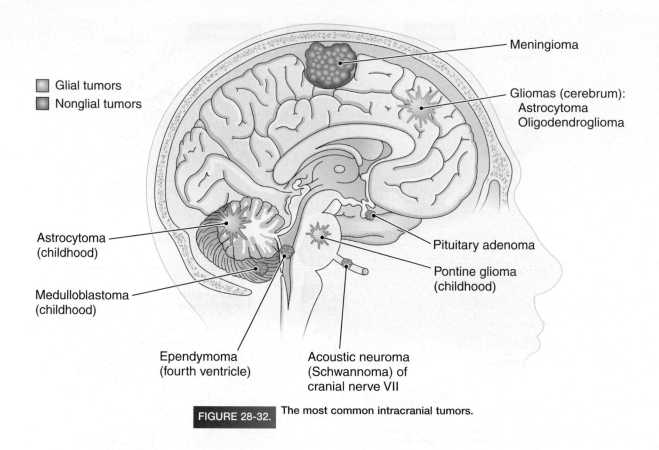

□ Glial tumors
■ Nonglial tumors

Meningioma

Gliomas (cerebrum):
Astrocytoma
Oligodendroglioma

Astrocytoma
(childhood)

Pituitary adenoma

Pontine glioma
(childhood)

Medulloblastoma
(childhood)

Ependymoma
(fourth ventricle)

Acoustic neuroma
(Schwannoma) of
cranial nerve VII

FIGURE 28-32. The most common intracranial tumors.

from the external granular layer of the cerebellum, which may explain why they are located almost exclusively in that location. Microscopically, medulloblastomas contain hyperchromatic, round to oval nuclei, and scant cytoplasm, typical of "small cell" neoplasms. The cells often crowd together and overlap, although rosette formation may be present. Immunostains for neurofilament protein and synaptophysin are positive. Multiple underlying molecular abnormalities have been identified, including c-myc amplification, isochromosome 17q formation, and loss of 17p heterozygosity. Patients often present with ataxia and signs of hydrocephalus. These lesions are highly sensitive to radiotherapy, but the 10-year survival rate is only 50% because of the highly infiltrative behavior of this neoplasm and its ability to disseminate within the CSF.

Meningioma is a Mesenchymally Derived Tumor

Meningiomas are benign tumors that arise from the meningothelium and often occur in the fourth or fifth decades, although young adults may also be affected. They account for 20% of all primary CNS neoplasms and most commonly occur in the parasagittal regions of the cerebral hemispheres, olfactory groove, and lateral sphenoid wing. *These lesions most commonly occur sporadically, although prior radiation treatment or association with a genetic disorder such as neurofibromatosis type 2 (NF2), may predispose to their development.*

Meningiomas grow as well-demarcated, firm, bosselated lesions attached to the meninges and often cause symptoms, such as seizures, by compression of adjacent brain parenchyma. Involvement of the meninges, which are innervated, may also cause headaches. The cut surface of meningiomas is gray and often demonstrates a homogeneous appearance. Microscopically,

these lesions are classically characterized by whorled patterns of meningothelial cells (Fig. 28-38) associated with psammoma bodies (laminated, spherical calcium deposits). Meningiomas are positive for epithelial membrane antigen and negative for GFAP and cytokeratin. Various morphological forms may occur, some of which appear to be more aggressive. Owing to their position, meningiomas may occasionally invade the skull, although this is not associated with a worsened prognosis. By contrast, local brain invasion portends a poorer outcome.

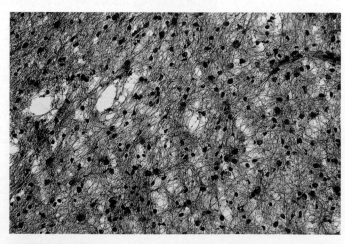

FIGURE 28-33. **Astrocytoma.** Moderately pleomorphic, neoplastic astrocytes infiltrate the white matter.

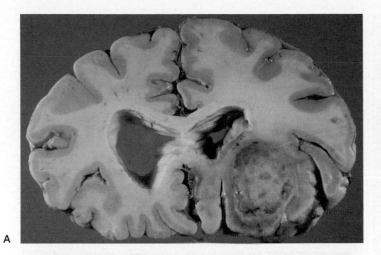

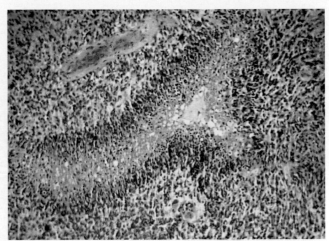

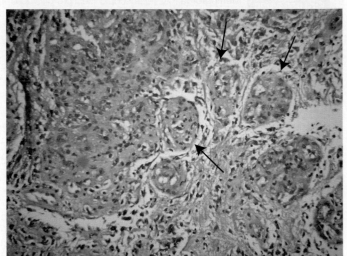

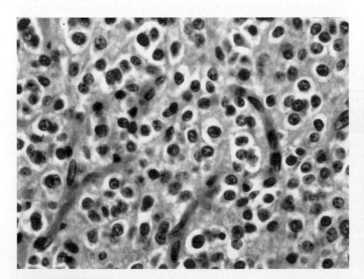

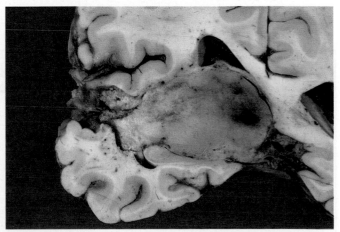

FIGURE 28-34. Glioblastoma multiforme. **A.** A coronal section of the brain shows a necrotic, hemorrhagic, expansile mass in the right hemisphere. **B**. Another area exhibits tumor necrosis, which is surrounded by pseudopalisaded tumor cells. **C**. A characteristic feature of glioblastoma multiforme is endothelial proliferation (*arrows*).

FIGURE 28-35. Oligodendroglioma. The tumor consists of sheets of uniform, small cells containing dark blue round nuclei (hematoxylin and eosin stain).

FIGURE 28-36. Ependymoma. This necrotic and hemorrhagic tumor arose in the lateral ventricle and infiltrates the surrounding parenchyma.

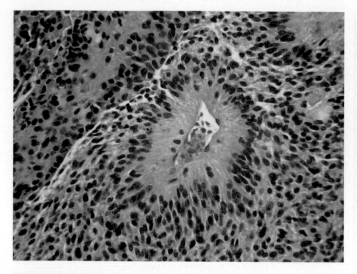

FIGURE 28-37. **Ependymoma.** A microscopic section shows a perivascular pseudorosette.

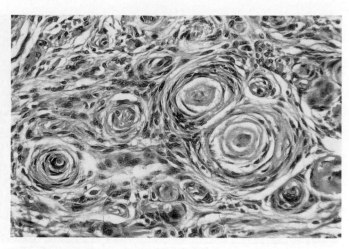

FIGURE 28-38. **Meningioma.** A microscopic section discloses a whorled arrangement of tumor cells, the so-called meningothelial appearance.

Schwannoma is Derived from the Nerve Sheath

Schwannomas are derived from Schwann cells, which produce both collagen and myelin. These lesions may occur at many locations, including spinal nerve roots and along the eighth cranial nerve, termed an acoustic neuroma. **Acoustic neuroma** arises in the internal auditory meatus and may cause tinnitus and deafness, as well as additional nerve compression if it has extended into the cerebellopontine angle. Microscopically, these lesions demonstrate interwoven fascicles of spindle cells, some of which form a parallel array termed a Verocay body. These lesions may occur in conjunction with NF2 gene deletion. Excision is usually curative. (See also Peripheral Nervous System below.)

Hereditary Diseases May be Associated with Intracranial Neoplasms

A variety of hereditary syndromes may be associated with the development of various CNS neoplasms. A listing of these disorders and associated genetic defects is presented in Table 28-7.

THE PERIPHERAL NERVOUS SYSTEM

The peripheral nervous system (PNS) is external to the brain and spinal cord and includes (1) cranial nerves, (2) dorsal and ventral spinal roots, (3) spinal nerves and their continuations, and (4) ganglia. Peripheral nerves carry somatic motor, somatic sensory, visceral sensory, and autonomic fibers. Somatic motor and preganglionic autonomic fibers arise from neuronal cell bodies within the CNS. The sensory and postganglionic autonomic fibers originate from neuronal cell bodies within ganglia located on cranial nerves, dorsal roots, and autonomic nerves. The neurons and satellite cells of the ganglia and all of the Schwann cells are derived from the neural crest. Peripheral nerve fibers are either myelinated or unmyelinated. Myelinated fibers range from 1 to 20 μm in diameter, whereas unmyelinated ones are considerably smaller, measuring 0.4 to 2.4 μm. Schwann cells ensheathe both myelinated and unmyelinated fibers. The axon determines whether the ensheathing Schwann cell differentiates into a myelin forming cell.

Table 28–7			
Hereditary Syndromes Associated with Intracranial Tumors			
Disease	**Chromosome Locus**	**Gene (Protein)**	**Nervous System Tumor(s)**
Neurofibromatosis 1	17q11	NF1 (neurofibromin)	Neurofibroma Malignant peripheral nerve sheath tumor Juvenile pilocytic astrocytoma of the optic nerves ("optic glioma")
Neurofibromatosis 2	22q12	NF2 (schwannomin/merlin)	Schwannoma Meningioma Ependymoma (spinal cord) Bilateral acoustic neuromas
Tuberous sclerosis	9q34 16p13.3	TSC1 (hamartin) TSC2 (tuberin)	Subependymal giant cell tumor Astrocytoma
von Hippel-Lindau syndrome	3p25	VHL	Hemangioblastoma

A. INTACT MYELINATED FIBER

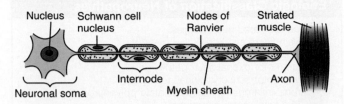

Nucleus Schwann cell
nucleus Nodes of
Ranvier Striated
muscle

Neuronal soma Internode Axon

Myelin sheath

B. DISTAL AXONAL DEGENERATION

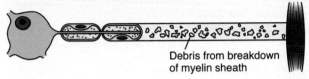

Debris from breakdown
of myelin sheath

**C. DEGENERATION OF CELL BODY
AND AXON**

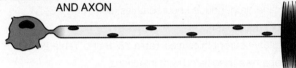

D. SEGMENTAL DEMYELINATION

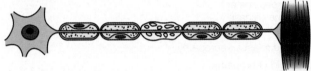

E. REMYELINATION

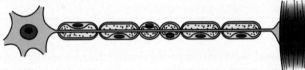

F. REGENERATING AXON

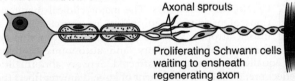

Axonal sprouts

Proliferating Schwann cells
waiting to ensheath
regenerating axon

G. REGENERATED NERVE FIBER

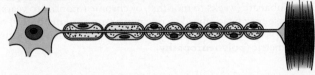

Reactions to Injury

Peripheral nerve fibers display only a limited number of reactions to injury (Fig. 28-39). The major types of nerve fiber damage are axonal degeneration and segmental demyelination. *Peripheral nerve fibers differ from CNS nerve fibers in having the capacity for functionally significant axonal regeneration and remyelination.*

FIGURE 28-39. **Basic responses of peripheral nerve fibers to injury.** **A.** Intact myelinated fiber. The axon is insulated by the Schwann cell-derived myelin sheaths. **B.** Distal axonal degeneration. The distal axon has degenerated, and myelin sheaths associated with the distal axon have secondarily degenerated. The striated muscle shows denervation atrophy. **C.** Degeneration of cell body and axon. Degeneration involves the neuronal cell body and its entire axon. The myelin sheaths associated with the axon have also degenerated. **D.** Segmental demyelination. The myelin sheath associated with one Schwann cell has degenerated, leaving a segment of axon uncovered by myelin. The underlying axon remains intact. **E.** Remyelination. Proliferating Schwann cells cover the demyelinated segment of the axon and elaborate new myelin sheaths. The remyelinating Schwann cells have short internodal lengths. **F.** Regenerating axon. Regenerating axons sprout from the distal end of the disrupted axon. Ideally, the regenerating axons reinnervate the distal nerve stump, where they will be ensheathed and myelinated by Schwann cells of the distal stump. **G.** Regenerated nerve fiber. The regenerated portion of the axon is myelinated by Schwann cells with short internodal lengths. The striated muscle is reinnervated.

Axonal Degeneration is Usually Restricted to the Distal Axon

Degeneration (necrosis) of the axon occurs in many neuropathies and reflects significant injury of the neuronal cell body or its axon. Axonal degeneration is quickly followed by breakdown of the myelin sheath and Schwann cell proliferation. Myelin degradation is initiated by Schwann cells and completed by macrophages, which infiltrate the nerve within 3 days after axonal degeneration. If the degeneration is restricted to the distal axon, regenerating axons may sprout within 1 week from the intact, proximal axonal stump. There are several types of axonal degeneration.

DISTAL AXONAL DEGENERATION: In many neuropathies axonal degeneration is initially restricted to the distal ends of the larger, longer fibers (see Fig. 28-39B). Peripheral neuropathies characterized by the selective degeneration of distal axons are known as **dying-back neuropathies (distal axonopathies)** and are typically seen as distal ("length-dependent" or "glove-and-stocking") neuropathies.

In distal axonal degeneration, the neuronal cell body and proximal axon remain intact. Therefore, axonal regeneration and return of nerve function may be possible if the cause of the distal axonal degeneration can be identified and removed. This must occur before the dying-back degeneration sufficiently extends centripetally to involve the proximal axon and kill the neuronal cell body. Recovery is limited in some dying-back neuropathies, because the distal axonal degeneration also affects centrally directed axons traveling in the dorsal columns of the spinal cord, which have little capacity for regeneration.

NEURONOPATHY: Axonal degeneration may result from death of the neuronal cell body, as occurs in an autoimmune dorsal root ganglionitis (see Fig. 28-39C). Neuropathies showing selective damage to the neuronal cell body are referred to as **neuronopathies** and are much less common than distal axonopathies. There is little potential for recovery of function in neuronopathy because death of the neuronal cell body precludes axonal regeneration.

WALLERIAN DEGENERATION: This term refers to the axonal degeneration that occurs in a nerve distal to a transection or crush of the nerve. If the transection is not too proximal, the nerve may regenerate.

Segmental Demyelination Reflects Direct Schwann Cell Injury or Underlying Axonal Abnormalities

Loss of myelin from one or more internodes (segments) along a myelinated fiber reflects Schwann cell dysfunction (see Fig. 28-39D). This condition may be caused by direct injury to the Schwann cell or myelin sheath (**primary demyelination**), or it may result from underlying axonal abnormalities (**secondary demyelination**). Loss of the myelin sheath is not accompanied by degeneration of the underlying axon. Macrophages infiltrate the nerve and clear the myelin debris. Degeneration of the internodal myelin sheath is followed sequentially by (1) Schwann cell proliferation, (2) remyelination of the demyelinated segments, and (3) recovery of function.

Peripheral Neuropathies

Peripheral neuropathy is a process that affects the function of one or more peripheral nerves. The disease may be restricted to the PNS, involve both the peripheral and central nervous systems, or affect multiple organ systems. Peripheral neuropathies are diverse in origin, are encountered in all age groups and may be hereditary or acquired (Table 28-8). Diabetic neuropathy is the most common neuropathy in the United States. Other common causes include hereditary disorders, alcoholism, renal failure, neurotoxic drugs, autoimmune diseases, monoclonal gammopathy, infections, and trauma.

PATHOLOGY: The pathologic findings in most neuropathies are mainly limited to axonal degeneration, segmental demyelination, or a combination of both.

TABLE 28–8
Etiologic Classification of Neuropathies

Immune-mediated neuropathies
  Guillain-Barré syndrome
    Acute inflammatory demyelinating polyneuropathy
  Acute motor axonal neuropathy
  Acute motor sensory axonal neuropathy
  Chronic inflammatory demyelinating polyneuropathy
    Multifocal motor neuropathy
  Dorsal root ganglionitis
  Neuropathy associated with monoclonal gammopathy
  Vasculitic neuropathy

Metabolic neuropathies
  Diabetic polyneuropathy and mononeuropathies
  Uremic neuropathy
  Critical illness polyneuropathy

Nutritional neuropathy (deficiency of vitamin B_1, B_6, B_{12}, or E)
Alcoholic neuropathy
Toxic and drug-induced neuropathies (see Table 28–7)
Amyloid neuropathy
Hereditary neuropathies (see Table 28–8 and Table 28–9)

Neuropathies associated with infections
  Leprosy
  Human immunodeficiency virus
  Cytomegalovirus
  Herpes zoster
  Lyme disease
  Diphtheria (toxin)

Paraneoplastic neuropathy
Sarcoid neuropathy
Radiation neuropathy
Traumatic neuropathy
Chronic idiopathic axonal neuropathy

When axonal degeneration predominates, the neuropathy is classified as an **axonal neuropathy**; when segmental demyelination is more prominent, the neuropathy is termed **demyelinating neuropathy**. *Most (80%–90%) neuropathies are axonal.*

CLINICAL FEATURES: The major clinical manifestations of peripheral neuropathy are muscle weakness, muscle atrophy, altered sensation, and autonomic dysfunction. Motor, sensory, and autonomic functions may be equally or preferentially affected. Sensory abnormalities may reflect predominant involvement of large-diameter fibers (position and vibration sense) or small-diameter fibers (pain and temperature). The tempo of the neuropathy may be acute (days to weeks), subacute (weeks to months), or chronic (months to years). The disease may be localized to one nerve (**mononeuropathy**) or several nerves (**mononeuropathy multiplex**), or it may be diffuse and symmetric (**polyneuropathy**).

Diabetic Neuropathy Has Several Clinical Presentations

Peripheral neuropathy is a common complication of diabetes mellitus. The neuropathy may manifest as a distal sensorimotor polyneuropathy, autonomic neuropathy, mononeuropathy, or mononeuropathy multiplex. The mononeuropathies may involve cranial nerves (cranial neuropathy), nerve roots (radiculopathy), or proximal peripheral nerves. *Distal, predominantly sensory, polyneuropathy is the most common form of diabetic neuropathy.*

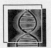 PATHOGENESIS: The pathogenesis of the nerve fiber injury in diabetes is unknown. It has long been held that the metabolic alterations of diabetes are responsible for the distal symmetric polyneuropathy, and that nerve ischemia caused by the small-vessel disease is responsible for the mononeuropathies. There is evidence, however, that local nerve ischemia may also play a significant role in the pathogenesis of the symmetric polyneuropathy.

 PATHOLOGY: The distal symmetric polyneuropathy of diabetes is characterized pathologically by a mixture of axonal degeneration and segmental demyelination, with axonal degeneration predominating. The axonal loss involves fibers of all sizes, but occasionally preferentially affects the large myelinated fibers (large-fiber neuropathy) or the small myelinated and unmyelinated fibers (small-fiber neuropathy).

Acute Inflammatory Demyelinating Polyneuropathy (Guillain-Barré Syndrome) is Immune-Mediated

Acute inflammatory demyelinating polyneuropathy (AIDP) is an acquired, immune-mediated neuropathy that often follows immunization or viral, bacterial, and mycoplasmal infections. It may also be sporadic or complicate surgery, cancer, or HIV infection. AIDP is the most common cause of the **Guillain-Barré syndrome**, in children and adults, and appears as an acute symmetric paralysis that begins distally and ascends proximally. Sensory and autonomic disturbances may also occur. The muscular paralysis may cause respiratory embarrassment, and the autonomic involvement may result in cardiac arrhythmias, hypotension, or hypertension. Resolution of the neuropathy begins 2 to 4 weeks after onset, and most patients make a good recovery. Lumbar puncture characteristically reveals an increased protein level in the CSF and no pleocytosis. The increased protein level is attributable to the inflammation of the spinal roots. Demyelination may be immunologically mediated, since plasmapheresis and intravenously administered gamma globulin have proven beneficial.

AIDP may involve all levels of the PNS, including spinal roots (polyradiculoneuropathy), ganglia, craniospinal nerves, and autonomic nerves. The distribution of the lesions varies from case to case. Involved regions show endoneurial infiltrates of lymphocytes and macrophages, segmental demyelination, and relative axonal sparing. The lymphoid infiltrates are often perivascular, but there is no true vasculitis. Macrophages are frequently found adjacent to degenerating myelin sheaths and have been observed to strip off and phagocytose the superficial myelin lamellae. Such macrophage-mediated demyelination is rarely observed in other neuropathies.

Chronic inflammatory demyelinating polyneuropathy (CIDP) is similar to AIDP but has a chronic course characterized by multiple relapses or a slow continuous progression. The nerves in CIDP may show numerous onion bulbs, owing to recurring episodes of demyelination, Schwann cell proliferation, and remyelination. Corticosteroid therapy is effective in CIDP but not in AIDP, suggesting that the two neuropathies have a different immune-mediated pathogenesis.

Toxic Neuropathy is Often Iatrogenic

A variety of environmental agents and industrial compounds cause peripheral neuropathy, but most cases of toxic neuropathy are caused by drugs. Almost all toxic neuropathies are characterized by axonal degeneration, usually of the dying-back type.

Hereditary Neuropathies are the Most Common Form of Chronic Neuropathy in Children

Peripheral neuropathy is a manifestation of a variety of inherited diseases. The neuropathy may be the sole manifestation of the hereditary disease or just one manifestation of a hereditary multisystem disease.

CHARCOT-MARIE-TOOTH DISEASE (CMT): *CMT is a genetically and pathologically heterogeneous group of slowly progressive distal sensorimotor polyneuropathies that manifest in childhood or early adult life.* It is the most common inherited neuropathy and among the most common inherited neurological disorders, with a prevalence of 1 in 2500. CMT may be broadly divided into demyelinating and axonal subtypes. **CMT1**, the most common subtype, has autosomal dominant inheritance and a chronic demyelinating polyneuropathy, with onion bulbs and axonal loss. The less common **CMT2** subtype also shows autosomal dominant inheritance and distal axonal degeneration. X-linked (**CMTX**) and autosomal recessive (**CMT4**) subtypes have also been described. The majority of cases of CMT are due to mutations in three genes: peripheral myelin protein 22 (*PMP22*), myelin protein zero (*MPZ*), and gap junction protein beta 1.

Tumors of the Peripheral Nervous System

Primary tumors of the PNS are of neuronal or nerve sheath origin. The neuronal tumors (e.g., neuroblastoma and ganglioneuroma) usually arise from the adrenal medulla or sympathetic ganglia. The common nerve sheath tumors are schwannoma and neurofibroma.

Schwannoma May Arise in Any Nerve

Schwannoma is a benign, slowly growing, typically encapsulated neoplasm of Schwann cells that originates in cranial nerves, spinal roots, or peripheral nerves. These tumors usually are seen in adults and only very rarely undergo malignant degeneration.

VESTIBULAR SCHWANNOMA (ACOUSTIC SCHWANNOMA): Intracranial schwannomas account for 8% of all intracranial tumors. Most arise from the vestibular branch of the eighth cranial nerve within the internal auditory canal or at the meatus and cause unilateral, sensorineural hearing loss, tinnitus, and vestibular dysfunction. The slowly growing tumor enlarges the meatus, extends medially into the subarachnoid space of the cerebellopontine angle (**cerebellopontine angle tumor**), and compresses the fifth and seventh cranial nerves, brainstem, and cerebellum. The posterior fossa mass may also lead to increased intracranial pressure, hydrocephalus, and tonsillar herniation. Most vestibular schwannomas are unilateral and are not associated with neurofibromatosis. Bilateral vestibular schwannomas are a defining feature of neurofibromatosis type 2.

INTRASPINAL AND PERIPHERAL SCHWANNOMAS: Intraspinal schwannomas are intradural, extra-axial tumors that arise most often from the dorsal (sensory) spinal roots. They produce radicular (root) pain and spinal cord compression. More peripherally located schwannomas usually originate on nerves of the head, neck, and extremities.

 PATHOLOGY: Schwannomas tend to be oval and well demarcated and vary in diameter from a few millimeters to several centimeters. The nerve of origin, if large enough, may be identifiable. The cut surface is firm and tan to gray, and often shows focal hemorrhage, necrosis, xan-

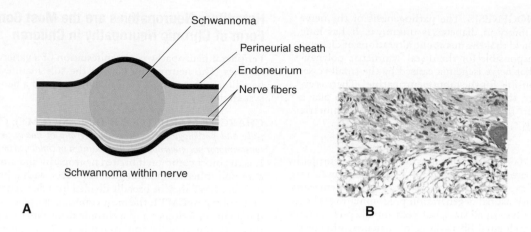

A Schwannoma within nerve

Schwannoma
Perineurial sheath
Endoneurium
Nerve fibers

B

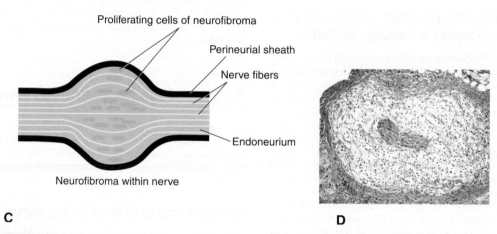

C Neurofibroma within nerve

Proliferating cells of neurofibroma
Perineurial sheath
Nerve fibers
Endoneurium

D

FIGURE 28-40. Growth patterns of schwannoma and neurofibroma within peripheral nerve. **A.** The cellular proliferation of the schwannoma is well-circumscribed and pushes surviving nerve fibers to the periphery of the tumor. **B.** A photomicrograph of a schwannoma shows the characteristically abrupt transition between the compact Antoni type A histologic pattern *(left)* and the spongy Antoni type B histologic pattern *(right).* **C.** The cellular proliferation of the neurofibroma is interspersed among the surviving nerve fibers. **D.** Photomicrograph of neurofibroma shows that the proliferating spindle-shaped Schwann cells form small strands that course haphazardly through a myxoid matrix.

thomatous change, and cystic degeneration. Microscopically, the proliferating Schwann cells form two distinctive histologic patterns (Fig. 28-40).

- **Antoni A pattern** is characterized by interwoven fascicles of spindle cells with elongated nuclei, eosinophilic cytoplasm, and indistinct cytoplasmic borders. The nuclei may palisade in areas to form structures known as **Verocay bodies**.
- **Antoni B pattern** features spindle or oval cells with indistinct cytoplasm in a loose, vacuolated background.

Degenerative changes in schwannomas are common and include collections of foam cells, recent or old hemorrhage, foci of fibrosis, and hyalinized blood vessels. Scattered atypical nuclei are frequently encountered in schwannomas, but mitotic figures are uncommon.

Neurofibroma Features Several Cell Types

Neurofibroma is a benign, slowly growing tumor of peripheral nerve composed of Schwann cells, perineurial-like cells, and fibroblasts. A distinction between neurofibroma and schwannoma is warranted because of the potential for sarcomatous transformation of the

former to malignant peripheral nerve sheath tumor. Schwann cells may be the neoplastic cells in neurofibroma.

Neurofibromas may be solitary or multiple and may arise on any nerve. They are found in both children and adults. Most commonly, neurofibromas involve the skin, major nerve plexuses, large deep nerve trunks, retroperitoneum, and gastrointestinal tract. Most **solitary cutaneous neurofibromas** occur outside the context of neurofibromatosis (NF1) and do not have the potential for sarcomatous transformation. The presence of multiple neurofibromas or one large plexiform neurofibroma is virtually diagnostic of NF1 and should prompt a careful search for other stigmata of the disease.

 PATHOLOGY: On gross examination, a neurofibroma arising in a large nerve appears as a poorly circumscribed, fusiform enlargement. The diffuse, intrafascicular growth of tumor within multiple nerve fascicles may so enlarge the fascicles that the nerve looks like a multistranded rope (**plexiform neurofibroma**). Cutaneous neurofibromas originate from dermal nerves and are seen as soft nodular or pedunculated skin tumors.

The cut surface of a neurofibroma is soft and light gray, and the greatly enlarged, individual nerve fascicles of the plexiform neurofibroma may be prominent. Microscopically, a tumor arising in a large nerve is characterized by an endoneurial proliferation of spindle cells with elongated nuclei, eosinophilic cytoplasm and indistinct cell borders (see Fig. 28-40 C, D). The proliferating spindle cells include Schwann cells, fibroblasts, and perineurial-like cells. There are also increased numbers of mast cells. The coursing of nerve fibers through the neurofibroma contrasts with the pattern in schwannoma, in which nerve fibers are pushed peripherally into the tumor capsule (see Fig. 28-40D). The neurofibromatous proliferation often extends beyond the nerve fascicle into the adjacent tissue. Some 5% of NF1-associated plexiform neurofibromas exhibit sarcomatous transformation to malignant peripheral nerve sheath tumor. The presence of increased cellularity and mitotic figures heralds malignant transformation.

Malignant Peripheral Nerve Sheath Tumor (Malignant Schwannoma, Neurofibrosarcoma)

Malignant peripheral nerve sheath tumor (MPNST) is a poorly differentiated, spindle cell sarcoma of peripheral nerve of uncertain histogenesis. The tumor may arise de novo or from malignant transformation of a neurofibroma. MPNST is most common in adults and typically arises in larger nerves of the trunk or proximal limbs. *About half of these sarcomas occur in patients with neurofibromatosis.* There is an increased incidence of MPNST at sites of previous irradiation. MPNST manifests grossly as an unencapsulated, fusiform enlargement of a nerve. Microscopically, the neoplasm resembles fibrosarcoma. The tumor is prone to local recurrence and blood-borne metastases.

29 The Eye

Gordon K. Klintworth

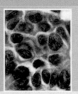
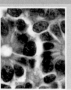
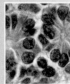
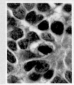

Disorders of the eye are common and many result in impairment of vision or blindness. The eyes are exposed to many injurious environmental agents including microorganisms, allergins, toxic chemicals, solar radiation, and, because of their unprotected position, traumatic injury. The eye is involved in numerous systemic diseases, and recognition of the associated ocular abnormalities aids in the diagnosis of such conditions.

The Orbit: Exophthalmos of Hyperthyroidism

The term **exophthalmos** is used mainly when the condition is bilateral; **proptosis** refers to a unilateral protrusion of the eye. Numerous conditions cause forward protrusion of the eye, and the most common is thyroid disease. Exophthalmos caused by Graves disease may precede or follow other manifestations of thyroid dysfunction. It usually occurs in early adult life, especially in women (female-to-male ratio, 4:1) and may be severe and progressive, particu-

larly in during middle age, when exophthalmos no longer correlates well with the state of thyroid function. The pathogenesis of the exophthalmos of hyperthyroidism is discussed in Chapter 21.

Complications of severe exophthalmos are potentially blinding and include corneal exposure with subsequent ulceration and optic nerve compression. Paradoxically, thyroidectomy may increase the incidence and severity of exophthalmos associated with hyperthyroidism.

The Cornea

Herpes Simplex Virus (HSV) Causes Corneal Ulcerations

HSV has a predilection for corneal epithelium, where it causes keratitis, but it can invade corneal stroma and occasionally other ocular tissues (see also Chapter 9).

PRIMARY INFECTION BY HSV TYPE 1: Subclinical or undiagnosed localized ocular lesions are caused by HSV type 1 in childhood. HSV type 2 rarely causes ocular infection except in newborns infected during birth. Such infections may produce widespread lesions of the cornea and retina. Most corneal lesions due to HSV are asymptomatic plaques of diseased epithelial cells that contain replicating virus. These lesions usually heal without ulceration, but an acute unilateral follicular conjunctivitis may occur.

REACTIVATION OF HSV INFECTION: Latent in the trigeminal ganglion, HSV may pass down the nerves and reactivate the infection. Reactivation disease is characterized by corneal ulceration and a more severe inflammatory reaction. Recurrence of corneal ulcers due to HSV may be precipitated by ultraviolet light, trauma, menstruation, emotional and physical stress, exposure to light or sunlight, vaccination, and other factors.

 PATHOLOGY: HSV causes multiple, minute, discrete, intraepithelial corneal ulcers (superficial punctate keratopathy). Although some of these lesions heal, others enlarge and eventually coalesce to form linear or branching fissures (**dendritic ulcers**, from the Greek, *dendron,* "tree"). The epithelium between the fissures desquamates, causing sharply demarcated, irregular geographical ulcers. The affected epithelial cells, which may become multinucleated, contain eosinophilic, intranuclear inclusion bodies (Lipschütz bodies). In reactivation infections, a central disc-shaped corneal opacity develops beneath the epithelium, due to edema and a minimal inflammatory cell infiltrate (**disciform keratitis**). The corneal stroma may become markedly thinned, and Descemet membrane may bulge into it (**descemetocele**). Corneal perforation can also occur.

Corneal Dystrophies Encompass Diverse Noninflammatory Genetic Corneal Disorders

Corneal dystrophies are a heterogeneous group of hereditary, noninflammatory, and degenerative diseases of the cornea. The corneal dystrophies have traditionally been classified according to the primary layer that is involved. However, many of the conditions relate to more than one layer.

EPITHELIAL DYSTROPHIES: The different epithelial dystrophies are characterized by a variety of distinct abnormalities, which include (1) microcysts or accumulations of anomalous material within the cytoplasm of the corneal epithelium, (2) defects in the epithelial basement membrane, and (3) deposition of a finely fibrillar substance in Bowman layer. In some epithelial dystrophies, faulty desmosomes may permit the separation of adjacent epithelial cells, leading to the accumulation of fluid-filled microcysts and painful, recurrent erosions that begin in early childhood. Although there may be a slow decrease in visual acuity, epithelial dystrophies do not ordinarily cause blindness. One epithelial dystrophy, **Meesmann dystrophy**, is associated with dominant mutations in the *KRT3* or *KRT12* genes, which encode keratin 3 and keratin 12. These mutations result in aggregations of abnormal cytokeratin filaments and severely impair cytoskeletal function in the affected cells.

STROMAL DYSTROPHIES: The stromal dystrophies are clear-cut entities in which different substances (e.g., amyloid, glycosaminoglycans, proteins, or a variety of lipids) accumulate within corneal stroma because of inherited metabolic disorders. Each stromal dystrophy causes a characteristic form of corneal opacification. The age of onset and rate of progression vary with the particular disorder. Several inherited corneal disorders, including the granular corneal dystrophies and most lattice corneal dystrophies, result from different mutations in the *TFGBI (BIGH3)* gene on chromosome 5 (5q31), which encodes keratoepithelin, a protein expressed in both the corneal epithelial and stromal keratocytes.

ENDOTHELIAL DYSTROPHIES: Several different endothelial dystrophies are recognized, usually accompanied by abnormalities in Descemet membrane, the basement membrane of the corneal endothelium. For example, missense mutations in *COL8A2*, the gene encoding the α_2 chain of type VIII collagen, have been identified in some patients with **early-onset Fuch dystrophy**, which affects the corneal endothelium and its basement membrane (Descemet membrane).

The Lens: Cataracts

Cataracts are opacifications in the crystalline lens that are a major cause of visual impairment and blindness throughout the world. They result from numerous conditions.

 PATHOGENESIS: Cataracts can be caused by diabetes or by deficiencies in riboflavin or tryptophan. Others are related to the actions of toxins, drugs, or physical agents (particularly ultraviolet light). A wide range of cataracts are inherited and some of them are associated with other ocular or systemic abnormalities. Cataracts can result from mutations in the heat shock transcription factor-4 *(HSF4)* gene, as well as in genes that encode specific lens proteins. However, the most common cataract in the United States is associated with aging (age-related cataract).

 PATHOLOGY: Age-related cataracts: Clefts appear between the lens fibers, and degenerated lens material accumulates in these spaces (morgagnian corpuscles, **incipient cataract**). The degenerated lens material exerts osmotic pressure, causing the damaged lens to swell by imbibing water. Such a swollen lens may obstruct the pupil and cause glaucoma (**phacomorphic glaucoma**).

In a **mature cataract** (Fig. 29-1), the entire lens degenerates, and its volume diminishes because lenticular debris escapes into the aqueous humor through a degenerated lens capsule (**hypermature cataract**). After becoming engulfed by macrophages, the extruded lenticular material may obstruct aqueous outflow and produce glaucoma (**phacolytic glaucoma**). Fortunately, cataractous lenses can be surgically removed, and optical devices can be provided to permit light to focus on the retina (spectacles, contact lenses, implantation of prosthetic lenses).

The Uvea

A variety of inflammatory conditions affect the uveal tract. Inflammation of the uvea (**uveitis**) also encompasses inflammation of the iris (**iritis**), the ciliary body (**cyclitis**), and the iris plus the ciliary body (**iridocyclitis**). Inflammation of the iris and ciliary body typically causes a red eye, photophobia, moderate pain, blurred vision, a pericorneal halo, ciliary flush, and slight miosis. Synechiae are complications of iritis and can cause glaucoma.

Posterior synechiae are adhesions that develop between the iris and the lens.

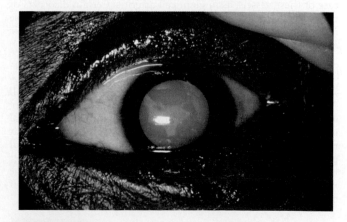

FIGURE 29-1. **Cataract.** The white appearance of the pupil in this eye is due to complete opacification of the lens ("mature cataract").

Peripheral anterior synechiae are adhesions between the peripheral iris and the anterior chamber angle.

Sympathetic Ophthalmitis is an Autoimmune Uveitis

In sympathetic ophthalmitis, the entire uvea develops autoimmune, granulomatous inflammation in response to an injury in the other eye. Perforating ocular injury and prolapse of uveal tissue often lead to a progressive, bilateral, diffuse, granulomatous inflammation of the uvea. This uveitis develops in the originally injured eye (exciting eye) and the uninjured eye (sympathizing eye) after a latent period of 4 to 8 weeks. Experimental studies suggest that the antigen responsible for sympathetic ophthalmitis resides in the photoreceptors of the retina.

Sarcoidosis Often Affects the Eye

Ocular involvement occurs in one fourth to one third of patients with sarcoidosis and is frequently the initial clinical manifestation. Ocular involvement is usually bilateral and most often takes the form of a granulomatous uveitis. Other ocular manifestations of sarcoidosis include calcific band keratopathy, cataracts, retinal vascularization, vitreous hemorrhage, and bilateral enlargement of the lacrimal and salivary glands (**Mikulicz syndrome**).

The Retina

Retinal Hemorrhage Has Different Causes

Among the causes of retinal hemorrhages are hypertension, diabetes mellitus, and central retinal vein occlusion. The appearance varies with the location. Hemorrhage in the nerve fiber layer spreads between axons and causes a flame-shaped appearance on funduscopy, whereas deep retinal hemorrhages tend to be round. When located between the retinal pigment epithelium and Bruch membrane, blood appears as a dark mass and clinically may resemble a melanoma. After accidental or surgical perforation of the globe, choroidal hemorrhages may detach the choroid and displace the retina, vitreous body, and lens through the wound.

Occlusive Retinal Vascular Disease is an Important Cause of Blindness

Vascular occlusion results from thrombosis, embolism, stenosis (as in atherosclerosis), vascular compression, intravascular sludging or vasoconstriction (e.g., in hypertensive retinopathy or migraine). Thrombosis of ocular vessels may accompany primary disease of these vessels, as in giant cell arteritis. Certain disorders of the heart and major vessels, such as the carotid arteries, predispose to emboli that lodge in the retina and are evident on funduscopic examination at points of vascular bifurcation.

 PATHOLOGY: The effect of vascular occlusion depends on the size of the vessel involved, the degree of resultant ischemia, and the nature of the embolus. Small emboli often do not interfere with retinal function, whereas septic emboli may cause foci of ocular infection. Retinal ischemia of any cause frequently leads to white fluffy patches that resemble cotton on ophthalmoscopic examination (**cotton-wool patches**, see Fig. 29-2). These round spots, which are seldom wider than the optic disc, consist of aggregates of swollen axons in the nerve-fiber layer of the retina. Cotton-wool spots are reversible if circulation is restored in time.

Central Retinal Artery Occlusion

Like neurons in the rest of the nervous system, those in the retina are extremely susceptible to hypoxia. Central retinal artery occlusion may follow thrombosis of the retinal artery, as in atherosclerosis, giant cell arteritis, or embolization to that vessel. Intracellular edema, manifested by retinal pallor, is prominent, especially in the macula, where ganglion cells are most numerous. The foveola, the center of the macula, stands out in sharp contrast as a prominent **cherry-red spot**, because of the underlying vascularized choroid. The lack of retinal circulation reduces retinal arterioles to delicate threads. *Permanent blindness follows central retinal artery obstruction, unless the ischemia is of short duration.* Unilateral blurred vision lasting a few minutes (**amaurosis fugax**) occurs with small retinal emboli.

Central Retinal Vein Occlusion

Central retinal vein occlusion results in flame-shaped hemorrhages in the nerve-fiber layer of the retina, especially around the optic disc. The hemorrhages reflect the high intravascular pressure that dilates and ruptures the veins and collateral vessels. Edema of the optic disc and retina occurs because of an impaired absorption of interstitial fluid.

Vision is disturbed but may recover surprisingly well. An intractable, closed-angle glaucoma, with severe pain and repeated hemorrhages, commonly ensues 2 to 3 months after central retinal vein occlusion. This distressing complication is caused by neovascularization of the iris and adhesions between the iris and the anterior chamber angle *(peripheral anterior synechiae)*.

Hypertensive Retinopathy Relates to the Severity of Hypertension

Increased blood pressure commonly affects the retina, causing changes that can readily be seen with the ophthalmoscope (Fig. 29-2).

 PATHOLOGY: In the eye, arteriolosclerosis accompanies long-standing hypertension and commonly affects the retinal and choroidal vessels. Lumina of the thickened retinal arterioles become narrowed, increasingly tortuous, and of irregular caliber. At sites where the arterioles cross veins, the latter appear kinked (**arteriovenous nicking**). The kinked appearance of the vein reflects sclerosis within the venous walls, because the retinal arteries and veins share a common adventitia at sites of arteriovenous crossings, rather than compression by a taut sclerotic artery. Small superficial or deep retinal hemorrhages often accompany retinal arteriolosclerosis. **Malignant hypertension** is characterized by a necrotizing arteriolitis with fibrinoid necrosis and thrombosis of the precapillary retinal arterioles.

Diabetic Retinopathy is Primarily a Vascular Disease

The eye is frequently involved in diabetes mellitus, and ocular symptoms occur in 20% to 40% of diabetics and may even be evident at the time diabetes is diagnosed. Virtually all patients with type 1 (insulin-dependent) diabetes and many of those with type 2 (non–insulin-dependent) diabetes develop some background retinopathy (see below) within 5 to 15 years of diabetes onset (Figs. 29-3 and 29-4). The more dangerous **proliferative retinopathy** does not appear until at least 10 years of diabetes, after which its incidence increases rapidly and remains high for many years. *The frequency of proliferative retinopathy correlates with the degree of glycemic control; patients whose diabetes is better controlled develop retinopathy less frequently.* Retinal ischemia can account for most features of diabetic retinopathy, including the cotton-wool spots, capillary closure, microaneurysms, and retinal neovascularization. Ischemia results from narrowing or occlusion of retinal arterioles (as from arteriolosclerosis or platelet and lipid thrombi) or from atherosclerosis of the central retinal or ophthalmic arteries.

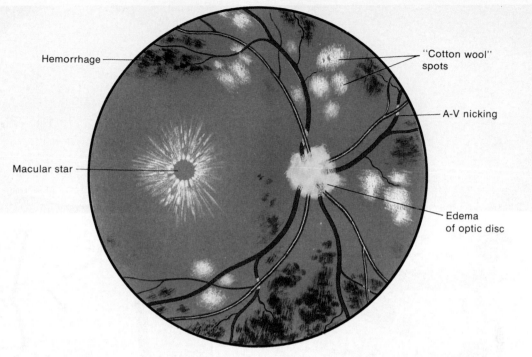

Hemorrhage

"Cotton wool" spots

A-V nicking

Macular star

Edema of optic disc

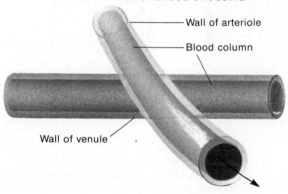

NORMAL ARTERIOVENOUS CROSSING

Wall of arteriole

Blood column

Wall of venule

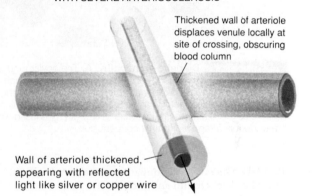

ARTERIOVENOUS CROSSING
WITH SEVERE ARTERIOSCLEROSIS

Thickened wall of arteriole displaces venule locally at site of crossing, obscuring blood column

Wall of arteriole thickened, appearing with reflected light like silver or copper wire

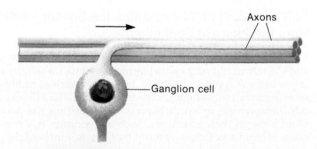

NORMAL NERVE FIBER LAYER OF RETINA

Axons

Ganglion cell

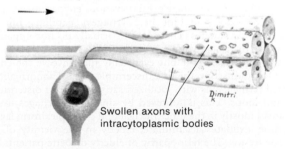

NERVE FIBER LAYER OF RETINA AT
CCOTTON WOOL SPOT

Dimitri
K

Swollen axons with intracytoplasmic bodies

FIGURE 29-2. **Hypertensive retinopathy.** Various abnormalities develop within the retina in hypertension. The commonly associated arteriolosclerosis affects the appearance of the retinal microvasculature. Light reflected from the thickened arteriolar walls mimics silver or copper wire. Blood flow through the retinal venules is not well visualized at the sites of arteriolar-venular crossings. This effect is due to a thickening of the venular wall rather than to an impediment to blood flow caused by compression; the column of blood proximal to the compression is not wider than the part distal to the crossing. Impaired axoplasmic flow within the nerve fiber layer, caused by ischemia, results in swollen axons with cytoplasmic bodies. Such structures resemble cotton on funduscopy ("cotton-wool spots"). Hemorrhages are common in the retina, and exudates frequently form a star around the macula.

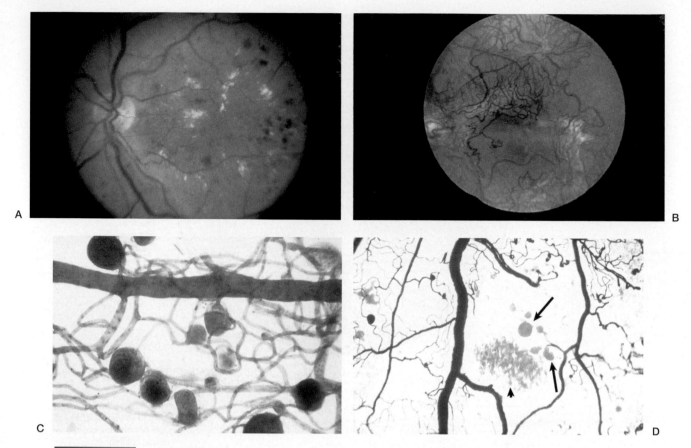

FIGURE 29-3. **Diabetic retinopathy. A.** The ocular fundus in a patient with background diabetic retinopathy shows several yellowish "hard," lipid-rich exudates, which are evident along with several relatively small retinal hemorrhages. **B.** A vascular frond has extended anterior to the retina in the eye with proliferative diabetic retinopathy. **C.** Numerous microaneurysms are present in this flat preparation of a diabetic retina. **D.** This flat preparation from a diabetic was stained with periodic acid-Schiff (PAS) after the retinal vessels had been perfused with India ink. Microaneurysms *(arrows)* and an exudate *(arrowhead)* are evident in a region of retinal nonperfusion.

 PATHOLOGY: The retinopathy of diabetes is characterized by background and proliferative stages.

BACKGROUND (NONPROLIFERATIVE) DIABETIC RETINOPATHY: This stage exhibits venous engorgement, small hemorrhages (dot and blot hemorrhages), capillary microaneurysms, and exudates. These lesions usually do not impair vision unless associated with macular edema. The retinopathy begins at the posterior pole but eventually may involve the entire retina. On funduscopy, the first discernible clinical abnormality is engorged retinal veins with localized sausage-shaped distentions, coils, and loops. This is followed by small hemorrhages in the same areas, mostly in the inner nuclear and outer plexiform layers. With time, exudates accumulate, chiefly in the vicinity of the microaneurysms. The retinopathy of elderly diabetic patients frequently displays numerous exudates (**exudative diabetic retinopathy**), which are not seen with type 1 diabetes. Because of the hyperlipoproteinemia of diabetics, the exudates are rich in lipid and thus appear yellowish (**waxy exudates**).

PROLIFERATIVE RETINOPATHY: After many years, diabetic retinopathy becomes proliferative. Delicate new blood vessels grow along with fibrous and glial tissue toward the vitreous body. Neovascularization of the retina is a prominent feature of diabetic retinopathy and of other conditions caused by retinal ischemia. Tortuous new vessels first appear on the surface of the retina and optic nerve head and then grow into the vitreous cavity. The newly formed friable vessels bleed easily, and resultant vitreal hemorrhages obscure vision. The proliferating fibrovascular and glial tissue contracts, often causing retinal detachment and blindness. Laser phototherapy and strict glycemic control early in the course of proliferative retinopathy have proved effective in controlling these complications.

Retinal Detachment Separates the Sensory Retina from the Pigment Epithelium

During fetal development, the space between the sensory retina and the retinal pigment epithelium is obliterated when these two layers become apposed. However, the sensory retina readily separates from the retinal pigment epithelium when fluid (liquid vitreous, hemorrhage, or exudate) accumulates within the potential space between these structures. Such a separation is a common cause of blindness. Laser treatment has greatly improved the prognosis for patients with detached retina.

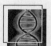 **PATHOGENESIS:** Factors predisposing to retinal detachment include retinal defects (due to trauma or certain retinal degenerations), vitreous traction, diminished pressure on the retina (e.g., after vitreous loss), and weakening of retinal fixation. The photoreceptors and retinal pigment epithelium normally function as a unit. After they separate in a retinal detachment, oxygen and nutrients that normally reach the outer retina from the choroid must diffuse across a greater distance. This situation causes the photoreceptors to degenerate, after which cyst-like extracellular spaces appear within the retina.

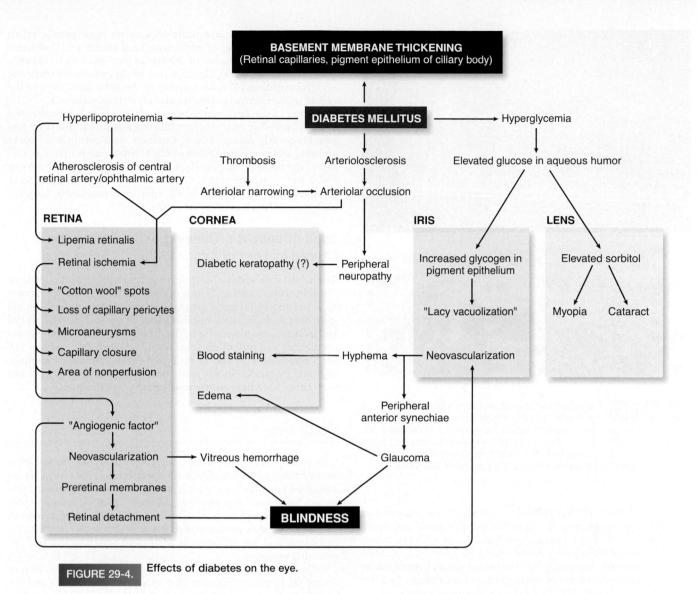

FIGURE 29-4. Effects of diabetes on the eye.

 PATHOLOGY: Three varieties of retinal detachment are recognized—rhegmatogenous, tractional, and exudative.

RHEGMATOGENOUS RETINAL DETACHMENT: This condition is associated with a retinal tear and often with degenerative changes in the vitreous body or peripheral retina. Retinal detachment follows intraocular hemorrhage (e.g., after trauma) and is a potential complication of cataract extractions and several other ocular operations.

TRACTIONAL RETINAL DETACHMENT: In some instances, the retina is detached by being pulled toward the center of the eye by adherent vitreoretinal adhesions, as occurs in proliferative diabetic retinopathy, in retinopathy of prematurity, and after intraocular infection.

EXUDATIVE RETINAL DETACHMENT: Accumulation of fluid in the potential space between the sensory retina and the retinal pigment epithelium causes a detached retina in disorders such as choroiditis, choroidal hemangioma, and choroidal melanoma.

Retinitis Pigmentosa is a Heritable Cause of Blindness

Retinitis pigmentosa (pigmentary retinopathy) is a generic term that refers to a variety of bilateral, progressive, degenerative retinopathies characterized clinically by night blindness and constriction of peripheral visual fields and pathologically by the loss of retinal photoreceptors (rods and cones) and pigment accumulation within the retina.

PATHOGENESIS: Retinitis pigmentosa is a misnomer because it does not feature inflammation of the retina. At least 39 genes and loci are associated with retinitis pigmentosa not associated with other systemic disorders. Because diverse mutations may lead to this disorder, a single defective protein cannot explain the death of photoreceptor cells that is characteristic of the condition. Presumably, the abnormal metabolic pathways that result from all mutations ultimately converge at a final common point.

 PATHOLOGY: In retinitis pigmentosa, destruction of rods and later cones is followed by migration of retinal pigment epithelial cells into the sensory retina (Fig. 29-5). Melanin appears within slender processes of spidery cells and accumulates mainly around small branching retinal blood vessels (especially in the equatorial portion of the retina), like spicules of bone. The retinal blood vessels then gradually attenuate, and the optic nerve head acquires a characteristic waxy pallor.

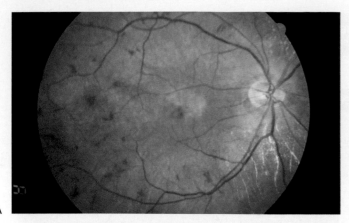

A

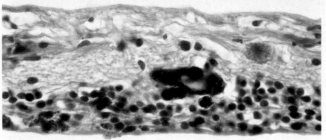

B

FIGURE 29-5. **Retinitis pigmentosa. A.** Fundus photograph of the retina of a patient with pigmentary retinopathy (retinitis pigmentosa) shows attenuated retinal vessels and foci of retinal pigmentation. **B.** Microscopic appearance of a severely degenerated retina in pigmentary retinopathy. Note the focal accumulations of pigmented cells (derived from retinal pigmented epithelium) within the retina.

 CLINICAL FEATURES: The clinical manifestations of retinitis pigmentosa, as well as the appearance and distribution of the retinal pigmentation, vary with the causes of the retinopathy. As the condition progresses, contraction of visual fields eventually leads to tunnel vision. Central vision is usually preserved until late in the course of the disease. In a few cases, the macula becomes involved, and blindness ensues.

Macular Degeneration is Mostly Age-Related

With aging, in certain drug toxicities (e.g., chloroquine) and in several inherited disorders, the macula degenerates, and central vision is impaired. *Age-related macular degeneration currently affects almost 2 million people in the United States and is the most common cause of blindness among persons of European descent older than 65 years of age.* Dry and wet forms of age-related macular degeneration are recognized. The wet variety of this disease is associated with subretinal fibrovascular tissue and sometimes bleeding into the subretinal space. Laser photocoagulation and other therapies are beneficial in this type of the disorder. A common missense variant of the CFH gene that encodes for complement factor H is a risk factor for about 40% of age-related macular degeneration cases.

The Optic Nerve

Optic Nerve Head Edema Often Reflects Increased Intracranial Pressure

Optic nerve head (optic disc) edema refers to a swelling of the optic nerve head where it enters the globe. Optic nerve head edema can result from various causes, the most important of which is increased intracranial pressure. The term **papilledema**, which is still widely used as a synonym for optic

nerve head edema, is inaccurate because no optic papilla exists. Other important causes of optic nerve head edema are (1) obstruction to the venous drainage of the eye (as may occur with compressive lesions of the orbit), (2) infarction of the optic nerve (ischemic optic neuropathy), (3) inflammation of the optic nerve close to the eyeball (optic neuritis, papillitis), and (4) multiple sclerosis.

Edema of the optic nerve head is characterized clinically by a swollen optic disc that displays blurred margins and dilated vessels. Frequently, hemorrhages, exudates, and cotton-wool spots are seen, and concentric folds of the choroid and retina may surround the nerve head. Acutely, optic nerve head edema results in few, if any, visual symptoms. Over time, swelling of the optic nerve head enlarges the normal blind spot, and eventually atrophic changes lead to a loss of visual acuity.

Optic Atrophy is a Thinning of the Optic Nerve Caused by Loss of Axons Within Its Substance

The nerve axons within the optic nerve are lost in many conditions. Possible causes include (1) long-standing edema of the optic nerve head (see above), (2) optic neuritis, (3) optic nerve compression, (4) glaucoma, and (5) retinal degeneration. Drugs such as ethambutol and isoniazid can also cause optic atrophy. The optic nerve head is usually flat and pale in optic atrophy, but when this disorder follows glaucoma, the disc is excavated (**glaucomatous cupping**). Multiple mutations in the mitochondrial genome are associated with **Leber hereditary optic neuropathy (see Chapter 6).**

Glaucoma

Glaucoma, the most common cause of preventable blindness in the United States, refers to a collection of disorders that feature an optic neuropathy accompanied by a characteristic excavation of the optic nerve head and progressive loss of visual field sensitivity. In most cases, glaucoma is produced by increased intraocular pressure (**ocular hypertension**); however, increased intraocular pressure does not necessarily cause glaucoma, and not all patients with glaucoma have elevated intraocular pressure.

After being produced by the ciliary body, the aqueous humor enters the posterior chamber (the space between the iris and the zonules) before passing through the pupil to the anterior chamber (between the iris and the cornea). From that site, it drains into veins by way of the trabecular meshwork and Schlemm canal (Fig. 29-6). A delicate balance between the production and drainage of the aqueous humor maintains intraocular pressure within its physiologic range (10 to 20 mm Hg). *In certain pathologic states, aqueous humor accumulates within the eye, and intraocular pressure increases.* Temporary or permanent impairment of vision results from pressure-induced degenerative changes in the retina and optic nerve head and from corneal edema and opacification. The changes include degeneration of the ganglion cell and nerve fiber layers of the retina, with sparing of the outer retina. Optic atrophy, with loss of axons, gliosis, and thickening of the pial septa, follows the retinal degeneration and damage to the nerve fibers at the optic disc.

Mechanical obstruction of aqueous drainage by a congenital or acquired lesion of the anterior segment of the eye almost always results in glaucoma. The obstruction may be located between the iris and lens, in the angle of the anterior chamber, in the trabecular meshwork, in Schlemm canal, or in the venous drainage of the eye. Glaucoma can be classified into several different types.

Congenital Glaucoma (Infantile Glaucoma, Buphthalmos) Results from Developmental Anomalies

Congenital glaucoma is caused by obstruction to aqueous drainage by developmental anomalies. The disorder develops although intraocular

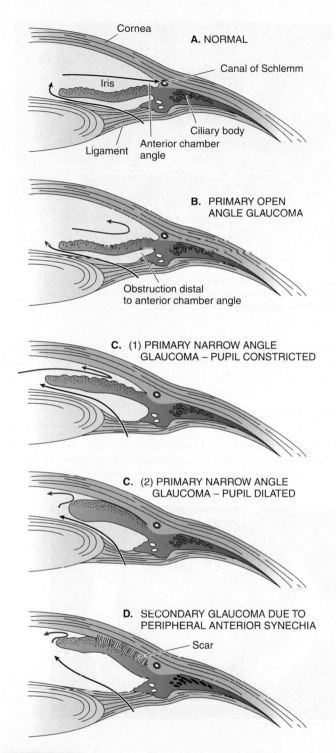

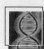

FIGURE 29-6. **Pathogenesis of glaucoma.** The anterior segment of the eye is affected differently in various forms of glaucoma. **A.** Structure of the normal eye. **B.** In primary open-angle glaucoma, the obstruction to the aqueous outflow is distal to the anterior chamber angle, and the anterior segment resembles that of the normal eye. **C.** In primary narrow-angle glaucoma, the anterior chamber angle is open but narrower than normal when the pupil is constricted **(C1)**. When the pupil becomes dilated in such an eye, the thickened iris obstructs the anterior chamber angle **(C2)**, causing increased intraocular pressure. **D.** The anterior chamber angle can become obstructed by a variety of pathological processes, including an adhesion between the iris and the posterior surface of the cornea (peripheral anterior synechiae).

pressure may not increase until early infancy or childhood. Most (65%) cases of congenital glaucoma occur in boys, and an X-linked recessive mode of inheritance is common. The developmental anomaly usually involves both eyes and, although often limited to the angle of the anterior chamber, may be accompanied by a variety of other ocular malformations. Several genes for congenital glaucoma have been identified.

Primary Open-Angle Glaucoma is the Most Frequent Type of Glaucoma

Primary open-angle glaucoma is the most frequent type of glaucoma and a major cause of blindness in the United States. It affects 1% to 3% of the population older than 40 years of age and occurs principally in the sixth decade. The intraocular pressure increases insidiously and asymptomatically, and although almost always bilateral, one eye may be affected more severely than the other. With time, damage to the retina and optic nerve causes an irreversible loss of peripheral vision.

PATHOGENESIS: Primary glaucoma is subdivided into **open-angle glaucoma**, in which the anterior chamber angle is open and appears normal, and **closed-angle glaucoma**, in which the anterior chamber is shallower than normal, and the angle is abnormally narrow (see Fig. 29-6B and below). In primary open-angle glaucoma, there is increased resistance to aqueous humor outflow in the vicinity of Schlemm canal. Individuals with diabetes mellitus and myopia have an increased risk of primary open-angle glaucoma. The condition has been mapped to several loci on many chromosomes.

Primary Closed-Angle Glaucoma is Associated With a Shallow Anterior Chamber

Primary closed-angle glaucoma occurs after 40 years of age.

PATHOGENESIS: The disorder afflicts individuals whose peripheral iris is displaced anteriorly toward the trabecular meshwork, thereby creating an abnormally narrow angle. When the pupil is constricted (miotic), the iris remains stretched so that the chamber angle is not occluded. However, when the pupil dilates (mydriasis), the iris obstructs the anterior chamber angle, thereby impairing aqueous drainage and resulting in sudden episodes of intraocular hypertension. This obstruction is accompanied by ocular pain, and halos or rings are seen around lights. In such individuals, intraocular pressure may also increase if the pupil becomes blocked (e.g., by a swollen lens) and aqueous humor accumulates in the posterior chamber.

CLINICAL FEATURES: *Acute closed-angle glaucoma is an ocular emergency, and it is essential to start ocular hypotensive treatment within the first 24 to 48 hours if vision is to be maintained.* The intraocular pressure is normal between attacks, but after many episodes, adhesions form between the iris and the trabecular meshwork as well as the cornea (peripheral anterior synechiae) and accentuate the block to the outflow of aqueous humor.

Secondary Glaucoma is Usually Unilateral

There are many causes of secondary glaucoma and include inflammation, hemorrhage, and neovascularization of the iris and adhe-

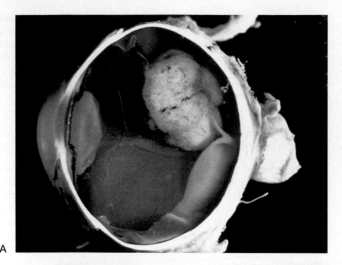

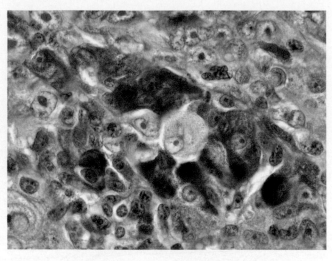

FIGURE 29-7. **Malignant melanoma. A.** A mushroom-shaped melanoma of the choroid is present in this eye. Choroidal melanomas commonly invade through Bruch membrane and result in this appearance. **B.** Photomicrograph of a heavily pigmented melanoma of the choroid depicting epithelioid tumor cells with prominent nucleoli.

sions. In secondary glaucoma, anterior chamber angles may be open or closed. Because the underlying disorder is usually limited to one eye, secondary glaucoma tends to be unilateral.

Low-Tension Glaucoma is Not Associated with Increased Intraocular Pressure

Low-tension glaucoma refers to an entity in which the characteristic visual-field defect and all of the ophthalmoscopic features of chronic open-angle glaucoma occur without an increase in intraocular pressure. Although

some eyes may be hypersensitive to normal intraocular pressure, many cases of low-tension glaucoma probably represent optic nerve head infarction.

Ocular Neoplasms

The eye and adjacent structures contain a large number of cell types, and as one might expect, benign and malignant neoplasms arise from them. *Intraocular neoplasms arise mostly from immature reti-*

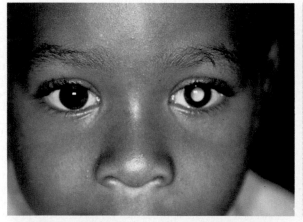

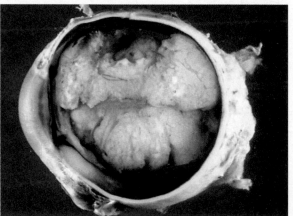

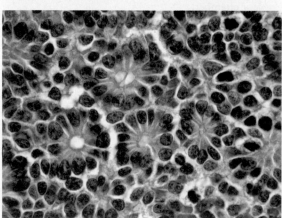

FIGURE 29-8. **Retinoblastoma. A.** The white pupil (leukocoria) in the left eye is the result of an intraocular retinoblastoma. **B.** This surgically excised eye is almost filled by a cream-colored intraocular retinoblastoma with calcified flecks. **C.** Light microscopic view of a retinoblastoma showing Flexner-Wintersteiner rosettes characterized by cells are that are arranged around a central cavity.

nal neurons (retinoblastoma) and uveal melanocytes (melanoma). Although the retinal pigment epithelium often undergoes reactive proliferation, it seldom becomes neoplastic.

Malignant Melanoma Arises from Melanocytes in the Uvea

Malignant melanoma is the most common primary intraocular malignancy. It may arise from melanocytes in any part of the eye, and the choroid is the most common site.

 PATHOLOGY: Choroidal melanomas are mostly circumscribed and invade Bruch membrane, causing a mushroom-shaped mass (Fig. 29-7). Some do not become apparent until extraocular dissemination has occurred. Aside from hematogenous spread, uveal melanomas disseminate by traversing the sclera to enter the orbital tissues, usually at sites where blood vessels and nerves pass through the sclera. Lymphatic spread does not occur because the eye has no lymphatic vessels. The usual treatment for most uveal melanomas is enucleation of the eye, but some cases are treated with other methods, such as radiotherapy or local excision. More than half of patients with uveal melanomas survive for 15 years after enucleation.

Retinoblastoma Originates from Immature Neurons

Retinoblastoma is the most common intraocular malignant neoplasm of childhood affecting 1:20,000 to 1:34,000 children. The tumor occurs most frequently within the first 2 years of life and may even be found at birth. Presenting signs include a white pupil (leukocoria), squint (strabismus), poor vision, spontaneous hyphema, or a red, painful eye. Secondary glaucoma is a frequent complication. Light entering the eye commonly reflects a yellowish color similar to that from the tapetum of a cat (cat's eye reflex). See also Chapter 5 for molecular details.

 PATHOLOGY: Retinoblastoma is a cream-colored tumor that contains scattered, chalky white, calcified flecks within yellow necrotic zones (Fig. 29-8), which may be detected radiologically. The tumors are intensely cellular and display several morphologic patterns. In some instances, densely packed, round neoplastic cells with hyperchromatic nuclei, scant cytoplasm, and abundant mitoses are randomly distributed. In other retinoblastomas, the cells are arranged radially around a central cavity (Flexner-Wintersteiner rosettes).

Retinoblastomas disseminate by several routes. They commonly extend into the optic nerve, from where they spread intracranially. They also invade blood vessels, especially in the highly vascular choroid, before metastasizing hematogenously throughout the body. Bone marrow is a common site of blood-borne metastases, but surprisingly, the lung is rarely involved.

 CLINICAL FEATURES: Retinoblastomas are almost always fatal if left untreated. However, with early diagnosis and modern therapy, the survival rate is high (about 90%). Patients with inherited retinoblastomas, presumably as a consequence of the loss of Rb gene function, have an increased susceptibility to other malignant tumors, including osteogenic sarcoma, Ewing sarcoma, and pinealoblastoma.

30 Cytopathology

Hormoz Ehya
Marluce Bibbo

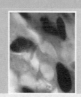

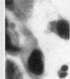

Cytopathology refers to diagnostic techniques that are used to examine cells from various body sites to determine the cause or nature of disease. In 1928, George Papanicolaou introduced a cytologic method for detecting malignant and precancerous lesions of the uterine cervix. The **"Pap" test** *has become widely accepted and proven to be the most successful cancer prevention method, saving millions of lives in the past 7 decades. Applications of cytopathology have been expanded to most body sites. Exfoliated cells and cells obtained by scraping, brushing, washing, and needle aspiration are routinely evaluated by cytopathologists to determine the nature of disease and surveillance of cancer. By applying imaging techniques to guide in placement, the uses of fine-needle aspiration have expanded greatly. Very small lesions (a few millimeters in size) can now be targeted.*

Cytopathology in the Early Detection of Cancer

The most important application of cytopathology in the area of cancer prevention is examination of scrapings and brushings from the uterine cervix. Widespread screening Pap smears has reduced the incidence of cervical cancer in the United States and many other countries by 70% (Figs. 30-1 and 30-2). Early cancers can also be detected in other organs, such as the bladder, stomach, lungs, esophagus, endometrium, and anus. Cytologic evaluation with radiologic guidance is particularly important when diagnosing tumors that may not be easily accessible or amenable to surgical treatment. Examples of such neoplasms include hepatocellular and pancreatic carcinomas, metastatic tumors, and small cell lung carcinoma.

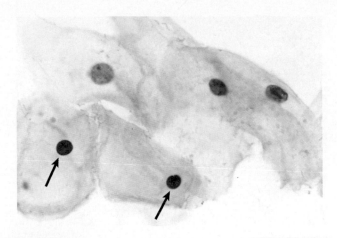

A

FIGURE 30-1. Normal cervical Papanicolaou (Pap) smear. Large squamous cells from the superficial and intermediate layers of the epithelium are illustrated. The cells have abundant cytoplasm that varies in staining from pink to blue. The nuclei are small, and the nuclear-cytoplasmic ratio is low. The most superficial cells have pyknotic nuclei (arrows).

Cytologic Methods

Specimens for cytopathological analysis are obtained by a variety of techniques depending on the site and nature of the lesion to be evaluated.

- **Exfoliative cytology** is used to evaluate cells spontaneously shed into body fluids such as sputum, urine, cerebrospinal fluid, and effusions in body cavities.
- **Abrasive cytology** uses endoscopic brushing, scraping, and washing (lavage) to dislodge cells from body surfaces, such as the gastrointestinal, respiratory, and urinary tracts.
- **Fine-needle aspiration cytology** allows virtually any organ to be sampled using suction through a thin (22- to 25-gauge) needle. Superficial lesions (such as nodules in the thyroid, breast, skin, and lymph nodes) are easily targeted (Fig. 30-3). Lesions in deep organs require guidance by fluoroscopy, computed tomography, or ultrasound (Fig. 30-4).

Morphologic Parameters in Cytologic Evaluation

Specimen Cellularity is Influenced by Various Factors

The type of tissue sampled greatly influences the cellularity of the specimen. Epithelial cells are generally detached more easily than are stromal cells or fibrous tissue. Malignant cells have lower cohesiveness than their benign counterparts and are more likely to exfoliate spontaneously or mechanically. Carcinomas tend to exfoliate cells more readily than do sarcomas.

Cell Arrangement is an Important Cytological Parameter

The relation between cells is a helpful criterion for cytologic diagnosis. Cells may appear singly, in small groups, in monolayer sheets, or in three-dimensional clusters. Several cells may fuse, forming a large formation termed a **syncytium**. Cell clusters may form:

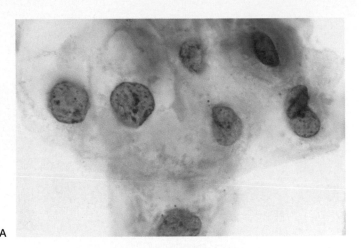

A

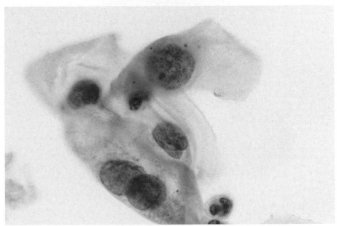

B

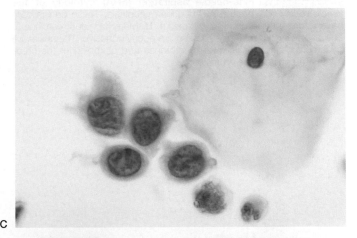

C

FIGURE 30-2. Spectrum of squamous intraepithelial lesions (SILs) in cervical smears. **A.** Low-grade SIL (mild dysplasia, cervical intraepithelial neoplasia [CIN]1). The dysplastic cells have abundant cytoplasm. The nucleus is enlarged and hyperchromatic. **B.** High-grade SIL (moderate dysplasia, CIN2). The dysplastic cells have a higher nuclear-cytoplasmic ratio than do mildly dysplastic cells. **C.** High-grade SIL (severe dysplasia, CIN3/carcinoma in situ). Multiple dysplastic squamous cells with scant cytoplasm and very high nuclear-cytoplasmic ratios are seen. Note the normal superficial squamous cell.

- **Papillary configurations** with fibrovascular cores (papillary urothelial carcinoma, papillary adenocarcinoma, malignant mesothelioma)
- **Glandular or tubular structures** (adenocarcinoma) (Fig. 30-5)
- **Follicles** (follicular neoplasms of the thyroid)
- **Rosettes** (neuroblastoma)
- **Pearls** (squamous cell carcinoma) (Fig. 30-6)

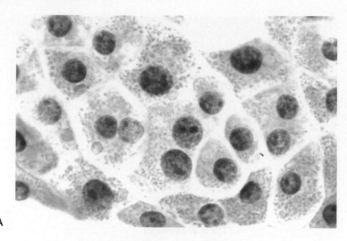

A

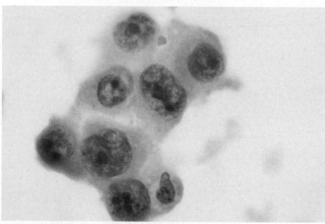

B

FIGURE 30-3. **Fine-needle aspiration (FNA) cytology of the breast. A.** Apocrine metaplasia. These benign cells have abundant and granular cytoplasm. **B.** Mammary duct carcinoma. The cells vary in size and shape and are poorly cohesive. The nuclei are hyperchromatic, with irregular membranes and clumping of the chromatin. The nucleoli are prominent.

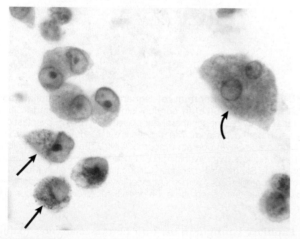

FIGURE 30-4. **Metastatic malignant melanoma in a fine-needle aspirate of the liver.** Poorly cohesive tumor cells exhibit eccentric nuclei and prominent nucleoli. The cytoplasm contains fine melanin granules *(straight arrows)*. A benign binucleated hepatocyte is evident *(curved arrow)*.

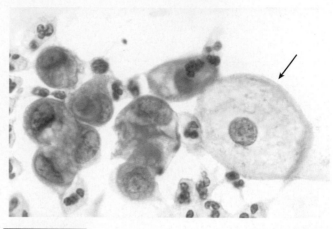

FIGURE 30-5. **Endometrial adenocarcinoma in a cervical smear.** A cluster of medium-sized malignant cells displays cytoplasmic vacuoles. The nuclei are eccentric and have irregular nuclear membranes and abnormally distributed chromatin. Note the benign squamous cell *(arrow)*.

Cell Size and Shape Characteristics Help to Identify Specific Neoplasms

The size of tumor cells varies greatly depending on the type of neoplasm. Small cell carcinoma of the lung, some types of lymphoma, and many childhood tumors are composed of small cells (compare dysplastic and normal cells in Fig. 30-2C). By contrast, squamous cell carcinoma, giant cell carcinoma, pleomorphic sarcomas, some endocrine carcinomas, and choriocarcinoma have very large cells. Cells are generally uniform (monomorphic) in normal tissues and benign neoplasms, whereas malignant tumors frequently exhibit significant variation in cell shape (**pleomorphism**) (see Fig. 30-6).

Cytoplasmic Features May Reveal the Tissue Origin or Etiology

The cytoplasm is evaluated for color, texture, presence of inclusions, vacuoles, pigments, and other cell products. With the Papanicolaou method of cell preparation, the cytoplasm assumes various shades of pink to blue; keratin stains orange (see Fig. 30-1). The presence of pigments (including melanin, hemosiderin, bile, lipofuscin, and carbon particles) is helpful in identifying the

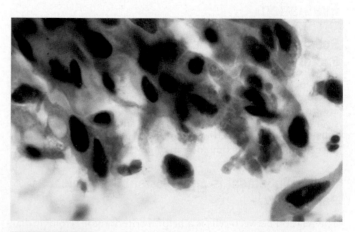

FIGURE 30-6. **Invasive squamous cell carcinoma of the cervix.** Pleomorphic elongated squamous cells, with enlarged, irregular and hyperchromatic nuclei.

cell type (see Fig. 30-4). Viral and chlamydial infections may produce inclusions in the cytoplasm. Squamous cells infected by human papillomavirus show characteristic changes called **koilocytotic atypia**, which consists of a large perinuclear halo and nuclear abnormalities.

The Most Important Features of Malignancy Reside in the Nucleus

The size and shape of the nucleus, alterations of nuclear membrane and chromatin, prominence of the nucleolus, and mitotic activity are important parameters in cytologic evaluation. Nuclei of normal cells vary little in size and shape (see Figs. 30-1 and 30-3A). Malignant cells usually exhibit significant nuclear enlargement, which is frequently disproportionate to the enlargement of the cell and results in an increased nuclear-to-cytoplasmic ratio (see Fig. 30-2C). In addition, significant variations and abnormalities in nuclear size (**anisokaryosis**), shape, and contour are common in malignant neoplasms (see Fig. 30-5). Molding of the nuclei against one another is seen in some tumors (classically in small cell carcinomas), probably due to a rapid growth rate and scanty cytoplasm.

Nuclei of cancer cells are usually darker (**hyperchromatic**) than those of normal cells, and the chromatin tends to be coarser and unevenly distributed (Fig. 30-3B). The nucleoli of cancer cells, particularly in poorly differentiated tumors, are often larger and more numerous than those in their benign counterparts. Although increased mitotic activity can occur in both benign and malignant tumors, cancer cells in general have a higher rate of mitosis. Additionally, the presence of abnormal mitoses (abnormal distribution of chromosomes or presence of more than two mitotic poles) is a reliable criterion for the diagnosis of malignancy.

Extracellular Material and Background Surround the Cells

The smear background is evaluated for the presence and type of inflammation, blood, various extracellular substances, cell products, necrotic debris, and microorganisms. Cell necrosis may occur in a variety of benign conditions but may also be a prominent feature of many malignant neoplasms. *When present in association with malignant cells, necrosis generally indicates an invasive cancer.*

Reporting Systems

Various methods have been used for reporting the results of cytologic tests. The **Bethesda system** is the standard for **gynecologic** cytology reports. This reporting system, with revisions, has been adopted by most laboratories in the United States (Table 30-1).

Advantages of Cytopathology

- Cytopathologic evaluation is invaluable from many different perspectives:
- **Less trauma** is involved in sampling by cytologic techniques than by biopsy.
- **A larger sampling surface** is available for cytologic methods. For example, in peritoneal and bladder washings, a very large area is sampled, whereas biopsy samples are limited to a few, small, grossly visible foci.
- **Tumors that are difficult to access by biopsy may be sampled by cytologic methods**. Cytopathology allows washing of a gastrointestinal tract stricture that does not permit passage of the biopsy instrument, and fine-needle aspiration of a periph-

TABLE 30–1
The 2001 Bethesda System
Specimen adequacy
Satisfactory for evaluation
Unsatisfactory for evaluation … (specify reason)
Interpretation/result:
Negative for intraepithelial lesion or malignancy
Other
Endometrial cells (in a woman ≥40 years of age)
Epithelial cell abnormalities
Squamous Cell:
ASC
ASC-US
Cannot exclude HSIL (ASC-H)
LSIL
Encompassing: HPV/mild dysplasia/CIN1
HSIL
Encompassing: moderate and severe dysplasia, CIS/CIN2, and CIN3
With features suspicious for invasion (if invasion is suspected)
Squamous cell carcinoma
Glandular Cell:
Atypical
Endocervical cells (NOS or specify in comments)
Endometrial cells (NOS or specify in comments)
Glandular cells (NOS or specify in comments)
Atypical
Endocervical cells, favor neoplastic
Glandular cells, favor neoplastic
Endocervical adenocarcinoma in situ
Adenocarcinoma
Endocervical
Endometrial
Extrauterine
NOS
Other malignant neoplasms (specify)

ASC, atypical squamous cells; ASC-US, of undetermined significance; CIN, cervical intraepithelial neoplasia; HPV, human papilloma virus; HSIL, high-grade squamous intraepithelial lesion; LSIL, low-grade squamous intraepithelial lesion; NOS, not otherwise specified.

eral carcinoma of the lung that is beyond the reach of a bronchoscope can be performed.
- **Rapid diagnosis** is one of the major advantages of cytologic methods. Results may be available for reading in minutes to less than an hour.
- **Greater convenience** is afforded by the collection of cytologic specimens than with biopsy. In most instances, no prior preparation of the patient is necessary, and the sampling is done as an office procedure.
- **Greater cost-effectiveness** of cytology for cancer detection has been amply demonstrated. Often, it eliminates needless tests, procedures, and surgical operations.

Limitations of Cytopathology

- **Classification of the tumor type** is generally more difficult with cytologic samples than with biopsy specimens due to the small size of cytologic samples and the loss of tissue pattern.

- **The extent and depth of invasion** cannot be assessed by cytologic methods.
- **Inadequate sampling** is a *major* cause of false-negative diagnoses in cytology. For example, in obtaining a sample of the uterine cervix, it is critical to include the transformation zone.

Accuracy of Cytologic Methods

The accuracy of cytologic diagnosis depends on several factors, including the experience of the specimen collector, the sampling method, the sample adequacy, the target organ, and the examiner's expertise. False-positive diagnoses are rarely made by experienced cytopathologists; thus, the specificity of a malignant diagnosis approaches 100%. The sensitivity of the test (a measure of false negatives), however, is in the range of 80% to 90% for most specimen types. *The absence of malignant cells in cytologic samples does not completely rule out the possibility of malignancy.* Unless a benign cause for a lesion can be established by cytologic examination (e.g., fibroadenoma of the breast, benign cyst of the thyroid, liver abscess, granuloma of the lung), further investigation, including histologic biopsy, is warranted.

New Trends in Cytopathology

Application of molecular tests to cytologic specimens is rapidly gaining importance as an adjunct to morphologic diagnosis. The clinical application of these methods include (1) classifying tumors, particularly hematopoietic and mesenchymal tumors; (2) establishing clonality, particularly in the diagnosis of non-Hodgkin lymphoma; (3) identifying minimal residual malignant disease and detecting recurrence after treatment; (4) assessing prognostic factors; and (5) providing guidance for targeted therapies.

Specific acknowledgment is made for permission to use the following material.

Chapter 1, Figure 1. Reprinted from Okazaki H, Scheithauer BW. *Atlas of Neuropathology.* New York: Gower Medical Publishing, 1988, with permission of the author.

Chapter 3, Figure 12. Reprinted from Okazaki H, Scheithauer BW. *Atlas of Neuropathology.* New York: Gower Medical Publishing, 1988, with permission of the author.

Chapter 5, Figure 3. Reprinted from Bullough PG, Vigorita VJ. *Atlas of Orthopaedic Pathology.* New York: Gower Medical Publishing, 1984, with permission from Elsevier.

Chapter 5, Figure 17. From US Mortality Public Use Data Tapes 1960–2002, US Mortality Volumes 1930–1959, National Center for Health Statistics, Centers for Disease Control and Prevention, 2005.

Chapter 6, Figure 30. Reprinted from Bullough PG, Vigorita VJ. *Atlas of Orthopedic Pathology.* New York: Gower Medical Publishing, 1988, with permission from Elsevier.

Chapter 7, Figure 1. Courtesy of UBC Pulmonary Registry, St. Paul's Hospital, Vancouver, British Columbia, Canada.

Chapter 7, Figure 6. Courtesy of Greg J. Davis, MD, Department of Pathology, University of Kentucky College of Medicine, Lexington, Kentucky.

Chapter 7, Figure 12. Courtesy of Ken Berry, MD, Department of Pathology, St. Paul's Hospital, Vancouver, British Columbia, Canada.

Chapter 9, Figures 28 and 40. Reprinted from Farrar WE, Wood MJ, Innes JA, et al. *Infectious Diseases Text and Color Atlas,* 2nd ed. New York: Gower Medical Publishing, 1992, with permission from Elsevier.

Chapter 12, Figure 15. Travis WB, Colby TV, Koss MN, et al. *Non-Neoplastic Disorders of the Lower Respiratory Tract.* Washington DC: American Registry of Pathology, 2002.

Chapter 12, Figure 25. Courtesy of the Armed Forces Institute of Pathology, Washington, DC.

Chapter 13, Figures 7B, 25, and 35. Reprinted from Mitros FA. *Atlas of Gastrointestinal Pathology.* New York: Gower Medical Publishing, 1988, with permission from Elsevier.

Chapter 18, Figure 27. Reprinted with permission of Stanley J. Robboy, MD, and Gynecologic Pathology Associates, Durham and Chapel Hill, North Carolina.

Chapter 18, Figures 4 and 9. Robboy SJ, Anderson MC, Russell P. *Pathology of the Female Reproductive Tract.* London: Churchill-Livingstone, 2002; 111–354.

Chapter 21, Figure 11. Sandoz Pharmaceutical Corporation, Princeton, New Jersey.

Chapter 24, Figures 3A, 8A, 9, 11A, 13A, 25A, 26, and 31A. Elder AD, Elenitsas R, Johnson BL, et al. *Synopsis and Atlas of Lever's Histopathology of the Skin.* Philadelphia: Lippincott Williams & Wilkins, 1999.

Chapter 26, Figures 20A, 20B, 51B, and 67A. Reprinted from Bullough PG. *Atlas of Orthopaedic Pathology,* 2nd ed. New York: Gower Medical Publishing, 1992, with permission from Elsevier.

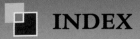

INDEX

Page numbers in *italic* denote figures.